CLINICAL Neuroanesthesia

SECOND EDITION

CLINICAL Neuroanesthesia

SECOND EDITION

Edited by

ROY F. CUCCHIARA, M.D.
Professor and Chairman
Department of Anesthesiology
University of Florida College of Medicine
Gainesville, Florida

SUSAN BLACK, M.D.
Associate Professor
Department of Anesthesiology
University of Florida College of Medicine
Gainesville, Florida

JOHN D. MICHENFELDER, M.D.
Professor Emeritus
Department of Anesthesiology
Mayo Medical School
Former Consultant
Department of Anesthesiology
Mayo Clinic
Rochester, Minnesota

CHURCHILL LIVINGSTONE

New York, Edinburgh, London, Madrid, Melbourne, San Francisco, Tokyo

Library of Congress Cataloging-in-Publication Data

A catalog record for this book is available from the Library of Congress.

Distributed in the United Kingdom by Churchill Livingstone, Robert Stevenson House, 1–3 Baxter's Place, Leith Walk, Edinburgh EH1 3AF, and by associated companies, branches, and representatives throughout the world.

Acquisitions Editor: *Michael J. Houston*
Assistant Editor: *Ann Ruzycka*
Production Editor: *Paul Bernstein*
Production Supervisor: *Sharon Tuder*
Cover Design: *Jeannette Jacobs*

Printed in the United States of America

First published in 1998 7 6 5 4 3 2 1

CONTRIBUTORS

ROBERT S. ALPHIN, M.D.

Assistant Professor, Department of Anesthesiology, University of North Carolina School of Medicine, Chapel Hill, North Carolina; Staff Anesthesiologist, Critical Care Systems of North Carolina, Wake Medical Center, Raleigh, North Carolina

JOSEPH F. ANTOGNINI, M.D.

Associate Professor, Department of Anesthesiology, University of California, Davis, School of Medicine, Davis, California

ALAN A. ARTRU, M.D.

Professor and Head of Research, Department of Anesthesiology, University of Washington School of Medicine; Chief of Neuroanesthesia, Department of Anesthesiology, University of Washington Medical Center, Seattle, Washington

JOHN L. D. ATKINSON, M.D.

Assistant Professor, Department of Neurosurgery, Mayo Medical School; Consultant, Department of Neurosurgery, Mayo Clinic, Rochester, Minnesota

SUSAN BLACK, M.D.

Associate Professor, Department of Anesthesiology, University of Florida College of Medicine, Gainesville, Florida

ROY F. CUCCHIARA, M.D.

Professor and Chairman, Department of Anesthesiology, University of Florida College of Medicine, Gainesville, Florida

DUDLEY H. DAVIS, M.D.

Associate Professor, Department of Neurosurgery, Mayo Medical School; Consultant, Department of Neurosurgery, Mayo Clinic, Rochester, Minnesota

ARTHUR L. DAY, M.D.

James and Newton Eblen Scholar and Professor, Department of Neurosurgery, University of Florida College of Medicine, Gainesville, Florida

RONALD J. FAUST M.D.

Professor, Department of Anesthesiology, Mayo Medical School; Consultant, Department of Anesthesiology, Mayo Clinic, Rochester, Minnesota

NEAL W. FLEMING, PH.D., M.D.

Associate Professor, Department of Anesthesiology, University of California, Davis, School of Medicine, Davis, California

ORLANDO G. FLORETE, JR., M.D.

Clinical Assistant Professor, Department of Anesthesiology, University of Florida Health Science Center, Jacksonville, Florida

NIKOLAUS GRAVENSTEIN, M.D.

Professor, Departments of Anesthesiology and Neurosurgery, University of Florida College of Medicine, Gainesville, Florida

GERALD A. GRONERT, M.D.

Professor, Department of Anesthesiology, University of California, Davis, School of Medicine, Davis, California

TERESE T. HORLOCKER, M.D.

Associate Professor, Department of Anesthesiology, Mayo Graduate School of Medicine; Consultant, Department of Anesthesiology, Mayo Clinic, Rochester, Minnesota

RORY S. JAFFE, M.D.

Associate Professor, Department of Anesthesiology, University of California, Davis, College of Medicine, Davis, California

PATRICK J. KELLY, M.D.
Professor and Chairman, Department of Neurological Surgery, New York University Medical Center, New York, New York

A. JOSEPH LAYON, M.D.
Associate Professor, Departments of Anesthesiology, Surgery, and Medicine, University of Florida College of Medicine; Chief, Division of Emergency Medicine and Associate Chief, Division of Critical Care Medicine, Burn Center, Shands Hospital of the University of Florida, Gainesville, Florida

THOMAS J. LOSASSO, M.D.
Consultant, Anesthesia Associates Duluth, Ltd., Duluth, Minnesota

MICHAEL E. MAHLA, M. D.
Associate Professor, Departments of Anesthesiology and Neurosurgery and Assistant Chair for Education, University of Florida College of Medicine, Gainesville, Florida

JOHN D. MICHENFELDER, M.D.
Professor Emeritus, Department of Anesthesiology, Mayo Medical School; Former Consultant, Department of Anesthesiology, Mayo Clinic, Rochester, Minnesota

J. PARKER MICKLE, M.D.
Professor, Department of Surgery, University of Florida College of Medicine, Gainesville, Florida

LESLIE NEWBERG MILDE, M.D.
Professor, Department of Anesthesiology, Mayo Medical School; Consultant, Department of Anesthesiology, Mayo Clinic, Scottsdale, Arizona

WILLIAM J. PERKINS, M.D.
Assistant Professor, Department of Anesthesiology, Mayo Medical School; Consultant, Department of Anesthesiology, Mayo Clinic, Rochester, Minnesota

RICHARD J. POLLARD, M.D.
Fellow, Division of Neuroanesthesia, Department of Anesthesiology, University of Florida College of Medicine, Gainesville, Florida

STEVEN N. ROPER, M.D.
Associate Professor, Department of Neurosurgery, University of Florida College of Medicine, Gainesville, Florida

DANIEL S. ROWE, JR., M.D.
Clinical Assistant Professor, Department of Anesthesiology, Univeristy of Floirda Health Science Center, Jacksonville, Florida

JOSEPH B. STACHNIAK, M.D.
Resident, Department of Neurosurgery, University of Florida College of Medicine, Gainesville, Florida

CHERI A. SULEK, M.D.
Assistant Professor, Department of Anesthesiology, University of Florida College of Medicine; Associate Director, Intraoperative Neurophysiologic Monitoring Laboratory, Department of Anesthesiology, Shands Hospital of the University of Florida, Gainesville, Florida

HIROSHI TAKESHITA, M.D.
Emeritus Professor, Department of Anesthesiology-Resuscitology, Yamaguchi University School of Medicine, Ube, Yamaguchi, Japan; Director and Senior Consultant, Departments of Anesthesiology and Intensive Care Medicine, Kokura Memorial Hospital, Kitakyushu, Japan

MARK F. TRANKINA, M.D.
Assistant Professor, Departments of Anesthesiology and Neurosurgery, University of Florida College of Medicine, Gainesville, Florida

PETER R. WILSON, M.D.
Associate Professor, Department of Anesthesiology, Mayo Medical School; Consultant, Department of Anesthesiology, Mayo Clinic, Rochester, Minnesota

PREFACE

Whereas the seven short years since the publication of the first edition of *Clinical Neuroanesthesia* have seen the retirement, death, or relocation of many of the original contributors, new authors have joined those remaining to expand the horizons of clinical neuroanesthesia. The second edition brings together contributors from the Mayo Clinic, in Rochester, Minnesota, and the University of Florida College of Medicine, in Gainesville, Florida. The links between these two centers exist on both an institutional and a personal level. Both are at the forefront of clinical research and practice in neurosurgery and neuroanesthesia, and both the Chairman of the Department of Anesthesiology and the Department of Neurosurgery at the University of Florida College of Medicine, together with members of the staff, were consultants at the Mayo Clinic for many years.

As in the first edition, topics are presented within two sections—Scientific Foundations and Clinical Applications—and are intended to cover all major aspects of the subspecialty. New to this edition are basic science chapters on neuroanatomy and brain fluid homeostasis, as well as in-depth coverage of anesthetic techniques in vertebral and spinal cord surgery, central nervous system trauma, and pediatric neurosurgery. We have also included a chapter on applications of transesophageal echocardiography in neurosurgery and neuroanesthesia.

The data presented in this book are from case volumes of the University of Florida College of Medicine and the Mayo Clinic.

The authors of this text are dedicated clinicians who care for neurosurgical patients as part of their daily work. The development of their approaches has been guided by scientific foundations and data, by constraints of the local and national medical environment, and, in the absence of data, by their own impressions of what is clinically effective. Some of the techniques use the application of basic skills in unique ways. Some are highly technical. All are practical.

Roy F. Cucchiara, M.D.
Susan Black, M.D.
John D. Michenfelder, M.D.

CONTENTS

SCIENTIFIC FOUNDATIONS

CLINICAL APPLICATIONS

1 CEREBRAL BLOOD FLOW AND METABOLISM

SUSAN BLACK
JOHN D. MICHENFELDER

This chapter reviews available basic information regarding cerebral blood flow (CBF) and cerebral metabolism (CMR) in normal brain, pathologic brain, hypothermic brain, and finally in the anesthetized brain. Armed with this information, it should be possible to arrive at rational conclusions regarding selection of anesthetic agents and techniques for the neurosurgical patient. The reader should be warned, however, that the information we possess, although considerable, might be viewed as a series of isolated blocks. The scientific process demands that we examine each intervention in as "pure" a manner as possible and in doing so we uncover individual blocks of information. However, when anesthetizing our patients, we combine these blocks in a bewildering array of shapes and sizes and assume that the individual effects remain operative even in various combinations. There is ample evidence that this is often not the case, and a number of examples of this will be given in this chapter. Furthermore, most of our information has been gleaned from studies of normal brain. The assumption that this information can be transferred to pathologic brain may not always be correct. Still, combined with healthy doses of clinical acumen and common sense, the information that is available can be put to good use in the care of our patients.

ANATOMIC CONSIDERATIONS

In humans the CBF is almost completely supplied by the internal carotid and vertebral arteries. The latter form the single basilar artery, which, along with the internal carotids, provide the input to the circle of Willis. Variability in the functional adequacy of the circle of Willis occurs because of variability in the development of the anterior and posterior communicating arteries. Normally there is no cross filling, but in the event of occlusion of a major input artery, the resulting pressure differential will cause cross filling of varying adequacy to the involved hemisphere. Blood is supplied from the circle of Willis by the paired anterior, middle, and posterior cerebral arteries and by the penetrating vessels. Overlap and anastomoses between terminal branches of the cortical vessels do occur (via the leptomeningeal vessels), but these are the most vulnerable regions in the event of reduced blood flow (so-called watershed zones). In the event of occlusion of one of the major cortical vessels, infarction is almost certain because of inadequate anastomotic connections, particularly in the depths of the brain structure. The cortical surface arteries are generally not considered to be resistance vessels. Rather the parenchymal arterioles branching from the penetrating vessels are believed to be the major resistance vessels.

Anatomically, there is a rich autonomic nervous supply to the cerebral vessels although the functional purpose of the system is controversial and largely unknown. There is evidence for two anatomically distinct noradrenergic systems. Extraparenchymal vessels down to the level of the conducting vessels in the pia are innervated by the cervical ganglia. The parenchymal microvasculature appears to be innervated from a system originating in the locus ceruleus. Parasympathetic supply comes primarily from the great superficial petrosal branch of the facial nerve.

The veins draining from the brain are thin walled and valveless. They eventually converge to enter the thick-walled, nonelastic dural sinuses. In order to maintain venous blood flow, the pressure in the cerebral veins must slightly exceed cerebral spinal fluid (CSF) pressure even in the circumstance of increasing intracranial pressure (ICP). In this event, venous pressure in the dural sinuses and the internal jugular vein is significantly less than that in the cerebral veins. This is accounted for by the development of constriction and increased resistance at the point where the cerebral veins enter the dural sinuses. Thus the perfusion pressure of the brain in the presence of increased ICP is virtually equal to the difference between mean arterial pressure and ICP. Within the venous circulation there is considerable but incomplete admixture of venous blood. A sample of jugular bulb blood will normally contain blood representative of the venous drainage of approximately two-thirds of the ipsilateral and one-third of the contralateral hemispheres. Additionally, extracerebral contamination of jugular bulb blood is usually present but is generally less than 5 percent.

METHODOLOGIES

With the exception of recent developments utilizing short-lived positron emitting isotopes in humans and autoradiographic techniques in experimental animals, we have relied primarily upon measurements of CBF for determining both cerebral hemodynamic and cerebral metabolic effects of anesthetics and other interventions. Cerebral metabolic rates for oxygen, glucose, and lactate are calculated as the product of measurements of CBF and arterial-venous differences in the individual substrate concentrations across the region of the brain in which CBF is measured.

Global Measurements

In humans these calculations are only valid when utilizing the classic original Kety-Schmidt methodology for measuring CBF with venous sampling at the jugular bulb.[1,2] This methodology relies upon inhalation of an inert freely diffusible indicator while determining the rate of saturation of the brain as a direct function of CBF. Alternatively, the rate of desaturation may be determined following equilibration of the indicator in the brain with the arterial blood concentration. The original indicator used by Kety and Schmidt was 15 percent N_2O; since then, both ^{85}Kr and ^{133}Xe have been used. The methodology requires either repetitive or continuous sampling of arterial and jugular bulb blood over a period of 10 to 14 minutes (preferably the latter) and requires knowledge of the blood-brain partition coefficient of the indicator for calculating CBF. The methodology yields a mean global value of CBF usually given in units of ml 100 g^{-1} min^{-1}. This multiplied by the arterial-jugular bulb blood substrate concentration differences will yield mean global values for cerebral oxygen consumption ($CMRO_2$), CMR glucose, or CMR lactate, usually given in units of ml · 100 g^{-1} · min^{-1}, mg · 100 g^{-1}, or μmol · 100 g^{-1} · min^{-1}, respectively. In those countries that have accepted the international system of units (SI), all three metabolic calculations are usually reported as μmol · 100 g^{-1} · min^{-1}. The Kety-Schmidt methodology is clumsy in that it requires up to 14 minutes for a single accurate determination and then only in the presence of a near steady state. Furthermore, jugular bulb blood is not exclusively representative of brain venous drainage with an average contamination by extracerebral tissue of about 5 percent. Still, the original values as reported by Kety and Schmidt in the 1940s have stood the test of time.[1,2]

Regional Measurements

In the 1960s Lassen et al. utilized the basic Kety-Schmidt methodology for measuring regional CBF in humans using ^{85}Kr.[3,4] With this technique, the freely diffusible indicator (now usually ^{133}Xe) is injected as a bolus in the internal carotid artery with almost immediate equilibration of the indicator in the brain. Thereafter, the rate of washout of the indicator is determined with one or more scintillation detectors placed about the ipsilateral hemisphere. With this method, the rate of washout can usually be characterized as a biexponential function yielding values for a fast-flow and a slow-flow compartment. These compartments are commonly assumed to be representative of the gray and white matter, respectively. This calculation also requires that washout be recorded for a 10 to 14-minute period. However, rapid determinations of CBF are possible if flow is calculated either from the initial slope of the washout or by a half-time calculation. These latter calculations are heavily weighted by the fast-flow compartment, which is usually the compartment of greatest interest. Such methodology is completely valid for comparing repetitive CBF measurements. Although, strictly speaking, repeat CBF measurements should await return of radioactivity to baseline, it is acceptable to repeat CBF measurements sooner by correcting for the baseline shift and extrapolating the rate of change in the baseline over the period of time used for the CBF calculation.

Although this method has been widely accepted as valid in many circumstances, there are deficiencies. In pathologic states, the phenomenon of *look-through* has been described wherein a region with little or no CBF may be missed because of gamma emission distal to the region that will be "seen" by the scintillation detector as normal. Furthermore, the blood-brain partition coefficient used for calculating CBF is only known for normal brain—changes are known to occur in certain pathologic states. Undoubtedly, the greatest deficiency in the method is the inability to validly sample venous blood which is exclusively representative of the region in which CBF is being measured. Although regional metabolic rates are commonly reported based upon jugular bulb blood samples in humans or sagittal sinus blood samples in animals, they cannot be accepted as necessarily valid and should be viewed with considerable caution.

In an effort to avoid the invasive nature of these measurements (i.e., jugular bulb or internal carotid artery puncture for global or regional measurements, respectively), methodologies have been described wherein the indicator (usually ^{133}Xe) is either inhaled or administered intravenously following which washout is measured with one or more scintillation detectors.[5] Although appealing because of both the relatively noninvasive requirements and because bilateral measurements are theoretically possible, the basic methodologies have never been widely accepted as quantitatively valid, particularly in low-flow states.[6,7] This is so because of several potential variables produced by the technique. A major deficiency is the unknown contribution of measured radioactivity from extracerebral tissues placed between the detector and the brain. Although this problem has been manipulated mathematically in a variety of ways, the offered solutions have failed to satisfy many critics. The problem of recirculation of the indicator is also introduced by these techniques, but this can be partially corrected for by measuring expired concentrations of the indicator. Finally, the radioactivity from air spaces near the detector (i.e., the nasal sinuses) must be shielded against to the degree possible. Given the inherent deficiencies of the method, reported measurements of regional CBF should be viewed with caution and then probably only as an index of CBF. Any calculations of regional metabolic rates using such measurements should probably be ignored.

In the very special circumstance where surgery requires exposure of the brain, it is possible to determine an accurate regional CBF by simple local application of the indicator (usually ^{133}Xe) followed by measurement of its washout with a single scintillation detector.[8]

PET and NMR Measurements

Positron emission tomography (PET) is a virtually noninvasive means of measuring both CBF and CMR in humans.[9] Unfortunately, in addition to the scanning equipment, the methodology requires the proximity of a cyclotron for producing short-lived isotopes of oxygen or metabolic substrates for injection into the subject to be studied. It is to be expected that this method will be used primarily to characterize cerebral vascular and metabolic states in a variety of pathologic conditions that are not amenable to study in experimental animals.

Nuclear magnetic resonance (NMR) spectroscopy provides a noninvasive means of measuring brain metabolites such as phosphocreatine and aderosine triphosphate (ATP) as well as brain pH in vivo in experimental animals and in humans.[10] To date, results have been reported primarily in experimental animals, and these have largely simply confirmed measurements previously made in vitro in whole brain or in brain biopsies.

Experimental Methodology

In addition to the methods available for measuring CBF (and calculating $CMRO_2$) in humans, there are a number`of invasive techniques that permit precise accurate measurements of CBF in experimental animals.

VENOUS OUTFLOW Rapela and Green first popularized a venous outflow technique in dogs that was based upon catheterizing the confluence of the sinuses and occluding the lateral sinuses.[11] The method did not prevent extracerebral contamination (or loss) via the emissary and diploic veins. Neither did the method yield flow values in units of ml · 100 g^{-1} · min^{-1}; as such it has never been validated. We described a method in dogs that virtually completely isolated the sagittal sinus outflow, yielded flow values in units of ml · 100 g^{-1} · min^{-1} and has been validated using two independent methods for measurement of CBF.[12,13]

In addition to providing accurate measurement of CBF from the cerebral hemispheres, the method inherently offers an almost foolproof means of calculating CMR. This is so because the venous effluent used to measure CBF is obviously exclusively representative of the region of the brain from which CBF is measured as regards substrate concentrations. Unfortunately, the method is not applicable to other species such as pigs and sheep because of anomalies in their venous anatomy that prevents isolation of the sagittal sinus flow.

OTHER METHODS A number of other methods for measuring CBF in experimental animals is available. The most popular methods include radioactive microspheres, hydrogen clearance, and autoradiographic techniques.[6,7,14] There are disadvantages to each of these. To begin with, none permit an accurate calculation of CMR with the possible exception of combining global hemispheric microsphere measurements with sagittal sinus blood measurements of substrates. Microsphere methodology is currently limited to a maximum of six measurements utilizing spheres with sufficiently different radioactive characteristics as to permit their separation on appropriate counting equipment. Microspheres are not accurate in measuring very low-flow states since a critical mass of spheres is required for accurate counting (400/cm^3). Hydrogen clearance is a variation on the original Kety-Schmidt method, requires the invasive placement of fine electrodes into the substance of the brain, and measures CBF only within millimeters of the electrode tip. As such, it requires several electrodes to be placed at different depths so as to provide a representative spectrum of flows from both fast-flow and slow-flow compartments. The autoradiographic technique using [^{14}C]iodantipyrine is extremely inefficient since it provides but one measurement of CBF per experimental animal and that measurement requires days of exposure to radiosensitive paper. Metabolic measurements are also possible using autoradiographic techniques. These include the [^{14}C]deoxyglucose method popularized by Sokoloff and related methods using [^{14}C]glucose.[15]

NORMAL BRAIN

The normal values for CBF and CMR are available for humans as well as a host of other species. A representative tabulation of reported values in humans is presented in Table 1.1.[1,16–19] It should be noted that in experimental animals the "normal" values may be distorted by background anesthetic drugs. Thus in my laboratory, "normal" canine values for CBF may be greatly exaggerated by the background of nitrous oxide analgesia whereas $CMRO_2$ values are only slightly affected.

In the absence of pathology or drugs, $CMRO_2$ in humans is remarkably stable between 3.0 and 3.8 ml · 100 g^{-1}· min^{-1}. This is maintained both during normal sleep or while engaged in intense mental activity. Measurements of regional CBF and PET measurements reveal shifting regional activity as different portions of the brain are activated, resulting in no major changes in global measurements. At normocarbia, CBF is likewise fairly stable at 45 to 65 ml · 100 g^{-1} · min^{-1} and is normally coupled to $CMRO_2$ with a ratio of approximately 15:1.

The primary controlling factors of CBF in normal brain are carbon dioxide levels, oxygen levels, and the cerebral perfusion pressure (Fig. 1.1). The most potent physiologic determinant of CBF is carbon dioxide. It is commonly (but not universally) accepted that it is the hydrogen ion concentration in the extracellular fluid of the vascular smooth muscle that mediates the response to $PaCO_2$. The potential magnitude of the response is impressive. A doubling of the normal $PaCO_2$ to 80 mmHg will approximately double the CBF; thereafter, CBF plateaus, presumably reflecting maximal vasodilation. Reducing the normal $PaCO_2$ by one-half to 20 mmHg will approximately halve the CBF; thereafter, CBF plateaus, presumably reflecting maximal vasoconstriction. At $PaCO_2$ values in excess of 80 mmHg, a reduction in $CMRO_2$ may occur reflecting the anesthetic effect of extreme hypercarbia. At $PaCO_2$ levels of 20 mmHg and below it is disputed whether cerebral ischemia can occur in normal brain. The evidence suggests that the brain will tolerate a 50 percent reduction in CBF without ischemic changes. However, this combined with the severe alkalosis produced by such hypocapnia may induce brain hypoxia secondary to the leftward shift of oxyhemoglobin dissociation, thus limiting the off-loading of oxy-

TABLE 1.1 *Normal values for CBF and $CMRO_2$ in humans (Kety-Schmidt method)*

REFERENCE	CBF ($ml \cdot 100\ g^{-1} \cdot min^{-1}$)	$CMRO_2$ ($ml \cdot 100\ g^{-1} \cdot min^{-1}$)	RATIO ($CBF/CMRO_2$)
Kety and Schmidt[1]	54	3.30	16
Schienberg and Stead[16]	65	3.81	17
Sokoloff et al.[17]	67	3.70	18
Lassen et al.[18]	50	3.50	14
Cohen et al.[19]	45	3.02	15

Abbreviations: CBF, cerebral blood flow; $CMRO_2$, cerebral metabolism

(From Michenfelder,[253] with permission.)

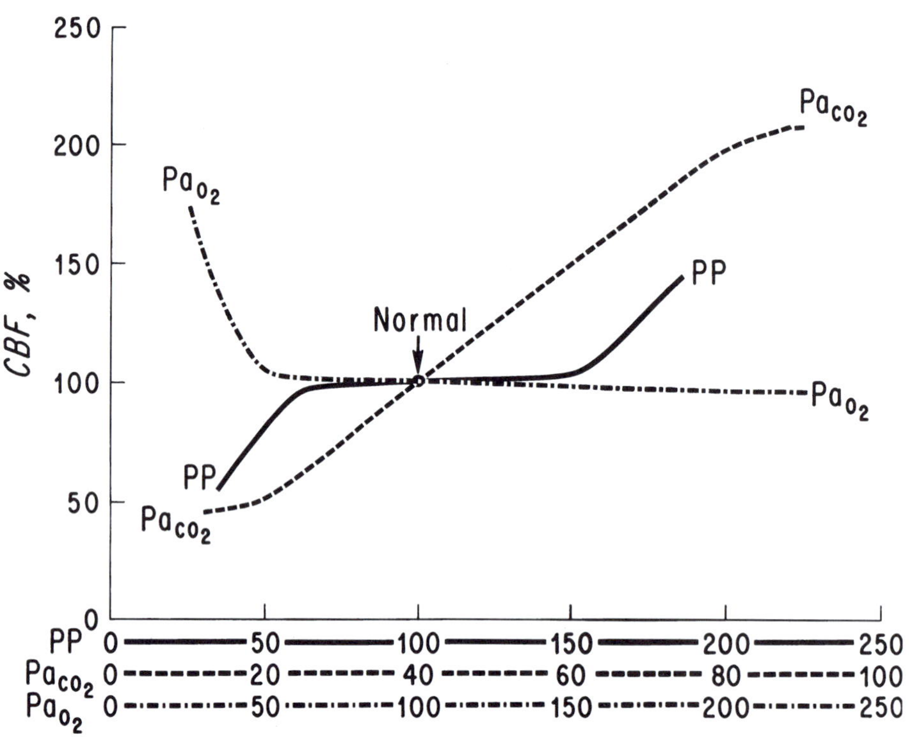

FIGURE 1.1 *Relationship of cerebral blood flow to perfusion pressure (PP), $PaCO_2$, and PaO_2. Units on abscissa are millimeters of Hg.*

gen at the capillary level.[20] It is also disputed whether the electroencephalogram (EEG) changes observed with extreme hypocapnia reflect brain hypoxia or simply the effect of alkalosis on neuroelectric activity.[21]

Most, if not all, abnormal or pathologic states will either attenuate or abolish normal CO_2 reactivity. An example of altered CO_2 reactivity occurs during hypotension at the lower limit of autoregulation. In this circumstance, autoregulation has imposed maximal vasodilation in order to maintain flow (see below), and the cerebrovasculature is unresponsive to induced hypocapnia (Fig. 1.2).[22] It is probably correct to generalize that any state that threatens the central nervous system (CNS) secondary to inadequate flow will render the involved vasculature unresponsive to hypocapnia.

Another extremely important feature of CBF control in normal brain is the phenomenon of autoregulation. Although unproven, it is generally assumed that a myogenic mechanism accounts for this phenomenon: thus when the muscle senses an increased pressure (stretch?), it responds with contraction and the opposite occurs in response to a decreased pressure. Whatever the mechanism, it is effective over a mean cerebral perfusion pressure of about 50 to 150 mmHg. Above this level, breakthrough occurs with hypertensive encephalopathy secondary to blood-brain barrier disruption, edema, and ischemia. At pressures below 50 mmHg, maximal vasodilation is assumed and flow becomes pressure passive. In fact there is evidence that background sympathetic tone prevents maximal vasodilation, and autoregulation can be extended below 50 mmHg by chemical or surgical sympathectomy.[23] The autoregulatory response is not instantaneous: following an abrupt change in blood pressure, 1 to 3 minutes may be required for the return of CBF to control levels. Autoregulation is affected by chronic hy-

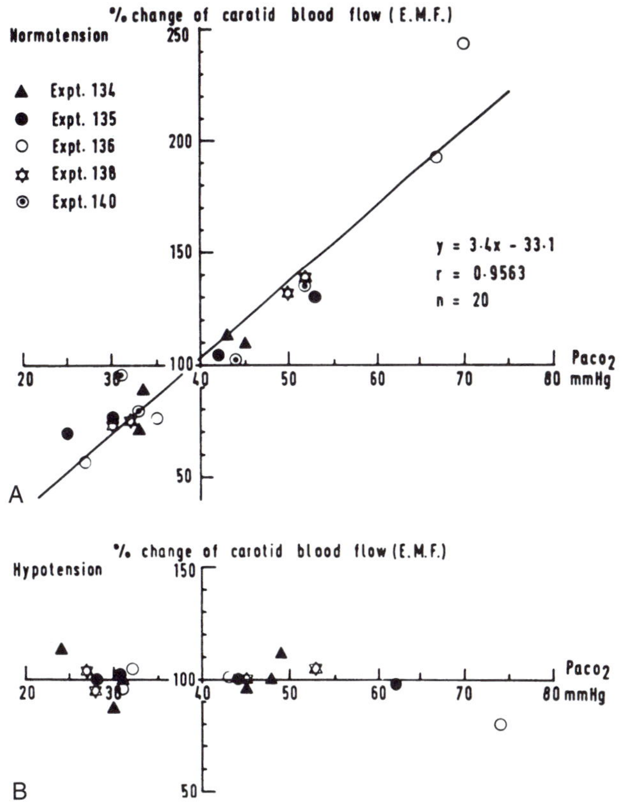

FIGURE 1.2 *The percentage changes of carotid blood flow in the baboon are plotted on the ordinate versus arterial blood* $PacO_2$ *on the abscissa. (A) The animals were normotensive, and* CO_2 *reactivity was intact and normal. (B) The animal were hypotensive at or beyond the autoregulatory range, and there was no response of cerebral blood flow to change in* $PaCO_2$*. (From Okuda et al.,[22] with permission).*

pertension such that the response is shifted to the right, presumably as a means of protecting against hypertensive encephalopathy. This in turn limits the safe level for reducing cerebral perfusion pressure. Following successful treatment of chronic hypertension, autoregulation returns toward control levels. In normal humans, cerebral perfusion pressure may be nearly equated to mean systemic arterial blood pressure (slightly less), but in the presence of increased ICP, it is approximately equal to mean arterial blood pressure minus ICP (actually slightly less since the draining venous channels must maintain a pressure slightly greater than ICP to prevent collapse).

Oxygen per se has little direct effect on CBF. At 1 atm, perhaps as much as a 10 percent decrease in CBF will occur. However, with hypoxia, there is a striking increase in CBF (assuming cerebral perfusion pressure is maintained). This increase is assumed to be secondary to acidic metabolic products—primarily lactic acid—that accumulate with severe hypoxia.

It is commonly assumed that CBF, cerebral blood volume (CBV), and ICP parallel one another, and under most circumstances this is usually so. Certainly on an acute basis CBF and ICP should change in tandem; however, CBF and CBV need not and do not always do so. For example, a drug such as nitroglycerin may dilate primarily the capacitance vessels of the brain with an increase in CBV and ICP but no increase in CBF. Similarly, at pressures below the autoregulatory range, CBF may be decreased while CBV is increased secondary to maximal vasodilation.

As has already been noted in the section on Methodologies, most in vivo cerebral metabolic determinations are limited to calculations of $CMRO_2$, CMR glucose, and CMR lactate from measurements of CBF and arterial-venous substrate concentration differences. In experimental animals in vitro, measurements in either whole brain or brain biopsies of cerebral metabolites are commonly done as a means of assessing the cerebral energy state. The most common measurements are those of the adenine nucleotides (ATP, adenosine diphosphate [ADP], and adenosine monophosphate [AMP]), phosphocreatine (PCr), lactate, pyruvate, and glucose. From measurements of the adenine nucleotides, the energy charge (EC) of the brain can be readily calculate[24]

$$EC = \frac{[ATP] + \frac{1}{2}[ADP]}{[ATP + ADP + AMP]}$$

Normal values for these variables in dogs, rats, and mice are summarized in Table 1.2.[25–27] In the event of cerebral hypoxia, the earliest changes in these variables are a decrease in PCr and an increase in lactate and the lactate:pyruvate ratio. A decrease in EC reflects a more serious degree of hypoxia. It should also be noted that following correction of an hypoxic event the cerebral energy state quickly returns toward normal even in the presence of irreversible functional brain damage. Measurement of brain metabolites has been used to determine the rate of energy utilization immediately after discontinuing substrate delivery to the brain. Such measured rates of energy consumption reflect those of nonfunctioning brain, because the EEG becomes isoelectric within seconds of discontinuing substrate delivery.

Also in experimental animals, autoradiographic measurements of regional glucose metabolism are possible using either [^{14}C] deoxyglucose or [^{14}C] glucose. Each method has its proponents and its critics.[28,29] Both methods have been used to "map" brain activity in response to various drugs or stimuli. A recurring criticism of such mapping is the inescapable fact that a region of increased glucose metabolism may result from either neural excitatory activity or neural inhibition of normal inhibitors, (i.e., disinhibition). Interpretation of such regional metabolic measurements is therefore limited.

HYPOTHERMIC BRAIN

Hypothermia has intrigued physiologists and clinicians since the mid-1950s as a potent nonpharmacologic means of reducing brain (and whole body) metabolism, limited only by the degree of hypothermia achieved. The relationship of temperature to metabolic rate is commonly expressed as the Q_{10} value, which is simply the ratio of two metabolic rates separated by 10°C; it defines a simple exponential relationship. Thus, if the Q_{10} value is 2.0, it follows that a 10°C decrease in temperature will result in a 50 percent decrease in metabolism. However, for function-

TABLE 1.2 *Normal brain metabolites in different species (μmol/g)*

REFERENCE	SPECIES	PCr	ATP	ADP	AMP	EC	LACTATE	L/P
Pontén et al.[25]	Rat	4.71	3.00	0.26	0.04	0.95	1.64	14
Pontén et al.[26]	Mouse	5.14	3.12	0.20	0.03	0.96	1.38	17
Roald et al.[27]	Dog	2.94	2.01	0.38	0.14	0.87	1.23	11

Abbreviations: PCr, phosphocreatine; ATP, ADP, AMP, adenosine triphosphate, diphosphate, monophosphate; EC, energy charge; L/P, lactate/pyruvate.

(From Michenfelder,[253] with permission.)

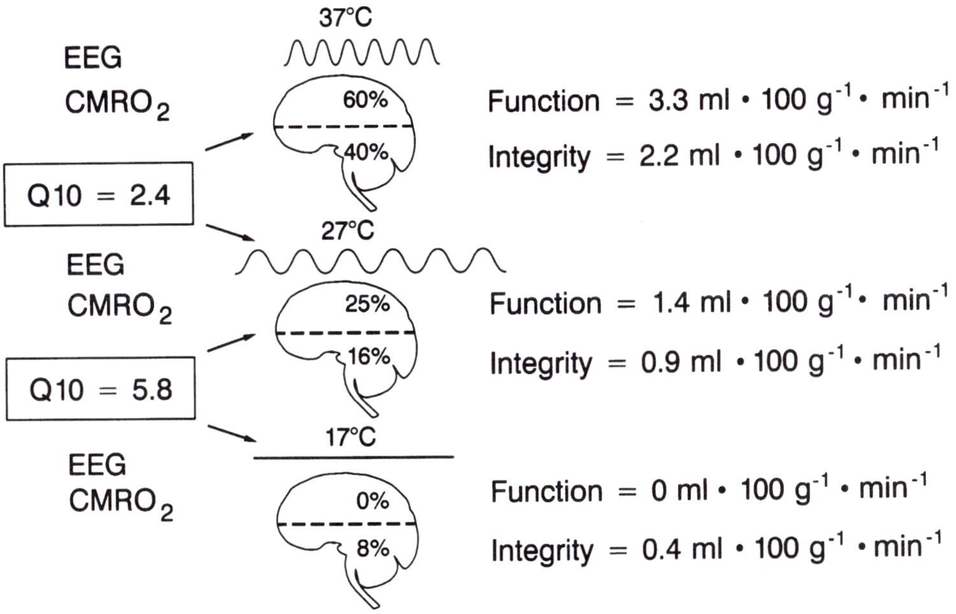

FIGURE 1.3 *Theoretical interaction of temperature, brain function, $CMRO_2$, and calculated Q_{10} values. In reducing temperature from 37 to 27°C, function is maintained, and both of the energy-consuming processes (i.e., function and integrity) are presumed to be affected equally with a slightly more than 50 percent reduction in $CMRO_2$, thus, generating a Q_{10} value of about 2.4. With a further 10° reduction in temperature to 17°C, function is abolished, resulting in a step decrease in $CMRO_2$ such that the calculated Q_{10} value is 5.0 or greater. At this point, the total oxygen consumed by the brain is reduced to less than 8 percent of the normothermic value.*

ing brain, the relationship is not a simple exponential one. In two canine studies, we observed Q_{10} values varying between approximately 2.0 and 5.0, depending on the temperature and the state of the brain function[30,31] (Fig. 1.3). Thus, between 27° and 37°C with continuous EEG activity, the Q_{10} was near 2.0. However, between 27° and 17°C during which the EEG becomes isoelectric, there is a presumed step decrease in $CMRO_2$, resulting in a calculated Q_{10} of near 5.0. Below 17°C, when EEG activity is minimal or absent, the Q_{10} returns to near 2.0.[32] In the absence of all EEG activity as maintained by deep barbiturate anesthesia, the Q_{10} remains near 2.0 over the entire temperature range.

To the degree that brain metabolic rate is diminished, hypothermia provides a measureable degree of brain protection as reflected by the brain's tolerance for ischemia. If normothermic brain will tolerate 5 minutes of total ischemia (estimates of as long as 15 to 17 minutes have been proposed based upon animal investigations), then at least 10 minutes will be tolerated at 27°C, whereas at 17°C this would be extended to 50 minutes or longer. These relationships were in part confirmed by demonstrating that the rate of energy depletion in canine brain upon discontinuing substrate delivery is reduced 50 percent at 27°C[33] (Fig. 1.4).

At moderate levels of hypothermia (i.e., above 27°C), both CO_2 reactivity and autoregulation are intact while CBF and $CMRO_2$ remain coupled. At lesser temperatures, this probably remains true, but studies are complicated by the needed presence of cardiopulmonary bypass, which introduces confounding variables that

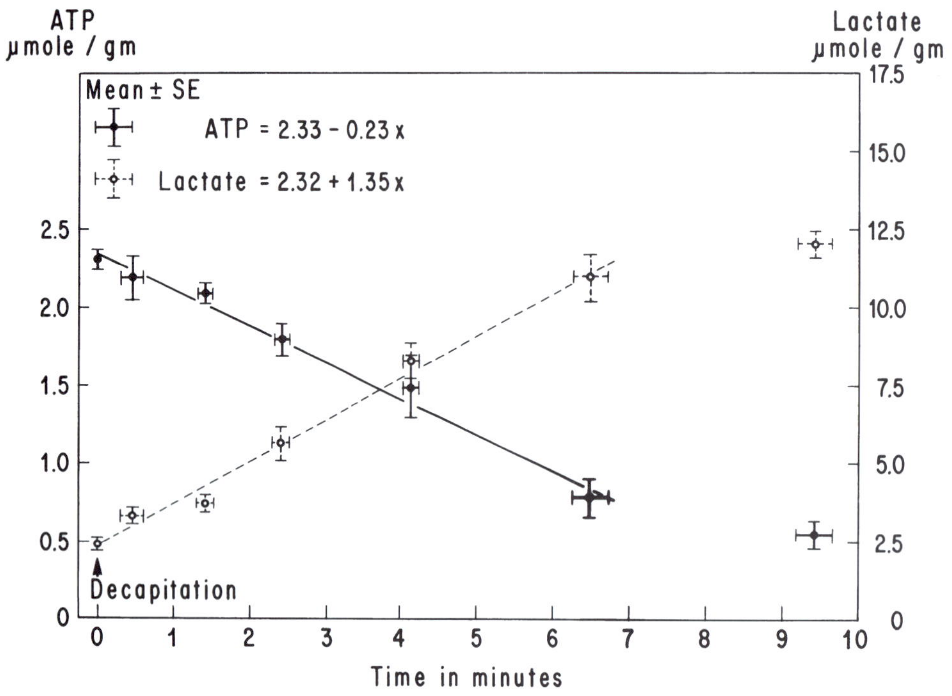

FIGURE 1.4 *Canine brain ATP and lactate values following decapitation at 30°C. The rates of ATP depletion and lactate accumulation following decapitation are depicted. These rates are about one-half those observed at normothermia. (From Michenfelder and Theye,[33] with permission).*

sometimes blur interpretation. From a physiologic standpoint, the limited available data suggest that uncorrected $PaCO_2$ values as measured at 37°C should be used for defining hypo or hypercarbia during hypothermia.[34,35]

PATHOLOGIC BRAIN

In the presence of brain pathology, almost any perturbation in the normal relationships between CBF, CMR, CBV, and ICP is possible. With the exception of discrete midbrain or brainstem lesions, the presence of intracranial pathology can be expected to reduce intracranial compliance such that the patient is at increased risk for significant ICP increases. In these circumstances, autoregulation is usually attenuated or absent, at least in the region of pathology, such that CBF (and ICP) may passively follow changes in cerebral perfusion pressure. Similary, CO_2 reactivity, although more robust than autoregulation, may be attenuated or absent in the region of pathology.[36] Accordingly, it is theoretically possible and experimentally demonstrable that hypercarbia may steal CBF from the region of pathology by dilating normal vessels, whereas hypocarbia may do the opposite (Robin Hood effect). Recognition that such phenomena can occur appears to have great appeal for certain pundits, even though the clinical relevance of such theoretical considerations is questionable at best.[37]

In many pathologic states, the normal tight coupling between CBF and CMR is absent or distorted. This may result in zones of luxury perfusion (CBF in excess of metabolic needs) or penumbral zones (regions of potentially viable tissue with marginal CBF). In the event of seizures, coupling between CBF and CMR is usually maintained such that both increase in the presence of an adequate cerebral perfusion pressure.

We are largely ignorant of the effect of anesthetics on CBF and CMR in pathologic brain. We assume that the volatile anesthetics may, like hypercarbia, steal CBF from pathologic regions by dilating normal vessels, but I know of no convincing experimental (or clinical) demonstration of such a phenomenon. It seems entirely probable that if the pathology is sufficient to abolish autoregulation and CO_2 reactivity, the normal effect of anesthetics will also be abolished or distorted. Hyperventilation is a commonly utilized intervention in the presence of brain pathology both in the operating room and in the intensive care unit. Its use assumes the presence of CO_2 reactivity sufficient to result in decreased CBF, CBV, and ICP. Logically, its application should be limited to a period of hours (as in the operating room) rather than days (as may occur in the intensive care unit). In the latter application, any effect of hypocarbia on CBF and ICP should be largely dissipated after 24 to 36 hours due to equilibration of CSF pH secondary to the slow egress of bicarbonate.[38] In this circumstance, an abrupt return to normocarbia will be interpreted by the cerebral vasculature as hypercarbia because of the abrupt decrease in CSF pH that will occur.

EFFECT OF ANESTHETICS

Before considering the cerebral effects of individual anesthetic drugs, some generalizations might be appropriate. An obvious but not easily answered question is, When is the brain anesthetized? There is no accepted definition. Mine is a simple one: the anesthetized brain is one incapable of self-awareness or subsequent recall. It is common to encounter arguments that anesthesia requires a minimum of 1 MAC of an inhalational anesthetic or its equivalent if using an intravenous or balanced technique. But 1 MAC defines that concentration at which 50 percent of subjects do not respond to a major noxious stimulus with some type of purposeful muscular movement. It has nothing to do with awareness or recall. There is a body of evidence that suggests that awareness and recall are lost at concentrations well less than 1 MAC. Thus in humans during induction of anesthesia with thiopental, there is an abrupt shift of EEG dominance to the anterior leads at about the same time as the subject ceases to respond to verbal commands. In subhuman primates, this anterior shift in EEG dominance is consistently observed to occur at about 0.5 MAC.[39] Also MAC awake in humans, (i.e., that expired concentration at which humans respond to simple verbal commands upon emerging from anesthesia) varies from 0.15 to 0.5 MAC.[40,41] In dogs the rate of change in $CMRO_2$ during induction of anesthesia is not linear; rather, there is an abrupt decrease in $CMRO_2$ at the same time as the EEG shifts from a stable "awake" pattern to a stable "anesthetic" pattern.[42] This occurs at MAC concentrations of 0.5 to 0.7 (Fig. 1.5). Finally, most patients will lapse into unconsciousness while breathing 50% nitrous oxide even though this is equivalent to only 0.48 MAC. Based upon these considerations, it is inappropriate to insist upon a minimum equivalent of 1.0 MAC of anesthesia for either our patients or for experimental animals.

Neither is the EEG a reliable indicator of anesthetic depth unless pushed to the point of burst suppression. At lighter EEG levels, various noxious stimuli can result in abrupt activation of the EEG yielding a pattern not unlike that of an awake EEG.

In the case of narcotics, there are isolated case reports that suggest that in some patients loss of recall is never achieved,[43,44] whereas in dogs even massive doses do not predictably prevent an arousal response to noxious stimuli.[45]

In practice we rely upon accurate vaporizers and flowmeters, expired gas concentrations, knowledge regarding the potency, pharmacokinetics, and pharmacodynamics of the drugs we administer, and a large dose of clinical experience in order to induce and maintain an ade-

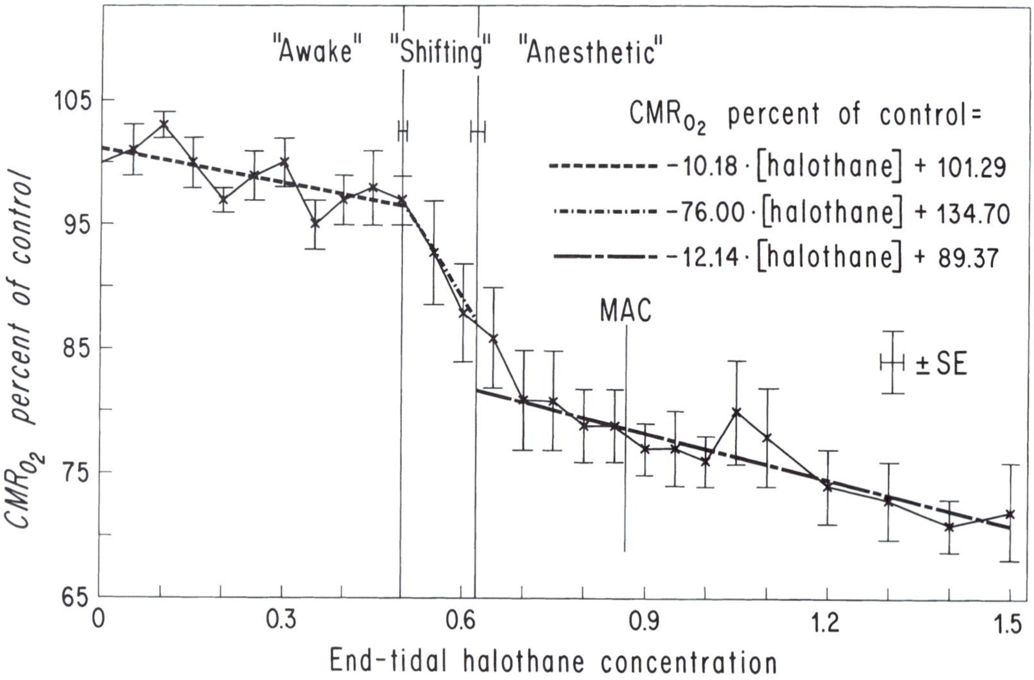

FIGURE 1.5 *The effects of halothane on $CMRO_2$ as a percentage of control. $CMRO_2$ is plotted versus end-tidal halothane concentration. Regression lines for changes in $CMRO_2$ are drawn for each EEG determined area. The pattern depicted here was characteristic for all of the anesthetics examined. (From Stullken et al.,[42] with permission.)*

quate anesthetic depth for our individual patients.

An important generalization regarding anesthetic effects is the relationship between their metabolic and functional effects. There is abundant evidence that anesthetics only alter cerebral metabolic rates to the degree that they alter cerebral function as reflected by the EEG. In the absence of EEG activity (whether produced by deep anesthesia, hypothermia, or ischemia), anesthetics are without effect on $CMRO_2$.[30,46,47] This relationship has important implications for the potential for brain protection by anesthetics. Thus, it was correctly predicted by some that barbiturates could not provide brain protection, at least on a metabolic basis, in the event of an isoelectric EEG such as occurs during and immediately following resuscitation from cardiac arrest. Similarly, it has been consistently demonstrable that anesthetics such as barbiturates can prolong the brain's tolerance for an ischemic or hypoxia insult so long as the insult is not sufficient to abolish EEG activity.

Inhalational Agents

NITROUS OXIDE Over the years nitrous oxide has enjoyed the status of near ubiquity, largely because it is an inexpensive, easily administered, nonexplosive potent analgesic. It has also been incorrectly characterized as being nontoxic and physiologically inert. Although of questionable relevance, toxicity secondary to prolonged administration is demonstrable as regards its effects on methionine synthetase.[48] Likewise, there is some circumstantial evidence of toxicity secondary to chronic exposure to trace concentrations of nitrous oxide.[49] More importantly, nitrous oxide is not physiologically inert. As regards the brain, it can have potential striking effects on CBF and ICP while affecting CMR little if any.

The literature is confusing regarding nitrous oxide effects on the brain primarily because of species differences in both response and potency and interactions with other drugs or interventions. As regards potency, the MAC for nitrous oxide varies from as little as 82 percent of an atmosphere for the toad[50] to as high as 275 percent of an atmosphere for mice[51]—more than a threefold difference. Unlike most drugs, this potency difference cannot be corrected for by adjusting doses (except in a hyperbaric chamber); thus we are often comparing the effects of 70 percent nitrous oxide in different species despite up to threefold differences in potential dose-response relationships.

In comparing the results reported in experimental animals, it becomes apparent that nitrous oxide has little or no effect on CBF and CMR in the rat, whereas it has potentially major effects on CBF in other species[52–73] (Table 1.3). Likewise, the evidence in humans strongly supports the conclusion that nitrous oxide is a potent cerebral vasodilator in the absence of other interventions (Table 1.4) and as such may cause ICP increases as well.[74–79] That this seems to be largely without clinical relevance is accounted for by the fact that nitrous oxide is rarely used in the absence of other interventions. When combined with barbiturates, narcotics, hypocarbia, or volatile anesthetics, the potential effects of nitrous oxide on CBF and ICP appear to be attenuated or abolished, at least in humans. Still it would seem prudent in the event of encountering a "tight" brain intraoperatively that discontinuation of nitrous oxide should be considered among possibly beneficial interventions.

HALOTHANE It is somewhat ironical that halothane for almost a decade (until 1969) enjoyed the status of the most commonly used anesthetic for neurosurgical procedures and that today it remains the most commonly condemned anesthetic for these same procedures. Although certain pundits tend to resist the facts, they are as follows: (1) halothane is a potent cerebral vasodilator; (2) as such it can cause striking increases in ICP; and (3) however, if preceded by hyperventilation to a $PaCO_2$ level of approximately 25 mmHg, these effects (i.e., 1 and 2) are obliterated. The conclusion from these facts should be that halothane may be used for neurosurgical procedures if used correctly rather than simple blind condemnation of its use.

The evidence in support of the above-identified facts is abundant. That halothane is a potent cerebral vasodilator resulting in increased CBF in the presence of normocarbia and a normal cerebral perfusion pressure has been repetitively demonstrated in a host of laboratories and subjects including humans.[80–87] Similarly, it is indisputable that under these same conditions (i.e., normocarbia and normal perfusion pressure) halothane will increase cerebral blood volume and in a brain rendered noncompliant by pathology will increase ICP, perhaps to a striking degree.

The above crystaline facts were blurred by the interpretation applied to a report published in 1969 by Jennett et al.[88] They described the effects of halothane, trichlorethylene, and methoxyflurane on ICP in patients with intracranial pathology. It was their intent to study patients at normocarbia, and as such it was to be fully expected that each of these volatile anesthetics would cause an increase in ICP in such patients and without exception. Such was the substance of their report. However, because their patients inadvertently became hypothermic (to less than 35°C)in most instances, the temperature-corrected values for $PaCO_2$ were consistently hypocarbic (by normothermic standards). As already stated, such temperature correction is probably not valid from a physiologic standpoint. In any case, an anonymous editorial in the *British Journal of Anaesthesia* followed this report and condemned volatile anesthetics for neurosurgical procedures, concluding that even hypocarbia did not prevent the potentially deleterious ICP effects.[89] Such remains the common perception today.

TABLE 1.3 *Effect of nitrous oxide on CBF and CMR in experimental animals*

REFERENCE	SPECIES	METHOD	NITROUS OXIDE CONCENTRATION (%)	SUPPLEMENTAL ANESTHESIA	MODIFIERS	CBF EFFECTS	CMR EFFECTS	OTHER EFFECTS
Carlsson et al.[52] (1976)	Rat	Kety-Schmidt	70		Adrenalectomy or beta block	None	None	Control values "stress free"
Carlsson et al.[53] (1976)	Rat	Kety-Schmidt	70	Diazepam		↓60%	↓60%	Diazepam alone had little effect on CBF and none on $CMRO_2$
Berntman et al.[54] (1976)	Rat	Kety-Schmidt	70		Adrenalectomy		Withdrawal of N_2O ↑ $CMRO_2$ 40–90% if not adrenalectomized only	Metabolites normal
Ingvar et al.[55] (1980)	Rat	[2-^{14}C]deoxyglucose	70				Little or no effect	
Dahlgren et al.[56] (1981)	Rat	[^{14}C]iodoantipyrine	70–80			No change in most structures		
Crosby et al.[58] (1983)	Rat	[2-^{14}C]deoxyglucose	70		Stimulation Saphenous nerve		↑ 10% in cortex with stimulation—no different from pentobarbital	
Crosby et al.[59] (1984)	Rat	[2-^{14}C]deoxyglucose	70				↑ 15–25% in most structures	
Sakabe et al.[60] (1985)	Rat	[2-^{14}C]deoxyglucose	67	Pentobarbital 30 and 125 mg/kg			↑ at 30 mg/kg; little effect at 125 mg/kg	
Seyde et al.[61] (1986)	Rat	Microspheres	70	Halothane 1.5%		↑ 15%		

Theye and Michenfelder[62] (1968)	Dog	Venous outflow	70	Halothane 0–1%	Spinal anesthesia	↑ 35%	↑ 11% without halothane; none with halothane	Sympathetics blocked (spinal)
Sakabe et al.[63] (1978)	Dog	Venous outflow	60	Halothane 0.2 and 0.8%	Reserpine	↑ 103% at 0.2% halothane ↑ 64% at 0.8% halothane	↑ 21% at 0.2% halothane ↑ 8% at 0.8% halothane	Not due to sympathetics
Oshita et al.[64] (1979)	Dog	Venous outflow and Kety-Schmidt	57	Halothane 0.18%		↑ 40%	↑ 17%	Validated CBF method
Fitzpatrick and Gilboe[65] (1982)	Dog	Isolated head	70		↓ CVR 16%	No effect		
Manohar and Parks[66] (1984)	Pig	Microspheres	50	Halothane 0–1.5 MAC		N_2O ↑ 100% at 1.0 MAC		
Manohar and Parks[67] (1984)	Pig	Microspheres	50	Isoflurane 0–1.5 MAC		N_2O ↑ 37% at 1.0 MAC		
Manohar and Parks[68] (1984)	Pig	Microspheres	50	Enflurane 0–1.5 MAC		N_2O ↑ 51% at 1.0 MAC		
Manohar[69] (1985)	Pig	Microspheres	50			↑ about 40% for 45 min		
Manohar[70] (1985)	Pig	Microspheres	70			↑ about 50% for 2 h in all structures		
Pelligrino et al.[71] (1984)	Goat	Direct	70			↑ 43%	↑ 70%	Plasma epinephrine and brain metabolites normal
Drummond et al.[72] (1987)	Rabbit	H_2 clearance	70	Halothane or isoflurane 0.5–1.0 MAC		↑ 20–100%		
Todd[73] (1987)	Rabbit	H_2 clearance	70	Halothane 1.0 MAC		↑ 40%		

Abbreviations: CBF, cerebral blood flow; CMR, cerebral metabolism; MAC

(From Michenfelder,[253] with permission.)

TABLE 1.4 *Effects of nitrous oxide on CBF, CMR, or ICP in humans*

REFERENCE	METHOD	NITROUS OXIDE CONCENTRATION (%)	MODIFIERS	EFFECTS	COMMENTS
Latinen et al.[74] (1967)	Cerebral impedance	75	Normocarbic; either no drugs or thiopental; patients without ↑ ICP	Impedance increased severalfold within 30 s, ICP ↑ simultaneously	Modifying effects of thoipental cannot be judged in this report
Henricksen and Jorgenson[75] (1973)	ICP measured	66	Pre-medicated with diazepam 2.5–10 mg; $PaCO_2$ 33–36 mmHg; minor BP changes	ICP ↑ from 13 to 40 mmHg within 60 s to 5 min; no patient excitation noted; Returned on withdrawal	Diazepam had no effect; effect blocked by hypocapnia to 29 mmHg
Sakabe et al.[76] (1976)	Measured C(a - v) O_2 across brain	60	Patients anesthetized with halothane 0.84%; $PaCO_2$ = 31–35 mmHg; BP stable	Threefold ↑ in CBF equivalent from 17 to 45; effect was nearly immediate and returned to control on withdrawal	Simple straightforward methods; either CBF ↑ 3 × or $CMRO_2$ ↓ 3 × or some combination
Phirman and Shapiro[77] (1977)	ICP measured	70	Case report in comatose patient with and without diazepam and thiopental $PaCO_2$ = 31 mmHg	ICP ↑ from 15 to 35 mmHg × 2; then blocked by diazepam (5 mg), thiopental (150 mg)	Cannot separate diazepam effects from thiopental effects
Jobes et al.[78] (1977)	Kety-Schmidt (volunteers)	70	N_2O plus morphine sulfate in dose of either 1 or 3 mg/kg; normocapnia; BP stable	No effects on CBF or $CMRO_2$	N_2O effects blocked by morphine sulfate
Moss and McDowall[79] (1979)	ICP measured	50	Head injury patients; no other drugs	Increased ICP a mean of 4 mmHg	Consistent response to N_2O was observed

Abbreviations: CBF, cerebral blood flow; CMR, cerebral metabolism; ICP, intracranial pressure; BP, blood pressure;

(From Michenfelder,[253] with permission.)

Still it has been shown that true hypocarbia (to a $PaCO_2$ of approximately 25 mmHg at normothermia) when induced prior to introducing 1 percent halothane consistently prevents any clinically relevant increase in ICP in patients with intracranial pathology[90] (Fig. 1.6). In that same study, it was shown that simultaneous introduction of hyperventilation and halothane did not consistently prevent a transient ICP increase. But even then, the increase (which occurred in one-third of the subjects) was usually moderate and always transient (less than 30

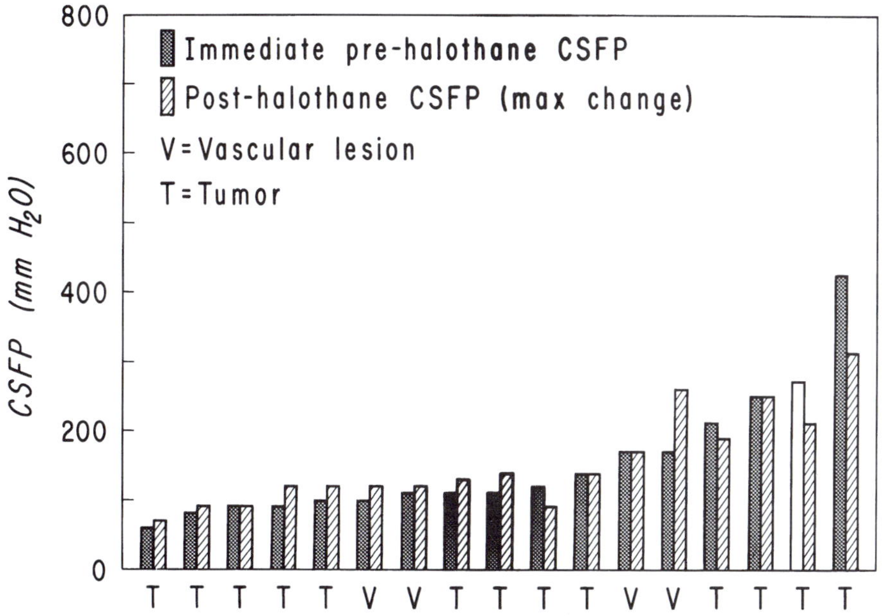

FIGURE 1.6 *Effect of halothane on cerebral spinal fluid pressure (CSFP) when administered 10 minutes after the onset of hyperventilation. Only small increases in pressure were observed in some patients after the use of halothane. The largest increase (90 mm water) occurred in a patient with a vascular lesion. There was no relationship between prehalothane CSFP and CSFP increases after halothane. (From Adams et al.,[90] with permission.)*

minutes in duration). There is simply no scientific basis for condemning the proper use of halothane or other volatile anesthetics in patients with intracranial pathology.

Other cerebral vascular effects of halothane include an apparent enhancement of CO_2 reactivity,[91,92] whereas autoregulation may be attenuated and, at concentrations exceeding 1.5 MAC, even abolished.[93,94] Qualitatively, these effects appear to be shared by all of the volatile anesthetics but to a varying degree quantitatively.

Another feature common to the volatile anesthetics is an apparent uncoupling of the relationship between CBF and $CMRO_2$. All tend to increase CBF while decreasing $CMRO_2$. The work of Smith suggests that coupling is not abolished but rather simply reset.[95] He showed for different volatile anesthetics (with and without nitrous oxide) that cerebral venous PO_2 was consistently increased above normal but at the same MAC equivalents was the same for all of the anesthetics. Furthermore, as dose increased so too did cerebral venous PO_2. The mechanism to account for such resetting is unknown: an optimist might conclude that the brain is "superoxygenated," whereas a pessimist might conclude that such resetting is a subclinical manifestation of toxicity such that the brain needs more oxygen. Smith and Wollman also pointed out that the ratio of CBF to $CMRO_2$ was the same for a variety of anesthetics at the same MAC equivalents and increased with increasing concentrations[96] (Fig. 1.7). Drummond et al. have expanded on these observations and suggest that the CBF response to an anesthetic is determined solely by the metabolic response.[97] It follows from this that halothane must be a more potent vasodilator than isoflurane because the latter is a more potent depressant of $CMRO_2$. Similarly, it has been shown that pentobarbital actually causes cerebral vasodilation when administered

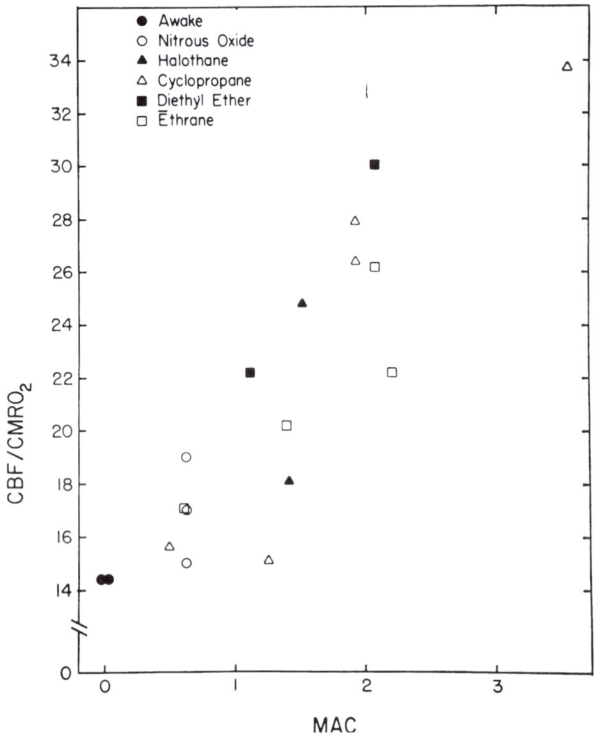

FIGURE 1.7 *Effect of various inhalational anesthetics on the ratio of CBF to $CMRO_2$. All of the inhalational anesthetics increased the ratio to a similar degree and do so in a dose-related fashion. (From Smith and Wollman,[96] with permission.)*

to an animal with an isoelectric EEG or burst-suppression as produced by deep isoflurane anesthesia.[98] In this circumstance, no further metabolic suppression by the barbiturate is possible, and thus the usually "coupled" vasoconstriction does not occur; rather the true vasodilator properties of barbiturates are unmasked (as is demonstrable in vitro).[99–103]

Within clinically relevant concentrations, halothane causes a moderate decrease in $CMRO_2$ (20 to 30 percent) without any evidence of toxicity as reflected by normal brain metabolites in experimental animals.[104] However, at end-expired concentrations exceeding 2.3 percent, evidence for toxicity exists both in vivo and in vitro. In the latter studies, state 3 of mitochondrial respiration was progressively disrupted,[105] whereas in vivo studies demonstrated progressive deterioration in the brain energy state with increased brain lactate[106] (Fig. 1.8). In the latter study, it was noteworthy that at blood halothane concentrations equivalent to 4.5 percent the EEG became isoelectric, but unlike the case for isoflurane and thiopental (see below), $CMRO_2$ did not plateau at this point but continued to decrease with increasing concentrations. This combined with the disruption of the cerebral energy state was considered incontrovertible evidence of toxicity. The latter was not related to either a reduction in CBF or to maldistribution of CBF.

The potential for halothane-induced cerebral toxicity is consistent with the fact that halothane has been reported to aggravate the effects of regional cerebral ischemia in experimental animals.[107,108] This of course might be explained by a simple unfavorable redistribution of CBF rather than any direct toxic effects. In any case, at concentrations used for clinical anesthesia, there is no evidence for cerebral toxicity induced by halothane.

ENFLURANE In large part because of concern regarding possible halothane-induced hepatotoxicity, enflurane enjoyed the status of the preferred volatile anesthetic for a few years until isoflurane became available in 1981–1982. Enflurane is a less potent cerebral vasodilator than halothane and a more potent suppressant of $CMRO_2$,[109] thus conforming to the already suggested relationships between CBF and $CMRO_2$ induced by anesthetics (see above). As with the other volatile anesthetics in use today, enflurane tends to augment CO_2 reactivity while attenuating autoregulation. At concentrations of 1.0 MAC or less, these potential effects are of only minimal clinical relevance.

A unique property for enflurane is its predictable capacity to induce seizures when administered in high concentrations (greater than 1.5 MAC) and particularly when combined with significant hypocapnia (less than 30 mmHg). In experimental animals (and presumably humans), this combination plus a loud auditory stimulus will consistently produce a burst of seizure activity on the EEG.[109] This is accompa-

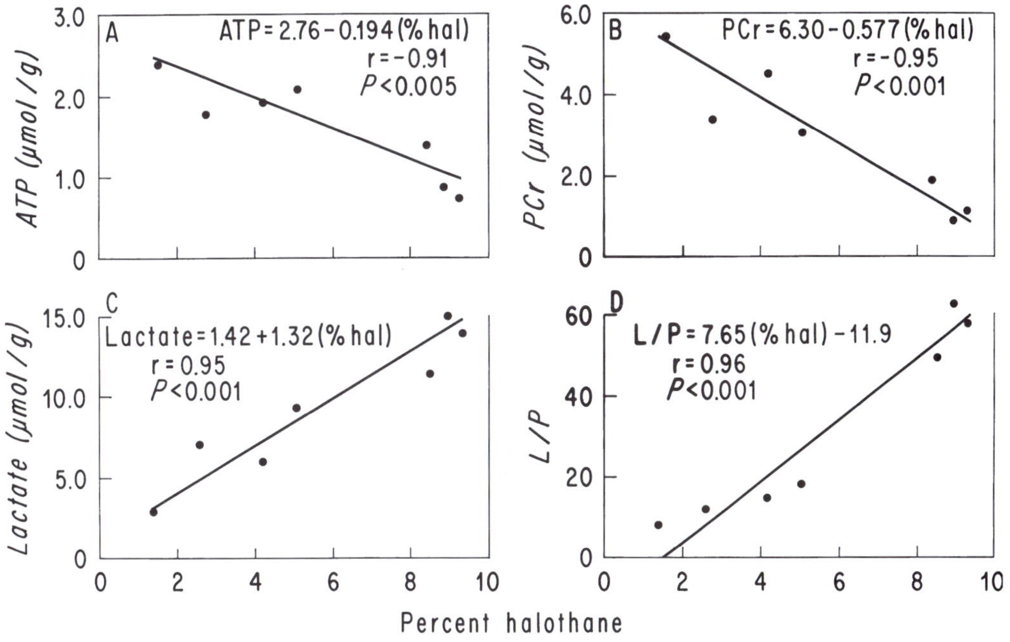

FIGURE 1.8 *Cerebral concentrations of ATP, PC and lactate and cerebral L/P plotted against blood halothane concentrations. A linear relationship is suggested for all with progressive decreases in ATP and PCR (A and B) and increases in lactate and L/P (C & D). (From Michenfelder and Theye,[106] with permission.)*

nied by an increase in $CMRO_2$ to that of control levels or greater as well as an appropriate increase in CBF (assuming maintenance of an adequate cerebral perfusion pressure). In volunteers such seizures resulted in no residual effects,[110] and to my knowledge none have been demonstrated in patients. Although controversial, there is no scientific evidence to support an opinion that enflurane should be avoided in patients with a seizure history. Granted, enflurane has been used to purposefully bring out a seizure focus in patients undergoing surgery for control of seizures, but at concentrations normally used for maintaining anesthesia (and assuming avoidance of extreme hypocapnia), seizures do not occur.

ISOFLURANE Isoflurane is the most popular of the volatile anesthetics in use today. Although an isomer of enflurane, its cerebral properties are strikingly different. Compared to halothane and enflurane, it is the least potent vasodilator and the most potent depressant of $CMRO_2$ (again conforming to the previously suggested relationship between CBF and $CMRO_2$ induced by anesthetics). Uniquely among all available volatile anesthetics, isoflurane has the capacity to induce an isoelectric EEG at concentrations that are tolerated hemodynamically by both humans and experimental animals[47] (approximately 2.0 MAC). Unlike the case with halothane, the onset of an isoelectric EEG in dogs is accompanied by a plateau effect on $CMRO_2$ (Fig. 1.9) similar to that seen with thiopental[46] (see below). Similarly, the cerebral energy state in the presence of even 4.0 MAC isoflurane is normal as is the case with high-dose thiopental, contrasting strikingly with that seen with high-dose halothane.

Like halothane, isoflurane has been shown in

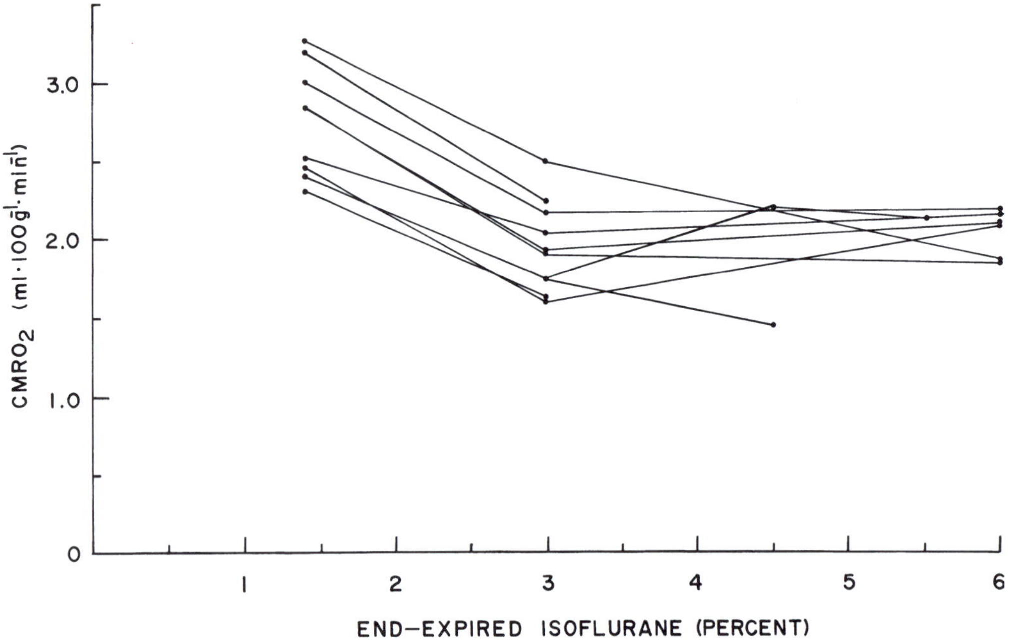

FIGURE 1.9 *Effect of high doses of isoflurane on $CMRO_2$. At 2 MAC isoflurane (3 percent), an isoelectric EEG was produced, and further increases in isoflurane concentration to as much as 4 MAC had no further affect on $CMRO_2$. (From Newberg et al.,[47] with permission.)*

humans to have the potential to increase ICP in patients with intracranial pathology, but this potential is completely obliterated by hyperventilation.[111] Unlike halothane, it is not necessary to induce hypocapnia prior to introducing the anesthetic. Rather, the simultaneous introduction of both hyperventilation and isoflurane will prevent any ICP increases. There is one study reported in humans wherein the authors arrived at a different conclusion.[112] In 14 patients with brain tumors given isoflurane plus moderate hyperventilation, 8 did not develop any increase in ICP. In the remaining 6, a modest increase in ICP was observed but was judged insufficient to require any change in protocol or discontinuation of isoflurane. Still, the authors concluded "isoflurane may not be a benign anesthetic in patients known to be at risk for increases in ICP." One must wonder why. I am unaware of any evidence to support such a conclusion.

The case for meaningful brain protection by isoflurane relative to the barbiturates remains unproven. Certainly the case for such protection relative to halothane and enflurane in patients undergoing carotid endarterectomy has been made.[113] For routine neurosurgical procedures, most practitioners have accepted isoflurane as an appropriate anesthetic if accompanied by hypocapnia. It has been a long, slow climb since 1969, when halothane was wrongly condemned, to today's perception by most (but certainly not all) that another volatile agent—isoflurane—is acceptable.

DESFLURANE Desflurane is a recently introduced volatile anesthetic for clinical use in the United States. It differs from isoflurane chemically by the substitution of fluorine for chlorine on the α-carbon of the ethyl group. It differs physically from the other available volatile anesthetics primarily because of its very low blood solubility (blood-gas partition coefficient equals 0.42 in humans), similar to that of nitrous oxide (0.47). This property ensures rapid emergence from the anesthetic state and makes the agent potentially valuable for use in outpatient surgery and in certain neurosurgical procedures where immediate postoperative neurological evaluation of the patient is considered desirable. In clinically used concentrations in humans, desflurane does not adversely affect ICP.[114]

The cerebral metabolic and vascular effects of desflurane are qualitatively and, for the most part, quantitatively similar to the effects of other volatile anesthetics previously described.[115] In canine studies at normocapnia, it has been shown that there is a dose-related decrease in CMR and, if blood pressure is maintained, increases in both CBF and ICP, at least up to concentrations of 2.0 MAC.[116] In that same study, it was observed that at 2.0 MAC an initial EEG pattern of burst-suppression reverted spontaneously to continuous activity with the passage of time. Such an effect has not been previously observed with the other volatile anesthetics and suggested the possibility of an acute tolerance phenomenon. In a subsequent study in swine, this reported canine EEG effect was specifically looked for but never observed.[117] Neither has this phenomenon been observed in humans.

In another canine study, it was shown that CO_2 reactivity of the cerebral vaculature remained intact in the presence of desflurane, at least up to concentrations of 1.5 MAC,[118] even in the presence moderate hypotension. Hypotension was deliberately induced in a subsequent canine study using desflurane concentrations of up to 2.4 MAC (17.1%) to maintain blood pressure at 40 mmHg for 1 hour.[119] Despite a 60% decrease in CBF, there was no indication of cerebral ischemia at the end of the hour as reflected by brain metabolite concentrations of PCR, ATP, ADP, AMP, lactate, and pyruvate. This presumably was accounted for by an accompanying 21% decrease in CMR.

SEVOFLURANE Sevoflurane has been recently approved for clinical use in the United States, although it has been used clinically in Europe for several years. It shares with desflurane a relatively low blood solubility (blood gas partition coefficient, 0.63). Its primary potential advantages include rapid onset and offset, which might offer advantages in some neurosurgical procedures. In addition, it has a less irritating effect on the airway compared to other volatile anesthetic agents, making it a popular agent for inhalation induction. Like isoflurane, sevoflurane causes little or no increase in ICP at concentrations up to 1.5 MAC both in normocapnic and hypocapnic animal models.[120,121]

The effects of sevoflurane on CBF and CMR most closely resemble those of isoflurane. In most animal models, both at normocarbia and hypocarbia, sevoflurane, like isoflurane, causes minimal changes in global CBF.[120,122,123] In dogs administered sevoflurane after prior institution of hyperventilation, sevoflurane caused no increase in ICP at concentrations up to 1.5 MAC, whereas in the same model, increases in ICP were observed with both halothane and enflurane.[121] However, the impact of simultaneous administration of sevoflurane and institution of hyperventilation was not studied, as has been done with isoflurane. In addition, it causes similar decreases in $CMRO_2$ when compared to isoflurane.[120,122] Sevoflurane in clinically useful concentrations can cause burst suppression (approximately 2 MAC).[122] In patients with ischemic cerebrovascular disease, the effect of sevoflurane on cerebral autoregulation and CBF response to changes in $PaCO_2$ was investigated. Cerebral autoregulation was found to be intact in the presence of sevoflurane at a concentration slightly below 1 MAC, and cerebral vascular responsiveness to changes in $PaCO_2$ was preserved although slightly blunted as compared to other volatile agents.[122] There is no evidence that acute tolerance or cerebral toxicity develops after prolonged exposure to higher concentrations.[125,126] In animal models, the addition of hyperventilation or hypotension resulting in significant decreases in CBF (>50% below control) resulted in depletion of brain energy stores in the presence of 4 MAC sevoflurane. However, in the absence of hyperventilation or hypotension, administration of 4 MAC sevoflurane did not result in abnormalities of brain energy stores. Lesser degrees of hyperventilation were tolerated during halothane administration.[126] In some animal models, sevoflurane appears to have proconvulsant effects similar to enflurane, whereas in other models this effect is not demonstrated.[122,125]

Intravenous Agents

BARBITURATES Thiopental and the other anesthetic barbiturates (primarily pentobarbital and methohexital) are commonly characterized as cerebral vasoconstrictors even though this may only be an effect secondary to metabolic suppression (see above). Regardless of cause and effect, the barbiturates do not uncouple CBF and $CMRO_2$, which therefore decrease in tandem with increasing doses of barbiturate up to the point of onset of an isoelectric EEG. As in the case of isoflurane, this is associated with a 50 to 60 percent decrease in $CMRO_2$ and, in experimental animals, no disruption in the normal cerebral metabolites or energy charge.[46]

The first study in humans of the effects of thiopental on CBF and $CMRO_2$ was reported in 1962 by Pierce et al.[127] They used large doses (10 to 55 mg/kg) and observed an approximate 50 to 55 percent decrease in both CBF and $CMRO_2$. With hyperventilation, they reported a further decrease in CBF but not $CMRO_2$. Thus in a single study, they reported the near maximal metabolic effects of thiopental (they did not correlate this with the EEG), the presence of coupling of CBF and $CMRO_2$, and the retention of CO_2 reactivity. In a host of subsequent animal investigations, these findings have been expanded upon and refined, but the basic information contained in that initial report remains unchallenged.

In a dog study we showed that even massive doses of thiopental do not induce any cerebral metabolic evidence of toxicity, whereas the maximum $CMRO_2$ effects were determined by the functional effects of the drug and not the dose given.[46] Thus with onset of an isoelectric EEG, $CMRO_2$ plateaued and was unaffected by additional large doses (Fig. 1.10). These results sup-

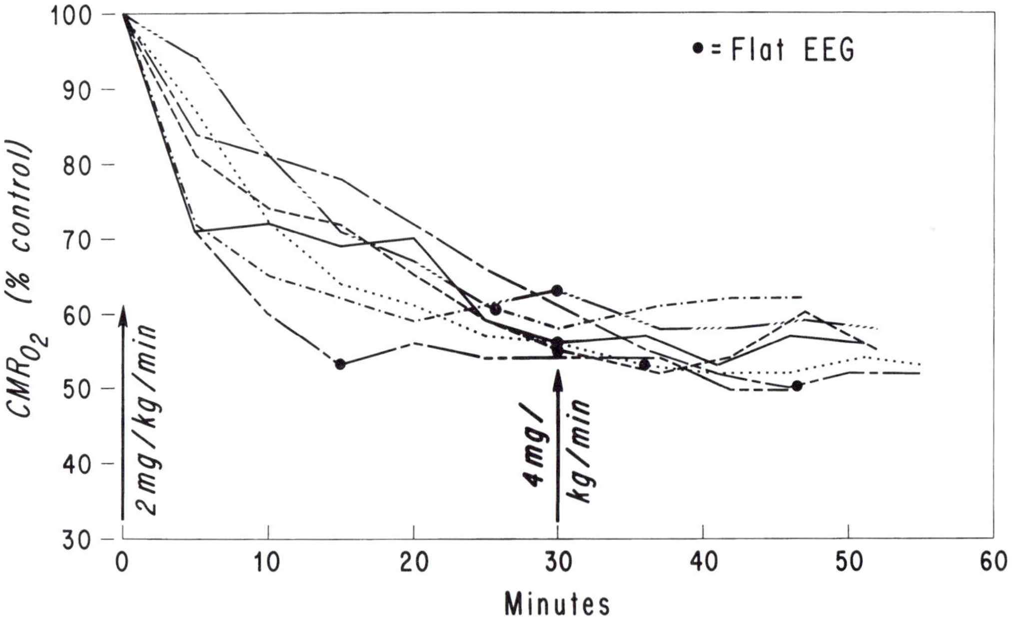

FIGURE 1.10 *Effect of massive doses of thiopental on $CMRO_2$. Individual $CMRO_2$ values are plotted as percentages of control values. In each dog $CMRO_2$ decreased progressively until the EEG became isoelectric. At this point $CMRO_2$ stabilized and despite continued infusion of thiopental did not decrease further. (From Michenfelder,[46] with permission.)*

port the hypothesis that in the absence of toxicity anesthetics only after brain metabolism to the degree that they alter brain function. Further, these results were the basis for predicting that barbiturates could not protect brain (on a metabolic basis) during or following complete global ischemia since the insult itself abolished the functional component. Finally, these results are consistent with the clinical reality that barbiturate "intoxication" is completely reversible if circulation and respiration can be supported.

In the clinical setting, if it is desirable to pursue near maximal brain metabolic suppression with thiopental for the purpose of protecting the brain, an end point of burst-suppression on the EEG should be sought. To strive for an isoelectric EEG introduces an increased risk of significant hemodynamic suppression with little further cerebral metabolic suppression. The use of barbiturates for the purpose of either protecting the brain or to reduce ICP will be dealt with in the chapters concerned with those topics.

NARCOTICS In terms of their cerebral functional effects narcotics are not true anesthetics, since their site of action is primarily subcortical rather than cortical. This presumably accounts for the recurrent case reports of patient recall even when very large doses have been used.[43,44] In dogs fentanyl doses ranging from 125 to 3,000 μg/kg failed to induce anesthesia consistently as judged by loss of response to a tail clamp.[45] Accordingly, narcotics are usually administered in combination with other anesthetics or with an amnestic drug such as diazepam or midazolam.

The effect of narcotics on CBF is not easy to characterize because of multiple conflicting reports in humans and experimental animals. When viewed in total an apparent pattern does emerge that largely accounts for the conflicts. As summarized in Table 1.5, the directional effects of narcotics on CBF seem to be dictated by the control circumstance.[128–148] Thus if a cerebral vasodilator such as nitrous oxide or halothane was used as the control anesthetic condition, narcotics consistently induced a decrease in CBF. If, however, a vasoconstricting anesthetic or no anesthesia was used during control measurements, narcotics either had no effect on CBF or caused an increase in CBF. The latter reported effect could not be accounted for either by the presence of seizures or hypercarbia.

A similar relationship appears to exist for the $CMRO_2$ effects of narcotics (Table 1.6). In the presence of nitrous oxide, narcotics consistently caused a decrease in $CMRO_2$, whereas in the absence of anesthetics, no change in $CMRO_2$ was reported.[128,130–137,141,142,146–151] The only exception was a study in awake humans reported in 1957 wherein morphine, 60 mg, caused a 40 percent decrease in $CMRO_2$.[148] There is no obvious explanation for this anomalous report. It should be noted that in those studies reporting metabolic suppression a plateau effect was commonly observed (suggesting complete receptor occupation), and when a narcotic antagonist was administered, the observed effect was immediately reversible. The latter observation leaves little doubt that the observed narcotic effects were not artifactual.

As used clinically, there is no evidence that narcotics induce major changes in cerebral hemodynamics. Except for one report in brain tumor patients of alfentanil-induced increases in ICP[152] and one report in head trauma patients of fentanyl- and sufentanil-induced increases in ICP,[153] there is no clinical evidence of meaningful ICP increases during craniotomy following narcotic administration,[154,155] rather narcotics (in the absence of hyperventilation) tend to cause either no change or a small decrease in ICP in patients with intracranial mass lesions. Because narcotics do not alter CO_2 reactivity, their use in combination with hypocapnia accounts for the resulting favorable effect upon brain bulk and ICP.

KETAMINE When first introduced, ketamine was touted as the ideal anesthetic for children requiring neurodiagnostic procedures: it could be given IM, the airway was protected, and the child could be rendered immobile. This was bolstered by an initial report in the German literature that ketamine caused a decrease in CBF.[156] However, in 1971 a report in the

TABLE 1.5 *Effect of narcotics on CBF*

REFERENCE	SPECIES	ANESTHETIC	NARCOTIC	DOSE	EFFECT ON CBF
Baughman et al.[128]	Rat	N_2O	Fentanyl	200 μg/kg	Decreased
Safo et al.[129]	Rat	N_2O	Fentanyl	100 or 400 μg/kg	Decreased
Naughton et al.[130]	Rat	N_2O	Fentanyl	25 and 100 μg/kg	Decreased
Carlsson et al.[131]	Rat	N_2O	Fentanyl	25–400 μg/kg	Decreased
Vernhiet et al.[132]	Man	N_2O + diazepam	Fentanyl	10 μg/kg	Decreased
Takeshita et al.[133]	Dog	N_2O	Morphine	Up to 3.0 mg/kg	Decreased
Michenfelder and Theye[134]	Dog	N_2O	Fentanyl	6 μg/kg	Decreased
Keykhah et al.[135]	Rat	N_2O	Sufentanil	5–160 μg/kg	Decreased
Jobes et al.[136]	Man	N_2O	Morphine	1 or 2 mg/kg	No effect compared with awake value
Matsumiya and Dohi[137]	Dog	Halothane	Morphine	1 mg/kg	Decreased
McPherson and Traystman[138]	Dog	Pentobarbital	Fentanyl	25 or 100 μ/kg	None
Freeman and Ingvar[139]	Cat	Phenobarbital	Fentanyl	20 μg/kg	None
Wahl[140]	Cat	α-Chloralose	Morphine	Up to 10^{-3} M	None or increased
Buchweitz et al.[141]	Cat	α-Chloralose	Morphine	1.5 mg/kg	None
Olsen et al.[142]	Fetal lamb	None	Morphine	60 $\mu g \cdot kg^{-1} \cdot min^{-1}$	None
Maekawa et al.[143]	Rat	None	Fentanyl	Enough to produce seizures	Increased
Koskinen and Bill[144]	Rabbit	None	Morphine	2 mg/kg	None
Vernhiet et al.[145]	Man	None	Fentanyl	1.9 or 16 μg/kg	None
Milde and Milde[146]	Dog	None	Sufentanil	2–200 μg/kg	Increased
Yaster et al.[147]	Neonatal lamb	None	Fentanyl	Up to 4.4 mg/kg	None
Freeman and Ingvar[139]	Cat	None	Fentanyl	Up to 20 μg/kg	Increased
Moyer et al.[148]	Man	None	Morphine	60 mg	None

Abbreviation: CBF, cerebral blood flow.

(From Michenfelder,[253] with permission.)

TABLE 1.6 *Effect of narcotics on CMR*

REFERENCE	SPECIES	ANESTHETIC	NARCOTIC	DOSE	EFFECT ON CMR
Baughman et al.[128]	Rat	N_2O	Fentanyl	200 μg/kg	Decreased
Naughton et al.[130]	Rat	N_2O	Fentanyl	25 or 100 μg/kg	Decreased
Carlsson et al.[131]	Rat	N_2O	Fentanyl	25–400 μg/kg	Decreased
Young et al.[149]	Rat	N_2O + 0.3% halothane	Sufentanil	40 or 160 μg/kg	Decreased
Keykhah et al.[135]	Rat	N_2O	Sufentanil	5–160 μg/kg	Decreased
Messick and Theye[150]	Dog	N_2O	Meperidine	5–160 μg/kg	Decreased
Matsuyima and Dohi[137]	Dog	Halothane	Morphine	1 μg/kg	Decreased
Takeshita et al.[133]	Dog	N_2O	Morphine	Up to 3.0 μg/kg	Decreased
Michenfelder and Theye[134]	Dog	N_2O	Fentanyl	6 μg/kg	Decreased
Vernhiet et al.[132]	Man	N_2O + diazepam	Fentanyl	10 μg/kg	Decreased
Jobes et al.[136]	Man	N_2O	Morphine	1 or 2 μg/kg	None compared with awake value
Buchweitz et al.[141]	Cat	α-Choralose	Morphine	1–5 mg/kg	None
Olsen et al.[142]	Fetal lamb	None	Morphine	60 μg/ $kg^{-1}\cdot min^{-1}$	None
Yaster et al.[147]	Neonatal lamb	None	Fentanyl	Up to 4.4 mg/kg	None
Levy et al.[151]	Rat	None	Morphine	Sufficient to decrease tail flick	None
Milde and Milde[146]	Dog	None	Sufentanil	2–200 μg/kg	None
Moyer et al.[148]	Man	None	Morphine	60 mg	Decreased

(From Michenfelder,[253] with permission.)

Japanese literature showed in humans that ketamine caused a significant increase in CBF,[157] whereas we showed a similar effect in the dog (Fig. 1.11).[158] In these and subsequent reports ketamine was found to have little or no effect on global $CMRO_2$.

Subsequent to the CBF reports, there were a host of reports of ketamine-induced increases in ICP in both normal subjects and patients with intracranial pathology.[159–167] Although there is anecdotal evidence that the ICP effects can be prevented by pretreatment with diazepam or thiopental, the evidence is not sufficient to justify any such recommendation. Certainly in dogs, pretreatment with thiopental completely blocks the otherwise striking CBF effects of ketamine.[158] Given the fact that there are many available alternatives to ketamine, it seems reasonable to avoid its use in patients at risk for increased ICP.

ETOMIDATE In terms of effects on CBF and $CMRO_2$, etomidate resembles thiopental in many respects. In large doses it induces a 50 to 60 percent decrease in $CMRO_2$ accompanied by a similar decrease in CBF.[168] In dogs an isoelec-

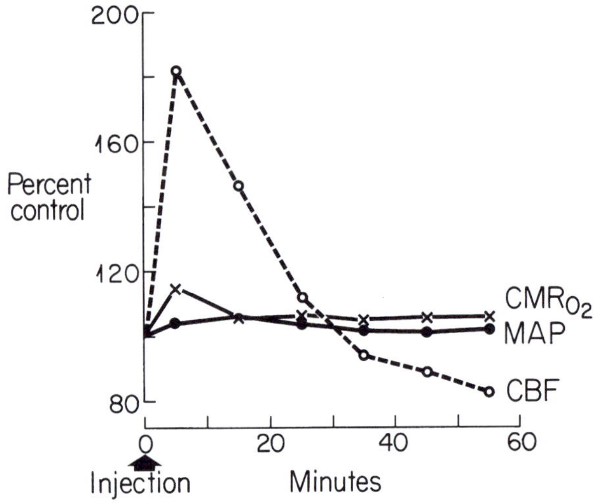

FIGURE 1.11 *Canine CBF, $CMRO_2$, and mean arterial pressure (MAP) after ketamine, 2 mg/kg. (From Dawson et al.,[158] with permission.)*

tric EEG can be induced, and as with thiopental and isoflurane, there is no evidence of toxicity as reflected by normal brain metabolites and energy charge. Compared to thiopental, there is only minimal hemodynamic suppression even at doses sufficient to abolish the EEG.

Despite these desirable effects, the drug has not gained wide acceptance for perhaps two reasons: there is a high incidence of vigorous myoclonus (not seizures) produced by the drug, and adrenal cortical suppression also occurs.[169] This latter effect is unimportant in most patients with intracranial mass lesions, because most of them are already receiving a high-dose regimen of steroids. The occurrence of myoclonus might be judged as little more than a nuisance that is easily controlled with muscle relaxants; however, in patients with intracranial pathology, the onset of myoclonus can easily be misinterpreted as the onset of a seizure and might result in inappropriate or unnecessary therapy.

BENZODIAZEPINES In terms of CBF and $CMRO_2$ effects, it is assumed that all of the benzodiazepines would be similar because, like narcotics, their site of action is thought to be receptor specific and saturable. Midazolam has gained favor as a possible induction agent because it is well tolerated when administered intravenously in doses sufficient to produce anesthesia. In humans an induction dose of midazolam (0.15 mg/kg), has a delayed onset of action of 1 to 3 minutes and causes a 30 percent decrease in CBF.[170–172] This effect as well as the sedative effects can be completely blocked by prior administration of the specific antagonist flumazenil. In dogs a continuous infusion of midazolam produced a 25 percent decrease in CBF and $CMRO_2$ in the absence of other anesthetic drugs.[173] This effect then plateaued, and despite large additional doses (up to 40 mg/kg in 1 hour), no further change in CBF and $CMRO_2$ was observed. This presumably reflected saturation of binding sites and was accompanied by a stable EEG pattern of mixed high-amplitude theta and delta activity. The effects were completely reversible with flumazenil, 1 mg/kg. Also, in dogs not reversed, the cerebral metabolites and energy charge were unaffected. Finally, in this study, the addition of nitrous oxide had no effect on $CMRO_2$ and only moderately increased CBF. The combined effect of nitrous oxide and a benzodiazepine has been reported to cause a significant decrease in $CMRO_2$ in the rat when using diazepam.[174] However, such an effect has not been reported in other species or with midazolam.

PROPOFOL Propofol is the most recently introduced potent intravenous anesthetic for clinical use in the United States. It is chemically unrelated to the other intravenous anesthetics; rather, it belongs to a series of alkyl phenols known to have anesthetic properties in animals. These compounds exist as oils at room temperature, and propofol requires unusual solubilizing agents for intravenous administration. The current preparation is solubilized in a soybean emulsion. Its anesthetic properties are characterized by rapid onset of action, short duration of action, a high therapeutic index, and a high clearance rate.[175] Propofol has proven useful for sedation, outpatient surgery, induction of anesthesia, and maintenance of anesthesia, even for major surgical procedures, particularly neurosurgical procedures, where rapid recovery may be desirable.[176]

The cerebral vasculature and metabolic effects of propofol resemble the effects of the barbiturates. In both experimental animals and humans, propofol induces a dose-related decrease in cerebral perfusion pressure, CBF, and CMR with no change in arterial-venous oxygen content across the brain, thus reflecting maintenance of coupling between blood flow and metabolic rate.[177–182] As is true for the barbiturates, propofol does not interfere with autoregulation[178] or CO_2 reactivity,[181,183] although the latter may be quantitatively attenuated. As with the barbiturates, propofol also has the potential for decreasing ICP, particularly when combined with hyperventilation. When combined with N_2O, the cerebrovascular and metabolic effects of propofol are unaffected.[181,183] When used for prolonged sedation in an intensive care setting, particular attention must be given to sterile technique, because the solubilizing agent for propofol provides an excellent growth media for contaminating bacteria.

Local Anesthetics

Local anesthetics rapidly cross the blood-brain barrier and because of their membrane stabilizing effects would be expected to exert an effect on cerebral function, CMR, and CBF. The biphasic CNS toxic manifestations of local anesthetics are well recognized, progressing from sedation to seizures and finally to severe CNS depression and death. In subtoxic doses, local anesthetics as represented by lidocaine in dogs cause a modest decrease in $CMRO_2$ (10 to 27 percent) accompanied by a similar transient decrease in CBF.[184] When pushed to the point of seizures, $CMRO_2$ immediately increased to 112 percent of control with a concomitant increase in CBF to 150 percent of control. Thus, as is the case for enflurane-induced seizures, oxygen delivery more than keeps pace with oxygen demand during seizures so long as perfusion pressure is maintained. This was confirmed in rats wherein lidocaine-induced seizures had no effect on the brain energy charge.[185]

Astrup et al. examined the cerebral metabolic effects of a massive dose of lidocaine (100 mg/kg) in the dog in which the EEG had been suppressed by pentobarbital with and without hypothermia.[186] They showed that despite an isoelectric EEG this dose of lidocaine caused a further 15 to 20 percent decrease in $CMRO_2$ and speculated that this reflected a specific membrane stabilizing effect that would potentiate the cerebral protective effects of barbiturates. They did not rule out a possible toxic effect to account for this observation. Milde and Milde produced an isoelectric EEG in dogs with isoflurane and then administered lidocaine, 15 mg/kg.[187] They observed no further decrease in $CMRO_2$ but instead observed a decrease in ATP and the energy charge with an increase in AMP. This suggests a toxic effect similar to that seen with high-dose halothane and might explain the observation of Astrup et al. regarding the effect of high-dose lidocaine.[186] This is consistent with the in vitro observation that lidocaine is a potent uncoupler of oxidative phophorylation, which blocks electron transport at the reduced form of nicotinamide adenine dinucleotide (NADH) dehydrogenase level.[188]

EFFECT OF ANCILLARY DRUGS

Muscle Relaxants

Although muscle relaxants do not cross the blood-brain barrier, secondary effects are possible. These might be expected secondary to histamine release, systemic hemodynamic effects, effects of metabolites, or altered cerebral afferent input from muscle spindles.

d-Tubocurarine is known to release histamine and was reported in dogs and cats when given as a bolus to cause an increase in CBF.[189] This effect was then shown to be attenuated by pretreatment with diphendydramine. In humans a bolus dose of 0.6 mg/kg caused a transient (1 to 2 minutes) modest increase in CSF pressure (from 10 to 18 mmHg) simultaneous with a decrease in blood pressure and increase in heart rate.[190] This effect was assumed to be secondary to histamine release. Given that demonstration of this modest response requires a relatively large dose of *d*-tubocurarine administered as a bolus, there is little justification for condemning the use of this muscle relaxant in patients at risk for increased ICP. By simply avoiding large bolus doses, any undesirable ICP effects should be avoidable.

Pancuronium has been reported to decrease the MAC of halothane by 25 percent in humans.[191] This is assumed to be secondary to decreased cerebral afferent input from paralyzed muscle spindles. Despite this, we were unable to demonstrate any effect of pancuronium (0.1 or 0.2 mg/kg) on canine CBF, $CMRO_2$, ICP, or EEG in animals maintained at 1 MAC halothane.[192] A potentially undesirable side effect of pancuronium is that of hypertension and tachycardia. In patients with intracranial pathology and defective autoregulation, such a response will induce increases in CBF and ICP. This hemodynamic response can usually be minimized by avoiding bolus doses of pancuronium but remains somewhat unpredictable such that alternative relaxants should be sought for patients at risk for increased ICP.

Atracurium can cause histamine release but to a considerably lesser degree than that possible with *d*-tubocurarine and is not usually a matter for concern. Of greater interest is one of its metabolites produced by Hoffman elimination, laudanosine. This metabolite readily crosses the blood-brain barrier and in large enough doses can cause seizures in experimental animals.[193–196] In dogs maintained at less than 1.0 MAC halothane (0.69 percent end-expired), a cumulative dose of atracurium of 3.5 mg/kg consistently produced EEG arousal but not measureable changes in CBF, $CMRO_2$, or ICP.[192] At halothane concentrations of 1.0 MAC, even the EEG arousal response is absent in most dogs. Thus in clinically relevant doses, the potential cerebral effects of laudanosine are modest indeed.

Vecuronium appears to be without any cerebral effects whatsoever. It does not release histamine, it has no cerebrally active metabolites, and it has no effect on systemic hemodynamics. Predictably, it has been reported to have no effects on ICP.[197,198]

The cerebral effects of succinylcholine have been controversial primarily because of inconsistent and even contradictory reports regarding its effects on ICP in experimental animals and in patients.[199–207] Lanier et al. clarified much of this by demonstrating in dogs that succinylcholine can cause impressive increases in CBF (and ICP) that appear to be secondary to increased muscle spindle activity (and thus increased cerebral afferent input) concomitant with the onset of fasciculations and persisting for as long as 30 minutes.[208] This is consistent with reports in patients that succinylcholine-induced increases in ICP can be attenuated or blocked by vecuronium or by defasciculating doses of metocurine.[206]

Vasoactive Drugs

In considering the effects of drugs used to induce hypotension on CBF (and ICP), it becomes difficult or impossible to separate direct effects of the drug from those secondary to normal autoregulation, which may in turn be attenuated or abolished by some anesthetics. Thus in normal humans, a decrease in blood pressure within the autoregulatory range (no matter how produced) should result in cerebral vasodilation with no change in CBF. In theory, at least, this should result in an increase in CBV and possibly ICP if intracranial compliance is decreased. Thus, unless a hypotensive drug causes an absolute increase in CBF, it is impossible to determine whether cerebral vasodilation observed during hypotension induced by that drug is secondary to the drug, autoregulation, or to some combination of the two.

In the case of sodium nitroprusside (SNP), it is commonly characterized as a cerebral vasodilator, yet most of the available data are at best only suggestive of such an effect and rely primarily upon ICP measurements rather than CBF effects. In both humans and subhuman primates, SNP-induced hypotension is consistently associated with an increase in ICP and either no change or a decrease in CBF[209–224] (Table 1.7). Of itself, this defies interpretation regarding the direct effects of SNP on the cerebral vasculature. However, in several of these studies, the effects of hypotension induced by a different means were compared to that observed with SNP. Consistently in these studies, the ICP effects of SNP were greater than that induced by the alternative means. This clearly implies SNP-induced vasodilation beyond that imposed by autoregulation and by implication (since CBF is unchanged or decreased) dilation of capacitance rather than resistance vessels.

In a canine study, we demonstrated that SNP-induced hypotension in the presence of isoflurane caused a decrease in CBF and no change in ICP (unpublished data). However, when the same dose of SNP was given without hypotension (by partial aortic occlusion), we observed increases in both CBF and ICP. This implies that SNP in the presence of isoflurane dilates resistance vessels but that isoflurane attenuates autoregulation such that CBF in fact decreases during hypotension. When the same experiment was repeated in the absence of isoflurane, SNP-induced hypotension had no effect on either CBF or ICP. However, when blood pressure was maintained, CBF was unaffected by SNP while ICP was increased. This implies that in the absence of isoflurane SNP dilates capacitance vessels, a conclusion consistent with the bulk of the reported experimental data.

Nitroglycerin-induced hypotension has also been reported to cause increased ICP in humans and is commonly assumed to dilate capacitance vessels.[225–230] As is the case for SNP, there are no direct observations of such an effect, but the available data do support such a conclusion.

The reported cerebral effects of epinephrine

TABLE 1.7 *Effect of sodium nitroprusside in primates*

REFERENCE	SPECIES	MAP	ICP EFFECT	CBF EFFECT
Henriksen et al.[209]	Man	↓	NM	None
Henriksen et al.[210]	Man	↓	NM	↓
Henriksen and Paulsen[211]	Man	↓	NM	↓
Larsen et al.[212]	Man	↓	NM	None
Griswold et al.[213]	Man	↓	↑	NM
Marsh et al.[214]	Man	↓	↑	NM
Cottrell et al.[215]	Man	↓	↑	NM
Turner et al.[216]	Man	↓	↑	NM
Brown et al.[217]	Man	↓	NM	↓
Bunemann et al.[218]	Man	↓	NM	None
Griffiths et al.[219]	Man	↓	NM	None
Sivarajan et al.[220]	Monkey	↓	NM	None
Candia et al.[221]	Monkey	↓	↑	None
Brown et al.[222]	Monkey	↓	NM	↓
Crockard et al.[223]	Monkey	↓	NM	↓
Keaney et al.[224]	Baboon	↓	NM	↓

Abbreviations: MAP, mean arterial pressure: ICP, intracranial pressure; CBF, cerebral blood flow; NM, not measured.

(From Michenfelder,[253] with permission.)

and norepinephrine are variable in both humans and experimental animals.[231–238] This appears to be accounted for by variable effects on blood pressure, autoregulation, and the blood-brain barrier. It is probably correct to generalize that if these drugs do not cross the blood-brain barrier, they do not affect $CMRO_2$. Similarly, if autoregulation is intact and not exceeded, these drugs should not have any sustained effect on CBF. If, however, the catecholamines cross the blood-brain barrier, striking increases in $CMRO_2$ and CBF may be observed.

Naloxone

Naloxone received considerable attention when it was first reported in gerbils that it could reverse or prevent stroke secondary to carotid occlusion while morphine aggravated or induced stroke findings.[239,240] This work has never been reproduced,[241–243] although intermittent anecdotal reports of positive effects of naloxone on ischemic stroke in patients continue to appear.[244,245] Likewise, the reported effects of naloxone on CBF are variable. We found no effect of naloxone, 10 mg/kg, in dogs[246] on CBF while Turner et al. reported increased CBF in dogs unless deeply anesthetized with pentobarbital.[247–250] It has also been reported that naloxone increases CBF in various animal models of induced ischemia or anoxia.[251,252]

Despite early promising reports, it is now generally agreed that regardless of possible transient effects naloxone has no positive effect on outcome following a cerebral ischemic event.

CONCLUSION

In the past 25 years the available information about CBF and $CMRO_2$ has grown in almost exponential fashion. Certainly this has been true as regards our anesthetic drugs and techniques. It is tempting to conclude that we have now learned all we need learn about this subject and may therefore turn our attention to other matters. However, for the most part, we have only addressed the question of What happens? when we anesthetize our patients and not Why? Certainly it is important, for example, to know that some anesthetics alter the way in which CBF and $CMRO_2$ are normally coupled. This information assists us in selecting the proper anesthetic and adjuncts for the management of our individual patients. But to understand why this occurs may provide insight into a host of basic mechanisms including perhaps the very nature of the anesthetized state.

Uncovering mechanisms is a far greater challenge than simply uncovering phenomena, but the latter must be characterized before the former can be intelligently explored. We have largely accomplished the easy part of this task. In theory, at least, determining mechanisms should permit intelligent design of drugs and techniques to accomplish specific purposes without introducing undesirable side effects. This is no where more apparent than when considering the potential for protecting the brain from ischemia or hypoxia with drugs or other interventions. In this arena, to understand a drug's effect on cerebral metabolism and blood flow is an obvious requirement, but it is little more than a first step.

Another requirement for the future is to explore drug-drug interactions and drug-disease interactions. As already noted, we possess a host of individual blocks of information, but they are often in isolation from the reality of clinical practice and from one another. As an example, it is a fact that succinylcholine can cause an increase in ICP. Taken in isolation, this would lead many to conclude that succinylcholine is contraindicated in any patient at risk for increased ICP. However, in the reality of clinical practice, this has never been recognized by most practitioners to be an important problem, undoubtedly because of various drug-drug interactions.

References

1. Kety SS, Schmidt CF: The determination of cerebral blood flow in man by the use of nitrous oxide in low concentrations. Am J Physiol 143:53, 1945

2. Kety SS, Schmidt CF: The nitrous oxide method for the quantitative determination of cerebral blood flow in man: theory, procedure, and normal values. J Clin Invest 27:476, 1948
3. Lassen NA, Ingvar DH: Blood flow of the cerebral cortex determined by radioactive krypton 85. Experientia (Basel) 17:42, 1961
4. Ingvar DH, Lassen NA: Regional blood flow of the cerebral cortex determined by krypton 85. Acta Physiol Scand 54:325, 1962
5. Obrist WE, Thompson HK, Wang HS, Wilkinson WE: Regional cerebral blood flow estimated by ^{133} xenon inhalation. Stroke 6:245, 1975
6. Betz E: Cerebral blood flow: its measurement and regulation. Physiol Rev 52:595, 1972
7. Posner JB: Newer techniques of cerebral blood flow measurement. Stroke 3:227, 1972
8. Eintrei C, Leszniewski W, Carlsson C: Local application of ^{133}xenon for measurement of regional cerebral blood flow (rCBF) during halothane, enflurane, and isoflurane anesthesia in humans. Anesthesiology 63:391, 1985
9. Raichle ME: Quantitative in vivo autoradiography with positron emission tomography. Brain Res Rev 1:47, 1979
10. Chance B, Clark BJ, Nioka S et al: Phosphorous nuclear magnetic resonance spectroscopy in vivo. Circulation 72:IV103, 1985
11. Rapela CE, Green HD: Autoregulation of canine cerebral blood flow. Circ Res XIV & XV:205, 1964
12. Michenfelder JD, Messick JM Jr, Theye RA: Simultaneous cerebral blood flow measured by direct and indirect methods. J Surg Res 8:475, 1968
13. Artru AA, Michenfelder JD: Effects of hypercarbia on canine cerebral metabolism blood flow with simultaneous direct and indirect measurement of blood flow. Anesthesiology 52:466, 1980
14. Marcus ML, Busija DW, Bischof CJ, Heistad DD: Methods for measurement of cerebral blood flows. Fed Proc 40:2306, 1981
15. Sokoloff L: Relation between physiological function and energy metabolism in a central nervous system. J Neurochem 29:13, 1977
16. Schienberg P, Stead EA: The cerebral blood flow in male subjects as measured by the nitrous oxide technique: normal values for blood flow, oxygen utilization, glucose utilization, and peripheral resistance with observations on the effect of tilting and anxiety. J Clin Invest 28:1163, 1949
17. Sokoloff L, Perland S, Kornetsky C, Kety SS: The effects of D-lysergic acid diethylamide on cerebral circulation and overall metabolism. Ann NY Acad Sci 66:468, 1957
18. Lassen NA, Feinberg I, Lane MH: Bilateral studies of cerebral oxygen uptake in young and aged normal subjects and in patients with organic dementia. J Clin Invest 39:491, 1960
19. Cohen PJ, Alexander SC, Smith FC et al: Effects of hypoxia and normocarbia on cerebral blood flow and metabolism in conscious man. J Appl Physiol 23:183, 1967
20. Michenfelder JD, Theye RA: The effects of profound hypocapnia and dilutional anemia on canine cerebral metabolism and blood flow. Anesthesiology 31:449, 1969
21. Paulson OB, Sharbrough FW: Physiologic and pathophysiologic relationship between the electroencephalogram and the regional cerebral blood flow. Acta Neurol Scand 50:194, 1974
22. Okuda Y, McDowall DG, Ali MM, Lane JR: Changes in CO_2 responsiveness and in autoregulation of the cerebral circulation during and after halothane induced hypotension. J Neurol Neurosurg Psychiatry 39:221, 1976
23. Fitch W, Mackenzie ET, Harper AM: Effects of decreasing arterial blood pressure on cerebral blood flow in the baboon. Circ Res 37:550, 1975
24. Atkinson DE: The energy charge of the adenylate pool as a regulatory parameter. Interaction with feedback modifiers. Biochemistry 7:4030, 1968
25. Pontén U, Ratcheson RA, Salford LG, Siesjö BK: Optimal freezing conditions for cerebral metabolites in rats. J Neurochem 21:1127, 1973
26. Pontén U, Ratcheson RA, Siesjö BK: Metabolic changes in the brains of mice frozen in liquid nitrogen. J Neurochem 21:1121, 1973
27. Roald OK, Steen PA, Stangland K, Michenfelder JD: The effects of triazolam on cerebral blood flow and metabolism in the dog. Acta Anaesthesiol Scand 30:223, 1986
28. Hawkins R: Potential pitfalls in measuring regional cerebral glucose utilization. Anesthesiology 58:290, 1983
29. Crosby G, Sokoloff L: In reply. Anesthesiology 58:292, 1983
30. Steen PA, Newberg LA, Milde JH, Michenfelder JD: Hypothermia and barbiturates: individual and combined effects on canine cerebral oxygen consumption. Anesthesiology 58:527, 1983
31. Michenfelder JD, Milde JH: The relationship among canine brain temperature, metabolism,

and function during hypothermia. Anesthesiology 75:130, 1991
32. Michenfelder JD, Milde JH: The effect of profound levels of hypothermia (below 14°C) on canine cerebral metabolism. J Cereb Blood Flow Metab 12:877, 1992
33. Michenfelder JD, Theye RA: The effects of anesthesia and hypothermia on canine cerebral ATP and lactate during anoxia produced by decapitation. Anesthesiology 33:430, 1970
34. Rahn H: Body temperature and acid-base regulation (a review article). Pneumonologie 151:87, 1974
35. Ream AK, Reitz BA, Silverberg G: Temperature correction of P_cO_2 and pH in estimating acid-base status: an example of the emperior's new clothes? Anesthesiology 56:41, 1982
36. Christopherson TJ, Milde JH, Michenfelder JD: Cerebral vascular autoregulation and CO_2 reactivity following onset of the delayed postischemic hypoperfusion state in dogs. J Cereb Blood Flow Metab 13:260, 1993
37. Waltz AG, Sundt TM, Jr, Michenfelder JD: Cerebral blood flow during carotid endarterectomy. Circulation 45:1091, 1972
38. Severinghaus JW, Chiodi H, Eger EI et al: Cerebral blood flow in man at high altitude: the role of cerebral spinal fluid pH and normalization of flow in chronic hypocapnia. Circ Res 19:274, 1966
39. Tinker JH, Sharbrough FW, Michenfelder JD: Anterior shift of the dominant EEG rhythm during anesthesia in the Java monkey: correlation with anesthetic potency. Anesthesiology 46:252, 1977
40. Stoelting RK, Longnecker DE, Eger EI II: Minimum alveolar concentrations in man on awakening from methoxyflurane, halothane, ether, and fluroxene anesthesia: MAC awake Anesthesiology 33:5, 1970
41. Gross TB, Alexander CM: Awakening concentrations of isoflurane are not affected by analgesic doses of morphine. Anesth Analg 67:27, 1988
42. Stullken EH Jr, Milde JH, Michenfelder JD, Tinker JH: The non-linear responses of cerebral metabolism to low concentrations of halothane, enflurane, isoflurane and thiopental. Anesthesiology 46:28, 1977
43. Mummaneni N, Rao TLK, Montoya A: Awareness and recall with high dose fentanyl oxygen anesthesia. Anesth Analg 59:948, 1980
44. Hilgenberg JC: Intraoperative awareness during high dose fentanyl oxygen anesthesia. Anesthesiology 54:341, 1981
45. Bailey PL, Port JD, McJames S et al: Is fentanyl an anesthetic in the dog? Anesth Analg 66:542, 1987
46. Michenfelder JD: The in vivo effects of massive concentrations of anesthetics on canine cerebral metabolism. p. 537. In Fink BR (ed): Molecular Mechanisms of Anesthesia. Raven Press, New York, 1975
47. Newberg LA, Milde JH, Michenfelder JD: The cerebral metabolic effects of isoflurane at and above concentrations that suppress cortical electrical activity. Anesthesiology 59:23, 1983
48. Nunn JF, Chonarin I: Nitrous oxide inactivates methionine synthetase. p. 211. In Eger EI II (ed): Nitrous Oxide. Elsevier, New York, 1985
49. Baden JM: Motorgenicity, carcinogenicity, and teratogenicity of nitrous oxide. p. 235. In Eger EI II (ed): Nitrous Oxide. Elsevier, New York, 1985
50. Shim CU, Anderson MB: The effect of oxygen on minimal anesthetic requirements in the toad. Anesthesiology 34:333, 1971
51. Deady JE, Koblin DD, Eger EI II et al: Anesthetic potencies and the unitary theory of narcosis. Anesth Analg 60:380, 1981
52. Carlsson C, Hagerdal M, Siesjö BK: The effect of nitrous oxide on oxygen consumption and blood flow in the cerebral cortex of the rat. Acta Anaesthesiol Scand 20:91, 1976
53. Carlsson C, Hagerdal M, Kasik AE, Siesjö BK: The effects of diazepam on cerebral blood flow and oxygen consumption in rats and its synergistic interaction with nitrous oxide. Anesthesiology 45:319, 1976
54. Berntman L, Carlsson C, Hagerdal M, Siesjö BK: Cerebral metabolic state after discontinuation of nitrous oxide supply in artificially ventilated rats. Acta Physiol Scand 98:248, 1976
55. Ingvar M, Abdul-Rahman A, Siesjö BK: Local cerebral glucose consumption in the artificially ventilated rat: influence of nitrous oxide analgesia and of phenobarbital anesthesia. Acta Physiol Scand 109:177, 1980
56. Dahlgren N, Ingvar M, Yokoyama H, Siesjö BK: Influence of nitrous oxide on local cerebral blood flow in awake minimally restrained rats. J Cereb Blood Flow Metab 1:211, 1981
57. Ingvar M, Siesjö BK: Effect of nitrous oxide on local cerebral glucose utilization in rats. J Cereb Blood Flow Metab 2:481, 1982
58. Crosby G, Crane AM, Jehle J, Sokoloff L: The lo-

cal metabolic effects of somatosensory stimulation in the central nervous system of rats given pentobarbital or nitrous oxide. Anesthesiology 58:38, 1983
59. Crosby G, Crane AM, Sokoloff L: A comparison of local rates of glucose utilization in spinal cord and brain in conscious and nitrous oxide or pentobarbital treated rats. Anesthesiology 61:434, 1984
60. Sakabe T, Tsutsui T, Maekawa T et al: Local cerebral glucose utilization during nitrous oxide and pentobarbital anesthesia in rats. Anesthesiology 63:262, 1985
61. Seyde WC, Ellis JE, Longnecker DE: The addition of nitrous oxide to halothane decreases renal and splanchnic flow and increases cerebral blood flow in rats. Br J Anaesth 58:63, 1986
62. Theye RA, Michenfelder JD: Effect of nitrous oxide on canine cerebral metabolism. Anesthesiology 29:1119, 1968
63. Sakabe T, Kuramoto T, Inou ES, Takeshita H: Cerebral effects of nitrous oxide in the dog. Anesthesiology 48:195, 1978
64. Oshita S, Ishikawa T, Tokutsu Y, Takeshita H: Cerebral circulatory and metabolic stimulation with nitrous oxide in the dog. Reconfirmation by the simultaneous measurement of cerebral blood flow using direct and Keyt-Schmidt methods. Acta Anaesthesiol Scand 23:177, 1979
65. Fitzpatrick JH Jr, Gilboe DV: Effects of nitrous oxide on the cerebral vascular tone, oxygen metabolism, and electroencephalogram of the isolated perfused canine brain. Anesthesiology 57:480, 1982
66. Manohar M, Parks C: Porcine regional brain and myocardial blood flows during halothane-O_2 and halothane-N_2O anesthesia: comparisons with equipotent isoflurane anesthesia. Am J Vet Res 45:465, 1984
67. Manohar M, Parks C: Regional distribution of brain and myocardial perfusion in swine while awake and during 1.0 and 1.5 MAC isoflurane anesthesia produced without or with 50 percent nitrous oxide. Cardiovasc Res 18:344, 1984
68. Manohar M, Parks CM: Porcine brain and myocardial perfusion during enflurane anesthesia without and with nitrous oxide. J Cardiovasc Pharmacol 6:1092, 1984
69. Manohar M: Regional distribution of porcine brain blood flow during 50 percent nitrous oxide administration. Am J Vet Res 46:831, 1985
70. Manohar M: Impact of 70 percent nitrous oxide administration on regional distribution of brain blood flow in unmedicated healthy swine. J Cardiovasc Pharmacol 7:463, 1985
71. Pelligrino DA, Miletich DJ, Hoffman WE, Albrecht RF: Nitrous oxide markedly increases cerebral cortical metabolic rate and blood flow in the goat. Anesthesiology 60:405, 1984
72. Drummond JC, Scheller MS, Todd MM: The effect of nitrous oxide on cortical cerebral blood flow during anesthesia with halothane and isoflurane with and without morphine in the rabbit. Anesth Analg 66:1083, 1987
73. Todd MM: The effects of $PaCO_2$ on the cerebral vascular response to nitrous oxide in the halothane anesthetized rabbit. Anesth Analg 66:1090, 1987
74. Laitinen LV, Johansson GG, Tarkkanen L: The effect of nitrous oxide on pulsatile cerebral impedence and cerebral blood flow. Br J Anaesth 39:781, 1967
75. Henricksen HG, Jorgensen PB: The effect of nitrous oxide and intracranial pressure in patients with intracranial disorders. Br J Anaesth 45:486, 1973
76. Sakabe T, Kuramoto T, Kumagae S, Takeshita H: Cerebral responses to the addition of nitrous oxide to halothane in man. Br J Anaesth 48:957, 1976
77. Phirman JR, Shapiro HM: Modification of nitrous oxide-induced intracranial hypertension by prior induction of anesthesia. Anesthesiology 46:150, 1977
78. Jobes DR, Kennel EM, Bush GL, et al: Cerebral blood flow and metabolism during morphine-nitrous oxide anesthesia in man. Anesthesiology 47:16, 1977
79. Moss E, McDowall DG: ICP increases with 50 percent nitrous oxide in oxygen in severe head injuries during controlled ventilation. Br J Anaesth 51:757, 1979
80. Alexander SC, Wollman H, Cohen PJ et al: Cerebral vascular response to $PaCO_2$ during halothane anesthesia in man. J Appl Physiol 19:561, 1964
81. Wollman H, Alexander SC, Cohen PJ et al: Cerebral circulation in man during halothane anesthesia. Anesthesiology 25:180, 1964
82. McDowall DG: The effects of clinical concentrations of halothane on the blood flow and oxygen uptake of the cerebral cortex. Br J Anaesth 39:186, 1967
83. Smith AL, Wollman H: Cerebral blood flow and

metabolism: effect of anesthetic drugs and techniques. Anesthesiology 36:378, 1972
84. Theye RA, Michenfelder JD: Effect of halothane on canine cerebral metabolism. Anesthesiology 29:1113, 1968
85. Scheller MS, Todd MM, Drummond JC: Isoflurane, halothane, and regional cerebral blood flow at various levels of $PaCO_2$ in rabbits. Anesthesiology 64:598, 1986
86. Manohar M, Geats TE: Cerebral, renal, adrenal, intestinal, and pancreatic circulation in conscious ponies and during 1, 1.5, and 2.0 minimal alveolar concentrations of halothane-O_2 anesthesia. Am J Vet Res 46:2492, 1985
87. Eintrei C, Leszniewski W, Carlsson C: Local application of ^{133}xenon for measurement of regional cerebral blood flow (rCBF) during halothane, enflurane, and isoflurane anesthesia in humans. Anesthesiology 63:391, 1985
88. Jennett WB, Barker J, Fitch W, McDowall DG: Effect of anesthesia on intracranial pressure in patients with space occupying lesions. Lancet 1:61, 1969
89. Anonymous: Halothane and neurosurgery (editorial). Br J Anaesth 41:277, 1969
90. Adams RW, Gronert GA, Sundt TM Jr, Michenfelder JD: Halothane, hypocapnia and cerebrospinal fluid pressure in neurosurgery. Anesthesiology 37:510, 1972
91. Drummond JC, Todd MM: The response of feline cerebral circulation to $PaCO_2$ during anesthesia with isoflurane and halothane and during sedation with nitrous oxide. Anesthesiology 62:268, 1985
92. Wollman H, Alexander SC, Cohen PJ et al: Cerebral circulation during general anesthesia and hyperventilaton in man. Anesthesiology 26:329, 1965
93. Miletich DJ, Ivankovich AD, Albrecht RF et al: Absence of autoregulation of cerebral blood flow during halothane and enflurane anesthesia. Anesth Analg 55:100, 1976
94. Morita H, Nemoto EM, Bleyaert AL, Stezoski SW: Brain blood flow autoregulation and metabolism during halothane anesthesia in monkeys. Am J Physiol 233:H670, 1977
95. Smith AL: Dependence of cerebral venous oxygen tension on anesthetic depth. Anesthesiology 39:291, 1973
96. Smith AL, Wollman H: Cerebral blood flow and metabolism: effects of anesthetic drugs and techniques. Anesthesiology 36:378, 1972
97. Drummond JC, Todd MM, Scheller MS, Shapiro HM: A comparison of the direct cerebral vasodilating potencies of halothane and isoflurane in the New Zealand white rabbit. Anesthesiology 65:462, 1986
98. Scheller MS, Smith RC, Todd MM, Drummond JC: Isoflurane influences the effects of barbiturates on CBF. Anesthesiology 67:A406, 1987
99. Altura BT, Altura BM: Effects of barbiturates, phencyclidine, ketamine, and analogues on cerebral circulation and cerebral vascular muscle. J Microcirculation Endothelium Lymphatics 1:169, 1984
100. Wendling WW, Harakal C: Comparative actions of pentobarbital and verapamil on canine cerebral and peripheral arteries in vitro. Res Commun Chem Pathol Pharmacol 49:189, 1985
101. Sanchez-Ferrer CF, Merin J, Salaices M, Rico ML, Munoz-Blanco JL: Interference of pentobarbital and thiopental with the vascular contraction and noredrenaline release in human cerebral arteries. Gen Pharmacol 16:469, 1985
102. Edvinsson L, McCulloch J: Effects of pentobarbital on contractive response of feline cerebral arteries. J Cereb Blood Flow Metab 1:437, 1981
103. Merin G, Lobato RD, Rico ML et al: Effect of pentobarbital on the reactivity of isolated human cerebral arteries. J Neurosurg 54:521, 1981
104. Theye RA, Michenfelder JD: Effect of halothane on canine cerebral metabolism. Anesthesiology 29:1113, 1968
105. Cohen PJ, Marshall BE: Effects of halothane on respiratory control and oxygen consumption of rat liver mitochondria. p. 24. In Finck BR (ed): Toxicity of Anesthetics. Williams & Wilkins, Baltimore, 1968
106. Michenfelder JD, Theye RA: In vivo toxic effects of halothane on canine cerebral metabolic pathways. Am J Physiol 229:1050, 1975
107. Smith AL, Hoff JT, Nelsen SL, Larson CP: Barbiturate protection in acute focal cerebral ischemia. Stroke 51:1, 1974
108. Michenfelder JD, Milde JH: Influence of anesthetics on metabolic, functional and pathological responses to regional cerebral ischemia. Stroke 6:405, 1975
109. Michenfelder JD, Cucchiare RF: Canine cerebral oxygen consumption during enflurane anesthesia and its modification during induced seizures. Anesthesiology 40:575, 1974
110. Wollman H, Smith AL, Hoffman JC: Cerebral blood flow and oxygen consumption in man dur-

ing electroencephalographic seizure patterns induced by anesthesia with ethrane. Fed Proc 28:356, 1969
111. Adams RW, Cucchiara RF, Gronert GA et al: Isoflurane and cerebrospinal fluid pressure in neurosurgical patients. Anesthesiology 54:97, 1981
112. Grosslight K, Foster R, Colohan AR, Bedford RF: Isoflurane for neuroanesthesia: risk factors for increases in intracranial pressure. Anesthesiology 63:533, 1985
113. Michenfelder JD, Sundt TM, Fode N, Sharbrough FW: Isoflurane when compared to enflurane and halothane decreases the frequency of cerebral ischemia during carotid endarterectomy. Anesthesiology 67:336, 1987
114. Muzzi DA, Losasso TJ, Dietz NM, et al: The effect of desflurane and isoflurane on cerebral spinal fluid pressure in humans with supratentorial mass lesions. Anesthesiology 76:720, 1992
115. Young WL: Effects of desflurane on the central nervous system. Anesth Analg 75:S32, 1992
116. Lutz LJ, Milde JH, Milde LN: The cerebral functional, metabolic, and hemodynamic effects of desflurane in dogs. Anesthesiology 73:125, 1990
117. Rampil IJ, Laster M, Dwyer RC et al: No EEG evidence of acute tolerance to desflurane in swine. Anesthesiology 74:889, 1991
118. Lutz LJ, Milde JH, Milde LN: The response of the canine cerebral circulation to hyperventilation during anesthesia with desflurane. Anesthesiology 74:504, 1991
119. Milde LN, Milde JH: The cerebral and systemic hemodynamic and metabolic effects of desflurane-induced hypotension in dogs. Anesthesiology 74:513, 1991
120. Scheller MS, Tateishi A, Drummond JC, Zornow MH: The effects of sevoflurane on cerebral blood flow, cerebral metabolic rate for oxygen, intracranial pressure, and the electroencephalogram are similar to those of isoflurane in the rabbit. Anesthesiology 68:548, 1988
121. Takahashi H, Murata K, Ikeda K: Sevoflurane does not increase intracranial pressure in hyperventilated dogs. Br J Anaesth 71:551, 1993
122. Scheller MS, Nakakimura K, Fleischer JE, Zornow MH: Cerebral effects of sevoflurane in the dog: comparison with isoflurane and enflurane. Br J Anaesth 65:388, 1990
123. Conzen PF, Volimer B, Habazettl H et al: Systemic and regional hemodynamics of isoflurane and sevoflurane in rats. Anesth Analg 74:79, 1992
124. Kitaguchi K, Ohsumi H, Kuro M et al: Effects of sevoflurane on cerebral circulation and metabolism in patients with ischemic cerebrovascular disease. Anesthesiology 79:704, 1993
125. Osawa M, Shingu K, Murakawa M et al: Effects of sevoflurane on central nervous system electrical activity in cats. Anesth Analg 79:52, 1994
126. Fujibayashi T, Sugiura Y, Yanagimoto M et al: Brain energy metabolism and blood flow during sevoflurane and halothane anesthesia: effects of hypocapnia and blood pressure fluctuations. Acta Anaesthesiol Scand 38:413, 1994
127. Pierce EC, Jr, Lambertsen CJ, Deutsch S et al: Cerebral circulation and metabolism during thiopental anesthesia and hyperventilation in man. J Clin Invest 41:1664, 1962
128. Baughman VL, Hoffman WE, albrecht RF, Miletich DJ: Cerebral vascular and metabolic effects of fentanyl and midazolam in young and aged rats. Anesthesiology 67:314, 1987
129. Safo Y, Young ML, Smith DS et al: Effects of fentanyl on local cerebral blood flow in the rat. Acta Anaesthesiol Scand 26:594, 1985
130. Naughton N, Hoffman WE, Larscheid P et al: A benzodiazepine antagonists inhibits the cerebral metabolic and respiratory depressant effects of fentanyl. Life Sci 36:2239, 1985
131. Carlsson C, Smith DS, Keykhah MM et al: The effects of high dose fentanyl on cerebral circulation and metabolism in rats. Anesthesiology 57:375, 1982
132. Vernhiet J, Renou AM, Orgogozo JM et al: Effects of diazepam-fentanl mixture on cerebral blood flow and oxygen consumption in man. Br J Anaesth 50:165, 1978
133. Takeshita H, Michenfelder JD, Theye RA: The effect of morphine and N-allylnormorphine on canine cerebral metabolism and circulation. Anesthesiology 37:605, 1972
134. Michenfelder JD, Theye RA: Effects of fentanyl, droperidol, and innovar on canine cerebral metabolism and blood flow. Br J Anaesth 43:630, 1971
135. Keykhah MM, Smith DS, Carlsson C et al: Influence of sufentanil on cerebral metabolism and circulation in the rat. Anesthesiology 63:274, 1985
136. Jobes DR, Kennell EM, Bush GL et al: Cerebral blood flow and metabolism during morphine-ni-

trous oxide anesthesia in man. Anesthesiology 47:16, 1977
137. Matsumiya N, Dohi S: Effects of intravenous subarachnoid morphine on cerebral and spinal cord hemodynamics and antagonism with naloxone in dogs. Anesthesiology 59:175, 1983
138. McPherson RW, Traystman RJ: Fentanyl and cerebral vascular responsivity in dogs. Anesthesiology 60:180, 1984
139. Freeman J, Ingvar DH: Effects of fentanyl on cerebral cortical blood flow and EEG in the cat. Acta Anaesthesiol Scand 11:381, 1967
140. Wahl M: Effects of enkephalins, morphine, and naloxone on pial arteries during perivascular microapplication. J Cereb Blood Flow Metab 5:451, 1985
141. Buchweitz E, Grandison L, Weiss HR: Effect of morphine on regional cerebral oxygen consumption and supply. Brain Res 291:301, 1984
142. Olsen JD, Hohimer AR, Mathis MD: Cerebral blood flow and metabolism during morphine induced stimulation of breathing movements in fetal lambs. Life Sci 33:751, 1983
143. Maekawa T, Tommasino C, Shapiro HM: Local cerebral blood flow with fentanyl induced seizures. J Cereb Blood Flow Metab 4:88, 1984
144. Koskinen LO, Bill A: Regional cerebral, occular, and peripheral vascular effects of naloxone and morphine in unanesthetized rabbits. Acta Physiol Scand 119:235, 1983
145. Vernhiet J, Macrez P, Renou AM et al: Effects of high doses of morphinomimetics on the cerebral circulation in normal subjects. Ann Anesthesiol Fr 18:803, 1977
146. Milde LN, Milde JH: Effects of sufentanil on cerebral circulation and metabolism in dogs. Anesth Analg 70:138, 1990
147. Yaster M, Koehler RC, Traystman RJ: Effects of fentanyl on peripheral and cerebral hemodynamics in neonatal lambs. Anesthesiology 66:524, 1987
148. Moyer JH, Pontius R, Morris G, Hirshberger R: Effect of morphine and N-allylnormorphine on cerebral hemodynamics and oxygen metabolism. Circulation 15:379, 1957
149. Young ML, Smith DS, Greenberg J et al: Effects of sufentanil on regional cerebral glucose utilization in rats. Anesthesiology 61:564, 1984
150. Messick JM, Jr, Theye RA: Effects of pentobarbital and meperidine on canine cerebral and total oxygen consumption rates. Can Anaesth Soc J 16:321, 1969
151. Levy RM, Fields HL, Stryker MP, Heinricher MM: The effect of analgesic doses of morphine on regional cerebral glucose metabolism in pain related structures. Brain Res 368:170, 1986
152. Jung R, Shah N, Reinsel R et al: Cerebrospinal fluid pressure in patients with brain tumors: Impact of fentanyl versus alfentanil during nitrous oxide-oxygen anesthesia. Anesth Analg 71:419, 1990
153. Sperry RJ, Bailey PL, Reichman MV et al: Fentanyl and sufentanil increase intracranial pressure in head trauma patients. Anesthesiology 77:416, 1992
154. From RP, Warner DS, Todd MM, Sokoll MD: Anesthesia for craniotomy: a double-blind comparison of alfentanil, fentanyl, and sufentanil. Anesthesiology 73:896, 1990
155. Todd MM, Warner DS, Sokoll MD et al: A prospective, comparative trial of three anesthetics for elective supratentorial craniotomy. Anesthesiology 78:1005, 1993
156. Kreuscher H, Grote J: Effect of the phencyclidine derivative ketamine (C1-581) on blood circulation and oxygen consumption of the dog brain. Anaesthesists 16:304, 1967
157. Sari A, Okuda Y, Takeshita H: Effect of ketamine on the cerebral circulation and metabolism. Masui 20:68, 1971
158. Dawson B, Michenfelder JD, Theye RA: Effects of ketamine on canine cerebral blood flow and metabolism: modification by prior administration of thiopental. Anesth Analg 50:443, 1971
159. Lockhardt CH, Jenkins JJ: Ketamine induced apnea in patients with increased intracranial pressure. Anesthesiology 37:92, 1972
160. Gardner AE, Olson BE, Lichtiger M: Cerebral spinal fluid pressure during dissociative anesthesia with ketamine. Anesthesiology 35:226, 1971
161. Wyte SR, Shapiro HM, Turner P, Harris AB: Ketamine induced intracranial hypertension. Anesthesiology 36:174, 1972
162. Gardner AE, Dannemiller FJ, Dean D: Intracranial cerebrospinal fluid pressure in man during ketamine anesthesia. Anesth Analg 51:741, 1972
163. Crumrine RS, Nulsen FE, Weiss MH: Alterations in ventricular fluid pressure during ketamine anesthesia in hydrocephalic children. Anesthesiology 42:758, 1975
164. Kaul HL, Jayalaxmi T, Gode GR, Mitra DK: Effects of ketamine on intracranial pressure in hydrocephalic children. Anesthesia 31:698, 1976

165. Wilson E, Marx M, Montaldo AM, Arana-Iniquez R: Effects of ketamine on the pressure of the cerebral spinal fluid. Variations of its effects. Acta Neurol Latinoam 22:10, 1976
166. Sari A, Okuda Y, Takeshita H: The effect of ketamine on cerebral spinal fluid pressure. Anesth Analg 51:560, 1972
167. Thorson T, Gran L: Ketamine/diazepam infusion anesthesia with special attention to the effect on cerebral spinal fluid pressure and arterial blood pressure. Acta Anaesthesiol Scand 24:1, 1980
168. Milde LN, Milde JH, Michenfelder JD: Cerebral functional, metabolic, and hemodynamic effects of etomidate in dogs. Anesthesiology 63:371, 1985
169. Longnecker DE: Stress free: to be or not to be. Anesthesiology 61:643, 1984
170. Forster A, Juge O, Louis M, Nahory A: Effects of specific benzodiazepine antagonist (Ro15-1788) on cerebral blood flow. Anesth Analg 66:309, 1987
171. Forster A, Juge O, Morel D: Effects of midazolam on cerebral hemodynamics and cerebral vasomotor responsiveness to carbon dioxide. J Cereb Blood Flow Metab 3:246, 1983
172. Forster A, Juge O, Morel D: Effects of midazolam on cerebral blood flow in human volunteers. Anesthesiology 56:453, 1982
173. Fleischer JE, Milde JH, Moyer TP, Michenfelder JD: Cerebral effects of high-dose midazolam and subsequent reversal with Ro15-1788 in dogs. Anesthesiology 68:234, 1988
174. Carlsson C, Hagerdahl M, Kaasik AE, Siesjo BK: The effects of diazepam on cerebral blood flow and oxygen consumption in rats and its synergistic interaction with nitrous oxide. Anesthesiology 45:319, 1976
175. Sebel PS, Lowdon JD: Propofol: a new intravenous anesthetic. Anesthesiology 71:260, 1989
176. Smith I, White PF, Nathanson M, Gouldson R: Propofol: an update on its clinical use. Anesthesiology 81:1005, 1994
177. Vandesteene A, Trempont V, Engelman E et al: Effect of propofol on cerebral blood flow and metabolism in man. Anaesthesia 43:42, 1988
178. Van Hemelrijck J, Fitch W, Mattheussen M et al: Effect of propofol on cerebral circulation and autoregulation in the baboon. Anesth Analg 71:49, 1990
179. Pinaud M, Lelausque J-N, Chetanneau A et al: Effects of propofol on cerebral hemodynamics and metabolism in patients with brain trauma. Anesthesiology 73:404, 1990
180. Dam M, Ori C, Pizzolato G et al: The effects of propofol anesthesia on local cerebral glucose utilization in the rat. Anesthesiology 73:499, 1990
181. Eng C, Lam AM, Mayberg TS et al: The influence of propofol with and without nitrous oxide on cerebral blood flow velocity and CO_2 reactivity in humans. Anesthesiology 77:872, 1992
182. Alkire MT, Haier RJ, Barker SJ et al: Cerebral metabolism during propofol anesthesia in humans studied with positron emission tomography. Anesthesiology 82:393, 1995
183. Fox J, Gelb AW, Enns J, et al: The responsiveness of cerebral blood flow to changes in arterial carbon dioxide is maintained during propofol-nitrous oxide anesthesia in humans. Anesthesiology 77:453, 1992
184. Sakabe T, Maekawa T, Ishikawa T, Takeshita H: The effects of lidocaine on canine cerebral metabolism and circulation related to electroencephalogram. Anesthesiology 40:433, 1974
185. Maekawa T, Oshibuchi T, Takeshita H, Imamura A: Cerebral energy state and glycolytic metabolism during lidocaine infusion in the rat. Anesthesiology 54:278, 1981
186. Astrup J, Srensen PM, Srensen HR: Inhibition of cerebral oxygen and glucose consumption in the dog by hypothermia, pentobarbital, and lidocaine. Anesthesiology 55:263, 1981
187. Milde LN, Milde JH: The detrimental effect of lidocaine on cerebral metabolism measured in dogs anesthetized with isoflurane. Anesthesiology 67:180, 1987
188. Haschke RH, Fink BR: Lidocaine effects on brain mitochondrial metabolism in vitro. Anesthesiology 42:737, 1975
189. Weiss MH, Kurze T, Apuzzo ML, Heiden JS: Effect of curare on intracranial dynamics. Surg Forum 25:458, 1974
190. Tarkkanen L, Laitinen L, Johansson G: Effects of d-tubocurarine on intracranial pressure and thalamic electrical impedance. Anesthesiology 40:247, 1974
191. Forbes AR, Cohen NH, Eger EI II: Pancuronium reduces halothane requirement in man. Anesth Analg 58:497, 1979
192. Lanier WL, Milde JH, Michenfelder JD: The cerebral effects of pancuronium and atracurium in halothane-anesthetized dogs. Anesthesiology 63:589, 1985

193. Stenlake JB, Waigh RD, Urwin J et al: Atracurium: conception and inception. Br J Anaesth 55:3S, 1983
194. Hennis PJ, Fahey MR, Miller RD et al: Pharmacology of laudanosine in dogs. Anesthesiology 61:A305, 1984
195. Babel A: Etude comparative de la laudanosine et de la papaverine au point de vue pharmacodynamique. Rev Med Suisse Romande 19:657, 1899
196. Mercier J, Mercier E: Action de quelques alcaloides secondairess de l'opium sûur l'electrocorticogramme du chien. C R Soc Biol (Paris) 149:760, 1955
197. Rosa G, Sanfilippo M, Vilardi V et al: Effect of vecuronium bromide on intracranial pressure and cerebral perfusion pressure. A preliminary report. Br J Anaesth 58:437, 1986
198. Giffin JP, Hartung J, Cottrell J et al: Effect of vecuronium on intracranial pressure, mean arterial pressure, and heart rate in cats. Br J Anaesth 58:441, 1986
199. Haigh JD, Nemoto EM, DeWolff AM, Bleyaert AL: Comparison of the effects of succinylcholine and atracurium on intracranial pressure in monkeys with intracranial hypertension. Can Anaesth Soc J 33:421, 1986
200. Marsh ML, Dunlop BJ, Shapiro HM et al: Succinylcholine intracranial pressure effects in neurosurgical patients. Anesth Analg 59:550, 1980
201. McLeskey CH, Cullen BF, Kennedy RD, Galindo A: Control of cerebral perfusion pressure during induction of anesthesia in high risk neurosurgical patients. Anesth Analg 53:985, 1974
202. Pall WL, Bishko JR, Woodham B: Succinylcholine, d-tubocurarine, dimethyl tubocurarine, and intracranial pressure in dogs. Anesth Analg 60:269, 1981
203. Bormann BE, Smith RB, Bunegin L, Albin MS: Does succinylcholine raise intracranial pressure? Anesthesiology 53:S262, 1980
204. Cottrell JE, Hartung J, Giffin JP, Shwiry B: Intracranial hemodynamic changes after succinylcholine administration in cats. Anesth Analg 62:1006, 1983
205. Lam AM, Gelb AW: Succinylcholine and intracranial pressure — a cause for "pause." Anesth Analg 63:619, 1984
206. Minton MD, Grosslight K, Stirt JA, Bedford RF: Increases in intracranial pressure from succinylcholine. Prevention by prior non-depolarizing blockade. Anesthesiology 65:165, 1986
207. Stirt JA, Grosslight KR, Bedford RF, Vollmer D: "Defasciculation" with metocurine prevents succinylcholine induced increases in intracranial pressure. Anesthesiology 67:50, 1987
208. Lanier WL, Milde JH, Michenfelder JD: Cerebral stimulation following succinylcholine in dogs. Anesthesiology 64:551, 1986
209. Henriksen L, Thorshauge C, Harmson A et al: Controlled hypotension with sodium nitroprusside: effects on cerebral blood flow and cerebral venous blood gases in patients operated for cerebral aneurysms. Acta Anaesthesiol Scand 27:62, 1983
210. Henriksen L, Paulson OB, Lauritzen M: The effects of sodium nitroprusside on cerebral blood flow and cerebral venous blood gases. I. Observations in awake man during and following moderate blood pressure reduction. Eur J Clin Invest 12:383, 1982
211. Henriksen L, Paulson OB: The effects of sodium nitroprusside on cerebral blood flow and cerebral venous blood gases. II. Observations in awake man during successful blood pressure reduction. Eur J Clin Invest 12:389, 1982
212. Larsen R, Teichmann J, Hilfiker O et al: Nitroprusside hypotension: cerebral blood flow and cerebral oxygen consumption in neurosurgical patients. Acta Anaesthesiol Scand 26:327, 1982
213. Griswold WR, Reznik V, Mendoza SA: Nitroprusside induced intracranial hypertension. JAMA 246:2679, 1981
214. Marsh ML, Shapiro HM, Smith RW, Marshall LF: Changes in neurologic status and intracranial pressure associated with sodium nitroprusside administration. Anesthesiology 51:336, 1979
215. Cottrell JE, Patel K, Turndorf H, Ransohof J: Intracranial pressure changes induced by sodium nitroprusside in patients with intracranial mass lesions. J Neurosurg 48:329:1978
216. Turner JM, Powell D, Gibson RM, McDowall DG: Intracranial pressure changes in neurosurgical patients during hypotension induced with sodium nitroprusside or trimethaphan. Br J Anaesth 49:419, 1977
217. Brown FD, Hanlin K, Crockard HA, Mullen S: Effect of sodium nitroprusside on cerebral blood flow in conscious human beings. Surg Neurol 7:67, 1977
218. Bunemann L, Jensen K, Thomsen L, Riisager S: Cerebral blood flow and metabolism during controlled hypotension with sodium-nitroprusside

and general anesthesia for total hip replacement. Acta Anaesthesiol Scand 31:487, 1987
219. Griffiths DPG, Cummins BH, Greenbaum R et al: Cerebral blood flow and metabolism during hypotension induced with sodium nitroprusside. Br J Anaesth 46:671, 1974
220. Sivarajan M, Amory DW, McKenzie SM: Regional blood flows during induced hypotension produced by nitroprusside or trimethaphan in the rhesus monkey. Anesth Analg 64:759, 1985
221. Candia GJ, Heros RC, Lavyne MH et al: Effect of intravenous sodium nitroprusside on cerebral blood flow and intracranial pressure. Neurosurgery 3:50, 1978
222. Brown FD, Crockard HA, Johns LM, Mullen S: The effects of sodium nitroprusside and trimethaphan camsylate on cerebral blood flow in rhesus monkeys. Neurosurgery 2:31, 1978
223. Crockard HA, Brown FD, Mullin JF: Effects of trimethaphan and sodium nitroprusside on cerebral blood flow in rhesus monkeys. Acta Neurochir 35:85, 1976
224. Keaney NP, McDowall DG, Turner JM et al: The effects of profound hypotension induced with sodium nitroprusside on cerebral blood flow and metabolism in the baboon. Br J Anaesth 45:639, 1973
225. Hoffman WE, Albrecht RF, Miletich DJ: Nitroglycerin induced hypotension will maintain CBF in hypertensive rats. Stroke 13:225, 1982
226. Ghani GA, Sung YF, Weinstein NS et al: Effects of intravenous nitroglycerin on intracranial pressure and volume pressure response. J Neurosurg 58:562, 1983
227. Dohi S, Matsumoto M, Takahashi T: The effects of nitroglycerin on cerebral spinal fluid pressure in awake and anesthetized humans. Anesthesiology 54:511, 1981
228. Cottrell JE, Gupta B, Rappaport H et al: Intracranial pressure during nitroglycerin-induced hypotension. J Neurosurg 53:309, 1980
229. Burt DE, Verniquet AJ, Homi J: The response of canine intracranial pressure to systemic hypotension induced with nitroglycerin. Br J Anaesth 54:665, 1982
230. Rogers MC, Hamburger C, Owen K, Epstein MH: Intracranial pressure in the cat during nitroglycerin-induced hypotension. Anesthesiology 51:227, 1979
231. Olesen J: The effect of intracarotid epinephrine, norepinephrine, and angiotensin on the regional cerebral blood flow in man. Neurology 22:978, 1972
232. Greenfield JC Jr, Tindall GT: Effect of norepinephrine, epinephrine, and angiotensin on blood flow in the internal carotid artery in man. J Clin Invest 47:1672, 1968
233. King BD, Sokoloff L, Wechsler RL: The effects of L-epinephrine and L-norepinephrine upon cerebral circulation and metabolism in man. J Crit Invest 31:273, 1952
234. Berntman L, Dahlgren N, Siesjo BK: Influence of intravenously administered catecholamines on cerebral oxygen consumption and blood flow in the rat. Acta Physiol Scand 104:101, 1978
235. Abdul-Rahman A, Dahlgren N, Johansson BB, Siesjo BK: Increase in local cerebral blood flow induced by circulating adrenaline: involvement of blood-brain barrier dysfunction. Acta Physiol Scand 107:227, 1979
236. Dahlgren N, Rosen I, Sakabe T, Siesjo BK: Cerebral functional, metabolic, and circulatory effects of intravenous infusion of adrenaline in the rat. Brain Res 184:143, 1980
237. Lluch S, Reimann C, Glick G: Evidence for the direct effect of adrenergic drugs on the cerebral vascular bed of the unanesthetized goat. Stroke 4:50, 1973
238. Artru AA, Nugent M, Michenfelder JD: Anesthetics affect the cerebral metabolic response to circulatory catecholamines. J Neurochem 36:1941, 1981
239. Baskin DS, Hosobuchi Y: Naloxone reversal of ischemic neurological deficits in man. Lancet 2:272, 1981
240. Hosobuchi Y, Baskin DS: Reversal of induced ischemic neurologic deficit in gerbils by the opiate antagonist naloxone. Science 215:69, 1982
241. Christie-Pope BC, Palmer GC, Palmer SJ: Effects of naloxone and morphine on cerebral ischemia in gerbils. J Neurosci Res 16:683, 1986
242. Kastin AJ, Nissen C, Olson RD: Failure of MIF-1 or naloxone to reverse ischemic-induced neurologic deficits in gerbils. Pharmacol Biochem Behav 17:1083, 1982
243. Gaines C, Nehls DG, Suess DM et al: Effect of naloxone on experimental stroke in awake monkeys. Neurosurgery 14:308, 1984
244. Estanol B, Aguilar F, Croona T: Diagnosis of reversal versus irreversible cerebral ischemia by the intravenous administration of naloxone. Stroke 16:1006, 1985
245. Jabaily S, Davis SM: Naloxone administration

to patients with acute stroke. Stroke 15:36, 1984

246. Artru AA, Steen PA, Michenfelder JD: Cerebral metabolic effects of naloxone administered with anesthetic and subanesthetic concentrations of halothane in the dog. Anesthesiology 52:217, 1980
247. Turner DM, Kassell NF, Sasaki T et al: Cerebral and systemic vascular effects of naloxone in pentobarbital-anesthetized normal dogs. Neurosurgery 14:276, 1984
248. Turner DM, Kassell NF, Sasaki T et al: Effects of naloxone on cerebral blood flow and metabolism in isoflurane/nitrous oxide-anesthetized dogs. Neurosurgery 14:688, 1984
249. Turner DM, Kassell NF, Sasaki T et al: High dose naloxone produces cerebral vasodilation. Neurosurgery 15:192, 1984
250. Turner DM, Kassell NF, Sasaki T et al: Effects of naloxone during high dose barbiturate anesthesia. Neurosurgery 15:509, 1984
251. Phillis JW, DeLong RE, Towner JK: Naloxone enhances cerebral reactive hyperemia in the rat. Neurosurgery 17:596, 1985
252. Sandor P, Goto HF, Tomita M et al: Effects of a stable enkephalin analog (D-Met2, Pro5)-enkephalinamide, and naloxone on cortical blood flow and cerebral blood volume in experimental brain ischemia in anesthetized cats. J Cereb Blood Flow Metab 6:553, 1986
253. Michenfelder JD: Anesthesia and the Brain. Churchill Livingstone, New York, 1988

2 CEREBROSPINAL FLUID DYNAMICS

ALAN A. ARTRU

Early investigations of cerebrospinal fluid (CSF) physiology examined chiefly the discrete properties of the system — the anatomy of the spaces that contain the CSF; CSF formation, reabsorption, and composition; and the effects of pharmacologic intervention and systemic physiologic changes. More recent work has focused on the dynamic aspects of CSF physiology, that is, the interaction between the discrete properties of the CSF system and the manner in which they affect and are affected by CSF pressure. This recent work suggests that CSF dynamics may be a clinically relevant factor in the care of patients where CSF pressure is of concern: patients with intracranial tumors, hydrocephalus, head injury, and so on. Because such patients frequently require anesthesia for surgery, some of the recent investigations on CSF dynamics have sought to determine the effects of anesthetics and other treatments commonly used by neuroanesthetists.

This chapter reviews the anatomy, physiology, and pharmacology of the CSF system and CSF dynamics and also some of the more recent work relating these basic properties to neuroanesthesia. It is hoped that this material will provide a foundation for understanding the relative importance of CSF dynamics in each of the clinical situations in Chapters 8 to 21 and how CSF dynamics might best be managed in the current practice of neuroanesthesia.

ANATOMY OF THE CSF SPACES AND PROPERTIES OF CSF

Structure of the Spaces

CSF is a clear aqueous solution that is formed in the brain and circulates through macroscopic and interstitial spaces that are in continuity. The macroscopic spaces include the ventricles and subarachnoid space within and around the brain and spinal cord. The interstitial space is that which surrounds the neuronal and glial elements of the central nervous system (CNS). The macroscopic CSF volume ranges from 50 ml in infants to 140 to 150 ml in adults, with ventricular volume being approximately 23 ml in adult humans.[1] Brain interstitial volume is calculated to be 300 to 350 ml in adult humans.

THE MACROSCOPIC SPACES The macroscopic CSF spaces include two lateral ventricles, the third cerebral ventricle, the aqueduct of Sylvius, the fourth (cerebellar) ventricle, the central canal of the spinal cord, and the subarachnoid space. Penetrating arterioles from the subarachnoid space are surrounded by an invagination of the pia mater, creating a perivascular space (the Virchow-Robin space) that is contiguous with the subarachnoid space. The choroid plexuses of the lateral ventricles extend from the inferior horn to the central part. At the interventricular foramina, the choroid plexuses of the two lateral ventricles become continuous with each other and with that of the third ventricle. Each plexus is suspended within the ventricle on vascular invaginations of the pia mater called the *tela choroidea*. The blood vessels supplying the choroid plexuses in the body of the lateral ventricles, third ventricle, and temporal horns include the posterior choroidal, anterior choroidal, and superior cerebellar arteries, respectively. The choroid plexus of the fourth ventricle is supplied by the posterior inferior cerebellar arteries.[2] The nervous supply to the choroidal plexus includes branches of the vagus, glossopharyngeal, and sympathetic nerves.

A single layer of epithelial cells lines most of the macroscopic CSF spaces. Exceptions are the ventricles and central canal of the spinal cord, which are lined by ependyma, a ciliated, low columnar epithelium. There are tight junctions between epithelial cells where they cover the choroid plexuses but not elsewhere. The cisterns and sulci of the subarachnoid space are bounded by an "open" mesothelium that is formed inwardly by the pia and outwardly by a loose investment of arachnoid cells.

THE INTERSTITIAL SPACES The interstitial spaces of the brain and spinal cord, in contrast to those of other organs in the body, are small in diameter (180 Å). Exchange between these spaces and cerebral capillaries is limited because the capillary membrane is highly impermeable. This impermeable membrane constitutes the structural basis of the *blood-brain barrier* (BBB) and consists of three elements. First, the cells of the cerebral capillary endothelium are joined by tight junctions (zonulae occludentae) that are capable of restricting the intercellular movement of molecules having a diameter of 20 Å or more.[3] Second, several features of the endothelial cells restrict transcellular passage of substances (heterolytic vesicles, specific enzymes, facilitated transport of only certain substances, and only a small number of pinocytotic vesicles for transport). Third, these specialized capillary endothelial cells are circumferentially invested by astrocyte foot processes. This architecture is unique to the cerebral vasculature and is found in all areas of the brain except at the choroid plexus (and several other small regions). Beyond the BBB, the extracellular spaces of the brain and spinal cord consist of narrow, interconnecting channels that are anatomically continuous with the adjoining macroscopic CSF spaces.

Some have suggested that the interstitial spaces also communicate with lymphatic channels. Up to 30% of labeled CSF or tracers injected into the brain can be recovered in the deep cervical lymph system.[4–6] CSF may reach these lymphatics by flowing through the cribiform plate. The arachnoid of the plate joins with olfactory perineurium comprised of fibroblasts and large intercellular spaces.[7–9] CSF and its contents may pass directly into the nasal submucosa and thence via afferent ducts into the deep cervical lymph nodes.

Composition of CSF

Compared to plasma, CSF contains higher concentrations of sodium, chloride, and magnesium and lower concentrations of glucose, proteins, amino acids, uric acid, potassium, bicarbonate, calcium, and phosphate (Table 2.1). The concentration of CSF constituents in the macroscopic spaces varies according to the sampling site because diffusion of substances between CSF and brain interstitial fluid occurs as CSF passes through the ventricles and subarachnoid spaces.[1] That CSF is not simply an ultrafiltrate of plasma has been taken as evidence that active secretory processes are involved in its formation. Regional variations in potassium, urea, albumin, globulin, and amino acids have been taken as evidence that sites other than the choroid plexus are involved with transport of solutes into and out of the CSF.[10] For example, the concentration of chloride is greater and the concentrations of bicarbonate, potassium and calcium are lower in mixed CSF than in freshly formed CSF. In the case of calcium, its movement out of CSF is reported to occur by a trans-

TABLE 2.1 *Composition of CSF and plasma in humans*[a]

	MEAN CSF CONCENTRATION	MEAN PLASMA CONCENTRATION
CSF pressure, mmHg		
Children	3.0–7.5	—
Adults	4.5–13.5	—
Volume, ml		
Infants	40–60	—
Young children	60–100	—
Older children	80–120	—
Adults	100–160	—
Specific gravity	1.007	1.025
Osmolality, mOsm/kg H_2O	289	289
pH	7.31	7.40
PCO_2, mmHg	50.5	41.1
Sodium, meq/L	141	140
Potassium, meq/L	2.9	4.6
Calcium, meq/L	2.5	5.0
Magnesium, meq/L	2.4	1.7
Chloride, meq/L	124	101
Bicarbonate, meq/L	21	23
Glucose, mg/100 ml	61	92
Protein, mg/100 ml	28	7,000
Albumin	23	4,430
Globulin	5	2,270
Fibrinogen	0	300

Abbreviation: CSF, cerebrospinal fluid.

[a] Average values based on references 1, 167–170.

port mechanism and to be independent of the concentration of calcium in CSF.[11] The higher concentration of protein in lumbar CSF relative to cisternal CSF probably reflects net addition of CNS metabolites to the bulk circulation of CSF as it drains toward sites of absorption.[12]

Function of CSF

The functions of CSF are varied and complex. CSF supports and protects the brain. The low specific gravity of CSF (1.007) relative to brain (1.040) reduces the effective mass of a 1,400-g brain to only 47 g.[13,14] Alteration of CSF calcium, potassium, and magnesium produces changes in heart rate, blood pressure, autonomic responses, ventilation, muscle tone, and emotional state.[15] Alteration of CSF acid-base balance influences cerebral blood flow (CBF), brain metabolism, autoregulation of CBF, and ventilation. In continuity with the brain interstitial fluid, CSF provides a stable supply of substrates, primarily glucose, even though plasma concentrations of substrates are continuously changing. Recent work has examined the role of

CSF in intracerebral transport of β-endorphin and the hormones of the hypothalamus and pineal gland. It was found that specialized ventricular cells and neurons within the brain parenchyma secrete these neuroendocrine factors. The factors diffuse into CSF (from the brain parenchyma) or are released into CSF (from ventricular cells), where they are transported by CSF flow within the macroscopic spaces. These CSF-borne factors stimulate the dendritic processes of other "CSF-contacting neurons" or enter the hypophyseal portal system via specialized ependymal cells.[16]

CSF maintains a chemically precise environment necessary for neurotransmission and removes metabolic products, unwanted drugs, and pathologic substances resulting from CNS injury. Accumulation of metabolites and substances in brain extracellular fluid (ECF) is prevented by their passage into CSF, cerebral veins, or cervical lymphatics. Although passage into CSF may occur by two mechanisms, net diffusion and bulk flow of ECF, bulk flow accounts for the majority of passage of many substrates of different molecular weights. Bulk flow is reported to account for clearance of substances entering the brain as well as substances synthesized by the brain. It is particularly important for clearing lipid-insoluble substances such as inulin, mannitol, sulfanilic acid, urea, albumin, globulin, dopamine, homovanillic acid, serotonin, and norepinephrine.[17] For other substances, less than 20% of solute clearance from the ECF is accounted for by drainage into CSF. Many of these substances, such as penicillin, methotrexate, and neurotransmitter acid metabolites, are absorbed into the veins of the choroid plexus using a probenecid-sensitive transport mechanism.[17] Prolactin is taken up and bound by the choroid plexus. This may reflect a role for prolactin in regulating CSF composition, or it might serve to transport prolactin from blood to CSF, permitting prolonged delivery of prolactin to hypothalamic receptor neurons.[17]

In contrast to substances that are cleared from brain ECF into choroid plexus veins, other substances entering the brain are cleared primarily by passage back across the BBB into cerebral vessels. Dual infusion of valproate intravenously and [^{3}H]valproate into the cerebral venticles coupled with intravenous infusion of probenecid (to block organic anion transporters at brain capillaries), infusion of probenecid into the cerebral ventricles (to block organic anion transporters at the choroid plexus) or infusion of silicone oil into the cerebral ventricles (to block nonprobenecid-sensitive transporters at the choroid plexus) was used to examine efflux of valproate from brain ECF.[18,19] Pharmacokinetic analysis of brain and CSF concentrations of valproate and [^{3}H]valproate indicated that valproate efflux from the brain occurs mainly via probenecid-sensitive transport at the brain capillary endothelium.

MOVEMENT OF CSF AND ITS CONSTITUENTS

CSF Formation

CSF in humans is formed at a rate of 0.35 to 0.40 ml/min or 500 to 600 ml/day. Approximately 0.25% of total adult CSF volume is replaced by freshly formed CSF each minute. Total CSF volume is replaced every 5 to 7 hours or 4 times per day.[20] About 40 to 70% of CSF formation occurs at the choroid plexus whereas 30 to 60% enters the macroscopic spaces across the ependyma and pia.[21–23]

CSF FORMATION AT THE CHOROID PLEXUS The capillary endothelium of the choroid plexus does not possess tight junctions between its cells as does the capillary endothelium of most of the rest of the brain. Instead, the capillary endothelium of the choroid plexus is fenestrated. Blood entering the plexus is filtered across these capillaries and forms a protein-rich fluid within the choroidal stroma, not unlike interstitial fluid in other tissues of the body. However, the choroid plexus epithelial cells, which separate the choroid stroma from the macroscopic CSF spaces, contain apical tight junctions that restrict passive solute exchange.[24] At the choroid plexus epithelium, selected constituents of the stromal fluid are transported across the relatively impermeable choroidal epithelium by the combined processes of ultrafiltration and secretion.[25,26] These epithelial cell tight junctions constitute a *blood-CSF barrier* at the choroid plexus. Also contributing to this barrier are (1) a system of epithelial cell enzymes that are involved with the active, bidirectional transport of substances between plasma and CSF[12,25–27] and (2) a system of pinocytotic vesicles and lysosomes.[28]

The ultrafiltrate of the choroidal stroma enters clefts between the choroid plexus epithelial cells due to hydrostatic pressure and bulk flow (Fig. 2.1). Adenosine triphosphate (ATP)-dependent "sodium-potassium pumps" on the cleft move sodium ions into the cell and potassium and hydrogen ions into the stroma as counter ions. Chloride ions move into the cell coupled with sodium ions. The local osmolar gradient created by this pump draws water into the cell

FIGURE 2.1 *Some of the processes involved in CSF formation at the choroid plexus are shown in schematic form. ATP-dependent membrane "pumps" transport Na^+ across the abluminal surface to within the choroid plexus cell and across the secretory surface, into the macroscopic CSF space, in exchange for K^+ and H^+. Water moves from the stroma into CSF as it follows the concentration gradient produced by the ionic "pumps". Author's drawing based on references 26, 29, 49, 167, and 171–175*

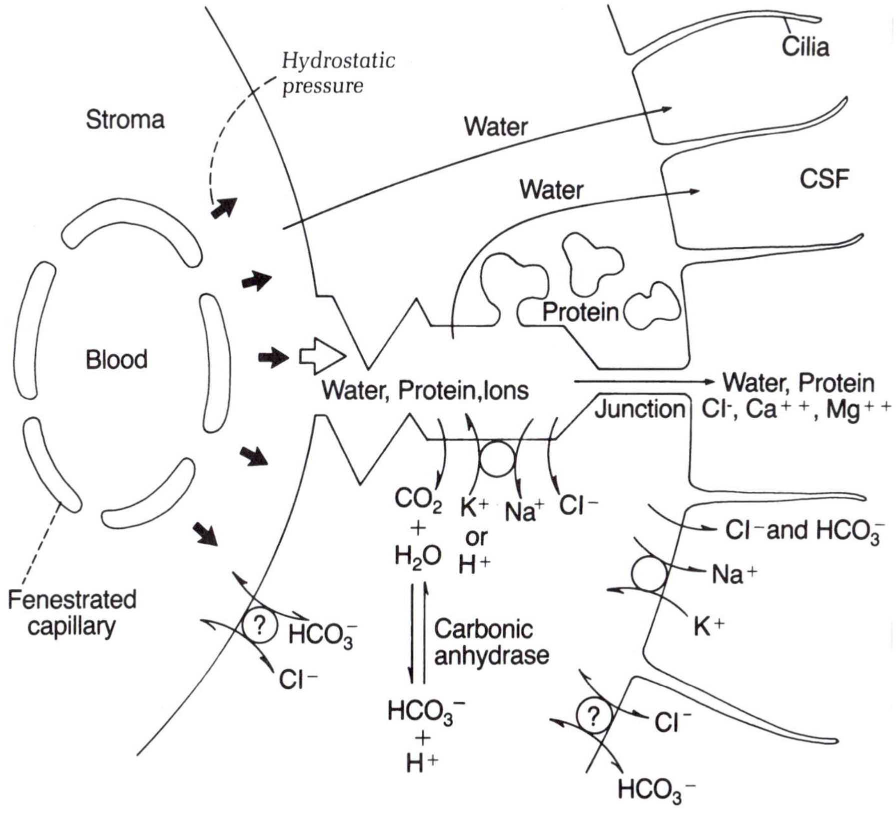

from the stroma. Bicarbonate and hydrogen ions within the epithelial cell result from the action of carbonic anhydrase on carbon dioxide that diffuses into the cell or is created within the cell as a result of cellular metabolism. ATP-dependent sodium-potassium pumps on the ventricular surface of the cell move sodium ions into the CSF and potassium ions in the direction of the stroma. It appears that water migrates across epithelial cells into the ventricle via the osmotic gradient established by active sodium secretion. Chloride and bicarbonate anions in the epithelial cell move passively into the CSF along an electrochemical gradient. In addition, water may move into the CSF from the stroma via "leaky" tight junctions. Some chloride anions and the ions found in low concentrations in the CSF (such as calcium and magnesium) also pass through leaky tight junctions.

EXTRACHOROIDAL CSF FORMATION Of the 30 to 60% of CSF formation occurring at extrachoroidal sites, 60% is estimated to be derived from oxidation by the brain of glucose and 40% from ultrafiltration from cerebral capillaries.[21,23,29] In most of the brain, the distinctive architecture and function of the vessels and perivascular space restrict passage of most large and polar molecules in and out of the brain across the "blood-brain (ECF)" interface. Characteristics features of the BBB include tight junctions between capillary endothelial cells, a paucity of pinocytotic vesicles within the endothelial cells, specialized heterolytic vesicles and specific enzyme systems within the cells to prevent transcellular passage of certain substances, facilitated transport systems allowing transcellular passage of certain substances but not others, and investment of the vessels by astrocyte foot processes. Water, electrolytes, urea, lipid-soluble materials, glucose, amino acids, and a number of small nonelectrolytes pass more freely across this interface.[30] Some of these substances may diffuse into the brain ECF, whereas others may be actively transported by the astrocyte layer that surrounds the capillary endothelium.[31] A relatively glucose-rich and protein poor "lymph" is formed that flows by diffusion through the narrow perivascular and intracellular spaces of the brain interstitium toward the macroscopic CSF spaces. In addition, beyond the capillary-glial complex, downstream from the blood-brain ECF interface, lie a number of transport systems that further modify the chemical composition of substances entering into the macroscopic CSF spaces. These systems include not only the sodium and potassium pumps associated with neurons[32] but also specialized transport mechanisms possessed by the ventricular ependyma.[30,33]

Movement of Glucose

The concentration of glucose in both mixed CSF and freshly formed CSF at the choroid plexus is approximately 60% of that in blood.[34] This ratio remains constant until blood glucose is elevated to more than 15 to 20 mM. Glucose moves from blood into CSF by a facilitated transport mechanism that allows glucose to cross more rapidly than would be predicted on the basis of its lipid solubility.[35] The rate of glucose transport into CSF is directly related to the serum glucose concentration and independent of the serum-to-CSF glucose concentration gradient.[36] Kinetic studies indicate that the transport mechanism is saturable. It is questionable whether significant amounts of glucose at normoglycemia are transferred from blood by simple diffusion.[37] The influx of glucose into CSF is maintained independently of the rate of CSF formation (V_f) by the downhill glucose concentration gradient between blood and CSF needed for facilitated diffusion.

Glucose also is transported from the cerebral ventricles into the surrounding brain and blood by oubain-sensitive and -insensitive fluxes and diffusion.[38] One transport site may be located at the choroid plexus.[39] Half of the glucose in CSF is cleared and metabolized by periventricular tissue.[36] As glucose is cleared from the CSF, it is replaced by glucose from serum in an amount that is about 25% of the serum glucose concentration.

Movement of Protein

CSF protein concentrations are normally 0.5% or less of the respective plasma or serum concentrations. Although proteins within blood are reported to enter CSF at the choroid plexus as well as extrachoroidal sites, the exact entry rates are uncertain.[1,24,40] Because a structural barrier between the brain interstitial space and the macroscopic CSF space does not exist, proteins that slowly enter the brain ECF are drained from the extracellular space into the macroscopic CSF space by bulk flow. Proteins entering the macroscopic space either from the interstitial space or from the choroid plexus are transported along with CSF through the macroscopic pathways and are discharged into dural venous sinuses. This "sink effect" of flowing CSF helps to keep the concentration of proteins in both CSF and brain low and far from equilibrium with blood.[1,29,41] In normal infants and adult humans, a concentration gradient of protein exists from a low level in the ventricles (about 26 mg/100 ml), to an intermediate level in the cisterna magna (about 32 mg/100 ml), and to the highest level in the lumbar sac (42 mg/100 ml).[42] Between ventricular and lumbar CSF, there is a 2.2-fold increase in albumin concentration, a 2.6-fold increase in Ig G concentration, but a decrease in the concentration of prealbumin by a factor of 0.7. Albumin and immunoglobulin G (IgG) in CSF appear to derive entirely from blood, whereas prealbumin is produced in part by nervous tissue or is transported actively into CSF. The increase of CSF protein concentration as CSF flows through the macroscopic space is suggested to be related to decreased CSF flow and washout rate in the lumbar subarachnoid compartment (56% of total CSF compartment volume) as compared to the ventricular and cisternal compartments (26 and 18% of total volume, respectively).[43]

About 60% of CSF protein enters CSF at the choroid plexus under normal conditions.[44] One route may be passage between epithelial cells. The apical tight junctions of choroid plexus epithelial cells are less restrictive than most cerebrovascular tight junctions and may permit protein passage.[45,46] A second route may be vesicular transport across the choroid epithelium.[47] A third route may be passage around the choroid plexus. At the edge of the plexus, a functional leak exists at the border between choroidal epithelium and ventricular ependyma that may permit protein passage.[47] Heterogeneous membrane models, allowing for two modes of protein entry into CSF (via pores of different radii or via a single set of pores plus vesicles) account for the CSF-to-blood protein concentration relationship better than do homogeneous models in which either a single set of pores or only pinocytotic vesicles contribute to protein transport. A model of aqueous pores with a 117-Å radius as well as transfer by pinocytotic vesicles with an assumed radius of 25 Å has been proposed as the most likely.[48]

Effects of Increased ICP on CSF Formation

There is a negative but poor correlation between $\dot{V}_f$ and increased intracranial pressure (ICP).[49] The correlation improves when V_f is evaluated relative to cerebral perfusion pressure (CPP). $\dot{V}_f$ diminishes when CPP decreases below approximately 70 mmHg whether CPP is reduced solely by arterial hypotension or by combining arterial hypotension with increased ICP. Increase of ICP to 20 mmHg with preservation of CPP greater than approximately 70 mmHg produces no change in $\dot{V}_f$.[50,51]

These effects of CPP on $\dot{V}_f$ are consistent with reported changes in CBF, lateral ventricle choroid plexus blood flow, and fourth ventricle choroid plexus blood flow caused by alteration of CPP.[49] Reduction of CPP to 70 mmHg by combining arterial hypotension and increased ICP reduces CBF and choroid plexus blood flows. Further reduction of CPP to 50 mmHg causes an additional decline in choroid plexus flows when CPP is reduced by a further increase in ICP but no additional decline in choroid plexus flow when CPP is reduced solely by arterial hypotension. It was suggested that the greater decrease of choroid plexus flow when CPP was lowered by combining arterial hypotension with increased ICP as compared to lowering CPP solely by arterial hypotension was due to an increase in choroidal vascular resistance (due to choroid plexus compression) as well as changes in hydrostatic forces within the choroidal vascular bed.[49] Both these factors reduce filtration from choroid plexus capillaries.

Circulation of CSF

Several mechanisms contribute to the movement of CSF within the macroscopic spaces. CSF is formed at a hydrostatic pressure of 15 cm H_2O, and the flow of CSF where it is freshly formed provides a force for CSF movement.[1] Cilia on ependymal cells produce currents that propel CSF toward the fourth ventricle and its foramina into the subarachnoid spaces.[52] Respiratory variations and vascular pulsations emanating from the choroid plexuses and cerebral arteries cause the ventricles to pulsate, supplying additional momentum for CSF movement. Mean CSF pressure in humans is 15 cm H_2O, whereas the pressure in the superior sagittal sinus is 9 cm H_2O, providing a 6-cm H_2O pressure gradient for passage of CSF across the arachnoid villi.[12,20,53] A suction-pump action that depends on the high velocity of the central blood flow through the fixed diameter of the sinuses and the low intraluminal pressure that develops at the circumference of the sinus wall where the arachnoid villi enter may explain how the circulation of the CSF continues through a wide range of postural pressures.[20]

CSF passes from the two lateral ventricles through the paired interventricular foramina of Monro into the midline third ventricle. From the third ventricle, CSF flows caudally through the aqueduct of Sylvius and fourth ventricle and from the fourth ventricle into the subarachnoid space by one of three exits. Two exits are the paired lateral foramina of Luschka, from which CSF flows around the brainstem into the cerebellopontine angle and prepontine cisterns. The third exit is the midline foramen of Magendie, from which fluid passes through the vallecula into the cisterna magna. A small volume of fluid may also exit through the central canal of the spinal cord.[54]

There are three courses that CSF may follow out of the cisterna magna. One route is for the CSF to pass superiorly into the subarachnoid space surrounding the cerebellar hemisphere. A second route is for the CSF to travel downward into the spinal subarachnoid space. Here CSF flows in a caudal direction behind the cord (posterior to the dentate ligaments) to the lumbar theca and then in a cephalad direction in front of the cord to the basilar cisterns.[20,54] A third route is for cisternal CSF to move cephalad into the premedullary, pontine, and interpeduncular cisterns. From these cisterns, known collectively as the *basilar cisterns*, CSF flows forward along two courses. One pathway is inferiorly through the interpeduncular cistern, through the Sylvian fissure and prechiasmatic cisterns, to the subarachnoid space that surrounds the lateral and frontal aspects of the cerebral hemisphere. A second pathway follows a dorsomedial route through the ambient cisterns and cisterna venal magnae cerebri to the subarachnoid space that surrounds the medial and posterior aspects of the cerebral hemispheres. The last step in CSF circulation occurs at the dural sinuses, located (1) at spinal dural sinusoids on dorsal nerve roots and (2) along the superior sagittal sinus, where absorption takes place across the arachnoid villi (Fig. 2.2).

Radioisotope studies show that labelled CSF flows from the ventricles to the basal cisterns within a few minutes and begins to pass through the anterior subarachnoid spaces and Sylvian fissures at 2 hours to collect along the superior sagittal sinus area at 12 to 24 hours.[55] Labelled CSF reaches the low cervical-high thoracic region in 10 to 20 minutes, the thoracolumbar area in 30 to 40 minutes, and the lumbosacral cul de sac in 60 to 90 minutes.[56] Ascent of CSF in the spinal subarachnoid space is slower than descent. Labelled CSF moves from the lumbar sac to the basal cisterns in approximately 1 hour. About 20 to 33% of the labelled CSF reaches the intracranial cavity within 12 hours. At 12 to 24 hours, most of the labelled lumbar CSF is de-

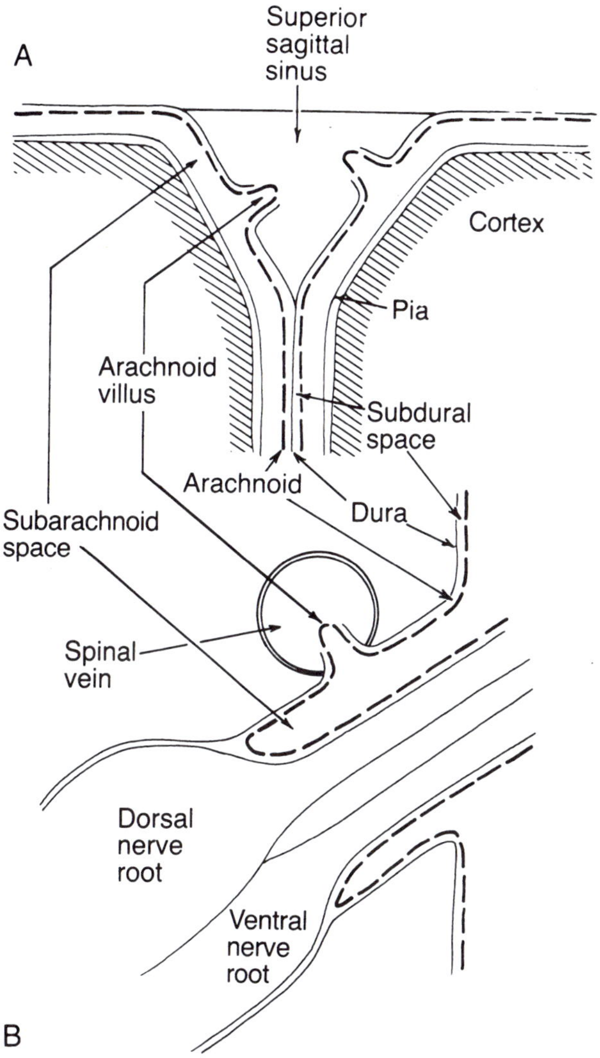

FIGURE 2.2 *CSF is reabsorbed via arachnoid villi at the sagittal sinus (A) and at spinal veins on dorsal nerve roots (B). Author's drawing based on references 29, 63, 70, 165, 176, 177.*

tectable along the superior sagittal sinus. The circulatory pattern of CSF is not altered by posture or ambulation, although physical activity is known to disturb CSF concentration gradients by promoting CSF mixing,[57] and coughing causes all spinal CSF to flow toward the cisterna magna.[58]

Clearance of Brain Interstitial Fluid

NORMAL ICP Under normal physiologic conditions, there is relatively little bulk flow across cerebral capillaries and through the parenchyma of the brain.[59] Molecules in the brain interstitial space move through that space primarily by diffusion. The distance traveled by these molecules relates to molecular size, tissue concentration gradients, and the ability of molecules to cross the BBB and reenter the vascular system.

CEREBRAL EDEMA Vasogenic brain edema is caused by damage to cerebral vessels. This type of edema frequently is associated with tumors, trauma, and infection. As a result of cerebral vascular injury, cerebrovascular permeability increases, allowing serum constituents to pass into the surrounding interstitial space under the hydrostatic pressure of the systemic circulation. During the formation and spread of vasogenic brain edema, fluid movement through the white matter is not by diffusion, but by bulk flow, with molecules of significantly different sizes all moving at the same rate for the same distance.[60] This bulk flow movement is controlled by the hydraulic conductivity of the cerebral blood vessels and increases in the tissue extracellular space.

One reported mechanism for clearance of vasogenic edema is movement of edema fluid into ventricular CSF. One factor favoring fluid movement out of the interstitial space is the pressure gradients between edematous brain tissue and CSF. A second factor favoring fluid movement out of the interstitial space is the sink action of CSF.[60,61] Extravasated serum proteins are cleared by intraglial uptake, and this protein clearance is believed to play a major role in the resolution of vasogenic brain edema.[62] Clearance of edema fluid was reported to increase when intracranial pressure was lowered, presumably due to an increase in the pressure gradient between edematous brain tissue and CSF.[63]

Reabsorption of CSF

CSF is reabsorbed from the macroscopic spaces through microscopic arachnoid villi and macroscopic arachnoid granulations. In the cranial CSF space, arachnoid villi are located within the dural wall bordering the superior sagittal sinus and venous lacunae, and in the spinal CSF space arachnoid villi are located within the dural wall bordering the dural sinusoids on dorsal nerve roots.[7,64] Under normal physiologic circumstances, 85 to 90% of CSF is reabsorbed at the superior sagittal sinus and 10 to 15% of CSF is reabsorbed at the dural sinusoids on dorsal nerve roots.

The arachnoid villus usually appears as a flask-shaped protrusion of arachnoid cells extending from the subarachnoid space into and through the wall of an adjacent venous sinus (Fig. 2.3). Except at the arachnoid granulations, the arachnoid membrane that covers the subarachnoid space is made up of several layers of arachnoid cells. The arachnoid cell layers adjacent to the dura are joined by tight junctions, thereby forming a barrier that prevents the transfer of CSF from the subarachnoid space into the dura.[65] At the arachnoid granulations large spaces are present between the inner layers of arachnoid cells, and this loose arrangement does not constitute an effective barrier. CSF flows easily from the subarachnoid space into the spaces within the villus. The core, or central

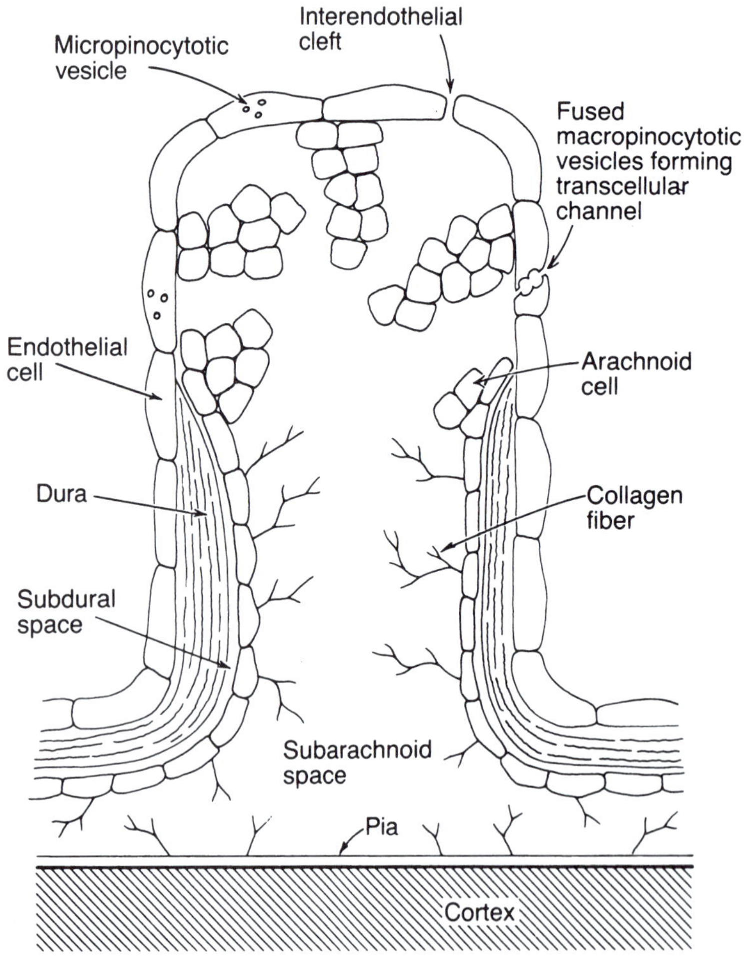

FIGURE 2.3 *Schematic drawing of the microscopic anatomy of an arachnoid villus. (Adapted from Upton and Weller,[176] with permission.)*

cavity, of the villus contained within the dural pocket is formed by a maze of loosely arranged arachnoid cells and intercellular spaces. Individually, these arachnoid cells are structurally similar to those of the rest of the subarachnoid space.[65] The open spaces between those loosely arranged arachnoid cells contain collagen fibers either singly or, more frequently, in bundles. Additionally, occasional myelinated and unmyelinated nerves are present within those spaces. The outer layer of arachnoid cells covering the villus remains joined by tight junctions, and under normal conditions, this endothelial covering of the villus is always preserved. In adults, multiple layers of endothelial cells may cover the villus.

NORMAL ICP The endothelial membrane covering the villus serves as a rate-limiting CSF-blood barrier for the movement of CSF and solute into venous blood. The rate at which CSF passes through the villi is determined by (1) the transvillus hydrostatic pressure gradient between CSF and the venous sinuses and (2) a pressure-sensitive resistance to CSF outflow at the arachnoid villus. The high permeability of the endothelial membrane suggests that osmotic differences across the barrier normally are not an important determinant of CSF movement through arachnoid villi.

Two pathways for CSF transport across the villus endothelium have been described, one extracellular and one intracellular. Although the endothelial cells are connected by tight junctions, occasional interendothelial clefts are observed in which there are no areas of membrane fusion or significant focal narrowing of the intercellular space.[66] These intercellular spaces thus seem to be open channels extending from the abluminal to the luminal surface of the cell and may serve as an extracellular pathway whereby CSF diffuses from the subarachnoid space into blood. The endothelial cells of the arachnoid villi also contain pinocytotic vesicles and transcellular openings formed by chains of fused vesicles extending from the abluminal to the luminal surface.[67,68] These vesicles transport fluid as well as macromolecular tracers from CSF to blood. At resting CSF pressure, micropinocytotic vesicles appear to be the primary route of CSF transport. The functional status of both pathways contributes to the total resistance to CSF outflow.

INCREASED ICP The rate of reabsorption of CSF ($\dot{V}_a$) increases with increasing CSF pressure. Resistance to reabsorption of CSF (R_a) remains close to "normal" as CSF pressure increases to above 30 cm H_2O. Thereafter, with further increases in CSF pressure, R_a declines.[69] Studies of arachnoid villus endothelium at normal and increased CSF pressures show little change in endothelial vesicles as CSF pressure is increased from 9 to 30 cm H_2O other than a small increase in their size and number.[66,70] When the villus endothelium from animals with CSF pressures greater than 30 cm H_2O was examined, increasing numbers of transcellular channels were present concurrent with progressive increases in steady-state pressures and decreases in R_a. Thus, comparison of the outflow-resistance curve (as a function of increasing CSF pressure) with corresponding changes in villus endothelial vesicles suggests that the decrease in R_a at the arachnoid villus is structurally characterized by the formation of open transcellular channels. This transition from micropinocytotic vesicles to larger pinocytotic vesicles and transendothelial channel formation associated with increasing CSF pressure may represent an alternative pressure-dependent form of vesicle transport that functions to transfer a proportionately greater volume of fluid across the endothelium with progressively increased steady-state pressure. By this sequence of events, cytoplasmic vesicles may also serve as a *mobile membrane reserve* capable of forming transcellular channels in response to increased CSF pressure.[71] In addition, increased CSF pressure may increase CSF flow in the villus by facilitating passage through existing open intercellular clefts and by opening closed intercellular spaces that, at resting pressure, appear occluded by tight junctions.

Methods of Determining V_f and R_a

EXPERIMENTAL ANIMALS Three commonly used methods for determining CSF dynamics in animals are ventriculocisternal perfusion, manometric infusion, and volume injection/withdrawal. Ventriculocisternal perfusion was first described by Pappenheimer, Heisey, and colleagues in 1962.[72,73] The method requires placement of cannulae in a lateral ventricle and in the cisterna magna. Labeled, mock CSF is infused into the ventricular cannula, and a mixture of labeled, mock CSF and native CSF is collected from the cisterna magna. The substance choosen to label mock CSF is one of large molecular weight and low lipid solubility and whose concentration in the mixed outflow solution can be accurately determined, such as blue dextran. The osmolality of mock CSF should be matched to that of native CSF, the pH of mock CSF should be buffered (usually by bubbling through 5% CO_2 in oxygen) to equal that of native CSF, and the composition of mock CSF should be consistent with the species of animal used. Labeled, mock CSF is usually infused into the ventricle at a rate of 2 to 10-fold greater than $\dot{V}_f$ according to the animal species. Mixed mock-native CSF from the cisternal cannula is collected and the volume of the outflow sample determined. The concentration of the label in the outflow sample is measured, and the time over which the sample was obtained is noted. $\dot{V}_f$. is calculated according to the formula

$$\dot{V}_f = \dot{V}_i\,(C_i - C_o/C_o)$$

where $\dot{V}_f$. is the inflow rate of labeled, mock CSF; C_i is the concentration of the label in mock CSF, and C_o is the concentration of the label in the mixed outflow solution. $\dot{V}_a$ is calculated either by the formula

$$\dot{V}_a = (\dot{V}_i\,C_o - \dot{V}_o C_o)/C_o$$

where $\dot{V}_f$ is the rate of outflow of mock and native CSF from the cisternal cannula, or by the formula

$$\dot{V}_a = \dot{V}_i + \dot{V}_f - \dot{V}_o$$

R_a is a reciprocal measure of the slope relating $\dot{V}_a$ to CSF pressure. Thus, in order to calculate R_a, $\dot{V}_a$ must be determined at several CSF pressures. If the slope relating $\dot{V}_a$ to CSF pressure at these several CSF pressure is linear, one R_a value is calculated. If the $\dot{V}_a$/CSF pressures slope is not linear, multiple R_a values are calculated as the inverse of tangents to the $\dot{V}_a$/CSF pressure slope.

Manometric infusion, as it is currently used, was described by Maffeo, Mann, and colleagues in the late 1970s.[74,75] The method requires placement of a manometric infusion device into the spinal or supracortical subarachnoid space. This device permits infusion of mock CSF into the subarachnoid space and measurement of CSF pressure at the same site as the infusion. As above, CSF osmolality, pH, and composition should be matched to that of the animal being studied. Five to eight infusions of mock CSF are made at infusion rates ranging from 2- to 100-fold greater than $\dot{V}_f$ according to the animal species. In animals, infusions are continued for 1 to 8 minutes until one of two possible CSF pressure patterns is observed. With lower infusion rates, CSF pressure increases during the first 0.2 to 2.0 minutes, then plateaus at a steady state where the sum of $\dot{V}_i$ and $\dot{V}_f$ equals $\dot{V}_a$. At higher infusion rates, CSF pressure increases with no apparent tendency toward stabilization. Only the data from the lower infusion rates (usually three to six of the five to eight infusions) are used to calculate $\dot{V}_f$ and R_a. The first step of the calculations is to pair each steady-state CSF pressure (P_s) achieved at lower infusion rates with its associated $\dot{V}_i$. Next, each pair of $\dot{V}_i$:P_s values is plotted on a semilog plot of $\dot{V}_i$ versus P_s, where each $\dot{V}_i$:P_s pair defines one data point. A linear slope is then fit through the three to six data points. To determine $\dot{V}_f$, the semilog plot is extrapolated toward the origin (to the left). The $\dot{V}_i$ value at resting CSF pressure (P_0), (i.e., the $\dot{V}_i$ value corresponding to the intersection of a perpendicular from P_0 and the extrapolated semilog plot), is considered to be $\dot{V}_f$. R_a is derived from additional calculations of two species-dependent parameters M (transport capacity) and P_R (pressure at maximum resistance). These species-dependent parameters are calculated based on the formula

$$\dot{V}_i = (1/M)e^{P_s/P_R}$$

Simultaneously, solving this equation for the several pairs of $\dot{V}_i$:P_s values used to calculate $\dot{V}_f$ yields one unique pair of M and P_R values. R_a is then calculated based on the formula

$$R_a = MPe^{-P_s/P_R}$$

In addition the compliance (C) of the CSF compartment can be calculated according to the formula

$$C = \dot{V}_i/(\triangle P/\triangle t)$$

where P is CSF pressure, t is time and, $\triangle P/\triangle t$ is the slope of the linear rise in CSF pressure during infusion of mock CSF.

Volume injection/withdrawal was described by Marmarou and colleagues and Miller in the mid-1970s.[17,76,77] The method requires placement of a ventricular or spinal subarachnoid catheter. The catheter allows injection or withdrawal of CSF and measurement of the CSF pressure change that accompanies injection/withdrawal. As above, CSF should match that of the animal being studied. P_0 is determined, then a known volume of CSF ($\triangle V$) is injected into (or withdrawn from) the catheter while a timed recording of CSF pressure is made. One method of calculating R_a is to first calculate the pressure volume index (PVI) as follows:

$$PVI = \triangle V/(\log P_p/P_0)$$

where P_p is the peak CSF pressure (increase following volume injection, decrease following volume withdrawal). R_a is then calculated based on the formula

$$R_a = t \cdot P_0/(PVI.\log_{10}[P_2(P_p - P_0)/P_p(P_2 - P_o)])$$

where P_2 is the CSF pressure measured sometime between P_p and the return of CSF pressure to P_0, and t is the time from volume injection/withdrawal to P_2. $\dot{V}_f$ is calculated based on the formula

$$P_0 = P_v - (R_a . \dot{V}_f)$$

which can be rewritten

$$\dot{V}_f = (P_v - P_0)/R_a$$

where P_v is the venous blood pressure of the sagittal sinus. C is calculated based on the formula

$$C = (0.4343 \cdot PVI)/P_0$$

HUMANS Ventriculocisternal perfusion and manometric infusion have also been used to calculate $\dot{V}_f$, R_a, and C in patients.[75,78] For ventriculocisternal perfusion, the outflow catheter may be placed in the lumbar subarachnoid space, and ventricular and spinal CSF pressures are closely monitored to be sure that CSF pressure does not increase to unacceptable levels due to obstructed perfusion. For manometric infusion, the number of infusions is reduced and infusion rates are limited to 1.5- to 15-fold greater than $\dot{V}_f$. Infusions are restricted to 20 to 60 seconds, being terminated at CSF pressures of 60 to 70 cm H_2O if a rapid rise in CSF pressure with no apparent tendency toward stabilization is observed. The procedures and formulas for calculation of $\dot{V}_f$, R_a, and C are the same as those for experimental animals.

Because of the hazards associated with sustained infusion of mock CSF, ventriculocisternal perfusion and manometric infusion are less commonly used in patients than is volume injection/withdrawal. An obvious advantage of this latter methods is that when ICP is of concern, CSF withdrawal is therapeutic as well as effective for calculating $\dot{V}_f$, R_a, and C. The system can remain completely closed, minimizing the risk of infection from infusion of mock CSF. For repeated testing, CSF can be alternately withdrawn, then injected, with the net change of CSF volume being made according to the patient's ICP responses. In addition, CSF dynamics can be calculated from a single change of CSF volume and pressure lasting for several minutes as opposed to a ventriculocisternal perfusion that may require more than 1 hour for tracer equilibration or the manometric technique that requires multiple infusions.

REGULATION OF CSF DYNAMICS

Neurogenic Regulation

STRUCTURAL ASPECTS The choroid plexus is supplied by adrenergic, cholinergic, and peptidergic nerves. These nerve fibers form networks around the small arteries and veins of the plexus. The distal portions of these nerves are located between the choroid plexus endothelium and the underlying fenestrated capillaries.

Adrenergic nerve density is greatest in the third ventricle, intermediate in the lateral ventricles, and least in the fourth ventricle. For the most part, these adrenergic nerves originate in the superior cervical ganglia, although some fibers in the plexus of the fourth ventricle may arise from lower ganglia.[79,80] Innervation of the lateral ventricles is unilateral, whereas innervation of the midline ventricles is bilateral. The plexus of the third ventricle is richly supplied by cholinergic nerves, whereas the fourth ventricle is almost devoid of cholinergic innervation.[81] The origin of the cholinergic nerve supply to the choroid plexus is uncertain. The density of peptidergic nerves is less than that of adrenergic and cholinergic nerves.[82,83] Some peptidergic nerves contain vasoactive intestinal peptide, a potent dilator of cerebral vessels. Others contain substance P, also a cerebral vasdilator.

FUNCTIONAL ASPECTS The adrenergic system appears to play a role in regulating choroid plexus blood flow. Norepinephrine, phenylephrine, and isoproterenol, in that order of potency, produced weak contractions of isolated anterior choroidal arteries.[84] The α-adrenergic receptor nature of this response was supported on the basis of inhibition of contraction by phentolamine. In vessels in which active tone was first induced by prostaglandin F2α, it was reported that isoproterenol, norepinephrine, epinephrine, and terbutaline, in that order of potency, produced relaxation. The β-adrenergic receptor nature of this response was supported on the basis of inhibition of relaxation by propranolol. The adrenergic system also appears to exert a functional influence on choroid epithelial cells. Sympathectomy achieved by surgical removal of the superior cervical ganglion or injection of reserpine increased carbonic anhydrase activity by 125 to 150% in plexus homogenate.[85] In another study, sympathetic denervation altered epithelial cell transport of organic acids and bases in isolated choroid plexuses.[86]

In addition, the adrenergic system is reported to alter $\dot{V}_f$. Intermittent electrical stimulation of the cervical sympathetic trunks was reported to reduce $\dot{V}_f$ by 32%.[80,87,88] Bilateral excision of the superior cervical ganglia resulted in a 33% increase in $\dot{V}_f$.[89] Intraventricular perfusion with norepinephrine at low concentrations caused a small reduction in $\dot{V}_f$, whereas higher concentrations reduced $\dot{V}_f$ by about 35%.[88] Intraventricular perfusion with phentolamine, propranolol, or intravenous infusion of phentolamine reversed the effect of norepinephrine. In contrast, intravenous infusion of propranolol potentiated the reduction of $\dot{V}_f$. It was suggested that the norepinephrine-induced reduction of $\dot{V}_f$ seen at low concentrations represents a β-adrenoreceptor-mediated effect on the secretory epithelium, whereas the reduction at high concentrations represents α-adrenoreceptor-mediated choroid vasoconstriction. In additional studies, intraventricular perfusion with a β_1-adrenoreceptor-stimulator decreased CSF formation rate, whereas intraventricular perfusion with a β_2-adrenoreceptor stimulator or intravenous infusion with either a β_1 or β_2 stimulator had little or no effect. Thus, the β-adrenoreceptor-induced decrease of $\dot{V}_f$ appears to derive from a direct, inhibitory action on the choroid epithelium via β_1-adrenoreceptors.

The cholinergic system also is reported to alter $\dot{V}_f$. Intraventricular perfusion with carbacholine or with acetylcholine in the presence of the cholinesterase inhibitor neostigmine reduced $\dot{V}_f$ by 25 to 55%.[90] Cholinergic receptors appear to be muscarinic in type because the effect of carbachol is blocked by atropine but is not altered by hexamethonium. The site of action of cholinergic agonists or antagonists is uncertain. It is believed that they act on the choroid epithelium rather than on the choroid vasculature because carbacholine has no vasomotor effect on isolated anterior choroidal arteries.[91]

Pharmacologic Alteration of CSF Dynamics

DIURETICS Diuretics have long been known to decrease $\dot{V}_f$. Acetazolamide reduces $\dot{V}_f$ by up to 50%.[92,93] Acetazolamide inhibits carbonic anhydrase, the enzyme that catalyzes the hydration of intracellular carbon dioxide. One view is that acetazolamide reduces $\dot{V}_f$ by decreasing the amount of hydrogen ions available for exchange with sodium on the abluminal border of the epithelial cell.[94] Another view is that acetazolamide exerts an indirect action on ion transport mediated by an effect on bicarbonate.[95] Yet another view is that acetazolamide causes constriction of choroid plexus arterioles, reducing choroid plexus blood flow.[96] Methazolamide, another carbonic anhydrase inhibitor, is reported to reduce $\dot{V}_f$ by up to 50%.[97] The reduction of $\dot{V}_f$ caused by carbonic anhydrase inhibitors is additive with that produced by drugs that work by other mechanisms. For example, the combination of acetazolamide and ouabain is reported to cause a 95% reduction of $\dot{V}_f$.[98]

Ethacrynic acid decreases $\dot{V}_f$, presumably by inhibiting the exchange of sodium into epithelial cells and potassium or hydrogen ions out of the cells at the abluminal border of the cell.[98] Spironolactone and amiloride decrease $\dot{V}_f$, probably by impairing the entry of sodium into cells at the abluminal transport site.[99] Furosemide decreases $\dot{V}_f$ either by reducing chloride transport (which is linked to sodium transport on the abluminal surface but follows the electrochemical gradient on the luminal surface)[100] or sodium transport.[101] Mannitol decreases $\dot{V}_f$, with the decrease resulting from both a reduction in choroid plexus output and a reduction of interstitial fluid flow from cerebral tissue to the macroscopic CSF compartment.[102] The effects of mannitol are dose related. A dose of 0.75 g/kg increased R_a and did not significantly change $\dot{V}_f$, whereas a dose of 2.0 g/kg decreased $\dot{V}_f$ (by about 50%) and did not significantly change R_a.[103]

STEROIDS A variety of steroids are reported to alter R_a and $\dot{V}_f$. Whereas R_a was increased due to pneumococcal meningitis, methylprednisolone was reported to reduce R_a to a value that was intermediate between control and untreated animals.[104] It was speculated that methylprednisolone improved CSF flow in the supracortical subarachnoid space and/or arachnoid villi. Where R_a was increased due to pseudotumor cerebri, prednisone was reported to reduce R_a to a value that was intermediate between pretreatment and normal values for patients.[105] Improved reabsorption of CSF was felt to be due, in part, to reversal of either impaired transport across arachnoid epithelial cells or metabolically induced changes in the structure of the villi. Cortisone was reported to decrease $\dot{V}_f$.[106] Because radioactive-labeled hydrocortisone is rapidly taken up in the choroid plexus, it is believed that cortisone exerts its action at the plexus rather than at extrachoroidal sites.[107] Dexamethosone decreases $\dot{V}_f$ by up to 50%.[108,109] presumably by inhibition of sodium-potassium-ATPase, which impedes the action of the sodium-potassium pump at the choroid epithelial membrane.

ANESTHETICS Anesthetics also influence many aspects of CSF dynamics (Tables 2.2 to 2.4). Early studies reported that enflurane (1

TABLE 2.2 *Effects of inhaled anesthetics on CSF dynamics*

	$\dot{V}_f$	R_a	PREDICTED EFFECT ON ICP
Desflurane	0, +[a]	0	0, +[a]
Enflurane			
Low concentration	0	+	+
High concentration	+	0	+
Halothane	−	+	+
Isoflurane			
Low concentration	0	0, +[b]	0, +[b]
High concentration	0	−	−
Nitrous oxide	0	0	0
Sevoflurane	−	+	?

Abbreviations: CSF, cerebrospinal fluid; V_f, rate of CSF formation; R_a, resistance to reabsorption of CSF; ICP, intracranial pressure; +, increase; 0, no change; −, decrease; ?, uncertain.

[a] Effect occurs only during hypocapnia combined with increased CSF pressure.

[b] Effect dependent on dose.

MAC) increases $\dot{V}_f$ by 50 to 80% upon initial exposure.[110,111] $\dot{V}_f$ gradually returns to normal over a period of several hours. Enflurane also increases R_a.[111,112] This effect does not reverse when administration of enflurane is continued for several hours. Enflurane produced these alterations of CSF dynamics when administered with either nitrogen (60 to 70%) or nitrous oxide (60 to 70%) in oxygen. More recent studies with enflurane reported that its effects on $\dot{V}_f$ and R_a are dose related. High concentrations of enflurane (2.6 and 3.5% end-expired) increased $\dot{V}_f$ (by about 40% when corrected for the effects of time), whereas low concentrations (0.9 and 1.8%) did not.[113] Conversely, low concentrations increased R_a, but high concentrations did not. Halothane (1 MAC) generally is reported to decrease $\dot{V}_f$[114–116] and increase R_a.[114,117] In a "closed" cranium model, it was concluded that the expansion of CSF volume caused by halothane-induced increase of R_a was greater than the contraction of CSF volume caused by halothane-induced decrease of $\dot{V}_f$.[118] In addition, halothane enhances transport of glucose into brain[119] and movement of albumin, immunoglobulin (IgG),[120,121] and sodium, chloride, and water into CSF.[122,123] Nitrous oxide (66%) is reported to produce no change in R_a or $\dot{V}_f$[124,125] and to decrease brain glucose influx and efflux.[126] Early studies reported that isoflurane (1 MAC) decreases R_a and causes no change in $\dot{V}_f$.[112,127] More recent studies with isoflurane reported that its effects on R_a are dose related. R_a

TABLE 2.3 *Effects of sedative-hypnotics and other intravenous drugs on CSF dynamics*

	$\dot{V}_f$	R_a	PREDICTED EFFECT ON ICP
Etomidate			
Low dose	0	0	0
High dose	−	0, −[a]	−
Flumazenil			
Low dose	0	0	0
High dose	0	−	−
Ketamine	0	+	+
Midazolam[b]			
Low dose	0	+, 0[a]	+, 0[a]
High dose	−	0, +[a]	−, ?[a]
Pentobarbital	0	0	0
Propofol	0	0	0
Thiopental			
Low dose	0	+, 0[a]	+, 0[a]
High dose	−	0, −[a]	−

Abbreviations: CSF, cerebrospinal fluid; V_f, rate of CSF formation; R_a, resistance to reabsorption of CSF; ICP, intracranial pressure; +, increase; 0, no change; −, decrease; ?, uncertain.

[a] Effect dependent on dose.

[b] Partial reversal with flumazenil causes CSF dynamics similar to lowest dose of midazolam; complete reversal with flumazenil causes CSF dynamics similar to premidazolam (control) values.

TABLE 2.4 *Effects of opioids and local anesthetics on CSF dynamics*

	$\dot{V}_f$	R_a	PREDICTED EFFECT ON ICP
Alfentanil			
Low dose	0	−	−
High dose	0	0	0
Fentanyl			
Low dose	0	−	−
High dose	−	0, +	−,?
Lidocaine			
Low dose	0	0	0
High dose	−	0	−
Sufentanil			
Low dose	0	−	−
High dose	0	+,0	+,0

Abbreviations: CSF, cerebrospinal fluid; V_f, rate of CSF formation; R_a, resistance to reabsorption of CSF; ICP, intracranial pressure; +, increase; 0, no change; −, decrease; ?, uncertain.

was normal at 0.6% (end-expired) isoflurane, increased at 1.1%, and decreased at 1.7 and 2.2%.[113] At 2% (inspired) isoflurane, the BBB transfer coefficient for small hydrophilic molecules was decreased.[128] Sevoflurane (1 MAC) is reported to decrease $\dot{V}_f$ by about 40% and to increase R_a as compared with a comparison group of cats anesthetized with 50% nitrous oxide in oxygen.[129] Studies with desflurane reported that its effects on $\dot{V}_f$ are related to CSF pressure and P_aCO_2. At normocapnia and normal CSF pressure, normocapnia and increased CSF pressure, and hypocapnia and normal CSF pressure, both 0.5 and 1 MAC desflurane caused no change in $\dot{V}_f$ or R_a.[130] However, at hypocapnia and increased CSF pressure, both concentrations of desflurane increased $\dot{V}_f$.

Ketamine (40 mg.kg^{-1}.h^{-1}) increases R_a but does not alter $\dot{V}_f$.[111] In addition, ketamine (150 mg/kg) decreases the transport of small hydrophilic molecules across the BBB.[131] Low doses of etomidate (0.86 mg/kg followed by 0.86 or 1.72 mg.kg^{-1}.h^{-1}) do not alter R_a or $\dot{V}_f$, whereas high doses (2.58 or 3.44 mg.kg^{-1}.h^{-1}) decrease both R_a and $\dot{V}_f$.[132] Low doses of thiopental (6 mg/kg followed by 6 or 12 mg.kg^{-1}.h^{-1}) increase or do not alter R_a and do not alter $\dot{V}_f$, whereas high doses (18 or 24 mg.kg^{-1}.h^{-1}) decrease both R_a and $\dot{V}_f$.[132] Thiopental (100 μg/ml but not 25 or 50 μg/ml) but not methohexital (10 to 50 μg/ml) increases the permeability of brain microvascular endothelial cells to α-aminoisobutyric acid but not to sucrose or Evans blue albumin.[133] Propofol (6 mg/kg followed by 12, 24, and 48 mg.kg^{-1}.h^{-1}) and pentobarbital (40 mg/kg IP) produce no change in R_a or $\dot{V}_f$.[111,134] In addition, pentobarbital decreases transport of glucose,[135] amino acids,[136] and small hydrophilic molecules[131] into brain. Among the sedative-hypnotic drugs, the effects of midazolam appear to be the most variable. Low doses of midazolam (1.6 mg/kg followed by 0.5 mg.kg^{-1}.h^{-1}) increase R_a and do not alter $\dot{V}_f$, intermediate doses (1.0 to 1.5 mg.kg^{-1}.h^{-1}) cause no change, and high doses (2.0 mg.kg^{-1}.h^{-1}) increase R_a and decrease $\dot{V}_f$.[132] The benzodiazepine antagonist flumazenil caused no change in $\dot{V}_f$ when given to dogs receiving midazolam (1.6 mg/kg followed by 1.25 mg.kg^{-1}.h^{-1}) or dogs not receiving midazolam.[137] Low-dose flumazenil (0.0025 mg/kg) caused no change in R_a and high-dose flumazenil (0.16 mg/kg) decreased R_a. In dogs receiving midazolam, low-dose flumazenil increased R_a (perhaps due to partial reversal of midazolam so that CSF dynamics approximated those of low-dose midazolam), whereas after high-dose flumazenil, R_a returned to normal (that is, to values characteristic of dogs not receiving midazolam).

Early studies reported that fentanyl (3.0 μg.kg^{-1}.min^{-1} for 20 minutes followed by 0.2 μg.kg^{-1}.min^{-1}) decreases R_a[117] and does not alter $\dot{V}_f$.[115] More recent studies reported that the effects of opioids on $\dot{V}_f$ and R_a are dose related. High doses of fentanyl decreased $\dot{V}_f$, whereas low doses did not.[125] R_a was decreased at the two low doses, normal at one high dose, and increased at the highest dose. Fentanyl (25 to 100 ng/ml) causes no change in the permeability of brain microvascular endothelial cells to α-aminoisobutyric acid, sucrose, or Evans blue albumin.[133] All doses of sufentanil studied caused no change in $\dot{V}_f$.[125] R_a was decreased at the two low doses, increased at one high dose, and normal at the highest dose. In addition, sufentanil (0.5 μg/kg followed by 0.1 $\mu g.kg^{-1}.h^{-1}$) combined with thiopental (2 to 5 mg/kg followed by 1 to 4 $mg.kg^{-1}.h^{-1}$) caused no increased movement of albumin or IgG into CSF.[121] None of the doses of alfentanil studied caused a change in $\dot{V}_f$.[125] R_a was decreased at the two low doses and normal at the two high doses. High doses of lidocaine (4.5 mg/kg followed by 9.0 $\mu g.kg^{-1}.min^{-1}$) decrease $\dot{V}_f$ without changing R_a, whereas low doses of lidocaine (0.5 mg/kg followed by 1.0 $\mu g.kg^{-1}.min^{-1}$ or 1.5 mg/kg followed by 3.0 $\mu g.kg^{-1}.min^{-1}$) produce no change of $\dot{V}_f$ or R_a.[138]

The mechanism(s) by which inhalational and intravenous anesthetics alter CSF dynamics is uncertain. Increase of $\dot{V}_f$ with enflurane may result from an enflurane-induced increase of choroid plexus metabolism.[139] Decrease of $\dot{V}_f$ with halothane may result from halothane-induced stimulation of vasopressin receptors.[140]

OTHER DRUGS A number of other drugs are reported to alter $\dot{V}_f$ and R_a. Hypertonic (3%) saline in a low dose (100 mg/kg followed by 34 $mg.kg^{-1}.h^{-1}$) decreased $\dot{V}_f$ by 30% and increased R_a. In a high dose (300 mg/kg followed by 70 $mg.kg^{-1}.h^{-1}$) it decreased $\dot{V}_f$ by 30% and caused no significant change of R_a.[141] Vasopressin decreases $\dot{V}_f$. One view is that $\dot{V}_f$ decreases due to vasoconstriction of choroidal blood vessels.[99] However, others have argued that physiologic doses of vasopressin provide insufficient choroid vascular effect to explain the observed reduction of CSF formation.[142,143] Theophylline increases $\dot{V}_f$, presumably due to inhibition of phosphodiesterase, leading to elevation of choroid plexus cyclic adenosine 3′, 5′-monophosphate levels and stimulation of the choroid epithelial sodium-potassium pump.[143] Dinitrophenol decreases $\dot{V}_f$ probably as a result of its action to uncouple oxidation phosphorylation, thereby reducing the energy available for active secretory and transport processes such as the ATP-dependent sodium-potassium pumps.[17] Digoxin[98] and oubain[144] decrease $\dot{V}_f$ by inhibition of the sodium-potassium-ATPase of the choroid epithelial sodium-potassium pump.

In contrast to the aforementioned drugs, continuous infusion of succinylcholine, vecuronium, or adenosine (in a commercial preparation of 5.3 mg/ml solution in 5% mannitol) produced no change in $\dot{V}_f$ or R_a.[145,146]

Metabolic Regulation

Alterations in metabolism or physiologic status influence $\dot{V}_f$ and $\dot{V}_a$. Hypothermia decreases $\dot{V}_f$ probably by reducing the activity of active secretory and transport processes and by reducing cerebral blood flow.[1] $\dot{V}_f$ decreases by 11% with each 1°C reduction in temperature between 41°C and 31°C.[147] Hypercapnia increases $\dot{V}_f$ to normal values if it was decreased at normocapnia but does not change $\dot{V}_f$ if it was normal at normocapnia and does not change $\dot{V}_a$.[148] It was suggested that normalization of $\dot{V}_f$ by hypercapnia resulted from improved choroid plexus blood flow. Hypocapnia acutely decreases $\dot{V}_f$ either due to reduced choroid plexus blood flow or reduced hydrogen ion availability for exchange with sodium at the abluminal surface of the choroidal epithelial cells.[149] However, $\dot{V}_f$ is not different from normal after several hours of hypocapnia.[150,151] Although metabolic acidosis does not change $\dot{V}_f$, metabolic alkalosis decreases $\dot{V}_f$ presumably due to a pH effect unrelated to ion or substrate availability.[152]

Reduced osmolarity of ventricular CSF[153] or increased osmolarity of serum[154] decreases $\dot{V}_f$. Similarly, increased osmolarity of ventricular CSF or reduced osmolarity of serum increases $\dot{V}_f$.[153–155] The effect of change in serum osmolarity was four-fold greater than a comparable change in ventricular fluid osmolarity. It was suggested that the changes in $\dot{V}_f$ due to altered ventricular fluid osmolarity occurred at the choroid plexus, whereas the changes in formation rate due to altered serum osmolarity occurred at extrachoroid sites.

CSF DYNAMICS AND ICP

Equilibrium Between CSF Formation and Reabsorption

Providing that CPP is not reduced below approximately 70 mmHg, $\dot{V}_f$ is relatively constant over a wide range of ICPs. Thus, $\dot{V}_f$ remains normal whether ICP is 2 or 22 cm H_2O (Fig. 2.4). In contrast, $\dot{V}_a$ varies as ICP changes. At ICPs less than about 7 cm H_2O, minimal reabsorption occurs. At ICPs greater than 7 cm H_2O, $\dot{V}_a$ increases directly as ICP increases. This relationship is linear for ICPs up to about 30 cm H_2O. The ICP at which the plots of $\dot{V}_f$/ICP and $\dot{V}_a$/ICP intersect is the equilibrium pressure for the CSF system. At that pressure, $\dot{V}_f$ equals $\dot{V}_a$ and no net change in CSF volume occurs.

Anesthetic- and Drug-Induced Changes in ICP

Treatments that alter either $\dot{V}_f$, $\dot{V}_a$, or both will alter ICP. For example, theophylline is reported to increase $\dot{V}_f$.[143] If reabsorption characteristics are not affected, the plots of $\dot{V}_f$/ICP and $\dot{V}_a$/ICP following administration of theophylline are seen to intersect at an ICP value that is higher than normal (Fig. 2.5, top). Stated another way, following the administration of theophylline, $\dot{V}_f$ increases so that the volume of CSF formed each minute exceeds the volume reabsorbed each minute. A net increase of CSF volume occurs, causing ICP to increase. ICP continues to increase as CSF volume expands, and as ICP increases, it provides an increasingly greater "driving force" for reabsorption of CSF. Once ICP is sufficiently elevated, $\dot{V}_a$ will have been increased to equal $\dot{V}_f$. A new equilibrium state is achieved where formation and reabsorption are equal and no net change in CSF volume occurs. The net effect of these changes is that by increasing $\dot{V}_f$, theophylline should cause an increase of ICP providing other CSF dynamics are not altered.

Ketamine is reported to increase R_a.[111] R_a is defined as the inverse of the slope of the relationship between $\dot{V}_a$ and ICP. So, increased R_a translates to a flattening of the $\dot{V}_a$/ICP regression line. If $\dot{V}_f$ is not affected, the plots of $\dot{V}_f$/ICP and $\dot{V}_a$/ICP following administration of ketamine are seen to intersect at an ICP that is higher than normal (Fig. 2.5, bottom). Stated another way, following administration of ketamine, $\dot{V}_a$ is reduced because normal ICP does not provide sufficient driving force to cause usual amounts of CSF to be reabsorbed now that R_a has increased.

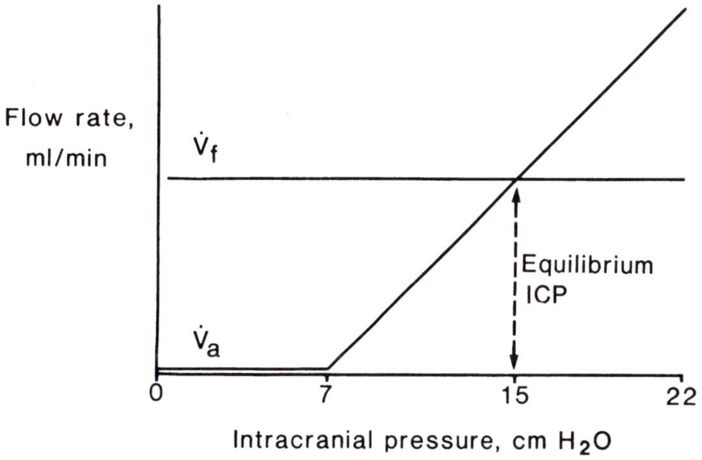

FIGURE 2.4 *The rate of CSF formation ($\dot{V}_f$) and rate of reabsorption of CSF ($\dot{V}_a$) are plotted as a function of ICP. So long as CPP remains above ~70 mm Hg, $\dot{V}_f$ is unaffected by ICP. At ICP <7 cm H2O, $\dot{V}_a$ is minimal. At 7 cm H_2O < ICP < 25–30 cm H_2O, resistance to reabsorption of CSF (R_a) is relatively constant and $\dot{V}_a$ is linearly related to ICP. ICP stabilizes at a value where $\dot{V}_f$ equals $\dot{V}_a$.*

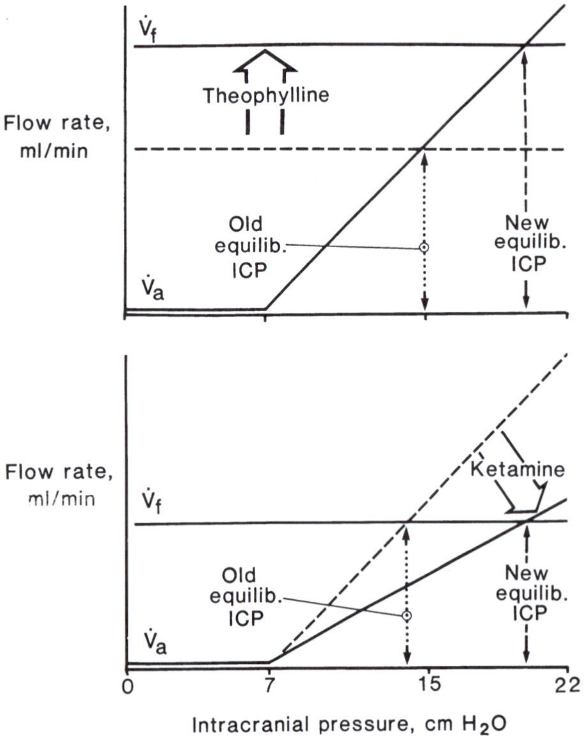

FIGURE 2.5 *Theophylline increases $\dot{V}_f$ ("elevating" the $\dot{V}_f$/ICP slope) (A) and ketamine increases R_a ("flattening" the $\dot{V}_a$/ICP slope) (B). With both treatments $\dot{V}_f$ equals $\dot{V}_a$ at increased ICP.*

As a result, the volume of CSF formed each minute exceeds the volume reabsorbed each minute. A net increase of CSF volume occurs, causing ICP to increase. ICP continues to increase as CSF volume expands, and as ICP increases, it provides a progressively greater driving force for reabsorption of CSF. Once ICP is sufficiently increased, $\dot{V}_a$ will have been increased to equal $\dot{V}_f$. A new equilibrium state is achieved where formation and reabsorption are equal and no net change in CSF volume occurs. The net effect of these changes is that by increasing R_a ketamine should cause an increase of ICP, providing other CSF dynamics are not altered.

Furosemide is an example of a treatment with the opposite effect on ICP. Furosemide decreases $\dot{V}_f$, lowering the $\dot{V}_f$/ICP regression line (Fig. 2.6, top).[100] Initially, normal $\dot{V}_a$ exceeds reduced $\dot{V}_f$, resulting in a contraction of CSF volume and reduction of ICP. ICP continues to decrease providing a lesser driving force for reabsorption of CSF. Once ICP has decreased enough, $\dot{V}_a$ is lowered to the point where it matches the reduced $\dot{V}_f$, and a new equilibrium between formation and reabsorption is achieved at that reduced ICP. Low doses of fentanyl decrease R_a, resulting in a steeper $\dot{V}_a$/ICP regression line (Fig. 2.6, bottom).[125] Initially, enhanced $\dot{V}_a$ exceeds normal $\dot{V}_f$, resulting in a contraction of CSF volume and reduction of ICP. ICP continues to decrease, providing a lesser driving force for reabsorption of CSF. Once ICP has decreased enough, $\dot{V}_a$ is lowered to the point where it matches normal $\dot{V}_f$, and a new equilibrium between formation and reabsorption is achieved at that reduced ICP. High doses

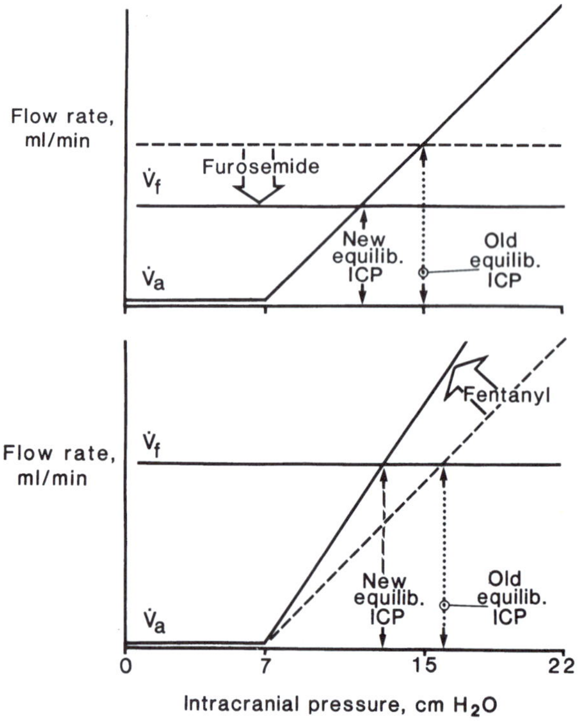

FIGURE 2.6 *Furosemide decreases $\dot{V}_f$ ("lowering" the $\dot{V}_f$/ICP slope), and fentanyl in low doses decreases R_a (steepening the $\dot{V}_a$/ICP slope). With both treatments, $\dot{V}_f$ equals $\dot{V}_a$ at decreased ICP.*

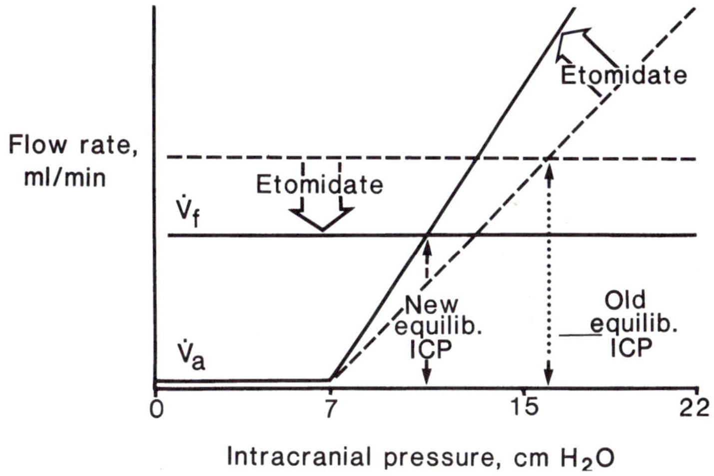

FIGURE 2.7 *Etomidate in high doses decreases both $\dot{V}_f$ ("lowering" the $\dot{V}_f$/ICP slope) and R_a ("steepening" the $\dot{V}_a$/ICP slope). As a result $\dot{V}_f$ equals $\dot{V}_a$ at decreased ICP.*

of etomidate reduce ICP by combined effects on $\dot{V}_f$ and R_a.[132] Etomidate decreases both so that the $\dot{V}_f$/ICP regression line is lowered and the $\dot{V}_a$/ICP regression line becomes steeper (Fig. 2.7). CSF volume contracts, because initially, enhanced $\dot{V}_a$ exceeds reduced $\dot{V}_f$. ICP decreases to a low value, because when R_a is reduced, only a small ICP is needed to provide a driving force for reabsorption of CSF.

CSF Volume Change to Compensate for Intracranial Volume Change

When intracranial volume increases, CSF volume contracts by translocation of intracranial CSF to the spinal subarachnoid space and by reabsorption of CSF. Conversely, when intracranial volume decreases, CSF volume expands by cephalad translocation and a temporary decrease in $\dot{V}_a$. These changes in CSF volume are easily illustrated using the $\dot{V}_f$/ICP and $\dot{V}_a$/ICP relationships as discussed above. For example, subdural hematoma adds volume to the intracranial contents, thereby increasing ICP (Fig. 2.8, top). Increased ICP (*A*) provides a driving force for reabsorption of CSF at a rate (*B*) in excess of $\dot{V}_f$ (which does not change). Consequently, the volume of CSF reabsorbed each minute exceeds the volume of CSF formed each minute. Gradually, CSF volume contracts. As it does, total intracranial volume decreases, and ICP decreases (*C*) from its increased level. As ICP approaches normal, the impetus for reabsorption of CSF at a rate in excess of $\dot{V}_f$ becomes progressively reduced. When ICP returns to prehematoma values, $\dot{V}_f$ and $\dot{V}_a$ once again are in equilibrium, and no further change of CSF volume or ICP occurs. The net result of these changes is that ICP and total intracranial volume are much the same as prior to the subdural hematoma, but cerebral blood volume (CBV) (part of it in the form of the hematoma) is increased and CSF volume is decreased.

Conversely, surgical removal of brain tissue reduces intracranial volume, thereby decreasing ICP (Fig. 2.8, bottom). Reduced ICP (*D*) provides only a weak driving force for reabsorption of CSF so that $\dot{V}_a$ (*E*) is less than $\dot{V}_f$ (which does not change). Consequently, the volume of CSF reabsorbed each minute is less than the volume formed each minute. Gradually, CSF volume expands. As it does, total intracranial volume increases and ICP increases (*F*) from its reduced level. As ICP approaches normal, the impetus for reabsorption of CSF progressively increases. When intracranial pressure reaches presurgical values, $\dot{V}_f$ and $\dot{V}_a$ once again are in equilibrium, and no further change of CSF volume or ICP occurs. The net result of these changes is that ICP and total intracranial volume is much the same

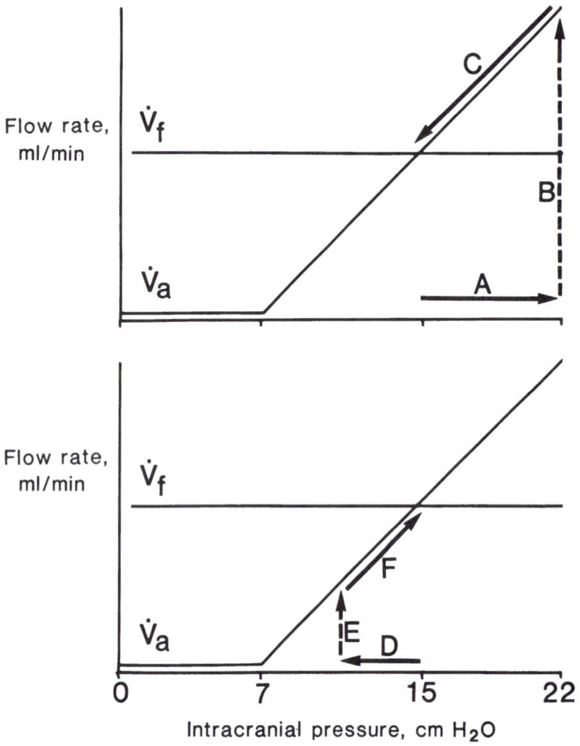

FIGURE 2.8 *The plots of $\dot{V}_f$/ICP and $\dot{V}_a$/ICP show how CSF volume changes to offset changes in intracranial volume, thereby minimizing ICP changes. In the top diagram, increase of intracranial volume increases ICP (A). At increased ICP, $\dot{V}_a$ (B) exceeds $\dot{V}_f$, so CSF volume decreases. As CSF volume decreases, ICP decreases (C) until $\dot{V}_f$ equals $\dot{V}_a$. If $\dot{V}_f$ and R_a are not altered, ICP returns to normal. In the bottom diagram, decrease of intracranial volume decreases ICP (D). At decreased ICP, $\dot{V}_a$ (E) is less than $\dot{V}_f$, so CSF volume increases. As CSF volume increases, ICP increases (F) until $\dot{V}_f$ equals $\dot{V}_a$. If $\dot{V}_f$ and R_a are not altered, ICP returns to normal.*

as prior to surgical removal of brain tissue, but brain tissue volume is decreased and CSF volume is increased.

In the same way that drugs and treatments that alter $\dot{V}_f$ and/or $\dot{V}_a$ will alter ICP, they will also alter the expansion or contraction of CSF volume in response to a change of intracranial volume. Thus, hypercapnia, which may increase $\dot{V}_f$, or low doses of thiopental, which may increase R_a, will oppose the contraction of CSF volume that occurs in response to a subdural hematoma. Mannitol, which decreases $\dot{V}_f$, will enhance the contraction of CSF volume. Conversely, acetazolamide, which also decreases $\dot{V}_f$, will oppose the expansion of CSF volume that occurs following surgical removal of brain tissue.

Limits to Linear Modelling of CSF Dynamics

Although these linear models of CSF dynamics offer a convenient way to understand the equilibrium between $\dot{V}_f$ and $\dot{V}_a$, CSF volume contraction and expansion, and the manner in which drugs and treatments affect these aspects of CSF physiology, they are not accurate predictors of ICP in all circumstances. There are several reasons for this. One reason is that concurrent treatments or conditions may themselves alter CSF dynamics. For example, in dogs it was reported that inflation of an intracranial epidural balloon increased R_a.[156] Thus, in the example of the epidural hematoma given above, increased R_a caused by the hematoma may prohibit adequate CSF volume contraction, and ICP may, therefore, not be restored to prehematoma levels.

Another reason that these linear models may not accurately predict ICP is that treatments or conditions may have a certain effect on $\dot{V}_f$ and/or $\dot{V}_a$ when these latter values are normal but have a quite different effect when these values are not normal. As an illustration, as noted above, hypercapnia had no effect on $\dot{V}_f$ when $\dot{V}_f$ was normal prior to hypercapnia but increased $\dot{V}_f$ when $\dot{V}_f$ was low prior to hypercapnia.[148]

A third reason that these linear models of CSF dynamics may not accurately predict ICP is that when ICP is substantially increased, the relationship between ICP and both $\dot{V}_f$ and $\dot{V}_a$ changes. $\dot{V}_f$, which is constant and independent of ICP when ICP is low, becomes inversely related to ICP when ICP becomes high enough to reduce CPP below approximately 70 mmHg. The ICP value at which CPP falls below approximately 70 mmHg depends, of course, on mean

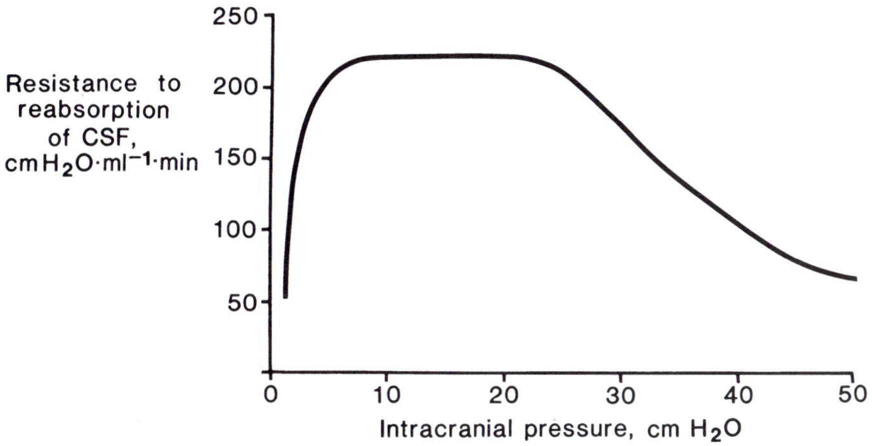

FIGURE 2.9 *Resistance to reabsorption of CSF (R_a) is plotted as a function of ICP. R_a is relatively constant at normal ICP but decreases as ICP increases above 25 to 30 cm H_2O. As a result, the $\dot{V}_a$/ICP slope no longer is linear but assumes more of the characteristics of an exponential curve.*

arterial blood pressure (MAP). R_a, which is constant and independent of MAP and ICP when ICP is low, decreases as ICP increases above 25 to 30 cm H_2O (Fig. 2.9).[157] This decrease in R_a corresponds with formation of macropinocytotic vesicles and transcellular channels across the arachnoid villus endothelium as well as pressure-facilitated diffusion of CSF through (1) occasional open interendothelial clefts and (2) transient opening of closed intercellular spaces that, at resting ICP, are functionally occluded by tight junctions. As a result, the slope of the $\dot{V}_a$/ICP regression line increases severalfold at intracranial pressures of 25 to 50 cm H_2O.

CONDITIONS WHERE ALTERED CSF DYNAMICS CHANGE ICP

Responses to Increased ICP

Recent work in animal models and in clinical studies demonstrates how $\dot{V}_f$ and R_a affect CSF volume and contribute to ICP change in clinically relevant ways.

INTRACRANIAL MASS One such animal study examined $\dot{V}_f$, R_a, CSF volume, CBV, and brain tissue composition in dogs.[156] Three groups were examined during administration of low concentrations of halothane in nitrous oxide (66%). Group 1 was examined during hypocapnia (P_aCO_2 20 mmHg), with no intracranial mass being present. Group 2 was examined with an intracranial mass present (epidural balloon, ICP 35 cm H_2O), but no hypocapnia. In group 3 an intracranial mass was present, and hypocapnia was used to lower ICP.

In group 1, hypocapnia initially reduced CBV from 3.4 to 2.4 ml. With continued hypocapnia, CBV reexpanded to 3.4 ml by 4 hours. $\dot{V}_f$ and R_a were not changed, allowing CSF volume to change reciprocally with CBV. As a result, ICP remained constant. In group 2, the intracranial mass reduced CBV to 2.7 ml. During 4 hours normocapnia CBV remained steady. $\dot{V}_f$ was not changed, but R_a increased. Consequently, CSF volume fell only slightly and ICP remained elevated. In group 3, the intracranial mass reduced CBV to 2.8 ml. Subsequent hypocapnia initially reduced CBV from 2.8 to 2.2 ml, and ICP decreased from 35 to 19 cm H_2O. With continued hypocapnia, CBV reexpanded to 2.8 ml by 4 hours. $\dot{V}_f$ was unchanged, and R_a was intermediate between normal and the increased value seen in group 2. As a result, CSF volume decreased from 6.1 to 5.0 ml, and ICP remained below the level initially produced by inflation of the intracranial epidural balloon. Net intracranial reabsorption of CSF did not exceed net intracranial CSF formation, suggesting that CSF volume decreased in group 3 because hypocapnia improved access of intracranial CSF to spinal sites of CSF reabsorption. Brain tissue composition was not different between groups. These results indicate that hypocapnia decreases an increased ICP initially by decreasing CBV. This ICP-lowering effect is sustained (despite reexpansion of CBV) by a further reduction of CSF volume.

EFFECTS OF ANESTHETICS Laboratory studies also demonstrate how anesthetics alter $\dot{V}_f$ and R_a and how these alterations of CSF dynamics affect CSF volume and ICP in clinically relevant ways.[122] Studied along with the above three groups were dogs anesthetized with inhalational or intravenous agents while an intracranial mass was present, and hypocapnia was used to decrease ICP. With enflurane anesthesia, hypocapnia initially reduced CBV from 2.8 to 2.2 ml, and ICP decreased from 33 to 19 cm H_2O. With continued hypocapnia, CBV reexpanded to 2.5 ml. $\dot{V}_f$ and R_a were high so that CSF volume did not contract as CBV reexpanded. Instead, CSF volume also expanded (to 6.3 ml). As a result, ICP did not remain at the low value initially achieved with hypocapnia, but increased to 43 cm H_2O. The intracranial volume increase that occurred during the 4-hour hypocapnia and enflurane anesthesia was comprised chiefly of CSF. With halothane anesthesia, hypocapnia initially reduced CBV from 2.8 to 2.3 ml, and ICP decreased from 34 to 17 cm H_2O. With continued hypocapnia, CBV reexpanded to 3.3 ml. $\dot{V}_f$ was low and R_a was high so that the magnitude of CSF volume contraction was less than the magnitude of CBV expansion. As a result, ICP did not remain at the low value initially achieved with hypocapnia but increased to 50 cm H_2O. When isoflurane, fentanyl, or thiopental were used for anesthesia, hypocapnia initially reduced CBV from 2.7–2.8 ml to 2.2 ml, and ICP decreased from 33–35 cm H_2O to 18 cm H_2O. With continued hypocapnia, CBV reexpanded (not significant with fentanyl) by 4 hours. $\dot{V}_f$ was normal, and R_a was similar to that during 4 hours of hypocapnia in dogs with an intracranial mass that were anesthetized with low concentrations of halothane in nitrous oxide (66%), so that CSF volume contracted as CBV expanded. As a result, ICP remained at the low value initially achieved with hypocapnia. These results indicate that anesthetics modify the ICP response to 4 hours of hypocapnia when hypocapnia is used to lower increased ICP. Anesthetics exert their effects both by altering the pattern of CBV reexpansion and by altering the magnitude of CSF volume contraction as CBV reexpands. The effect of anesthetics on CSF volume contraction results from the influence of anesthetics on $\dot{V}_f$ and/or R_a.

Causes for Increased ICP

Recent laboratory and clinical studies demonstrate the role of altered $\dot{V}_f$ and/or R_a in clinical conditions where ICP is increased.

ACUTE SUBARACHNOID HEMORRHAGE Acute subarachnoid hemorrhage frequently is accompanied by increased ICP. To examine the effect of blood components on $\dot{V}_f$ and $\dot{V}_a$ and to determine the effect of these CSF dynamics on ICP, animals were given intrathecally (1) heparinized whole blood, (2) plasma, (3) dialysate of plasma, (4) serum (fibrinogen free), and (5) saline.[75,158] CSF dynamics were determined by manometic infusion, and brain tissue was sampled for examination. Whole blood and plasma were found to increase ICP and to produce a 3- to 10-fold increase in R_a. Electron microscopic examination showed a marked reduction in the number of transendothelial channels within the arachnoid villi endothelium and fibrin deposits within the arachnoid villi.

CHRONIC CHANGES AFTER SUBARACHNOID HEMORRHAGE Hydrocephalus frequently follows subarachnoid hemorrhage. Scanning electron microscopic studies of the CSF pathways and arachnoid villi of both animals and human specimens examined at various time intervals after subarachnoid hemorrhage show most clearly the extensive fibrosis resulting from blood within these spaces.[159–161] On the basis of these observations, chronic obstruction to CSF outflow after subarachnoid hemorrhage as well as other clinical conditions in which leptomeningeal scarring exists appear to be directly related to functional narrowing or blockage of CSF outflow pathways.[153] By this mechanism, R_a is increased within both the subarachnoid space and the arachnoid villi.

BACTERIAL MENINGITIS Bacterial meningitis frequently is accompanied by increased ICP. To examine the effect of meningitis on $\dot{V}_f$, $\dot{V}_a$, and ICP on animals were given intrathecally (1) *Streptococci pneumoniae* or (2) *Escherichia coli.*[104] CSF dynamics were determined before innoculation, 16 to 24 hours after innoculation, and after therapy. ICP was increased in both groups, and R_a was increased 25-fold with *Streptococci pneumoniae* and 36-fold with *E-scherichia coli.* Antibiotic therapy sterilized the CSF and prevented mortality, but at 2 weeks posttreatment, R_a still was elevated. Addition of methylprednisolone reduced R_a to a value that was intermediate between control and infected animals.

PSEUDOTUMOR CEREBRI It has been speculated that the increased ICP seen in pseudotumor cerebri results from either (1) increased R_a, (2) increased $\dot{V}_f$, (3) increased water movement into brain across cerebral capillaries, (4) increased CBF and CBV, or (5) glial and/or neuronal cellular edema.[105] At present, the bulk of evidence favors altered CSF dynamics as the primary mechanism leading to increased ICP.[162] Recent manometric studies have examined CSF dynamics in both control patients and patients with pseudotumor cerebri.[163] Resting ICP was 33 cm H_2O in patients with P. *cerebri* and 14 cm H_2O in controls. Maximal R_a was increased 10-fold in the *P. cerebri* patients, whereas R_a at resting ICP was sixfold greater than in controls. $\dot{V}_f$ was decreased 39% in the *P. cerebri* patients compared to controls. These results support the view that impaired CSF reabsorption is a principle mechanism leading to increased ICP in these patients and are comparable to results previously reported by others.[164,165] Treatment with prednisone reduced R_a to a value that was intermediate between controls and untreated patients with *P. cerebri.*

HEAD INJURY Head injury frequently results in increased ICP. In a recent study, the PVI was used to determine CSF dynamics and their contribution to increased ICP in patients with head injuries.[166] It was found that R_a was increased, but $\dot{V}_f$ was within normal limits for 75% of the patients studied. The percentage of ICP increase attributable to CSF dynamics was about 20% as calculated by the product of $\dot{V}_f$ and R_a.

CONCLUSION

CSF dynamics are regulated by neurogenic, pharmacologic, and metabolic factors. CSF dynamics are intimately involved in a multitude of processes including neuroendocrine function, regulation of the neuronal milieu, and clearance of brain tissue water and pathologic substances. The importance of these aspects of CSF dynamics to neurologic outcome and the possibilities for meaningful therapeutic intervention remain largely unknown.

In contrast, our knowledge of the effects of anesthetics on CSF dynamics has grown tremendously over the last 15 years. Some of these recent investigations provide examples of how anesthetic-induced changes in CSF dynamics may be clinically relevant. The graphs of $\dot{V}_f$ vs. ICP and $\dot{V}_a$ vs. ICP are convenient ways to illustrate the roles of $\dot{V}_f$ and R_a in ICP regulation and how anesthetics alter $\dot{V}_f$ and R_a. Because this field of research is relatively new, a great number of questions remain unanswered. It is hoped that these questions will stimulate further research in this area and that such research will lead to improved care of patients with neurologic disease who require anesthesia for surgery.

References

1. Davson H: Physiology of Cerebrospinal Fluid. Churchill, London, 1967
2. Milhorat TH: Pediatric neurosurgery. p. 91. In Plum F, McDowell FH (eds): Contemporary Neurology Series. Vol. 16. FA Davis, Philadelphia, 1978
3. Feder N, Reese TS, Brightman MW: Microperoxidase, a new tracer of low molecular weight: a study of the interstitial compartments of the mouse brain. J Cell Biol 43:35A, 1969
4. Bradbury MWB: Lymphatic and the central nervous system. Trends Neurosci 4:100, 1981
5. Cserr HF, Cooper DM, Milhorat TJ: Flow of cerebral interstitial fluid as indicated by the removal of extracellular markers from rat caudate nucleus. Exp Eye Res, suppl. 25:461, 1977
6. Cserr HF, Cooper DM, Suri PK, Patlak CS: Efflux of radiolabeled polyethylene glycols and albumin from rat brain. Am J Physiol 240:F319, 1981
7. Brierley JB, Field EJ: The connexions of the spinal subarachnoid space with the lymphatic systems. J Anat 82:153, 1948
8. Maren TH: Ion secretion into cerebrospinal fluid. Exp Eye Res, suppl. 25:157, 1977
9. Weed LH: Studies on cerebrospinal fluid. III. The pathways of escape from the subarachnoid spaces with particular reference to the arachnoid villi. J Med Res 31:51, 1914
10. Franklin GM, Dudzinski DS, Cutler RWP: Amino acid transport into the cerebrospinal fluid of the rat. J Neurochem 24:367, 1975
11. Edvinsson L, Hakanson M, Lindvall M et al: Ultrastructural and biochemical evidence for a sympathetic neural influence on the choroid plexus. Exp Neurol 48:241, 1975
12. Milhorat TH: The third circulation revisited. J Neurosurg 42:628, 1975
13. Cserr HF: Physiology of the choroid plexus. Physiol Rev 51:273, 1971
14. Livingstone RB: Cerebrospinal fluid. p. 950. In Fulton JF (ed): A Textbook of Physiology. WB Saunders, Philadelphia, 1955
15. Leusen I: Regulation of cerebrospinal fluid composition with reference to breathing. Physiol Rev 52:1, 1972
16. Gross PM, Weindl A: Peering through the windows of the brain. J Cereb Blood Flow Metabol 7:663, 1987
17. Artru AA: Cerebrospinal fluid. p. 93. In Cottrell JE, Smith DS (eds): Anesthesia and Neurosurgery. CV Mosby, St. Louis, 1994
18. Adkison KDK, Artru AA, Powers KM, Shen DD: Contribution of probenecid-sensitive anion transport processes at the brain capillary endothelium and choroid plexus to the efficient efflux of valproic acid from the central nervous system. J Pharmacol Exp Ther 268:797, 1994
19. Adkison KDK, Artru AA, Powers KM et al: Role of choroid plexus epithelium in the removal of valproic acid from the central nervous system. Epilepsy Res 20:185, 1995
20. Milhorat TH: Hydrocephalus and the Cerebrospinal Fluid. Williams & Wilkins, Baltimore, 1972
21. Pollay M, Curl F: Secretion of cerebrospinal fluid by the ventricular ependyma of the rabbit. Am J Physiol 213:1031, 1967
22. Sahar A: Choroidal origin of cerebrospinal fluid. Isr J Med Sci 8:594, 1972
23. Sato O, Bering EA: Extra-ventricular formation of cerebrospinal fluid. Brain Nerve 19:883, 1967
24. Brightman MW, Reese TS, Feder N: Assessment with the electron microscope of the permeability to peroxidase of cerebral endothelium and epithelium in mice and sharks. p. 468. In Crone C, Lassen NA (eds): Capillary Permeability. Academic Press, New York, 1970
25. Milhorat TH, Davis DA, Hammock MK: Localization of ouabain-sensitive N^a-K-ATPase in frog, rabbit, and rat choroid plexus. Brain Res 99:170, 1975
26. Wright EM: Mechanisms of ion transport across the choroid plexus. J Physiol (Lond) 226:545, 1972
27. Becker NH, Sutton CH: Histochemistry of the choroid plexus. p. 67. In Netsky MB, Shuangshoti S (eds): The Choroid Plexus in Health and Disease. University of Virginia Press, Charlottesville, 1975
28. Davis DA, Milhorat TH: The blood-brain barrier of the rat choroid plexus. Anat Rec 181:779, 1975
29. Rapoport SI: Blood-Brain Barrier in Physiology and Medicine. Raven Press, New York, 1976
30. Katzman R, Pappius HM: Brain Electrolytes and Fluid Metabolism. Williams & Wilkins, Baltimore, 1973
31. Pappenheimer JR: On the location of the blood-barrier. p. 66. In Proceedings of the Wales Symposium on the Blood-Brain Barrier. Oxford University Press, London, 1970
32. Hamberger A, Blomstrand C, Lehninger AL:

Comparative studies on mitochondria isolated from neuron-enriched and glia-enriched fractions of rabbit and beef brain. J Cell Biol 45:221, 1970
33. Milhorat TH: Structure and function of the choroid plexus and other sites of cerebrospinal fluid formation. Int Rev Cytol 47:225, 1976
34. Sadler K, Welch K: Concentration of glucose in new choroidal cerebrospinal fluid of the rabbit. Nature 215:884, 1967
35. Hochwald GM, Gandhi M, Goldman S: Transport of glucose from blood to cerebrospinal fluid in the cat. Neuroscience 10:1035, 1983
36. Hochwald GM, Magee J, Ferguson V: Cerebrospinal fluid glucose: turnover and metabolism. J Neurochem 44:1832, 1985
37. Atkinson AJ, Weiss MF: Kinetics of blood-cerebrospinal fluid glucose transfer in the normal dog. Am J Physiol 216:1120, 1969
38. Bronsted HE: Ouabain-sensitive carrier-mediated transport of glucose from the cerebral ventricles to surrounding tissue in the cat. J Physiol (Lond) 209:187, 1970
39. Bronsted HE: Transport of glucose, sodium, chloride and potassium between the cerebral ventricles and surrounding tissues in cats. Acta Physiol Scand 79:523, 1970
40. Rapoport SI: A mathematical model for vasogenic brain edema. J Theor Biol 74:439, 1978
41. Felgenhauer K: Protein size and cerebrospinal fluid composition. Klin Wochenschr 52:1158, 1974
42. Weisner B, Bernhardt W: Protcin fractions of lumbar, cisternal and ventricular cerebrospinal fluid. J Neurol Sci 37:205, 1978
43. Lups S, Haan AMFH: The Cerebrospinal Fluid. Elsevier, Amsterdam, 1954
44. Hochwald GM, Wallenstein MC: Exchange of albumin between blood, cerebrospinal fluid and brain in the cat. Am J Physiol 212:1199, 1967
45. Bouldin TW, Krigman MR: Differential permeability of cerebral capillary and choroid plexus to lanthanum ion. Brain Res 99:444, 1975
46. Castel M, Sahar A, Erlij D: The movement of lanthanum across diffusion barriers in the choroid plexus of the cat. Brain Res 67:178, 1974
47. Brightman MW: Ultrastructural characteristics of adult choroid plexus: relation to the blood-cerebrospinal fluid barrier to proteins. p. 86. In Netsky MG, Shuangshoti S (eds): The Choroid Plexus in Health and Disease. University Press of Virginia, Charlottesville, 1975
48. Rapoport SI: Passage of proteins from blood to cerebrospinal fluid: model for transfer by pores and vesicles. p. 233. In Wood JH (ed): Neurobiology of Cerebrospinal Fluid 2. Plenum, New York, 1983
49. Pollay M, Stevens FA, Roberts PA: Alteration in choroid-plexus blood flow and cerebrospinal fluid formation by increased ventricular pressure. p. 687. In Wood JH (ed): Neurobiology of Cerebrospinal Fluid 2. Plenum, New York, 1983
50. Carey ME, Vela AR: Effect of systemic arterial hypotension on the rate of CSF formation in dogs. J Neurosurg 41:350, 1974
51. Weiss MH, Wertman N: Modulation of CSF production by alterations in cerebral perfusion pressure. Arch Neurol 35:527, 1978
52. Cathcart RS, Worthington WC: Ciliary movement in the rat cerebral ventricles, clearing action and directions of currents. J Neuropathol Exp Neurol 23:609, 1964
53. Bradley KC: Cerebrospinal fluid pressure. J Neurol Neurosurg Psychiatry 33:387, 1970
54. DiChiro G: Observations on the circulation of the cerebrospinal fluid. Acta Radiol Diagn 5:988, 1966
55. DiChiro G: Movement of the cerebrospinal fluid in human beings. Nature 204:290, 1964
56. DiChiro G, Hammock MK, Bleyer WA: Spinal descent of cerebrospinal fluid in man. Neurology 26:1, 1976
57. Post RM, Allen FH, Ommaya AK: Cerebrospinal fluid flow and iodide-131 transport in the spinal subarachnoid space. Life Sci 14:1885, 1974
58. Williams B: Cerebrospinal fluid pressure changes in response to coughing. Brain 99:331, 1976
59. Fenstermacher JD, Patlak CS: The movement of water and solutes in the brain of mammals. p. 87. In Pappius HM, Feindel W (eds): Dynamics of Brain Edema. Springer-Verlag, New York, 1976
60. Reulen HJ, Graham R, Spatz M, Klatzo I: Role of pressure gradients and bulk flow in dynamics of vasogenic brain edema. J Neurosurg 46:24, 1977
61. Reulen HJ, Kreysch KG: Measurement of brain tissue in cold induced cerebral edema. Acta Neurochir 29:29, 1973
62. Klatzo I, Chui E, Fujiwara K, Spatz M: Resolution of vasogenic brain edema (VBE). Adv Neurol 28:359, 1980
63. Reulen HJ, Prioleau GR, Tsuyumu M, Fenske A: Clearance of edema fluid into cerebrospinal

fluid: mechanisms for resolution of vasogenic brain edema. p. 777. In Wood JH (ed): Neurobiology of Cerebrospinal Fluid 2. Plenum, New York, 1983
64. Welch MH, Pollay M: The spinal arachnoid villi of the monkeys cercopithecus aethiops sabaeus and macacairus. Anat Rec 145:43, 1963
65. Nabeshima S, Reese TS, Landis DMD, Brightman MW: Junctions in the meninges and marginal glia. J Comp Neurol 164:127, 1975
66. Mann JD, Butler AB, Johnson RN, Bass NH: Clearance of macromolecular and particulate substances from the cerebrospinal fluid system of the rat. J Neurosurg 50:343, 1979
67. Simionescu N, Simionescu M, Palade GE: Permeability of muscle capillaries to small hemepepetides: evidence for the existence of patent transendothelial channels. J Cell Biol 64:586, 1975
68. Simionescu N, Simionescu M, Palade GE: Structural basis of permeability in sequential segments of the microvasculature of the diaphragm. II. Pathways followed by microperoxidase across the endothelium. Microvasc Res 15:17, 1978
69. Johnson RN, Maffeo CJ, Butler AB et al: Intracranial hypertension in experimental animals and man: quantitative approach to system dynamics of circulatory cerebrospinal fluid. p. 697. In Wood JH (ed): Neurobiology of Cerebrospinal Fluid 2. Plenum, New York, 1983
70. Butler AB, Mann JD, Maffeo CJ et al: Mechanisms of cerebrospinal fluid absorption in normal and pathologically altered arachnoid villi. p. 707. In Wood JH (ed): Neurobiology of Cerebrospinal Fluid 2. Plenum, New York, 1983
71. Wolff JR: Ultrastructure of the terminal vascular bed as related to function. p. 95. In Kaley G, Altura BM (eds): Microvascular Circulation. Vol. I. University Park Press, Baltimore, 1977
72. Pappenheimer JR, Heisey SR, Jordan EF, Downer JdeC: Perfusion of the cerebral ventricular system in unanesthetized goats. Am J Physiol 203:763, 1962
73. Heisey SR, Held D, Pappenheimer JR: Bulk flow and diffusion in the cerebrospinal fluid system of the goat. Am J Physiol 203:775, 1962
74. Maffeo CJ, Mann JD, Butler AB et al: Constant flow perfusion of the cerebrospinal fluid system of rat, dog, and man: a mathematical model. p. 447. In Saha S (ed): Proceedings of the Fourth New England Bioengineering Conference. Pergamon Press, New York, 1976
75. Mann JD, Butler AB, Rosenthal J et al: Regulation of intracranial pressure in rat, dog, and man. Ann Neurol 3:156, 1978
76. Marmarou A, Shapiro K, Shulman K: Isolating factors leading to sustained elevations of the ICP. p. 33. In Beks JWF, Bosch DA, Brock M (eds): Intracranial Pressure III. Springer-Verlag, New York, 1976
77. Miller JD: Intracranial pressure-volume relationships in pathological conditions. J Neurosurg Sci 20:203, 1976
78. Sullivan HG, Mote PS, Allison JD, Becker DP: Intracranial pressure monitoring and interpretation. p. 54. In Cottrell JE, Turndorf H (eds): Anesthesia and Neurosurgery. CV Mosby, St. Louis, 1986
79. Lindvall M: Fluorescence histochemical study on regional differences in the sympathetic nerve supply of the choroid plexus from various laboratory animals. Cell Tissue Res 198:261, 1979
80. Lindvall M, Edvinsson L, Owman C: Sympathetic nervous control of cerebrospinal fluid production from the choroid plexus. Science 201:176, 1978
81. Lindvall M, Edvinsson L, Owman C: Histochemical study on regional differences in the cholinergic nerve supply of the choroid plexus from various laboratory animals. Exp Neurol 55:152, 1977
82. Larsson L-I, Edvinsson L, Fahrenkrug J et al: Immunohistochemical localization of a vasodilatory peptide (VIP) in cerebrovascular nerves. Brain Res 113:400, 1976
83. Lindvall M, Alumets J, Edvinsson L et al: Peptidergic (VIP) nerves in the mammalian choroid plexus. Neurosci Lett 9:77, 1978
84. Edvinsson L, Lindvall M: Autonomic vascular innervation and vasomotor reactivity in the choroid plexus. Exp Neurol 62:394, 1978
85. Edvinsson L, Hakanson R, Lindvall M et al: Ultrastructural and biochemical evidence for a sympathetic neural influence on the choroid plexus. Exp Neurol 48:241, 1975
86. Winbladh B, Edvinsson L, Lindvall M: Effect of sympathectomy on active transport mechanisms in choroid plexus in vitro. Acta Physiol Scand 102:85A, 1978
87. Haywood JR, Vogh BP: Some measurements of autonomic nervous system influence on production of cerebrospinal fluid in the cat. J Pharmacol Exp Ther 208:341, 1979
88. Lindvall M, Edvinsson L, Owman C: Effect of

sympathomimetic drugs and corresponding receptor antagonists on the rate of cerebrospinal fluid production. Exp Neurol 64:132, 1979
89. Edvinsson L, Nielson KC, Owman C, West KA: Adrenergic innervation of the mammalian choroid plexus. Am J Anat 139:299, 1974
90. Lindvall M, Edvinsson L, Owman C: Reduced cerebrospinal fluid formation through cholinergic mechanisms. Neurosci Lett 10:311, 1978
91. Edvinsson L, Owman C, West KA: Changes in continuously recorded intracranial pressure of conscious rabbits at different time periods after superior cervical sympathectomy. Acta Physiol Scand 83:42, 1971
92. Davson H, Luck CP: The effect of acetazoleamide on the chemical composition of the aqueous humour and cerebrospinal fluid of some mammalian species and on the role of turnover of ^{24}Na in these fluids. J Physiol (Lond) 137:279, 1957
93. Maren TH: Carbonic anhydrase: chemistry, physiology and inhibition. Physiol Rev 47:595, 1967
94. Tschirgi RC, Frost RW, Taylor JL: Inhibition of cerebrospinal fluid formation by a carbonic anhydrase inhibitor, 2-acetylamino-1,3,4-thiadiazole-5-sulfonamide (Diamox). Proc Soc Exp Biol Med 87:373, 1954
95. Vogh BP, Maren TH: Sodium, chloride and bicarbonate movement from plasma to cerebrospinal fluid in cats. Am J Physiol 228:673, 1975
96. Macri FJ, Politoff A, Rubin R et al: Preferential vasoconstrictor properties of acetazolamide on the arteries of the choroid plexus. Int J Neuropharmacol 5:109, 1966
97. Oppelt WW, Patlak CS, Rall DP: Effect of certain drugs on cerebrospinal fluid production in the dog. Am J Physiol 206:247, 1964
98. Smith RV, Roberts PA, Fisher RG: Alteration of cerebrospinal fluid production in the dog. Surg Neurol 2:267, 1974
99. Davson H, Segal MB: The effects of some inhibitors and accelerators of sodium transport on the turnover of ^{22}Na in the cerebrospinal fluid and the brain. J Physiol (Lond) 209:131, 1970
100. Domer FR: Effects of diuretics on cerebrospinal fluid formation and potassium movement. Exp Neurol 24:54, 1969
101. Buhrley LE, Reed DJ: The effect of furosemide on sodium-22 uptake into cerebrospinal fluid and brain. Exp Brain Res 14:503, 1972
102. Rosenberg GA, Kyner WT: Effect of mannitol-induced hyperosmolarity on transport between brain interstitial fluid and cerebrospinal fluid. p. 765. In Wood JH (ed): Neurobiology of Cerebrospinal Fluid 2. Plenum, New York, 1983
103. Donato T, Shapira Y, Artru AA, Powers KM: Effect of mannitol on cerebrospinal fluid dynamics and brain tissue edema. Anesth Analg 78:58, 1994
104. Dacey RG Jr, Scheld WM, Winn HR: Bacterial meningitis: Selected aspects of cerebrospinal fluid pathophysiology. p. 727. In Wood JH (ed): Neurobiology of Cerebrospinal Fluid 2. Plenum, New York, 1983
105. Mann JD, Johnson RN, Butler AB, Bass NH: Cerebrospinal fluid circulatory dynamics in pseudotumor cerebri and response to steroid therapy. p. 739. In Wood JH (ed): Neurobiology of Cerebrospinal Fluid 2. Plenum, New York, 1983
106. Garcia-Bengochea F: Cortisone and the cerebrospinal fluid of noncastrated cats. Am Surg 31:123, 1965
107. Schwartz ML, Tator CH, Hoffman HJ: The uptake of hydrocortisone in mouse brain and ependymoblastoma. J Neurosurg 36:178, 1972
108. Sato O, Hara M, Asai T et al: The effect of dexamethasone phosphate on the production rate of cerebrospinal fluid in the subarachnoid space of dogs. J Neurosurg 39:480, 1973
109. Weiss MH, Nulsen FE: The effect of glucocorticoids on CSF flow in dogs. J Neurosurg 32:452, 1970
110. Artru AA, Nugent M, Michenfelder JD: Enflurane causes a prolonged and reversible increase in the rate of CSF production in the dog. Anesthesiology 57:255, 1982
111. Mann JD, Mann ES, Cookson SL: Differential effect of pentobarbital, ketamine hydrochloride, and enflurane anesthesia on CSF formation rate and outflow resistance in the rat. p. 466. In Miller JD, Becker DP, Hochwald G et al (eds): Intracranial Pressure IV. Springer-Verlag, New York, 1980
112. Artru AA: Effects of enflurane and isoflurane on resistance to reabsorption of cerebrospinal fluid in dogs. Anesthesiology 61:529, 1984
113. Artru AA: Concentration-related changes in the rate of CSF formation and resistance to reabsorption of CSF during enflurane and isoflurane anesthesia in dogs receiving nitrous oxide. J Neurosurg Anesth 1:256, 1989

114. Mann ES, Cookson SL, Mann JD: Effects of enflurane and halothane on CSF dynamics in the rat. Anesthesiology 51, suppl. 3:54, 1979
115. Artru AA: Effects of enflurane and isoflurane on resistance to reabsorption of cerebrospinal fluid in dogs. Anesthesiology 61:529, 1984
116. Van Landingham KE, Maffeo CJ, Jackson H et al: Cerebrospinal fluid dynamics in the cat under halothane and pentobarbital anesthesia, abstracted. Soc Neurosci 7:89, 1981
117. Artru AA: Effects of halothane and fentanyl anesthesia on resistance to reabsorption of CSF. J Neurosurg 60:252, 1984
118. Artru AA: Relationship between cerebral blood volume and CSF pressure during anesthesia with halothane or enflurane in dogs. Anesthesiology 58:533, 1983
119. Nemoto EM, Stezoski SW, MacMurdo D: Glucose transport across the rat blood-brain barrier during anesthesia. Anesthesiology 49:170, 1978
120. Hannan CJ Jr, Kettler TM, Artru AA, Aronstam A: Blood-brain barrier permeability during hypocapnia in halothane-anesthetized monkeys. Ann NY Acad Sci 529:172, 1988
121. Pashayan AG, Mickle JP, Vetter TR et al: Blood-CSF barrier function during general anesthesia in children undergoing ventriculoperitoneal shunt placement. Anesth Rev 15:30, 1988
122. Artru AA: Reduction of cerebrospinal fluid pressure by hypocapnia: changes in cerebral blood volume, cerebrospinal fluid volume and brain tissue water and electrolytes. II. Effects of anesthetics. J Cereb Blood Flow Metabol 8:750, 1988
123. Schettini A, Furniss WW: Brain water and electrolyte distribution during the inhalation of halothane. Br J Anaesth 51:1117, 1979
124. Artru AA: Effects of halothane and fentanyl on the rate of CSF production in dogs. Anesth Analg 62:581, 1983
125. Artru AA: Dose-related changes in the rate of CSF formation and resistance to reabsorption of CSF during administration of fentanyl, sufentanil, or alfentanil in dogs. J Neurosurg Anesth 3:283, 1991
126. Alexander SC, Helmer PH, Ramirez O, Chong J: Effects of general anesthesia on canine blood-brain barrier glucose transport. p. 9.37. In Harper M, Jennett B, Miller O, Rowan J (eds): Blood Flow and Metabolism in the Brain. Churchill Livingston, Edinburgh, 1975
127. Artru AA: Isoflurane does not increase the rate of CSF production in the dog. Anesthesiology 60:193, 1984
128. Chi OZ: Effects of isoflurane anesthesia on the blood-brain barrier transport. Anesthesiology 73:A682, 1990
129. Sugioka S: Effects of sevoflurane on intracranial pressure and formation and absorption of cerebrospinal fluid in cats. Masui 41:1434, 1992
130. Artru AA: Rate of cerebrospinal fluid formation, resistance to reabsorption of cerebrospinal fluid, brain tissue water content, and electroencephalogram during desflurane anesthesia in dogs. J Neurosurg Anesth 5:178, 1993
131. Saija A, Princi P, DePasquale R, Costa G: Modifications of the permeability of the blood-brain barrier and local cerebral metabolism in pentobarbital- and ketamine-anesthetized rats. Neuropharmacology 28:997, 1989
132. Artru AA: Dose-related changes in rate of cerebrospinal fluid formation and resistance to reabsorption of cerebrospinal fluid following administration of thiopental, midazolam, and etomidate in dogs. Anesthesiology 69:541, 1988
133. Fischer S, Renz D, Schaper W, Karliczek GF: In vitro effects of fentanyl, methohexital, and thiopental on brain endothelial permeability. Anesthesiology 82:451, 1995
134. Artru AA: Propofol combined with halothane or fentanyl/halothane does not alter the rate of CSF formation or resistance to reabsorption of CSF in rabbits. J Neurosurg Anesth 5:250, 1993
135. Gjedde A, Rasmussen M: Pentobarbital anesthesia reduces blood-brain glucose transfer in the rat. J Neurochem 35:1382, 1980
136. Sage JI, Duffy TE: Pentobarbital anesthesia: Influence on amino acid transport across the blood-brain barrier. J Neurochem 33:963, 1979
137. Artru AA: The rate of CSF formation, resistance to reabsorption of CSF, and aperiodic analysis of the EEG following administration of flumazenil to dogs. Anesthesiology 72:111, 1990
138. Artru AA, Bernards CM, Mautz DM: Intravenous lidocaine decreases but cocaine does not alter the rate of CSF formation in anesthetized rabbits. p. 397. In Nagai H, Kamiya K, Ishii S (eds): Intracranial Pressure IX. Springer-Verlag, Tokyo, 1994
139. Meyer RR, Shapiro HM: Paradoxical effect of enflurane on choroid plexus metabolism: clinical implications, abstracted. p. 489. In Abstracts of the American Society of Anesthesiologists, Chicago, 1978

140. Maktabi MA, El Bokl FF, Todd MM: Effect of halothane anesthesia on production of cerebrospinal fluid: possible role of vasopressin V_1 receptors, abstracted. J Cereb Blood Flow Metabol 11:S268, 1991
141. Foxworthy JC IV, Artru AA: Cerebrospinal fluid dynamics and brain tissue composition following intravenous infusions of hypertonic saline in anesthetized rabbits. J Neurosurg Anesth 2:256, 1990
142. Wood JH, Bartelt D, James AE, Udvarhelyi GB: Normal-pressure hydrocephalus: diagnosis and patient selection for shunt surgery. Neurology 24:517, 1974
143. Wright EM: Transport processes in the formation of cerebrospinal fluid. Rev Physiol Biochem Pharmacol 83:1, 1978
144. Vates TS, Bonting SJ, Oppelt WW: Na-K-activated adenosine triphosphatase formation of cerebrospinal fluid in the cat. Am J Physiol 206:1165, 1964
145. Artru AA: Muscle relaxation with succinylcholine or vecuronium does not alter the rate of CSF production or resistance to reabsorption of CSF in dogs. Anesthesiology 68:392, 1988
146. Shapira Y, Artru AA, Lam AM: Changes in the rate of formation and resistance to reabsorption of cerebrospinal fluid during deliberate hypotension induced with adenosine or hemorrhage. Anesthesiology 76:432, 1992
147. Snodgrass SR, Lorenzo AV: Temperature and cerebrospinal fluid production rate. Am J Physiol 222:1524, 1972
148. Heisey SR, Adams T, Fisher MJ, Dang W: Effect of hypercapnia and cerebral perfusion pressure on cerebrospinal fluid production in cat. Am J Physiol 244:R224, 1983
149. Ames A III, Higashi K, Nesbett FB: Effects of $P_{CO}2$, acetazolamide and oubain on volume and composition of choroid-plexus fluid. J Physiol (Lond) 181:516, 1965
150. Artru AA, Hornbein TF: Prolonged hypocapnia does not alter the rate of CSF production in dogs during halothane anesthesia or sedation with nitrous oxide. Anesthesiology 67:66, 1987
151. Martins AN, Doyle TF, Newby N: $P_{CO}2$ and rate of formation of cerebrospinal fluid in the monkey. Am J Physiol 231:127, 1976
152. Oppelt WW, Maren TH, Owens ES, Rall DP: Effects of acid-base alterations on cerebrospinal fluid production. Proc Soc Exp Biol Med 114:86, 1963
153. Wald A, Hochwald GM, Malhan C: Relationship between osmolarity and formation of cerebrospinal fluid (CSF). Fed Proc Fed Am Soc Exp Biol 33:418, 1974
154. Hochwald GM, Wald A, DiMattio J, Malhan C: The effects of serum osmolarity on cerebrospinal fluid volume flow. Life Sci 15:1309, 1974
155. Wald A, Hochwald GM, Gandhi M: Evidence for the movement of fluid, macromolecules and ions from the brain extracellular space to the CSF. Brain Res 151:283, 1978
156. Artru AA: Reduction of cerebrospinal fluid pressure by hypocapnia: changes in cerebral blood volume, cerebrospinal fluid volume and brain tissue water and electrolytes. J Cereb Blood Flow Metab 7:471, 1987
157. Johnson RN, Maffeo CJ, Butler AB et al: Intracranial hypertension in experimental animals and man: quantitative approach to system dynamics of circulatory cerebrospinal fluid. p. 697. In Wood JH (ed): Neurobiology of Cerebrospinal Fluid. Vol. 2. Plenum, New York, 1983
158. Butler AB, Maffeo CJ, Johnson RN, Bass NH: Impaired absorption of CSF during experimental subarachnoid hemorrhage: effects of blood components on vesicular transport in arachnoid villi. p. 245. In Shulman K, Marmarou A, Miller JD et al. (eds): Intracranial Pressure. Vol. IV. Springer-Verlag, New York, 1980
159. Ishii M, Suzuki S, Julow J: Subarachnoid hemorrhage and communicating hydrocephalus: scanning electron microscopic observations. Acta Neurochir 50:265, 1979
160. Julow J, Ishii M, Iwabuchi I: Scanning electron microscopy of the subarachnoid macrophages after subarachnoid hemorrhage, and their possible role in the formation of subarachnoid fibrosis. Acta Neurochir 50:273, 1979
161. Julow J, Ishii M, Iwabuchi T: Arachnoid villi affected by subarachnoid pressure and hemorrhage: scanning electron microscopic study in the dog. Acta Neurochir 51:63, 1979
162. Johnston I: The definition of a reduced CSF absorption syndrome: A reappraisal of benign intracranial hypertension and related syndromes. Med Hypotheses 1:10, 1975
163. Mann JD, Johnson RN, Butler AB, Bass NH: Impairment of cerebrospinal fluid circulatory dynamics in pseudotumor cerebri and response to steroid treatment. Neurology 29:550, 1979
164. Johnston I, Paterson A: Benign intracranial hy-

pertension. II. CSF pressure and circulation. Brain 97:301, 1974
165. Martins AN: Resistance to drainage of cerebrospinal fluid: clinical measurement and significance. J Neurol Neurosurg Psychiatry 36:313, 1973
166. Becker DP: Isolation of factors leading to raised ICP in head-injured patients: a preliminary report, abstracted. In Annual Meeting of the American Association of Neurological Surgeons, 1985
167. Wood JH: Physiology, pharmacology, and dynamics of cerebrospinal fluid. p. 1. In Wood JH (ed): Neurobiology of Cerebrospinal Fluid. Vol. 1. Plenum, New York, 1980
168. Hochwald GM: Cerebrospinal fluid mechanisms. p. 33. In Cottrell JRE, Turndorf H (eds): Anesthesia and Neurosurgery. CV Mosby, St. Louis, 1986
169. Milhorat TH, Hammock MK: Cerebrospinal fluid as reflection of internal milieu of brain. p. 1. In Wood JH (ed): Neurobiology of Cerebrospinal Fluid. Vol. 2. Plenum, New York, 1983
170. Cerebrospinal fluid. p. 165. In Diem K, Lentner C (eds): Geigy Scientific Tables. Ciba-Geigy, Basel, 1981
171. Johanson CE: The choroid plexus-arachnoid membrane-cerebrospinal fluid system. p. 33. In Boulton AA, Baker GB, Walz W (eds): Neuromethods; The Neuronal Microenvironment. Human Press, Clifton, 1988
172. Johanson CE, Parandoosh Z, Smith QR: Chloride-bicarbonate exchange in the choroid plexus: analysis by the DMO method for cell pH. Am J Physiol 249:F470, 1985
173. Woodbury JW: An epilogue, an hypothetical model for CSF formation and blood-brain barrier function. p. 465. In Siesjo BK, Sorensen SC (eds): Ion Homeostasis of the Brain. Munksgaard, Copenhagen, 1971
174. Millen JW, Woollam DHM: The Anatomy of Cerebrospinal Fluid. Oxford University Press, London, 1962
175. Segal MB, Pollay M: The secretion of cerebrospinal fluid. Exp Eye Res, suppl. 25:127, 1977
176. Upton ML, Weller RO: The morphology of cerebrospinal fluid drainage pathways in human arachnoid granulations. J Neurosurg 63:867, 1985
177. Weed LH: The absorption of cerebrospinal fluid into the venous system. Am J Anat 31:191, 1923

3 INTRACRANIAL PRESSURE

CHERI A. SULEK

An appreciation of the fundamental principles governing intracranial pressure (ICP) and the influence of pharmacologic interventions and hemodynamic changes on ICP is essential for any physician providing care to a patient with intracranial pathology and abnormal intracranial elastance. The importance of early diagnosis and aggressive treatment of intracranial hypertension cannot be overemphasized. The basic goal of treatment is to improve cerebral perfusion pressure (CPP) to minimize cerebral ischemia and permanent neurologic injury with either medical management and/or surgical intervention. One of the greatest concerns for a clinician in this scenario is the development of uncontrollable intracranial hypertension resulting in herniation of brain tissue and ensuing death. With current monitoring modalities and aggressive therapy for increased ICP, it is now rare for a physician to observe the classic triad (hypertension, bradycardia, and respiratory irregularities) originally described by Cushing in the early 1900s.[1]

The structural components of the intracranial compartment that contribute to and limit expansion are well defined; however, the concept of abnormal ICP and management goals continue to evolve as we gain a better understanding of the pathophysiologic processes involved and improvement in complex monitoring of cerebral hemodynamics. It is now accepted that ICP is not always uniform within the craniospinal axis; for example, local differences in ICP and cerebral blood flow (CBF) often exist in regions of brain tumors or head injury.[2,3] As new anesthetic agents are introduced, anesthesiologists must recognize the impact of these agents on ICP to provide a safe intraoperative course and optimal operating conditions for the neurosurgeons. This pharmacologic knowledge is also important in those patients with suspected or documented elevated ICP undergoing non-neurosurgical procedures. In recent years more sophisticated monitoring of ICP and cerebral hemodynamics and oxygenation has significantly improved optimization of treatment. Treatment of head-injured patients has continued to evolve, reflecting increased awareness of the frequency of associated cerebral ischemia and the important role of secondary neuronal injury.

Treatment of a patient with abnormal intracranial elastance often involves the care and contributions from multiple disciplines working in concert to preserve CBF and minimize ischemia in the presence of elevated ICP. It is important for the neuroanesthesiologist, critical care medicine intensivist, and neurosurgeon to understand what determines ICP, how pathologic processes alter intracranial dynamics, and the influence of pharmacologic and hemodynamic manipulations on ICP to ensure that intervention has a favorable effect on CPP, ICP, and outcome. The goals of this chapter are to provide (1) a basic understanding of ICP, (2) the regulation of ICP and its impact on cerebral perfusion in normal and pathologic states, (3) the impact of anesthetic agents on ICP, and (4) the management of intracranial hypertension.

CEREBRAL PHYSIOLOGY

Contents of the Craniospinal Axis

An appreciation of the regulation of normal intracranial contents and pressure is imperative before introducing pathology that perturbs normal cerebral homeostasis. In the absence of pathology, the intracranial volume remains essentially constant within the neuraxis. The intracranial contents (brain, cerebrospinal fluid, blood, and meninges) are encased by the calvarium externally and separated internally by the tentorium into superior and inferior compartments communicating via the tentorial incisura. The cranial and spinal contents are also in continuity, communicating through the foramen magnum. The calvarium is generally regarded as a thick, bony, nondistensible, semiclosed container that strictly limits intracranial volume and any expansion by acute or chronic pathologic processes. However, this container is no longer closed in the presence of a fracture, during a craniotomy, or in infancy prior to suture and fontanelle closure.

Brain tissue alone accounts for 88% of the total intracranial volume; the meninges and brain tissue supporting structures contribute minimally and have limited distensibility. The normal brain weighs 1,400 g in air, but in the cranium, its weight is reduced to 50 g by the buoyancy of the cerebrospinal fluid (CSF).[4–6] Eighty percent of brain volume is water, 20% of which is sequestered in the extracellular space.[6] Under normal circumstances, the extracellular environment of the brain is closely regulated by an intact blood-brain barrier that only selectively permits diffusion and active transport of certain limited substances. Expansion of brain volume is either secondary to an increase in water content or growth of the solid substance itself. Disruption of the blood-brain barrier, by head injury or hypertensive hemorrhage, for example, causes an increase in extracellular fluid or brain water, resulting in global or localized edema depending upon the site and extent of injury. Initially a developing brain tumor often increases only the solid component, and as it enlarges, the integrity of the blood-brain barrier is lost with resultant peritumor edema.

Cerebrospinal fluid contributes 9 percent to the total intracranial volume.[7] The total CSF volume is 150 ml at any one time in a normal adult, and total production approximates 0.3 to 0.4 ml/min or 500 to 600 ml/day with replacement of volume at least every 8 hours.[8–10] Fifty percent of the total CSF volume (75 ml) is contained within the intracranial space of which 30 ml occupies the ventricular system with 8 ml in each lateral ventricle.[5,6,10] Cerebrospinal fluid is secreted primarily by the choroid plexus lining portions of the ventricular system. In the intact system, CSF communicates freely through the ventricular system circulating by the action of cilia and hydrostatic forces and exiting via the foramina of Luschka and Magendie into the subarachnoid space of the cranial and ultimately spinal canal. Cerebrospinal fluid is principally absorbed from the subarachnoid space into venous blood by bulk flow at the arachnoid granulations bordering the superior sagittal sinus; there is some contribution by the arachnoid granulations at the veins along the spinal nerve roots.[8,11] Eighty-four percent of the CSF is absorbed within the intracranial compartment with the remainder absorbed in the spinal compartment.[12] Obstructions of any portion of the ventricular system including the arachnoid granulations results in hydrocephalus and occasionally interstitial edema.

The blood in the vascular system of the brain is the smallest component of the intracranial space, contributing to only 2 to 3 percent of its volume.[7] The brain receives 15% of the cardiac output, which has a rapid transit time through the brain. The cerebral blood volume (CBV) is only 75 ml, the majority of which resides in the low-pressure venous system.[5] Only 25% of the blood is found within the arteries and arterioles.[13] Despite the small volume of the vascular compartment, it is an important determinant of ICP, and the parameter most commonly manipulated by an anesthesiologist in a patient with abnormal intracranial elastance.

The intracranial volume remains virtually constant until a new volume (i.e., hematoma) is added or expansion of an existing intracranial volume (i.e., tumor) occurs in the noncompressible system. In order to maintain a normal ICP, a mandatory, reciprocal reduction in volume of one of the intracranial components (i.e., blood or, CSF) must occur to offset the effects of the new volume added. These concepts embody the basic principles of the Monroe-Kellie doctrine and its modifications.[7,12,14]

Normal Intracranial Pressure

The normal ICP measured in adults in the horizontal position is 5 to 15 mmHg; lower values are recorded in infants and young children. In the horizontal position, pressures are considered equal within the craniospinal axis; lumbar subarachnoid pressures should reflect ICP when the two compartments freely communicate. When Langfitt and colleagues created an obstruction at the levels of the tentorium and foramen magnum in monkeys simulating tentorial and tonsillar herniation of brain tissue, a pressure gradient developed early cephalad and caudad to the level of obstruction reflecting discontinuity between the two spaces.[15] A similar observation was made by Takizawa et al. in cats utilizing an epidural balloon to create a transtentorial pressure gradient.[16] Even in the presence of local ICP elevations, as observed in the region of peritumor edema, lumbar pressure can be misleading since the "global" ICP is often in the normal range. Intracranial pressure is considered abnormal when levels exceed 15 to 20 mmHg. Transient, benign elevations in ICP normally occur with Valsalva and Queckenstedt maneuvers. Neurologic outcome, especially in head-injured patients, appears to correlate with degree and duration of intracranial hypertension.[17] Intracranial pressure exceeding 20 mmHg warrants aggressive treatment. However, some investigators recommend maintaining ICP as low as 15 mmHg. Sustained elevations in ICP that exceed 25 to 30 mmHg and are refractory to treatment are often fatal. The detrimental effects of elevated ICP result from cerebral ischemia and direct compressive effects contributing to neuronal injury and poor neurologic outcome.

Mechanisms of Spatial Compensation

Intracranial pressure is closely regulated even in the presence of a space-occupying lesion as long as compensatory mechanisms are operational and the pathologic process evolves slowly. Any increase in intracranial volume must be reciprocated by a reduction in volume of one of the other compartments to maintain normal ICP. If rapid volume expansion occurs in the rigid system (i.e., epidural hematoma), ICP rises acutely due to inadequate compensatory mechanisms. Conversely, a slow-growing tumor increases brain volume, but the chronicity of the disease process allows adequate reductions in both CBV and CSF volume to maintain normal intracranial dynamics until the mechanisms for spatial compensation are exhausted. Even though the blood volume of the cerebral vasculature only accounts for a small portion of the intracranial contents, the reduction of its volume can easily be manipulated and provides additional space for an expanding lesion. Because the majority of blood volume resides in the low-pressure venous system, it can be easily displaced by an enlarging mass. The CSF system has the greatest buffering capacity of the intracranial contents with the largest contribution from CSF absorption. Intracranial hypertension from a chronic pathologic process ensues when the buffering capacity of the CSF pathways is exhausted. The rate of CSF absorption increases in the presence of a mass lesion and lowers the intracranial volume; rate of CSF production is minimally affected. Marmarou et al. determined that brain edema in cats was predominantly cleared by CSF pathways via pressure-dependent bulk flow with only 11% clearance through the vasculature.[18] Slow expansion of a mass can result in brain atrophy reflecting chronic loss of water and electrolytes. The meninges and brain tissue supporting structures have limited distensibility and contribute minimally to the buffering capacity of the intracranial contents.

Pressure-Volume Curve

The intracranial pressure-volume curve was formally defined in 1965 by Langfitt et al., and their integral relationship is depicted in Figure 3.1.[19] During the period of compensation, ICP increases minimally even with relatively large changes in intracranial volume. When the buffering capacity of the intracranial space is exhausted, primarily when maximal CSF absorption occurs, small increases in volume are followed by abrupt rises in ICP. Ideally, the pressure-volume curve depicts the relationship between intracranial pressure and volume with slow volume expansion, allowing adequate time for compensation with minimal alterations in ICP. If a mass expands rapidly, as is often the case with an epidural hematoma, the additional volume cannot be accommodated and ICP rises acutely.

FIGURE 3.1 *Idealized intracranial pressure-volume curve. Points* A-B *represent spatial compensation with expanding intracranial volume. The elastance of the intracranial compartment is low. At point* C, *spatial exhaustion occurs as compensatory mechanisms fail. Between points* C *and* D, *the elastance of the intracranial space is increased and small changes in volume result in large changes in ICP.*

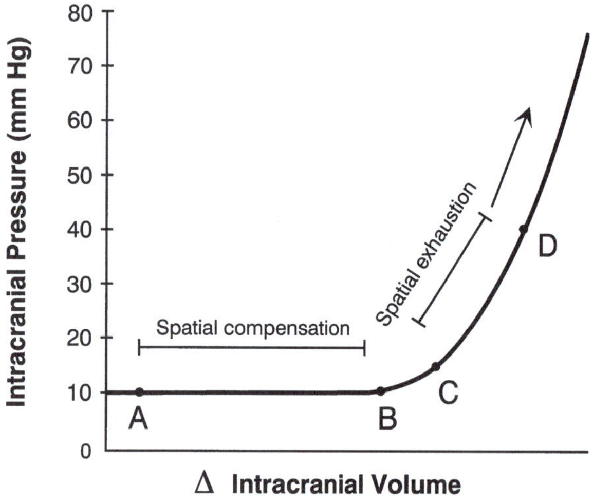

The slope dP/dV of the pressure-volume curve defines the elastance of the system and reflects its stiffness or the resistance to deformation exerted by the intracranial contents with the addition of volume.[20] Lofgren et al. determined that elastance increased 20-fold when an ICP of 15 mmHg was reached in dogs.[20] Many authors refer to the compliance, not elastance, of the system. The slope dV/dP defines compliance and reflects the distensibility of the intracranial space. Along the horizontal portion of the pressure-volume curve, the elastance of the intracranial compartment is low and compliance is high; the reverse relationship exists for the vertical portion of the curve.

Cerebral Perfusion Pressure

When elevated profoundly, ICP alters perfusion of cortical and subcortical structures. The relationship between ICP and CPP is classically defined as CPP = MAP – ICP (MAP = mean arterial pressure). The lower limit of CPP acceptable in adults is 50 mmHg and lower in infants. Cerebral ischemia occurs in dogs as CPP approaches 40 mmHg in the absence of cerebral protective measures. In the absence of intracranial pathology, ICP is low, usually 5 mmHg or less, and CPP changes reflect alterations in MAP. When ICP is unknown,central venous pressure has been substituted. In the presence of intracranial pathology, effective perfusion pressure declines as ICP rises. Historically, maintenance of a CPP greater than 50 mmHg was considered acceptable in head-injured patients. Rosner and other investigators now recommend maintaining CPP greater than 70 mmHg in head-injured patients to minimize cerebral ischemia and prevent the cascade of events that result from inadequate perfusion.[21,22] Either a decrease in MAP or an elevation in ICP will deleteriously alter the effective perfusion pressure.

Regulation of Cerebral Blood Flow

Cerebral autoregulation involves the maintenance of a constant CBF when MAP (or CPP if ICP is normal) is between 50 and 150 mmHg and is accomplished by adjustment of cerebrovascular resistance (CVR) (see Fig. 3.2). Autoregulation protects the brain from experiencing abrupt changes in blood pressure. As MAP decreases, the cerebral resistance vessels (arterioles) dilate increasing CBV to maintain a constant blood flow; conversely, CVR increases with acute hypertension to prevent abrupt rises in CBF.[23] Cerebral blood flow passively follows blood pressure when the limits of autoregulation have been exceeded or the mechanism is impaired. Autoregulation is often impaired globally or regionally after acute stroke, subarachnoid hemorrhage, or head injury or in association with arteriovenous malformations,tumors, hypoxia (PaO_2 less than 50 mmHg), extreme hypercarbia, or acidosis, and even iatrogenically with high doses of potent inhalational anesthetic agents.[24,25] In chronic hypertension, the autoregulatory curve is shifted to the right moving the upper and lower limits of CPP to higher levels (Fig. 3.2). In hypertensive individuals, cerebral ischemia can occur at a CPP that generally would ensure adequate CBF in normotensive individuals. With institution of antihypertensive therapy and restoration of normal blood pressure values, autoregulation rapidly shifts back toward normotensive limits. Intracranial hypertension alone does not appear to abolish autoregulation. Hauerberg and Juhler demonstrated that severe intracranial hypertension in rats shifted the lower limit of autoregulation to a lower CPP and may have reflected the brain's attempt to preserve CBF.[26] In awake humans, a decrease in blood pressure results in a change in CBF within 2 seconds or less when assessing middle cerebral artery blood flow velocity (V_{mca}) by transcranial Doppler (TCD).[24] Autoregulation of CBF occurs within seconds and at least in unanesthetized humans appears to depend on the underlying $PaCO_2$; the fastest autoregulatory response occurred with hypocapnia, implying that the status of the underlying vascular tone plays a role in response time.[24] The exact mechanism of autoregulation is not known, but it is speculated that resistance vessels may be responsive to the local metabolic environment or to transmural pressure.[26,27]

FIGURE 3.2 *Cerebral autoregulation curves in normotensive and chronic hypertensive states and with loss of autoregulation. CBF is unchanged when MAP ranges from 50 to 150 mmHg in normotensive individuals. The upper and lower limits of autoregulation shift to higher values when MAP is chronically elevated. With loss of autoregulatory capacity, CBF passively follows changes in MAP.(—), cerebral autoregulation in normotensive individual; (------), cerebral autoregulation chronic hypertensive individual; (×), loss of autoregulation.*

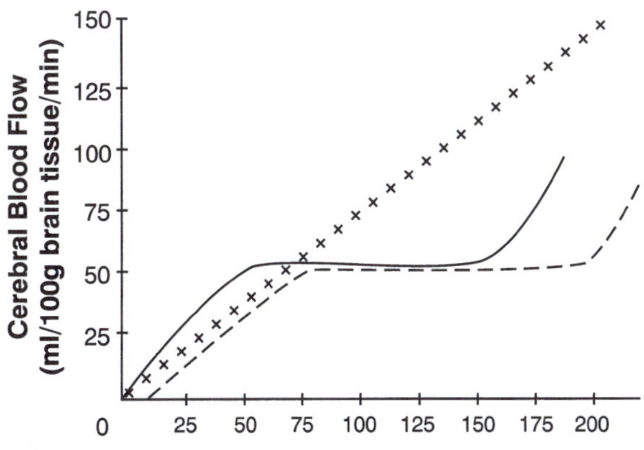

Normal global CBF is approximately 50 to 55 ml/100 g brain tissue/min.[28–30] Gray matter receives 75 ml/100 g/min (75% of CBF), whereas white matter, only 25 ml/100 g/min (25% of CBF), reflecting the increased metabolic activity of the gray matter.[28] Local increases in CBF in the nonpathologic state indicates the use a specific region of the cortex during a task or activity.[31] For example, the performance of a simple task with one hand results in increased blood flow and metabolic activity in the contralateral sensorimotor regions. Cerebral blood flow is normally tightly coupled to cerebral oxygen consumption ($CMRO_2$) and is expressed as $CMRO_2 = CBF \times AVDO_2$ (arteriovenous difference of oxygen).[22] Under normal circumstances, $CMRO_2$ is constant at 3.2 to 3.5 ml/100 g brain tissue/min.[22,28,29] $CMRO_2$ is decreased with coma, severe head injury, hypothermia, and many anesthetic agents (i.e., thiopental); increases are profound with seizure activity and certain drugs such as ketamine.[32] Cerebral blood flow and $CMRO_2$ do not always remain coupled, as observed often after head injury and during use of potent inhalational agents.[33]

Cerebral ischemia is manifested when CBF falls below a critical level required to meet the metabolic demands of the cerebral tissue. Under halothane anesthesia, ischemia manifests by electroencephalogram (EEG) when regional CBF (rCBF) falls below 18 ml/100 g/min.[34] During carotid endarterectomies using isoflurane, EEG changes consistent with ischemia were detected when rCBF decreased to less than 10 ml/100 g/min.[35] Cortical somatosensory-evoked potentials are abolished at a rCBF of less than 15 ml/100 g/min. At CBF levels of 15 ml/100 g/min, the EEG becomes isoelectric as synaptic transmission ceases.[36,37] Cellular integrity is preserved (i.e., membrane ion pumps and ion gradients) until much lower flows are reached; loss of electrical activity is a protective mechanism to reduce the energy expenditure of the cell. As flows approach 6 to 10 ml/100 g/min, extracellular potassium concentrations increase and cell death follows if rCBF is not restored.[36,37] The threshold for cerebral ischemia is increased under most general anesthetic techniques, especially isoflurane, and predominantly results from $CMRO_2$ reduction. Tolerance for ischemia is significantly reduced in the awake patient.

Factors Influencing CBF and CBV

Cerebral blood flow is influenced not only by pathology disrupting autoregulation, but by potent inhalational agents, IV anesthetics, and alterations in $PaCO_2$ and PaO_2. In general, changes in CBF are accompanied by parallel changes in CBV by a ratio of 7:1.[38] This relationship does not always exist, and each factor affecting CBF and CBV must be considered independently. For example, it is accepted that inhalational agents and hypercarbia produce elevations in CBF and CBV by cerebral vasodilation, but hypotension with a MAP of less than 50 mmHg results in a decreased CBF but increased CBV reflecting changes in the tone of the cerebral resistance vessels.

The cerebral resistance vessels, predominantly end arterioles, are exquisitely sensitive to alterations in $PaCO_2$ and rapidly alter ICP. Hypocapnia is characterized by vasoconstriction of arterioles resulting in decreased CBV, CBF, and ICP; hypercapnia influences the vascular tone in an opposite manner.[13,39,40] Cerebral blood flow is increased by approximately 2 ml/100 g brain tissue/min or a 4 percent change for each 1 Torr increase in $PaCO_2$[30,39] For each 1 Torr change in $PaCO_2$ the change in gray matter blood volume is 0.053 and 0.046 ml/100 g for white matter.[41] The pH of the extracellular fluid of the brain, determined acutely by hydrogen ion concentration, influences the tone of the cerebral vasculature, but within 24 to 36 hours the CSF pH begins to normalize despite elevated arterial pH during hyperventilation.[30,40,42] When hyperventilation is instituted for the treatment of intracranial hypertension, CBF, CBV, and ICP decrease as long as CPP is maintained. The effectiveness of hyperventilation diminishes with time as CBV, CBF, and ICP return toward prehyperventilation levels with normalization of CSF pH by adjustment of CSF bicarbonate concentrations. Responsiveness of the resistance vessels to CO_2 diminishes as the upper and lower limits of cerebral autoregulation are approached.[39,43] A linear relationship exists between CBF and $PaCO_2$ when $PaCO_2$ ranges from 20 to 80 mmHg.[43] Outside of this range, cerebrovascular tone is less responsive to changes in $PaCO_2$.[43] The potent inhalational anesthetic agents do not interfere with reactivity of the cerebral vasculature to carbon dioxide (CO_2) at 1.0 minimum alveolar concentration (MAC) of anesthesia. When inducing hyperventilation, $PaCO_2$ should be maintained above 25 mmHg to avoid cerebral ischemia that has been observed with values of 20 mmHg or less and corresponds to a CBF of approximately 20 ml/100 g/min. *Currently aggressive hyperventilation is not advocated for head-injured patients with potentially compromised blood flow.*

Cerebral blood flow is resistant to most changes in PaO_2 unless hypoxia or hyperoxia (hyperbaric oxygen) occurs. Cerebral blood flow is not affected until the PaO_2 falls below 50 mmHg and reflects a response to tissue acidosis.[30,42,44] Cerebral blood flow increases with the development of severe hypoxemia but rapidly reverses with correction of PaO_2.

DIAGNOSIS OF INTRACRANIAL HYPERTENSION

Clinical Diagnosis

The symptoms and signs of elevated ICP are relatively nonspecific and depend upon the chronicity and location of the underlying pathologic process. The clinical presentation of a slow-growing brain tumor is markedly different from an acute, rapidly expanding epidural hematoma with impending herniation. The development of symptomatology, although dependent upon elevation of ICP, reflects the direct or indirect distortion or ischemia of brain tissue secondary to the increased ICP. A multitude of disease processes may result in increased intracranial elastance (decreased compliance) and clinical manifestations of intracranial hypertension.

Disease Processes That Increase ICP

- Brain tumors
- Head injury
- Subdural or epidural hematomas
- Pseudotumor cerebri
- Subarachnoid hemorrhage
- Hepatic encephalopathy
- Eclampsia
- Hydrocephalus
- Stroke
- Venous sinus thrombosis
- Arteriovenous malformation
- Inflammatory processes
- Hypoxic injury
- Reye syndrome

Abbreviation: ICP, intracranial pressure.

The most classic clinical manifestations of elevated ICP are headache, nausea, vomiting, visual disturbances, altered mentation, papilledema, and ocular palsies.[4,19,45] Focal neurologic deficits reflect mass effect or ischemia of surrounding brain tissues by an expanding lesion. Elevation of ICP may be more difficult to assess in children but is most often manifested by irritability, somnolence, altered feeding habits, nausea, and vomiting. Headache is a common clinical manifestation that is often bifrontal or bioccipital in location, worse in the morning upon awakening, exacerbated by coughing or a Valsalva maneuver, paroxysmal in nature, and relieved by emesis.[45] Dural stretching or traction on vessels at the base of the brain caused by the mass lesion contribute to headache. Headache is highly suggestive of elevated ICP but is not diagnostic. Nausea and projectile vomiting occur usually in the morning or at night, and emesis often relieves headache. Papilledema is evident bilaterally 24 to 48 hours after ICP elevation and is postulated to result from axoplasmic stasis as ICP is transmitted through the subarachnoid space to the optic disc. Focal neurologic deficits may be evident if an intracranial mass lesion compresses or distorts underlying sensory, motor, or cranial nerve pathways.

The initial clinical presentation and progression of neurologic deterioration may depend on the location of the mass lesion. Deterioration of the neurologic exam progresses in a rostral-to-caudal fashion with supratentorial mass lesions; brainstem dysfunction is a late finding with a slowly expanding mass but occurs early with a rapidly enlarging mass signaling herniation.[4] However, the initial clinical manifestation of an infratentorial mass lesion may be brainstem dysfunction (i.e., cranial nerve palsy, cerebellar findings, or respiratory abnormalities) if compression of vital brainstem structures occurs.

Loss of consciousness associated with a supratentorial mass is an ominous finding in the absence of a metabolic etiology and implies bilateral cerebral hemispheric or diencephalic dysfunction. The degree of midline shift of the pineal body by computed tomography (CT) of the brain correlates with level of consciousness: alert with 0 to 3 mm shift, drowsy with 3 to 4 mm, stuporous with 6 to 8.5 mm, and comatose with 8 to 13 mm.[46] Mental status impairment with infratentorial lesions often results from development of noncommunicating hydrocephalus as the cerebral aqueduct or fourth ventricle is compressed but may be even more ominous, suggesting disruption or compression of the reticular activating system.

Assessment of brainstem function is the basis of the neurologic exam when the patient becomes comatose. Evaluation of brainstem reflexes documents progression of neurologic deterioration and confirms brain death (i.e., herniation of brain tissue) (Fig. 3.3). The neurologic evaluation of brainstem function primarily consists of assessment of pupil reactivity and size, respiratory pattern, oculomotor response, and motor response to painful stimuli.

Several herniation syndromes have been recognized, differing not only in presentation, but in mortality. Herniation represents maximal spatial exhaustion with an acute or chronic expansive pathologic process, is associated with marked intracranial hypertension until decompression occurs and usually denotes a poor prognosis unless corrected with aggressive ICP-

FIGURE 3.3 *Brainstem responses with progressive rostral-to-caudal herniation.* Abbreviations*: MLF, medial longitudinal fasciculus, EW, Edinger-Westphal nucleus. (From Shapiro,[4] with permission.)*

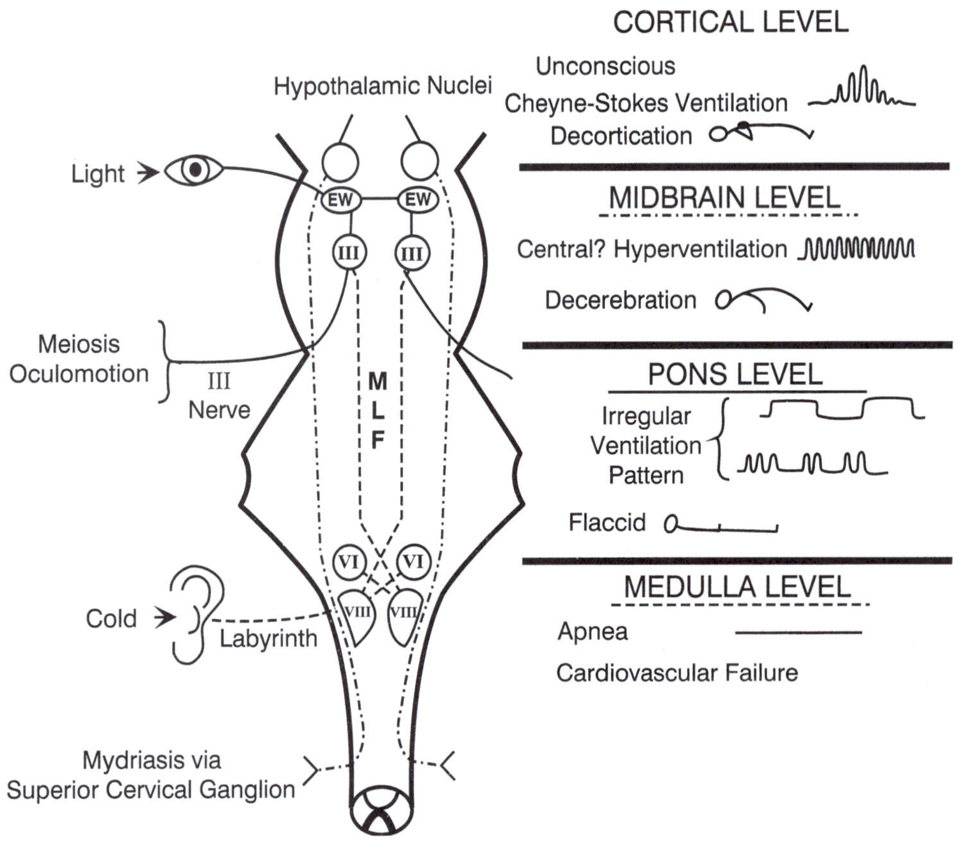

reducing measures. Herniation of brain tissue can occur downward or upward depending upon the site of the lesion and can even be transcalvarial if a bony defect exists (i.e., postoperative craniectomy site or, skull fracture) (Fig. 3.4). Neurologic deterioration from supratentorial lesions progresses in a rostral-to-caudal manner and if left untreated results in central, uncal, or tonsillar herniation. Expansion of infratentorial mass lesions causes tonsillar or upward cerebellar herniation. Subfalcine or cingulate herniation is associated with supratentorial lesions and is often asymptomatic unless the anterior cerebral artery is compromised; however, it can precede central (or transtentorial) herniation.

Central (or transtentorial) and uncal herniation are virtually indistinguishable once deterioration progresses to the pontine level. Central herniation differs from uncal herniation: (1) it often results from a more chronic pathologic process (i.e., tumor), and (2) it initially manifests with diencephalic dysfunction preceding midbrain involvement. Uncal herniation more commonly follows an acute injury, such as a rapidly expanding epidural hematoma, and involves either herniation of the medial uncus through the tentorial incisura or horizontal shifting of structures that may compromise or stretch the third cranial nerve, usually ipsilaterally, and the posterior cerebral artery.[47] Mental status is often impaired but is not a hallmark of early uncal herniation and reflects lateral displacement of the midbrain, not herniation.

FIGURE 3.4 *Sites of herniation.* A, *Subfalcine* B, *Transcalvarial (postoperative);* C, *Uncal;* D, *Tonsillar.*

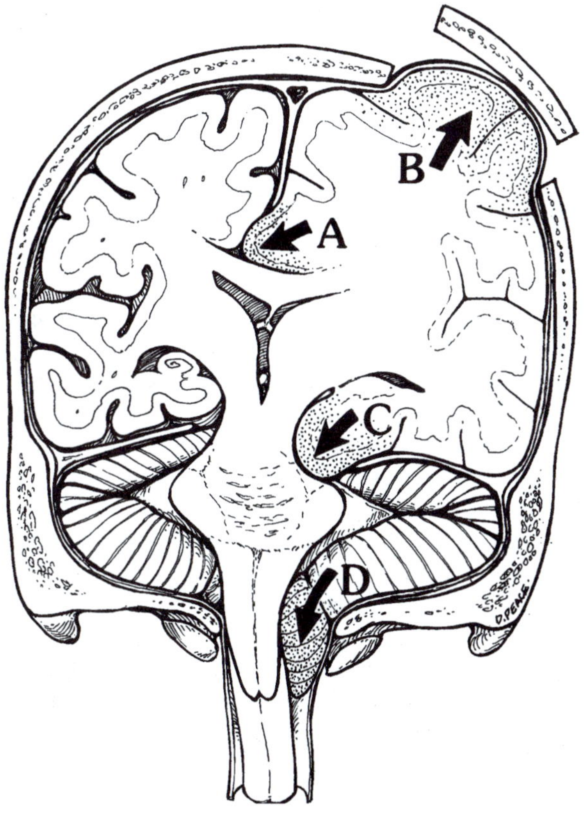

Diencephalic involvement occurs with central herniation as the structure is forced through the tentorial incisura and may be clinically detected by the development of diabetes insipidus from shearing of the pituitary stalk or blindness if the posterior cerebral arteries are compressed. There is early alteration of consciousness progressing to coma. The pupils are small but still minimally reactive, and gaze is conjugate as long as the brainstem is intact. The oculovestibular and oculocephalic reflexes remain intact, but upward gaze may become impaired as the superior colliculi and pretectum are compressed. A Cheyne-Stokes respiratory pattern predominates in the late diencephalic stage and is manifested as hyperpnea followed by apnea.[48] In the early diencephalic stage, the motor responses remain appropriate to painful stimuli but ultimately progress to decorticate posturing, usually contralateral to the mass lesion. As cerebral cortex function is lost, decorticate rigidity predominates, reflecting activity of the medullary reticulospinal tract.

The development of midbrain compression is associated with a poor prognosis with either central or uncal herniation, especially in the late stages. In central herniation, the pupils become dilated and fixed in midposition, reflecting impairment of the Edinger-Westphal nucleus comprised of parasympathetic fibers.[4] Pupillary findings are typically unilateral early in uncal herniation. With progressive third nerve compromise, a complete oculomotor nerve palsy occurs, resulting in unopposed fourth and sixth cranial nerves and a gaze that is typically described as "down and out." Early in midbrain compression, the oculovestibular and oculocephalic reflexes may be intact but are impaired or absent as herniation progresses. Testing of the oculocephalic reflex is contraindicated in patients with cervical spine injuries. A normal or Cheyne-Stokes respiratory pattern is replaced by hyperventilation at the midbrain level. True central neurogenic hyperventilation is rare and should only be a diagnosis of exclusion. In most instances, pulmonary dysfunction or shunting is responsible for hyperventilation in patients with neurologic injury. Central neurogenic hyperventilation is the result of a mesencephalic or pontine injury and reflects loss of descending inhibitory control of ventilation by the cerebral cortex.[48] In uncal herniation, hemiparesis ipsilateral to the cerebral lesion may occur as the contralateral cerebral peduncle is compressed (Kernohan's notch) and gives false localizing information to the physician.[49] Decorticate posturing is rare with uncal herniation, unlike central herniation. Decerebrate rigidity ultimately characterizes both central and uncal herniation. The input from the cerebral cortex and upper midbrain to the medullary reticulospinal tract is absent, rendering the activity of the pontine reticulospinal tract, with prominent effects on extensors, unopposed.

Central and uncal herniation are indistinguishable when deterioration to the pontine levels occurs (Fig. 3.3). Distortion of the pons is characterized by (1) pupils that are dilated and fixed in the midposition, (2) absence of oculovestibular and oculocephalic reflexes, and (3) flaccid motor response replaces bilateral decerebrate rigidity. Apneustic breathing, characterized by marked pauses at the end of inspiration, is common after pontine infarction but is rare with herniation.[48] Prognosis is grave as clinical deterioration progresses to the pontine level in either central or uncal herniation. Reversibility of herniation at this level depends upon the underlying pathologic process and the effectiveness of aggressive surgical or medical ICP-reducing maneuvers. For example, a rapidly expanding epidural hematoma may result in life-threatening herniation that can be reversed by emergent surgical decompression.

Medullary compression and distortion leads to terminal events. The pupils become fully dilated, and respiratory effort is irregular, marked by sighs or gasps ultimately replaced by apnea, reflecting compromise of the respiratory center. Hemodynamic instability manifested by hypertension, and tachycardia or bradycardia often precede cardiovascular collapse.

Significant hemodynamic alterations can occur as ICP rises and approaches the levels of diastolic blood pressure. Hemodynamic manifestations probably reflect brainstem compression or distortion secondary to elevated ICP but are not the direct result of intracranial hypertension alone. The triad of hypertension, bradycardia, and respiratory irregularities was first reported by Cushing in 1901, which he believed to be the sequelae of medullary ischemia.[1] The Cushing triad, as it has been termed, is rare and has most commonly been reported in association with infratentorial mass lesions. Its low incidence probably reflects earlier diagnosis of intracranial pathology and surgical intervention as well as improved monitoring techniques and aggressive treatment. Significant intracranial hypertension can be present without hemodynamic compromise.[50] The hemodynamic changes that can occur with intracranial hypertension are likely due to compression or distortion of the cardiovascular and respiratory centers of the medulla and not ischemia.

Tonsillar herniation from a supra or infratentorial lesion is a rapid, often fatal event if not immediately recognized and treated. The cerebellar tonsils descend through the foramen magnum compressing the lower brainstem resulting in fatal respiratory arrest. Tonsillar herniation is differentiated from central herniation by the rapidity of events and the narrow window of intervention to prevent death. Upward cerebellar herniation occurs with infratentorial lesions only and can be precipitated by supratentorial CSF drainage (decompression into a lower pressure compartment) or hyperventilation (similar principle to CSF drainage). The incidence of upward herniation with hyperventilation is probably very rare since the effects of hypocapnia are likely reflected equally in both supra- and infratentorial compartments. As the cerebellar vermis herniates upward through the incisura, the midbrain is compressed against the tentorial edges.

DIAGNOSTIC TESTING

Neuroradiologic Imaging

All patients with intracranial pathology and suspected intracranial hypertension undergo neuroradiologic imaging of the brain. Disease processes leading to abnormal intracranial elastance are detected by CT or magnetic resonance imaging (MRI) of the brain. Peritumor edema, diffuse cerebral edema, subarachnoid blood, hydrocephalus, compressed ambient cisterns, midline shift, and the presence of mass lesions only suggest elevated ICP but do not provide information quantifying the degree of ICP elevation (Fig. 3.5). In severely head-injured patients, the presence of midline shift and compressed ambient cisterns by CT imaging are highly predictive of increased ICP.[51] Herniation can be detected by radiologic imaging of the brain and is suggested by the obliteration of the ambient cisterns and may even occur through a skull defect if present (Figs. 3.6 and 3.7). When diagnosing herniation or degree of ICP elevation, correlation of CT or MRI findings with the neurologic exam is mandatory. A CT image may suggest elevated ICP (significant peritumor edema), but due to the chronicity of the disease process, the patient can be free of symptoms or signs suggestive of intracranial hypertension. A CT or MRI of the brain should only be used to diagnose underlying pathology and not for attempted quantitation of ICP.

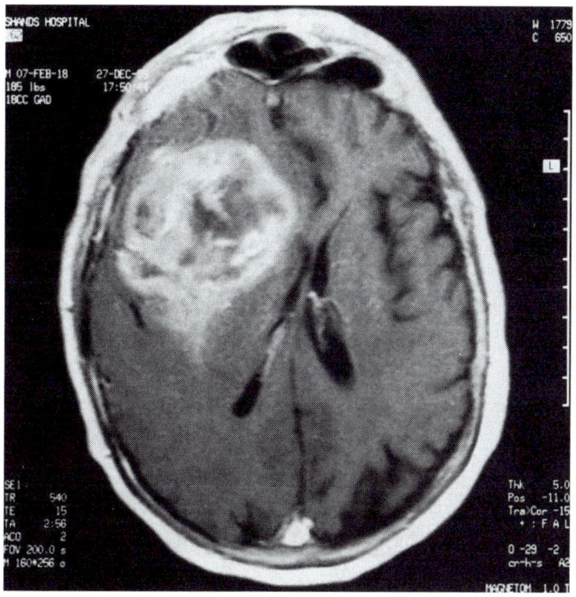

FIGURE 3.5 *T_1-weighted MRI of a glioblastoma multiforme of the frontal lobe with associated mass effect and subfalcine herniation.*

ICP Monitoring

The intraventricular catheter (or ventriculostomy) was introduced by Lundberg in 1960 and has remained the gold standard for ICP monitoring.[52] Over the subsequent years, newer monitoring modalities have been developed, and ICP can be recorded from an epidural, subdural, subarachnoid, ventricular, or intraparenchymal location depending upon the device used (Fig. 3.8). The monitoring devices in use include catheters, bolts, screws, and fiberoptic cables. Intracranial pressure monitoring is most often achieved from a supratentorial location and is less commonly employed in the posterior fossa due to the risk of cranial nerve or brainstem injury.[53] It is presumed that once the monitor is in position the ICP recorded is reflective of pressure in the supra- and infratentorial compartments in the absence of obstruction; however, global ICP may be in the normal range and local increases (i.e., surrounding a tumor) may exist. There must be communication between the two compartments for the ICP to be reflective of the other compartment. Rosenwasser et al. recorded simultaneous supra- and infratentorial pressures in 20 patients for 48 hours after surgical removal of a posterior fossa tumor.[53] Early in the postoperative period, pressure recorded in the infratentorial space exceeded that in the supratentorial compartment with equilibration

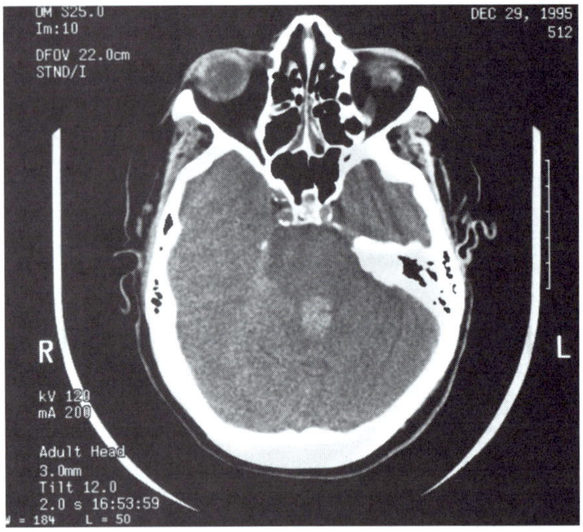

FIGURE 3.6 *Computed tomography scan of transtentorial herniation with obliteration of the pontine cisterns following a massive hemorrhagic stroke.*

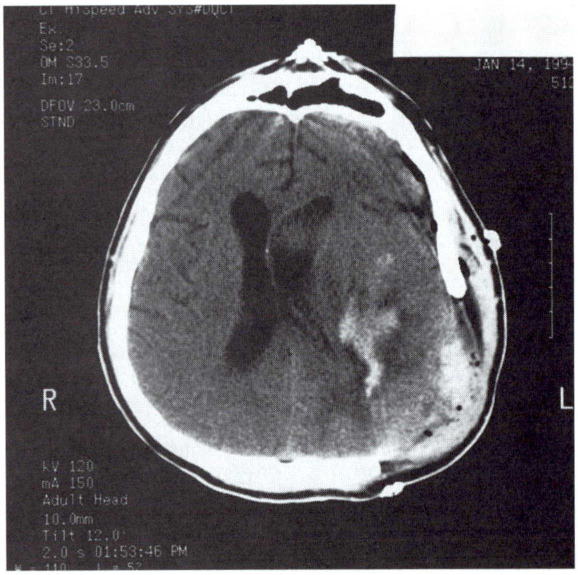

FIGURE 3.7 *Computed tomography scan of a large intracerebral hemorrhage following arteriovenous malformation resection with transcalvarial herniation.*

of pressure within 48 hours. Kaufmann and Clark observed a 10 mmHg pressure gradient between intraventricular and cervical subarachnoid recordings in comatose patients with transtentorial or tonsillar herniation documented at autopsy.[54]

An ICP monitor does not replace the neurologic exam but can guide treatment when the patient is comatose and intracranial hypertension is suspected. The Glasgow Coma Scale (GCS) is utilized to determine the appropriateness of ICP monitoring in head-injured patients (Table 3.1). A GCS of 8 or less in head-injured patients warrants consideration of the placement of a monitoring device.[55] Eisenberg et al. reported that 10 to 15% of patients with severe head injury and a relatively normal admission CT scan will develop evidence of intracranial hypertension.[51] O'Sullivan et al. documented intracranial hypertension at some time during hospitalization in seven of eight head-injured patients with a GCS of 8 or less and a normal admission CT scan.[55] Any therapeutic intervention that may elevate ICP (i.e., addition of positive end-expiratory pressure [PEEP]) in a patient with compromised intracranial elastance and coexisting medical illnesses (i.e., adult respiratory distress syndrome) warrants consideration of placement of an ICP monitor. Ventriculostomies are commonly placed in patients with aneurysmal subarachnoid hemorrhage with hydrocephalus or a Hunt-Hess grade of 3 or greater (with suspected ICP elevations without hydrocephalus) prior to aneurysm clipping (see Ch. 8). In this patient population, ventriculostomies are placed primarily to drain CSF and must be done so cautiously to avoid acute reductions in ICP that can alter the transmural pressure across the aneurysm, predisposing to rebleeding. ICP monitors may be placed prior to tumor resection for optimization of perioperative management. The presence of a coagulopathy precludes the placement of an ICP monitor in most scenarios at least until the bleeding diathesis has been adequately corrected. This issue has become even more relevant with the increased number of liver transplantations being performed, some of which will be done in encephalopathic patients with coexisting coagulopathy. Indications for ICP monitoring and the device utilized often reflect the bias and experience of the neurosurgeon and any institutional protocols that exist.

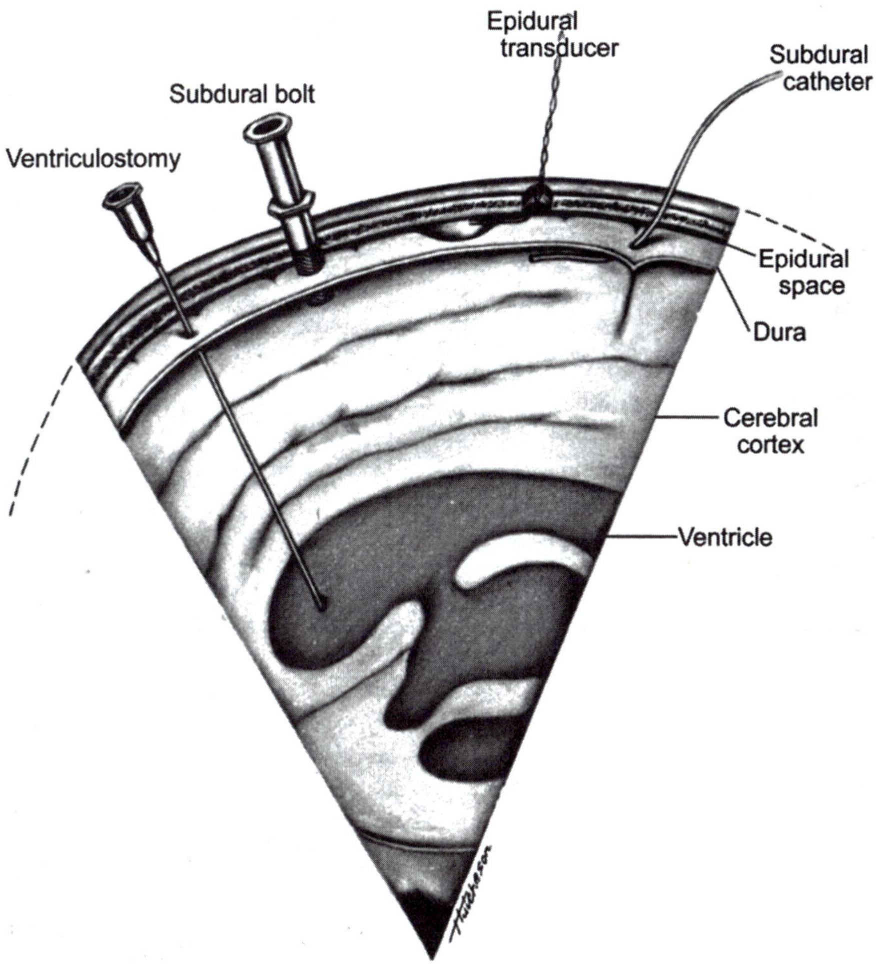

FIGURE 3.8 *Intracranial pressure monitoring sites with different devices. (From Cucchiara et al.,[252] with permission.)*

TABLE 3.1 *Glasgow Coma Scale*

POINTS	EYE OPENING	VERBAL RESPONSE	MOTOR RESPONSE
6			Obeys
5		Oriented	Localizes to pain
4	Spontaneous	Disoriented	Flexion withdrawal to pain
3	To speech	Inappropriate	Decorticate rigidity
2	To pain	Incomprehensible	Decerebrate rigidity
1	None	None or intubated	None

The intraventricular catheter has been the "gold standard" for the development of improved recording devices and has been used repeatedly to determine the accuracy of new monitors. In addition to recording ICP, an intraventricular catheter has the added therapeutic advantage of CSF drainage and can be used concurrently to treat intracranial hypertension. The drainage of CSF is a feature unique to the intraventricular catheter. Technical problems limit its use in patients with small or compressed ventricles as seen in pseudotumor cerebri or a large brain tumor. Placement of an intraventricular catheter requires more skill than with other monitoring devices, has been associated with a higher incidence of infection and has a greater potential to cause brain injury during placement.

The subarachnoid bolt or screw has also been popular over the last few years. It is associated with a lower incidence of infection and less potential for brain injury and requires less skill to place. Mollman et al. determined that the subarachnoid bolt was less accurate for ICP monitoring when compared to either a subarachnoid catheter or ventriculostomy technique.[56] The accuracy of the subarachnoid catheter paralleled that of the intraventricular catheter. When ICP is high, subarachnoid bolts are less reliable due to obstruction of the lumen of the bolt by brain tissue and produces falsely low readings.

Fiberoptic ICP monitoring systems have become popular over recent years. The monitor can be placed in the intraparenchymal, subdural, or intraventricular compartment. Fiberoptic monitors have proven to be reliable, accurate devices when compared to intraventricular monitors.[57] The devices have major drawbacks including significant drift, inability to recalibrate in vivo, expense of the monitor, and fragility of the fiberoptic catheter.[58] A cumulative drift of ± 6 mmHg over a 5-day period, maximum ± 2.5 mmHg/day, has been documented with fiberoptic systems.[58] It is generally recommended that these devices be replaced every 5 days to minimize false readings and infectious complications.

A new ICP monitor recently introduced utilizes a microchip pressure transducer and not a fiberoptic cable. From initial reports, these ICP systems provide distinct advantages over the fiberoptic device: (1) minimal drift and (2) increased durability since a fiberoptic cable is not utilized. The catheters are flexible, not prone to breakage and demonstrate accurate ICP waveforms. A less than 1 mmHg drift has been reported over 9 days in rabbits (Codman, Johnson and Johnson). Similar to the fiberoptic device, calibration must be performed prior to insertion into the patient.

The incidence of complications associated with ICP monitors ranges from approximately 1 to 7.7%.[53] Because placement of an ICP monitoring device is associated with risk and morbidity, a strong indication must be present for placement. A variety of complications have been reported and include infection, hemorrhage, brain injury, seizures, and CSF leaks.[52,53,57] Intracranial pressure monitoring of the posterior fossa poses additional risks to the brainstem and cranial nerves. Technical problems or malfunction of the device can be encountered and specifically include significant monitor drift, inability to recalibrate in vivo, fragility, and occlusion of the catheter.

INTRACRANIAL PRESSURE WAVEFORMS

The morphology of the physiologic ICP waveform is comprised of small pulsations corresponding to the systolic arterial pressure wave and the central venous A wave and is influenced by the normal respiratory pattern (Fig. 3.9).[59] The pulsations of the ICP waveform reflect transmission of the systemic blood pressure to the intracranial compartment. The initial, larger peak (or pulsation) of the ICP waveform is 1 to 2 mmHg in amplitude with a small dicrotic notch, correlates with the systolic arterial pressure wave, and increases in amplitude with an elevation in the systolic component of the systemic arterial pressure.[60] Smaller peaks follow the di-

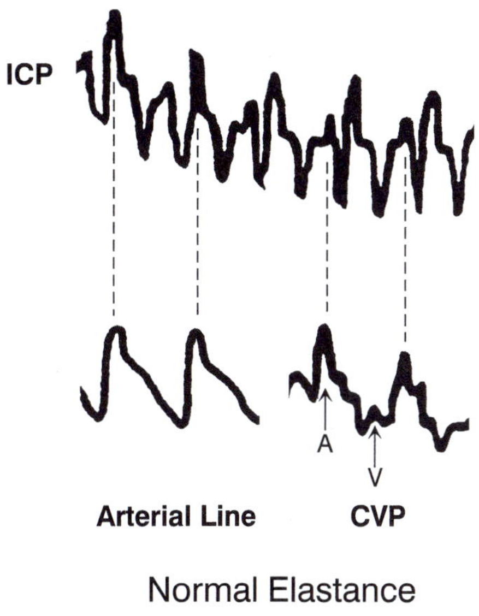

FIGURE 3.9 *Correlation of pulsations of the ICP waveform with components of the arterial and central venous pressure tracings. The initial peak of the ICP waveform corresponds to the systolic component of the systemic arterial waveform. The subsequent peak correlates to the central venous A wave from the right atrium.*

crotic notch, and their significance is unknown. A smaller, distinct peak follows the initial peak of the ICP waveform and has been termed the *central venous A wave*, originating from the right atrium.[59] When cannon A waves are observed on the central venous pressure tracing (i.e., junctional rhythms, heart block, and tricuspid atresia), the ICP waveform changes morphology becoming more venous appearing. The pulsations of the ICP waveform are superimposed on large background sinusoidal waves resulting from normal inspiration and expiration. Intracranial pressure increases with expiration during spontaneous ventilation, and the opposite effect is observed in mechanically ventilated patients and when CSF pressure is recorded in the lumbar subarachnoid space, which is influenced by pressure in the inferior vena cava. As ICP rises to 20 to 30 mmHg, the pulsations of venous origin disappear, and the morphology of the ICP waveform assumes an arterialized shape.[59] It is postulated that the cerebrovascular tone and elastance of the intracranial compartment influence the morphology of the ICP waveform during intracranial hypertension. Cerebral vasodilation allows the systemic arterial blood pressure to be more readily transmitted to the intracranial space. During hypoxemia, the ICP waveform has a prominent arterial shape presumably due to cerebral vasodilation; the waveform observed with hypoxemia mimics that detected with intracranial hypertension.

Pathologic pressure waves were first described by Lundberg in 1960 in patients with brain tumors and associated intracranial hypertension.[52] These waves have been named Lundberg A (plateau), B, and C waves. Plateau, or A waves, have the most clinical relevance in the setting of intracranial hypertension but are rarely seen with aggressive treatment of elevated ICP (Fig. 3.10).[60] Plateau waves are typically abrupt in appearance with an amplitude

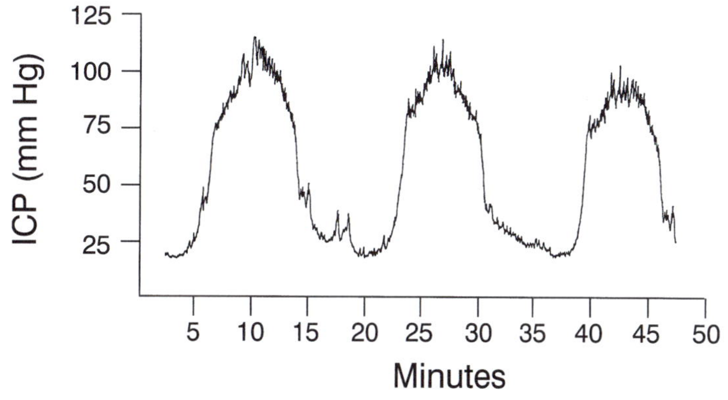

FIGURE 3.10 *The abrupt appearance of plateau waves in a patient with a brain tumor and intracranial hypertension.*

increase of 50 to 100 mmHg above baseline and duration of 5 to 20 minutes or longer.[52,60,61] The presence of plateau waves is an ominous finding, and if ICP is not aggressively treated, decompensation and death will ensue. It is generally accepted that plateau waves do not occur until spatial exhaustion has occurred, placing the patient on a tenuous portion of the pressure-volume curve. Plateau waves are often accompanied by headache, nausea, alteration in consciousness, hyperpnea, or decerebrate rigidity.[60] Systemic hypertension, although not invariably present, can accompany plateau waves.

The clinical significance, if any, of Lundberg B and C waves remains unclear. B waves, or 1/min waves, occur at a frequency of 0.5 to 2/min with an amplitude ranging from imperceptible to 50 mmHg and have been associated with abnormal respiratory patterns.[52,60–62] Newell and colleagues determined that B waves are the result of vasomotor waves producing transient alterations in CBV and CBF amplified in the ICP waveform, especially when intracranial elastance is increased.[62] Vasomotor waves are produced by constriction and dilation of small cerebral arteries by an unknown central regulating mechanism, causing fluctuations in V_{mca} (or CBF). They can occur under normal circumstances at a frequency of 0.5 to 2/minute. In this study, B waves were still present during mechanical ventilation, dispelling the notion that CO_2 may play some role in their etiology.[62]

Lundberg C waves have a frequency of 4 to 8/min with a lower amplitude (usually less than 30 mmHg) and may be related to Traube-Hering-Mayer variations of the systemic blood pressure.[60,61] C waves have been observed superimposed on the plateau wave and in this instance herald a terminal event.

Transcranial Doppler

Transcranial Doppler monitoring has become an increasingly important adjuvant for the diagnosis of elevated ICP and brain death when performed by an experienced technologist and utilized in conjunction with the clinical exam. Transcranial Doppler imaging provides an inexpensive, noninvasive bedside method to document severe intracranial hypertension, brain death, and cerebral vasospasm. It currently must be used in conjunction with the clinical exam (brainstem reflexes) to document brain death. Transcranial Doppler imaging is an ultrasound technique that is utilized to determine blood flow velocity and its direction through a major cerebral artery (anterior or posterior circulation) and reflects the status of the vascular resistance or tone of the vessel. As ICP increases, approaching diastolic arterial pressure levels, the diastolic flow velocity diminishes, approaches zero, and then reverses flow (Fig. 3.11).[63] In a series of 37 patients with intracranial hypertension studied by TCD, brain death was associated with one of three patterns: diastolic flow reversal, small systolic spikes, or absence of signal.[63] In a TCD study of comatose patients, the absence or reversal of diastolic flow or presence of systolic spikes in at least two vessels was 91.3% sensitive and 100% specific for the diagnosis of brain death.[64] An absent signal should be interpreted cautiously and verified in other vessels. A signal from the middle cerebral artery, for instance, can be difficult to detect in older women and when the temporal bone is ossified.

Somatosensory and Brainstem Auditory-Evoked Potentials

Multimodality-evoked potentials, including somatosensory and brainstem auditory-evoked potentials, can be used to diagnose brain death and neurologic outcome in comatose patients. Both evoked potential recording modalities are not accepted as diagnostic criteria alone and should be used with knowledge of the neurologic exam. In 41 children with a GCS of less than 8 studied with somatosensory and brainstem auditory-evoked potentials, patterns were described that predicted brain death and chronic vegetative states.[65] The absence of all waveforms except wave I in a brainstem auditory-evoked potential recording accompanied by absence of cortical somatosensory-evoked potentials (with preserved peripheral responses) reliably predicted

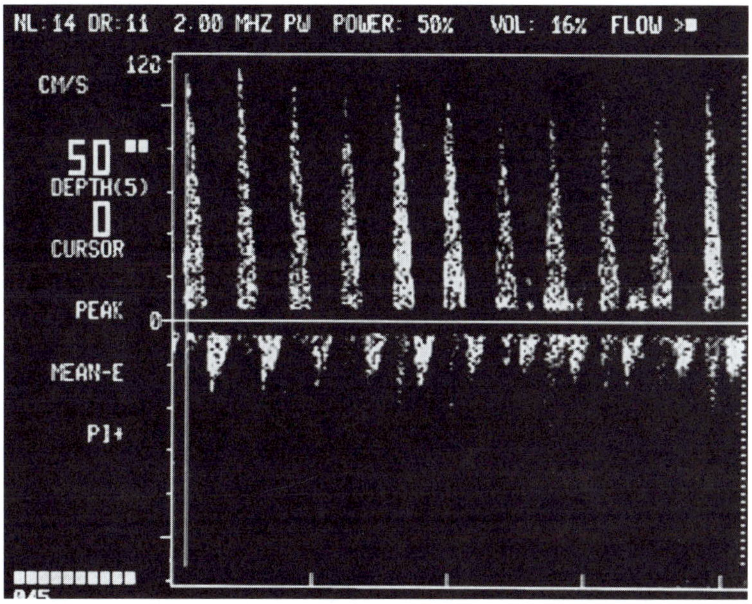

FIGURE 3.11 *Transcranial Doppler image depicting diastolic flow reversal in a patient with severe intracranial hypertension and ultimate brain death.*

brain death (Fig. 3.12) In some brain-dead patients, wave I may be absent secondary to destruction of the organ of Corti with cell loss in the cochlear nucleus. Ototoxic drug administration can also lead to loss of wave I. In the presence of normal or abnormal brainstem auditory-evoked potentials and absence of cortical somatosensory-evoked potentials, a persistent vegetative state is predicted. Some authors report that a prolonged I to V interpeak latency of the brainstem auditory-evoked potentials suggests elevated ICP and herniation; however, it is not cost-effective to employ multimodality-evoked potentials to diagnose intracranial hypertension unless brain death is suspected.[66]

EFFECTS OF ANESTHETICS AND DRUGS ON ICP

The selection of an anesthetic technique and supplemental drugs for a patient with intracranial hypertension should be tailored to meet the following goals: (1) maintenance of adequate CBF, (2) minimizing ICP elevations, (3) ability to provide cerebral protective measures if necessary to prevent further neurologic insult, and (4) ability to reduce ICP. It is important for the anesthesiologist to recognize the impact that anesthetic agents or pharmacologic interventions may have in improving or worsening primary underlying pathology. The use of agents to prevent or attenuate secondary neuronal injury following cerebral ischemia may become as important as treatment directed toward treatment of the primary injury.

Inhalational Agents

HALOTHANE In animals and humans, halothane is a potent cerebral vasodilator that increases CBF by a reduction in CVR and deleteriously affects ICP, especially in the presence of an intracranial mass.[67–69] It is well accepted that halothane increases CBF in a dose-related fashion, and most agree that it increases the ratio of CBF to $CMRO_2$ to a greater extent than other volatile agents in clinical use, reflecting its potent cerebral vasodilating properties.[70] There is, however, some evidence to suggest that halothane and isoflurane have similar influences on global CBF and only exhibit their differences

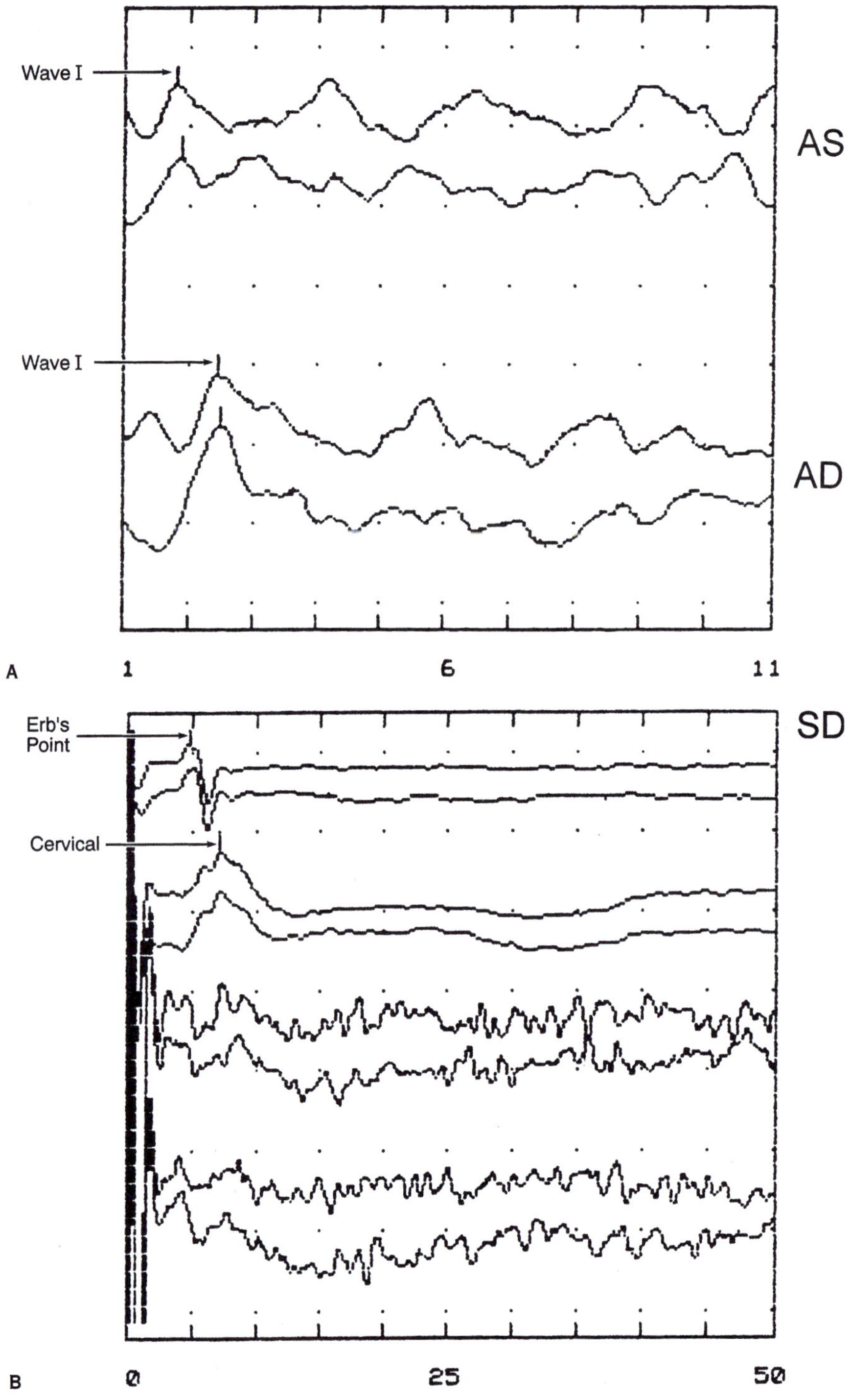

FIGURE 3.12 *Brainstem auditory evoked potentials from right and left ear stimulation (A) and somatosensory-evoked potentials from right (B)*

(Figure continues.)

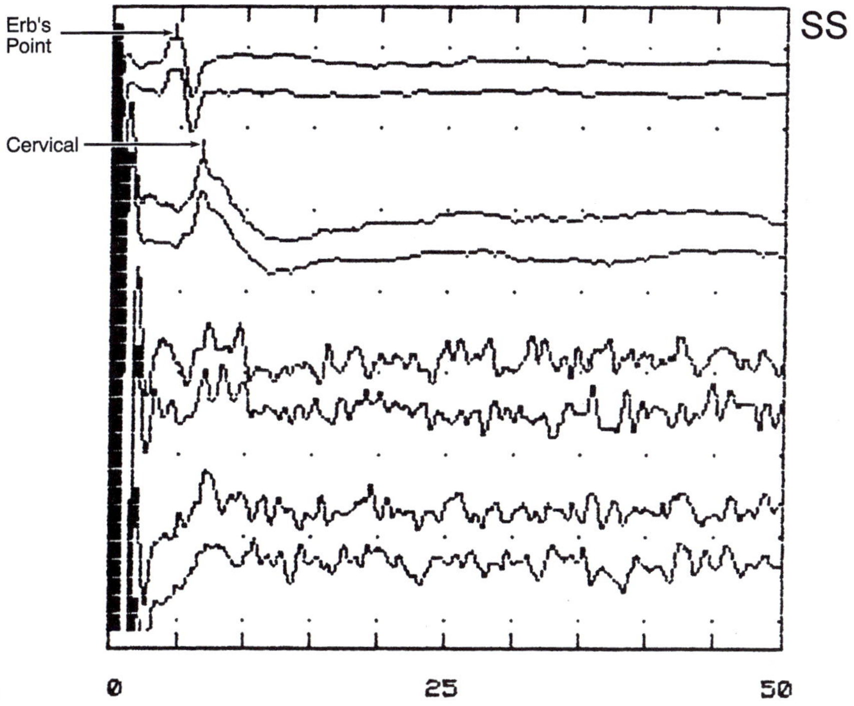

FIGURE 3.12 *(Continued) and left (C) median nerve stimulation consistent with brain death in a child with diffuse cerebral edema after a drowning episode. There is presence of wave I only bilaterally (A) with absent cortical somatosensory-evoked potentials (B&C).*

in blood flow regionally.[71–73] When comparing cerebrovascular and metabolic effects of volatile agents, interpretations and conclusions must account for differences in animal models, CBF techniques, and background anesthetics employed.

Halothane decreases $CMRO_2$, yet it has powerful vasodilating properties that predominate except at very low concentrations of agent. Most human and animal studies agree that the cerebral metabolic depressant effects of halothane are less pronounced than those induced by isoflurane when equipotent doses of anesthetic are compared.[74] The uncoupling of $CMRO_2$ and CBF characteristic of volatile agents is exaggerated with halothane use. Theye and Michenfelder reported an average reduction of 17% in $CMRO_2$ with clinically relevant doses of halothane (up to 1% halothane) in dogs and attributed this reduction to a direct metabolic depressant effect on the brain.[74] A dose-dependent biphasic flow pattern has been observed with halothane. In a study of normocapnic baboons administered halothane with phencyclidine and nitrous oxide as background anesthetics, $CMRO_2$ and CBF both declined at low concentrations of halothane, 0.375% or less.[75] The initial CBF decrease observed paralleled the reduction in $CMRO_2$. As halothane concentrations were increased in the presence of blood pressure support, $CMRO_2$ continued to decline, but the vasodilatory effects of the anesthetic predominated, resulting in increased CBF. Cerebral oxygen consumption decreases nonlinearly and reaches a plateau at 1.0 MAC of halothane without evidence of disruption of oxidative phosphorylation.[76,77] An isoelectric EEG is not produced until halothane concentrations of 4.5% are reached. As halothane concentrations exceed 2.3%, $CMRO_2$ decreases in a dose-related fashion irrespective of the presence of EEG activity or silence, unlike isoflurane or thiopental, with evidence of toxic effects on cerebral metabolic pathways.[78]

In most animal and human studies, administration of clinically relevant concentrations of halothane consistently increases CBF and CBV by lowering CVR. In craniectomized cats anesthetized with varying but equipotent concentrations of halothane, enflurane, or isoflurane, greater brain protrusion was observed with halothane than with either isoflurane or enflurane, (except enflurane at 0.5 MAC concentration).[70] When the arterial blood pressure was supported, the amount of cortical protrusion caused by halothane was even more profound when compared to isoflurane or enflurane. Adams et al. established that initiation of hyperventilation ($PaCO_2$ less than 30 mmHg) prior to institution of halothane attenuated or prevented elevations of CSF pressure (CSFP) in patients with intracranial pathology.[67] When hyperventilation and halothane were initiated simultaneously, increases in CSFP were not consistently prevented, and elevations were clinically significant. All elevations in CSFP occurred within 1 to 5 minutes of halothane administration and were transient, declining toward baseline values within 10 to 30 minutes. In the presence of intracranial pathology, a catastrophic reduction in CPP may result not only from elevations in ICP but from exacerbation by associated systemic hypotension with halothane use.

Recent animal studies suggest that halothane and isoflurane may have similar effects on global CBF, exerting their differences only on a regional level.[71,73] Similar hemispheric CBF was observed in rats hemodynamically supported during exposure to either 1.0 MAC of halothane or isoflurane.[71] Cortical CBF was consistently higher in those animals exposed to halothane. Isoflurane predominantly influenced blood flow in subcortical structures. Eintrei et al. reported a similar finding in humans with brain tumors anesthetized with a combined 1.5 MAC concentration of nitrous oxide and halothane, isoflurane, or enflurane.[72] Regional cerebral blood flow tripled (increase of 166%) with halothane; small or no changes in rCBF resulted from enflurane and isoflurane exposure, respectively. It is speculated that halothane and isoflurane may have different metabolic effects on cortical and subcortical structures.

Halothane's effect on ICP results from increased CBV, alterations of CSF dynamics, or a combination of the two. The mechanism of anesthetic-induced cerebral vasodilation is not well understood. Jensen et al. recently demonstrated that halothane remains a potent vasodilator even in vessels devoid of endothelium.[79] This study does not support a membrane-bound receptor or endothelium-dependent mechanism (i.e., endothelium-derived relaxing factor) for halothane-induced vasodilation. Direct smooth muscle relaxation or cerebral vessel relaxation in response to a second messenger, such as cyclic adenosine monophosphate, are also proposed mechanisms. Alteration of the normal CSF pathways probably contributes to the late sustained increase in CSFP that has been recorded with prolonged halothane exposure. Resistance to reabsorption of CSF has been observed in dogs anesthetized with halothane.[80] Any disruption in normal CSF dynamics increases CSF volume and in the presence of a space-occupying lesion elevates ICP.

The reactivity of the cerebral circulation to CO_2 is preserved with halothane at 1.0 MAC anesthesia. Reactivity to CO_2 is enhanced with isoflurane-nitrous oxide compared to a halothane-nitrous oxide technique.[81] Cerebral autoregulation is, however, impaired to a greater extent with halothane than with isoflurane or enflurane.[69,70,75] Autoregulation may be impaired but not abolished with halothane concentrations as low as 0.5%.[82] The duration of impairment during anesthesia is not known.

In neuroanesthesia practice, halothane should be utilized cautiously in patients with suspected or documented intracranial hypertension. Halothane can be administered relatively safely as long as low concentrations are employed and hyperventilation is established prior to its use. In current clinical practice, there are safer, alternative inhalational agents that can be substituted for halothane in patients with space-occupying lesions.

ENFLURANE Enflurane has cerebral metabolic depressant activity similar to halothane, although its cerebral vasodilating properties are significantly weaker. Enflurane produces a nonlinear, dose-dependent reduction in $CMRO_2$ attaining maximal supression at 1.0 MAC anesthetic levels.[76,77] Minimal changes are evident beyond 1.0 MAC enflurane. Enflurane possesses epileptogenic activity when used in high doses in combination with extreme levels of hypocapnia. In dogs anesthetized with 1.5 MAC enflurane, Michenfelder and Cucchiara documented reproducible seizure activity precipitated by hyperventilation (to $PaCO_2$ 20 mmHg) and auditory stimuli.[76] During the seizure activity, $CMRO_2$ rose by 48% and was accompanied, as anticipated, by a parallel increase in CBF.

Animal studies demonstrate that enflurane is a cerebral vasodilator increasing CBF and CBV in a dose-dependent fashion, although these effects are less pronounced when compared to halothane.[70,76,83] The CBF changes with enflurane, as seen with halothane and isoflurane, can be augmented by maintenance of arterial blood pressure. Enflurane caused brain surface protrusion in cats similar to isoflurane (except at 0.5 MAC concentrations) and was exaggerated with blood pressure support, albeit, protrusion was significantly less than that caused by halothane.[70] Enflurane's effects on human cerebral vasculature is less clear than in animals. In humans, enflurane is a cerebral vasodilator and likely increases CBF but to a significantly lesser extent than halothane. Similar to halothane, enflurane has regionally selective effects on CBF. Eintrei et al. documented a 35% increase in rCBF (or cortical) with a 1.5 MAC combination of enflurane and nitrous oxide.[72]

Intracranial pressure elevation has been reported in animals and humans with enflurane anesthesia, especially with high concentrations of agent and in the presence of intracranial pathology.[83–85] In the absence of pathology, ICP elevations are relatively small and insignificant. When lower concentrations of volatile agent are utilized, ICP elevations, even in patients with mass lesions, are small.[86] In normocapnic dogs with baseline intracranial hypertension secondary to epidural balloon inflation, 3% enflurane use caused significant increases in ICP and clinical signs of herniation (unilateral dilated pupil) in two animals.[84] Establishment of hyperventilation concurrent with enflurane use can prevent or attenuate elevations in ICP. Cerebrovascular reactivity to CO_2 is well preserved with the use of enflurane anesthesia at near MAC levels, allowing appropriate CBF changes with alterations in CO_2. Intracranial pressure elevations are proposed to result from increased CBV and disruption of CSF homeostasis. Artru reported an increased resistance to reabsorption and rate of production of CSF in dogs exposed to prolonged enflurane anesthesia.[87]

Enflurane is an acceptable volatile anesthetic for intracranial procedures as long as low concentrations of agent are used and hyperventilation is initiated to prevent ICP increases. The combination of high concentrations of enflurane and aggressive hyperventilation should be avoided to prevent precipitating seizure activity and associated deleterious increases in $CMRO_2$ and CBF. The availability of alternative inhalational agents without epileptogenic properties have made enflurane an unpopular volatile agent in clinical neuroanesthesia.

ISOFLURANE Isoflurane has profound nonlinear (at less than 1.0 MAC anesthesia), dose-related cerebral metabolic depressant properties when compared to halothane or enflurane at equipotent doses. With 2.0 MAC isoflurane in dogs, an isoelectric EEG is produced at which point $CMRO_2$ reduction is maximal.[88,89] Increasing anesthetic depth (up to 4.0 MAC) is not accompanied by further reductions in $CMRO_2$ and is not associated with disruption of the cerebral metabolic pathways.[89] Because of its potent metabolic effects, isoflurane has been used as a cerebral protective agent during temporary arterial occlusion for complicated aneurysm clipping and during carotid endarterectomies.[35,90] It is becomingly increasingly apparent, though, that a drug's ability to produce an isoelectric EEG does not always equate to cerebral protection. A drug's ability to convey cerebral protection is probably multifactorial, involving not only $CMRO_2$ reduction, but perhaps the ability to scavenge free radicals, inhibit release of excitatory amino acids, or interfere with calcium influx into the cell. In a recent study by Drummond et al., the extent of brain injury in rats subjected to focal cerebral ischemia was significantly greater when cerebral protection was provided by isoflurane or etomidate titrated to EEG burst suppression.[91] Thiopental titrated to EEG burst suppression afforded the greatest cerebral protection. It was speculated by these investigators that the vasodilation produced by high-dose isoflurane increased ICP, reduced effective CPP during MCA occlusion, and ultimately worsened extent of injury and outcome. Of interest, the control group of animals anesthetized with 1.2 MAC halothane had less brain injury than either the isoflurane or etomidate group.

Isoflurane is a moderate cerebral vasodilator increasing CBF in a dose-related manner in dogs.[88,92] As observed with halothane and enflurane, a decline in CVR accounts for the change in CBF and CBV. In humans, minimal CBF changes occur with isoflurane concentrations of 1 to 2%.[93–95] Profound changes have been observed, however, when nitrous oxide is substituted for an equipotent concentration of isoflurane.[93,96,97] In humans with intracranial disease, Lam et al. found that the combination of nitrous oxide and isoflurane (0.5 MAC isoflurane and 0.6 MAC nitrous oxide) resulted in a higher V_{mca} and metabolic rate ($AVDO_2$) than an equipotent concentration of isoflurane.[93] A similar study was published earlier by Algotsson and colleagues, reporting similar results except no change in $CMRO_2$ with nitrous oxide administration.[96] Both studies validate concerns that nitrous oxide is a potent cerebral vasodilator. Nitrous oxide is often used clinically to reduce the concentration of isoflurane, but its substitution for an equipotent dose of volatile agent is probably contraindicated in patients with intracranial pathology where changes in CBF are likely to alter ICP in a deleterious fashion. In humans and animals, isoflurane selectively affects subcortical and lower brain structure CBF possibly reflecting preferential metabolic changes in those areas of the brain.[71–73]

Isoflurane, given its cerebral vasodilating properties, may elevate ICP, especially in patients with increased intracranial elastance. Establishing hyperventilation ($PaCO_2$ 25 to 30 mmHg) simultaneously with introduction of isoflurane consistently prevented elevations in CSFP in patients with intracranial pathology.[98] Unlike halothane, hyperventilation does not need to be initiated prior to isoflurane administration. When nitrous oxide and isoflurane are utilized together, hyperventilation does not consistently prevent increases in CBF.[96] Relative to halothane, the effect of isoflurane on ICP is small and is the preferred agent for use in individuals with space-occupying lesions. Increases in ICP in response to isoflurane result from cerebral vasodilation alone. Resistance to reabsorption of CSF is lowered and the rate of CSF production is unaffected with isoflurane, both of which enhance spatial compensation.[87,99]

Cerebrovascular reactivity to CO_2 is also well preserved with isoflurane anesthesia in animals and humans. Cerebral blood flow response to alterations in $PaCO_2$ is appropriate at 1.0 and 2.0 MAC of isoflurane in dogs.[88,92] Cerebral autoregulation remains intact at 1.0 MAC of isoflurane but is significantly attenuated or abolished at 2.0 MAC of isoflurane.[73,92] In rats, autoregulation is attenuated at low doses of isoflurane, but this observation has not been validated in humans.[82] Hoffman et al. found that autoregulation is impaired at 1.0 MAC of isoflurane in the midbrain and spinal cord but preserved at cortical and subcortical levels in rats.[73] At 2.0 MAC of isoflurane, impairment was evident in all brain regions with the most substantial attenuation in the midbrain and spinal cord.

Isoflurane remains a safe volatile agent for use in intracranial procedures. Isoflurane is a cerebral vasodilator; however, hyperventilation initiated concurrently with introduction of isoflurane readily prevents elevation in ICP. The replacement of isoflurane by an equipotent dose of nitrous oxide has significant effects on CBF when compared to the use of the same MAC concentration of isoflurane alone. In patients with existing intracranial disease, the combination of nitrous oxide and isoflurane should be avoided since elevations in CBF in this scenario cannot be consistently prevented with hyperventilation.

SEVOFLURANE Sevoflurane is a new ether inhalational anesthetic possessing a low blood:gas partition coefficient that provides for a rapid induction and emergence, both of which are ideal for neurosurgical patients. In limited animal studies available, sevoflurane has metabolic and cerebrovascular effects strikingly similar to isoflurane.

Sevoflurane causes minimal effects on CBF with even high doses (1.5, 2.0, 2.5 MAC).[100,101] In three rabbits anesthetized with 0.5 or 1.0 MAC end-tidal concentrations of sevoflurane, sagittal sinus CBF was significantly elevated but was not reflected regionally in cortical CBF values.[100]

Reduction in $CMRO_2$ appears dose related and is reported to decline by 50% at 1.0 MAC end-tidal concentrations.[100] Burst suppression of the EEG is observed at 2.15 MAC sevoflurane in dogs. Sevoflurane may have epileptogenic activity similar to enflurane, a property that would make this agent undesirable in neurosurgical patients. Scheller et al. were not able to elicit seizure activity clinically or by EEG in hyperventilated dogs anesthetized with concentrations up to 2.5 MAC even with auditory stimuli.[101] In this study, one normocapnic animal had evidence of seizures with 2.0 MAC sevoflurane that could not be reproduced with the inition of hyperventilation and auditory stimuli. In contrast, a recent study by Osawa et al. demonstrated reproducible seizure activity in 2 of 13 cats exposed to 5% sevoflurane, hyperventilation ($PaCO_2$ 29 to 31 mmHg), and peripheral stimulation.[102] At this depth of anesthesia, amplitude of the cortical somatosensory-evoked potential was augmented, similar to the effects of etomidate, when compared to responses at 3% sevoflurane. At 5% sevoflurane, EEG activity was still present in structures of the limbic system, whereas the neocortex was isoelectric. From preliminary studies, sevoflurane may possess epileptogenic properties that are weaker and elicited by higher concentrations than enflurane.

Intracranial pressure elevations have been reported resulting from alterations in CBV and can be prevented by establishing hypocapnia that, in animals, was initiated prior to anesthetic administration.[103] If sevoflurane behaves similarly to isoflurane, ICP elevations can probably be prevented by simultaneous introduction of hyperventilation and sevoflurane use. Cerebrovascular reactivity to CO_2 and cerebral autoregulation are preserved in humans at 0.88 MAC levels of sevoflurane.[104] There are limited data defining the anesthetic depth at which cerebral autoregulation is attenuated or abolished.

Sevoflurane closely resembles isoflurane in its effects on CBF, $CMRO_2$, and CBV. The data are conflicting: sevoflurane may precipitate seizure activity at high anesthetic concentrations but has less propensity to evoke than does enflurane.

DESFLURANE Desflurane is another new volatile anesthetic with a blood:gas partition coefficient resembling nitrous oxide, allowing for rapid emergence to the evaluate the neurologic status of the patient. Desflurane is a potent cerebral vasodilator and thus has the potential to produce adverse effects on CBF and CBV particularly when intracranial elastance is abnormal.[105–108] Cerebral blood flow increases in a dose-dependent manner and is augmented by hemodynamic support in dogs.[106] Reductions in $CMRO_2$ following EEG changes are similar to isoflurane. At 2.0 MAC desflurane, EEG activity is suppressed with polyspiking, often seen with isoflurane, and there is no alteration of oxidative phosphorylation with high concentrations of anesthetic.[106] The response of the cerebral vasculature to CO_2 is intact in dogs and humans at clinically relevant concentrations of desflurane.[107,109]

Desflurane's effect on ICP is controversial, particularly in humans. Intracranial pressure elevations have been documented in canine studies and are similar to those reported under isoflurane anesthesia in the absence of pathology.[106,107] It is speculated that the ICP elevations are attributable to an elevated CBV reflecting desflurane's potent vasodilating properties. Muzzi and colleagues studied the effects of 1.0 MAC desflurane or isoflurane on CSFP in patients with supratentorial lesions with mass effect hyperventilated ($PaCO_2$ 24 to 28 mmHg) prior to administration of the volatile agent.[105] A progressive increase in CSFP was documented in the group under desflurane anesthesia, and no significant change was seen in the isoflurane group. In contrast, Ornstein et al. found no significant difference in CBF values in hyperventilated patients receiving equipotent doses of either desflurane or isoflurane.[109] Until additional studies are available, desflurane should be used cautiously in patients with abnormal intracranial elastance.

NITROUS OXIDE For years nitrous oxide has been widely used as a supplemental anesthetic during neurosurgical procedures and was previously considered to be safe with minimal effects on CBF and ICP. Cerebral blood flow studies have often been difficult to interpret due to species differences, CBF technique, or the use of supplemental anesthetics with the potential to profoundly effect the cerebral vasculature and metabolism. There is now substantial evidence to suggest that nitrous oxide has powerful cerebral vasodilating properties.

Cerebral blood flow has been consistently shown to increase with nitrous oxide alone or in combination with volatile anesthetics in both animals and humans.[110–113] Nitrous oxide alone can substantially elevate CBF; however, some investigators have speculated that increases may be due to light anesthesia and are not a reflection of direct cerebral vasodilation.[110,113] In rats nitrous oxide increases blood flow in both cortical and subcortical regions, but in humans, flow is enhanced in all brain regions except the cerebellum and pons.[113] The combination of nitrous oxide and isoflurane produces a greater elevation in CBF than an equipotent dose of the volatile agent alone in humans and animals.[93,96,97] The combination of nitrous oxide and halothane results in CBF levels that are similar to equipotent concentrations of halothane alone.[97]

The effects of nitrous oxide on CBF are caused by direct vasodilatory actions or indirectly by changes in $CMRO_2$ and may, in part, depend upon the depth of anesthesia. Theye and Michenfelder reported an increase in $CMRO_2$ with nitrous oxide alone in dogs.[114] Lam et al. found that a higher metabolic rate and CBF were associated with combinations of nitrous oxide and isoflurane when compared to an equipotent dose of isoflurane alone.[93] Other studies have found no relationship between CBF changes and $CMRO_2$. It is postulated that the vasodilatory activity of nitrous oxide predominates at increased depths of anesthesia when $CMRO_2$ is maximally suppressed by the volatile agent in use.

Intracranial pressure elevations have been reported in patients with abnormal elastance.[115,116] Henriksen and Jörgensen observed ICP elevations in all patients with intracranial pathology exposed to nitrous oxide and was effectively reduced with moderate hyperventilation.[116] Over the years it was generally agreed that nitrous oxide-induced ICP increases could be prevented or abolished by the administration of concurrent drugs (i.e., thiopental) and hyperventilation. Recent studies have demonstrated that hyperventilation does not consistently prevent increases in CBF even if established prior to nitrous oxide administration.[96,112,113] The administration of nitrous oxide is contraindicated in the presence of an existing pneumocephalus because its use in this scenario can elevate ICP and precipitate a life-threatening tension pneumocephalus. Domino et al. reported no difference in ICP or volume of intracranial air postoperatively between those patients receiving nitrous oxide until the conclusion of surgery and those with discontinuation of the agent at dural closure.[117] If nitrous oxide is to be utilized during a craniotomy, the agent should be initiated at the onset of surgery and not added after dural closure so as to avoid expansion of a pneumocephalus.

Nitrous oxide is an acceptable anesthetic for neurosurgical procedures as long as intracranial elastance is normal. Nitrous oxide is a potent cerebral vasodilator, the effects of which cannot be reliably prevented by hypocapnia. The combination of nitrous oxide and isoflurane, in particular, appear to increase CBF and should probably be used with great care when ICP is elevated.

Intravenous Anesthetics

BARBITURATES Barbiturates display powerful effects on the cerebral vasculature and metabolism that, unlike potent inhalational agents, are coupled. Thiopental is the most widely used barbiturate in anesthesia practice; however, pentobarbital is commonly utilized in the intensive care unit (ICU) to lower ICP and establish barbiturate coma. Due to the similarity of cerebral effects among the barbiturates, thiopental will be concentrated on in this section.

Thiopental has been consistently shown to lower CBF and $CMRO_2$ in a dose-dependent fashion in animals and humans.[77,118,119] The effects of thiopental are not exclusive to the cerebral circulation with spinal cord blood flow similarly affected.[120] Methohexital, predominantly in small doses, possesses epileptogenic properties that can increase CBF and $CMRO_2$. Cerebral oxygen consumption is reduced by 55% when the EEG becomes isoelectric with thiopental.[118] At this point, no further reductions in $CMRO_2$ are observed and ATP, lactate, pyruvate, and phosphocreatine concentrations are normal even with massive doses of thiopental. Similar dose-dependent $CMRO_2$ reductions have been reported with phenobarbital and pentobarbital in rats.[121,122] The combination of pentobarbital and hypothermia lowered $CMRO_2$ by 70% in dogs, a greater effect than with either one alone.[123] Thiopental suppresses neuronal synaptic transmission but preserves metabolic function required to maintain cellular integrity and homeostasis.

Intracranial pressure is consistently and effectively lowered with thiopental in patients with intracranial hypertension.[124] Horsley was among the first to report reductions in CSFP with barbiturates in human volunteers.[125] Barbiturates have minimal effect on ICP in individuals with normal elastance. Barbiturates are utilized to treat ICP elevations especially when intracranial hypertension is intractable and more conventional measures have failed. Eisenberg et al. determined that the institution of high-dose pentobarbital with conventional treatment was more effective in treating intracranial hypertension in severely head-injured patients than aggressive conventional treatment alone.[126] Reduction in ICP with barbiturates did not improve mortality or outcome. Prophylactic barbiturates employed in severe head injury have also not been shown to improve outcome or mortality.[127] When barbiturates are used to control intracranial hypertension, the drug is titrated to maintain 90% suppression of total EEG activity. Systemic hypotension is common especially with high doses and requires aggressive vasopressor treatment to maintain adequate CPP.

Barbiturates provide cerebral protection during focal but not global ischemia, especially when administered prior to the ischemic event.[91,128,129] Pentobarbital significantly reduced the incidence of stroke and neurologic deficits when compared to untreated monkeys after permanent MCA occlusion.[128] In a recent study of rats subjected to temporary MCA occlusion, thiopental-treated animals were found to have the least amount of brain injury relative to animals treated with etomidate or isoflurane.[91] Nussmeier and colleagues evaluated the effectiveness of thiopental in reducing neuropsychiatric complications in cardiac patients undergoing open-ventricle procedures.[129] Barbiturates limited cerebral infarct size and minimized permanent neurologic deficits. The cerebral protective effects of barbiturates are not solely related to $CMRO_2$ reduction but likely involve attenuation of secondary neuronal injury (i.e., free radical scavenging or alteration of fatty acid metabolism).

ETOMIDATE Etomidate lowers $CMRO_2$ and CBF, but in contrast to barbiturates, blood flow changes are independent of changes in metabolism.[130–132] With an etomidate infusion, CBF decreased earlier and more rapidly than did reductions in $CMRO_2$ that were maximal with the onset of an isoelectric EEG in dogs.[130] No further suppression of neuronal function or alteration of cerebral metabolic pathways was observed despite continuous etomidate administration after achieving electrical silence.[130] The drug has been reported to preferentially suppress cortical structures. Etomidate has the potential to induce seizure activity; it consistently augments the amplitude of the cortical somatosensory-evoked potential perhaps by preferentially affecting inhibitory postsynaptic potentials, leaving excitatory postsynaptic potentials unopposed.

Etomidate effectively lowers ICP, reflecting its powerful vasoconstrictive effects on CBF.[133] Because CBF changes occur more rapidly than $CMRO_2$ reductions, it is theoretically possible for ischemia to occur. Even though etomidate reduces $CMRO_2$ and produces an isoelectric EEG, it has not been proven to provide cerebral protection during focal ischemia.[91] Cerebrovascular response to CO_2 remains intact with etomidate anesthesia.[131,132]

Etomidate is not commonly used in neuroanesthesia practice in patients with abnormal elastance, because barbiturates effectively control ICP, provide cerebral protection, and do not precipitate seizure activity. Although etomidate is associated with greater hemodynamic stability than thiopental, it has several undesirable side effects including myoclonic activity during induction and prolonged use, adrenocortical suppression, and epileptogenic properties. Etomidate should be used cautiously, if at all, in patients with seizure disorders.

PROPOFOL Limited data exist on the cerebral effects of propofol. In humans, propofol has been reported to decrease both CBF and $CMRO_2$; its ability to reduce CBF has been attributed to parallel changes in metabolism.[134,135] Propofol can suppress neuronal function to produce a burst-suppressed or isoelectric EEG with clinically relevant doses much like barbiturates, etomidate, or isoflurane. It is not known whether propofol has direct toxic effects on the cerebral metabolic pathway.

Propofol reduces or has minimal effects on ICP. The largest reductions in ICP have been observed in patients with intracranial hypertension and to a lesser extent when elastance is normal.[134,136] Significant reductions in MAP, even in young healthy patients, are seen clinically with anesthetic doses of propofol. It is thus imperative to treat significant declines in MAP to prevent deleterious reductions in CPP that can augment intracranial hypertension by compensatory vasodilatory mechanisms. It has been questioned by some investigators if propofol's effect on ICP is a reflection of decreased CBF and $CMRO_2$ or merely a result of decreased CPP. More definitive studies are needed before conclusions can be made.

Kochs and colleagues evaluated the cerebral protective effects of propofol in normothermic, normocarbic rats subjected to temporary common carotid artery occlusion and systemic hypotension by comparing three groups: (1) propofol titrated to EEG burst suppression, (2) fentanyl-nitrous oxide, and (3) propofol and glucose load.[137] The propofol-treated animals (with or without glucose) had less brain injury and better neurologic outcomes than the fentanyl-nitrous oxide group. Propofol has not been compared to barbiturates, which are considered to be the gold standard for cerebral protection. Until further data becomes available, propofol should not be utilized in scenarios in which cerebral protection is warranted.

Preliminary studies suggest that propofol may have metabolic effects that resemble barbiturates but with more profound effects on systemic blood pressure. It is currently used in neuroanesthesia primarily for sedation in the operating room and ICU and for short-duration procedures for cost-effective reasons. Patients receiving propofol have a clearer sensorium postoperatively when compared to their counterparts receiving traditional inhalational anesthetics. Propofol is currently not advocated for cerebral protection until more definitive data are available and should be used cautiously in patients with elevated ICP, avoiding dangerous reductions in MAP.

LIDOCAINE Lidocaine is an amide local anesthetic that has been used in neuroanesthesia during induction and prior to placement of the pinion system, extubation, or endotracheal suctioning. Lidocaine has a biphasic effect on CBF and $CMRO_2$. At low doses sufficient to produce sedation and general anesthesia, $CMRO_2$ and probably CBF are reduced; however, at higher doses seizures are precipitated, causing dramatic rises in $CMRO_2$ and CBF. In dogs, IV lidocaine (3 mg/kg) decreased $CMRO_2$ by 10% and by 30% at higher doses prior to onset of seizure activity (27 mg/kg).[138]

Lidocaine has been reported to either decrease or have no effect on ICP.[139,140] Bedford et al. reported that lidocaine (1.5 mg/kg) was as effective as thiopental (3 mg/kg) in reducing ICP in patients with brain tumors and was associated with greater hemodynamic stability.[139] In subsequent studies, lidocaine has been shown to only prevent, not reduce, elevations in ICP if used prior to placement of the pinion system, intubation, or endotracheal suctioning. Intratracheal lidocaine may be more effective than intravenous lidocaine, given in similar doses, in attenuating ICP elevations during endotracheal suctioning.[140] Intratracheal lidocaine anesthetizes the tracheobronchial mucosa, although initial administration can be associated with increases in ICP. The cerebral protective effects of lidocaine, at this point, are inconclusive.

KETAMINE Ketamine is a phencyclidine derivative with *N*-methyl-D-asparatate (NMDA) antagonist properties that has potent cerebral stimulant properties demonstrated by its propensity to induce hallucinations (in as many as 30% of adult patients) and seizure activity.[141–143] Ketamine causes marked increases in both CBF and $CMRO_2$. Dawson et al. reported an increase in CBF by 80% and $CMRO_2$ by 16% after ketamine administration in dogs.[141] Similar CBF elevations not accompanied by alterations in $CMRO_2$ have been observed in humans.[144] The CBF changes result from direct vasodilating activity by reducing CVR and perhaps from accompanying metabolic alterations. The vasodilating properties of ketamine may, in part, be the result of an alteration in transmembrane movement of calcium.[145] Cerebral blood flow changes produced by ketamine are regionally selective and may reflect stimulation of specific brain regions. In humans, ketamine selectively increases CBF in the frontotemporal and parieto-occipital regions of the brain.[146]

Ketamine consistently elevates ICP or CSFP, changes that are substantial when used as the primary anesthetic agent in patients with normal and abnormal elastance.[147,148] Ketamine-induced ICP elevations can be attenuated or prevented by thiopental administration and hyperventilation.[141,147] In a recent study by Mayberg et al., ketamine (1 mg/kg) was administered to mildly hyperventilated neurosurgical patients with abnormal elastance and background anesthesia of isoflurane and nitrous oxide.[149] No significant changes in ICP or V_{mca} by TCD were detected and were attributed to a nullifying effect of background anesthesia and controlled ventilation. The use of ketamine should be restricted in neurosurgical patients with documented intracranial hypertension or suspected increased intracranial elastance. If hemodynamic instability is present in head-injured patients, etomidate is a viable alternative for induction of anesthesia.

Recent interest has focused on ketamine's NMDA antagonist properties and use in scenarios in which ischemia is likely to occur (i.e., head injury). During ischemia, the excitatory amino acid glutamate is released and stimulates NMDA receptors, resulting in calcium influx into the cell and ultimately death if the process is not interrupted. Antagonism of this reaction would attenuate the extent of secondary neuronal injury that may be more important in determining the extent of neuronal injury and outcome than the primary injury. Shapira et al. evaluated the effects of intraperitoneal ketamine administered 1, 2, and 4 hours after closed head injury in rats.[150] In those animals treated with ketamine 1 and 2 but not 4 hours after injury, the neurologic severity score at 48 hours was improved and extent of hemorrhagic necrosis was less. In the future, ketamine or a similar agent without the adverse effects on CBF, $CMRO_2$ and ICP may have a role in attenuation of secondary injury.

BENZODIAZEPINES Benzodiazepines have been commonly used in anesthesia for sedation, anxiolysis, and treatment of seizures but vary in their duration of action. The cerebral effects of benzodiazepines are variable depending on the animal model, background anesthetic, and neurologic status of the subject. In general, benzodiazepines can be regarded as metabolic depressants possessing vasoconstrictive properties that are less potent than barbiturates. Intravenous diazepam administered in sedating or general anesthetic doses in rats decreased CBF by 20 to 30% without significant changes in $CMRO_2$[151] In this animal model, the addition of 70% nitrous oxide reduced CBF and $CMRO_2$ by an additional 30 to 40%. In dogs, $CMRO_2$ is unchanged or reduced with diazepam and CBF is consistently lowered.[152–154] Reductions in $CMRO_2$ and CBF have been reported in humans.[155–156] Tateishi et al. observed no significant change in ICP in neurosurgical patients treated with diazepam (0.25 mg/kg) despite presumed alterations in CBF and $CMRO_2$[157] Diazepam appears to preserve the reactivity of the cerebral vasculature to CO_2[155]

Midazolam is a short-acting benzodiazepine commonly used for sedation and anxiolysis and is readily reversed by flumazenil, a benzodiazepine antagonist. Midazolam decreases $CMRO_2$ and CBF in humans and animals.[153,158,159] In rats, midazolam reduced $CMRO_2$ by 55% with concomitant reductions in CBF by 40 to 45%; however, with the addition of nitrous oxide, $CMRO_2$ reduction was attenuated.[159] The cerebral effects of benzodiazepines in the presence of nitrous oxide appears to be variable. In healthy human volunteers administered midazolam (0.15 mg/kg), CVR rose by 52% and was accompanied by a 39% reduction in CBF.[158] Cerebral oxygen consumption was not measured in this study, but its reduction was suggested as the mechanism of lowered CBF. There appears to be a ceiling effect on CBF and $CMRO_2$ changes with benzodiazepines that may reflect maximal occupancy of benzodiazepine receptors.

The response of ICP to midazolam is variable and may depend on the neurologic status of the patient and whether the drug is given as a large bolus or by infusion.[160,161] Intracranial pressure did not change in patients with intracranial tumors induced with midazolam (mean total dose 0.32 mg/kg) alone.[161] In contrast, Papazian et al. reported a dual effect of midazolam (0.15 mg/kg) on ICP in severely head-injured patients.[160] In 5 of 12 patients with an ICP 18 mmHg or greater, a mild decrease in ICP was noted; however, in 7 to 12 patients with ICP less than 18 mmHg, elevations were reported and in some cases were significant. Significant reductions in MAP occurred with midazolam boluses in the majority of patients, resulting in a dangerously low CPP that may have elevated ICP in some patients studied. In severely head-injured patients, 30% will have CBF levels consistent with ischemia and require a higher CPP (recommended greater than 70 mmHg) than previously considered adequate.[3,21,162,163] Benzodiazepines may have cerebral protectant effects during periods of ischemia that are greater with midazolam than diazepam but significantly less than afforded by barbiturates.[153]

Benzodiazepines are safe when administered to neurosurgical patients as long as hemodynamics are supported but should be used cautiously in unventilated patients, because respiratory depression and hypercapnia can occur alone or in combination with other anesthetics. Benzodiazepines are often unpopular with the neurosurgeons because of their potential to alter mental status. Flumazenil is now available for benzodiazepine reversal but must be used with caution in patients with a seizure disorder or at risk for seizure development.

Narcotics

The effects of narcotics on CBF, $CMRO_2$ and ICP are highly variable, and their response may depend on the following: (1) animal model, (2) background anesthetic, (3) use of supraclinical doses, (4) administration of the drug (bolus vs.

infusion), (5) intracranial elastance, (6) presence or absence of neuromuscular blockade, and (7) ventilation (spontaneous vs. controlled). Of recent concern are reports of ICP and CBF elevations in both non-neurosurgical and neurosurgical patients after administration of the synthetic opioids fentanyl, sufentanil, and alfentanil. Narcotics, especially the synthetic opioids, remain an important component of the anesthetic management of neurosurgical patients due to their hemodynamic stability and association with a rapid, smooth emergence.

MORPHINE Morphine has been reported to produce significant reduction in $CMRO_2$ and CBF in normocapnic dogs anesthetized with 0.1% halothane, and the cerebral effects are readily reversed by nalorphine.[164] The changes in CBF reflect corresponding alterations in $CMRO_2$. During morphine-nitrous oxide anesthesia in normocarbic healthy volunteers, no significant changes in CBF or $CMRO_2$ were observed and may have reflected a nullifying effect on cerebral hemodynamics caused by the vasodilating properties of nitrous oxide.[165] High doses of morphine sulfate should be avoided in patients with abnormal elastance due to potential histamine release and subsequent hypotension that may lower CPP.

FENTANYL Conflicting studies have been published regarding the safety of fentanyl in neuroanesthesia use. Fentanyl used alone in normocarbic dogs with a nitrous oxide background decreased $CMRO_2$ and CBF significantly.[166] Droperidol is a potent vasoconstrictor producing profound effects on CBF but no alteration in $CMRO_2$.[166] When the two drugs are combined (Innovar), the vasoconstrictor properties of droperidol predominate. The combination of fentanyl and droperidol does not elevate ICP in patients with intracranial masses but has been associated with dangerous reductions in CPP.[167]

Fentanyl may have either no effect or increase ICP in humans.[168–173] Marx et al. did not detect any elevations in CSFP when fentanyl (5 μg/kg) was administered to normocapnic neurosurgical patients with intracranial tumors anesthetized with nitrous oxide.[171] Although the actual numerical changes in CSFP were small with both sufentanil and alfentanil, sufentanil administration (1 μg/kg) was associated with the largest percentage increase in CSFP. In a similar study in patients with brain tumors, CSFP was unaffected by fentanyl-nitrous oxide as compared to a 30% increase in CSFP with alfentanil-nitrous oxide.[170] Brain retractor pressure was unaltered by the use of fentanyl, sufentanil, or alfentanil in neurosurgical patients anesthetized with isoflurane.[172] Similar findings were reported by From et al. after evaluation of brain conditions with dural opening after fentanyl, sufentanil, or alfentanil administration, and there was no difference in outcome among the groups.[173] In contrast, Trindle and colleagues observed elevations in V_{mca} by TCD with fentanyl and sufentanil in normocapnic volunteers.[174] A recent study by Sperry et al. demonstrated ICP elevations of similar magnitude with both fentanyl (3 μg/kg) and sufentanil (0.6 μg/kg) boluses in severely head-injured patients despite ongoing therapeutic measures to lower ICP.[169] The mechanism of ICP elevation may be secondary to increases in CBF and perhaps increased resistance to reabsorption of CSF at high narcotic doses.[175] Fentanyl, in high doses, can precipitate seizure activity with adverse effects on CBF, $CMRO_2$, and ICP.

SUFENTANIL Sufentanil has been found to decrease $CMRO_2$ and to either increase or decrease CBF in dogs.[176,177] Sufentanil administered alone in supraclinical doses (10 to 200 μg/kg) caused transient, marked elevations in CBF not accompanied by ICP elevations in dogs and without apparent seizure activity.[177] Cerebral oxygen consumption was reduced, and no toxic effects on the cerebral metabolic pathways were noted. When sufentanil (20 μg/kg) was given in dogs anesthetized with isoflurane and nitrous oxide, both $CMRO_2$ and CBF were reduced in a parallel fashion.[176] Sufentanil has been observed to have either no effect or increase CBF in healthy human subjects.[174,178]

Sufentanil has been reported to produce inconsistent effects on ICP. Sufentanil has been used safely in neurosurgical patients with abnormal intracranial elastance without associated elevations in ICP, brain retractor pressure, or adverse brain conditions upon dural opening.[172,173,179] Marx et al. were among the first to document CSFP increases in neurosurgical patients with sufentanil use that were significantly greater than with alfentanil or fentanyl.[171] The numerical changes in CSFP with sufentanil, albeit statistically significant, were relatively small (4.4 ± 1.1 mmHg). Sperry and colleagues also observed ICP elevations in severely head-injured patients after a sufentanil bolus despite aggressive ongoing measures to reduce ICP.[169] Recently, Albanese et al. demonstrated similar results with sufentanil (1 μg/kg and infusion of 0.005 μg/kg/min) in head-injured patients sedated with propofol and relaxed with vecuronium.[180] The ICP elevations were transient, lasting less than 15 minutes, and were accompanied by marked reductions in MAP and CPP that remained decreased during the 30-minute study period. The transient effects on ICP did not appear to adversely effect outcome in the population studied.

ALFENTANIL Conflicting studies documenting the cerebral effects of alfentanil also exist. In neurosurgical patients and non-neurosurgical patients anesthetized with isoflurane and nitrous oxide, low or high doses of alfentanil decreased or had no effect on V_{mca} by TCD.[181] As with fentanyl and sufentanil, brain retractor pressure was unaffected by alfentanil in neurosurgical patients undergoing craniotomies.[172] During ventriculoperitoneal shunt revisions in pediatric patients, alfentanil did not elevate ICP, although significant reductions in CPP were documented.[182] Cerebrospinal fluid pressure elevations have been documented with alfentanil administration in patients with brain tumors.[170,171] Marked reductions in MAP often result from alfentanil and warrant aggressive treatment, especially when intracranial elastance is abnormal.

REMIFENTANIL Limited studies are available documenting the cerebral effects of remifentanil but is expected to behave similar to the other synthetic opioids. In dogs anesthetized with nitrous oxide, low and high doses of remifentanil decreased CBF in a regionally selective manner and reduced ICP.[183] Of interest, as the opioid was metabolized, a rebound effect occurred with ICP elevation above baseline values.

CONCLUSIONS Narcotics have a longstanding history of safety in neurosurgical patients; however, recent studies contend that fentanyl, sufentanil, and alfentanil may cause ICP elevations. The narcotic-induced ICP increases may be attributable to one of the following: (1) use of supraclinical doses, (2) influence of background anesthetic, (3) opioid-induced chest wall rigidity, (4) use of large bolus doses, or (5) associated hypotension reducing CPP. The mechanism of these ICP elevations are unclear. When increases in ICP occur, they appear to be transient and not associated with an adverse outcome. Narcotics are likely still safe for use in the presence of space-occupying lesions as long as large bolus doses are avoided, systemic hypotension is aggressively treated and use is concurrent with other anesthetic agents and hyperventilation.

Neuromuscular Blockade Agents

SUCCINYLCHOLINE The use of succinylcholine consistently causes dramatic elevations in CBF and ICP in both humans and animals even in the absence of fasciculations.[184–187] In dogs anesthetized with halothane, succinylcholine, (1.0 mg/kg) produced marked increases in CBF that were accompanied by EEG arousal.[185] It is speculated that succinylcholine-induced increases in CBF and ICP reflect (1) afferent muscle spindle activation with stimulation of portions of the motor and somatosensory cortex and (2) secondary increases in $PaCO_2$ from enhanced muscle oxygen consumption.[184,185] Pretreatment with a defasciculating dose of nondepolarizing muscle relaxant may prevent fasciculations but does not prevent CBF elevations unless intubating doses of nondepolarizing agents are used as pretreatment.[186] Succinylcholine causes significant ICP elevations in patients with both normal and abnormal intracranial elastance. In a recent study by Kovarik et al., succinylcholine (1.0 mg/kg) had no effect on V_{mca}, ICP, or EEG in patients with neurologic insults and intracranial hypertension.[188] Absence of ICP changes in response to succinylcholine may have reflected the inability of a severely injured brain to react to afferent muscle spindle activity.

Succinylcholine should be avoided, if possible, in patients with intracranial hypertension or space-occupying lesions. If succinylcholine is used when intracranial elastance is abnormal, pretreatment with a nondepolarizing muscle relaxant (i.e., d-tubocurarine) is recommended and use of lidocaine may attenuate, not prevent, elevations in ICP. The use of barbiturates for induction of anesthesia and rapid control of the airway and hyperventilation may also attenuate the ICP elevations that occur with succinylcholine. The increases in ICP with succinylcholine are transient and less profound than those produced by laryngoscopy. The loss of an airway or aspiration of gastric contents resulting in hypoxemia and hypercarbia would have more deleterious effects on ICP than one dose of succinylcholine. If a patient with intracranial hypertension presents with a full stomach or a difficult airway, the use of succinylcholine is justified. The newer nondepolarizing muscle relaxants, rocuronium and mivacurium, are viable alternatives to succinylcholine use when rapid intubating conditions are required.

NONDEPOLARIZING MUSCLE RELAXANTS *d*-Tubocurarine has been replaced by newer muscle relaxants with fewer systemic effects but is still commonly used for pretreatment prior to succinylcholine use. *d*-Tubocurarine has been observed to increase CSFP in neurosurgical patients.[189] It is postulated that histamine release produces cerebral vasodilation; however, the systemic hypotension that often occurs may decrease CPP and cause a compensatory cerebral vasodilation.

Vecuronium has no effect on ICP in neurosurgical patients; rocuronium would be expected to have similar cerebral and systemic hemodynamic effects.[190,191] Pancuronium, (0.1 mg/kg) caused no changes in CBF, $CMRO_2$, ICP, or EEG in dogs anesthetized with halothane.[192] Although pancuronium can elevate heart rate and blood pressure, narcotics are commonly used concurrently and appear to blunt the hemodynamic effects of the nondepolarizing agent.

Atracurium administered in clinically relevant doses (0.5 mg/kg) produced no significant change in ICP in patients with intracranial pathology.[193,194] Atracurium-induced histamine release is related to high doses and rapid administration of the drug. In high doses administered to dogs, EEG arousal was seen but not accompanied by changes in $CMRO_2$, CBF, or ICP.[192] The metabolite, laudanosine, can precipitate seizures and may be directly responsible for cerebral stimulation.

Vasoactive Agents

The cerebral vasculature is highly innervated by α- and β-receptors, but their role in the brain is not clear. No significant changes in CBF, $CMRO_2$, or CVR occur with phenylephrine, epinephrine, or norepinephrine use. These vasopressors do not constrict the cerebral vessels and thus are safe for use in patients with cerebral ischemia (i.e., head injury and cerebral vasospasm). The cerebral vasculature is unaffected by α or β blockade; reactivity to CO_2 and autoregulation remain intact despite blockade.[195–197] The cerebral vasculature is likely affected predominantly by local metabolic and transmural pressure changes.

Nitroglycerin is an antihypertensive, antianginal agent contraindicated for use in neurosurgical patients with abnormal elastance due to its potent venodilating effects. Nitroglycerin produces deleterious increases in ICP in humans and animals in the absence or presence of space-occupying lesions within minutes of administration.[198–200] Nitroglycerin appears to have greater effects on ICP than does sodium nitroprusside.

Intracranial pressure elevations result from dilation of venous capacitance vessels, causing increases in CBV. Barbiturates do not attenuate nitroglycerin-induced ICP changes.[199] Unlike with sodium nitroprusside, CBF is not preserved when CPP reaches 50 mmHg.

Sodium nitroprusside is an antihypertensive commonly utilized in neuroanesthesia that causes significant ICP elevations similar to but less profound than with nitroglycerin. It is a popular IV antihypertensive due to its rapid profound effects on blood pressure and ability to tightly control the blood pressure. Sodium nitroprusside consistently elevates ICP in humans and animals by dilating capacitance, not resistance, vessels.[201–206] Even with significant levels of hypotension, CBF is preserved.[205,207] Adverse effects resulting from sodium nitroprusside administration include ICP elevations, cyanide toxicity, metabolic acidosis, and tachyphylaxis. Sodium nitroprusside does not mask the hemodynamic signs of intracranial hypertension (i.e., postoperative posterior fossa hemorrhage); tachyphylaxis to the drug is often seen when ICP increases.

Calcium channel antagonists may elevate ICP by dilating pial vessels. Nifedipine caused small but statistically significant increases in ICP in cats with normal and elevated ICP.[208] Nimodipine is routinely used prophylactically to treat cerebral vasospasm following subarachnoid hemorrhage. Calcium channel antagonists, especially the dihydropyridine derivatives, may have cerebral protectant effects during ischemia by preventing calcium influx into cells.

Nitroglycerin and sodium nitroprusside are potent dilators of capacitance vessels and thus are unsafe in patients with abnormal elastance. If a patient is on a tenuous portion of the pressure-volume curve, the dramatic rise in CBV caused by nitroglycerin or sodium nitroprusside use would be catastrophic, resulting in spatial exhaustion and intracranial hypertension. Nitroglycerin increases CBV to a greater extent than sodium nitroprusside but does not make sodium nitroprusside a safer drug in patients with mass lesions. Sodium nitroprusside is an appropriate drug for the induction of hypotension during aneurysm clipping or arteriovenous malformation resection, situations that warrant systemic hypotension with preservation of CBF until CPP is less than 50 mmHg. Trimethaphan, phentolamine, and β blockade agents (such as labetalol) are acceptable antihypertensives that have minimal effects on the cerebral vasculature. The prophylactic use of calcium channel antagonists, especially nimodipine, may be beneficial in patients at risk for cerebral ischemia (i.e., head injury with traumatic subarachnoid hemorrhage).

ANESTHETIC MANAGEMENT OF PATIENTS WITH INTRACRANIAL HYPERTENSION

Anesthetizing a patient with suspected or documented intracranial hypertension mandates an understanding of the pathophysiology of the underlying disease process and the effects of anesthetic agents, mechanical ventilation, and hemodynamic manipulations on ICP. Patients with intracranial pathology may present for neurosurgical intervention or for non-neurosurgical procedures, as often occurs with head injury and concomitant injuries (i.e., orthopedic and abdominal). Regardless of the surgical procedure, an anesthetic plan should be tailored to maintain effective perfusion pressures and cerebral oxygenation and minimize alterations in ICP. Of utmost importance is the avoidance of ischemia or any event that promotes secondary injury initiating free radical production, glutamate release, lipolysis of fatty acids, intracellular acidosis, and transmembrane influx of calcium. These events, if not corrected, lead to neuronal death. The outcome of head-injured patients has not only been correlated to GCS but to concomitant cerebral ischemia, the number of hypotensive and hypoxic events, and the duration and degree of ICP elevations.

Anesthetic Considerations

Minimal or no premedication
Maintenance of anticonvulsant and steroids
Euvolemia
Placement of ICP monitor
Ventriculostomy/CSF drainage
Voluntary hyperventilation
Neutral, 30° head elevation
Maintain CPP > 70 mmHg
Mechanical ventilation with hyperventilation
Mannitol, loop diuretics
Low concentrations of inhaled anesthetics
Barbiturates

Abbreviations: ICP, intracranial pressure; CSF, cerebrospinal fluid; CPP, cerebral perfusion pressure.

A detailed history of the current disease process and baseline neurologic exam are essential to document symptoms of intracranial hypertension and to aid in the diagnosis of new neurologic deficits on emergence from anesthesia. Not every patient with space-occupying lesions will manifest overt symptoms of elevated ICP. A CT or MRI of the brain localizes intracranial pathology and although not diagnostic may suggest elevated ICP. Midline shift and obliteration of the ambient cisterns strongly suggest intracranial hypertension.[51] Diffuse cerebral edema, hydrocephalus, subarachnoid blood, and peritumor edema also suggest abnormal elastance.

The need for ICP monitoring and/or CSF drainage should be established preoperatively by the neurosurgeon and anesthesiologist. The use of a ventriculostomy may be preferred in some cases not only to assess the impact of anesthetic and hemodynamic interventions on ICP, but to provide a therapeutic measure to actively lower ICP. For a non-neurosurgical procedure, placement of an ICP monitoring device may be helpful in the management of patients with a closed head injury and a GCS of 8 or less because the neurologic exam is lost after induction of general anesthesia. Regional anesthesia would be ideal in selected non-neurosurgical cases, such as orthopedics, and allow frequent assessment of the neurologic exam. Regional anesthesia is often not a viable alternative to general anesthesia for the following reasons: (1) the patient is uncooperative; (2) the presence of an intracranial mass precludes spinal anesthesia, (3) presence of hemodynamic instability due to concomitant injuries, (4) presence of coagulopathy, and (5) an unprotected airway if the neurologic status deteriorates. As the number of liver transplants increase in encephalopathic patients with coexisting coagulopathy, the decision to place an ICP monitor to improve perioperative management must be made carefully against the risk of intracranial hemorrhage. Invasive intraoperative monitoring should include placement of an arterial catheter either prior to induction or as soon as feasible. Additional monitoring (i.e., central venous access) is mandated by the underlying intracranial pathology, any concurrent injuries, or coexisting medical illnesses. Maintenance of anticonvulsants and steroids preoperatively is mandatory. Premedication with anxiolytics or narcotics should be titrated very carefully to avoid oversedation that can result in hypoventilation and hypercarbia. Benzodiazepines are unpopular with the neurosurgeons and are often avoided so that emergence is not delayed and mental status is not altered, especially when the procedure is of short duration.

Anesthetizing an infant or child with intracranial pathology and associated intracranial hypertension can be challenging but warrants the same considerations as an adult patient. Intracranial pressure elevation is possible even in infants with open fontanelles and sutures and should be suspected if the fontanelles are bulging or tense with palpation. As with adults, sedation should be administered cautiously to avoid hypoventilation. Premedication with benzodiazepines or narcotics is often avoided in children and adults with elevated ICP, but each case should be individualized. The anesthesiologist must also decide whether to proceed with placement of an IV catheter prior to induction or to proceed with mask induction. The neurosurgeon is often able to provide valuable information pertaining to the suspected degree of ICP elevation that may guide the induction technique. Intravenous catheter insertion, even after local anesthetic cream application, often results in crying and transient elevation in ICP, which can be exacerbated by difficult IV placement. Mask induction with halothane will also elevate ICP but poses the additional risk of laryngospasm or loss of the airway prior to securing an IV line. Many neuroanesthesiologists prefer to place an IV prior to induction in infants or children with intracranial hypertension. If a mask induction technique is chosen, then rapid IV placement after induction, administration of thiopental and muscle relaxant, and control of the airway with hyperventilation are recommended.

Prior to induction of anesthesia, the patient should be positioned with the head neutral and elevated 30° to facilitate venous return from the cerebral circulation. The arterial line and ICP monitor, if in place, should be zeroed at the level of the external auditory canal to reflect accurately CPP and ICP. Voluntary hyperventilation can be initiated prior to induction of anesthesia in cooperative children and adults.

Selection of the induction technique should be made with the following goals: (1) maintenance of hemodynamic stability to preserve CPP and minimize ICP elevations, (2) rapid airway control and initiation of hyperventilation, and (3) laryngoscopy time less than 15 seconds when feasible. Barbiturates are the induction agents of choice when the patient is hemodynamically stable; etomidate may be preferable in the presence of myocardial dysfunction or hypovolemia. Ketamine should be avoided in patients with space-occupying lesions. Despite reports of ICP elevations with synthetic opioids, they are an important adjunct for induction and maintenance of anesthesia. Sufentanil and fentanyl are the preferred opioids for procedures of long duration. Narcotics are probably safe for use in patients with increased intracranial elastance as long as (1) large bolus doses are avoided, (2) chest wall rigidity is attenuated by pretreatment with priming doses of neuromuscular blockade agents, (3) hypotension associated with their administration is aggressively treated, (4) barbiturates are used concurrently during induction, and (5) hyperventilation is instituted.

The choice of neuromuscular blockade agent depends upon the urgency of the procedure, NPO (nothing by mouth) status of the patient, airway examination, and presence of concomitant facial or cervical injuries. Succinylcholine can be utilized if a difficult airway is anticipated or a rapid sequence induction is warranted. If succinylcholine is used, pretreatment with a defasciculating dose of a nondepolarizing muscle relaxant is recommended in conjunction with barbiturates and initiation of hyperventilation after the airway is secured. Intravenous lidocaine may also attenuate ICP elevations in response to intubation. Succinylcholine transiently elevates ICP but is safer and less detrimental to the ICP than loss of the airway, resulting in hypercarbia and hypoxemia. If cervical spine injuries are suspected or documented, neutral head position *without inline traction* controlled by the neurosurgeon is now recommended. Intubation should not be attempted until full relaxation occurs to avoid precipitous rises in ICP associated with coughing and bucking during endotracheal tube placement. Laryngoscopy time should be kept to less than 15 seconds to minimize hemodynamic response to intubation. If a difficult airway is anticipated or facial injuries preclude the placement of an endotracheal tube under general anesthesia, awake intubation is acceptable as long as the airway is well topicalized with local anesthesia and sedation is administered judiciously. Any maneuvers that compromise venous return from the cerebral circulation should be avoided including final positioning with the head in extreme flexion or lateral rotation or taping the endotracheal tube circumferentially around the neck.

Maintenance of anesthesia in patients with abnormal elastance should be performed with the same goals for induction. Halothane should be used cautiously in patients with intracranial hypertension, and hyperventilation should be established prior to its administration. The use of low concentrations of isoflurane has minimal effects on CBF and is safe in conjunction with simultaneous hyperventilation. A continuous infusion of narcotics is preferable in long duration cases to promote hemodynamic stability, ensure steady-state plasma levels, and provide a smooth emergence at the conclusion of surgery. Neuromuscular blockade is maintained to prevent movement in the pinion system that can result in scalp lacerations or cervical spine injuries. Ventilation is controlled, maintaining mild to moderate hypocarbia until time of dural closure unless ICP is still elevated at that time. Hyperventilation may have detrimental effects on CBF in head-injured patients, and many trauma centers across the country now maintain $PaCO_2$ in the low to midthirties to avoid worsening cerebral ischemia if present. Frequent arterial blood gas determinations are mandatory to evaluate the end-tidal-to-arterial gradient of CO_2. Addition of PEEP to maintain oxygenation increases dead space ventilation mandating frequent evaluation of $PaCO_2$. When ICP monitoring is not available or utilized, MAP should be maintained close to preoperative values. Hypotension should always be aggressively treated; marked hypertension is treated unless it is suspected that elevations are a protective measure to maintain CPP. Hypertension is often associated with placement of the pinion system and during surgical opening until the bone flap is removed and can be attenuated or prevented by the administration of supplemental narcotics, barbiturates, inhalational agent, or β-blockade agents (i.e., esmolol). Phentolamine or trimethaphan can also be utilized and are often done so in combination with β-blockade to attenuate the reflex tachycardia commonly observed with these antihypertensive agents. Trimethaphan produces ganglionic blockade and results in mydriasis that interferes with a vital part of the neurologic exam.

A plan should be formulated preoperatively to address ICP elevations that occur intraoperatively. If an ICP monitor is not in place, the dura and brain can be inspected for tenseness when the bone flap is removed. Even though ICP is zero after the dura is open, the brain can still protrude through the craniotomy site resulting in ischemia or difficult closure. Mannitol 20% (0.5 to 1.0 g/kg) is routinely administered prior to removal of the bone flap. If the response to mannitol is not adequate, furosemide may be useful, especially when antidiuretic hormone levels are elevated secondary to stress. Furosemide should only be administered as long as the patient is relatively euvolemic and hemodynamically stable. If ICP remains elevated despite hyperventilation and mannitol, the following should be considered intraoperatively: (1) additional hyperventilation if ischemia is not suspected avoiding $PaCO_2$ of less than 25 mmHg, (2) consider furosemide only if patient is not hypovolemic, (3) verify head position and absence of neck compression, (4) increase head elevation as long as the blood pressure is stable; (5) maintenance of CPP greater than 70 mmHg with IV fluids or vasopressors, (6) treatment of hypertension as long as it is not a protective mechanism, (7) CSF drainage if ventriculostomy in place, (8) barbiturates, or (9) administration of hypertonic saline.

Intraoperative fluid management is directed toward maintenance of a euvolemic state. Hypovolemia is no longer recommended due to the danger of associated hypotension. Hypotension below autoregulatory levels causes a compensatory vasodilation, leading to elevation of ICP and ultimately worsening CPP. Isotonic fluids are the mainstay of fluid replacement. Hypertonic saline consistently reduces ICP and may be a useful adjunct to decrease cerebral edema while maintaining hemodynamic stability.[209–214] Glucose-containing solutions are avoided, especially when a risk of cerebral ischemia exists.

At the conclusion of surgery, the CO_2 should be normalized so as to minimize the degree of pneumocephalus that can be large after CSF drainage and after posterior fossa procedures and to prevent reaccumulation of blood that can occur with subdural hematomas. In any case where ICP elevations are expected to persist or develop postoperatively, controlled ventilation with hyperventilation may be necessary. The addition of nitrous oxide is contraindicated after dural closure to prevent enlargement of a pneumocephalus. The emergence period often requires the use of antihypertensives to control blood pressure elevations during light planes of anesthesia. Nitroglycerin and sodium nitroprusside are still not recommended after the mass lesion has been removed because edema may occur postoperatively. The anesthesiologist should tailor the anesthetic to provide a rapid, smooth emergence to expedite performance of the neurologic exam. Extubation is planned at the conclusion of surgery unless hyperventilation is planned to lower ICP, mental status is impaired, neurologic exam is significantly changed, or large doses of barbiturates have been administered during the case.

MANAGEMENT OF INTRACRANIAL HYPERTENSION

The management of intracranial hypertension involves aggressive surgical intervention if warranted and medical therapy in the ICU. Once the primary injury has occurred (i.e., closed head injury, hematoma, or tumor), it is important to minimize secondary neuronal injury that is often precipitated by ischemic or traumatic brain injury. Recently, attention and treatment has been directed toward prevention of secondary injury because it appears to play a significant role in the extent of neurologic injury and ultimate neurologic outcome. Most of the therapy used to treat secondary injury is still experimental but may prove to be beneficial in improving outcome for patients in the future. The primary treatment of ICP has evolved with improvements in monitoring (i.e., jugular bulb venous oxygen saturation [S_{jv} O_2]) and a better understanding of the pathophysiology of head injury.

Cerebral ischemia (CBF less than 18 ml/100 g/min) occurs either globally or regionally in approximately 30% of head-injured patients when CBF measurements are made within 4 to 6 hours after injury.[3,162] The incidence would likely be higher if CBF measurements were determined earlier after injury. Bouma et al. confirmed ischemia in these patients rather than a low cerebral metabolic state by measurement of high $AVDO_2$.[162] Diffuse cerebral swelling and hematomas are more likely to be associated with low CBF.[3] It is speculated that ischemia may result from vasospasm that has been demonstrated radiographically or by TCD in as many as 40% of patients after head injury.[162,215] It is not clear if vasospasm is accompanied by traumatic subarachnoid hemorrhage as occurs with aneurysmal subarachnoid hemorrhage. Within 24 hours of injury, a relative or absolute hyperemia occurs in select patients and is often uncoupled from $CMRO_2$ ($AVDO_2$ is low). An uncoupling of CBF and $CMRO_2$ can occur early after injury but is most pronounced within 24 hours of head injury.[33] Autoregulation is intact in 60 to 70% of head-injured patients.[25,216] Because CBF and metabolic status cannot reliably be predicted after head injury, ICP and $S_{jv}O_2$ (with $AVDO_2$) monitoring are vital to guide therapy and perhaps predict outcome. A $S_{jv}O_2$ less than 50% for longer than 5 minutes is indicative of ischemia, warranting treatment and may be the result of elevated ICP, hypotension, aggressive hyperventilation, hypoxia, or anemia. Guidelines for the treatment of head-injured patients will soon be released nationwide.

Treatment is generally initiated when ICP is 20 mmHg or greater; however, some investigators recommend maintaining ICP less than 15 mmHg. There are still others that place more importance on maintenance of CPP at greater than 70 mmHg at the expense of higher ICPs (often greater than 20 mmHg). At least 50% of patients with severe head injury will develop intracranial hypertension at some point during the course of hospitalization.[217] Historically, hyperventilation was the mainstay of treatment for lowering ICP; however, the trend now is to maintain mild hypocapnia ($PaCO_2$ in the low to midthirties). Hyperventilation acutely lowers CBF by vasoconstriction of the end arterioles and is effective until CSF pH normalizes within 1 or 2 days after initiation. It is common to observe a rebound in ICP elevation after discontinuation of hyperventilation that is related to CSF pH changes. Cerebrovascular reactivity to CO_2 initially may be attenuated after head injury but is restored within the first 24 hours after injury. Hyperventilation can reduce CBF even further when cerebral ischemia is present after head injury. Unless $S_{jv}O_2$ measurement is available, aggressive hyperventilation should be avoided and only instituted if there is no evidence of ischemia. Muizelaar and colleagues evaluated the effects of hyperventilation ($PaCO_2$ 25 mmHg) ± tromethamine (THAM) on the neurologic outcome of severely head-injured patients.[218] A worse neurologic outcome at 3 and 6 months was documented in patients with motor scores of 4 to 5 treated with hyperventilation without THAM. An inverse steal phenomena has been observed in head-injured patients with disrupted autoregulation.[219] Hypocapnia results in vasoconstriction of reactive cerebrovascular beds and inadvertently diverts blood flow to brain regions lacking autoregulation augmenting flow and increasing edema.[219] If all other measures fail and no evidence of cerebral ischemia exists, $PaCO_2$ can be lowered cautiously with the guidance of $S_{jv}O_2$ monitoring. The addition of THAM may attenuate the degree of acidosis that accompanies prolonged hyperventilation.

Concomitant pulmonary injuries (including aspiration, contusions, and adult respiratory distress syndrome) often accompany head injury resulting in hypoxemia warranting the use of PEEP. When PEEP of 10 cm H_2O or less is utilized with frequent determinations of $PaCO_2$, no significant elevations in ICP occur.[220] With increasing PEEP levels, deadspace ventilation rises increasing $PaCO_2$ and elevating ICP if not corrected by adjusting ventilatory parameters. When a PEEP of greater than 10 cm H_2O is employed, ICP elevations result not only from increased deadspace ventilation, but obstruction of venous return from the cerebral circulation as central venous pressures rises. Low levels of PEEP can be used safely as long as $PaCO_2$ levels are followed closely. If oxygenation worsens, requiring increasing PEEP levels, hypoxemia should be aggressively treated by increasing PEEP levels or pressure control inverse ratio ventilation regardless of effects on ICP. It is well known that hypoxemia prior to initial resuscitation and during hospitalization adversely affects neurologic outcome (for further discussion of PEEP and ICP, see Ch. 19).

Mannitol is a hypertonic, hyperosmolar agent that effectively reduces brain water by establishing an osmotic gradient that favors the movement of water from the brain interstitium into the vasculature. Mannitol is only effective in areas of intact blood-brain barrier, and onset is within 10 to 20 minutes of administration. Within minutes of administration, ICP rises in response to direct vasodilation followed by a decrease in ICP and rise in CPP that often lasts up to 90 minutes.[221] In rats subjected to intracranial hemorrhage, edema formation was maximal within 24 hours of injury, validating initiation of mannitol early in the course of treatment for head injury.[222] Duration of mannitol use is limited by serum osmolality (315 mOsm/kg or less). The combination of mannitol and furosemide has an additive effect on ICP reduction and duration of diuresis.[223] There is danger of profound hypovolemia if the two drugs are administered in combination. Mannitol may also have the added benefit of free radical scavenging activity.

Aggressive treatment of hypotension is of paramount importance to maintain CPP. If autoregulation is intact, hypotension lowers CPP, causing cerebral vasodilation and exacerbation of intracranial hypertension, which in turn lowers CPP, initiating a vicious cycle. In contrast, CBF falls dramatically with systemic hypotension in the absence of autoregulation. Rosner and Coley advocate the maintenance of CPP above 70 mmHg with volume expansion and vasopressors to ensure adequate cerebral perfusion even if ICP increases above 20 mmHg.[21,163] In most trauma centers, CPP is maintained higher than 50 mmHg, which was previously considered adequate for effective perfusion in head-injured patients.

Head elevation, usually at 30° with neutral position has been a standard of care for lowering ICP and improving cerebral venous drainage. Elevation of the head has been challenged by Rosner and Coley, who recommend that the head be maintained at 0° to improve CPP by maintenance of MAP.[163] A greater reduction in CPP relative to ICP was found for every 10° change in head elevation. Feldman et al., in contrast, determined that head elevation to 30° decreased ICP without a significant reduction in CPP.[224] Until more data become available, the head should be elevated and kept in a neutral position. Intracranial pressure monitors are zeroed at the level of the external auditory canal and the same should be done with arterial pressure monitoring to accurately reflect CPP.

Sedation, pain control, and neuromuscular blockade can be utilized as part of the global treatment of ICP. Agitation or pain may commonly contribute to elevations in ICP and can be treated with sedation or narcotics. Sedation is frequently accomplished with propofol to ensure rapid emergence for neurologic assessments. If neuromuscular blockade is instituted for agitation, the use of a twitch monitor is mandatory to minimize prolonged blockade and ensure reversibility. Neuromuscular blockade should be accompanied by sedation; it should not be instituted until other measures fail since the neurologic exam, except for pupillary findings, is lost.

The drainage of CSF can improve spatial compensation and can be highly effective in reducing ICP. A ventriculostomy must be utilized to provide both ICP monitoring and CSF drainage. In the presence of a space-occupying lesion, lumbar CSF drainage is contraindicated. Rosner and Daughton routinely employ the use of a ventriculostomy and CSF drainage as a primary treatment to lower ICP.[21]

Maintenance of euvolemia is now advocated for head-injured patients. Historically, volume restriction was employed to reduce brain water but often resulted in hypotension, especially in patients with concomitant injuries and bleeding. In the intact brain, the movement of fluid across the brain is dictated by the plasma osmolality and not plasma oncotic pressure.[225] Isotonic crystalloid (i.e., normal saline) is safe for use in head-injured patients. Normal saline use did not promote increases in brain water in rats with cryogenic lesions even though plasma oncotic pressure was significantly reduced.[226] Even though colloids increase plasma oncotic pressure, there was no difference in brain water content between animals with cryogenic injury treated with lactated Ringer's solution or 6% dextran-70.[227] Hypotonic fluids (including lactated Ringer's) exacerbate cerebral edema by lowering plasma osmolality and should not be used in patients with intracranial hypertension. Hypertonic saline has been shown to lower ICP consistently with reductions similar to mannitol, improve rCBF, and improve cardiovascular status during early resuscitation without the use of large volumes of fluid.[209–214] Hypertonic saline ideally can be used in patients with severe head injury and hemorrhage to reduce ICP and stabilize hemodynamics. Adverse effects from hypertonic saline include significant hypernatremia and hyperchloremic metabolic acidosis. The rapid elevation of serum sodium from previously normal levels has not been associated with pontine myelinolysis.

Hyperglycemia should be aggressively treated when the risk of cerebral ischemia is present. Elevated plasma glucose levels provide substrate for anaerobic metabolism during periods of ischemia, which elevate lactate levels and worsen intracellular acidosis leading to neuronal injury. Lam et al. documented that head-injured patients with a GCS of 8 or less had a worse neurologic outcome if postoperative glucose levels exceeded 200 mg/dl.[228] Higher glucose levels were also recorded on admission and postoperatively in patients who died or remained in a persistent vegetative state. A better outcome was reported for those patients with glucose levels less than 150 mg/dl either on admission or postoperatively. Monkeys receiving dextrose prior to global ischemia had a worse neurologic outcome than their counterparts receiving lactated Ringer's solution.[229] Serum glucose should be maintained at 200 mg/dl or less; more aggressive control can easily result in hypoglycemia that also has detrimental effects on the brain.

The efficacy of mild hypothermia in lowering ICP and reducing secondary neuronal injury appears promising from preliminary trials, but further trials with large numbers of patients are needed to validate its cerebral protectant effects. Hypothermia has several potential advantages: lowering $CMRO_2$ and CBF, inhibition of excitatory amino acid release, and membrane stability. The volume of cerebral infarction was lower in hypothermic rats (24°C) with permanent MCA occlusion compared to normothermic controls.[230] In this study, hypothermia was initiated prior to initiation of ischemia. Mild hypothermia (32 to 33°C) initiated within 30 minutes of focal cerebral ischemia decreased the extent of infarct in rats compared to normothermic animals.[231] Hypothermia established at 60 minutes of ischemia was not protective. Marion et al. evaluated the efficacy of mild hypothermia (32 to 33°C, brain) instituted within 10 hours of injury (mean time) in improving neurologic outcome in patients with severe head injury.[232] At 3 months after injury, a trend toward a better neurologic outcome, not statistically significant, was seen in the hypothermia group compared to normothermic controls. Deep hypothermia is associated with numerous complications, including cardiac dysrhythmias and coagulopathy. Mild hypothermia may be cerebral protective, but a large clinical study is warranted to study its efficacy in ICP treatment and improvement in outcome.

Initial clinical trials utilizing calcium channel antagonists have not yielded promising results. Calcium channel antagonists, especially the dihydropyridine derivatives, are hypothesized to improve outcome and decrease infarct volume by improving blood flow (predominantly through pial vessels) and attenuating secondary injury by preventing calcium influx. A randomized placebo-controlled trial of nimodipine in 852 patients with severe head injury initiated within 12 hours of injury did not demonstrate improved outcome for treated patients.[233] Nimodipine-treated patients with traumatic subarachnoid hemorrhage had a better outcome than placebo-treated patients with subarachnoid hemorrhage, but results did not reach statistical significance. A large clinical trial assessing outcome with nimodipine use in traumatic subarachnoid hemorrhage patients is planned. AT877 is a calcium channel antagonist that prevents release of intracellular calcium and has been used in rats during focal cerebral ischemia.[234] In animals pretreated with AT877, volume of cerebral injury was less and neurologic outcome was better at 24 hours compared to control animals. Until further data are available, calcium channel antagonists do not appear useful in head injury unless they can be shown to provide benefit to a specific group of patients.

Early surgical intervention to evacuate mass lesions is mandatory to lower ICP, increase CPP, and improve neurologic outcome. The presence of a mass lesion amenable to surgical intervention is the treatment of choice early in injury and should be done so expeditiously to avoid worsening outcome (i.e., rapidly expanding epidural hematoma with impending herniation). Many patients sustaining head injury do not have operable lesions and require medical treatment to control ICP. If ICP is uncontrollable with maximum medical therapy, a lobectomy may be considered to lower ICP by surgical decompression. Surgical removal of brain tissue to lower ICP is considered an option for treatment only when other measures have failed.

Clinical trials utilizing THAM to lower ICP and minimize acidosis associated with prolonged hyperventilation have not yielded positive results. Muizelaar et al. determined that neurologic outcome was improved in head-injured patients treated with hyperventilation ($PaCO_2$ 25 ± 2 mmHg) and THAM or normocarbia than those treated with hyperventilation alone.[218] In a subsequent study, Wolf et al. evaluated the effectiveness of THAM in improving neurologic outcome in severely head-injured patients.[235] Despite lower ICPs and less requirements for barbiturate coma in the THAM-treated group, no difference in neurologic outcome was detected even at 1 year between the THAM-treated and control group. THAM may be useful in treating metabolic acidosis when the serum sodium is elevated and sodium bicarbonate is not a viable option; otherwise, it appears to have no role in head injury.

Barbiturates are often instituted when conventional measures to lower ICP have failed. Barbiturates are highly effective in reducing ICP by lowering $CMRO_2$ and CBF but can be associated with significant systemic hypotension, especially when large doses or continuous infusions are employed. Pentobarbital is the most common barbiturate utilized to induce barbiturate coma in the ICU. Barbiturates are titrated to 90% suppression of total EEG activity in an attempt to control the amount of drug administered; $CMRO_2$ reduction from 90% EEG suppression to isoelectricity is not clinically significant. Vasopressors are often needed to maintain adequate CPP. Once barbiturates are administered, neurologic assessments are impossible and monitoring modalities such as somatosensory-evoked potentials may be difficult to interpret. Declaration of brain death cannot be determined until barbiturates are fully metabolized determined by following urine barbiturate levels. In focal cerebral ischemia, barbiturates convey cerebral protection by reduction in $CMRO_2$ and probably by attenuating secondary injury. Ward et al. (the Richmond Study) studied the effects of prophylactic pentobarbital in severely head-injured patients treated regardless of ICP.[127] The use of prophylactic barbiturates did not improve neurologic outcome or consistently lower ICP and was associated with significant systemic hypotension. Eisenberg and colleagues evaluated the effectiveness of barbiturates in reducing ICP in head-injured patients.[126] Although ICP was more effectively controlled in the barbiturate-treated group, morbidity and short-term outcome did not differ between barbiturate-treated and control groups. In dogs with and without intracranial hypertension, hyperventilation alone (to $PaCO_2$ 25 mmHg) was as effective in reducing ICP as the combination of hyperventilation and barbiturates despite further declines in CBF with the addition of barbiturates.[236] Barbiturates are effective in lowering ICP but in limited studies available do not appear to improve outcome in head-injured patients.

Hyperbaric oxygen therapy has been suggested as an adjunct to treat ICP and improve neurologic outcome. Hyperoxia produced with hyperbaric oxygen administration causes vasoconstriction reducing CBF and ultimately ICP. It is also postulated that hyperbaric oxygen may improve glucose utilization. Rockswold and colleagues found that hyperbaric oxygen treatment in closed head injury patients did not significantly lower ICP or improve neurologic outcome.[237] The mortality rate was significantly lower in the treated group when compared to the control group. Currently hyperbaric oxygen treatment does not have a role in the treatment of head injury.

Treatment of head-injured patients in the future promises to focus on the cascade of events that contribute to secondary neuronal injury. Secondary neuronal injury may follow traumatic or ischemic brain injury. Excitatory amino acids are liberated after ischemia or traumatic brain injury (i.e., concussion with diffuse depolarization) and mediate their effects through activity at the NMDA receptor ultimately resulting in transmembrane influx of calcium, cell edema, and death. Ketamine, MK-801, CGS 19755, and D-CPP-ene are NMDA antagonists that have been utilized in animal trials to assess cerebral protectant properties of these agents. Cerebrospinal fluid glutamate levels are significantly elevated in patients with severe head injury.[238] Rats with acute subdural hematoma treated with the NMDA antagonists, MK-801, CGS 19755, and D-CPP-ene, had significantly smaller areas of ischemic injury than did their untreated counterparts.[239] These competitive NMDA antagonists had no effect on ICP. The cerebral protective effects of MK-801 and mild hypothermia were evaluated in rats subjected to permanent focal cerebral ischemia.[240] Rats treated with hypothermia alone and MK-801 alone demonstrated smaller areas of infarct, but no additive effect was seen with the two used in combination. Human clinical trials are warranted to assess the efficacy of NMDA antagonists in reducing stroke rate and improving neurologic outcome in head-injured patients. Ischemic injury with reperfusion leads to the generation of the free radicals, the most important of which is the superoxide anion. The superoxide anion generates additional free radicals that are responsible for lipid peroxidation, endothelial injury, and calcium influx. The use of free radical scavengers, such as polyethylene glycol-conjugated superoxide dismutase (PEG-SOD), has recently been evaluated in a phase II trial. Superoxide dismutase scavenges free radicals and inhibits the oxidation of nitric oxide by superoxide anion. Muizelaar et al. demonstrated a trend toward a better outcome, not statistically significant, in severely head-injured patients treated with PEG-SOD (two different doses) than their placebo counterparts.[241] A larger phase III trial is anticipated. The 21-aminosteroid tirilazad (U74006F) inhibits iron-mediated lipid peroxidation and has shown encouraging results in reducing stroke rate and improving outcome after cerebral vasospasm in patients with aneurysmal subarachnoid hemorrhage. From preliminary trials, tirilazad does not appear to have a role in the treatment of head-injured patients.

Steroids have a beneficial role in reducing edema associated with brain tumors and are a mainstay of treatment. Steriods do not, however, improve outcome or lower ICP in head-injured patients. Two independent studies have validated the failure of dexamethasone to alter the neurologic outcome of head-injured patients.[242,243] Gudeman and colleagues found no significant reductions in ICP when high-dose methylprednisolone was administered in severely head-injured patients.[244] Steriods are associated with significant complications including hyperglycemia, infections, and gastrointestinal bleeding; they should only be utilized to manage edema formation of a space-occupying lesion.

Treatment of intracranial hypertension is likely to be directed toward prevention of secondary injury in the future. New guidelines from the Consortium for Brain Injury for treatment of head-injured patients will be released nationwide soon. Most agents to treat secondary neuronal injury are still experimental and await validation in human trials.

OUTCOME

The outcome of patients with intracranial hypertension largely depends upon the underlying pathologic process and its chronicity. With operable hematomas, prognosis may be favorable if evacuation is expedited. The prognosis of patients with brain tumors depends upon the pathology of the lesion. The outcome of head-injured patients is predicted by the following: (1) age of the patient, (2) intracranial pathology, (3) initial GCS, (4) the number of episodes of hypoxemia and hypotension, (5) degree and duration of ICP elevations, (6) $CMRO_2$, and (7) presence of ischemia.[17,162,245–247] The frequency of hypoxemia and hypotension, especially during resuscitation, worsens neurologic outcome and may lead to diffuse cerebral swelling that independently alters prognosis.[248] Children with diffuse swelling have a higher mortality than their adult counterparts.[248] Mortality increases with CT evidence of a midline shift more than 3 mm, compressed ambient cisterns, masses of more than 15 cc, and the presence of an extracerebral mass.[51] The presence of cerebral ischemia at any time during the hospital course or the persistence of a low flow state is associated with increased morbidity and mortality.[162,249] A persistently low $AVDO_2$ predicts a chronic vegetative state. Secondary injury is postulated to profoundly influence not only the extent of injury but overall outcome. Patients often continue to improve after discharge; functional status 6 months after injury correlates well with final neurologic outcome.[250] The most common neurobehavioral finding at 1 year after injury is impairment of memory and information processing.[251] Although the neurologic outcome of patients with intracranial hypertension, especially when associated with head injury, has improved, the morbidity and mortality is still high for this patient population. Improvement in neurologic outcome depends upon understanding the pathophysiologic processes involved in producing intracranial hypertension and ischemia, avoidance of cerebral ischemia, aggressive surgical intervention, aggressive monitoring and treatment, and perhaps in the future the use of agents to prevent or attenuate secondary neuronal injury.

The fundamental processes controlling normal intracranial dynamics have not significantly changed over time but our understanding of the impact of pathologic processes on global or local CBF, cerebral autoregulation, and potentiation of injury after the primary insult has continued to evolve at a rapid pace. With improvements in ICP and cerebral hemodynamic monitoring, medical therapy can be more accurately directed toward providing beneficial not detrimental effects on ICP and ultimately neurologic outcome. To prevent further neurologic insult the anesthesiologist must understand not only the underlying intracranial pathology but the impact that anesthetic agents, pharmacologic interventions, and hemodynamic manipulations have on ICP and promotion of secondary neuronal injury. In the future, improved monitoring techniques that can accurately and continuously assess CBF are likely to become available to improve perioperative management and perhaps influence outcome. Medical therapy is likely to be directed not only toward the primary brain injury, but toward active prevention of secondary injury that may have a greater impact upon stroke rate and neurologic outcome than the initial insult. Ultra-early intervention directed toward attenuation or prevention of secondary injury may become part of routine therapy if human trials validate their effectiveness.

References

1. Cushing H: Concerning a definite regulatory mechanism of the vaso-motor centre which controls blood pressure during cerebral compression. Bull Johns Hopkins Hospital 12:290, 1901
2. Marion DW, Darby J, Yonas H: Acute regional cerebral blood flow changes caused by severe head injuries. J Neurosurg 74:407, 1991
3. Bouma GJ, Muizelaar JP, Stringer WA et al: Ultra-early evaluation of regional cerebral blood flow in severely head-injured patients using xenon-enhanced computerized tomography. J Neurosurg 77:360, 1992
4. Shapiro HM: Intracranial hypertension: therapeutic and anesthetic considerations. Anesthesiology (review article). 43:445, 1975
5. Fishman RA: Brain edema. N Engl J Med 293:706, 1975
6. Rowland LP, Fink ME, Rubin L: Cerebrospinal fluid: blood-brain barrier, brain edema, and hydrocephalus. p. 1050. In Kandel ER, Schwartz JH, Jessell TM (eds): Principles of Neural Science. 3rd Ed. Elsevier, New York, 1991
7. Wilkinson HA: Intracranial pressure. p. 662. In Youmans JR (ed): Neurological Surgery. 3rd Ed. Vol. 2. WB Saunders, Philadelphia, 1990
8. Pollay M: Review of spinal fluid physiology: production and absorption in relation to pressure. Clin Neurosurg 24:254, 1976
9. Cutler RWP, Page L, Galicich J, Watters GV: Formation and absorption of cerebrospinal fluid in man. Brain 91:707, 1968
10. Wright EM: Transport processes in the formation of the cerebrospinal fluid. Rev Physiol Biochem Pharmacol 83:1, 1978
11. Heisey SR, Held D, Pappenheimer JR: Bulk flow and diffusion in the cerebrospinal fluid system of the goat. Am J Physiol 203:775, 1962
12. Marmarou A, Shulman K, LaMorgese J: Compartmental analysis of compliance and outflow resistance of the cerebrospinal fluid system. J Neurosurg 43:523, 1975
13. Smith AL, Neufeld GR, Ominsky AJ, Wollman H: Effect of arterial CO_2 tension on cerebral blood flow, mean transit time, and vascular volume. J Appl Physiol 31:701, 1971
14. Kuncz A, Dóczi T, Bodosi M: The effect of skull and dura on brain volume regulation after hypo- and hyperosmolar fluid treatment. Neurosurgery 27:509, 1990
15. Langfitt TW, Weinstein JD, Kassell NF, Simeone FA: Transmission of increased intracranial pressure. I. Within the craniospinal axis. J Neurosurg 21:989, 1964
16. Takizawa H, Gabra-Sanders T, Miller JD: Analysis of changes in intracranial pressure and pressure-volume index at different locations in the craniospinal axis during supratentorial epidural ballon inflation. Neurosurgery 19:1, 1986

17. Jaggi JL, Obrist WD, Gennarelli TA, Langfitt TW: Relationship of early cerebral blood flow and metabolism to outcome in acute head injury. J Neurosurg 72:176, 1990
18. Marmarou A, Hochwald G, Nakamura T et al: Brain edema resolution by CSF pathways and brain vasculature in cats. Am J Physiol 267:H514, 1994
19. Langfitt TW, Weinstein JD, Kassell NF: Cerebral vasomotor paralysis produced by intracranial hypertension. Neurology 15:622, 1965
20. Löfgren J, von Essen C, Zwetnow NN: The pressure-volume curve of the cerebrospinal fluid space in dogs. Acta Neurol Scand 49:557, 1973
21. Rosner MJ, Daughton S: Cerebral perfusion pressure management in head injury. J Trauma 30:933, 1990
22. Muizelaar JP, Schröder ML: Overview of monitoring of cerebral blood flow and metabolism after severe head injury. Can J Neurol Sci 21:S6, 1994
23. Forbes HS: The cerebral circulation. I. Observation and measurement of pial vessels. Arch Neurol Psych 19:751, 1928
24. Aaslid R, Lindegaard KF, Sorteberg W, Nornes H: Cerebral autoregulation dynamics in humans. Stroke 20:45, 1989
25. Bouma GJ, Muizelaar JP, Bandoh K, Marmarou A: Blood pressure and intracranial pressure-volume dynamics in severe head injury: relationship with cerebral blood flow. J Neurosurg 77:15, 1992
26. Hauerberg J, Juhler M: Cerebral blood flow autoregulation in acute intracranial hypertension. J Cereb Blood Flow Metab 14:519, 1994
27. Aaslid R, Newell DW, Stooss R et al: Assessment of cerebral autoregulation dynamics from simultaneous arterial and venous transcranial Doppler recordings in humans. Stroke 22:1148, 1991
28. Lassen NA, Feinberg I, Lane MH: Bilateral studies of cerebral oxygen uptake in young and aged normal subjects and in patients with organic dementia. J Clin Invest 39:491, 1960
29. Lassen NA, Munck O: The cerebral blood flow in man determined by the use of radioactive krypton. Acta Phys Scand 33:30, 1954
30. Lassen NA, Christensen MS: Physiology of cerebral blood flow. Br J Anaesth 48:719, 1976
31. Roland PE, Larsen B, Lassen NA, Skinhoj E: Supplementary motor area and other cortical areas in organization of voluntary movements in man. J Neurophysiol 43:118, 1980
32. Plum F, Posner JB, Troy B: Cerebral metabolic and circulatory responses to induced convulsions in animals. Arch Neurol 18:1, 1968
33. Muizelaar JP, Marmarou A, DeSalles AAF et al: Cerebral blood flow and metabolism in severely head-injured children. J Neurosurg 71:63, 1989
34. Sharbrough FW, Messick JM, Sundt TM: Correlation of continuous electroencephalograms with cerebral blood flow measurements during carotid endarterectomy. Stroke 4:674, 1973
35. Messick JM, Casement B, Sharbrough FW et al: Correlation of regional cerebral blood flow (rCBF) with EEG changes during isoflurane anesthesia for carotid endarterectomy: critical rCBF. Anesthesiology 66:344, 1987
36. Morawetz RB, Crowell RH, DeGirolami U et al: Regional cerebral blood flow thresholds during cerebral ischemia. Fed Proc 38:2493, 1979
37. Astrup J, Siesjö BK, Symon L: Thresholds in cerebral ischemia—the ischemic penumbra. Stroke 12:723, 1981
38. Risberg J, Ancri D, Ingvar DH: Correlation between cerebral blood volume and cerebral blood flow in the cat. Exp Brain Res 8:321, 1969
39. Grubb RL, Raichle ME, Eichling JO, Ter-Pogossian MM: The effects of changes in $PaCO_2$ on cerebral blood volume, blood flow, and vascular mean transit time. Stroke 5:630, 1974
40. Severinghaus JW, Chiodi H, Eger EI, II et al: Cerebral blood flow in man at high altitude. Circ Res 19:274, 1966
41. Greenberg JH, Alavi A, Reivich M et al: Local cerebral blood volume response to carbon dioxide in man. Circ Res 43:324, 1978
42. Kogure K, Scheinberg P, Reinmuth OM et al: Mechanisms of cerebral vasodilation in hypoxia. J Appl Physiol 29:223, 1970
43. Grubb RL, Raichle ME, Phelps ME, Ratheson RA: Effects of increased intracranial pressure on cerebral blood volume, blood flow, and oxygen utilization in monkeys. J Neurosurg 43:385, 1975
44. Cohen PJ, Alexander SC, Smith TC et al: Effects of hypoxia and normocarbia on cerebral blood flow and metabolism in conscious man. J Appl Physiol 23:183, 1967
45. Brain WR: A clinical study of increased intracranial pressure in sixty cases of cerebral tumour. Brain 48:105, 1925
46. Ropper AH: Lateral displacement of the brain

and level of consciousness in patients with an acute hemispheral mass. N Engl J Med 314:953, 1986
47. McKissock W, Taylor JC, Bloom WH, Till K: Extradural haematoma: observations on 125 cases. Lancet 2:167, 1960
48. Hodge CJ, Primrose D: Physiological considerations. p. 1574. In Apuzzo MLJ (ed): Brain Surgery. Complication Avoidance and Management. Churchill Livingstone, New York, 1993
49. Adams RD, Victor M: Intracranial neoplasms. p. 521. In Adams RD, Victor M (eds): Principles of Neurology. McGraw-Hill. New York, 1989
50. Browder J, Meyers R: Observations on behavior of the systemic blood pressure, pulse and spinal fluid pressure following craniocerebral injury. Am J Surg 31:403, 1936
51. Eisenberg HM, Gary HE, Aldrich EF et al: Initial CT findings in 753 patients with severe head injury. J Neurosurg 73:688, 1990
52. Lundberg N: Continuous recording and control of ventricular fluid pressure in neurosurgical practice. Acta Psych Neurol Scand, suppl. 149:1, 1960
53. Rosenwasser RH, Kleiner LI, Krzeminski JP, Buchheit WA: Intracranial pressure monitoring in the posterior fossa: a preliminary report. J Neurosurg 71:503, 1989
54. Kaufmann GE, Clark K: Continuous simultaneous monitoring of intraventricular and cervical subarachnoid cerebrospinal fluid pressure to indicate development of cerebral or tonsillar herniation. J Neurosurg 33:145, 1970
55. O'Sullivan MG, Statham PF, Jones PA et al: Role of intracranial pressure monitoring in severely head-injured patients without signs of intracranial hypertension on initial computerized tomography. J Neurosurg 80:46, 1994
56. Mollman HD, Rockswold GL, Ford SE: A clinical comparison of subarachnoid catheters to ventriculostomy and subarachnoid bolts: a prospective study. J Neurosurg 68:737, 1988
57. Chambers IR, Mendelow AD, Sinar EJ et al: A clinical evaluation of the camino subdural screw and ventricular monitoring kits. Neurosurgery 26:421, 1990
58. Crutchfield JS, Narayan RK, Robertson CS, Michael LH: Evaluation of a fiberoptic intracranial pressure monitor. J Neurosurg 72:482, 1990
59. Hamer J, Alberti E, Hoyer S, Wiedemann K: Influence of systemic and cerebral vascular factors on the cerebrospinal fluid pulse waves. J Neurosurg 46:36, 1977
60. Kjällquist A, Lundberg N, Pontén U: Respiratory and cardiovascular changes during rapid spontaneous variations of ventricular fluid pressure in patients with intracranial hypertension. Acta Neurol Scand 40:291, 1961
61. Lundberg N, Troupp H, Lorin H: Continuous recording of the ventricular-fluid pressure in patients with severe acute traumatic brain injury. J Neurosurg 22:581, 1965
62. Newell DW, Aaslid R, Stooss R, Reulen HJ: The relationship of blood flow velocity fluctuations to intracranial pressure B waves. J Neurosurg 76:415, 1992
63. Feri M, Ralli L, Felici M et al: Transcranial Doppler and brain death diagnosis. Crit Care Med 22:1120, 1994
64. Petty GW, Mohr JP, Pedley TA et al: The role of transcranial Doppler in confirming brain death: sensitivity, specificity, and suggestions for performance and interpretation. Neurology 40:300, 1990
65. Goodwin SR, Friedman WA, Bellefleur M: Is it time to use evoked potentials to predict outcome in comatose children and adults? Crit Care Med 19:518, 1991
66. Barelli A, Valente MR, Clemente A, et al: Serial multimodality-evoked potentials in severely head-injured patients: diagnostic and prognostic implications. Crit Care Med 19:1374, 1991
67. Adams RW, Gronert GA, Sundt TM, Michenfelder JD: Halothane, hypocapnia, and cerebrospinal fluid pressure in neurosurgery. Anesthesiology 37:510, 1972
68. Albrecht RF, Miletich DJ, Rosenberg R, Zahed B: Cerebral blood flow and metabolic changes from induction to onset of anesthesia with halothane or pentobarbital. Anesthesiology 47:252, 1977
69. Albrecht RF, Miletich DJ, Madala LR: Normalization of cerebral blood flow during prolonged halothane anesthesia. Anesthesiology 58:26, 1983
70. Drummond JC, Todd MM, Toutant SM, Shapiro HM: Brain surface protrusion during enflurane, halothane, and isoflurane anesthesia in cats. Anesthesiology 59:288, 1983
71. Hansen TD, Warner DS, Todd MM et al: Distribution of cerebral blood flow during halothane versus isoflurane anesthesia in rats. Anesthesiology 69:332, 1988
72. Eintrei C, Leszniewski W, Carlsson C: Local ap-

plication of [133]xenon for measurement of regional cerebral blood flow (rCBF) during halothane, enflurane, and isoflurane anesthesia in humans. Anesthesiology 63:391, 1985
73. Hoffman WE, Edelman G, Kochs E et al: Cerebral autoregulation in awake versus isoflurane-anesthetized rats. Anesth Analg 73:753, 1991
74. Theye RA, Michenfelder JD: The effect of halothane on canine cerebral metabolism. Anesthesiology 29:1113, 1968
75. Brüssel T, Fitch W, Brodner G et al: Effects of halothane in low concentrations on cerebral blood flow, cerebral metabolism, and cerebrovascular autoregulation in the baboon. Anesth Analg 73:758, 1991
76. Michenfelder JD, Cucchiara RF: Canine cerebral oxygen consumption during enflurane anesthesia and its modification during induced seizures. Anesthesiology 40:575, 1974
77. Stullken EH, Milde JH, Michenfelder JD, Tinker JH: The nonlinear responses of cerebral metabolism to low concentrations of halothane, enflurane, isoflurane, and thiopental. Anesthesiology 46:28, 1977
78. Michenfelder JD, Theye RA: In vivo toxic effects of halothane on canine cerebral metabolic pathways. Am J Physiol 229:1050, 1975
79. Jensen NF, Todd MM, Kramer DJ et al: A comparison of the vasodilating effects of halothane and isoflurane on the isolated rabbit basilar artery with and without intact endothelium. Anesthesiology 76:624, 1992
80. Artru AA: Effects of halothane and fentanyl anesthesia on resistance to reabsorption of CSF. J Neurosurg 60:252, 1984
81. Drummond JC, Todd MM: The response of the feline cerebral circulation to $PaCO_2$ during anesthesia with isoflurane and halothane and during sedation with nitrous oxide. Anesthesiology 62:268, 1985
82. Lee JG, Hudetz AG, Smith JJ et al: The effects of halothane and isoflurane on cerebrocortical microcirculation and autoregulation as assessed by laser-Doppler flowmetry. Anesth Analg 79:58, 1994
83. Artru AA: Relationship between cerebral blood volume and CSF pressure during anesthesia with halothane or enflurane in dogs. Anesthesiology 58:533, 1983
84. Boop WC, Knight R: Enflurane anesthesia and changes of intracranial pressure. J Neurosurg 48:228, 1978
85. Stullken EH, Sokoll MD: Anesthesia and subarachnoid intracranial pressure. Anesth Analg 54:494, 1975
86. Moss E, Dearden NM, McDowall DG: Effects of 2% enflurane on intracranial pressure and cerebral perfusion pressure. Br J Anaesth 55:1083, 1983
87. Artru AA: Effects of enflurane and isoflurane on resistance to reabsorption of cerebrospinal fluid in dogs. Anesthesiology 61:529, 1984
88. Cucchiara RF, Theye RA, Michenfelder JD: The effects of isoflurane on canine cerebral metabolism and blood flow. Anesthesiology 40:571, 1974
89. Newberg LA, Milde JH, Michenfelder JD: The cerebral metabolic effects of isoflurane at and above concentrations that suppress cortical electrical activity. Anesthesiology 59:23, 1983
90. Meyer FB, Muzzi DA: Cerebral protection during aneurysm surgery with isoflurane anesthesia. J Neurosurg 76:541, 1992
91. Drummond JC, Cole DJ, Patel PM, Reynolds LW: Focal cerebral ischemia during anesthesia with etomidate, isoflurane, or thiopental: a comparison of the extent of cerebral injury. Neurosurgery 37:742, 1995
92. McPherson RW, Brain JE, Traystman RJ: Cerebrovascular responsiveness to carbon dioxide in dogs with 1.4% and 2.8% isoflurane. Anesthesiology 70:843, 1989
93. Lam AM, Mayberg TS, Eng CC et al: Nitrous oxide-isoflurane anesthesia causes more cerebral vasodilation than an equipotent dose of isoflurane in humans. Anesth Analg 78:462, 1994
94. Bisonnette B, Leon JE: Cerebrovascular stability during isoflurane anaesthesia in children. Can J Anaesth 39:128, 1992
95. Algotsson L, Messeter K, Nordström CH, Ryding E: Cerebral blood flow and oxygen consumption during isoflurane and halothane anesthesia in man. Acta Anaesthesiol Scan 32:15, 1988
96. Algotsson L, Messeter K, Rosen I, Holmin T: Effects of nitrous oxide on cerebral haemodynamics and metabolism during isoflurane anaesthesia in man. Acta Anaesthesiol Scand 36:46, 1992
97. Hansen TD, Warner DS, Todd MM, Vust LJ: Effects of nitrous oxide and volatile anaesthetics on cerebral blood flow. Br J Anaesth 63:290, 1989
98. Adams RW, Cucchiara RF, Gronert GA et al: Isoflurane and cerebrospinal fluid pressure in

neurosurgical patients. Anesthesiology 54:97, 1981
99. Artru AA: Isoflurane does not increase the rate of CSF production in the dog. Anesthesiology 60:193, 1984
100. Scheller MS, Tateishi A, Drummond JC, Zornow MH: The effects of sevoflurane on cerebral blood flow, cerebral metabolic rate for oxygen, intracranial pressure, and the electroencephalogram are similar to those of isoflurane in the rabbit. Anesthesiology 68:548, 1988
101. Scheller MS, Nakakimura K, Fleischer JE, Zornow MH: Cerebral effects of sevoflurane in the dog: comparison with isoflurane and enflurane. Br J Anaesth 65:388, 1990
102. Osawa M, Shingu K, Murakawa M et al: Effects of sevoflurane on central nervous system electrical activity in cats. Anesth Analg 79:52, 1994
103. Takahashi H, Murata K, Ikeda K: Sevoflurane does not increase intracranial pressure in hyperventilated dogs. Br J Anaesth 71:551, 1993
104. Kitaguchi K, Ohsumi H, Kuro M et al: Effects of sevoflurane on cerebral circulation and metabolism in patients with ischemic cerebrovascular disease. Anesthesiology 79:704, 1993
105. Muzzi DA, Losasso TJ, Dietz NM et al: The effect of desflurane and isoflurane on cerebrospinal fluid pressure in humans with supratentorial mass lesions. Anesthesiology 76:720, 1992
106. Lutz LJ, Milde JH, Milde LN: The cerebral functional, metabolic, and hemodynamic effects of desflurane in dogs. Anesthesiology 73:125, 1990
107. Lutz LJ, Milde JH, Milde LN: The response of the canine cerebral circulation to hyperventilation during anesthesia with desflurane. Anesthesiology 74:504, 1991
108. Young WL: Effects of desflurane on the central nervous system. Anesth Analg 75:S32, 1992
109. Ornstein E, Young WL, Fleischer LH, Ostapkovich N: Desflurane and isoflurane have similar effects on cerebral blood flow in patients with intracranial mass lesions. Anesthesiology 79:498, 1993
110. Baughman VL, Hoffman WE, Miletich DJ, Albrecht RF: Cerebrovascular and cerebral metabolic effects of N_2O in unrestrained rats. Anesthesiology 73:269, 1990
111. Drummond JC, Scheller MS, Todd MM: The effect of nitrous oxide on cortical cerebral blood blow during anesthesia with halothane and isoflurane, with and without morphine, in the rabbit. Anesth Analg 66:1083, 1987
112. Kaieda R, Todd MM, Warner DS: The effects of anesthetics and PaCO2 on the cerebrovascular, metabolic, and electroencephalographic responses to nitrous oxide in the rabbit. Anesth Analg 68:135, 1989
113. Reinstrup P, Ryding E, Algotsson L et al: Effects of nitrous oxide on human regional cerebral blood flow and isolated pial arteries. Anesthesiology 81:396, 1994
114. Theye RA, Michenfelder JD: The effects of nitrous oxide on canine cerebral metabolism. Anesthesiology 29:1119, 1968
115. Phirman JR, Shapiro HM: Modification of nitrous oxide-induced intracranial hypertension by prior induction of anesthesia. Anesthesiology 46:150, 1977
116. Henriksen HT, Jörgensen PB: The effect of nitrous oxide on intracranial pressure in patients with intracranial disorders. Br J Anaesth 45:486, 1973
117. Domino KB, Hemstad JR, Lam AM et al: Effect of nitrous oxide on intracranial pressure after cranialdural closure in patients undergoing craniotomy. Anesthesiology 77:421, 1992
118. Michenfelder JD: The interdependency of cerebral functional and metabolic effects following massive doses of thiopental in the dog. Anesthesiology 41:231, 1974
119. Pierce EC, Lambertsen CJ, Deutsch S et al: Cerebral circulation and metabolism during thiopental anesthesia and hyperventilation in man. J Clin Invest 41:1664, 1962
120. Hitchon PW, Kassell NF, Hill TR et al: The response of spinal cord blood flow to high-dose barbiturates. Spine 7:41, 1982
121. Hodes JE, Soncrant TT, Larson DM et al: Selective changes in local cerebral glucose utilization induced by phenobarbital in the rat. Anesthesiology 63:633, 1985
122. Nilsson L, Siesjö BK: The effect of phenobarbitone anaesthesia on blood flow and oxygen consumption in the rat brain. Acta Anaesth Scand, suppl. 57:18, 1975
123. Lafferty JJ, Keykhah MM, Shapiro HM et al: Cerebral hypometabolism obtained with deep pentobarbital anesthesia and hypothermia (30°C). Anesthesiology 49:159, 1978
124. Shapiro HM, Galindo A, Wyte SR, Harris AB: Rapid intraoperative reduction of intracranial

pressure with thiopentone. Br J Anaesth 45:1057, 1973
125. Horsley JS: The intracranial pressure during barbital narcosis. Lancet 232:141, 1937
126. Eisenberg HM, Frankowski RF, Contant CF et al: High-dose barbiturate control of elevated intracranial pressure in patients with severe head injury. J Neurosurg 69:15, 1988
127. Ward JD, Becker DP, Miller JD et al: Failure of prophylactic barbiturate coma in the treatment of severe head injury. J Neurosurg 62:383, 1985
128. Michenfelder JD, Milde JH, Sundt TM: Cerebral protection by barbiturate anesthesia: use after middle cerebral artery occlusion in java monkeys. Arch Neurol 33:345, 1976
129. Nussmeier NA, Arlund C, Slogoff S: Neuropsychiatric complications after cardiopulmonary bypass: cerebral protection by a barbiturate. Anesthesiology 64:165, 1986
130. Milde LN, Milde JH, Michenfelder JD: Cerebral functional, metabolic, and hemodynamic effects of etomidate in dogs. Anesthesiology 63:371, 1985
131. Renou AM, Vernhiet J, Macrez P et al: Cerebral blood flow and metabolism during etomidate anaesthesia in man. Br J Anaesth 50:1047, 1978
132. Cold GE, Eskesen V, Eriksen H et al: CBF and $CMRO_2$ during continuous etomidate infusion supplemented with N_2O and fentanyl in patients with supratentorial cerebral tumour. Dose-response study. Acta Anaesthesiol Scand 29:490, 1985
133. Prior JGL, Hinds CJ, Williams J, Prior PF: The use of etomidate in the management of severe head injury. Intensive Care Med 9:313, 1983
134. Pinaud M, Lelausque JN, Chetanneau A et al: Effects of propofol on cerebral hemodynamics and metabolism in patients with brain trauma. Anesthesiology 73:404, 1990
135. Vandesteene A, Trempont V, Engelman E et al: Effect of propofol on cerebral blood flow and metabolism in man. Anaesthesia, suppl. 43:42, 1988
136. Ravussin P, Thorin D, Guinard JP, Freeman J: Effect of propofol on cerebrospinal fluid pressure in patients with and without intracranial hypertension. Anesthesiology 71:A120, 1989
137. Kochs E, Hoffman WE, Werner C et al: The effects of propofol on brain electrical activity, neurologic outcome, and neuronal damage following incomplete ischemia in rats. Anesthesiology 76:245, 1992
138. Sakabe T, Maekawa T, Ishikawa T, Takeshita H: The effects of lidocaine on canine cerebral metabolism and circulation related to the electroencephalogram. Anesthesiology 40:433, 1974
139. Bedford RF, Persing JA, Pobereskin L, Butler A: Lidocaine or thiopental for rapid control of intracranial hypertension? Anesth Analg 59:435, 1980
140. Yano M, Nishiyama H, Yokota H et al: Effect of lidocaine on ICP response to endotracheal suctioning. Anesthesiology 64:651, 1986
141. Dawson B, Michenfelder JD, Theye RA: Effects of ketamine on canine cerebral blood flow and metabolism: modification by prior administration of thiopental. Anesth Analg 50:443, 1971
142. Kayama Y, Iwama K: The EEG, evoked potentials, and single-unit activity during ketamine anesthesia in cats. Anesthesiology 36:316, 1972
143. Ferrer-Allado T, Brechner VL, Dymond A et al: Ketamine-induced electroconvulsive phenomena in the human limbic and thalamic regions. Anesthesiology 38:333, 1973
144. Takeshita H, Okuda Y, Sari A: The effects of ketamine on cerebral circulation and metabolism in man. Anesthesiology 36:69, 1972
145. Fukuda S, Murakawa T, Takeshita H, Toda N: Direct effects of ketamine on isolated canine cerebral and mesenteric arteries. Anesth Analg 62:553, 1983
146. Hougaard K, Hansen A, Brodersen P: The effect of ketamine on regional cerebral blood flow in man. Anesthesiology 41:562, 1974
147. Sari A, Okuda Y, Takeshita H: The effect of ketamine on cerebrospinal fluid pressure. Anesth Analg 51:560, 1972
148. Gibbs JM: The effect of intravenous ketamine on cerebrospinal fluid pressure. Br J Anaesth 44:1298, 1972
149. Mayberg TS, Lam AL, Matta BF et al: Ketamine does not increase cerebral blood flow velocity or intracranial pressure during isoflurane/nitrous oxide anesthesia in patients undergoing craniotomy. Anesth Analg 81:84, 1995
150. Shapira Y, Lam AM, Eng CC et al: Therapeutic time window and dose response of the beneficial effects of ketamine in experimental head injury. Stroke 25:1637, 1994
151. Carlsson C, Hagerdal M, Kaasik AE, Siesjö BK: The effects of diazepam on cerebral blood flow

and oxygen consumption in rats and its synergistic interaction with nitrous oxide. Anesthesiology 45:319, 1976
152. Maekawa T, Sakabe T, Takeshita H: Diazepam blocks cerebral metabolic and circulatory responses to local anesthetic-induced seizures. Anesthesiology 41:389, 1974
153. Nugent M, Artru AA, Michenfelder JD: Cerebral metabolic, vascular and protective effects of midazolam maleate. Anesthesiology 56:172, 1982
154. Roald OK, Steen PA, Milde JH, Michenfelder JD: Reversal of the cerebral effects of diazepam in the dog by the benzodiazepine antagonist Ro15-1788. Acta Anaesthesiol Scand 30:341, 1986
155. Vernhiet J, Renou AM, Orgogozo JM et al: Effect of a diazepam-fentanyl mixture on cerebral blood flow and oxygen consumption in man. Br J Anaesth 50:165, 1978
156. Cotev S, Shalit MN: Effects of diazepam on cerebral blood flow and oxygen uptake after head injury. Anesthesiology 43:117, 1975
157. Tateishi A, Maekawa T, Takeshita H, Wakuta K: Diazepam and intracranial pressure. Anesthesiology 54:335, 1981
158. Forster A, Juge O, Morel D: Effects of midazolam on cerebral blood flow in human volunteers. Anesthesiology 56:453, 1982
159. Hoffman WE, Miletich DJ, Albrecht RF: The effects of midazolam on cerebral blood flow and oxygen consumption and its interaction with nitrous oxide. Anesth Analg 65:729, 1986
160. Papazian L, Albanese J, Thirion X et al: Effect of bolus doses of midazolam on intracranial pressure and cerebral perfusion pressure in patients with severe head injury. Br J Anaesth 71:267, 1993
161. Giffin JP, Cottrell JE, Shwiry B et al: Intracranial pressure, mean arterial pressure, and heart rate following midazolam or thiopental in humans with brain tumors. Anesthesiology 60:491, 1984
162. Bouma GJ, Muizelaar P, Choi SC et al: Cerebral circulation and metabolism after severe traumatic brain injury: the elusive role of ischemia. J Neurosurg 75:685, 1991
163. Rosner MJ, Coley IB: Cerebral perfusion pressure, intracranial pressure, and head elevation. J Neurosurg 65:636, 1986
164. Takeshita H, Michenfelder JD, Theye RA: The effects of morphine and N-allylnormorphine on canine cerebral metabolism and circulation. Anesthesiology 37:605, 1972
165. Jobes DR, Kennell EM, Bush GL et al: Cerebral blood flow and metabolism during morphine-nitrous oxide anesthesia in man. Anesthesiology 47:16, 1977
166. Michenfelder JD, Theye RA: Effects of fentanyl, droperidol, and innovar on canine cerebral metabolism and blood flow. Br J Anaesth 43:630, 1971
167. Misfeldt BB, Jörgensen PB, Spotoft H, Ronde F: The effects of droperidol and fentanyl on intracranial pressure and cerebral perfusion pressure in neurosurgical patients. Br J Anaesth 48:963, 1976
168. Tobias JD: Increased intracranial pressure after fentanyl administration in a child with closed head trauma. Pediatr Emerg Care 10:89, 1994
169. Sperry RJ, Bailey PL, Reichman MV et al: Fentanyl and sufentanil increase intracranial pressure in head trauma patients. Anesthesiology 77:416, 1992
170. Jung R, Shah N, Reinsel R et al: Cerebrospinal fluid pressure in patients with brain tumors: impact of fentanyl versus alfentanil during nitrous oxide-oxygen anesthesia. Anesth Analg 71:419, 1990
171. Marx W, Shah N, Long C et al: Sufentanil, alfentanil, and fentanyl: impact on cerebrospinal fluid pressure in patients with brain tumors. J Neurosurg Anesth 1:3, 1989
172. Herrick IA, Gelb AW, Manninen PH et al: Effects of fentanyl, sufentanil, and alfentanil on brain retractor pressure. Anesth Analg 72:359, 1991
173. From RP, Warner DS, Todd MM, Sokoll MD: Anesthesia for craniotomy: a double-blind comparison of alfentanil, fentanyl, and sufentanil. Anesthesiology 73:896, 1990
174. Trindle MR, Dodson BA, Rampil IJ: Effects of fentanyl versus sufentanil in equianesthetic doses on middle cerebral artery blood flow velocity. Anesthesiology 78:454, 1993
175. Artru AA: Dose-related changes in the rate of CSF formation and resistance to reabsorption of CSF during administration of fentanyl, sufentanil, or alfentanil in dogs. J Neurosurg Anesth 3:283, 1991
176. Werner C, Hoffman WE, Baughman VL et al: Effects of sufentanil on cerebral blood flow, cerebral blood flow velocity, and metabolism in dogs. Anesth Analg 72:177, 1991
177. Milde LN, Milde JH, Gallagher WJ: Effects of sufentanil on cerebral circulation and metabolism in dogs. Anesth Analg 70:138, 1990
178. Mayer N, Weinstabl C, Podreka I, Spiss CK:

Sufentanil does not increase cerebral blood flow in healthy human volunteers. Anesthesiology 73:240, 1990
179. Weinstabl C, Mayer N, Richling B et al: Effect of sufentanil on intracranial pressure in neurosurgical patients. Anaesthesia 46:837, 1991
180. Albanese J, Durbec O, Viviand X et al: Sufentanil increases intracranial pressure in patients with head trauma. Anesthesiology 79:493, 1993
181. Mayberg TS, Lam AM, Eng CC et al: The effect of alfentanil on cerebral blood flow velocity and intracranial pressure during isoflurane-nitrous oxide anesthesia in humans. Anesthesiology 78:288, 1993
182. Markovitz BP, Duhaime AC, Sutton L et al: Effects of alfentanil on intracranial pressure in children undergoing ventriculoperitoneal shunt revision. Anesthesiology 76:71, 1992
183. Hoffman WE, Cunningham F, James MK et al: Effects of remifentanil, a new short-acting opioid, on cerebral blood flow, brain electrical activity, and intracranial pressure in dogs anesthetized with isoflurane and nitrous oxide. Anesthesiology 79:107, 1993
184. Lanier WL, Iaizzo PA, Milde JH: Cerebral function and muscle afferent activity following intravenous succinylcholine in dogs anesthetized with halothane: the effects of pretreatment with a defasciculating dose of pancuronium. Anesthesiology 71:87, 1989
185. Lanier WL, Milde JH, Michenfelder JD: Cerebral stimulation following succinylcholine in dogs. Anesthesiology 64:551, 1986
186. Minton MD, Grosslight K, Stirt JA, Bedford RF: Increases in intracranial pressure from succinylcholine: prevention by prior nondepolarizing blockade. Anesthesiology 65:165, 1986
187. Cottrell JE, Hartung J, Giffin JP, Shwiry B: Intracranial and hemodynamic changes after succinylcholine administration in cats. Anesth Analg 62:1006, 1983
188. Kovarik WD, Mayberg TS, Lam AM et al: Succinylcholine does not change intracranial pressure, cerebral blood flow velocity, or the electroencephalogram in patients with neurologic injury. Anesth Analg 78:469, 1994
189. Tarkkanen L, Laitinen L, Johansson G: Effects of d-tubocurarine on intracranial pressure and thalamic electrical impedance. Anesthesiology 40:247, 1974
190. Stirt JA, Maggio W, Haworth C et al: Vecuronium: effect on intracranial pressure and hemodynamics in neurosurgical patients. Anesthesiology 67:570, 1987
191. Rosa G, Sanfilippo M, Vilardi V et al: Effects of vecuronium bromide on intracranial pressure and cerebral perfusion pressure. Br J Anaesth 58:437, 1986
192. Lanier WL, Milde JH, Michenfelder JD: The cerebral effects of pancuronium and atracurium in halothane-anesthetized dogs. Anesthesiology 63:589, 1985
193. Rosa G, Orfei P, Sanfilippo M et al: The effects of atracurium besylate (Tracrium) on intracranial pressure and cerebral perfusion pressure. Anesth Analg 65:381, 1986
194. Minton MD, Stirt JA, Bedford RF, Haworth C: Intracranial pressure after atracurium in neurosurgical patients. Anesth Analg 64:1113, 1985
195. Hoff JT, Sengupta D, Harper M, Jennett B: Effect of alpha-adrenergic blockade on response of cerebral circulation to hypocapnia in the baboon. Lancet 2:1337, 1972
196. Waltz AG, Yamaguchi T, Regli F: Regulatory responses of cerebral vasculature after sympathetic denervation. Am J Physiol 221:298, 1971
197. Van Aken H, Puchstein C, Schweppe ML, Heinecke A: Effect of labetalol on intracranial pressure in dogs with and without intracranial hypertension. Acta Anaesthesiol Scand 26:615, 1982
198. Cottrell JE, Gupta B, Rappaport H et al: Intracranial pressure during nitroglycerin-induced hypotension. J Neurosurg 53:309, 1980
199. Dohi S, Matsumoto M, Takahashi T: The effects of nitroglycerin on cerebrospinal fluid pressure in awake and anesthestized humans. Anesthesiology 54:511, 1981
200. Rogers MC, Hamburger C, Owen K, Epstein MH: Intracranial pressure in the cat during nitroglycerin-induced hypotension. Anesthesiology 51:227, 1979
201. Marsh ML, Aidinis SJ, Naughton KVH et al: The technique of nitroprusside administration modifies the intracranial pressure response. Anesthesiology 51:538, 1979
202. Marsh ML, Shapiro HM, Smith RW, Marshall LF: Changes in neurologic status and intracranial pressure associated with sodium nitroprusside administration. Anesthesiology 51:336, 1979
203. Cottrell JE, Patel K, Turndorf H, Ransohoff J: Intracranial pressure changes induced by sodium

nitroprusside in patients with intracranial mass lesions. J Neurosurg 48:329, 1978
204. Turner JM, Powell D, Gibson RM, McDowall DG: Intracranial pressure changes in neurosurgical patients during hypotension induced with sodium nitroprusside or trimetaphan. Br J Anaesth 49:419, 1977
205. Michenfelder JD, Milde JH: The interaction of sodium nitroprusside, hypotension, and isoflurane in determining cerebral vasculature effects. Anesthesiology 69:870, 1988
206. Tabaddor K, Tavares A, Marmarou A, Shulman K: Intracranial pressure and cerebral compliance during hypotension induced by sodium nitroprusside. Acta Neurol Scand, suppl, 56:310, 1977
207. Candia GJ, Heros RC, Lavyne MH et al: Effect of intravenous sodium nitroprusside on cerebral blood flow and intracranial pressure. Neurosurgery 3:50, 1978
208. Giffin JP, Cottrell JE, Hartung J, Shwiry B: Intracranial pressure during nifedipine-induced hypotension. Anesth Analg 62:1078, 1983
209. Ducey JP, Mozingo DW, Lamiell JM et al: A comparison of the cerebral and cardiovascular effects of complete resuscitation with isotonic and hypertonic saline, hetastarch, and whole blood following hemorrhage. J Trauma 29:1510, 1989
210. Walsh JC, Zhuang J, Shackford SR: A comparison of hypertonic to isotonic fluid in the resuscitation of brain injury and hemorrhagic shock. J Surg Research 50:284, 1991
211. Battistella FD, Wisner DH: Combined hemorrhagic shock and head injury: effects of hypertonic saline (7.5%) resuscitation. J Trauma 31:182, 1991
212. Prough DS, Whitley JM, Taylor CL et al: Regional cerebral blood flow following resuscitation from hemorrhagic shock with hypertonic saline. Anesthesiology 75:319, 1991
213. Schmoker JD, Zhuang J, Shackford SR: Hypertonic fluid resuscitation improves cerebral oxygen delivery and reduces intracranial pressure after hemorrhagic shock. J Trauma 31:1607, 1991
214. Freshman SP, Battistella FD, Matteucci M, Wisner DH: Hypertonic saline (7.5%) versus mannitol: a comparison for treatment of acute head injuries. J Trauma 35:344, 1993
215. DeBray JM, LeJeune JJ, Pourcelot L et al: ^{99}Tcm-HMPAO cerebral scintigraphy and transcranial pulsed Doppler in acute intracranial hypertension in rabbits. Br J Radiology 67:540, 1994
216. Muizelaar JP, Ward JD, Marmarou A et al: Cerebral blood flow and metabolism in severely head-injured children. J Neurosurg 71:72, 1989
217. Chan KH, Dearden NM, Miller JD et al: Multimodality monitoring as a guide to treatment of intracranial hypertension after severe brain injury. Neurosurgery 32:547, 1993
218. Muizelaar JP, Marmarou A, Ward JD et al: Adverse effects of prolonged hyperventilation in patients with severe head injury: a randomized clinical trial. J Neurosurg 75:731, 1991
219. Darby JM, Yonas H, Marion DW, Latchaw RE: Local "inverse steal" induced by hyperventilation in head injury. Neurosurgery 23:84, 1988
220. Cooper KR, Boswell PA, Choi SC: Safe use of PEEP in patients with severe head injury. J Neurosurg 63:552, 1985
221. Donato T, Shapira Y, Artru A, Powers K: Effect of mannitol on cerebrospinal fluid dynamics and brain tissue edema. Anesth Analg 78:58, 1994
222. Yang GY, Betz AZ, Chenevert TL et al: Experimental intracerebral hemorrhage: relationship between brain edema, blood flow, and blood-brain barrier permeability in rats. J Neurosurg 81:93, 1994
223. Pollay M, Fullenwider C, Roberts PA, Stevens FA: Effect of mannitol and furosemide on blood-brain osmotic gradient and intracranial pressure. J Neurosurg 59:945, 1983
224. Feldman Z, Kanter MJ, Robertson CS et al: Effect of head elevation on intracranial pressure, cerebral perfusion pressure, and cerebral blood flow in head-injured patients. J Neurosurg 76:207, 1992
225. Zornow MH, Prough DS: Fluid management in patients with traumatic brain injury. New Horizons 3:488, 1995
226. Zornow MH, Scheller MS, Todd MM, Moore SS: Acute cerebral effects of isotonic crystalloid and colloid solutions following cryogenic brain injury in the rabbit. Anesthesiology 69:180, 1988
227. Zhuang J, Shackford SR, Schmoker JD, Pietropaoli JA: Colloid infusion after brain injury: effect on intracranial pressure, cerebral blood flow, and oxygen delivery. Crit Care Med 23:140, 1995
228. Lam AM, Winn HR, Cullen BF, Sundling N: Hyperglycemia and neurological outcome in pa-

tients with head injury. J Neurosurg 75:545, 1991
229. Lanier WL, Stangland KJ, Scheithauer BW et al: The effects of dextrose infusion and head position on neurologic outcome after complete cerebral ischemia in primates: examination of a model. Anesthesiology 66:39, 1987
230. Onesti ST, Baker CJ, Sun PP, Solomon RA: Transient hypothermia reduces focal ischemic brain injury in the rat. Neurosurgery 29:369, 1991
231. Karibe H, Chen J, Zarow GJ et al: Delayed induction of mild hypothermia to reduce infarct volume after temporary middle cerebral artery occlusion in rats. J Neurosurg 80:112, 1994
232. Marion DW, Obrist WD, Carlier PM et al: The use of moderate therapeutic hypothermia for patients with severe head injuries: a preliminary report. J Neurosurg 79:354, 1993
233. The European Study Group on Nimodipine in Severe Head Injury: A multicenter trial of the efficacy of nimodipine on outcome after severe head injury. J Neurosurg 80:797, 1994
234. Ohtaki M, Tranmer B: Pretreatment of transient focal cerebral ischemia in rats with the calcium antagonist AT877. Stroke 25:1234, 1994
235. Wolf AL, Levi L, Marmarou A et al: Effect of THAM upon outcome in severe head injury: a randomized prospective clinical trial. J Neurosurg 78:54, 1993
236. Louis PT, Goddard-Finegold J, Fishman MA et al: Barbiturates and hyperventilation during intracranial hypertension. Crit Care Med 21:1200, 1993
237. Rockswold GL, Ford SE, Anderson DC et al: Results of a prospective randomized trial for treatment of severely brain-injured patients with hyperbaric oxygen. J Neurosurg 76:929, 1992
238. Baker AJ, Moulton RJ, MacMillan VH, Shedden PM: Excitatory amino acids in cerebrospinal fluid following traumatic brain injury in humans. J Neurosurg 79:369, 1993
239. Kuroda Y, Fujisawa H, Strebel S et al: Effect of neuroprotective N-methyl-D-aspartate antagonists on increased intracranial pressure: studies in the rat acute subdural hematoma model. Neurosurgery 35:106, 1994
240. Frazzini VI, Winfree CJ, Choudhri HF et al: Mild hypothermia and MK-801 have similar but not additive degrees of cerebroprotection in the rat permanent focal ischemia model. Neurosurgery 34:1040, 1994
241. Muizelaar JP, Marmarou A, Young HF et al: Improving the outcome of severe head injury with the oxygen radical scavenger polyethylene glycol-conjugated superoxide dismutase: a phase II trial. J Neurosurg 78:375, 1993
242. Dearden NM, Gibson JS, McDowall DG et al: Effect of high-dose dexamethasone on outcome from severe head injury. J Neurosurg 64:81, 1986
243. Cooper PR, Moody S, Clark WK et al: Dexamethasone and severe head injury: a prospective double-blind study. J Neurosurg 51:307, 1979
244. Gudeman SK, Miller JD, Becker DP: Failure of high-dose steroid therapy to influence intracranial pressure in patients with severe head injury. J Neurosurg 51:301, 1979
245. Hamm RJ, Jenkins LW, Lyeth BG et al: The effect of age on outcome following traumatic brain injury in rats. J Neurosurg 75:914, 1991
246. Cruz J: On-line monitoring of global cerebral hypoxia in acute brain injury. J Neurosurg 79:228, 1993
247. Sheinberg M, Kanter MJ, Robertson CS et al: Continuous monitoring of jugular venous oxygen saturation in head-injured patients. J Neurosurg 76:212, 1992
248. Aldrich EF, Eisenberg HM, Saydjari C et al: Diffuse brain swelling in severely head-injured children: a report from the NIH Traumatic Coma Data Bank. J Neurosurg 76:450, 1992
249. Sioutos PJ, Orozco JA, Carter LP et al: Continuous regional cerebral cortical blood flow monitoring in head-injured patients. Neurosurgery 36:943, 1995
250. Choi SC, Barnes TY, Bullock R et al: Temporal profile of outcomes in severe head injury. J Neurosurg 81:169, 1994
251. Levin HS, Gary HE, Eisenberg HM et al: Neurobehavioral outcome 1 year after severe head injury: experience of the Traumatic Coma Data Bank. J Neurosurg 73:699, 1990
252. Cucchiara RF, Black S, Steinkeler JA: Anesthesia for intracranial procedures. p. 853. In Barash PG, Cullen BF, Stoelting RK (eds): Clinical Anesthesia. Lippincott-Raven, Philadelphia, 1989

4 NEUROLOGIC MONITORING

MICHAEL E. MAHLA

Nervous system function can be readily assessed in the awake patient by physical examination supplemented by laboratory tests such as an electroencephalogram (EEG) or magnetic resonance imaging study. When abnormalities of the central nervous system (CNS) (e.g., aneurysms, tumors), its supporting structures (e.g., spondylitic myelopathy, scoliosis), or its blood supply (e.g., carotid artery arteriosclerosis, thoracoabdominal aortic or intracranial aneurysms) require surgery, nervous system function may be jeopardized. During surgery, the anesthetic used to prevent the patient from experiencing the pain associated with operation usually precludes "on-line" assessment of nervous system function, and until the 1970s, there were no commonly used intraoperative methods of assessing nervous system function in the anesthetized patient.

Over the past several decades, clinicians have begun to use tests previously used only in the diagnostic laboratory as continuous intraoperative monitors of various portions of the CNS and peripheral nervous system. This chapter explains the rationale for the use of each of the monitors and presents evidence for and against each monitor's efficacy in the perioperative period.

For a monitor of the nervous system to have maximum usefulness, it must meet the requirements set forth in the accompanying box. Close examination of these criteria raise the question frequently asked about other monitors, "Do these monitors accurately reflect the intraoperative condition of the patient and correctly predict outcome?" This is clearly an important question, and many insurance companies are now requiring evidence of usefulness to justify reimbursement for this and many other types of monitoring.

As clinicians decide what monitoring to use to help with patient management, neurologic monitoring should not be held to a higher standard than the remainder of the monitors used. In fact, no monitor in the operating room (OR) has been shown to change or reliably predict outcome.

Requirements for a Nervous System Monitor

Changes in monitored parameters should reflect changes in the function or the blood supply of the part of the nervous system that is at risk during surgery.

- The monitor should be used continuously if possible, particularly during periods of risk.
- The number of other factors affecting the monitored parameters should be minimal.
- There should be some possibility of intervention to correct damage detected during surgery.

TABLE 4.1 *Efficacy of neurologic monitors*

OPERATION/ PROCEDURE	NEUROLOGIC MONITOR	GOAL OF MONITORING	EFFICACY LEVEL	ANESTHETIC IMPACT	REFERENCES
Carotid endarterectomy	EEG	Reduce CVA risk	SOC	High	1, 8, 34
Cardiopulmonary bypass	EEG	Reduce CVA risk	EXP	High	2, 4, 21, 22
Posterior spinal fusion (scoliosis and others risking spinal cord)	SSEP	Reduce paraplegia risk	SOC	Moderate to high	1, 3, 7, 8, 27
Aortic vascular surgery	SSEP	Reduce paraplegia risk	EXP	Moderate to high	
Craniotomy for aneurysm	SSEP	Reduce CVA risk	CLIN	High	8, 9, 10
Carotid endarterectomy	SSEP	Reduce CVA risk	CLIN	Moderate to high	8, 19, 20
Resection acoustic neuroma	BAEP	Preserve hearing	SOC	Minimal	1, 8, 15
Microvascular decompression CN VII or V	BAEP	Preserve hearing	CLIN-SOC	Minimal	8, 25
Posterior spinal fusion (scoliosis)	Neurogenic MEPs	Reduce paraplegia risk	CLIN	Minimal	30
Posterior spinal fusion	Transcranial MEPs (electrical or magnetic)	Reduce paraplegia risk	EXP	High	5
Other spine operations	MEPs	Reduce paraplegia risk	EXP	High	35
Resection acoustic neuroma	Facial nerve EMG	Prevent facial weakness	CLIN	Muscle relaxants only	1, 8, 14, 18
Resection brainstem tumor or other lesion	Cranial nerve EMG (especially X)	Prevent loss of gag reflex, facial weakness	EXP	Muscle relaxants only	Abstracts only
Pedicle screw spine fixation	EMG	Prevent iatrogenic radiculopathy	CLIN	Muscle relaxants only	29
Selective dorsal rhizotomy	EMG	Determine which nerve roots to cut	SOC	High	16, 26
Carotid endarterectomy	TCD	Reduce CVA risk	CLIN	None	12, 13, 17
Cardiopulmonary bypass	TCD	Reduce postoperative neuropsychiatric abnormalities	EXP	None	
Brain death determination	TCD	Simplify determination	CLIN	None	31
Head trauma monitoring	Jugular vein O_2 saturation	Optimize BP, ventilation	EXP	Effects on $CMRO_2$	28, 33
Carotid endarterectomy	$Xenon^{133}$ cerebral blood flow	Determine need for shunting	CLIN	Effects on CBF	
Carotid endarterectomy	Near-infrared spectroscopy	Reduce CVA risk	EXP	Effects on $CMRO_2$	6, 23, 24
Carotid endarterectomy	Awake patient	Reduce CVA risk	SOC	Reduce specificity	32
Posterior spinal fusion (scoliosis)	Wake-up test	Reduce paraplegia risk	SOC (if EP monitoring not used)	High	3, 11

Abbreviations: EXP, experimental use justified; CLIN, considerable experimental and clinical data to support efficacy, not yet standard of care; SOC, meets standard of care for monitoring.

The electrocardiogram (ECG) used in the OR can detect only a small fraction of myocardial ischemia that occurs during surgery, even if it is watched continuously (which it is not!). Certainly, patients with intraoperatively ECG-detected ischemia have a higher likelihood of perioperative myocardial infarction (MI),[1,2] but ECG detection of intraoperative ischemia does not reliably predict MI nor does its absence guarantee that an MI subsequently will not occur. Likewise, a prospective study of 20,000 patients failed to demonstrate an outcome advantage to the routine use of intraoperative pulse oximetry.[3] Even in the absence of such studies, both ECG monitoring and pulse oximetry are the standard of care according to the American Society of Anesthesiologists.

Most clinicians who routinely use neurologic monitoring have become convinced of its usefulness, not because of scientific studies but rather, like other monitors, by cases in which major changes in therapy guided by monitoring have resulted in good outcome. In a recent study at the University of Florida, 13 percent of all intracranial aneurysm clipping procedures monitored by somatosensory evoked potentials (SSEP) had evoked potential (EP) changes that caused alterations in management including changes in clip positioning, complete removal of clip and wrapping of the aneurysm, and changes in blood pressure.[4] Most clinicians using neurologic monitoring would be totally unwilling at this point in time to participate in prospective studies designed to test the usefulness of neurologic monitoring, just as many anesthesiologists would be uncomfortable testing the usefulness of pulse oximetry, capnometry, and blood pressure monitoring. Definitive outcome studies proving the worth of neurologic monitoring are *unlikely* to be published in the near future.

Numerous retrospective studies have examined the question as to whether intraoperative monitoring accurately reflects nervous system function. Most of these studies used either EEG, SSEP, or brainstem auditory evoked potentials (BAEP), and the results are very impressive. In a series originally of more than 1,000 (now more than 5,000) patients undergoing carotid endarterectomy (CEA) at the Mayo Clinic, no patient awakened with a new neurologic deficit that was not detected by EEG.[5] EP monitoring has accumulated a similar accuracy record for monitoring during scoliosis surgery and is now considered by many to be a standard of care during this operation.[6–10] However, a few cases have been reported in which neurologic monitoring was used and adverse neurologic outcome occurred despite no change in the monitored parameters ("false-negative" results).[11–14] Indeed, it would be extremely surprising if such cases were not reported!

Even if all the reported false-negative cases are valid (most are not), the number of such events is exceedingly small compared with the total number of cases monitored. Many of these cases were generated by an inappropriate use of the monitor, in which the monitored pathway did not correspond to the part of the nervous system at risk from the operation, or by inadequate quality control resulting in technical problems with the recordings. Some of these reports, however, did reflect true false-negatives and have improved our understanding of how well the function of the monitored pathway predicts function of adjacent areas of the brain and spinal cord.[13] Thus, we are better able to define the limitations of neurologic monitoring.

Cases in which a perceived or real failure of the monitor occurred must be kept in perspective. When used carefully and appropriately, intraoperative neurologic monitoring appears to be useful in the early detection of a change in monitored function, and the initiation of therapeutic interventions to prevent permanent neurologic injury.

Table 4.1 represents a summary of most monitors of the nervous system that were in common use in 1996 as well as the most common reported use of each monitor. The next to last column in this table presents my opinion as to the usefulness of each neurologic monitor in a particular application. This opinion is based on a synthesis of my clinical experience, currently available literature (all referenced during the course of the chapter), and the opinions of other experts and consensus panels. The remainder of the chapter is organized around this table. The table is divided into sections by monitor type. Monitor types discussed include both monitors of function (EEG, EPs, awake examination) and blood flow (cerebral blood flow [CBF], transcranial Doppler [TCD], jugular venous O_2 saturation [$S_{jv}O_2$], and cerebral oximetry). Each monitor will be discussed according to the following general outline:

A. Theoretical basis for the monitor
B. Procedures in which this monitor is used
   1. Rationale for the monitor's use in this procedure
   2. Evidence for the monitor's efficacy in this procedure
   3. Limitations of the monitor in this procedure

MONITORS OF FUNCTION

The Neurologic Examination: The Wake-up Test and Continuous Examination

The neurologic examination may be used intraoperatively either intermittently (the wake-up test) or continuously (during local or regional anesthesia). Continuous assessment of the awake patient is extremely useful in any situation with potentially unstable CNS function. Under local or regional anesthesia, patients with an unstable neck (e.g., rheumatoid arthritis or cervical myelopathy secondary to degenerative arthritis) may be positioned awake and neurologic examination followed during surgery. A patient with compromised blood supply to the head (e.g., severe carotid stenosis) may be assessed continuously to make certain that the cerebral perfusion pressure is adequate to supply the brain's needs. Neurologic function may be monitored similarly in carotid surgery during application of a carotid cross-clamp. This type of neurologic monitoring, when feasible, is becoming increasingly popular in this era of cost-containment. It requires no special equipment or technologists to operate the equipment, but it does require special skill on the part of the anesthesiologist in selecting the right patient, placing the blocks properly, and coaching patients through difficult times during the operation.

Awake neurologic monitoring may be difficult during lengthy procedures. A 3-hour limit is probably a good cutoff. Patients often become uncomfortable from lying in the same position for a prolonged period and may require analgesics and sedation to tolerate the procedure. At some point, such therapy may decrease the sensitivity and specificity of the neurologic examination to detect injury. This type of monitoring has not found extensive use in spine surgery to date. However, with new, relatively noninvasive techniques on the horizon, awake neurologic monitoring may play an increased role in the future, particularly during endoscopic disc surgery.

Intermittent neurologic monitoring (the wake-up test) is used to test neurologic function following a *reversible* surgical manipulation that has the potential to cause neurologic damage. The test is most commonly used after distraction of the spinal column during surgery for correction of kyphoscoliosis. The wake-up test has been considered for many years to be the "gold standard" for assessment of spinal cord function during scoliosis surgery. *However, its sensitivity is open to question*. First, the test is applied only intermittently. During most of the operation, nervous system function is unknown. Thus, the effects of induced hypotension, which potentially risks spinal cord function (particularly when distraction is applied to the spinal column), are not assessed except during the test performance. The appropriate time(s) to apply the wake-up test is also not clear. The spinal cord and brain have both gray and white matter. Gray matter has a higher metabolic need for O_2 and will stop functioning within seconds after a complete interruption in blood supply. White matter, which consumes much less O_2, may continue to function for many minutes after a complete interruption. Partial interruption of blood supply to white matter may take much longer (possibly hours) to manifest loss of function. Thus, a wake-up test applied immediately after spinal column distraction may fail to detect loss of blood flow to white matter pathways in the mid-thoracic spinal cord (the area at highest risk for ischemia) and, therefore, cannot reliably detect partial loss of blood flow that may later become critical.

In summary, the wake-up test can evaluate both motor and sensory function at the time it is applied, but it cannot assess function at other times. Ideally, the test should be applied in conjunction with other less dangerous and more continuous forms of neurologic function monitoring. Despite these shortcomings, results of the wake-up test seem to correlate well with neurologic outcome. I know of only two cases in which the patient demonstrated a neurologic deficit postoperatively that was not detected by an intraoperative wake-up test; one published case and one from my own personal experience.

CNS Electrical Activity

GENERAL THEORETICAL BASIS When O_2 delivery to the brain falls below a level sufficient to meet the cerebral metabolic rate (requirement) for oxygen ($CMRO_2$) required, function fails. Because function is disrupted *before* cellular integrity is lost, monitors of function provide early warning of inadequate O_2 supply and provide opportunity to correct this problem before irreversible damage occurs. Such monitors can be used to guide therapy when CNS O_2 supply may be compromised during surgery and to detect surgically induced structural damage that produces changes in function.

The function of some motor and sensory pathways (motor and sensory EPs), as well as the spontaneous electrical activity of the cerebral cortex (EEG), is easily monitored during general anesthesia. These pathways and spontaneous electrical activity of the cerebral cortex, however, reflect the function of only a portion of the entire nervous system. Changes in one monitored parameter may *imply* damage to other nearby areas of the nervous system; however, damage to unmonitored portions of the nervous system may occur without detection. Thus, when areas of the nervous system that cannot currently be monitored are at risk during surgery, false-negative monitoring patterns should be expected.

THE ELECTRO-ENCEPHALOGRAM

Theoretical Basis

The EEG recorded from the scalp is a summation of excitatory (EPSP) and inhibitory (IPSP) postsynaptic potentials produced in the pyramidal layer of the cerebral cortex. EPSPs or IPSPs are produced when a small amount of neurotransmitter (insufficient to cause depolarization of the postsynaptic membrane in the case of an EPSP) is released from the presynaptic nerve terminal. These electrical signals range in amplitude from less than 10 μV to about 100 μV (larger in children and adolescents).

As with recording of the ECG, EEG electrodes are placed in a standardized fashion so that tracings from one individual may be compared either with later tracings from the same individual or with those of other individuals. The International Ten-Twenty Electrode System (Fig. 4.1) places EEG or EP recording electrodes over specific areas of the cerebral cortex and is based on measurements made between pairs of specific sites on the patient's head.[15] Each recording point is designated with a letter and a number and can often be associated with underlying CNS structures; for example, C3, Cz, and C4 are all associated with the motor cortex. By convention, recording electrodes placed over the right hemisphere are even-numbered and those

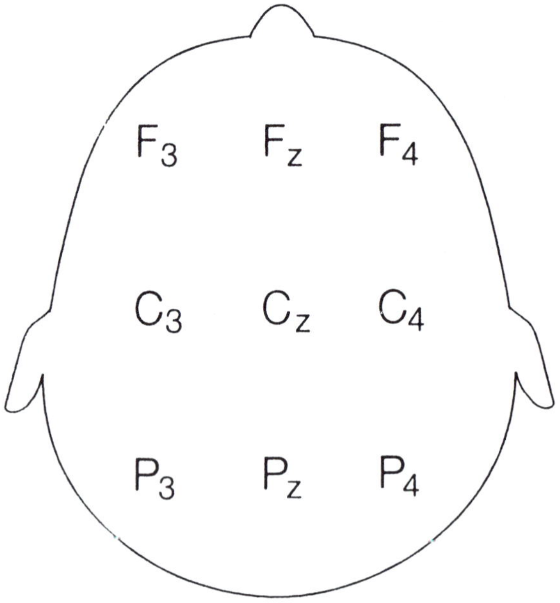

FIGURE 4.1 *International 10–20 System of EEG electrode placement. (From Mahla,[125] with permission.)*

placed over the left are odd-numbered. Midline electrodes are designated by a "z" subscript.

These electrodes are connected in pairs to a differential amplification system (Fig. 4.2), and the output is displayed, just as the ECG, as a plot of voltage versus time. Each EEG channel represents the electrical activity of one electrode pair. The recording of multiple EEG channels simultaneously on paper moving at speeds up to 3 cm-sec^{-1} creates a large amount of on-line data (Fig. 4.3). It is not practical for the anesthesiologist to monitor these data in addition to all other tasks, and a neurophysiologist (e.g., Ph.D., or a physician—neurologist or anesthesiologist), with or without a technician, must monitor the EEG output continuously for maximal usefulness.

Reduction in the number of channels or simplification and suitable formatting of data may enable anesthesiologists with appropriate training to use the EEG for intraoperative monitoring without the aid of a technologist or neurologist. The display can be simplified through signal processing techniques, which include power spectrum analysis, frequency analysis, filtering, and rectification, and displayed in time-compressed formats such as compressed spectral array and density spectral array (Fig. 4.4). Functionally, most of these displays convert the standard plot of voltage versus time to a plot of frequency versus time. Of extreme importance, however, is the retention of access to the real-time unprocessed EEG. Except for gross artifact rejection by voltage criteria, these simplified monitors do not yet have the ability to distinguish brain activity from other biologic signals (e.g., ECG) or noise. Noise is processed just as if it were electrical brain activity.

It is not clear just how much data reduction can occur before the sensitivity of EEG monitoring is compromised. The largest clinical se-

FIGURE 4.2 *Schematic of a differential amplification system. The differential amplifier accepts input from two separate electrodes. The (–) input is subtracted from the (+) input, and the difference is amplified. If a signal is present in both inputs, differential amplification will cancel out this signal. This amplification characteristic is very useful when recording signals in a hostile electrical environment because noise will be present in both channels and not amplified.*

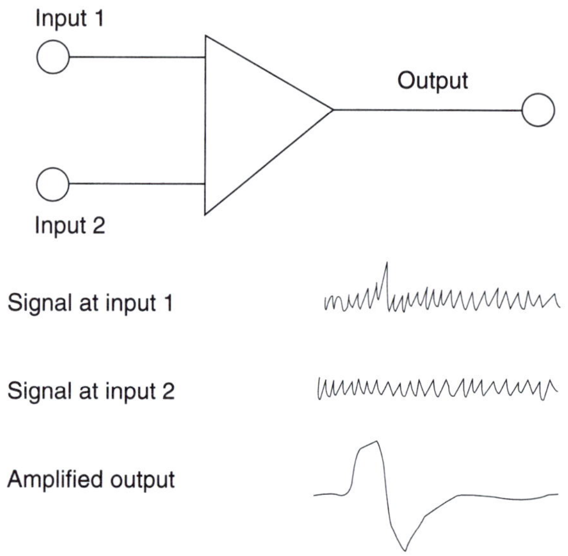

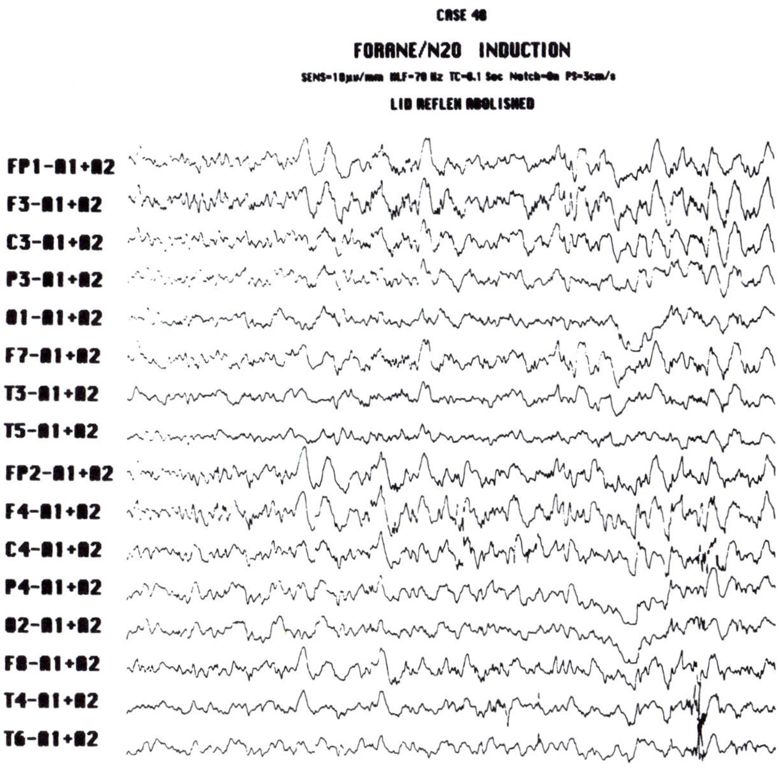

FIGURE 4.3 *Unprocessed 16-channel EEG. Continuous monitoring of unprocessed EEG generates a very large amount of on-line data for analysis.*

ries that examined the usefulness of EEG monitoring during carotid surgery used 16 channels of acquired data for analysis.[5] Although no carefully performed studies have compared lesser numbers of channels systematically with the 16-channel unprocessed recordings, data suggest fewer numbers of channels may be very useful. Two separate studies compared two or four-channel computer-processed EEG with 16-channel hard-copy EEG monitored by a trained technician and a neurologist. In both cases, the processed monitor was able to identify about 75 percent of the significant EEG changes seen on the 16-channel EEG.[16,17] These studies suggest that even two or four channels are very useful for monitoring a carotid endarterectomy. At least two channels (one on each hemisphere) help to differentiate EEG changes caused by global factors such as anesthetic drugs from changes caused by more regional factors such as carotid cross-clamping. A recent study suggests that strategic placement of the electrodes over the watershed distribution of the middle cerebral and anterior cerebral arteries can improve the sensitivity of EEG monitoring to more than 90 percent even when only four channels are used.[18]

For pattern recognition in the EEG, the complex waveforms are described in terms of frequency (cycles × sec^{-1} = Hz) and amplitude (voltage). Four basic EEG rhythms or frequency patterns are analyzed (Fig. 4.5): delta (0 to 4 Hz); theta (4 to 8 Hz); alpha (8 to 13 Hz); and beta (greater than 13 Hz). Delta rhythm or marked slowing occurs during deep sleep, deep anesthesia, and many pathologic states such as ischemia, drug overdose, or severe metabolic derangements. Theta rhythm or moderate slowing is commonly seen during general anesthesia and may occur during the same pathologic states as delta rhythm. Alpha rhythm can be recorded, mainly over the occipital region, in an alert, relaxed patient whose eyes are closed. During lighter surgical planes of anesthesia, this 8- to

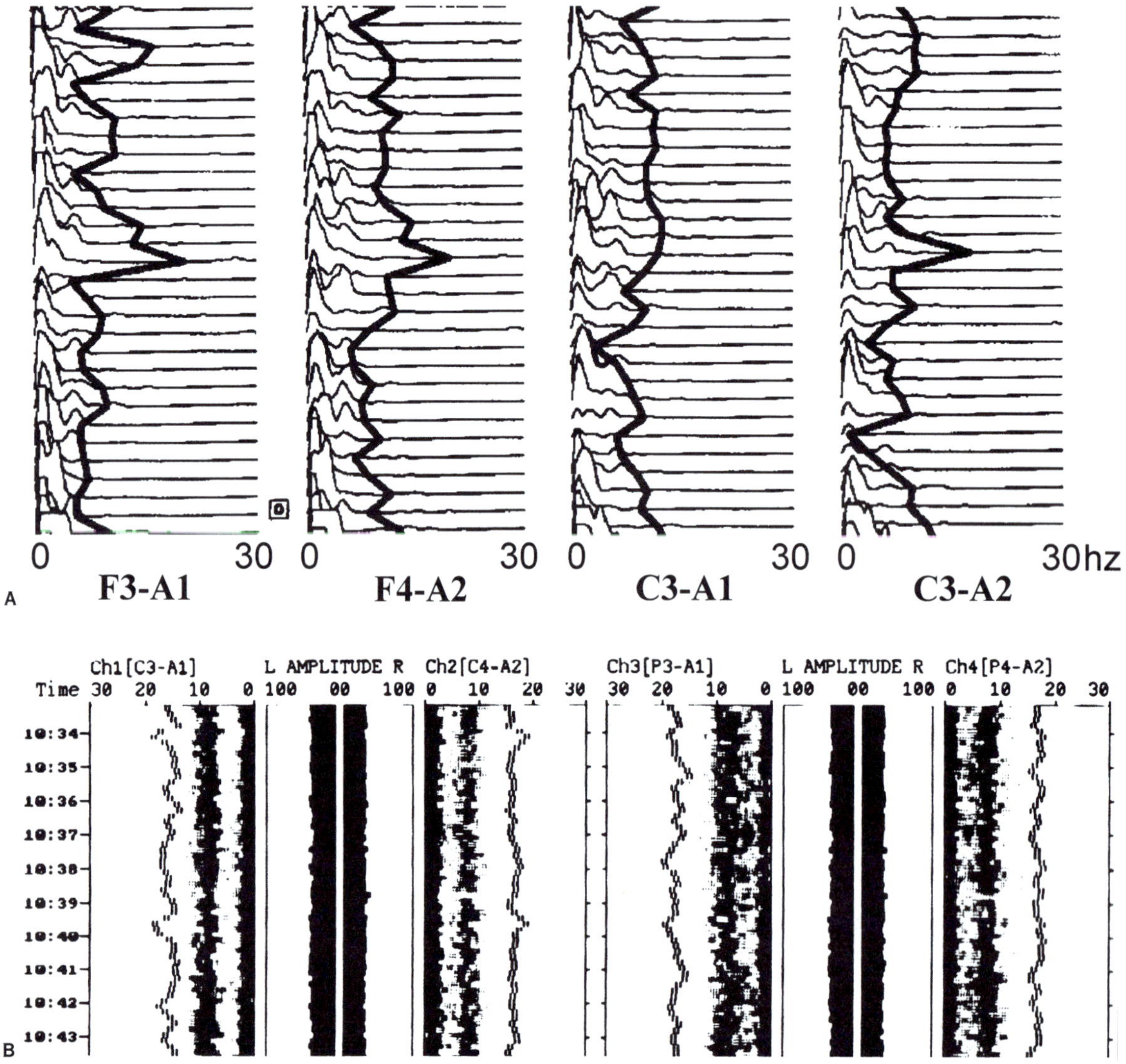

FIGURE 4.4 *Processed EEG. The most common types of processed EEG are compressed spectral array (A) and density spectral array (B) In A, height of "mountain indicates power at a given frequency. In B, dot density indicated power at a given Frequency. (From Mahla,[125] with permission.)*

13-Hz activity can be recorded over much of the cortex but especially in the anterior leads. Beta rhythm accompanies mental concentration or may be induced with low doses of many sedative/hypnotic drugs such as barbiturates or benzodiazepines. Deep anesthesia, ischemia, or other pathologic states abolish both alpha and beta frequencies, after which slower frequencies predominate.

Changes in EEG amplitude normally result from synchronization or desynchronization of cortical electrical activity. Larger, synchronized EEG activity is seen during sleep or surgical anesthesia. However, very deep levels of anes-

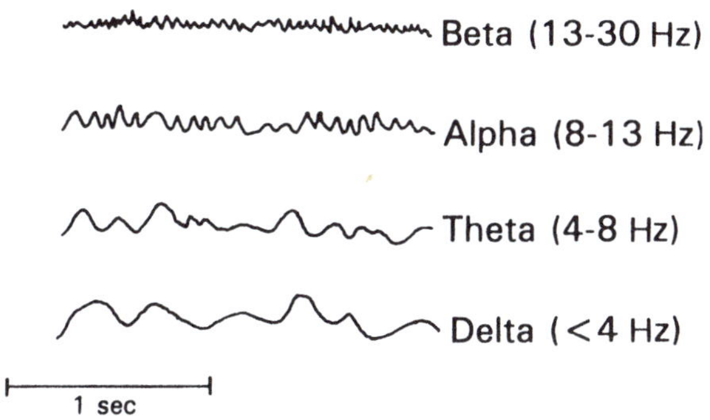

FIGURE 4.5 *Basic EEG frequency patterns: Beta (greater than 13 Hz), alpha (8 to 13 Hz), theta (4 to 8 Hz), and delta (less than 1 to 4 Hz).*

thesia cause a loss in EEG amplitude secondary to direct depression of cortical neuronal activity. Awakening usually desynchronizes the EEG and produces a decrease in amplitude, with the appearance of higher frequency patterns such as beta. In general, more complex (higher) function is represented by faster, less synchronized (lower voltage) activity. For example, mental concentration is accompanied by the appearance of beta frequencies.

General Rationale for Intraoperative Use of EEG

EEG activity (i.e., cortical electrical activity) requires about 50 percent of the total O_2 consumed by the brain; the remaining 50 percent is needed to maintain cellular integrity. When O_2 delivery is compromised by either hypoxemia or decreased blood supply, O_2 that ordinarily would be used to produce electrical activity will instead be diverted to maintain cellular integrity. Slowing of EEG activity thus reflects decreased O_2 delivery (Fig. 4.6). Interventions based on recognition of these patterns may be made in much the same fashion as interventions are made after recognition of ECG changes.

In a large series of patients undergoing CEA at the Mayo Clinic, the EEG was compared with regional CBF by using the ^{133}Xenon washout method. This study validated the EEG as an indicator of the adequacy of regional CBF.[5] Normal gray/white CBF averages 50 $ml \cdot 100\ g^{-1} \cdot min^{-1}$. With most anesthetic techniques, the EEG begins to become abnormal when CBF falls to 20 $ml \cdot 100\ g^{-1} \cdot min^{-1}$.[5] The threshold for EEG changes appears to be much lower (8 to 10 $ml \cdot 100\ g^{-1} \cdot min^{-1}$), however, when isoflurane is used.[19] Cellular survival is not threatened until CBF falls to 12 $ml \cdot 100\ g^{-1} \cdot min^{-1}$ (lower with isoflurane). Thus, a margin of safety is present between the time at which the EEG becomes abnormal and that at which cellular damage begins to occur. Severe anemia and decreases in O_2 saturation also decrease O_2 delivery. The EEG activity becomes abnormal once increased blood flow cannot compensate for decreased arterial O_2 content.

Unfortunately, changes in EEG frequency and amplitude may be caused by administration of anesthetic drugs as well as changes in anesthetic depth. Low doses of potent inhalation agents with N_2O produce an active EEG with alpha and beta frequencies present. Steady-state anesthesia, regardless of the agent used, usually produces a stable EEG pattern. *Be aware that deep anesthesia and ischemia produce similar EEG changes* (Fig. 4.7A, ischemia; Fig. 7B, effects of adding N_2O to a Forane anesthetic). In both cases, fast activity is replaced by slower, larger EEG waveforms. As anesthesia is further deepened or ischemia worsens, additional slowing occurs, and the EEG amplitude decreases,

FIGURE 4.6 *EEG patterns seen in cerebral ischemia.*

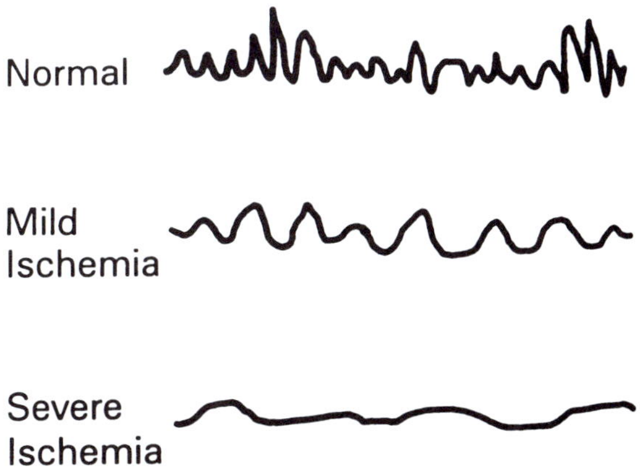

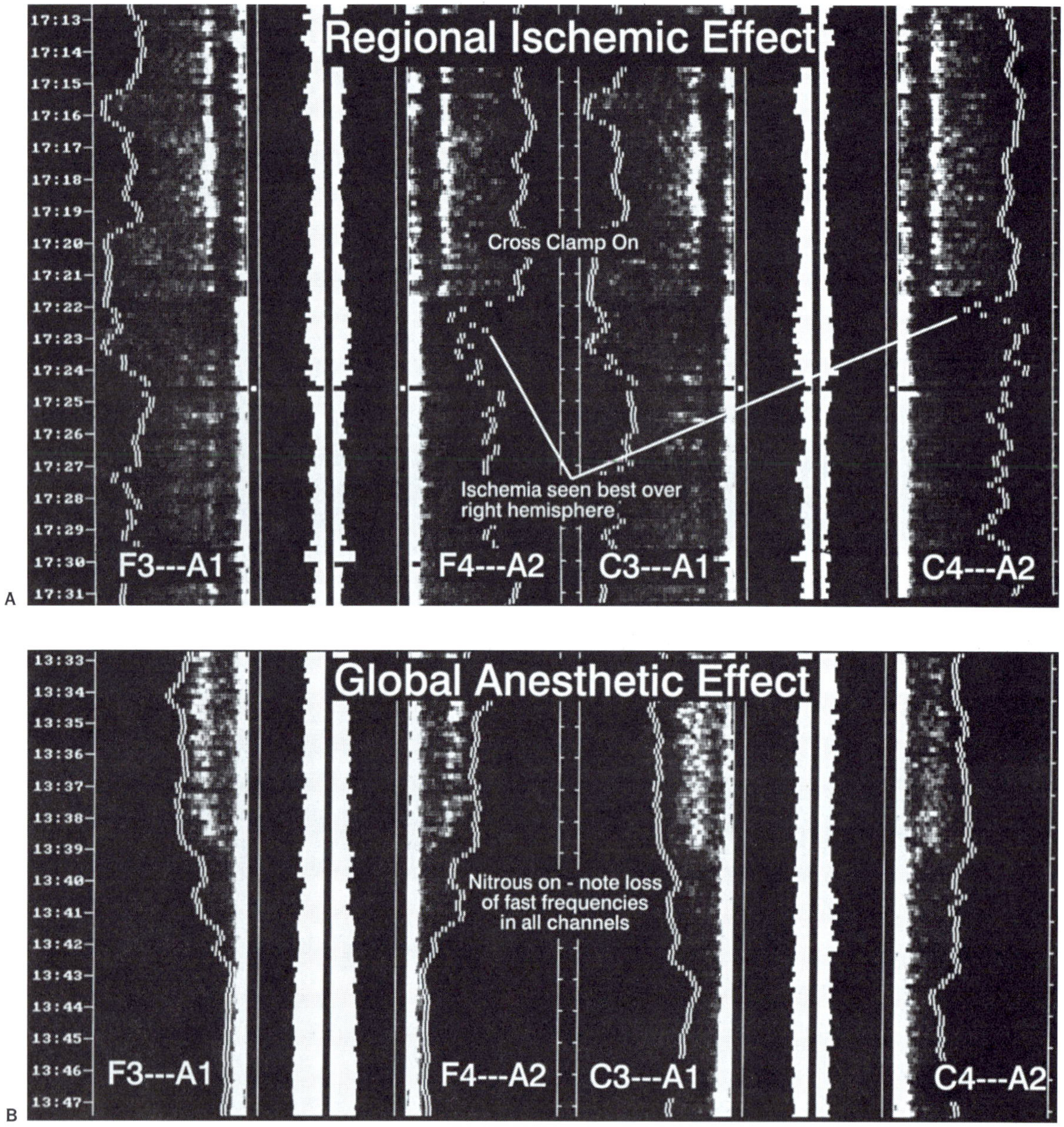

FIGURE 4.7 *Density spectral array view: ischemia versus anesthetic effect. (A) EEG change primarily in one channel associated with carotid cross-clamping. (B) EEG change associated with a dramatic change in anesthetic technique. Note that the anesthetic effect is global, whereas in this (but not all) case, the ischemic effect is only regional.*

ultimately becoming flat (isoelectric). Boluses of anesthetic drugs may produce large EEG changes indistinguishable from those seen during ischemia.

EEG during Carotid Endarterectomy

If monitoring of the EEG could be proved scientifically to reduce the incidence of stroke, the question of EEG monitoring during carotid surgery would require no discussion. Such data, however, do not exist. There are no prospective, randomized controlled trials proving that EEG monitoring improves outcome during carotid surgery. What information is available is strongly suggestive that EEG monitoring is useful. In a large series of patients undergoing CEA with selective shunting who were monitored with 16-channel unprocessed EEG, no patient awakened with a new neurologic deficit not predicted by EEG. Transient, correctable EEG changes were not associated with stroke. Persistent changes were associated with stroke.[5] The most commonly reported use of the EEG during CEA is to determine the need for placement of an intraoperative shunt. Because, under stable anesthetic conditions, EEG patterns correlate with CBF,[5] EEG can be used to determine when CBF falls to a level that could threaten cellular survival. A shunt may then be inserted to improve CBF.[20] Although there are no adequate prospective studies proving that stroke is more likely with EEG changes during cross-clamping than when EEG changes do not occur, a large retrospective series suggests that strokes *do not* occur in the absence of persistent EEG changes during cross-clamping when a shunt was not inserted.[5] Thus, when selective shunting is used, the clinician is left with a persuasive logical argument favoring EEG use based on the relationship of EEG to CBF and on the fact that during a very large clinical series, there has never been a patient who awakened with a neurologic deficit not detected by EEG monitoring.

More difficult to prove is that EEG monitoring is useful when all patients are shunted during carotid clamping. EEG monitoring has detected correctable shunt malfunction (personal experience). A retrospective analysis of 3,328 CEAs in 46 institutions showed a statistically significant reduction in stroke rate in patients who were monitored and selective shunting used compared with patients who were not monitored.[21] A recent multicentered study of 1,495 CEAs supports selective shunting and provides convincing data that shunting of patients without evidence of decreased cerebral perfusion actually increases the incidence of perioperative stroke by more than sixfold.[22] In the absence of properly designed outcome studies, these data suggest that optimal results during carotid surgery will be obtained with selective shunting guided by EEG monitoring.

Ideally, EEG use during CEA should be continuous, yet it has been described most frequently as a spot check to determine the need for shunt placement after carotid cross-clamping in anesthetized patients. This short-term use, however, detects only a small portion of the neurologic injuries that can occur during and after carotid surgery. Most strokes, in fact, occur after repair of the carotid stenosis. Critical carotid luminal narrowing risks cerebral hypoperfusion during hypotension or positioning.[23,24] Shunt malfunction has also been detected by EEG monitoring (personal experience). All these problems would be missed if the EEG is not monitored continuously. Serious intraoperative reduction in cerebral O_2 supply may also result from nonsurgical factors that the anesthesiologist can correct. Reduction in CBF produced by hyperventilation or hypotension may be corrected by reducing ventilation and restoring normal blood pressure. Because the EEG correlates with adequacy of CBF, it serves as a monitor of the effectiveness of therapy instituted to correct ischemia.

Without EEG monitoring, blood pressure decreases occurring during surgery are treated empirically according to a predetermined "lower limit" of mean blood pressure. Elevation of blood pressure with a vasopressor is known to increase the likelihood of myocardial ischemia during carotid surgery.[25] Monitoring of the EEG helps to determine whether hypotension actually produces a reduction in CBF that requires treatment, and in one study, limitation of the use of vasopressors for treatment of hypotension to those episodes in which EEG changes were present did not increase the incidence of perioperative myocardial ischemia.[24] Thus, it would seem logical that treatment of hypotension should only be undertaken when a documented need for treatment, such as EEG or ECG changes, exists.

In summary, based on available evidence, the EEG is a useful monitor of the adequacy of CBF during carotid surgery. The overwhelming consensus of many experts is that EEG monitoring meets the standard of care for monitoring neurologic function during carotid surgery.[26,27] As discussed below, however, it is not the only method that can be used for monitoring the brain.

EEG during Cardiopulmonary Bypass

EEG has been monitored by clinicians during cardiopulmonary bypass for more than 30 years. However, EEG monitoring has not yet attained either standard of care status or widespread acceptance for monitoring the brain during cardiopulmonary bypass. Some clinicians would go so far as to say that EEG monitoring has no role during cardiopulmonary bypass at all.[28] The most likely reason for this problem is that EEG monitoring during bypass fails one of the important requirements for a nervous system monitor to have maximum usefulness—the number of other factors affecting the monitor should be minimal. The types of drugs commonly used during cardiac operations as well as the induced hypothermia have profound effects on the EEG that are difficult to distinguish from changes associated with ischemia.[29,30] In addition, unlike for CEA, little standardization of monitoring techniques exists among institutions using EEG monitoring during cardiopulmonary bypass. A systematic normative database for EEG changes during cardiopulmonary bypass under standard, interinstitutional conditions controlling for EEG monitoring technical parameters as well as anesthetic technique simply does not yet exist.

Nonetheless, several studies in the literature have attempted to establish a relationship between EEG monitoring during bypass and postoperative neurologic outcome. Most of the more recent studies used some variation of "quantitative EEG." Quantitative EEG monitors multiple channels (usually at least eight, but most commonly 16 or 32 channels) of information. Sophisticated computer analysis breaks the complex EEG patterns down into frequency bands. Comparison is then made to a baseline study either visually or numerically or by a computer estimate of the probability that the current data are actually different from the baseline data in each channel of information. Intraoperative EEG changes were then compared with postoperative neurologic findings (usually obtained by detailed neuropsychiatric testing). Several small series showed a good correlation between intraoperative data and postoperative neurologic outcome. A few series attempted to alter intraoperative management based on EEG findings to improve outcome. None of these series were large enough to have significant statistical power to show a difference in outcome, but several appear promising,[31,32] as does at least one animal study.[33] Other series, particularly in children, were unable to show any consistent intraoperative pattern that predicted postoperative outcome.[34]

On an individual case basis, the EEG is clearly useful. I am personally aware of three cases, and there are anecdotal published reports of EEG monitoring detecting unsuspected serious intraoperative problems with cerebral perfusion during bypass.[35,36] Most of these patients were able to have CBF restored before permanent damage occurred.

Finally, EEG monitoring during bypass may be used to monitor levels of burst suppression if thiopental is given for cerebral protection. As explained below, the dose of thiopental may thus be minimized.

In summary, EEG monitoring may be useful during cardiopulmonary bypass. However, there are no compelling scientific studies supporting its routine use or even strongly suggesting clinical usefulness at this time. Such a status likely awaits development of standardized monitoring protocols and normative databases. Much further work needs to be done, and EEG monitoring during cardiopulmonary bypass, while anecdotally useful, must still be considered largely experimental at this time.

Other Uses of EEG

BARBITURATE SUPPRESSION OF THE $CMRO_2$ The EEG may be used to monitor cerebral O_2 demand. Barbiturates are commonly administered to either lower intracranial pressure (ICP) or to reduce cerebral metabolism and presumably increase tolerance to ischemia. Monitoring barbiturate levels to guide therapy is impractical at most centers. Because barbiturates and other drugs that depress cerebral metabolism, almost without exception, are cardiovascular depressants, the minimum dose of drug necessary for the intended effect on $CMRO_2$ should be given. Barbiturates lower ICP and $CMRO_2$ by depressing cortical electrical activity. Thus, the EEG would be a logical monitor of barbiturate effect. Once cortical electrical activity is abolished, barbiturates cannot further reduce $CMRO_2$, CBF, or ICP. Hence, the EEG may be used to determine the minimum dose of drug necessary to obtain what we currently believe to be the maximal effect (i.e., near-total EEG suppression).

INDUCED HYPOTENSION Monitoring cerebral cortical function during induced hypotension is a logical extension of EEG use in carotid surgery. There are no carefully controlled studies in the literature describing the use of EEG for these purposes, but there are both human and laboratory studies that suggest that EEG correlates well with the adequacy of cerebral O_2 delivery in the setting of induced hypotension.[37–42] Use of EEG for this purpose remains experimental.

Information Not Provided by EEG Monitoring

EEG monitoring provides information about the overall electrical functioning of the cerebral cortex but not much about the subcortical brain, spinal cord, or cranial and peripheral nerves. The functioning of CNS sensory or motor pathways that may be at risk during surgical procedures is monitored by sensory EPs and motor evoked potentials (MEP), and individual cranial or peripheral nerves may be monitored with spontaneous and evoked electromyography (EMG).

EVOKED POTENTIALS

General Theoretical Concepts

The EEG records *spontaneous* electrical activity produced by the CNS. EPs consist of CNS electrical activity that is evoked by sensory (electrical, auditory, visual) or motor (electrical, magnetic) stimuli. Sensory EPs are of three types: (1) peripheral or cranial nerve, (2) subcortical, and (3) cortical. MEPs are responses of the nervous system to electrical or magnetic stimuli applied directly to the motor cortex or spinal cord and may be recorded from spinal cord, peripheral nerve, and muscle. Sensory EPs are usually quite small in amplitude. Signal averaging must frequently be used to detect EPs because background EEG and other types of biologic noise are much larger than these evoked responses. MEPs are generally much larger and frequently do not require averaging to be readily recorded.

Signal Averaging

The EP signals produced by a single stimulus are small and can be easily obscured by background activity including electrical or surgeon-generated noise, EEG, EMG, or ECG activity. Intraoperative electrical noise generated from equipment or by the surgeon can be especially problematic and interfere with monitoring of the EP responses of clinical interest. Signal averaging is used to improve the quality of EP monitoring by reducing or eliminating random background activity such as EEG, EMG, or electrical noise to allow identification of time-locked EP responses that are not random. The signal-to-noise ratio is improved by the square root of the number of epochs (or events) averaged (Fig. 4.8). The required number of epochs in the average is related to the amplitude of the EP response. A response that is small in amplitude requires a greater number of averaged responses to obtain an identifiable reproducible response. SSEP recordings are generally obtained by averaging 1,000 responses. BAEPs are smaller, subcortically generated signals that may require averaging of at least 2,000 responses to obtain an adequate recording. There are also other methods to improve the quality of the EP response intraoperatively including (1) selection of a stimulus repetition rate that is not synchronized with background activity (i.e., 60-cycle electrical noise); (2) selection of appropriate high and low cut filters; (3) acceptable electrode impedance levels; and (4) elimination of background biologic activity when possible (i.e., administration of muscle relaxant to abolish EMG activity).

FIGURE 4.8 *Signal averaging. The very small evoked potential (arrow) is obscured by background EEG signal. Signal averaging, however, improves the signal-to-noise ratio by averaging out random background EEG, leaving only the evoked response, which is time locked to the stimulus.*

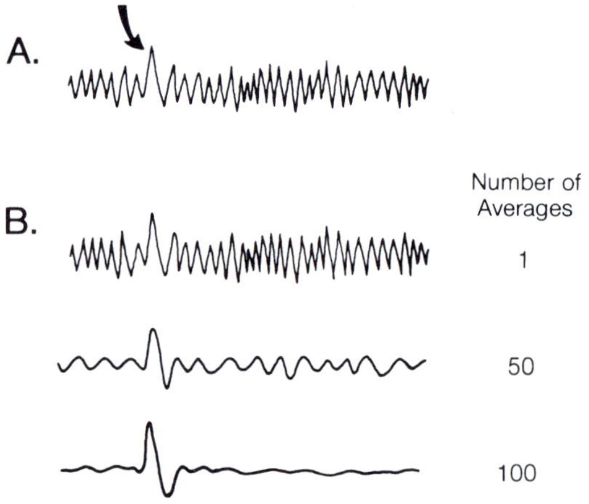

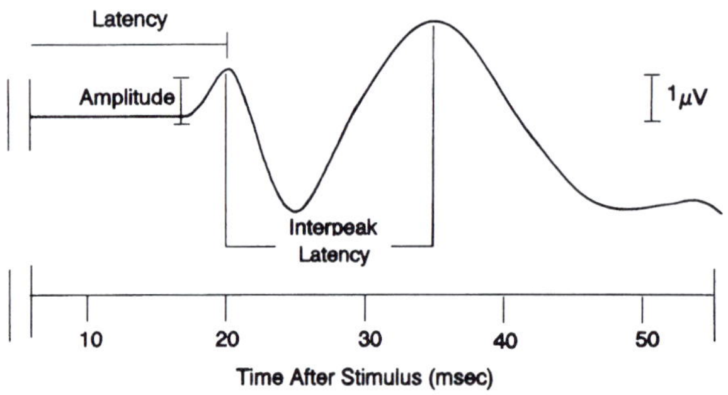

FIGURE 4.9 *Evoked potentials are described in terms of latency (time from delivery of stimulus to onset of response) and amplitude (size in microvolts).*

Descriptive Terms

EPs are described in terms of latency and amplitude (Fig. 4.9). Latency is the time measured from the application of the stimulus to the point of maximum amplitude of the EP. Some types of EPs have more than one peak. Latency measured between EP peaks (interpeak latency) measures transit time between signal generators along the pathway being stimulated and is often important clinically. Amplitude is defined as the voltage difference between two peaks of opposite polarity or between an EP peak and a reference level representing zero potential.

SOMATOSENSORY EVOKED POTENTIALS

Theoretical Concepts

SSEPs monitor the function of the somesthetic sensory system, which extends throughout the peripheral nervous system and CNS. Thus peripheral nerve, spinal cord, subcortical, and cortical structures in the brain may be monitored. The somesthetic system carries sensory infor-

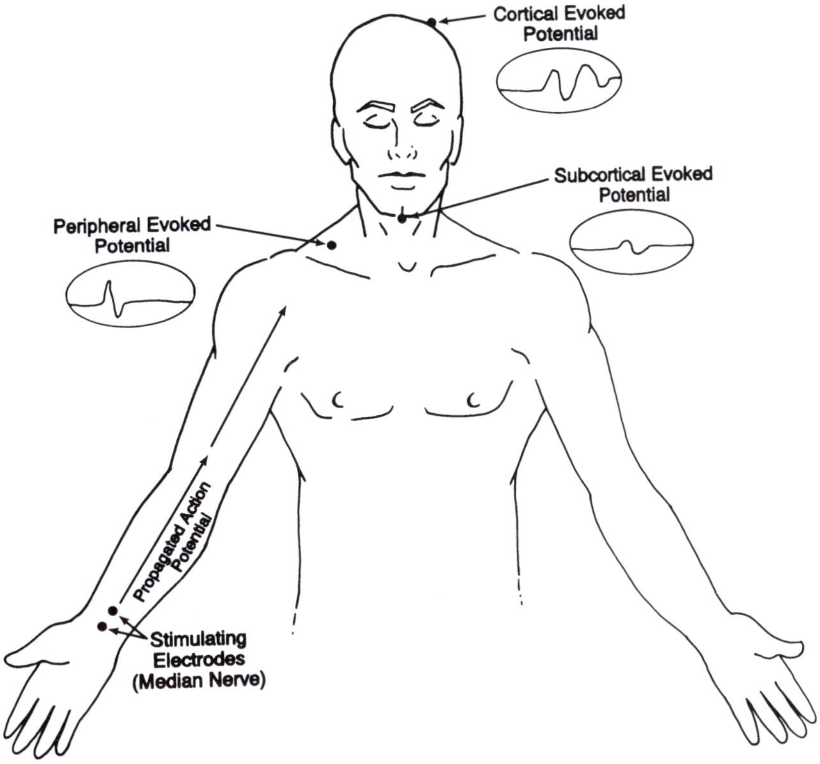

FIGURE 4.10 *Somatosensory evoked potentials may be recorded anywhere in the nervous system but most commonly over peripheral nerve, spinal cord, and cortex.*

mation including vibration, proprioception, and light touch. A SSEP is generated when repetitive electrical stimuli are applied to a peripheral nerve, and many single responses are averaged together to produce the evoked response. Responses may be recorded over the peripheral nerve, nerve plexus, spinal cord, brainstem, and cerebral cortex (Fig. 4.10). Recording sites are related directly to the somesthetic pathway.

As with the EEG, cortical recording electrode locations are based on the ten-twenty system[15] of electrode placement. The number of recording channels will vary with the type of case being monitored. In an ideal situation, recordings should be made over each peripheral nerve being stimulated, the spinal cord rostral to the nerve's entry, the second cervical vertebrae, and the opposite cerebral cortex. In addition, if possible, a portion of the somatosensory system not at risk from surgery should be monitored as well to help differentiate surgically induced changes in SSEPs produced by global factors such as anesthetic drugs or metabolic abnormalities. Thus, for example, during a right CEA, cortical responses from both left and right median nerve stimulation should be recorded. During surgery correcting thoracolumbar scoliosis, responses from both posterior tibial nerves as well as from at least one median nerve (above the level of surgery) are desirable. Generally, these requirements translate into at least four channels of data.

The most important use of peripheral nerve recordings is to make certain that a stimulus is actually reaching the CNS. If the SSEP disappears during a surgical procedure, one must ensure that the cause is not failure to stimulate adequately. A peripheral nerve response rules out this technical failure.

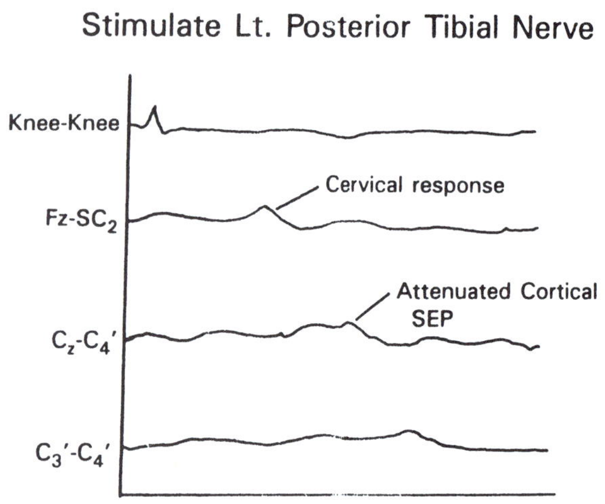

FIGURE 4.11 *Somatosensory evoked responses generated subcortically are more resistant to the effects of anesthetic drugs than cortically generated responses.*

Recordings over the spinal cord also provide insurance against technical failure. In addition, they monitor spinal cord function below the level of electrode placement. In the case of operations on the spinal cord or on the spinal column, if recordings over the spinal cord rostral to the operative site can be made, cortical recordings become less important. This fact is important to the anesthesiologist, because recordings made over the spinal cord are much less sensitive to the effects of anesthetic drugs than recordings made over the cortex (Fig. 4.11). Reliance on spinal recordings allows the anesthesiologist much greater freedom in drug choice. Spinal recordings, however, give little information about cortical function except to show that a stimulus has reached the CNS.

Because factors other than surgery may alter the SSEP signal, the clinician must be able to decide when a change is significant and requires treatment. Based on many clinical series (not studies!) and on studies looking at the effects of different anesthetic agents on the SSEP, many experts quote a 50 percent decrease in amplitude or a 10 percent increase in latency as the degree of change that should provoke concern. Amplitude changes are considered the more important factor. In an environment in which factors known to influence the SSEP such as anesthetic drugs, temperature, or $PaCO_2$ cannot be carefully controlled, these guidelines may be appropriate. If tight control of these factors can be maintained, in my opinion, any amount of *event-related change or sudden change in the SSEP should be considered significant*. In the absence of any observable event occurring around the time of an SSEP change, I use the aforementioned latency and amplitude criteria to help decide when a change needs to be investigated urgently.

Somatosensory Pathway

SSEPs monitor the function of the somatosensory system, which carries sensory information including vibration, proprioception, and light touch and extends throughout the peripheral nervous system and CNS. Electrical stimuli have been shown to activate the largest peripheral nerve sensory fibers (group I) preferentially, which mediate primarily vibratory and proprioceptive sensation. The peripheral nerves most commonly used for stimulation include the median nerve, ulnar nerve, common peroneal nerve, and posterior tibial nerve, depending on which portion of the nervous system is being monitored.

The propagated nerve action potential elicited by electrical stimulation can easily be recorded more proximally over the peripheral nerve (e.g., at Erb's point over the supraclavicular brachial plexus or in the popliteal fossa over the tibial nerve). These signals are usually very large and easy to record. Most evidence indicates that upper extremity EPs are conducted rostrally in the spinal cord via dorsal column pathways (fasciculus cuneatus). The response is conducted across a synapse in the nucleus cuneatus, just above the cervicomedullary junction. This signal usually cannot be recorded near the cells or pathways producing EP. Instead, it is recorded from the skin overlying the spinal cord and brainstem and thus has a smaller amplitude.

After the synapse, the pathway crosses and projects onto the ventral posterolateral nucleus of the thalamus. From there, the response is conducted via the thalamocortical radiations to the postcentral gyrus (somatosensory cortex). Cortical EPs are produced by the summation of excitatory and inhibitory postsynaptic potentials in the pyramidal layer of the cerebral cortex and also have a very small amplitude. These EPs are recorded from scalp electrodes over the cerebral cortex. The amplitude of spontaneous background EEG activity is generally much larger than either subcortical or cortical EPs and easily obscures these smaller signals. This problem is solved through filtering and signal averaging techniques as explained previously.

In the case of the somatosensory response to lower extremity stimulation, much data suggest that SSEPs are not entirely conducted by the posterior columns but at least partially if not substantially by the lateral funiculus.[43–46] Stimulation of the posterior tibial nerve or common peroneal nerve at or above motor threshold activates group I fibers that synapse and travel rostrally through the dorsal spinocerebellar tract. After synapsing in nucleus Z at the spinomedullary junction, the pathway crosses and travels similarly to the SSEP from upper extremity stimulation. Studies with dogs, cats, and monkeys support the concept that lower extremity sensory EPs are conducted in all quadrants of the spinal cord but primarily in the dorsal lateral funiculus. This difference is quite important. One of the scenarios in which SSEPs may give a false-negative monitoring pattern is when damage occurs to the circulation of the anterior spinal artery. If the SSEP is carried solely by the posterior columns, they would not be sensitive to damage to the anterior spinal artery. If, however, the SSEP is carried in the lateral funiculus, which is supplied by the anterior spinal artery, sensitivity should be good.

In summary, then SSEPs monitor the function of the somesthetic sensory system, which extends throughout the peripheral nervous system and CNS. Thus, peripheral nerve, spinal cord, subcortical, and cortical structures in the brain may be monitored. The somesthetic system carries sensory information including vibration, proprioception, and light touch. An SSEP is generated when repetitive electrical stimuli are applied to a peripheral nerve, and many single responses are averaged to record the evoked response. Responses may be recorded over the peripheral nerve, nerve plexus, spinal cord (posterior columns, lateral funiculus), brainstem (medial lemniscus), and cerebral cortex (somatosensory area). SSEPs, therefore, directly monitor the function of the peripheral nerve sensory fibers, the posterolateral portion of the spinal cord, about 5 to 10 percent of the cross-sectional area of the brainstem, and a limited area of subcortical white matter and cortical gray matter. Nearby motor pathways or pathways related to consciousness are monitored only by assuming that changes in sensory function will reflect changes in postoperative level of consciousness or in motor function.

There are multiple factors other than surgical damage that may also alter the SSEP and confuse the intraoperative picture. Intraoperative depression of SSEPs can result from decreased body temperature, cold irrigation to the surgical field, hypoxemia, variations in $PaCO_2$, and anesthetic agents. Of these, changes in anesthetic drug dose are the most important[47–57] (Table 4.2). Most of these factors can be kept constant during SSEP monitoring by an anesthesiologist with a good basic understanding of the requirements for good quality monitoring.

SSEP Monitoring in Spine and Spinal Cord Surgery

Spinal cord monitoring is the most widely applied intraoperative use of SSEPs, particularly during spinal instrumentation for the treatment of kyphoscoliosis. This mode of monitoring has also been used, but to a lesser extent, during other operations on the spinal cord and its supporting structures, such as resection of spinal cord tumors or vascular malformations, discectomies, and stabilization procedures for trauma or degenerative disease.

The incidence of postoperative paraplegia fol-

TABLE 4.2 *Anesthetics and somatosensory evoked potentials*

ANESTHETIC DRUG	EFFECT ON PERIPHERAL NERVE POTENTIAL	EFFECT ON SUBCORTICAL POTENTIAL	EFFECT ON CORTICAL POTENTIAL LATENCY	EFFECT ON CORTICAL POTENTIAL AMPLITUDE
Barbiturates	None	None	1 to 2+ D	1 to 3− D
Nitrous oxide	None	None	1+	1 to 2− D
Halothane Enflurane Isoflurane Desflurane Sevoflurane[a]	None	None	1 to 4+ D	1 to 4− D
Narcotics	None	None	±	±
Benzodiazepines	None	None	1+	1 to 2−
Etomidate	None	None	1+	2 to 4+ D
Ketamine	None	None	1+	1 to 2+
Propofol	None	None	1 to 2+ D	1 to 2− D
Muscle relaxants	May clarify if EMG noise is a problem	May clarify if EMG noise is a problem	None; may clarify if EMG present	None; may clarify if EMG present

Abbreviations: 1+ = >10% inc; 2+ = >20% inc; 3+ = >50% inc; 4+ = 100% or more inc; 1− = >10% dec; 2− = >20% dec; 3− = >50% dec; 4− = incompatible with monitoring; D, dose related.

[a] Expected result, not adequately studied.

lowing posterior spinal fusion for scoliosis ranges from less than 1 percent to 10 percent, depending on the type of instrumentation. Most cases of spinal cord injury from scoliosis surgery are caused by disruption of radicular blood flow when the spinal column is distracted. Because the reduction in blood flow is likely to be global in these cases, SSEP loss *should* reflect loss of motor function. Preservation of the SSEP should reflect preserved motor function. Direct spinal cord trauma from instrumentation or bony manipulation is also possible. The highest incidence of injury occurs when sublaminar wires are used, as in the Luque fusion. In these cases, either global or more segmental damage with mainly individual nerve roots being involved is possible.

Intraoperative SSEPs have replaced the wake-up test in many centers, including the University of Florida, for assessing lower extremity motor function intraoperatively. When EPs clearly indicate neurologic damage, the distraction may be removed or reduced without performing a wake-up test. The wake-up test may be used for confirmation, if desired, but this is not necessary. The wake-up test should be used when changes in SSEPs are equivocal or when good-quality waveforms cannot be obtained. In addition, when changes in EPs occur that appear to be unrelated to surgery, the wake-up test may be used to confirm changes in neurologic function.

Early results of monitoring SSEPs during orthopaedic and neurosurgical operations were later confirmed in a study of SSEP monitoring for 300 spinal procedures.[8] In this later study, three neurologic deficits were detected intraoperatively and confirmed on postoperative neurologic examination. In four cases of altered

SSEPs, surgical corrective action improved the EPs and no postoperative deficit occurred. There were no deficits unpredicted by SSEPs.

The SSEP generated from lower extremity nerve stimulation is carried in the spinal cord primarily by the lateral funiculus and the posterior columns.[43–46] The SSEP, therefore, does not *necessarily* reflect motor function. Interestingly, however, SSEP monitoring during posterior spinal fusion has correlated very well with postoperative sensory *and* motor neurologic outcome. There are case reports, however, in which SSEPs were unaffected during surgery and patients awakened with motor deficits (false-negative results).[11,12,14] These cases are rare, and most are controversial. Even if all reported cases are valid, the reported false-negative rate is still much less than 1 percent, a record not approached by any other intraoperative monitor. I have never personally observed a case involving spinal column surgery in which a patient awakened with a deficit not predicted by SSEP monitoring. There are, however, one reported case and one case in my personal experience in which the SSEP predicted a postoperative motor deficit ***not*** predicted by an intraoperative wake-up test.[58] MEPs *may* be useful in overcoming this limitation of SSEPs.

Occasionally, technically satisfactory waveforms cannot be obtained either secondary to preexisting patient pathology or to an unfavorable anesthetic technique. In such cases, the wake-up test must be used, if feasible, to monitor spinal cord function.

SSEPs have also been used during resection of spinal cord tumors. Many patients with spinal cord tumors, however, cannot be monitored with SSEPs because the lesion itself severely distorts or abolishes the SSEPs. It must also be remembered that, because the sensory and motor pathways are physically separated by distances measured in millimeters, microoperative dissection may allow selective damage to motor components of the spinal cord without damaging sensory components. Thus, occasionally resection of tumor will not affect or even improve SSEPs but will cause complete or partial loss of motor function. More commonly, complete loss of SSEPs follows myelotomy secondary to direct damage to or retraction on the somatosensory pathway. Motor function is frequently preserved in this case. This pattern contrasts sharply with use of monitoring during scoliosis or vascular surgery, in which the risk to the spinal cord is more global. Changes in SSEPs in these cases correlate well with changes in motor function.

In summary, for spinal operations that risk global damage to the spinal cord (e.g., for scoliosis repair), SSEP monitoring meets the standard of care for monitoring neurologic function. For other operations that risk focal areas of the spinal cord or nerve roots, SSEP monitoring may be useful, but false-negative monitoring patterns will clearly occur. Supplementation of SSEP monitoring with other monitoring modalities such as MEP monitoring or EMG monitoring may be useful in these cases.

Dermatomal SSEPs in Spine Surgery

There are numerous reports of using *dermatomal* SSEPs to monitor individual nerve root function.[59–62] Stimulating electrodes are placed directly on the skin in the appropriate dermatome rather than over a peripheral nerve. An electrical stimulus is applied, for example, to the web space between the first and second toes to stimulate the L5 dermatome. Dermatomal stimulation generally yields smaller and later cortical responses than mixed nerve stimulation, presumably because smaller caliber nerve fibers are involved. Spinal or subcortical potentials usually cannot be recorded after dermatomal stimulation probably for the same reason. Abnormalities in dermatomal sensory EPs may not always correlate to clinical abnormalities. There is likely a population variability in peripheral innervation patterns of the dorsal nerve roots that accounts for the discrepancy between dermatomal sensory EPs, which are produced with standard stimulating electrode placement, and the actual clinical examination.[60] In my experience, these responses are difficult to produce during anesthesia and are only poorly reproducible. In a recent study of pedicle screw fixation procedures, an operation that risks damage to the sensory and motor nerve roots (n = 81), dermatomal sensory EPs were reliably obtained from nearly all patients during anesthesia.[59] Intraoperative alterations of these EPs, however, were not helpful in guiding the surgeon. Prediction of outcome depended only on responses obtained at closing and not those during surgery. For example, dermatomal sensory EPs were suppressed in one case for a prolonged period during instrumentation but returned during closure. There was no detectable deficit postoperatively. Dermatomal SSEPs have not been shown to be clearly useful during intraoperative monitoring and must be considered experimental at this time.

SSEP Monitoring during Aortic Vascular Surgery

SSEPs have been used to monitor spinal cord function during operations on the thoracic aorta (aneurysm or coarctation correction); results have been variable.[63–71] Careful examination of the blood supply of the spinal cord explains the variable findings. The single anterior spinal artery (ASA) arises from the vertebral arteries. In the cervical cord, the ASA is richly supplied from other sources. In the mid-thoracic cord, however, only a few radicular branches of the aorta provide additional blood. No significant further blood supply comes from the aorta until the artery of Adamkiewicz, a branch of the aorta, enters the spinal cord anywhere from T8 to L1. There is thus a large segment of the anterior two-thirds of the spinal cord (supplied by the ASA) from about T4 to T8 that is highly susceptible to ischemia. By contrast, the paired posterior spinal arteries also arise from the vertebral arteries. These arteries are supplied with radicular branches at nearly every level in the thoracic spinal cord. The area of the spinal cord (posterior one-third) supplied by these arteries is, at least theoretically, less susceptible to ischemia. In this case of aortic vascular surgery, a normal SSEP at the conclusion of the operation clearly ***does not*** guarantee normal postoperative motor function. The most important factor in predicting ultimate outcome with SSEP monitoring is the duration of time over which the SSEP is lost during aortic cross-clamping. Restoration of a normal SSEP after aortic cross-clamp release does not assure a good outcome if the EP was lost for more than 14 minutes during cross-clamping.[72,73] Loss of SSEPs for less than 14 minutes, with subsequent return to normal, is associated with good outcome at least during aortic coarctation repair. The reason for this observation is explained by the blood supply of the spinal cord. If ischemia is maintained long enough, the better supplied posterior spinal cord is able to recover function as evidenced by a normal SSEP, but the anterior spinal cord does not (paraplegia).

Changes in the SSEP during surgery may be corrected by a trial of clamp reposition, shunting, induced hypertension, spinal fluid drainage, or intercostal reimplantation in an attempt to reestablish adequate spinal cord blood flow. Well-documented reports indicate that if normal SSEPs are continuously monitored and remain unchanged throughout surgery, major new neurologic deficits will not occur. Japanese investigators have found that reimplanting critical intercostal branches may improve outcome even when prolonged SSEP changes occur.[65]

In summary, SSEP monitoring during aortic vascular surgery may be clinically useful in some circumstances but clearly should not be considered the standard of care for monitoring these cases. As yet, no neurologic monitor has been proved effective for monitoring spinal cord function during descending aortic vascular surgery (see MEP discussion below).

SSEPs during Intracranial Aneurysm Surgery

The supraspinal portion of the somatosensory pathway may be at risk during intracranial aneurysm clipping. In response to posterior tibial or median nerve stimulation, the SSEP is conducted rostrally from nucleus Z or the dorsal column nuclei in the medulla via the medial lemniscus to the ventral posterolateral nucleus of the thalamus. The response is then conducted to the somatosensory cortex via the thalamocortical radiations, which pass through the posterior limb of the internal capsule.[74] Resulting cortical sensory EPs are a summation of EPSP and IPSP. Generating SSEPs is an energy-requiring process that will fail if any part of the pathway receives inadequate blood flow. If gray matter is involved (the somatosensory cortex), loss of response occurs rapidly when blood flow becomes less than 15 $ml.100.min^{-1}$.[75–77] If white matter with its lower metabolic requirement for O_2 is involved (most of the subcortical somatosensory pathway), failure may occur more slowly depending on the degree of blood flow reduction. Theoretically, sensory EPs would be useful during aneurysm surgery if the vessel(s) involved with the aneurysm supplies blood to either the cortex generating the sensory EPs or to a portion of the subcortical SSEP pathway.

The following criteria are generally accepted as constituting a significant change in the cortical sensory EP: decrease in amplitude by 50 percent or increase in latency by 1 ms. These criteria were not developed statistically but rather from empiric observations. Most likely, these criteria became necessary because amplitude and latency of the cortical sensory EPs vary substantially with nonsurgical factors, such as depth of anesthesia, temperature, and amplitude of the spontaneous EEG. One important way of minimizing the likelihood that EP changes caused by nonsurgical factors will be incorrectly attributed to surgical manipulations is to monitor an area of the nervous system not at risk from surgery during the same time period. Nonsurgical factors should cause changes in EPs regardless of which hemisphere or which part of the same hemisphere generates the response. Thus, for example, during the clipping of a left middle cerebral artery aneurysm, the left and right median nerve are sequentially stimulated, thus producing responses from each hemisphere. Only responses generated from right median nerve stimulation should be affected by surgery, but factors such as anesthesia and metabolic factors should affect both responses. Provided there is good control of other factors affecting the SSEP, based on my clinical experience only, I recommend the following criteria for interpreting a change in cortical sensory EPs as significant and requiring investigation:

- Any change related to a surgical event, even if the change is slight, particularly if there is no change in the EP on the opposite hemisphere
- Decreases in amplitude more than 50 percent or increases in latency more than 1 s without any obvious surgical or medical deterioration of the patient (e.g., hypotension), especially if there is no change in the response on the opposite hemisphere

Cortical SSEPs are generated only from certain areas of the cortex. The primary somatosensory cortex receives blood from either the middle or anterior cerebral artery. The area of the somatosensory cortex that responds to median nerve stimulation is supplied by the middle cerebral artery. The somatosensory cortex producing the response to posterior tibial nerve stimulation is supplied by the anterior cerebral artery. The thalamocortical radiations are supplied by the lenticulostriate arteries arising from the proximal middle cerebral artery. To monitor aneurysm clipping with sensory EPs, the vascular areas of the brain at risk of surgically induced injury must be identified (Fig. 4.12). In theory, the best use of sensory EP monitoring would be for anterior circulation aneurysms. If the clipping of a proximally located anterior circulation aneurysm reduces blood flow to the cerebral cortex supplied by either the anterior or middle cerebral artery, the sensory EPs generated from lower and upper extremity stimulation, respectively, will be attenuated or lost. Because most aneurysms are proximally located on these vessels, all sections of cortex supplied by the artery will be equally affected, and loss of sensory EPs will correlate with loss of motor function as well.

As expected from the anatomy of the somatosensory pathway and its blood supply, mul-

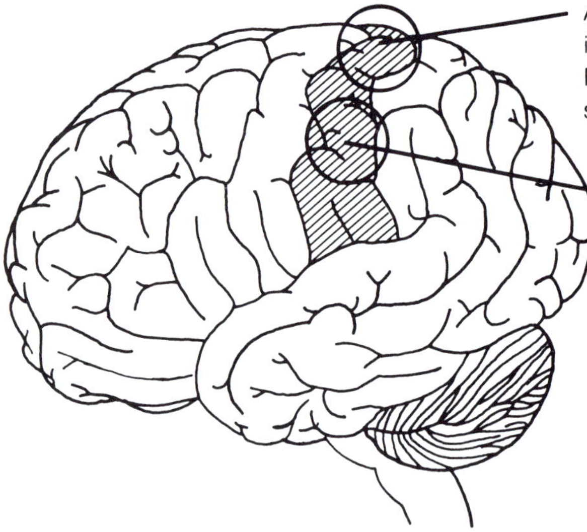

FIGURE 4.12 *The vascular territory of the middle cerebral artery includes the cortex that generates the somatosensory evoked response from median nerve stimulation. The vascular territory of the anterior cerebral artery includes the cortex that generates the somatosensory evoked response from posterior tibial nerve stimulation. Shaded area shows somatosensory cortex.*

tiple studies have documented the usefulness of sensory EP monitoring during clipping of anterior circulation cerebral aneurysm.[78–81] Results are not as good during posterior circulation aneurysm clipping.[82] The posterior circulation does provide blood via perforating vessels to the somatosensory pathway as it ascends through the brainstem to the thalamus. This same circulation, however, also supplies blood via other perforating vessels to large portions of the brain not involved with the somatosensory pathway. Examples of these areas include the descending motor pathways and the reticular activating system. Damage to tiny perforating blood vessels supplying motor pathways and the reticular formation may result in motor deficit, global depression of consciousness, or both without affecting sensory EPs.[82]

A recent retrospective study reviewed all intracranial aneurysm repairs (n = 277) monitored with cortical SSEPs at the University of Florida from January 1990 through February 1994.[4] A significant intraoperative SSEP change caused a change in treatment in 37 patients (13.4 percent). Interventions in response to sensory EP change were of three types: repositioning or removing the clip after its placement, increasing systemic blood pressure, or adjusting retractor position. Blood pressure adjustment, which most commonly occurred after temporary vessel occlusion, appeared to be related to vasospasm in some cases. In two cases, the aneurysms could not be clipped without substantially affecting SSEPs and were wrapped instead. In one case, the cranium was reopened after closure before emergence from anesthesia. Removal of retraction had caused the shifting brain to displace the clip, which partially kinked the middle cerebral artery and altered the cortical SSEPs (Fig. 4.13). For anterior circulation aneurysms with sensory EP changes, if intervention rapidly restored the sensory EPs to baseline, outcome was clearly better, and SSEP monitoring was useful to both the surgeon and the anesthesiologist. During clippings of posterior circulation aneurysms, when EPs changed, outcome tended to be poor even if intervention restored sensory EPs to baseline. This observation confirms the limitation of SSEP monitoring in predicting function in areas of the brain not involved with the somatosensory pathway.

In summary, use of SSEP monitoring during aneurysm surgery cannot yet be considered a standard of care but appears to be clinically very useful. Surgeons and anesthesiologists who use this modality to monitor patients undergoing aneurysm clipping are clearly convinced of its usefulness. There are clearly limitations of this monitoring modality that are not yet totally defined. Once enough clinical experience has been gained to better define these limitations, this monitor will likely achieve standard-of-care status.

Carotid Endarterectomy

SSEPs are not firmly established for monitoring during CEA. Both laboratory investigations[75,76] and theoretical considerations based on the generators of the cortical SSEPs, however, suggest that SSEP monitoring would be useful for this purpose. Monitoring during carotid artery surgery has been compared in two different studies between SSEPs and the EEG, a monitor with established efficacy. The results of these studies are conflicting. One study showed that both modalities were about equivalent[83] in detecting cerebral ischemia, and the other study showed SSEP monitoring to be much less sensitive.[84] Both studies involved fewer than 100 patients, and there were no patients in either series with a permanent new neurologic deficit postoperatively.

In the laboratory, changes in the EEG precede changes in SSEPs as CBF decreases below 20 $ml \cdot 100\ g \cdot min^{-1}$.[5,85] In addition, when multiple channels are used during EEG monitoring, the area of the monitored cerebrovascular territory is much larger than SSEPs can monitor. Cortical SSEPs can only measure function of the somatosensory cortex and the subcortical somatosensory pathway. Thus, at least theoretically, EEG should be a better monitor of cortical function *but not subcortical areas at risk during carotid vascular surgery*.

The question of which monitor is better during carotid surgery—EEG or sensory EPs?—remains largely unanswered, and either monitor may be used. On a purely practical basis, SSEP monitoring, when performed properly, requires a technician to monitor the data continuously. EEG monitoring, particularly when a limited number of processed EEG channels is being used (four or less), may be performed without a technician provided that the anesthesiologist or surgeon is adequately trained. However, SSEPs are less sensitive to anesthesia and metabolic changes and may even be recorded after administration of enough barbiturate to render the EEG isoelectric.[48] The waveform is simpler to interpret, and interpretation does not require the presence of an electroencephalographer in the OR. SSEPs are clinically useful during CEA. There are not yet enough data to determine whether SSEP monitoring is as effective as EEG monitoring for CNS monitoring during CEA.

Coma Evaluation

When used in combination with BAEPs, investigators at the University of Florida as well as in other institutions have found SSEPs to be very helpful in the management of comatose patients.[86–94] In general, if both BAEPs and cortical SSEPs are intact at presentation and remain intact, ultimate outcome is good. A relatively good outcome may occur in this case even if all clinical signs indicate a very poor prognosis.[87] If the cortical SSEPs at presentation are absent and the BAEPs are present, the best outcome expected is a chronic vegetative state. If both cortical SSEPs and all BAEP waves beyond wave I are absent, brain death is very likely. Drug overdose will not eliminate either the BAEP or the early and intermediate latency components of the SSEP. Although the EEG may be entirely absent in the case of drug overdose (or therapy such as in barbiturate coma), the BAEP and SSEP should be present if the patient has brain function.

SSEPS AND NEUROLOGIC INJURY DURING SURGERY

As with other monitors, no carefully controlled studies prove that SSEP monitoring improves outcome after neurologic surgery. Lack of such outcome studies, however, should not prevent clinicians from using this monitoring modality. It has an *excellent overall correlation* with neurologic outcome. Feedback to the surgeon is rapid, which, in turn, enables rapid intervention, either surgical or anesthetic, to prevent permanent neurologic deficit. In Figure 4.13, note that the cortical SSEP disappeared after middle cerebral artery aneurysm clipping after removal of retraction from the frontal and temporal lobes. The brain then shifted, causing the clip to kink the middle cerebral artery. Retractors were again placed, and the clip position was adjusted so that no further problems occurred. Prompt feedback prevented a major neurologic injury that would not otherwise have been detectable. There were no concomitant vital sign changes.

Provided other factors affecting SSEPs are kept constant, increases in latency and decreases in amplitude are ominous signs; surgical causes should be sought and corrected rapidly if possible. Changes in SSEPs usually reflect damage to motor pathways as well. However, because motor and sensory pathways are located in different parts of the brain and spinal cord, and in some places have a different blood supply, the SSEP will not always reflect motor function. SSEP monitoring is most effective when a large area of brain or spinal cord or its blood supply is threatened during surgery.

BRAINSTEM AUDITORY EVOKED POTENTIALS

Theoretical Concepts

The brainstem auditory pathway encompasses the cochlear hair cells, spiral ganglion, eighth cranial nerve, cochlear nuclei, superior olivary complex, lateral lemnisci, inferior colliculus,

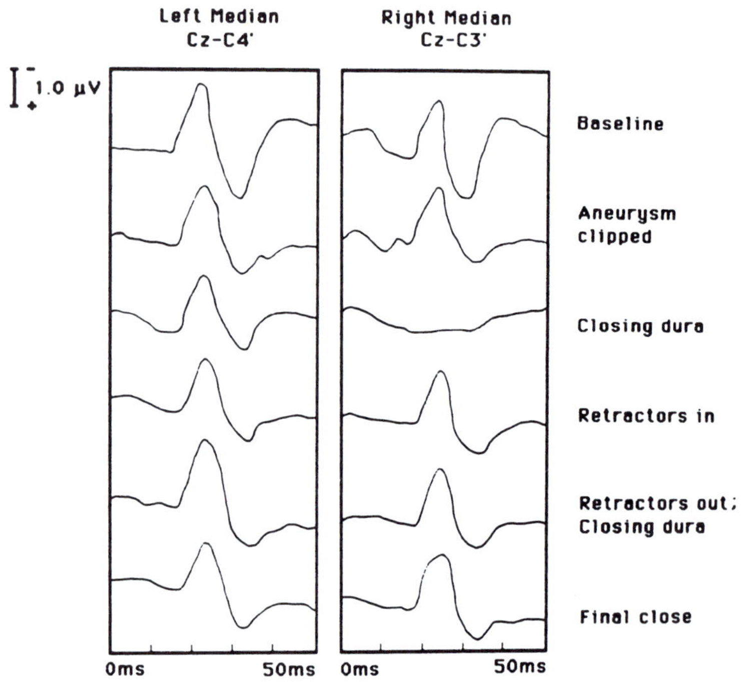

FIGURE 4.13 *Retractor-related SSEP changes. There were no changes in the evoked response during this clipping of a middle cerebral artery aneurysm until the retractors were removed before closure. Removal of retraction caused the clip to move and kink the middle cerebral artery, resulting in a loss of the cortical response. Only the cortical responses are shown here. (From Mahla,[125] with permission.)*

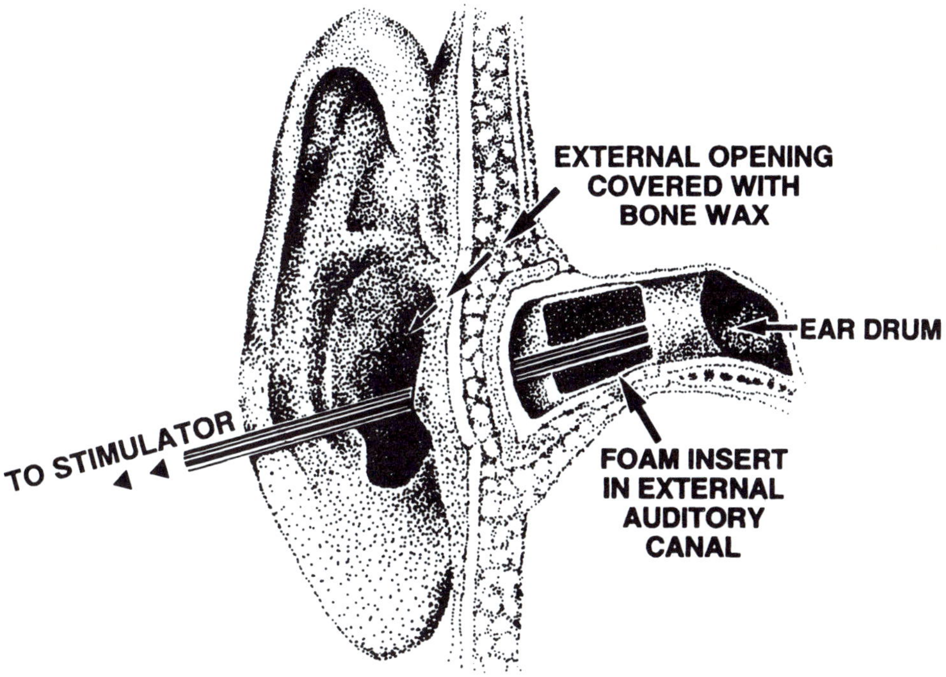

FIGURE 4.14 *Schematic of the stimulator for brainstem auditory evoked responses.*

and medial geniculate thalamic nuclei. The stimulus is a loud repetitive click delivered to the patient by small ear inserts placed in the external auditory canal (Fig. 4.14). Because recording electrodes cannot be placed close to the brainstem, the BAEP is recorded from the scalp far from the generating structures. This far-field potential is thus very small, and as many as 2,000 repetitions may be required to produce a good averaged response. The typical waveform is composed of six or seven positive waveforms when recorded from the vertex, all within 10 m of the stimulus presentation (Fig. 4.15).

In an ideal situation, recording electrodes should be placed on the skin overlying each earlobe, the seventh cervical vertebrae, and the vertex. A typical montage would be

Channel 1: C_z–ipsilateral ear

Channel 2: C_z–contralateral ear

Channel 3: C_z–seventh cervical vertebrae

Channel 4: Ipsilateral ear–contralateral ear

The channel likely to provide the most information, showing all waves, is channel 1 (C_z–ipsilateral ear). The C_z–contralateral ear shows the responses from the auditory pathway that has crossed to the opposite side of the brainstem and may help identify wave V. Channel 3 will often also emphasize wave V of the response and may be used when wave V is only poorly seen in channel 1. Occasionally, wave I will not be well visu-

FIGURE 4.15 *Typical BAEP waveform. Note that there are usually six to seven positive waves in a typical response.*

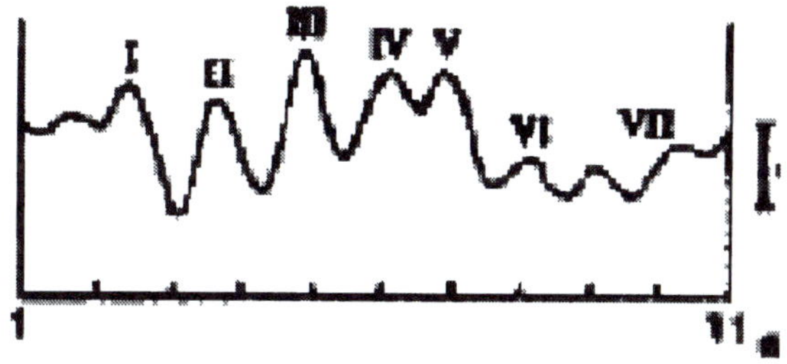

alized in channel 1 and may be better seen in channel 4.

Wave I must be adequately visualized to make certain that a stimulus is actually reaching the cochlea. If wave I is well seen, changes in the auditory EP are unlikely to be caused by failure of adequate stimulation.

Auditory Pathway

Initially, investigators thought that each component of the BAEP represented the activity of a distinct structure along the brainstem auditory pathway. The sites of origin of each wave were thought to be as follows: wave I—eighth cranial nerve, wave II—cochlear nucleus, wave III—superior olivary complex, wave IV—lateral lemniscus, wave V—inferior colliculus, wave VI—medial geniculate, and wave VII—primary auditory cortex. This schema seemed to hold up rather well when abnormalities of the potentials were compared with locations of clinical lesions.[95,96] For example, lesions of the midbrain were reported to correlate well with abnormalities of waves IV and V. Lesions in the pons altered wave III. Lesions of the eighth cranial nerve itself were associated with loss of the entire potential or prolongation of the latency of all components after wave I. Unfortunately, the types of lesions encountered in clinical situations usually involve more than one auditory structure and may also have remote effects via pressure or edema. Limitations in clinical correlation between anatomic lesions and BAEP abnormalities have led to both human and animal experimentation. Animal experimentation in which recordings were made directly from brainstem structures suggests that, during most of the EP, high-amplitude fields occur throughout the brainstem. This observation led to the conclusion that most of the BAEP waves are generated in multiple auditory structures. Many different discrete brainstem lesions in animals decrease the amplitude of but have no effect on the latency of the BAEP waveforms. Only with lesions of the eighth cranial nerve were all BAEP components suppressed. Large lesions elsewhere generally led to attenuation, but not loss, of these components. The BAEP waveforms beyond wave I thus likely represent a highly complex interaction between multiple structures[97–102] (Fig. 4.16).

Several studies have involved recording from human brainstem structures during posterior fossa explorations. The compound eighth cranial nerve action potential latency recorded from the eighth nerve just proximal to the internal auditory meatus occurred midway between surface-recorded waves II and III.[103] This finding indicated that the eighth cranial nerve plays a major role in the generation of both waves I and II. Potentials recorded near the cochlear nucleus have corresponded to the surface-recorded wave III.[104] Although the precise generators of the various components of the BAEPs remain controversial, most investigators agree that longer latency components are generated in structures located progressively more rostrally along the brainstem auditory pathway. This schema continues to have great clinical usefulness.

BAEPs assume an adult configuration in early childhood.[105] Many factors will affect their latencies and amplitudes, including head size, body temperature, anesthetic drugs, and especially, auditory acuity. Interpeak latencies (usually I to III and I to V), which tend to be less affected by these factors than are absolute latencies, are therefore the preferred measures of normality.

Compared with SSEPs or visual evoked potentials (VEP), intraoperative factors other than surgical damage are relatively *unlikely* to seriously alter the BAEP. They may be recorded successfully during any anesthetic technique. Intravenous anesthetic agents, even in very high doses, have no significant effects on the BAEP. Although both the absolute and interpeak latencies of the later components of the BAEP will be increased by potent inhalation anesthetics, the degree of increase is not clinically significant. Changes in anesthetic technique are unlikely to produce a change in the waveform that will be mistaken for a surgically induced change (Table 4.3).

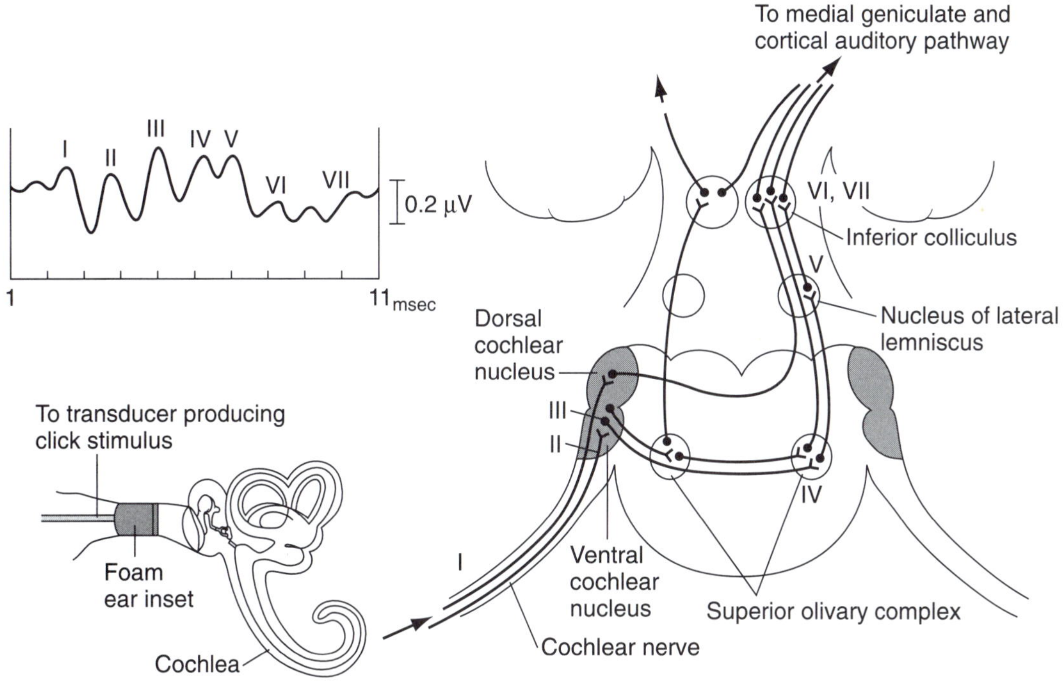

FIGURE 4.16 *BAEP waveform and associated structures that are thought to generate each wave.*

TABLE 4.3 *Anesthetics and brainstem auditory evoked potentials*

ANESTHETIC DRUG	EFFECT ON I-V INTERPEAK LATENCY	EFFECT ON AMPLITUDE OF WAVE V	CLINICAL SIGNIFICANCE[a]
Barbiturates	Increases	Decreases	None
Nitrous oxide	Minimal	Minimal	None
Halothane	Increases	Decreases	Minimal
Enflurane			
Isoflurane			
Desflurane[b]			
Sevoflurane[b]			
Narcotics	None	None	None
Benzodiazepines	Minimal	Minimal	Minimal
Etomidate	Minimal	Minimal	None
Ketamine			
Propofol			
Muscle relaxants (all types)	None	None	None

[a] Clinical significance is based on criteria for significant changes at the University of Florida.

[b] Presumed effect; not studied adequately.

As discussed, factors other than surgically induced may alter the BAEP signal to a mild degree. The clinician must be able to decide when a change is significant and requires treatment. The degree of intraoperative alteration in the BAEP waveform that is acceptable is controversial. Some neurophysiologists warn the surgeon about alterations in the BAEPs with as little as a 1-ms increase in the I to V interpeak latency.[106,107] In a study of BAEP alterations during 21 microvascular decompressions,[108] cerebellar retraction for exposure of the cerebellopontine angle significantly prolonged the I to V interpeak latency in all cases. In four cases, all waveforms beyond wave I were completely lost for various periods. In this series, the I to V interpeak latency increased more than 1 ms in all cases, but the surgeon was warned only in the case of disappearance of all waves beyond wave I. Clearly, postoperative hearing dysfunction would not be expected in all these cases. The BAEPs appear to be an exquisitely sensitive monitor of auditory function. *False-positive results will likely be frequent when latency is the only criterion used for warning the surgeon.* At my institution, the surgeon is warned and retraction altered only if gross changes in the BAEPs cause complete or impending loss of wave V. With this criterion, there have still been no cases of clinically detectable hearing loss postoperatively despite major increases in I-V interpeak latency in more than 200 patients. Hearing loss has only occurred in those cases in which wave V was lost immediately after placement of retraction and adjustment of retraction was unable to restore it.

Microvascular Decompression of the Fifth or Seventh Cranial Nerve (Jannetta Procedure)

The incidence of complete ipsilateral hearing loss after microvascular decompression for trigeminal neuralgia has been reported to be between 1 and 4 percent.[108] Up to 20 percent of patients may have partial hearing loss. Microvascular decompression of the facial nerve for hemifacial spasm risks hearing function more because of the immediate proximity of the eighth cranial nerve. Intraoperative monitoring of BAEPs may minimize the likelihood of this complication. Placement of cerebellar retraction to expose the fifth or seventh cranial nerve root entry zone may stretch the eighth cranial nerve between its attachment to the brainstem and its entry into the internal auditory meatus. Stretching of the nerve produces ischemia, which slows conduction and desynchronizes the action potential of the eighth nerve produced in response to an auditory click stimulus. Thus, the waveform definition beyond wave I deteriorates, and the I-V interpeak latency increases (Fig. 4.17). Many studies in the literature document the efficacy of BAEP monitoring during microvascular decompression.[106,107] Complete and irreversible loss of the BAEPs during operation has been correlated with postoperative deafness. There are also numerous reports of transient loss of potentials in patients without postoperative hearing deficit. In these cases, after cerebellar retraction was released, nerve function recovered either immediately after notification of the surgeon or after the procedure was completed. The duration of insult to the nerve was insufficient to produce permanent damage. Postoperative deafness in a patient with normal intraoperative BAEPs after microvascular decompression has never been reported. (This pattern would, however, be possible in a patient who developed a postoperative hematoma of the eighth nerve or a similar problem.)

As discussed above, the *degree* of intraoperative alteration in the BAEP waveform that is acceptable is controversial, but based on the data in the literature, BAEP monitoring for prevention of hearing loss during microvascular decompression is clearly clinically useful and probably approaching standard of care.

Resection of Acoustic Neuroma

BAEPs have also been used during resection of acoustic neuromas to help the surgeon preserve

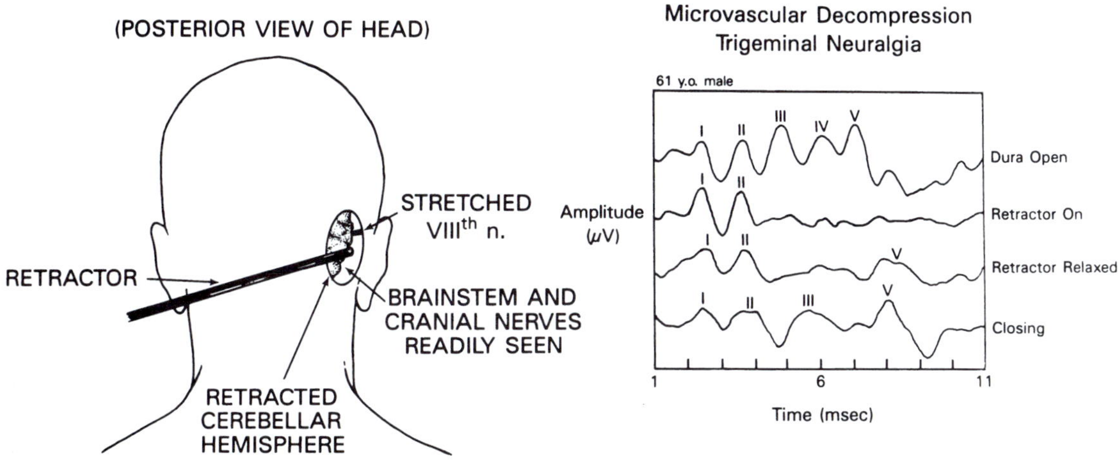

FIGURE 4.17 *Cerebellar retraction resulted in complete loss of all waves beyond wave I. Adjustment of retraction restored nerve function and resulted in a good outcome.*

hearing.[109–111] Damage to the auditory pathway during this operation may occur by one of four mechanisms: brainstem compression, direct operative trauma to the eighth nerve, damage to the blood supply to the eighth nerve and cochlea, and again, stretching of the eighth nerve caused by cerebellar retraction needed to expose the tumor in the cerebellopontine angle. Stretching the nerve and brainstem compression are the only potentially reversible mechanisms of the four. Both direct nerve damage and interruption of the blood supply usually cause permanent loss of both the BAEPs and hearing. In one series, hearing preservation after acoustic neuroma resection was compared between 90 consecutive patients who had BAEP monitoring and 90 historical control patients matched for tumor size and preoperative hearing status who did not have EP monitoring. With tumors smaller than 2 cm, BAEP monitoring was associated with a higher rate of hearing preservation and a greater chance that the hearing preserved was clinically useful.[110] Changes in the BAEPs intraoperatively correlated well with postoperative hearing status. In a second study, authors reviewed hearing in 99 patients who were operated on via the suboccipital approach for acoustic neurinoma and who were not deaf before surgery. Hearing was preserved in 29 patients (29.3 percent), of whom 23 had neurinomas smaller than 30 mm and six had tumors exceeding 30 mm in size. Fifty-seven patients in this series were monitored with BAEPs, and the rate of postoperative hearing was higher in this group than in the 42 without monitoring ($P < .05$).[112] My experience is consistent with the above studies. I would add that if the tumor is larger than 2 cm in size, the usefulness of BAEP monitoring and the likelihood of hearing preservation after surgery are greatly reduced. For resection of acoustic neuroma in which hearing preservation is desired, BAEP monitoring is absolutely necessary and is a standard of care. However, with some tumors and some operative approaches to acoustic neuromas (e.g., translabyrinthine), hearing preservation is not possible, and BAEP monitoring is of no proven value.

Other Posterior Fossa Operations

BAEP monitoring during other posterior fossa operations has also been reported. During most of these applications, however, no changes in therapy resulted from monitoring. In addition, the BAEPs monitor only a small portion of the brainstem. Except when the entire brainstem is at risk, there will likely be a high incidence of cases in which BAEPs are unaffected intraoperatively and significant impairment in motor function or consciousness occurs postoperatively. This limitation is exemplified by surgery on the posterior cerebral circulation (basilar artery and its branches). Because the auditory pathway occupies a relatively small cross-sectional area of the brainstem, vascular injury to other areas of the brainstem may occur without concomitant changes in BAEPs.[113] Occasionally, however, the brainstem may be compressed by a large lesion, and the BAEPs may be used to monitor global brainstem function. Reversible obliteration of the BAEPs has been reported to follow positioning of patients for removal of lesions in the cerebellopontine angle[114]; presumably the obliteration was caused by worsened brainstem compression after positioning.

Coma Evaluation

The declaration of brain death is usually based on clinical criteria or radiographic evidence of absence of CBF; neurophysiologic testing (EEG and EPs), however, is often supportive of this diagnosis.[86–94] For BAEPs to support the diagnosis of brain death, wave I must be evident. Although wave I is generated in the peripheral portion of the auditory nerve, the blood supply to the nerve and to the cochlea itself (i.e., the labyrinthine artery) often has an intracranial origin. Thus, increased ICP, with resultant decreases in blood flow, can lead to cochlear damage and loss of wave I. If no components of the BAEP are evident, it is consistent with but not diagnostic of brain death. Other possibilities include preexistent deafness or hearing loss, temporal bone fracture with resultant hearing loss, fluid in the middle ear, high doses of aminoglycoside antibiotics, and technical malfunction. Only if wave I is evident do we know that the auditory system has actually been stimulated. SSEP testing may also be helpful in this situation (see above).

VISUAL EVOKED POTENTIALS

VEPs reflect the function of the visual pathway, which extends from the optic nerve, through the chiasm, to the visual cortex. The VEP is generated primarily by the visual cortex. Intraoperatively, the stimulus is usually applied by goggles that deliver a repetitive bright flash through closed eyelids. Contact lenses containing light-emitting diodes also have been applied directly to the cornea. This arrangement takes up less space and is less likely to interfere with surgical exposure; also, when contact lenses are used, a closed eyelid does not interfere with delivery of the stimulus as it does with goggles. Recordings are from scalp electrodes placed over the calcarine cortex.

Use during Surgery

VEPs are not widely used during surgery. They have been used for visual function monitoring in operations near the optic nerve and chiasm (most commonly during pituitary surgery). They can also be monitored during resection of intracranial tumors such as meningiomas involving or compressing the optic nerve.

Correlation between changes in VEPs and outcome has not been evaluated in a large series of patients. Which VEP changes during manipulation of the optic nerve and chiasm are normal and which are ominous have not been identified. The major reasons for this lack of data are difficulties with stimulus application and the exquisite sensitivity of the VEP to anesthetic agents. Some investigators believe that VEPs are too variable intraoperatively to be of any clinical use.

MOTOR EVOKED POTENTIALS

There is great interest in intraoperative use of MEPs because of the theoretical limitations of SSEPs in monitoring motor function. Although

MEPs are not technically difficult to produce in the awake patient, the lack of widespread use of MEPs in the OR suggests that the intraoperative use of MEPs may not be as simple as it seems.

Theoretical Basis

The same type of system that is used to monitor sensory EPs may also be used to monitor the motor system. The stimulus to the motor system is either electrical or magnetic in nature. Both of these types of stimuli have been used at several different stimulus sites: the motor cortex, the spinal cord (any level), or the peripheral nerve. The technology for recording MEPs (i.e., types of recording electrodes, preamplification, computer averaging, etc.) is identical to that used for recording SSEPs. Table 4.4 summarizes the possible stimulus and recording sites. MEPs recorded from peripheral nerves and spinal cord are called neurogenic MEPs. These potentials are relatively small and usually require some signal averaging to be readily seen. MEPs recorded from muscle are called myogenic MEPs. These potentials are much larger and frequently do not require averaging.

One of the major difficulties with MEPs, whether the stimulus is applied transcranially to the motor cortex or directly to the spinal cord, is an uncertainty as to which structures are being activated by the stimulus and which structures are producing the recorded waveforms.[115–123] Transcranial electrical stimulation of the motor cortex produces a responses that can be recorded at medullary, spinal cord, peripheral nerve, and muscle levels. At the medullary and spinal cord levels, a series of waves is produced. The earliest wave is called a D or direct wave. The subsequent waveforms are called I or indirect waves. The D-wave can be produced by stimulation of subcortical white matter after the cortex is ablated, but the I-waves seem to require intact gray matter.[115] Given the scope of this chapter, it should be assumed that the corticospinal tract carries the descending response evoked from transcranial electrical stimulation. It is likely, however, that other descending tracts are also involved.[116,122] The major portion of the corticospinal tract in humans crosses at the pyramidal decussation at the level of the foramen magnum and forms the lateral corticospinal tract. A smaller uncrossed portion forms the ventral corticospinal tract. The descending D- and I-waves cause activation of the spinal motor neurons. The resulting action potential is conducted via the ventral nerve root to the peripheral nerve. The impulse then crosses the neuromuscular junction and produces a recordable compound muscle action potential. Thus, with transcranial electrical stimulation, responses may be recorded over the spinal cord, peripheral nerve, and muscle. Transcranial magnetic stimulation produces MEPs that show longer latency onset as well as longer central conduction times than those recorded after transcranial electrical stimulation.[124] Because electrical and magnetic stimulation of the cervi-

TABLE 4.4 *Stimulus and recording sites for MEPs*

STIMULUS SITE→ RECORDING SITE ↓	TRANSCRANIAL	SPINAL CORD	PERIPHERAL NERVE
Spinal cord	X	X (caudal)	
Peripheral nerve	X	X	X (distal)
Muscle	X	X	X

cal spinal cord produce myogenic MEPs with similar latencies, differences in MEPs produced by transcranial stimulation must arise more rostrally in the CNS. One plausible explanation would be that the longer latency MEP produced by transcranial magnetic stimulation is produced by activation of the cortical motor neurons themselves, whereas the shorter latency MEP produced by transcranial electrical stimulation is produced by additional activation of the subcortical pyramidal tract. A recent study in cats, however, suggests that transcranial magnetic stimulation may activate subcortical portions of the motor pathway as well.[125] This type of MEP may also be recorded over the spinal cord, peripheral nerve, and muscle.

MEPs may also be produced by stimulation of the spinal cord. Direct electrical stimulation of the spinal cord has been used to produce a myogenic potential recorded from a muscle group distal to the site of surgery.[126] Direct electrical spinal cord stimulation has also been used to produce a neurogenic potential recorded from a peripheral nerve caudal to the site of surgery.[127,128] This type of recording represents by far the most common use of MEPs and has a major advantage for intraoperative applications. Neuromuscular blockade that would prevent the myogenic response may (and in fact *must*) be used. Use of neuromuscular blockade will prevent gross movement in response to stimulation, which may be problematic during more delicate surgery. Spinal cord stimulation is produced by needles placed in the base of the spinous processes of two adjacent vertebrae or by stimulating electrodes placed into the epidural space (Fig. 4.18).

Collision studies and lesioning studies in animals support the view that the neurogenic response is, in fact, mediated by activation of motor pathways.[129] This optimistic view is not shared by all investigators, however. Some investigators believe that the neurogenic response may not be mediated solely by motor pathway activation. Because there is no synapse in the somatosensory pathway between the dorsal columns and the peripheral nerve, electrical stimulation of the dorsal columns would be expected to produce a recordable electrical potential in a peripheral nerve. Thus, electrical stimu-

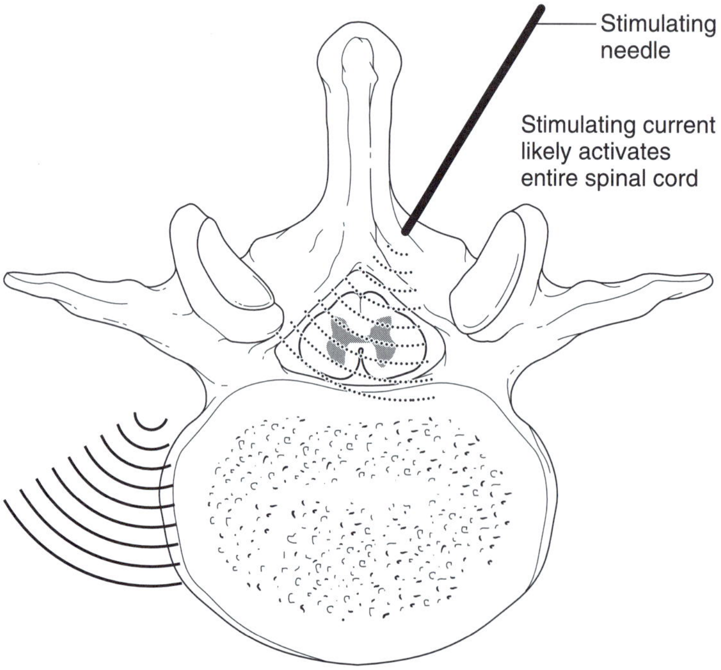

FIGURE 4.18 *Schematic of spinal cord electrical stimulation used to produce the neurogenic motor evoked potential. Current is passed between two needles imbedded in the base of the spinous process of two adjacent vertebrae.*

lation of the spinal cord may produce a mixed response mediated by both sensory and motor tract stimulation. One study conducted in animals strongly suggests that the neurogenic response is produced primarily by activation of sensory pathway.[130] If recordings after spinal cord stimulation are made from muscle rather than nerve, purely motor tract function is monitored.

Many investigators hoped that MEPs would be more useful during surgery that risks the vascular supply of the spinal cord. Several clinical series report excellent results.[127,128,131–134,] Laboratory studies, however, suggest that there will be a similar incidence of false-negative monitoring results with MEPs, at least during aortic vascular surgery, as there is with SSEP monitoring. In a dog model in which aortic cross-clamping produced a 90 percent incidence of poststudy paraplegia, spinally recorded MEPs at the lumbosacral cord level produced by transcranial electrical stimulation were intact in most animals despite paraplegia.[135,136] This observation would suggest that descending anterolateral white matter motor tracts remain intact after spinal cord ischemia. The spinal motor neurons with their higher metabolic rate, however, likely did not survive the ischemic insult. More distal monitoring that would detect damage to the motor neurons is not possible during aortic clamping because both the peripheral nerve and especially muscle become ischemic rapidly after interruption of blood supply.

Some types of MEPs are surprisingly susceptible to anesthetic agents. MEP responses produced by electrical stimulation of the spinal cord are resistant to the effects of anesthesia and require no special anesthetic considerations other than the need for muscle relaxants to prevent gross movements. However, MEPs produced by either transcranial magnetic or electrical stimulation using single stimuli *cannot be recorded during general anesthesia using virtually any commonly used anesthetic drug*[137–142] (Table 4.5). Electrically produced MEPs are slightly more resistant to anesthetics than magnetically produced MEPs. Halothane, enflurane, isoflurane, and (presumably) desflurane and sevoflurane cannot be used at all during MEP recordings. N_2O when given in combination with narcotics cannot be used in concentrations greater than 50 percent. However, a relatively high dose of narcotic in combination with N_2O in concentrations up to 50 percent have been successfully used. Benzodiazepines and sodium pentothal, when given in bolus doses, abolish the MEP. Although the nitrous/narcotic-based technique is familiar to many anesthesiologists, many clinicians think that avoidance of all benzodiazepines or potent inhalation agents will produce an unacceptable risk of awareness during surgery. Interestingly, two newer hypnotic drugs, etomidate and propofol, may be used during MEP recordings. Total intravenous anesthesia using infusions of etomidate or propofol in combination with a narcotic infusion allows stable MEP recordings. Propofol may also be used

TABLE 4.5 *Anesthetics and motor evoked potentials: transcranial magnetic and electrical*

ANESTHETIC DRUG	MUSCLE POTENTIAL (EMG)
Barbiturate	P
Nitrous oxide	P (D)
Halothane	P
Enflurane	
Isoflurane	
Desflurane[a]	
Sevoflurane[a]	
Narcotics	A
Benzodiazepines	P
Ketamine	A
Etomidate	A
Propofol	?P[b]
Muscle relaxant	A (provided 1–2 twitches maintained)

Abbreviations: A, Acceptable; P, prohibitive in clinically used concentrations <1 MAC.

[a] Presumed effect; not studied adequately.

[b] Conflicting data in literature.

without narcotics either alone or in combination with N_2O in concentrations up to 50 percent. Total intravenous anesthesia based on an infusion of ketamine is also compatible with stable recordings. None of these MEP. compatible anesthetic techniques is commonly used by anesthesiologists, and many clinicians would be uncomfortable with these techniques. Use of propofol is increasing, and if subsequent studies confirm that propofol may be used during MEP recordings, this technique will likely be the technique of choice for most anesthesiologists.

Recently, several techniques for facilitation of motor responses evoked from transcranial electrical or magnetic stimulation in the awake patient have been applied intraoperatively. These techniques include facilitation by peripheral sensory stimulation and temporal summation of responses by short interval sequential stimulation. Preliminary results show that these techniques may overcome some of the anesthetic-related difficulties with MEPs.[143,144]

Muscle relaxants, because of their blocking effects at the neuromuscular junction, may also alter the myogenic MEP. Surprisingly, however, they may be used in amounts that will suppress most gross motor movement associated with stimulation. Several studies, both in animals and humans, report that neuromuscular blockade resulting in a 70 percent or less reduction in the height of the response to ulnar nerve stimulation, *is* compatible with MEP monitoring.[142] All these studies used quantitative neuromuscular blockade monitoring. Most anesthesiologists use the more readily available and inexpensive "blockade monitors" to monitor gross motor response to a nonstandardized electrical stimulus. These monitors are ***not*** suitable for MEP monitoring because they are unable to accurately quantify either the amount of stimulus given to the nerve or the amount of muscular response produced. I have been very successful titrating the new ultrashort-acting nondepolarizing relaxants to a twitch height of about 25 percent of control. Unless MEP monitoring can be clearly demonstrated to be superior to SSEP monitoring during surgery, most anesthesiologists will be reluctant to provide the relatively unfamiliar anesthetic techniques needed for motor monitoring.

MEP Monitoring during Spine Operations

MEP monitoring has been used during many types of spine operations. Most experience has been reported during scoliosis operations and during surgery to remove spinal cord tumors. Zentner[133,134] has reported a relatively large series of patients monitored during spinal cord surgery with MEPs produced by transcranial electrical stimulation. Other than the abovementioned anesthetic susceptibility of the responses, this group reported good success, with no false-negative response patterns. Edmonds and colleagues[131] have reported a series of patients undergoing scoliosis correction who were monitored with MEPs produced by transcranial magnetic stimulation as well as SSEPs. This group also reported good success with this technique. However, in this and in other published studies like it, there are no reports of a false-negative SSEP monitoring pattern that was detected by MEP monitoring!

Perhaps the largest series of patients monitored with MEPs has been reported by Owen and colleagues[127–129] using neurogenic MEP responses from stimulation of the rostral spinal cord. They report excellent correlation of monitored responses with neurologic outcome during scoliosis surgery, spinal cord surgery, and aortic vascular surgery despite the theoretical limitation that the neurogenic response is likely not a pure motor response. Single stimulus transcranial magnetic stimulation has recently been approved by the FDA as a low-risk procedure. However, neither transcranial electrical stimulation (singly or in trains) nor transcranial magnetic stimulation when used in trains has been approved for use in humans. Given the technical difficulties in producing the MEP and the lack of studies proving that motor monitoring is superior to SSEP monitoring, transcranial MEP monitoring should still be considered largely experimental. There is now considerable experience with electrical stimulation of the spinal cord. Although the precise pathways involved with the neurogenic MEP are controversial, this monitoring method appears to be as effective and safe as SSEP monitoring.

ELECTROMYOGRAPHY: FACIAL NERVE MONITORING

Some operations in the posterior fossa, particularly those involving resection of acoustic neuromas and tumors near the base of the skull, may result in damage to the facial nerve (VII). Postoperative weakness or paralysis of the facial nerve produces serious morbidity. First, eye closure may be incomplete, producing corneal drying and damage, and muscles of facial expression can fail to function, with resulting serious disfigurement.

Methods of Facial Nerve Monitoring

DIRECT OBSERVATION The simplest method involves direct observation of the face while the surgeon uses a nerve stimulator to locate the facial nerve in the surgical field. This method is limited for several reasons. First, the facial nerve is not assessed except when the surgeon attempts to locate it with a nerve stimulator. Serious damage that will not be detected can occur at other times during surgery (e.g., during exposure of an acoustic tumor over which the facial nerve has been stretched). Second, the face may not be readily visible for direct observation. For example, during procedures conducted in the three-quarter prone position, commonly used for posterior fossa explorations, the face cannot be seen except by crawling under the table and shining a light on it.

For facial nerve monitoring, EMG recording needles are placed in the orbicularis oculi and orbicularis oris muscles (Fig. 4.19). To locate the facial nerve, a repetitive electrical stimulus is applied, and EMG activity is recorded from these muscles. The EMG response is displayed on a screen and converted to an audio signal that gives immediate direct feedback to the surgeon. If the surgeon stimulates a structure that is thought to be the facial nerve or near the facial nerve, evoked EMG activity recorded from the ipsilateral orbicularis oculi or orbicularis oris muscles is confirmatory. The absence of evoked activity indicates either that the structure is not the facial nerve or that damage to the nerve has already occurred. When the surgeon electrically stimulates a nerve, if the stimulus exceeds threshold voltage for activating the nerve, a regular EMG signal is produced. The size of the EMG signal is proportional to the amount of nerve activated. If the nerve is already stretched or damaged, the threshold voltage for activation of the nerve is higher. When the surgeon is close enough to a nerve that the resultant EMG signal reaches a user definable threshold voltage, an auditory signal is produced providing immediate feedback to the operating team.

The other type of EMG activity that may be monitored intraoperatively is spontaneous EMG activity. If a nerve root or cranial nerve becomes irritated or is touched intraoperatively, spontaneous EMG activity will occur that may alert the operative team that a nerve is very close to the area where the surgeon is working. There is a spectrum of spontaneous muscle activity than can be encountered during passive nerve monitoring.[145,146] (Fig. 4.20). The most benign type, called a "popcorn" discharge, is quite common and is caused by a brief mechanical stimulus of the nerve. The EMG discharge that results is not sustained. This type of discharge serves to warn the surgeon that contact or near contact with the nerve has occurred. It does not, however, signify any type of significant nerve damage. More sustained muscle activity indicates more serious irritation of the nerve. The most serious type of discharge, a neurotonic discharge, causes prolonged continuous muscle activity, and indicates serious trauma to the nerve is occurring. Several prospective studies have demonstrated that increasing numbers of neurotonic discharges during an operation decreases the likeli-

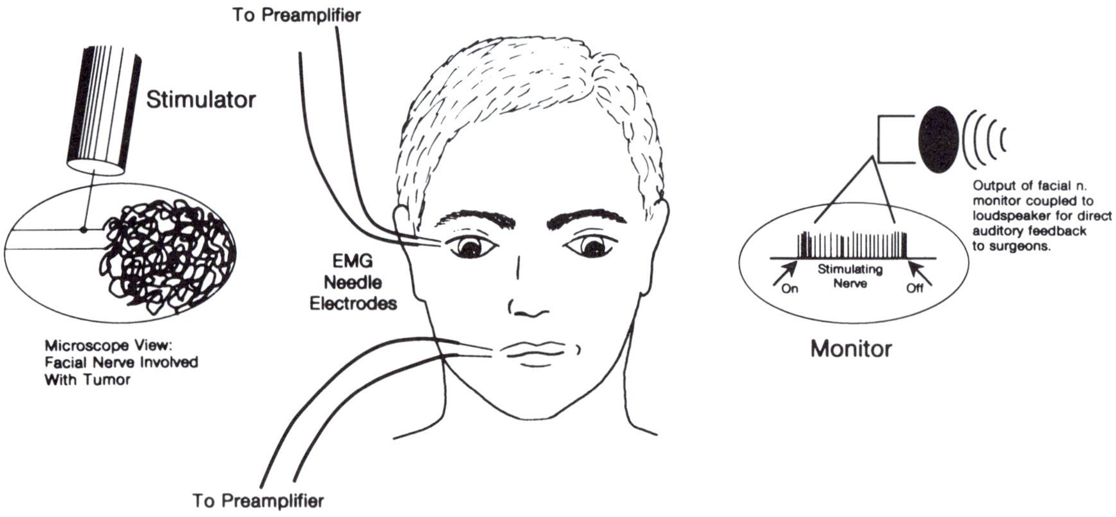

FIGURE 4.19 *Schematic of facial nerve monitor. (From Mahla,[125] with permission.)*

hood of useful nerve function 1 year after surgery.[147] A word of caution is needed, however. If the patient is lightly anesthetized during nerve monitoring (especially facial nerve), spontaneous EMG activity caused by slight movements may become apparent. Some of this activity may mimic neurotonic activity.

Because the neuromuscular junction is a part of the pathway being tested by using EMG monitoring, the use of muscle relaxants by the anesthesiologist can potentially interfere both with active and passive monitoring of nerve function. Because movement of a patient fixed in a head pinion during delicate neurologic microsurgery could produce catastrophic results, most anesthesiologists would prefer to completely block the neuromuscular junction to prevent movement and possible injury to the patient. *The effects of muscle relaxants on EMG monitoring has not been adequately studied*. It is clear that a given dose of muscle relaxant has different effects on different muscle groups. For example, the diaphragm is much more resistant to the effects of muscle relaxants than the muscles in the hand. One study tested the effects of partial neuromuscular blockade on the EMG response to direct intracranial facial nerve stimulation. This study found no significant effects provided that the muscle twitch response to peripheral nerve stimulation was at least 50 percent of the control amplitude.[148] Greater degrees of neuromuscular blockade and the effect of partial neuromuscular blockade on passive EMG monitoring were not tested. The effects of neuromuscular blockade on both active and passive EMG monitoring of spinal nerve roots have not been studied. As a result, our practice is not to paralyze patients during the time EMG monitoring is used. A short-acting muscle relaxant is given during induction. This relaxant will wear off before completion of exposure, and no further relaxant is given until closure begins.

Summary

These techniques are much more reliable than mere observation for facial twitching. Facial nerve monitoring leads to improved facial nerve function after acoustic tumor removal.[147,149–153] The EMG is also safer than facial observation because the anesthesiologist does not have to disturb the arrangement of equipment, personnel, or drapes to see the face. Facial nerve mon-

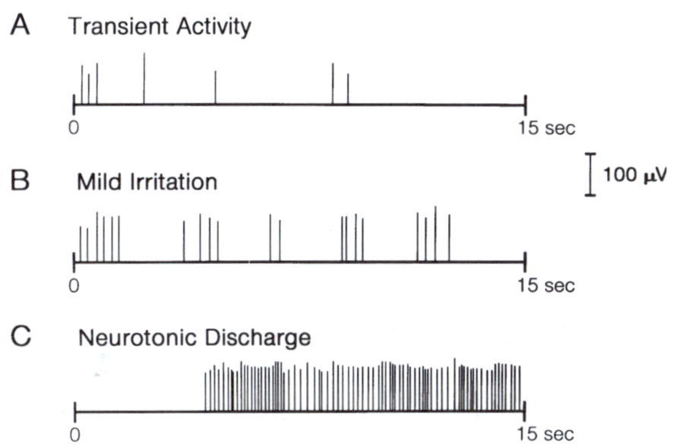

FIGURE 4.20 *Types of spontaneous EMG discharges. (A) Popcorn discharge. This response is generated by simple contact with the nerve. No damage is done. (B) Train of responses. This response is generated by mild irritation of the nerve. The abnormal response is not sustained, and this type of response is not associated with serious damage to the nerve. (C) Neurotonic discharge. This type of response is produced by serious irritation of the nerve. The more of these responses that are seen during surgery, the more likely that permanent damage to the nerve will be present after surgery.*

itoring is clearly the standard of care[154] during acoustic neuroma surgery and during other surgery that risks facial nerve function (e.g., parotid surgery). The motor component of cranial nerves III, IV, VI, X, XI, and XII[155,156] also can be monitored in a similar fashion to detect surgical trauma in the posterior fossa. Injury to these cranial nerves will produce significant disability to the patient in many areas including phonation, swallowing, and vision. Experience with EMG monitoring of cranial nerves other than VII is relatively limited, and the use of monitoring to prevent injuries to these nerves is not widespread nor universally accepted.

SPINAL NERVE ROOT MONITORING

Spontaneous or evoked EMG may be recorded from any muscle in the upper or lower extremities. Muscles are chosen for monitoring based on the nerve root(s) at greatest risk from surgery. For example, the gastrocnemius muscle is innervated primarily by the S1 nerve root. Surgery that puts this nerve root at risk (e.g., L5–S1 discectomy) could potentially benefit from EMG monitoring of this muscle. Some investigators have reported success in detecting impending damage to spinal nerve roots using this monitoring technique.[157–160] When pedicle screws are used as part of a stabilization procedure, the nerve root may be damaged if the screw does not remain within the pedicle as it is placed into the vertebral body. Spontaneous EMG may be monitored during screw placement to detect trauma to the nerve. After final placement of the screw, the hardware itself may be used to stimulate the nerve root. In one recent study in animals,[158] the investigators found that if EMG activity could be produced with a stimulus voltage of 5.5 V or less, the pedicle screw had likely migrated outside the pedicle. Also, a sudden burst of spontaneous EMG activity may warn the surgeon of potential nerve root trauma.

MONITORING CEREBRAL BLOOD FLOW

All the previously discussed monitors are monitors of nervous system function. When function fails, they do not necessarily give information about the *mechanism* of nervous system damage. One of the most common mechanisms of CNS and peripheral nerve damage is inadequate blood flow. The remainder of this chapter examines those methods that are available to monitor CBF. These methods have not been applied to the spinal cord in most cases.

Direct CBF Measurement

Direct measurements of regional CBF (rCBF) are not used commonly. The only "practical" intraoperative measurement involves injection of a radioactive isotope of xenon into the carotid artery, followed by measurement of the radioactivity washout with a gamma detector placed over a specific area of the brain (Fig. 4.21). This method cannot measure CBF over other areas of the brain and cannot distinguish flow at different depths (gray and white matter). Rather, rCBF measurements reflect average gray/white matter flow. The technique is not continuous; therefore, during most of the operation, CBF is unknown. Despite its shortcomings, this method has been used at a few major centers[5] in combination with other forms of continuous monitoring, particularly during CEA. It has not achieved widespread usage largely because of technical limitations and the need for radioactive material.

Transcranial Doppler Ultrasound

An easy-to-apply, direct, continuous, and noninvasive monitor of CBF uses TCD ultrasound. It has found increasing application as a monitor in the OR and intensive care unit.

THEORETICAL BASIS Ultrasound waves are used to measure the velocity of blood flow in the basal arteries of the brain. These waves are transmitted through the relatively thin temporal bone (Fig. 4.22). When they contact moving red blood cells, they are reflected at a changed frequency through the brain and skull back to a detector. The change in frequency as blood cells move toward or away from the ultrasound trans-

FIGURE 4.21 *Schematic of ^{133}Xe cerebral blood flow measurement.*

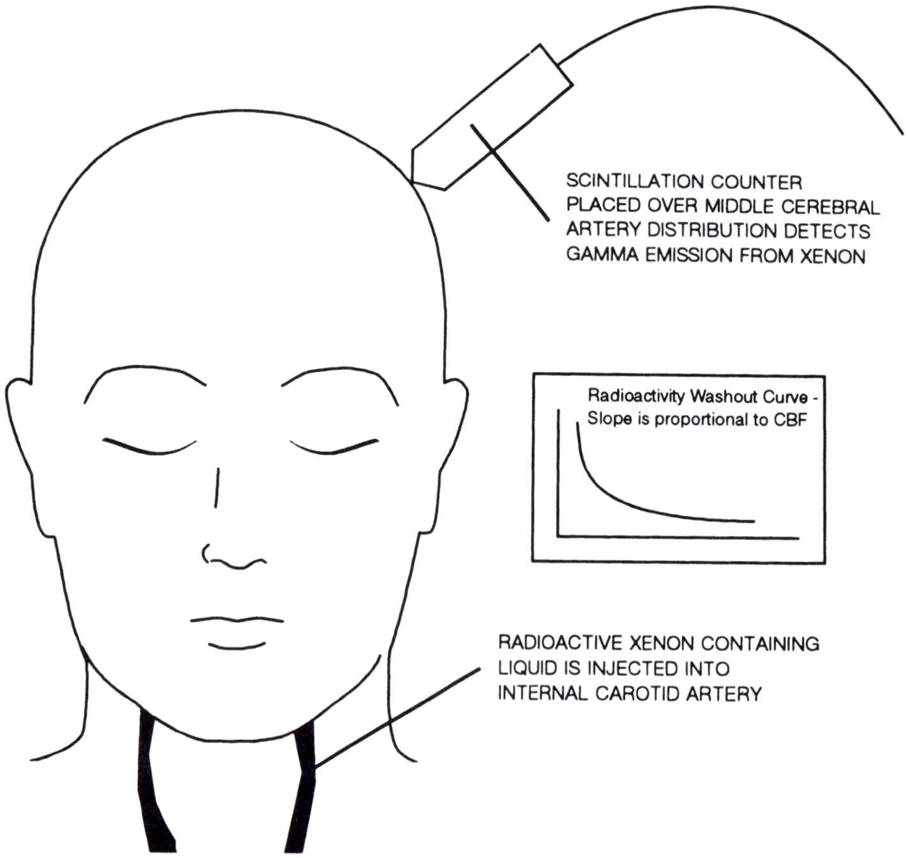

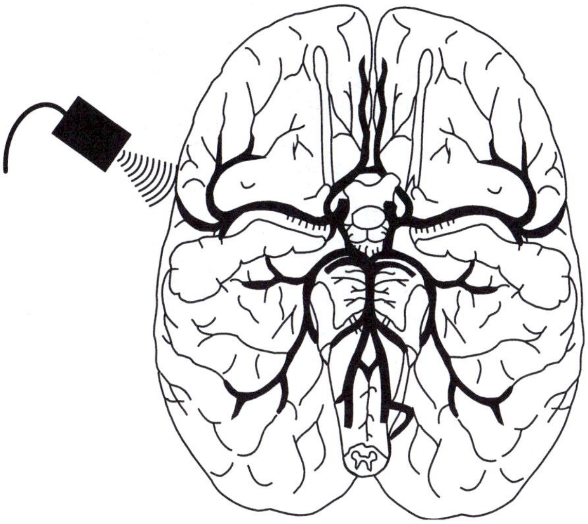

FIGURE 4.22 *Schematic of transcranial Doppler ultrasound. Sound waves are passed through the thin temporal bone and are reflected off the moving red blood cells in the arteries at the base of the brain. The change in frequency of the reflected sound waves is related to the velocity and direction of the blood flow.*

mitter and detector is an example of the Doppler effect and is related to the velocity and direction of flow. Velocity increases during systole and decreases during diastole; blood in the center of the lumen moves faster than that near the vessel wall, producing a spectrum of flow velocities. This spectrum resembles the shape of the waveform produced by an intra-arterial pressure transducer (Fig. 4.23).

TCD flow velocity measurements are most commonly and easily made in the middle cerebral (MCAv) and internal carotid arteries but may also be measured in other vessels including the anterior cerebral, anterior communicating, posterior cerebral, posterior communicating, and basilar arteries. Two assumptions must be made for TCD measured blood flow velocity to have a direct relationship to CBF. First, flow and flow velocity are directly related only if the diameter of the artery at the point of flow velocity measurement and the measurement angle of the Doppler probe (angle of insonation) remain constant. The angle of insonation may be kept constant by rigidly mounting the TCD probe on the patient's head with a headset. Second, the blood flow in the basal arteries of the brain must be directly related to cortical CBF.

Neither of these assumptions has been proved. TCD technology, in my opinion, has not been adequately validated in a large series of intraoperative cases against established monitors of CBF such as the EEG or against direct cortical CBF measurements.

TCD During Carotid Endarterectomy

The major reported intraoperative use of the TCD involves testing CBF adequacy while the carotid artery is cross-clamped during CEA. A study comparing radioactive xenon-measured CBF with TCD-derived MCAv did not demonstrate a good correlation.[161] In addition, the period of carotid cross-clamping is only a small portion of the time that the patient with carotid disease is at risk for ischemia; most strokes occur at other times during or after surgery. Little data are available about the nature and degree of acceptable TCD changes during the remainder of the operation.

Normal variations in blood flow velocities during surgery in patients without cerebrovascular disease appear to be large (Pashayan and Mahla, unpublished data). Thus, in 1997, recommending TCD ultrasound as the optimal monitor of CBF during carotid surgery is probably premature. However, I have found TCD to be very useful in the detection of emboli. Because the most probable cause of perioperative stroke in the patient undergoing carotid surgery is embolic, this monitor has the potential to detect the occurrence of emboli before irreversible brain damage occurs. When used in combination with EEG, TCD may have a supplementary role in the detection of emboli and changes in subcortical blood flow during CEA. TCD may also have a significant role in the preoperative evaluation of patients with cerebrovascular disease. When used in conjunction with vasodilating challenges

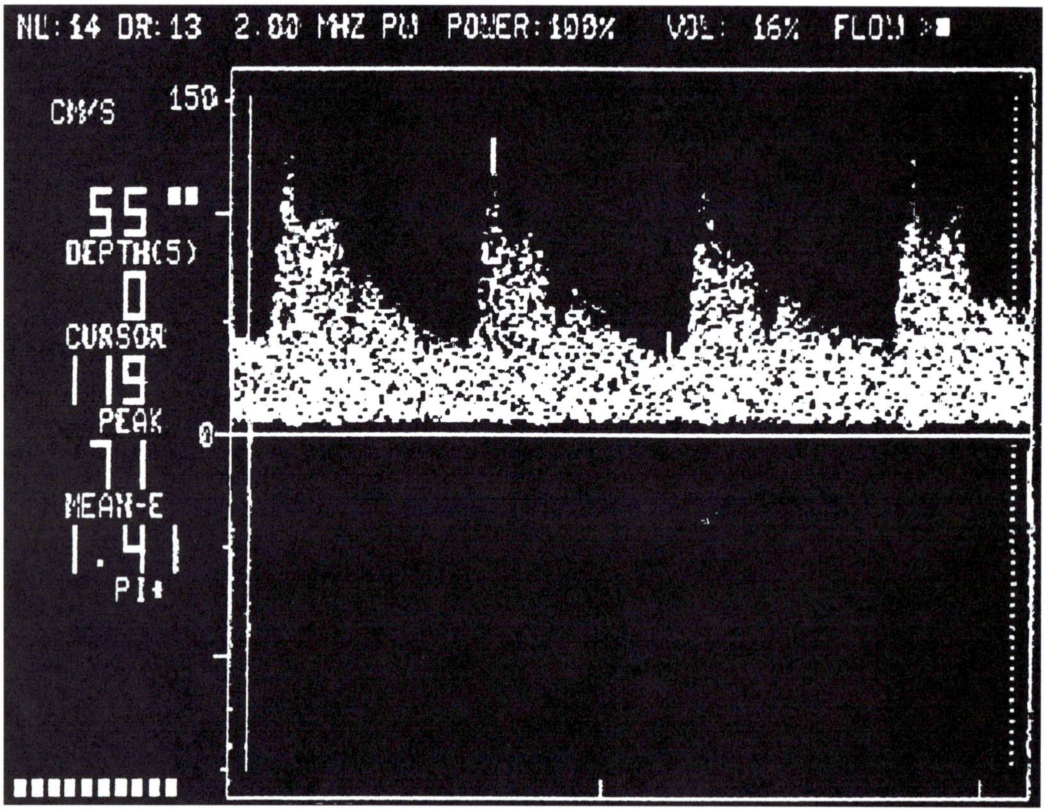

FIGURE 4.23 *Normal TCD waveform. Note the close resemblance to an arterial waveform.*

(e.g., inhaled CO_2 or intravenous acetazolamide), TCD measurements may assist the clinician in determining cerebrovascular reserve.

TCD DURING CARDIOPULMONARY BYPASS TCD measurements also have been made during cardiopulmonary bypass to assess CBF and to detect emboli. Based on a limited number of studies involving a small number of patients, correlation between CBF and TCD measurements appears to be poor during cardiopulmonary bypass.[162,163] Emboli are readily detected, but studies determining whether the incidence and severity of Doppler-detected emboli correlate with neurologic outcome have not yet been completed, although several, including one at my institution, are underway. If the number and type (air versus particulate) of emboli or duration of embolic periods can be shown to correlate with neurologic outcome, this type of monitoring would give the opportunity to intervene in some instances to prevent further embolization once emboli are detected.

DETECTION OF CEREBRAL VASOSPASM Measurements of CBF have found much greater and more successful uses in the intensive care unit. Detection and documentation of the severity of vasospasm after subarachnoid hemorrhage (SAH) is possible.[164–170] As the diameter of the arterial lumen decreases with vasospasm, the velocity of blood flowing through the narrowed vessel must increase if flow is to be maintained (Fig. 4.24A [normal] and 4.24B [vasospasm]). If studies involving greater numbers of patients confirm reasonable sensitivity and specificity, TCD measurement will facilitate the

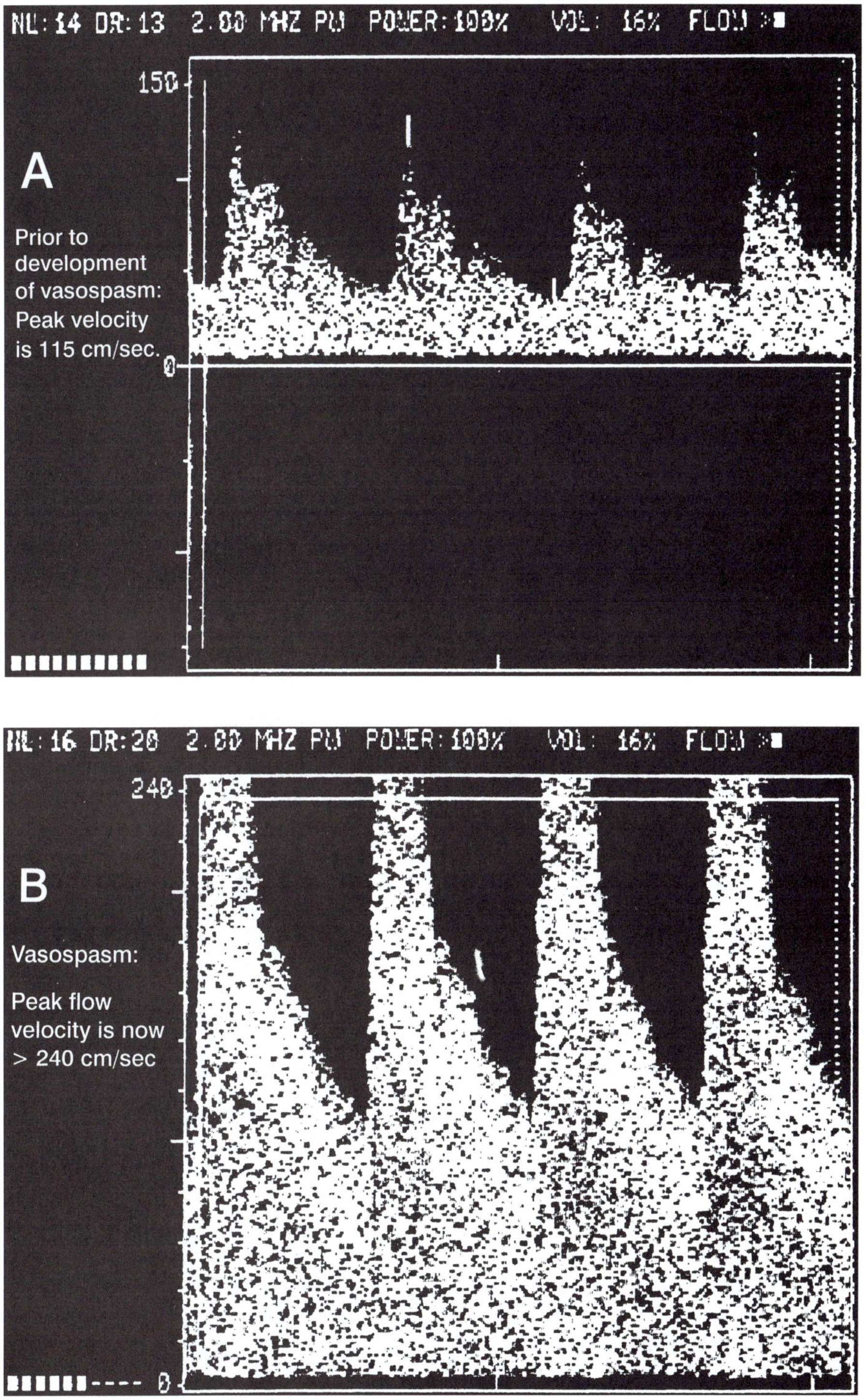

FIGURE 4.24 *(A) Normal TCD waveform. (B) Waveform from the same patient after development of cerebral vasospasm. Note the greatly increased flow velocity of the blood traveling through the narrowed vessel.*

detection of vasospasm in patients who are still asymptomatic. Early detection will allow prophylactic treatment and close monitoring. In addition, preoperative evidence of vasospasm in asymptomatic patients with SAH can alert the anesthesiologist to the patient who may be at greater risk for ischemia during hypotension if it is needed for aneurysm clipping.

CONFIRMATION OF BRAIN DEATH

Studies have demonstrated a characteristic blood flow velocity pattern in patients who are clinically brain dead (Fig. 4.25).[171–175] There is a short systolic inflow of blood followed by an exit of blood (flow direction reverses) from the cranium during diastole. Measurements are easily performed at the bedside, and in a few centers the TCD method is used to determine whether definitive studies to document brain death need to be performed. For example, if the TCD does *not* show the flow velocity pattern characteristic of brain death, angiographic or radioactive xenon blood flow studies are *unlikely* to show absent cortical CBF. Transport of these critically ill patients for CBF studies is thus unnecessary. However, if the TCD study does show the pattern characteristic of brain death, the patient can be transported for definitive blood flow studies without further delay or expenditure of resources. Further studies documenting the sensitivity and specificity of this test in the diagnosis

FIGURE 4.25 *TCD tracing associated with brain death. Blood moves forward during systole. Because blood flow has ceased in the microvascular bed, flow reverses during diastole. There is no net forward blood flow. (From Mahla,[125] with permission.)*

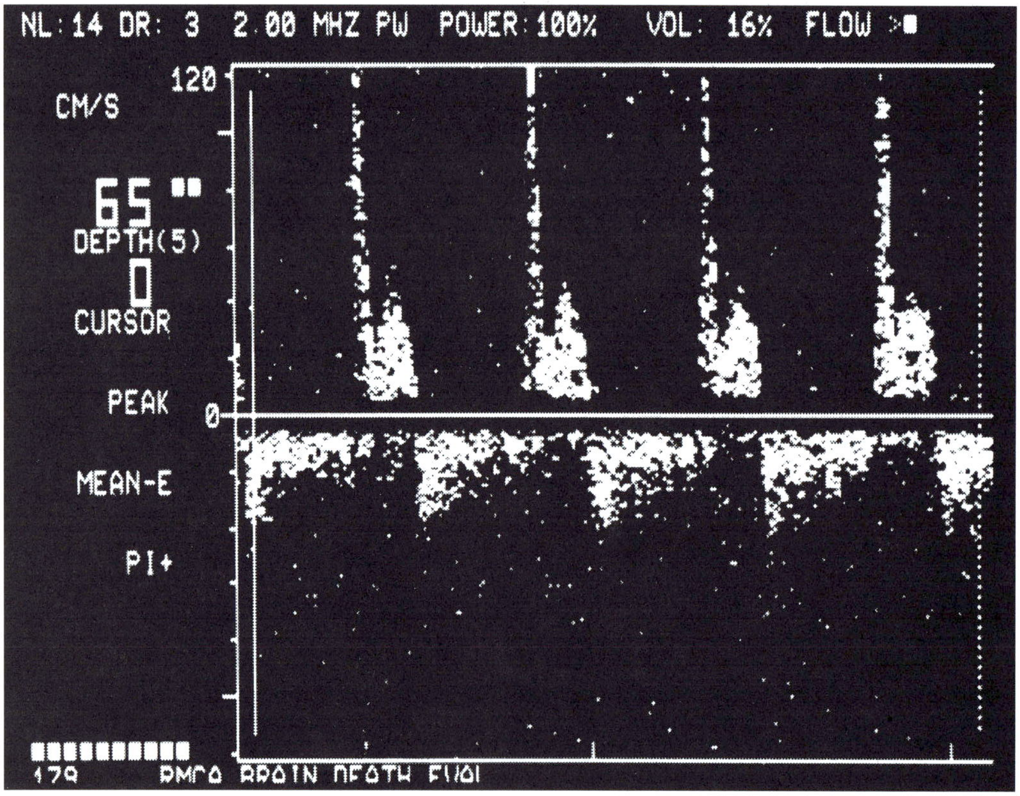

of brain death are needed before this test can be used as part of the criteria for brain death.

TCD SUMMARY Technically satisfactory recordings cannot be obtained in some patients (particularly elderly women), rendering TCD diagnosis or monitoring useless. When recordings can be made, TCD is very attractive because of its continuous and easy-to-use characteristics. TCD **may** have important roles during CEA and cardiopulmonary bypass, and it clearly is of benefit in the laboratory evaluation of patients with cerebrovascular disease.

Cerebral Oxygen Supply/Demand Balance: Jugular Bulb Oxygen Saturation

Cerebral O_2 demand (requirement) varies with changing CNS conditions. Reduction of brain temperature by 5°C may reduce O_2 needs by 35 percent or more. CBF may be adequate for cerebral function and cellular integrity at 32°C but inadequate at 37°C. Cerebral O_2 delivery varies with CBF and O_2 content. Cerebral function is determined by the *balance* between cerebral O_2 demand and supply. Thus numerical values of CBF, taken alone, do not guarantee either preservation or loss of function; they must be interpreted with regard to O_2 demand and supply. Clinically applicable direct measurements of O_2 demand are not available at this time. The EEG can be used to assess O_2 demand indirectly. Generation of spontaneous electrical activity uses about 50 percent of the total O_2 consumed by the brain. As a corollary, if drugs are given to totally suppress spontaneous electrical activity, the O_2 demand will be reduced by about 50 percent.

THEORETICAL BASIS Measurements that reflect the balance between O_2 supply and demand, however, can be made directly by measuring the O_2 saturation in the jugular venous blood (SvO_2) returning from the brain. A catheter is advanced retrograde under fluoroscopic guidance in the jugular vein until its tip lies in the jugular bulb. Blood can then be aspirated and saturation measured. When cerebral O_2 delivery falls (as a result of decreased blood O_2 content, decreased CBF, or both), cerebral O_2 extraction increases. This change results in decreased SvO_2 of venous blood returning from the brain. Measurement also can be made continuously by using a small fiberoptic catheter similar to those used to measure mixed venous O_2 saturation in the pulmonary artery.

JUGULAR BULB OXYGEN SATURATION MONITORING IN HEAD TRAUMA PATIENTS[177–185] Most reported uses of jugular bulb oxygen saturation (JvO_2) monitoring involve management of severely head-injured patients. It has been used primarily in head trauma patients who require control of increased ICP with hyperventilation, barbiturates, or both. Jugular SvO_2 appears to be helpful in detecting cerebral ischemia associated with excessive hyperventilation. Although hyperventilation may lower ICP, the accompanying decrease in CBF can cause O_2 delivery to fall below demand. Falling JvO_2 suggests that another technique to control ICP e.g., barbiturate coma, ventriculostomy or lumbar catheter with CSF drainage might be safer. In addition, outcome differences are apparent when comparing patients who have episodes of jugular venous O_2 desaturation with those who do not.

There are several theoretical problems with this technique. Blood in a single jugular bulb comes from sources on both sides of the brain (70 percent ipsilateral, 30 percent contralateral). This measurement technique evaluates the *global* balance between cerebral O_2 supply and demand. Inadequate CBF to a small area of cortex may be masked by blood that has a higher SvO_2 from areas of adequately perfused brain in either hemisphere. Thus, a high saturation can be falsely reassuring. More important, placement of a catheter in the jugular vein may block jugular outflow or cause thrombosis after prolonged use. Even unilateral placement sometimes impedes jugular outflow sufficiently to raise ICP in patients with decreased intracranial compliance. These theoretical concerns have prevented widespread use of such monitoring, but use of JvO_2 monitoring is becoming more common in the 1990s with the increased efforts being made to look for ways of improving outcome in head injured patients. Many neurointensivists strongly believe that this monitor is very helpful in the care of the patient with brain damage from any cause including trauma, SAH and intracerebral hemorrhage.

Cerebral Oxygen Supply/Demand Balance: Cerebral Oximetry

The cerebral oximeter was developed as a noninvasive assessment of the adequacy of CBF based on technology similar in concept to that for pulse oximetry.[186] The probe is usually placed on the skin overlying the frontopolar portion of the cerebral cortex (forehead). The basic rationale for use of this type of device is that when CBF falls, O_2 extraction from the blood will increase, and cerebral venous O_2 saturation will fall. A schematic of the most commonly used cerebral oximeter is shown in Figure 4.26. Photodetector 1 detects infrared light absorption of scalp/extracranial blood. Photodetector 2 detects infrared light absorption of both cerebral and extracranial blood. Cerebral oxygenation is calculated by subtracting absorption measured at detector 1 from that measured at detector 2.

There are now good studies in the literature that have attempted to validate this monitor as an accurate measurement of the adequacy of CBF.[186–191] These studies have allowed the FDA to recently grant approval for the use of the device to monitor cerebral O_2 saturation.

One recent study compared measurements made with the cerebral oximeter to simultaneously recorded TCD and jugular bulb venous oxygen saturation.[192] Although neither of these monitors is currently considered a gold standard for the measurement of the adequacy of CBF, the relationships demonstrated were interesting. In this study, falls in cerebral O_2 saturation were accompanied by significant falls in MCAv. The converse was not always true, however. Significant falls in MCAv could occur without any change in O_2 saturation at all, suggesting the presence of collateral circulation. There was also a strong correlation between JvO_2 and cerebral O_2 saturation. The degree of change in the two monitors was not necessarily similar, however. Placement of the probe over the parietal cortex produced a more similar degree of change in the two monitors than the standard frontal placement. A second study demonstrated a significant influence of external carotid artery blood saturation on the cerebral O_2 saturation reading[193] In this study, scalp ischemia induced by a pneumatic tourniquet was able to reduce the measured intracranial O_2 saturation by 13 percent. Finally, data are not clear as to how low the cerebral O_2 saturation can fall before one should become concerned. In one study in awake patients undergoing CEA, changes associated with clamping the internal carotid artery varied from +2.6 to −26.8 percent of the control value.[194] None of the patients became clinically symptomatic. This finding could perhaps be explained by probe placement over the frontopolar region of cortex. Function of this area of the brain would be difficult to assess intraoperatively. In another study, cerebral O_2 saturation was compared with EEG during controlled episodes of ventricular fibrillation in human.[195] These investigators found a good correlation between EEG evidence ischemia of cerebral O_2 saturation and determined a threshold value for development of EEG ischemia of 47 percent (patients were under general anesthesia).

Perhaps the greatest limitation of this monitor is the lack of multichannel capability. There

FIGURE 4.26 *Schematic of the cerebral oximeter.*

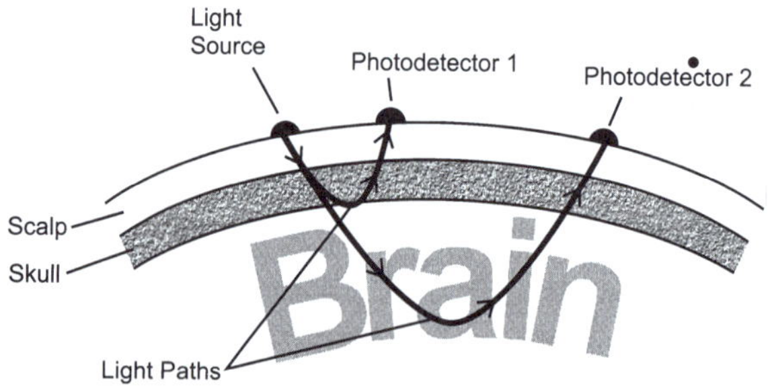

is no reason to expect that O_2 saturation in one portion of the brain would reflect O_2 saturation in other areas of the brain. Indeed, EEG changes during carotid surgery are sometimes limited to a few channels. Even with the limitations of the monitor and unresolved questions about extracranial tissue contribution to the saturation reading, this monitor shows great promise. I fully expect significant developments in this area in the next 5 years.

CONCLUSIONS

Neurologic monitoring, both of function and blood flow, has gained much more widespread use during the past decade. Many of these monitors are now considered a standard of care during certain types of surgery that risk neurologic injury. Over the past 20 years, anesthesiologists have begun to use devices for monitoring the cardiovascular system that previously were used only by cardiologists (i.e., pulmonary artery catheters and transesophageal echocardiography). Monitoring expertise is a highly developed skill in anesthesiologists that can be applied equally well to neurologic monitoring. As advocates of patient safety, we can no longer ignore neurologic monitoring as something that gets in our way. We must be at least facilitatory participants, if not actively involved, in neurologic monitoring if it is to achieve its maximal potential.

References

1. Smith RC, Leung JM, Mangano DT: Postoperative myocardial ischemia in patients undergoing coronary artery bypass graft surgery. S.P.I. Research Group. Anesthesiology 74:464, 1991
2. Cheng DC, Chung F, Burns RH et al: Postoperative myocardial infarction documented by technetium pyrophosphate scan using single-photon emission computed tomography: significance of intraoperative myocardial ischemia and hemodynamic control. Anesthesiology 71:818, 1989
3. Moller JT, Johannessen NW, Espersen K et al: Randomized evaluation of pulse oximetry in 20,802 patients: II. Perioperative events and postoperative complications. Anesthesiology 78:445, 1993
4. Clark RK, Mahla ME, Day AL: Evoked potential monitoring of aneurysms: does it matter? abstracted. Anesthesiology 81:A216, 1994
5. Sundt TW, Sharbrough FW, Piepgras DG et al: Correlation of cerebral blood flow and electroencephalographic changes during carotid endarterectomy: with results of surgery and hemodynamics of cerebral ischemia. Mayo Clin Proc 56:533, 1981
6. Nash CL, Lorig RA, Schatzinger LA, Brown RH: Spinal cord monitoring during operative treatment of the spine. Clin Orthop 126:100, 1977
7. Grundy BL: Monitoring of sensory evoked potentials during neurosurgical operations: methods and applications. Neurosurgery 11:556, 1982
8. Brown RH, Nash CL, Berilla JA, Amaddio MD: Cortical evoked potential monitoring. Spine 9:256, 1984
9. Bradshaw K, Webb JK, Fraser AM: Clinical evaluation of spinal cord monitoring in scoliosis surgery. Spine 9:636, 1984
10. Nuwer MR, Dawson EG, Carlson LG et al: Somatosensory evoked potential spinal cord monitoring reduces neurologic deficits after scoliosis surgery: results of a large multicenter survey. Electroencephalogr Clin Neurophysiol 96:6, 1995
11. Ginsburg HH, Shetter AG, Raudzens PA: Postoperative paraplegia with preserved intraoperative somatosensory evoked potentials: a case report. J Neurosurg 63:296, 1985
12. Lesser RP, Raudzens PA, Lüders H et al: Postoperative neurological deficits may occur despite unchanged somatosensory evoked potentials. Ann Neurol 19:22, 1986
13. Little JR, Lesser RP, Luders H: Electrophysiological monitoring during basilar aneurysm operation. Neurosurgery 20:421, 1987
14. Dawson EG, Sherman JE, Kanim LE, Nuwer MR: Spinal cord monitoring. Results of the Scoliosis Research Society and the European Spinal Deformity Society survey. Spine 16:S361, 1991
15. Jasper HH: The ten-twenty electrode system of the International Federation. Electoencephalogr Clin Neurophysiol 10:371, 1958
16. Kearse LA Jr, Martin D, McPeck K, Lopez-Bresnahan M: Computer-derived density spectral array in detection of mild analog electroencephalographic ischemic pattern changes during carotid endarterectomy. J Neurosurg 78:884, 1993
17. Spackman TN, Faust RJ, Cucchiara RF et al: A

comparison of aperiodic analysis of the EEG with standard EEG and cerebral blood flow for the detection of ischemia. Anesthesiology 66:229, 1987
18. Craft RM, Losasso TJ, Perkins WJ et al: EEG monitoring for cerebral ischemia during carotid endarterectomy (CEA): how much is enough? abstracted. J Neurosurg Anesth 6:301, 1994
19. Messick JM Jr, Casement B, Sharbrough FW et al: Correlation of regional cerebral blood flow (rCBF) with EEG changes during isoflurane anesthesia for carotid endarterectomy: critical rCBF. Anesthesiology 66:344, 1987
20. Messick JM Jr, Sharbrough F, Sundt TJ: Selective shunting on the basis of EEG and regional CBF monitoring during carotid endarterectomy. Int Anesthesiol Clin 22:137, 1984
21. Fode NC, Sundt TM Jr, Robertson JT et al: Multicenter retrospective review of results and complications of carotid endarterectomy in 1981. Stroke 17:370, 1986
22. Halsey JH Jr: Risks and benefits of shunting in carotid endarterectomy. The international transcranial Doppler collaborators. Stroke 23:1583, 1992
23. Silbert BS, Koumoundouros E, Davies MJ, Cronin KD: Comparison of the processed electroencephalogram and awake neurological assessment during carotid endarterectomy. Anaesth Intensive Care 17:298, 1989
24. Modica PA, Tempelhoff R, Rich KM, Grubb RL Jr: Computerized electroencephalographic monitoring and selective shunting: influence on intraoperative administration of phenylephrine and myocardial infarction after general anesthesia for carotid endarterectomy. Neurosurgery 30:842, 1992
25. Smith JS, Roizen MF, Cahalan MK et al: Does anesthetic technique make a difference? Augmentation of systolic blood pressure during carotid endarterectomy: effects of phenylephrine versus light general anesthesia and of isoflurane versus halothane on the incidence of myocardial ischemia. Anesthesiology 69:846, 1988
26. Nuwer MR, Daube J, Fischer C et al: Neuromonitoring during surgery. Report of an IFCN Committee. Electroencephalogr Clin Neurophysiol 87:263, 1993
27. Nuwer MR: Intraoperative electroencephalography. J Clin Neurophysiol 10:437, 1993
28. Bashein G, Nessly ML, Bledsoe SW et al: Electroencephalography during surgery with cardiopulmonary bypass and hypothermia. Anesthesiology 76:878, 1992
29. Levy WJ: Intraoperative EEG patterns: implications for EEG monitoring. Anesthesiology 60:430, 1984
30. Levy WJ: Quantitative analysis of EEG changes during hypothermia. Anesthesiology 60:291, 1984
31. Edmonds HL Jr, Griffiths LK, van der Laken J et al: Quantitative electroencephalographic monitoring during myocardial revascularization predicts postoperative disorientation and improves outcome. J Thorac Cardiovasc Surg 103:555, 1992
32. Arom KV, Cohen DE, Strobl FT: Effect of intraoperative intervention on neurological outcome based on electroencephalographic monitoring during cardiopulmonary bypass. Ann Thorac Surg 48:476, 1989
33. Arroyo S, Lesser RP, Gillinov AM et al: EEG and prognosis of neurologic recovery of dogs under profound hypothermic circulatory arrest. Electroencephalogr Clin Neurophysiol 87:242, 1993
34. Newburger JW, Jonas RA, Wernovsky G et al: A comparison of the perioperative neurologic effects of hypothermic circulatory arrest versus low-flow cardiopulmonary bypass in infant heart surgery. N Engl J Med 329:1057, 1993
35. Salerno TA, Lince DP, White DN et al: Monitoring of electroencephalogram during open-heart surgery. A prospective analysis of 118 cases. J Thorac Cardiovasc Surg 76:97, 1978
36. Bolsin SN: Detection of neurologic damage during cardiopulmonary bypass. Anaesthesia 41:61, 1986
37. Myers RR, Stockard JJ, Saidman LJ: Monitoring of cerebral perfusion during anesthesia by time-compressed Fourier analysis of the electroencephalogram. Stroke 8:331, 1977
38. Sullivan HG, Keenan RL, Isrow L, Feria AW: The critical importance of PaCO2 during intracranial aneurysm surgery. Case report. J Neurosurg 52:426, 1980
39. Graham DI, McGeorge A, Fitch W et al: Ischaemic brain damage induced by rapid lowering of arterial pressure in hypertension. J Hypertens 2:297, 1984
40. Artru AA: Cerebral metabolism and EEG during combination of hypocapnia and isoflurane-induced hypotension in dogs. Anesthesiology 65:602, 1986
41. Artru AA, Wright K, Colley PS: Cerebral effects of hypocapnia plus nitroglycerin-induced hypotension in dogs. J Neurosurg 64:924, 1986
42. Dong WK, Bledsoe SW, Chadwick HS et al: Electrical correlates of brain injury resulting from

severe hypotension and hemodilution in monkeys. Anesthesiology 65:617, 1986
43. Cohen AR, Young W, Ransohoff J: Intraspinal localization of the somatosensory evoked potential. Neurosurgery 9:157, 1981
44. Ealand-Snyder BG, Holliday TA: Pathways of ascending evoked spinal cord potentials of dogs. Electroencephalogr Clin Neurophysiol 58:140, 1984
45. Gaines R, York DH, Watts C: Identification of spinal cord pathways responsible for the peroneal-evoked response in the dog. Spine 9:810, 1984
46. York DH: Somatosensory evoked potentials in man: differentiation of spinal pathways responsible for conduction from the forelimb vs hindlimb. Progr Neurobiol 25:1, 1985
47. Sebel PS, Ingram DA, Flynn PJ et al: Evoked potentials during isoflurane anaesthesia. Br J Anaesth 58:580, 1986
48. Drummond JC, Todd MM, U HS: The effect of high dose sodium thiopental on brainstem auditory and median nerve somatosensory evoked responses in humans. Anesthesiology 63:249, 1985
49. McPherson RW, Sell B, Traystman RJ: Effects of thiopental, fentanyl and etomidate on upper extremity somatosensory evoked potentials in humans. Anesthesiology 65:584, 1986
50. McPherson RW, Mahla ME, Johnson R et al: Effects of enflurane, isoflurane and nitrous oxide on somatosensory evoked potentials during fentanyl anesthesia. Anesthesiology 62:626, 1985
51. Schubert A, Drummond JC, Peterson DO et al: The effect of high-dose fentanyl on human median nerve somatosensory-evoked responses. Can J Anaesth 34:35, 1987
52. Sloan TB, Ronai AK, Toleikis JR et al: Improvement of intraoperative somatosensory evoked potentials by etomidate. Anesth Analg 67:582, 1988
53. Koht A, Schütz W, Schmidt G et al: Effects of etomidate, midazolam, and thiopental on median nerve somatosensory evoked potentials and the additive effects of fentanyl and nitrous oxide. Anesth Analg 67:435, 1988
54. Maurette P, Simeon F, Castagnera L et al: Propofol anaesthesia alters somatosensory evoked cortical potentials. Anaesthesia, 43, suppl:44, 1988
55. Haghighi SS, Sirintrapun SJ, Johnson JC et al: Suppression of spinal and cortical somatosensory evoked potentials by desflurane anesthesia. J Neurosurg Anesthesiol 8:148, 1996
55a. Schindler E, Thiel A, Muller M et al: Changes in somatosensory evoked potentials after sevoflurane and isoflurane. A randomized phase III study. Anaesthesist, 45, suppl. 1:S52, 1996
55b. Drummond JC, Todd MM, Schubert A et al: Effect of the acute administration of high dose pentobarbital on human brainstem auditory and median nerve somatosensory evoked responses. Neurosurgery 20:830, 1987
56. DuBois MY, Sato S, Chassy J et al: Effects of enflurane on brainstem auditory evoked responses in humans. Anesth Analg 61:898, 1982
57. Manninen PH, Lam AM, Nicholas JF: The effects of isoflurane and isoflurane-nitrous oxide anesthesia on brainstem auditory evoked potentials in humans. Anesth Analg 64:43, 1985
58. Ben-David B, Taylor PD, Haller GS: Posterior spinal fusion complicated by posterior column injury. A case report of a false-negative wake-up test. Spine 12:540, 1987
59. Toleikis JR, Carlvin AO, Shapiro DE, Schafer MF: The use of dermatomal evoked responses during surgical procedures that useintrapedicular fixation of the lumbosacral spine. Spine 18:2401, 1993
60. Owen JH, Bridwell KH, Lenke LG: Innervation pattern of dorsal roots and their effects on the specificity of dermatomalsomatosensory evoked potentials. Spine 18:748, 1993
61. Dumitru D, Newton BY, Dreyfuss P: Segmental v dermatomal somatosensory-evoked potentials. Normal intertrial variation and side-to-side comparison. Am J Phys Med Rehabil 72:75, 1993
62. Owen JH, Padberg AM, Spahr Holland L et al: Clinical correlation between degenerative spine disease and dermatomal somatosensory-evoked potentials in humans. Spine 16:S201, 1991
63. Crawford ES, Mizrahi EM, Hess KR et al: The impact of distal aortic perfusion and somatosensory evoked potential monitoring on prevention of paraplegia after aortic aneurysm operation. J Thorac Cardiovasc Surg 95:357, 1988
64. McNulty S, Arkoosh V, Goldberg M: The relevance of somatosensory evoked potentials during thoracic aorta aneurysm repair. J Cardiothorac Vasc Anesth 5:262, 1991
65. Maeda S, Miyamoto T, Murata H, Yamashita K: Prevention of spinal cord ischemia by monitoring spinal cord perfusion pressure and somatosensory evoked potentials. J Cardiovasc Surg 30:565, 1989
66. Kaplan BJ, Gravenstein N, Friedman WA et al: Thoracic aortic occlusion: somatosensory evoked potential monitoring and neurologic outcome in a canine mode. Surg Neurol 28:351, 1987

67. Svensson LG, Patel V, Robinson MF et al: Influence of preservation or perfusion of intraoperatively identified spinal cord blood supply on spinal motor evoked potentials and paraplegia after aortic surgery. J Vasc Surg 13:355, 1991
68. Krieger KH, Spencer FC: Is paraplegia after repair of coarctation of the aorta due principally to distal hypotension during aortic cross-clamping? Surgery 97:2, 1985
69. Laschinger JC, Cunningham JN, Cooper MM et al: Monitoring of somatosensory evoked potentials during surgical procedures on the thoracoabdominal aorta. I. Relationship of aortic cross-clamp duration, changes in somatosensory evoked potentials and incidence of neurologic dysfunction. J Thorac Cardiovasc Surg 94:260, 1987
70. Laschinger JC, Cunningham JN, Baumann FG et al: Monitoring of somatosensory evoked potentials during surgical procedures on the thoracoabdominal aorta. II. Use of somatosensory evoked potentials to assess adequacy of distal aortic bypass and perfusion after thoracic aortic cross-clamping. J Thorac Cardiovasc Surg 94:266, 1987
71. Cunningham JN, Laschinger JC, Spencer FC: Monitoring of somatosensory evoked potentials during surgical procedures on the thoracoabdominal aorta. IV. Clinical observations and results. J Thorac Cardiovasc Surg 94:275, 1987
72. Kaplan BJ, Friedman WA, Alexander JA, Hampson SR: Somatosensory evoked potential monitoring of spinal cord ischemia during aortic operations. Neurosurgery 19:82, 1986
73. Pollock JC, Jamieson MP, McWilliam R: Somatosensory evoked potentials in the detection of spinal cord ischemia in aortic coarctation repair. Ann Thorac Surg 41:251, 1986
74. York DH: Somatosensory evoked potentials in man: differentiation of spinal pathways responsible for conduction from the forelimb vs hindlimb. Progr Neurobiol 25:1, 1985
75. Branston NM, Ladds A, Symon L, Wang AD: Comparison of the effects of ischaemia on early components of the somatosensory evoked potential in brainstem, thalamus, and cerebral cortex. J Cereb Blood Flow Metab 4:68, 1984
76. Branston NM, Symon L: Depression of the cortical evoked potential with reduction of local blood flow in baboons. J Physiol (Lond) 24:98P, 1974
77. Branston NM, Symon L, Crockard HA, Pasztor E: Relationship between the cortical evoked potential and local cortical blood flow following acute middle cerebral artery occlusion in the baboon. Exp Neurol 45:195, 1974
78. Friedman WA, Chadwick GM, Verhoeven FJS et al: Monitoring of somatosensory evoked potentials during surgery for middle cerebral artery aneurysms. Neurosurgery 29:83, 1991
79. Schramm J, Koht A, Schmidt G et al: Surgical and electrophysiologic observations during clipping of 134 aneurysms with evoked potential monitoring. Neurosurgery 26:61, 1990
80. Mooji JJA, Buchtal A, Belopavlovic: Somatosensory evoked potential monitoring of temporary middle cerebral artery occlusion during aneurysm operation. Neurosurgery 21: 492, 1987
81. Buchthal A, Belopavlovic M, Mooih JJA: Evoked potential monitoring and temporary clipping in cerebral aneurysm surgery. Acta Neurochir (Wien) 93:28, 1988
82. Little JR, Lesser RP, Lüders H: Electrophysiological monitoring during basilar aneurysm operation. Neurosurgery 20:421, 1987
83. Lam AM, Manninen PH, Ferguson GG, Nantau W: Monitoring electrophysiologic function during carotid endarterectomy: a comparison of somatosensory evoked potentials and conventional electroencephalogram. Anesthesiology 75:15, 1991
84. Kearse LA Jr, Martin D, McPeck K, Lopez-Bresnahan M: Computer-derived density spectral array in detection of mild analog electroencephalographic ischemic pattern changes during carotid endarterectomy. J Neurosurg 78:884, 1993
85. Symon L: The relationship between CBF, evoked potentials and the clinical features in cerebral ischaemia. Acta Neurol Scand (Suppl) 78:175, 1980
86. Goodwin SR, Friedman WA, Bellefleur M: Is it time to use evoked potentials to predict outcome in comatose children and adults? Crit Care Med 19:518, 1991
87. Goodwin SR, Toney KA, Mahla ME: Sensory evoked potentials accurately predict outcome from prolonged coma caused by strangulation. Crit Care Med 21:631, 1993
88. Greenberg RP, Mayer DJ, Becker DP, Miller JD: Evaluation of brain function in severe human head trauma with multimodality evoked potentials. Part 1. J Neurosurg 47:150, 1977
89. Greenberg RP, Becker DP, Miller JD, Mayer DJ: Evaluation of brain function in severe human head trauma with multimodality evoked potentials. Part 2. J Neurosurg 47:163, 1977
90. Greenberg RP, NeWlon PG, Becker DP: The somatosensory evoked potential in patients with severe head injury: outcome prediction and

monitoring of brain function. Ann NY Acad Sci 388:683, 1982

91. Greenberg RP, Newlon PG, Hyatt M et al: Prognostic implications of early multimodality evoked potentials in severely head-injured patients. J Neurosurg 55:227, 1981
92. Machado C: Multimodality evoked potentials and electroetinography in a test battery for an early diagnosis of brain death. J Neurosurg Sci 37:125, 1993
93. Machado C, Valdes P, Garcia-Tigera J et al: Brainstem auditory evoked potentials and brain death. Electroencephalogr Clin Neurophysiol 80:392, 1991
94. Mackey-Hargadine JR, Hall JW: Sensory evoked responses in head injury. CNS Trauma 2:187, 1985
95. Starr A, Hamilton AE: Correlation between confirmed sites of neurological lesions and abnormalities of far-field auditory brainstem responses. Electroencephalogr Clin Neurophysiol 41:596, 1976
96. Stockard JJ, Stockard JE, Sharbrough FW: Detection and localization of occult lesions with brainstem auditory responses. Mayo Clin Proc 52:761, 1977
97. Achor LJ, Starr A: Auditory brain stem responses in the cat. I. Intracranial and extracranial recordings. Electroencephalogr Clin Neurophysiol 48:154, 1980
98. Achor LJ, Starr A: Auditory brain stem responses in the cat. II. Effects of lesions. Electroencephalogr Clin Neurophysiol 48:174, 1980
99. Buchwald JS, Huang CM: Far-field acoustic response: Origins in the cat. Science 189:382, 1975
100. Greenberg RP, Stablein DM, Becker DP: Noninvasive localization of brain-stem lesions in the cat with multimodality evoked potentials. J Neurosurg 54:740, 1981
101. Sherg M, von Cramon D: A new interpretation of the generators of BAEP waves I-V: results of a spatio-temporal dipole model. Electroencephalogr Clin Neurophysiol 62:290, 1985
102. Starr A, Achor LJ: Anatomical and physiological origins of auditory brain stem responses (ABR). p. 415. In Lehmann D, Calloway E (eds): Human Evoked Potentials: Applications and Problems. Plenum Press, New York 1979
103. Møller AR, Jannetta PJ, Møller MB: Neural generators of brainstem evoked potentials results from human intracranial recordings. Ann Otol 90:591, 1981
104. Møller AR, Jannetta PJ: Auditory evoked potentials recorded from the cochlear nucleus and its vicinity in man. J Neurosurg 59:1013, 1983
105. Starr A, Amlie RN, Martin WH, Sanders S: Development of auditory function in newborn infants revealed by auditory brainstem potentials. Pediatrics 60:831, 1977
106. Grundy BL, Jannetta PJ, Procopio PT et al: Intraoperative monitoring of brain-stem auditory evoked potentials. J Neurosurg 57:674, 1982
107. Møller AR, Møller MB: Does intraoperative monitoring of auditory evoked potentials reduce incidence of hearing loss as a complication of microvascular decompression of cranial nerves. Neurosurgery 24:257, 1989
108. Friedman WA, Kaplan BJ, Gravenstein D, Rhoton AL: Intraoperative brain-stem auditory evoked potentials during posterior fossa microvascular decompression. J Neurosurg 62:552, 1985
109. Fischer G, Fischer C, Remond J: Hearing preservation in acoustic neurinoma surgery. J Neurosurg 76:910, 1992
110. Harper CM, Harner SG, Slavit DH et al: Effect of BAEP monitoring on hearing preservation during acoustic neuroma resection. Neurology 42:1551, 1992
111. Watanabe E, Schramm J, Strauss C et al: Neurophysiologic monitoring in posterior fossa surgery. II. BAEP-waves I and V and preservation of hearing. Acta Neurochir Wien 98:118, 1989
112. Fischer G, Fischer C, Remond J: Hearing preservation in acoustic neurinoma surgery. J Neurosurg 76:910, 1992
113. Manninen PH, Patterson S, Lam AM et al: Evoked potential monitoring during posterior fossa aneurysm surgery: a comparison of two modalities. Can J Anaesth 41:92, 1994
114. Grundy BL, Procopio PT, Janetta PJ, Doyle E: Evoked potential changes produced by positioning for retromastoid craniectomy. Neurosurgery 10:766, 1982
115. Cracco RQ: Evaluation of conduction in central motor pathways: techniques, pathophysiology, and clinical interpretation. Neurosurgery 20:199, 1987
116. Kawai N, Nagao S: Origins and conducting pathways of motor evoked potentials elicited by transcranial magnetic stimulation in cats. Neurosurgery 31:520, 1992
117. Kitagawa H, Takano H, Takakuwa K et al: Origins and conducting pathways of motor evoked potentials elicited by transcranial stimulation of the motor cortex in cats. Neurosurgery 28:358, 1991
118. Levy WJ: Spinal evoked potentials from the motor tracts. J Neurosurg 58:38, 1983

119. Levy WJ, McCaffrey M, York DH, Tanzer F: Motor evoked potentials from transcranial stimulation of the motor cortex in cats. Neurosurgery 15:214, 1984
120. Levy WJ, York DH: Evoked potentials from the motor tracts in humans. Neurosurgery 12:422, 1983
121. Levy WJ, York DH, McCaffrey M, Tanzer T: Motor evoked potentials from transcranial stimulation of the motor cortex in humans. Neurosurgery 15:287, 1984
122. York DH: Review of descending pathways involved with transcranial stimulation. Neurosurgery 20:70, 1987
123. Zappulla RA, Hollis P, Ryder J et al: Noncortical origins of the spinal motor evoked potential in rats. Neurosurgery 22:846, 1988
124. Caramia MD, Pardal AM, Zarola F, Rossini PM: Electric vs magnetic trans-cranial stimulation of the brain in healthy humans: a comparative study of central motor tracts "conductivity" and "excitability." Brain Res 479:98, 1989
125. Kawai N, Nagao S: Origins and conducting pathways of motor evoked potentials elicited by transcranial magnetic stimulation in cats. Neurosurgery 31:520, 1992
126. Machida M, Weinstein SL, Yamada T et al: Spinal cord monitoring: electrophysiologic measures of sensory and motor function during spinal surgery. Spine 5:407, 1985
127. Owen JH, Bridwell KH, Grubb R et al: The clinical application of neurogenic motor evoked potentials to monitor spinal cord function during surgery. Spine 16:S385, 1991
128. Owen JH, Laschinger J, Bridwell K et al: Sensitivity and specificity of somatosensory and neurogenic motor evoked potentials in animals and humans. Spine 13:1111, 1988
129. Owen JH, Jenny AB, Naito M et al: Effects of spinal cord lesioning on somatosensory and neurogenic-motor evoked potentials. Spine 14: 673, 1989
130. Fukui Y: An experimental and clinical study of peripheral nerve potentials evoked by stimulating the spinal cord. Nippon Seikeigeka Gakkai Zasshi 67:427, 1993
131. Edmonds HL Jr, Paloheimo MP, Backman MH et al: Transcranial magnetic motor evoked potentials for functional monitoring of motor pathways during scoliosis surgery. Spine 14:683, 1989
132. Herdmann J, Lumenta CB, Huse KO: Magnetic stimulation for monitoring of motor pathways in spinal procedures. Spine 18:551, 1993
133. Zentner J: Noninvasive motor evoked potential monitoring during neurosurgical operations on the spinal cord. Neurosurgery 24:709, 1989
134. Zentner J: Motor evoked potential monitoring during neurosurgical operations on the spinal cord. Neurosurg Rev 14:29, 1991
135. Elmore JR, Gloviczki P, Harper CM et al: Failure of motor evoked potentials to predict neurologic outcome in experimental thoracic aortic occlusion. J Vasc Surg 14:131, 1991
136. Reuter DG, Tacker WA Jr, Badylak SF et al: Correlation of motor-evoked potential response to ischemic spinal cord damage. J Thorac Cardiovasc Surg 104:262, 1992
137. Zentner J, Albrecht T, Heuser D: Influence of halothane, enflurane, and isoflurane on motor evoked potentials. Neurosurgery 31:298, 1992
138. Jellinek D, Platt M, Jewkes D et al: Effects of nitrous oxide on motor evoked potentials under total anesthesia with intravenously administered propofol. Neurosurgery 29:558, 1991
139. Ghaly RF, Stone JL, Levy WJ et al: The effect of etomidate on motor evoked potentials induced by transcranial magnetic stimulation in the monkey. Neurosurgery 27:936, 1990
140. Zentner J, Kiss I, Ebner A: Influence of anesthetics—nitrous oxide in particular—on electromyographic response evoked by transcranial electrical stimulation of the cortex. Neurosurgery 24:253, 1989
141. Kalkman CJ, Drummond JC, Ribberink AA et al: Effects of propofol, etomidate, midazolam, and fentanyl on motor evoked responses to transcranial electrical or magnetic stimulation in humans. Anesthesiology 76:502, 1992
142. Kalkman CJ, Drummond JC, Kennelly NA et al: Intraoperative monitoring of tibialis anterior muscle motor evoked responses to transcranial electrical stimulation during partial neuromuscular blockade. Anesth Analg 75:584, 1992
143. Kalkman CJ, Ubags LH, Been HD et al: Improved amplitude of myogenic motor evoked responses after paired transcranial electrical stimulation during sufentanil/nitrous oxide anesthesia. Anesthesiology 83:270, 1995
144. Taniguchi M, Cedzich C, Schramm J: Modification of cortical stimulation for motor evoked potentials under general anesthesia: technical description. Neurosurgery 32:219, 1993
145. Prass RL, Luders H: Acoustic (loudspeaker) facial electromyographic monitoring: part 1. Evoked electromyographic activity during acoustic neuroma resection. Neurosurgery 19:392, 1986

146. Prass RL, Kinney SE, Hardy RW et al: Acoustic (loudspeaker) facial EMG monitoring: II. Use of evoked EMG activity during acoustic neuroma resection. Otolaryngol Head Neck Surg 97:541, 1987
147. Harner SG, Daube JR, Ebersold MJ et al: Improved preservation of facial nerve function with use of electrical monitoring during removal of acoustic neuromas. Mayo Clin Proc 62:92, 1987
148. Lennon RL, Hosking MP, Daube JR et al: Effect of partial neuromuscular blockade on intraoperative electromyography in patients undergoing resection of acoustic neuromas. Anesth Analg 75:729, 1992
149. Dickins JR, Graham SS: A comparison of facial nerve monitoring systems in cerebellopontine angle surgery. Am J Otol 12:1, 1991
150. Kartush JM, Lundy LB: Facial nerve outcome in acoustic neuroma surgery. Otolaryngol Clin North Am 25:623, 1992
151. Møller AR, Jannetta PJ: Monitoring of facial nerve function during removal of acoustic tumor. Am J Otol 5:27, 1985
152. Møller AR, Jannetta PJ: Preservation of facial function during removal of acoustic neuromas. J Neurosurg 61:757, 1984
153. Prasad S, Hirsch BE, Kamerer DB et al: Facial nerve function following cerebellopontine angle surgery: prognostic value of intraoperative thresholds. Am J Otol 14:330, 1993
154. Acoustic neuroma. Consensus Statement 9:1, 1991
155. Schaefer SD. Laryngeal electromyography. Otolaryngol Clin North Am 24:1053, 1991
156. Sterkers JM, Morrison GA, Sterkers O et al: Preservation of facial, cochlear, and other nerve functions in acoustic neuroma treatment. Otolaryngol Head Neck Surg 110:146, 1994
157. Blumenthal S, Gill K: Complications of the Wiltse Pedicle Screw Fixation System. Spine 18:1867, 1993
158. Calancie B, Ayyar DR, Eismont FJ: Myokymic discharges: prompt cessation following nerve root decompression during spine surgery. Electromyogr Clin Neurophysiol 32:443, 1992
159. Calancie B, Lebwohl N, Madsen P, Klose KJ: Intraoperative evoked EMG monitoring in an animal model. A new technique for evaluating pedicle screw placement. Spine 17:1229, 1992
160. Owen JH, Kostuik JP, Gornet M et al: The use of mechanically elicited electromyograms to protect nerve roots during surgery for spinal degeneration. Spine 19:1704, 1994
161. Halsey JH, McDowell HA, Gelmon S, Morawetz RB: Blood velocity in the middle cerebral artery and regional cerebral blood flow during carotid endarterectomy. Stroke 20:53, 1989
162. Nuttall GA, Cook DJ, Fulgham JR et al: The relationship between cerebral blood flow and transcranial Doppler blood flow velocity during hypothermic cardiopulmonary bypass in adults. Anesth Analg 82:1146, 1996
163. Weyland A, Stephan H, Kazmaier S et al: Flow velocity measurements as an index of cerebral blood flow. Validity of transcranial Doppler sonographic monitoring during cardiac surgery. Anesthesiology 81:1401, 1994
164. Grosset DG, Straiton J, du Trevou M, Bullock R: Prediction of symptomatic vasospasm after subarachnoid hemorrhage by rapidly increasing transcranial Doppler velocity and cerebral blood flow changes. Stroke 23:674, 1992
165. Grosset DG, Straiton J, McDonald I et al: Use of transcranial Doppler sonography to predict development of a delayed ischemic deficit after subarachnoid hemorrhage. J Neurosurg 78:183, 1993
166. Grosset DG, Straiton J, McDonald I et al: Angiographic and Doppler diagnosis of cerebral artery vasospasm following subarachnoid haemorrhage. Br J Neurosurg 7:291, 1993
167. Newell DW, Aaslid R: Transcranial Doppler: clinical and experimental uses. Cerebrovasc Brain Metab Rev 4:122, 1992
168. Newell DW, Winn HR: Transcranial Doppler in cerebral vasospasm. Neurosurg Clin North Am 1:319, 1990
169. Seckhar LN, Wechsler LR, Yonas H et al: Value of transcranial Doppler examination in the diagnosis of cerebral vasospasm after subarachnoid hemorrhage. Neurosurgery 22:813, 1988
170. Sloan MA, Haley EC, Kassell NF et al: Sensitivity and specificity of transcranial Doppler ultrasonography in the diagnosis of vasospasm following subarachnoid hemorrhage. Neurology 39:1514, 1989
171. Hassler W, Steinmetz H, Pirschel J: Transcranial Doppler study of intracranial circulatory arrest. J Neurosurg 71:195, 1989
172. Newell DW, Grady MS, Sirotta P, Winn HR: Evaluation of brain death using transcranial Doppler. Neurosurgery 24:500, 1989
173. Petty GW, Mohr JP, Pedley TA et al: The role of trnascranial Doppler in confirming brain death: sensitivity, specificity, and suggestions for performance and interpretation. Neurology 40:300, 1990

174. Petty GW, Wiebers DO, Meissner I: Transcranial Doppler ultrasonography: clinical applications in cerebrovascular disease. Mayo Clin Proc 65:1350, 1990
175. Zurynski Y, Dorsch N, Pearson I, Choong R: Transcranial Doppler ultrasound in brain death: experience in 140 patients. Neurol Res 13:248, 1991
176. Cruz J: Cerebral oxygenation: monitoring and management. Acta Neurochir (Suppl) 59:86, 1993
177. Dearden NM, Midgley S: Technical considerations in continuous jugular venous oxygen saturation measurement. Acta Neurochir (Suppl) 59:91, 1993
178. Matta B, Menon D: Severe head injury in the United Kingdom and Ireland: a survey of practice and implications for management. Crit Care Med 24:1743, 1996
179. Robertson CS, Gopinath SP, Goodman JC et al: $S_{jv}O_2$ monitoring in head injured patients. J Neurotrauma 12:891, 1995
180. Murr R, Schurer L: Correlation of jugular venous oxygen saturation to spontaneous fluctuations of cerebral perfusion pressure in patients with severe head injury. Neurol Res 17:329, 1995
181. Schneider GJ, von Helden A, Lanksch WR, Unterberg A: Continuous monitoring of jugular bulb oxygen saturation in comatose patients—therapeutic implications. Acta Neurochir Wien 134:71, 1995
182. Muizelaar JP, Schroder ML: Overview of monitoring of cerebral blood flow and metabolism after severe head injury. Can J Neurol Sci 21:S6, 1994
183. Gopinath SP, Robertson CS, Contant CF et al: Jugular venous desaturation and outcome after head injury. J Neurol Neurosurg Psychiatry 57:717, 1994
184. Chan KH, Dearden NM, Miller JD et al: Multimodality monitoring as a guide to treatment of intracranial hypertension after severe brain injury. Neurosurgery 32:547, 1993
185. McCormick PW, Stewart M, Goetting MG et al: Noninvasive cerebral optical spectroscopy for monitoring cerebral oxygen delivery and hemodynamics. Crit Care Med 19:89, 1991
186. Pollard V, Prough DS, DeMelo AE et al: Validation in volunteers of a near-infrared spectroscope for monitoring brain oxygenation in vivo. Anesth Analg 82:269, 1996
187. Duncan LA, Ruckley CV, Wildsmith JA: Cerebral oximetry: a useful monitor during carotid artery surgery. Anaesthesia 50:1041, 1995
188. McCormick PW, Stewart M, Lewis G et al: Intracerebral penetration of infrared light. Technical note. J Neurosurg 76:315, 1992
189. Ausman JI, McCormick PW, Stewart M et al: Cerebral metabolism during hypothermic circulatory arrest in humans. J Neurosurg 79:810, 1993
190. Slavin KV, Dujovny M, Ausman JI et al: Clinical experience with transcranial cerebral oximetry. Surg Neurol 42:531, 1994
191. Williams IM, Picton A, Farrell A et al: Light-reflective cerebral oximetry and jugular bulb venous oxygen saturation during carotid endarterectomy. Br J Surg 81:1291, 1994
192. Germon TJ, Young AE, Manara AR, Nelson RJ: Extracerebral absorption of near infrared light influences the detection of increased cerebral oxygenation monitored by near infrared spectroscopy. J Neurol Neurosurg Psychiatry 58:477, 1995
193. Samra SK, Dorje P, Zelenock GB, Stanley JC: Cerebral oximetry in patients undergoing carotid endarterectomy under regional anesthesia. Stroke 27:49, 1996
194. Levy WJ, Levin S, Chance B: Near-infrared measurement of cerebral oxygenation. Correlation with electroencephalographic ischemia during ventricular fibrillation. Anesthesiology 83:738, 1995
195. Mahla ME: Monitoring the nervous system. In Kirby RR, Gravenstein W (eds): Clinical Anesthesia Practice. WB Saundera, Philadelphia, 1994

5 CEREBRAL PROTECTION

LESLIE NEWBERG MILDE

This chapter reviews normal cerebral physiology and biochemistry, discusses the present knowledge of pathophysiologic and biochemical changes that occur during and after cerebral ischemia, and presents current therapeutic measures for preventing or attenuating the consequences of cerebral ischemia, irreversible cell damage, and death.

CELLULAR STRUCTURE

The brain consists of a complex neuronal network surrounded by glial cells and a blood-brain barrier (BBB) that selectively limits the transfer of substances between blood and brain. Neurons, because they contain axons and dendrites, are unique in their ability to transmit impulses of depolarization in a nondecremental manner. The electric activity of neurons results from the presence in their surface membranes of ion-selective and voltage-sensitive channels.[1] The voltage-sensitive channels are controlled by changes in membrane potential that open the channels, allowing rapid movement of ions down their concentration gradient. This results in depolarization. Other ion-selective channels in the cell membrane are controlled by receptors sensitive to neurotransmitters.

The neuron has an outer limiting membrane, a nucleus, and cellular organelles including rough and smooth endoplasmic reticulum; Golgi apparatus; lysosomes responsible for degradation of cellular waste; lipofuscin granules; mitochondria responsible for oxidative phosphorylation; neurotubules and neurofilaments; and ribosomes.[2]

The cell membrane is a bimolecular phospholipid layer. Intercollated in the matrix of this are proteins including the adenosine triphosphatases (ATPases), adenylate cyclases, and cytochrome oxidases.[3] Enzymatic conversion of one phospholipid into another can alter membrane fluidity, which can influence the opening of channels to specific ions. Membrane phospholipid conversion can be stimulated by receptor agonists, neurotransmitters active in the normal state or induced during ischemia, or by calcium ion-activated phospholipases, which degrade phospholipids to lysophospholipids and free fatty acids (FFAs).[3] This latter reaction occurs during ischemia and may be an important step in the destruction of cell membranes leading to irreversible cell death. The high-energy source ATP is needed to replenish these membrane phospholipids.

CELLULAR FUNCTION

Ion Homeostasis

SODIUM AND POTASSIUM During cell depolarization, sodium ion (Na^+) influx occurs rapidly by passive diffusion down its large extracellular-to-intracellular concentration gradient.

During the recovery phase, sodium is actively pumped out of the cell and potassium ions (K^+) are reaccumulated inside the cell against their concentration and electrochemical gradients. This is achieved by a membrane-associated energy-requiring sodium pump (Na^+-K^+-ATPase) that maintains the normal sodium and potassium gradients across the cell membrane. Outward transport of sodium exceeds inward potassium transport, producing a difference in potential across the cell membrane, with the inside of the cell being negative relative to the outside. The activity of this sodium pump is stimulated by increases in intracellular sodium or extracellular potassium, that is, by the ionic changes associated with depolarization.[4] The energy required for the sodium pump is provided by the hydrolysis of ATP to adenosine diphosphate (ADP) and inorganic phosphate (P_i). The ADP that is produced activates the energy-producing reactions in the cell: glycolysis via the Embden-Meyerhof pathway in the cytosol and the tricarboxylic acid cycle in the mitochondria to produce more ATP.

CALCIUM Calcium has a ubiquitous role in the transmission of information from the external environment to the cell interior where the calcium ion (Ca^{2+}) acts as a second messenger to alter membrane function and gene expression.[5] Calcium is necessary for cell excitation and transmitter release; it can inhibit some intracellular enzymes such as the sodium pump and the glycolytic enzymes and it can stimulate other enzymes either directly or through the action of calmodulin, a calcium-dependent soluble modulator protein.[4]

External free Ca^{2+} concentration is approximately 10^{-3} mol/L, which is about the same as the total intracellular calcium concentration. However, 10^{-4} mol/L intracellular Ca^{2+} is stored within the cell on internal membranes, in the endoplasmic reticulum, in calcium-binding proteins, and in the mitochondria, leaving a free intracellular Ca^{2+} concentration of 10^{-7} to 10^{-8} mol/L. This produces a free Ca^{2+} concentration gradient of 10,000 to 1 between the extracellular fluid and the cytosol.[3,4] This large gradient together with diffusion and drift causes Ca^{2+} to enter the cell.[6] Calcium ions enter the cell through three mechanisms: (1) by a voltage-dependent entry activated by an increase in extracellular K^+ or an increase in intracellular Na^+ (i.e., cell depolarization), (2) by changes in membrane fluidity and (3) when an agonist such as excitatory amino acid neurotransmitters (glutamate or aspartate), norepinephrine, acetylcholine, or 5-hydroxytryptamine bind to a membrane receptor to open specific calcium channels[3] (Fig. 5.1).

The high concentration gradient of Ca^{2+} across the plasma membrane is maintained by the active removal of calcium from the cytosol. There are four energy-dependent calcium transport systems (Fig. 5.1). There are two calcium ion pumps in the plasma membrane: an ATP- and magnesium-dependent Ca^{2+}-ATPase translocase containing calmodulin that pumps calcium out of the cell and a Ca^{2+}-Na^+ exchange mechanism in which three Na^+ ions are exchanged for one Ca^{2+} ion. The energy for this Ca^{2+}-Na^+ exchange is provided by the inward movement of Na^+.[4] Because this Na^+ influx is regulated by the energy-requiring sodium pump (Na^+-K^+-ATPase), the Ca^{2+}-Na^+ exchange mechanism is ultimately also energy dependent. A third calcium transport system moves calcium into the endoplasmic reticulum facilitated by a transmembrane hydrogen ion (H^+) gradient using energy from ATP.[4] Calcium can also be bound to the calcium-binding proteins, the calmodulins, and to membrane phospholipids.[7] Only when the intracellular Ca^{2+} concentration is increased despite the other three removal mechanisms does the fourth transport mechanism become operative. Mitochondria are capable of removing excess Ca^{2+} from the cytosol. In mitochondrial membranes, Ca^{2+} is exchanged for H^+ using energy obtained from mitochondrial oxidative phosphorylation, energy that would otherwise be stored as ATP. Calcium ion release from the mitochondria occurs via a Ca^{2+}-Na^+ exchange mechanism and does not require energy.[4] In summary, calcium influx into the cell across the cell membrane and calcium release from the mitochondria are spontaneous

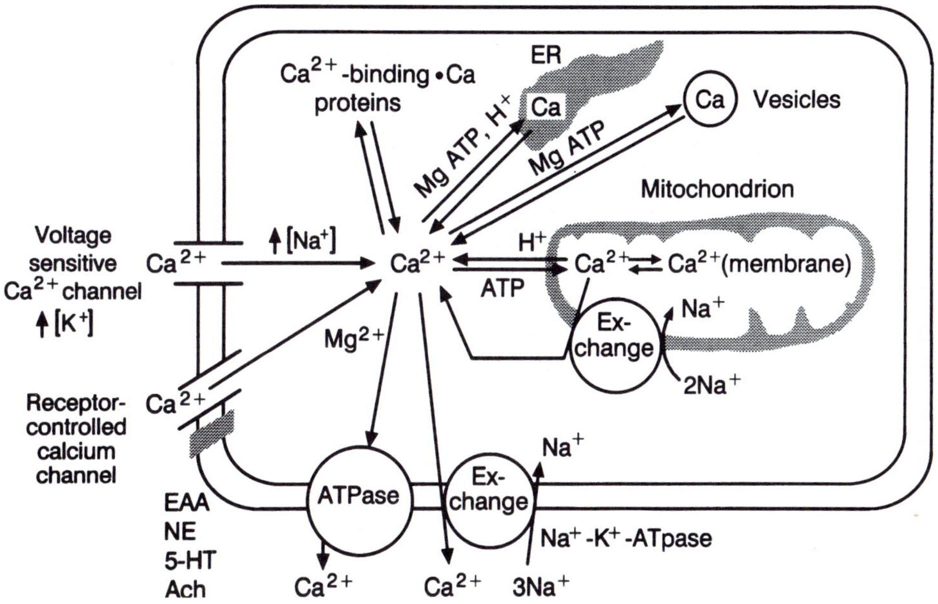

FIGURE 5.1 *Calcium transport processes. Calcium influx through cell membranes is passive down a concentration gradient through voltage-sensitive and NMDA receptor-controlled Ca^{2+} channels. Calcium efflux is via a Ca^{2+} translocase and a Na^{+}–Ca^{2+} exchange mechanism, both of which require energy. Calcium uptake into cellular organelles (endoplasmic reticulum, vesicles, mitochondria) requires energy.*

processes and occur freely during ischemia, whereas the active transport of Ca^{2+} out of the cell and sequestration of Ca^{2+} by the mitochondria require energy and are inhibited during ischemia.

HYDROGEN Normal intracellular brain pH values range from 6.94 to 7.06.[8] Intracellular H^{+} concentration is a result of passive H^{+} entry into the cell, intracellular metabolism, and fluxes of the ionized forms of weak bases and acids. Mechanisms for the neutralization of intracellular acid include chemical buffering, consumption of nonvolatile acids by the cell, and transfer of acid or alkali between the cytosol and the intracellular organelles, particularly the mitochondria. At the end of the electron transport chain of mitochondrial oxidative phosphorylation, two electrons are donated to each oxygen atom, which then combines with two H^{+} ions to form water (H_2O). Some of the energy produced by the electron transport chain is used to pump H^{+} out of the mitochondria. This results in an electrochemical gradient of H^{+} that drives the synthesis of ATP during the downhill reentry of H^{+} into the mitochondria via membrane-bound ATP synthetase.[9] In the long term, restoration of a normal intracellular pH requires extrusion of acid from the cell. This is accompanied by Na^{+} influx and efflux of chloride (Cl^{-}) ion. The energy needed for acid extrusion may come either from the entry of Na^{+} down its electrochemical gradient or from ATP.[8]

Metabolism

The energy requirements of the neuron can be viewed as normally subserving two components. Energy needed for neuronal function, that is, synaptic transmission of nerve action potentials (that indicated by electric activity on the electroencephalogram [EEG]), is termed *activation metabolism*.[10] Most of the activation energy is used for Na^+ and K^+ transport to restore ion gradients after action potentials.[7] The energy needed for the preservation of cellular integrity, which includes such processes as membrane stabilization, ion pumping to maintain ion concentration gradients across cell membranes; the synthesis and handling of neurotransmitters, proteins, nucleic acids, and lipids; and the initial steps in glucose metabolism,[11] has been termed *residual metabolism*.[10] Residual metabolism supports the cellular processes that continue to function after synaptic transmission has been abolished (isoelectric EEG). Approximately 55 percent of the total energy requirements of the neuron is needed for synaptic transmission and 40 to 45 percent is needed to maintain cellular integrity.[11]

The high energy demands of the neurons are supplied by the utilization of ATP, which is produced by the oxidation of glucose through the Embden-Meyerhof pathway in the cytosol and the tricarboxylic acid cycle in the mitochondria (Fig. 5.2). In the presence of oxygen, glucose is initially metabolized to pyruvate in the cytosol, which produces 2 moles of ATP per mole of glucose metabolized. Pyruvate is then metabolized to carbon dioxide and water within the mitochondria via the tricarboxylic acid cycle. This produces 36 moles of ATP. Eighty-nine percent of cellular ATP is generated from mitochondrial oxidative phosphorylation. The brain has low stores of high-energy phosphate compounds, no oxygen and minimal glucose or glycogen substrate stores. Therefore, it is very dependent on its circulation for substrate delivery[12] to maintain the energy requirements of neuronal function and cellular integrity.

FIGURE 5.2 *Embden-Meyerhof pathway of glycolysis. During ischemia pyruvate is metabolized to lactate to replenish the NAD+ supply for glycolysis.*

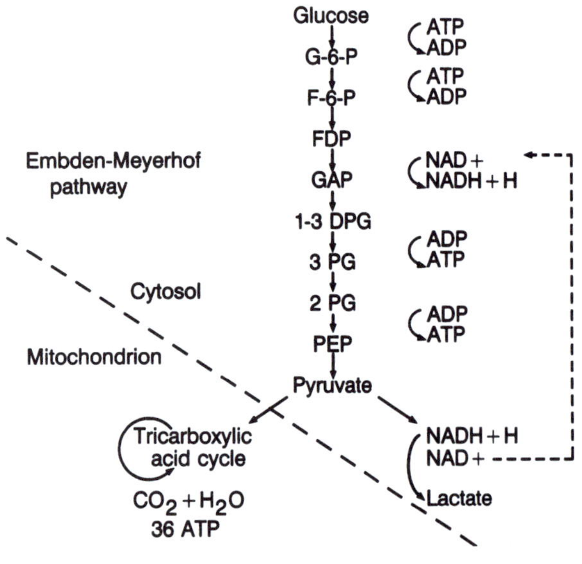

Glucose

The brain depends on glucose as the sole source of its energy and biosynthetic functions. Glucose is transported into neurons primarily via a stereospecific carrier-mediated mechanism. This carrier-mediated transport is affected by four variables: (1) the blood glucose concentration and the intracellular glucose concentration forming a glucose gradient across the membrane, (2) the affinity between glucose and the carrier, (3) the maximal flux rate of glucose that is achieved when the carrier is saturated, and (4) the rate of glucose utilization within the cell.[13] The higher the glucose metabolism within the cell, the higher the transport of glucose must be to supply substrate because there are minimal glucose stores within the neurons. Changes in glucose transport from blood to brain to match neuronal metabolic requirements affect blood-to-brain glucose concentration ratios. The factor limiting intracellular glucose concentration is the maximal flux rate of glucose. Because several factors affect glucose transport into cells, there is not a linear relationship between blood glucose and intracellular brain glucose.[14] As blood glucose increases, brain glucose reaches a threshold.

Insulin affects glucose transport primarily into muscle.[15,16] It can increase the uptake of glucose into spinal cord by approximately 10 to 15 percent.[17] However, insulin has little effect on glucose transport into brain,[18–21] although insulin does affect glucose transport out of brain cells. The administration of insulin can lower brain glucose only by increasing the uptake of glucose into muscle cells, thereby lowering blood glucose. This produces a glucose concentration gradient with intracellular brain glucose being higher than blood glucose, such that glucose will leave the cell. This explains the time delay between the administration of insulin with a decrease in blood glucose and the observed decrease in intracellular brain glucose.[22]

Oxidative Phosphorylation

Mitochondria function as metabolic compartments separated from the cytosol by a membrane that selectively allows passage of metabolites and ions, thereby providing control over mitochondrial metabolism.[23] Mitochondria metabolize pyruvate (produced in the cytosol through glycolysis) through a series of intermediates to ATP, carbon dioxide, and water. The mitochondrial multienzyme complex, pyruvate dehydrogenase, controls the entry of pyruvate into the tricarboxylic acid cycle by converting it to acetylcoenzyme A (acetyl-CoA). This is the rate-limiting step in oxidative phosphorylation.[23] Pyruvate dehydrogenase is inhibited by hypoxia and ischemia.[23] such that pyruvate is unable to enter the tricarboxylic acid cycle but instead must be converted to lactate, in the cytosol, a process that replenishes nicotinamide adenine dinucleotide (NAD^+) which is needed to continue glycolysis[23] (Fig. 5.2).

ISCHEMIA

Ischemia results when a decrease in tissue perfusion exceeds the tissue's ability to increase oxygen extraction from the blood and consists of inadequate oxygen delivery, inadequate carbon dioxide removal, increased intracellular lactic acid production, decreased stores of high-energy phosphates (phosphocreatine and ATP), decreased production of ATP, release of excitatory amino acid neurotransmitters, and disruption of the BBB.[12,24]

> *Components of Ischemia*
> - Decreased tissue perfusion
> - Increased oxygen extraction
> - Inadequate delivery of oxygen
> - Inadequate removal of carbon dioxide
> - Anaerobic metabolism
> - Increased intracellular lactic acid production
> - Decreased stores of high-energy phosphates
> - Decreased production of high-energy phosphates
> - Release of excitatory amino acid neurotransmitters
> - Disruption of the blood-brain barrier

Ischemia can be global, affecting the whole brain, or focal. Global ischemia may be complete or incomplete, whereas focal ischemia is incomplete. Complete global ischemia occurs with cardiac arrest and results in the cessation of oxidative phosphorylation (aerobic metabolism) within 15 to 20 seconds. Anaerobic metabolism with glycolysis supplying ATP will continue until the cellular stores of glucose have been depleted. Anaerobic glycolysis produces lactic acid, causing a decrease in intracellular pH, which peaks 2 to 3 minutes after the onset of ischemia. Free fatty acid content, primarily arachidonic acid, continues to increase throughout the period of ischemia and produces changes in membrane structure and function.[7] When glycolysis ceases and ATP concentrations have been depleted, all energy-requiring reactions of the neurons cease and cells soon die.

Incomplete ischemia may be more damaging than *short* periods of complete ischemia because the oxygen supply will be inadequate, resulting in anaerobic metabolism, whereas the continued, albeit reduced, supply of glucose will be metabolized to lactic acid, producing greater intracellular acidosis.[25,26]

In focal ischemia the residual cerebral blood flow (CBF) depends on the existence of collateral vessels and local perfusion pressure.[10] The relative oxygen availability of the blood is much lower than that of glucose under normal conditions. This deficiency is exacerbated during ischemia. It is hypothesized that a topographic gradient of ischemia exists in which a center of dense ischemia can be surrounded by areas of variable levels of perfusion, the ischemic penumbra.[27] These penumbral areas are potentially viable if blood flow to them can be increased.[28,29] Hemodynamic manipulation to support or increase perfusion to these areas during ischemia can decrease the amount of neurologic damage occurring as a result of the ischemia.

Flow Thresholds

The functional state of the neuron depends on adequate CBF for the delivery of oxygen and glucose. When CBF decreases below a certain threshold, neuronal function becomes impaired.[30] Ischemic flow thresholds[27,30] refer to the level of blood flow at which energy-requiring functions of the cell fails. Descriptions of such flow thresholds must include not only blood flow (supply), but also the functional and metabolic state of the cell (demand). The upper ischemic flow threshold is that flow at which neuronal function or electrical activity ceases. At this flow, neurons may become electrically silent, but they remain intact structurally. If CBF increases above this upper ischemic threshold, there is full recovery of all neuronal function. The lower ischemic threshold is that flow at which there is ATP depletion causing membrane and mitochondrial failure. This lower threshold is associated with cell death.[27,30]

The ischemic flow threshold for cessation of electrical activity depends on the metabolic demands of the cell. The lower the cerebral metabolic demand, the lower the CBF that can be tolerated before signs of ischemia (electrical silence) occur. Metabolic demands can be decreased by some anesthetics and by hypothermia. Therefore there is not an absolute value of CBF that is the ischemic flow threshold for electrical activity. The CBF at which signs of ischemia occur on the EEG (the upper ischemic flow threshold) has been measured in patients undergoing carotid endarterectomy. In awake humans, EEG signs of ischemia occur at a CBF of 25 $ml \cdot min^{-1} \cdot 100\ g^{-1}$. Under halothane-nitrous oxide anesthesia EEG signs of ischemia occur when the CBF decreases to 18 to 20 $ml \cdot min^{-1} \cdot 100\ g^{-1}$.[31] With enflurane-nitrous oxide or Innovar-nitrous oxide anesthesia, a slightly lower CBF (15 to 18 $ml \cdot min^{-1} \cdot 100\ g^{-1}$) occurs before there are signs of ischemia.[32] Under isoflurane-nitrous oxide anesthesia, the CBF at which signs of ischemia occur on the EEG is significantly lower than that with the other agents (8 to 10 $ml \cdot min^{-1} \cdot 100\ g^{-1}$).[33] It is believed that the extent to which each anesthetic decreases cerebral metabolic demand roughly correlates with the CBF that is tolerated before signs of ischemia occur. In primate studies of middle cerebral artery occlusion (MCA_o), it has been shown that the lower ischemic threshold for membrane failure is 6 to 8 $ml \cdot min^{-1} \cdot 100\ g^{-1}$.[29,34]

These ischemic blood flow thresholds have been correlated to neurologic outcome in animal studies.[35] When CBF decreased below 23 $ml \cdot min^{-1} \cdot 100\ g^{-1}$, reversible paralysis occurred. When CBF decreased below 8 to 9 $ml \cdot min^{-1} \cdot 100\ g^{-1}$, paralysis was permanent.

The differences in absolute blood flow between the two ischemic thresholds can be small such that any increase in CBF may improve neurologic outcome significantly or small decreases in CBF may cause irreversible death to what were potentially viable cells. In addition, the differences in vulnerability to ischemia among different types of neurons makes prevention or treatment of ischemia even more difficult. Ideally, the ischemic damage of the most sensitive cells must be prevented.

Selective Vulnerability

Neurologic recovery is not predictable after prolonged ischemia, and both ischemic injury and reperfusion injury may affect recovery. The concept of selective vulnerability applies to the *range* of responses by various regions of the brain that occur in response to the same ischemic insult. Regions especially vulnerable to ischemic damage include the limbic system, primarily the pyramidal cells of the CA_1 region of the hippocampus, Purkinje cells of the cerebellum, and small and medium-sized neurons of the striatum and layers 3, 5, and 6 of the cortex.[36] Damage to these selectively vulnerable neurons impairs cognition, motor function, coordination, recent memory, emotion, and drive. This explains the poor functional neurologic outcome of some survivors of cardiac arrest.[37] It is hypothesized that the selective vulnerability of neurons may be due to a combination of specific neuroanatomical connections, synaptic organization, membrane properties, anatomical patterns of neurotransmitters and receptors,[36] altered mitochondrial function, and disturbed signal transduction and protein synthesis,[38] which result in altered energy metabolism[39] in these vulnerable areas. There is a 24 to 72 hour delay between the ischemic insult and the occurence of irreversible cell damage, which allows a therapeutic window. Several drugs are under investigation to determine their ability to prevent damage to these areas if given during this window.

Secondary Consequences of Ischemia

Ischemic injury may occur as a result of the ischemia itself or during the period of reperfusion following ischemia (postischemic or reperfusion injury) (Fig. 5.3). The secondary consequences of ischemia are those that occur during this reperfusion period. These include extracellular events such as tissue edema, vasospasm, and red cell sludging, all of which can reduce blood flow, causing postischemic hypoperfusion. Intracellular secondary events also occur as a result of intracellular acidosis, the release of excitatory amino acid neurotransmitters; increased catecholamine release, increased metabolism, secondary depression of previously recovered metabolic activity, recovery of oxygen metabolism and high energy phosphates but prolonged depression of glucose metabolism, intracellular calcium overload initiating calcium-mediated processes, changes in normal chelation and compartmentalization of free metals, and altered oxygen metabolism leading to the production of free radicals, initiating free radical damage and lipid peroxidation.[36,39,40] These specific biochemical disturbances are believed to contribute to the ultimate neurologic damage following ischemia.[41]

If much of the tissue injury does not take place until the time of reperfusion, then the therapeutic implications could be profound. Drugs presently under investigation for their ability to block reperfusion injury include calcium entry blockers, excitatory amino acid neurotransmit-

Secondary Consequences of Ischemia

VASCULAR CHANGES

Vasospasm

Red cell sludging

Hypoperfusion

NEURONAL CHANGES

Intracellular acidosis

Release of excitatory amino acid neurotransmitters

Intracellular calcium overload

Calcium-mediated processes

Arachidonic acid cascade

Changes in chelation and compartmentalization of free metals

Altered oxygen metabolism

Production of free radicals

(Free radical damage)

Lipid peroxidation

Nitric oxide-mediated processes

Secondary depression of metabolism

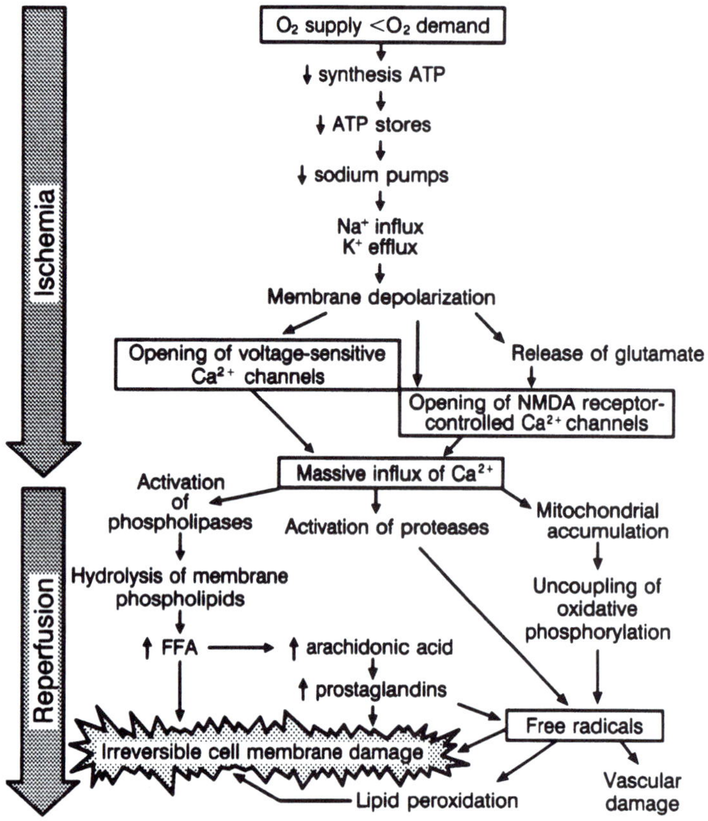

FIGURE 5.3 *Ischemic/reperfusion injury. Two components of tissue injury contribute to the ultimate neurologic damage. The ischemic component includes the processes of tissue damage occurring during ischemia. Cell death due to the ischemic component alone depends upon the severity and duration of ischemia. The secondary consequences of ischemia include the biochemical changes that take place at the time of reperfusion and reoxygenation following ischemia. The duration of these secondary processes and the extent to which they contribute to ultimate neurologic damage will determine the therapeutic window during which treatment administered after ischemia may be effective.*

ter antagonists, free radical scavengers, antagonists to the arachidonic acid cascade, and agents that block the lipid peroxidation of cellular and mitochondrial membranes. In general, the utility of postischemic therapy for the treatment of tissue injury resulting from ischemia will be related to the proportion of injury that is due to reperfusion versus the proportion due to the ischemia per se.[42]

PATHOPHYSIOLOGY OF ISCHEMIA

Vascular Changes

Two types of vascular changes after cerebral ischemia have been described in the literature: the no-reflow phenomenon[43] and delayed postischemic hypoperfusion.[36]

The no-reflow phenomenon was believed to be the combined result of an increase in viscosity of the stagnant blood,[44] compression of the microcirculation by swollen perivascular glial cells (due to K^+ fluxes),[45] formation of endothelial microvilli, and disseminated intravascular aggregation of blood particles. The occurrence and the extent of the no-reflow phenomenon was believed to depend on the type and duration of ischemia.[46] However, this complete absence of blood flow is not seen.

More commonly, a different pattern of blood flow is observed. When the circulation is restored after complete global ischemia, there is a 15 to 20-minute period of reactive hyperemia. This occurs because the viscosity of the blood washing through the microcirculation is decreased relative to that of the stagnant blood[36] that had pooled in the vascular beds and because vascular tone is temporarily reduced by vasoactive substances released during ischemia. An increased metabolic rate to restore energy stores and ionic gradients occurs at this time and may also cause the increased blood flow. The postischemic hyperemia is heterogeneous, with areas of little flow and areas of markedly increased flow.[47] Postischemic hypoperfusion develops after this period of reactive hyperemia. The severity and duration of the postischemic hypoperfusion depends upon the severity and duration of the ischemic insult. It has been reported to last from 6 to more than 24 hours in animals and humans.[48] There is some evidence that this postischemic hypoperfusion period contributes to the ultimate neurologic damage and that postischemic hypoperfusion in areas of increased functional (and metabolic) activity contributes to the selective vulnerability of neurons in that area.[49–51]

It is hypothesized that this postischemic hypoperfusion is due in part to vasoconstriction caused by calcium ion activation of the contractile mechanisms in endothelial cells. An increase in intracellular calcium in vascular smooth muscle cells occurring during ischemia activates myosin light-chain kinase, which in turn catalyzes the phosphorylation of myosin. This increases the actin-myosin interaction, resulting in contraction.[52] Increased production of thromboxane A_2, a potent vasoconstrictor, made from arachidonic acid during reperfusion may also contribute to the hypoperfusion. This hypoperfusion cannot be influenced by sympathomimetic vasoconstrictors or sympatholytic, direct-acting, or ganglion-blocking vasodilators but can be ameliorated by some calcium entry blockers and inhibitors of prostaglandin synthesis.

Recent investigation has reported that a multitude of microvascular changes occur during ischemia and the subsequent reperfusion period.[53,54] These include activation of intracellular processes: polymorphonuclear (PMN) leukocyte activation, the elaboration of cytokines, endothelial cell responses, prostaglandin synthesis, platelet activation, coagulation system activation, microvascular reactivity, and peri-

Microvascular Changes During Ischemia and Reperfusion

INTRACELLULAR PROCESSES

Polymorphonuclear leukocyte activation

Elaboration of cytokines

Endothelial cell responses

Prostaglandin synthesis

Platelet activation

- Coagulation system activation
- Microvascular reactivity
- Perivascular astrocyte, neuron, and pericyte signaling

EXTRINSIC MECHANICAL COMPRESSION

Astrocyte foot process swelling

Perivascular cell swelling

Perivascular hemorrhage

Endothelial cell swelling

Red cell aggregation

Platelet aggregation

Polymorphonuclear leukocyte adhesion

Thrombosis

vascular astrocyte, neuron, and pericyte signaling. Extrinsic mechanical compression of the microvasculature can affect postischemic hypoperfusion. Extrinsic compression of the vasculature may be caused by swelling of astrocyte foot processes, causing perivascular edema; perivascular cell swelling caused by increased permeability due to widening of the interendothelial tight junctions; and perivascular hemorrhage. Obstruction within the microvasculature can be caused by endothelial cell swelling, red cell aggregation, platelet aggregation, PMN adhesion to endothelial cells, and thrombosis.

Membrane Changes

During complete cerebral ischemia, the high-energy phosphate stores of phosphocreatine are depleted within 1 minute, glucose and glycogen stores within 4 minutes, and ATP stores within 5 to 7 minutes.[3] This exhaustion of energy stores results in failure of the membrane sodium pumps, allowing influx of Na^+ and Cl^-, efflux of K^+, and membrane depolarization.[3,24] The influx of Na^+ and Cl^- ions is accompanied by water, which can produce cell swelling and death. When the extracellular K^+ concentration increases, changes in the plasma membrane potential open voltage-dependent Ca^{2+} channels and the increased extracellular concentrations of glutamate occurring in response to ischemia open receptor-controlled channels. This results in a massive intracellular influx of Ca^{2+}.[3,24,55] This failure of membranes to maintain normal ion gradients characterizes irreversible cell damage and death.

In focal ischemia membrane failure may be prevented by maintaining blood flow to the ischemic area above the ischemic flow threshold for membrane failure. In complete global ischemia, however, the development of membrane failure can only be delayed by blocking Na^+ or K^+ leakage across membranes or by enhancing anaerobic ATP production. Hypothermia can block the influx of Na^+ or efflux of K^+ across cell membranes.[56] In the normal brain, this is manifested by a decrease in oxygen consumption, whereas in the ischemic brain, this is manifested by a delay in the development of irreversible cell damage.

Mitochondrial Changes

Mitochondrial dysfunction also characterizes irreversible cell injury. The primary factors believed to cause mitochondrial damage during ischemia include intracellular lactic acidosis, Ca^{2+} activated degradative enzymes, mitochondrial Ca^{2+} overload, and free radical-induced membrane lipid peroxidation. Intracellular acidosis attenuates both mitochondrial oxidative phosphorylation and Ca^{2+} sequestration by the mitochondria.[57,58] The energy used for mitochondria sequestration of calcium prevents the synthesis of ATP. The remaining free Ca^{2+} is then buffered poorly by the calcium-binding proteins. The excess free intracellular calcium activates degradative enzymes, including phospholipases and proteases that destroy phospholipids and proteins within cell and mitochondrial membranes.

Glucose

During ischemia the cell must rely on both its dwindling store of ATP and glycolysis to produce ATP for energy. Rapid utilization of ATP for the active transport of ions depletes the ATP store within a few minutes. In order to continue glycolysis, pyruvate is converted to lactate to replenish the supply of NAD^+ (Fig. 5.2). The glycolytic conversion of glucose to lactate continues in an inefficient attempt to produce ATP necessary for cellular function until there is no further supply of glucose to the cell.

It is this production of lactate that underlies the most commonly proposed mechanism by which hyperglycemia aggravates ischemic cerebral injury. Intracellular lactic acid concentration is a function of several factors, including oxygen supply,[59] the glucose concentration in blood and brain,[60,61] and the rate of lactate efflux out of the cells.[62] Cerebral intracellular lactate concentration is therefore proportional to the cellular store of glucose at the time of ischemia during complete cerebral ischemia or to the cellular store plus the continued supply of glucose during incomplete cerebral ischemia. Because the supply of glucose could be greater during incomplete ischemia than during complete ischemia, intracellular concentrations of lactate can increase more during incomplete ischemia and the resultant cell damage may be greater.[26,60,63–66] Intracellular lactate concentrations exceeding 20 μmol/g are associated with irreversible cell damage.[26,61,67] Intracellular pH remains stable until intracellular lactate concentration reaches 17 μmol/g at which point the pH decreases as lactate concentration increases.[68,69] The decrease in intracellular pH may be responsible for the increased ischemic damage associated with high lactate levels[70,71] The molecular basis by which the increased intracellular acid produces irreversible cell damage is unknown. It has been suggested that the acid medium causes reduction of ferric to ferrous iron, and its subsequent release from organic stores may catalyze the generation of free radicals, which destroy cell membranes.[72]

As commonly as the mechanism of hyperglycemia-enhanced ischemic injury is proposed to be due to a rise in lactate production and concomitant tissue acidosis,[73,74] it remains controversial whether acidosis even plays a role in the hyperglycemic enhancement of ischemic brain damage because it has been reported that chronic hyperglycemia actually improves recovery of intracellular pH following ischemia.[75] An alternate theory suggests that hyperglycemia enhances ischemic injury by attenuating an increase in adenosine.[76,77] Adenosine, a purine nucleotide, blocks some of the secondary effects of ischemia through cerebral vasodilation, inhibition of the release of excitatory amino acid neurotransmitters,[78] and modulation of the production of free radicals.[79–81] It has also been suggested that hyperglycemia may aggravate ischemic brain injury by increasing the excitatory neurotransmitters released during ischemia. Although increased glucose does not directly increase glutamate concentration, it does increase the extracellular concentration of glycine, a neurotransmitter that binds on the *N*-methyl-D-aspartate (NMDA) receptor to amplify the receptor's activation by glutamate.[80]

Mechanisms of Hyperglycemia-Enhanced Ischemic Injury

- Tissue acidosis
- Attenuation of adenosine concentration
- Increase in excitatory neurotransmitter release
- Reduction in cerebral blood flow

A third alternative theory suggests that hyperglycemia significantly worsens the degree of acute BBB disruption that occurs during ischemia.[81] Fourthly, Hyperglycemia is associated with a significantly reduced CBF and increased heterogeneity of regional cerebral blood flow (rCBF) during the postischemic period.[59,82–84] This heterogeneity associated with hyperglycemia is unlike the more regionally uniform alteration of flow caused by ischemia alone.[82] It can be concluded that preischemic blood glucose concentration, to the extent that it reflects intracellular glucose, lactate concentration, and pH and to the extent that it decreases adenosine concentration, increases excitatory amino acid neurotransmitters, or worsens rCBF, can significantly influence neurologic outcome following cerebral ischemia.

Detrimental effects of increased blood glucose vary with the type of cerebral ischemia and the presence of diabetes mellitus.[85] Animal studies of the effect of blood glucose concentration during complete cerebral ischemia report that hyperglycemia or the use of glucose-containing solutions is associated with a significantly greater neurologic or histopathologic injury and increased death rate even when the preischemic blood glucose levels are only moderately increased or are similar to control levels.[74,86–89] Treatment with insulin even after the ischemic insult has been shown to attenuate this neurologic injury and death rate.[89,90]

Clinical studies correlating blood glucose and neurologic outcome after complete cerebral ischemia have been retrospective.[91,92] In patients resuscitated from cardiac arrest, awakening from coma without neurologic deficits was associated with a lower blood glucose (262 ± 7 mg/100 ml) than in those remaining comatose (341 ± 13 mg/100 ml). The authors concluded that a high blood glucose level is an independent risk factor for increased neurologic injury after cardiac arrest and recommended that glucose infusions be avoided during and immediately after resuscitation from cardiac arrest unless a low blood glucose level could be documented.[91] This recommendation has now been expanded to include all patients with altered mental status presenting to the emergency room.[93]

There is less consensus of opinion regarding the effect of hyperglycemia during focal cerebral ischemia, although the majority of studies cite an association between increased blood glucose and worsening neurologic outcome.[94–102] The only human study of the effect of blood glucose concentration on neurologic outcome in focal ischemia was a retrospective study of patients suffering from stroke.[95] Diabetic patients with a mean blood glucose level of 259 ± 125 mg/100 ml had significantly worse neurologic outcome and higher death rates than did nondiabetic patients (blood glucose 106 ± 19 mg/100 ml). A separate group of nondiabetic patients were analyzed prospectively. Nondiabetic patients with blood glucose levels greater than 120 mg/100 ml had significantly worse neurologic outcome than patients with blood glucose levels less than 120 mg/100 ml.[95]

From these observations, it has been concluded that high blood glucose levels before and/or during an ischemic event in patients at risk for cerebral ischemia may be deleterious and actually worsen neurologic function.[102] Such patients include those resuscitated from cardiac arrest, those suffering from severe dysrhythmias or shock, those undergoing cardiac or cerebrovascular surgery, those with vascular disease, or those with evolving strokes. It is recommended that blood glucose levels be routinely monitored in these patients and that solutions containing glucose not be used unless there is a risk of hypoglycemia. The physiologic stress of anesthesia and surgery or the stress of stroke or cardiac arrest will increase blood glucose levels, and exogenously administered glucocorticoids will increase blood glucose. It remains to be studied whether aggressive therapy to normalize blood glucose levels before a potentially ischemic event (i.e., cardiopulmonary bypass or temporary clamping of a major cerebral artery during surgery) will improve neurologic recovery. Clearly, additional studies need to be done to delineate the effects and timing of insulin treatment on blood glucose, intracellular glucose, lactate, and pH, infarct size, and ultimate neurologic outcome in situations of focal ischemia or cardiac arrest. However, even without these studies, it has become common practice to treat with insulin blood glucose levels greater than 150 mg/dl.

Calcium

During ischemia, Ca^{2+} enters the cells through voltage-dependent channels, through agonist receptor-controlled channels, and when a reversal of the Na^{+}-Ca^{2+} exchange pump occurs (Fig. 5.1). Calcium ions then accumulate in the cytosol because both outward transport and mitochondrial sequestration of calcium require energy. This intracellular Ca^{2+} overload appears to be one of the pathways leading to irreversible cell damage and death[103] (Figs. 5.4 and 5.5). Calcium influx activates destructive proteases that destroy cell membranes, resulting in receptor dysfunction and the failure of intracellular transport mechanisms.[5] Proteolysis cleaves the cytoskeleton, which prevents intracellular communication via axoplasmic transport, and destroys proteins that normally anchor the plasma membrane to the cytoskeleton, resulting in "blebbing" of the plasma membrane.[5]

Increased intracellular Ca^{2+} also activates phospholipases A_1, A_2, and C, which hydrolyze phospholipids within mitochondrial and cell membranes, to physically disrupt these membranes, altering their permeability and function. These enzymes do not require oxygen or energy and so may continue to function during or after

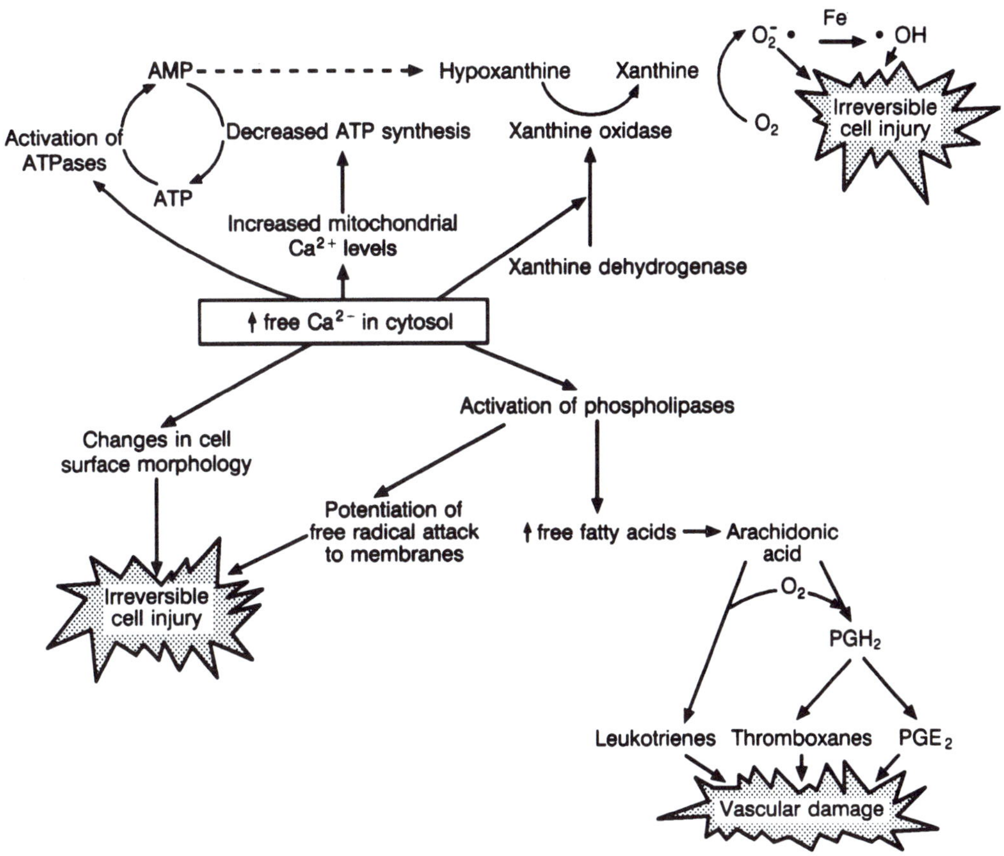

FIGURE 5.4 *Relationship between energy supply, cellular calcium regulation, the arachidonic acid cascade, the formation of prostaglandins, and the formation of free radicals. During ischemia, cellular stores of ATP are metabolized to AMP and ultimately to hypoxanthine. Increased cellular concentrations of Ca^{2+} activate proteases converting xanthine dehydrogenase to xanthine oxidase which catalyzes the metabolism of hypoxanthine to xanthine with superoxide radicals (•O_2) as a byproduct. Increased intracellular [Ca^{2+}] also activates phospholipases to release FFAs from cell membranes. During the reperfusion period with the presence of oxygen, primary FFA, arachidonic acid, is metabolized to prostaglandins and leukotrienes. Free radicals and prostaglandins are responsible for cell injury following ischemia.*

ischemia. Hydrolysis of the membrane phospholipids releases FFAs that have detergent properties that can destroy the lipid portions of cellular and mitochondrial membranes. The major FFA is arachidonic acid, which can be metabolized to free radicals, prostaglandins, and leukotrienes,[24,104] which can produce further changes in membrane permeability and ion distribution.[24,105] The normal mechanisms for control of intracellular Ca^{2+} concentration include the cell membrane ATP-dependent Ca^{2+} translocase, the cell membrane Ca^{2+}-Na^+ exchange pump, the ATP-dependent Ca^{2+} uptake into the endoplasmic reticulum, and the sequestration of Ca^{2+}

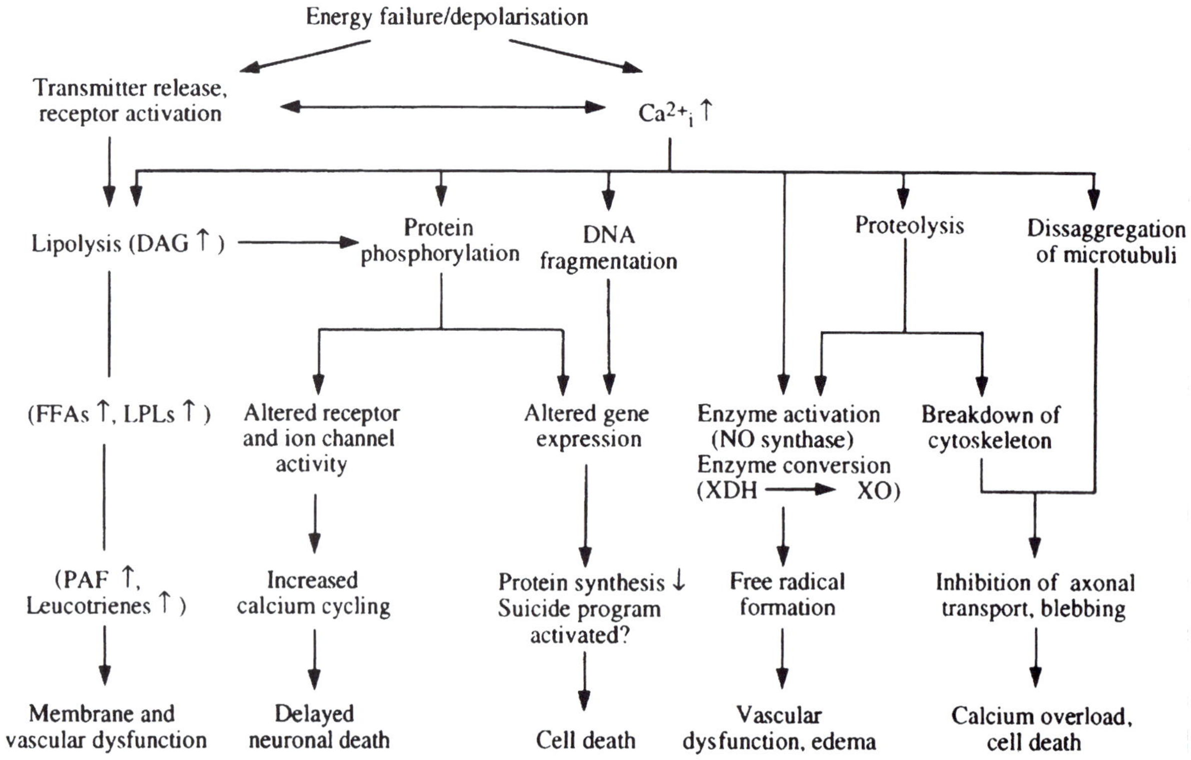

FIGURE 5.5 *Overview of calcium-triggered reactions that may lead to irreversible cell damage and death. (From Siesjö et al.,[103] with permission.)*

into the mitochondria at the expense of oxidative phosphorylation.[3] All require energy and will consume any ATP stores or prevent further ATP synthesis.

Following ischemia, protein synthesis recovers slowly. The increase in intracellular Ca^{2+} occurring during ischemia triggers the transcription of new genes (c-*fos*, c-*jun*) that promote the production of growth factors and heat shock and stress proteins.[5,106] The greatest level of protein production occurs in cells that have suffered ischemic damage but are salvageable.[106]

Prostaglandins

Prostaglandins are products of the interaction between molecular oxygen and FFAs. Phospholipids in cell membranes can be converted by hydrolysis to FFAs by phospholipase A_2, which is activated by a surface stimulus or by the influx of Ca^{2+} into the cell, which occurs during ischemia. FFAs are normally converted to acyl-CoA by an ATP-dependent lipase and then enter into the tricarboxylic acid cycle. However, during ischemia, this metabolism cannot take place because of the depletion of ATP so that the concentration of FFAs increases. High concentrations of FFAs may be deleterious to mitochondrial function because they uncouple oxidative phosphorylation, cause efflux into the cytosol of K^+ and Ca^{2+} stored within the mitochondria, and increase prostaglandin synthesis.

The most common FFA is arachidonic acid, the precursor of the prostaglandins. The concentration of arachidonic acid in normal tissues is negligible. An increase in arachidonic acid concentration can be stimulated by a variety of conditions including ischemia, trauma, hypoxia, severe hypoglycemia, pyrogen fever, convulsions, and tissue dissection.[107]

During ischemia, arachidonic acid accumulates and can then serve as a substrate during the early recirculation and reoxygenation phase for the production of prostaglandins via the prostaglandin endoperoxides (Fig. 5.6). When reperfusion and reoxygenation occur after ischemia, arachidonic acid is converted by cyclooxygenase to endoperoxides, which are short-lived intermediates and the precursors of prostacyclin made in vascular endothelial cells and thromboxane A_2 synthesized in platelets. Arachidonic acid is also converted by lipoxygenase in leukocytes to leukotrienes, which are the slow reactive substances of anaphylaxis and by lipoxygenase in platelets to hydroperoxy acids and peroxy acids.[108] It is hypothesized that during and immediately following ischemia, the endoperoxides inactivate prostacyclin synthetase in the wall of the ischemic cerebral vessels so that relatively less prostacyclin, a potent vasodilator, is made.[109] Thromboxane synthetase is less affected by the endoperoxides because only a small fraction of total platelet content is in the brain during ischemia. The reduced synthesis of prostacyclin can result in increased synthesis of thromboxane A_2,[110–112] a potent vasoconstrictor that may contribute to postischemic hypoperfusion.

Arachidonic acid, the endoperoxides, and thromboxane A_2 are potent platelet aggregators that can contribute to hypoperfusion. The endoperoxides are also potential free radicals, and an increase in their production may elicit a cascade of harmful reactions, including cross-linking reactions of membrane phospholipids and proteins and peroxidation of the polyunsaturated fatty acids in cell membranes. These reactions have the potential to irreversibly change cell structure such that cell and mitochondrial membrane function is adversely affected.[113]

It has been hypothesized that inhibitors of arachidonic acid metabolism might, with the production of these vasoconstrictors, attenuate postischemic hypoperfusion, thereby ameliorating neuronal damage following ischemia. The production of prostaglandins can be blocked by the cyclo-oxygenase inhibitors, indomethacin or ibuprofen, if given prior to the ischemic event such that hypoperfusion is prevented.[114–119] Postischemic treatment by indomethacin has no effect on hypoperfusion or neurologic outcome.[115,116] It has been assumed that pretreat-

FIGURE 5.6 *Role of arachidonic acid in the production of leukotrienes, endoperoxides, hydroperoxy acids, and prostaglandins with reperfusion and reoxygenation following ischemia.*

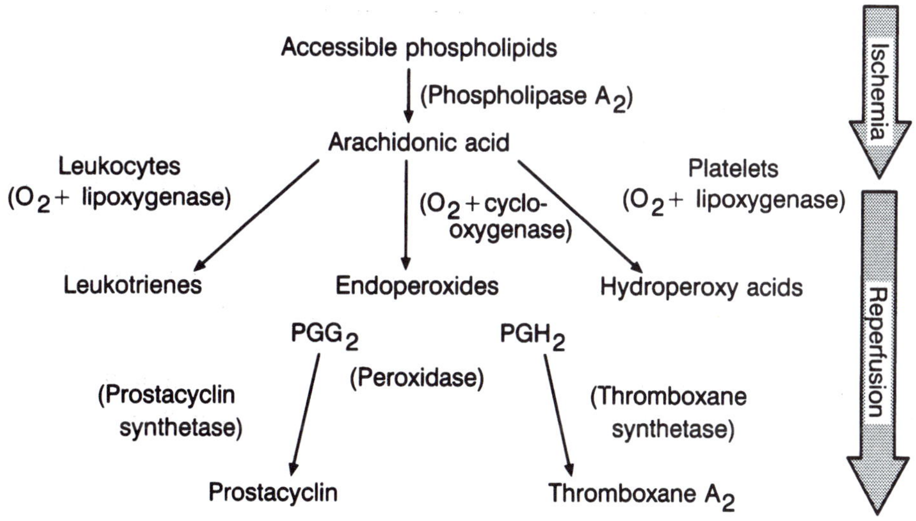

ment with cyclo-oxygenase inhibitors attenuates the postischemia hypoperfusion by inhibiting thromboxane A_2 synthesis more than prostacyclin synthesis, allowing increased production of prostacyclin. If postischemic hypoperfusion were the result of the imbalance between prostacyclin and thromboxane A_2 in favor of thromboxane A_2, then specifically inhibiting the synthesis of thromboxane A_2 might attenuate the postischemic hypoperfusion. However, a specific inhibitor of thromboxane A_2 synthetase failed to attenuate postischemic hypoperfusion.[119]

The above-cited studies indicate that treatment with inhibitors of prostaglandin synthesis before ischemia can affect the postischemic CBF. If this hypoperfusion does contribute to the ultimate neurologic damage suffered after ischemia, then further studies should be done to determine whether inhibitors of specific prostaglandin pathways can influence neurologic outcome.

Free Radicals

Most molecules have chemical bonds consisting of paired electrons. The two electrons spin in opposite directions, thereby canceling each other's magnetic field, resulting in a low energy state. Free radical molecules with an odd number of electrons are formed by a break in a covalent bond. The bond splits symmetrically, and both fragments retain a single electron. This unpaired electron has a magnetic field that produces a high energy state, making the molecule highly reactive and unstable, resulting in a very short half-life. Because of this, free radicals exist only in very low concentration and do not travel far from their site of formation. Such molecules react with adjacent nonradical molecules to produce a stable molecule and a new free radical. This starts a chain reaction of free radical generation until it is terminated by the random collision of two free radicals to form a molecule with a stable bond or by a reaction with a free radical scavenger, an antioxidant enzyme, that forms a stable molecule.

Free radicals are normally generated in small amounts during oxidative phosphorylation in which production of ATP is linked to the reduction of molecular oxygen to water.[120] Under normal conditions, four electrons are gained at once to reduce O_2 to H_2O. However, leaks in the mitochondrial electron transport system allow the acceptance of single electrons. If the four electrons are acquired singly, a series of free radical intermediates are formed (superoxide, $^{\bullet}O_2$; hydrogen peroxide, H_2O_2, and the hydroxyl radical, $^{\bullet}OH$).[120] These free radicals usually remain tightly bound within the mitochondrial membrane so that they can donate electrons further down the mitochondrial electron transport system, and normally they present no threat to the cell. Any small leak of free radicals that does occur is controlled by scavenging mechanisms. Free radicals can also be produced during the synthesis of prostaglandins, by auto-oxidation of small molecules including the catecholamines, and by the microsomal cytochrome *P*-450 reductase system.[121]

Superoxide is the first free radical formed by the addition of a single electron to molecular oxygen. Under normal conditions, superoxide radicals will dismutate spontaneously to hydrogen peroxide.[122] Hydrogen peroxide is a weak oxidizing agent and can react catalytically with transitional metals (iron and copper) to form the hydroxyl radical in a reaction known as the Fenton reaction.[123] Hydroxyl radicals are the most reactive of the free radicals and will react with almost any intracellular molecule: carbohydrates, lipids, proteins, or nucleic acid bases. Membrane polyunsaturated fatty acids are particularly susceptible to hydroxyl radical attack forming lipid radicals. This is the initial step in the chain reaction of lipid peroxidation.[124] Lipid radicals react with oxygen to form lipid hydroperoxides and other products (alkanes, alkenes, hydroxy and epoxy derivatives, ketones, and polyhydroperoxides). Most of these radical products are toxic to cells even in small quantities.

The brain may be especially vulnerable to free radical damage because of several biochemical, physiologic, and anatomic reasons.[125] These include high rate of oxidative metabolism; high concentration of substrate, membrane lipid polyunsaturated fatty acids; low concentration of antioxidant enzymes; endogenous generation of free radicals; specialized neuronal conduction and synaptic transmission; large membrane surface area to cellular volume; neural anatomic network vulnerable to disruption; and the inability of neurons to regenerate.

During ischemia, several events take place that augment the formation of free radicals (Fig. 5.4). Sources of free radicals include the enzyme xanthine oxidase, arachidonic acid metabolism, catecholamine oxidation, NO synthesis, amine oxidase activity, mitochondrial leakage, and activated white blood cells.[126,127] Ischemia stops the production of ATP, and the existing stores of ATP are rapidly metabolized for energy. With depletion of the cell's energy stores, transmembrane ion gradients cannot be maintained. This allows a massive influx of calcium. The metabolism of ATP also increases the cellular concentrations of AMP. AMP is metabolized to adenosine and inosine intermediates and then to hypoxanthine. The elevated cytosolic calcium concentration activates the protease calpain, which converts xanthine dehydrogenase to xanthine oxidase. In addition, sulfhydryl oxidation in ischemic tissues can convert xanthine dehydrogenase to xanthine oxidase. Xanthine oxidase converts the hypoxanthine that has accumulated in the cells during ischemia to xanthine, reducing O_2 to the superoxide radical as a byproduct. This appears to be the major source of superoxide radicals in postischemic tissues.

The formation of superoxide radicals is also increased during the reperfusion period following ischemia because of the abundance of reducing equivalents, such as nicotinamide adenine dinucleotide phosphate (NADPH), which is produced in excess during ischemia; the action of xanthine oxidase; and the availability of molecular oxygen.[128] Intracellular levels of free iron may increase during ischemia due to Ca^{2+}-mediated mitochondrial injury releasing stores of mitochondrial iron and due to the release of free iron from iron storage proteins, transferrin, and ferritin.[129] This increased free iron concentration catalyzes the conversion of the superoxide radicals to the more highly reactive and toxic hydroxyl radicals.[130,131] With reperfusion, free radicals can also be generated as by-products of the oxidation of arachidonic acid to prostaglandins and leukotrienes.

It is hypothesized that cellular damage that occurs following ischemia may be due in part to biochemical alterations produced by superoxide and hydroxyl radicals.[129] Neuronal membranes, rich in polyunsaturated fatty acids, are especially susceptible to attack by free radicals at carbon-carbon double bonds. Peroxidation of the polyunsaturated fatty acids in the membranes severely damages them. Potential consequences of damage to membranes include changes in fluidity and permeability and in the orientation of proteins embedded within the membranes, altering their function.[132,133] The end products of lipid peroxidation are aldehydes, hydrocarbon gases, and other residue that can cause cytotoxic and vasogenic cell edema, alter vascular endothelial and BBB permeability and produce inflammation, and chemotaxis.[134,135] Free radicals can cause point mutations, DNA cross-linkage, and DNA strand breaks in mitochondrial genes. This impairs mitochondrial respiration.[7] Superoxide radicals themselves can elicit an inflammatory response with a resultant influx of neutrophils, which will respond by secreting oxygen radicals of their own and by forming vascular plugs, thereby increasing cellular edema.[124]

The normal defense systems against free radical damage include the spatial separation of radical-generating reactions and target molecules, enzymatic systems that quench free radicals, and antioxidative enzymes that scavenge free radicals.[136] Free radical scavengers include the superoxide dismutases directed against superoxide; catalase and glutathione peroxidase directed against H_2O_2, and vitamin C, vitamin E, and ceruloplasmin directed against those radicals in lipid and aqueous phases. Uric acid can scavenge hydroxyl radicals and bind transitional metals to prevent hydroxyl radical formation. Transferrin can bind free iron, and plasma ceruloplasmin can convert free iron to ferric iron. It is the free iron that catalyzes the Fenton reaction to form hydroxyl radicals. Superoxide dismutases catalyze the conversion of two superoxide radicals to hydrogen peroxide and water. Catalase converts hydrogen peroxide into O_2 and H_2O, whereas glutathione peroxidase uses hydrogen peroxide to oxidize glutathione. The brain contains only small concentrations of the free radical scavengers: superoxide dismutase, catalase, glutathione peroxidase, and vitamin E. Therefore, during reperfusion following ischemia, superoxide dismutase and catalase, capable of destroying the superoxide radicals formed during normal aerobic metabolism, are overwhelmed. This results in an increased concentration of superoxide radicals, some of which are converted to hydroxyl radicals by iron-catalyzed reactions.[137]

Therapy designed to prevent ischemic damage by free radicals includes anoxic reperfusion to deliver free radical scavengers before reoxygenation, reduction in circulating leukocyte concentration, administration of specific free radical scavengers such as superoxide dismutase or catalase or the nonspecific scavenger vitamin E to scavenge free radicals and block the chain reaction formation of more free radicals, the binding of free iron by iron chelators such as desferoxamine to prevent the formation of hydroxyl radicals and the subsequent cell damage initiated by them, and inhibition of xanthine oxidase by allopurinol to block the formation of xanthine and the subsequent formation of superoxide radicals.[127,137–141] The efficacy of the administration of protective enzymes or free radical scavengers in ameliorating neurologic injury following cerebral ischemia is the subject of ongoing investigation. The beneficial effect, if any, of such use of scavenging agents will depend on the possibility of mediation of the pathology produced by free radicals, the biologic compatibility of the scavenging agents, the dosage used, and the ability to deliver the scavenger to the cellular site where the free radicals are causing injury.

Lipid Peroxidation

Lipid peroxidation, which is the destruction of phospholipids within cell and mitochondrial membranes, thereby destroying their structure and function, is believed to be a major cause of postischemic cell damage and death.[140,142] It is the end mechanism in the calcium cascade and arachidonic acid cascade and results from the peroxidative attack of membrane fatty acids by free radicals. Lipid peroxidation can be inhibited by steroids such as high-dose methylprednisolone and tirilazed mesylate, a 21-amino steroid (lazaroid) that lacks glucocorticoid activity. The lazaroids are potent inhibitors of oxygen free-radical-induced, iron-catalyzed lipid peroxidation. In animal studies, these agents have been reported to attenuate postischemic hypoperfusion, reduce postischemic brain edema and metabolic dysfunction, and improve survival.[126,127,138,139,143–145]

Excitatory Amino Acid Neurotransmitters

The dicarboxylic amino acids, glutamate and aspartate, are excitatory neurotransmitters in many brain regions.[146,147] Glutamate is normally stored in vesicles in presynaptic terminals of neurons and released when the cell is depolarized. Glutamate then acts at receptors on the postsynaptic neuron.[148,149] Normally the *extracellular* concentration of glutamate increases only very briefly during synaptic transmission because of cellular reuptake.[150,151] However, during cerebral ischemia, there is increased synaptic release and impaired cellular reuptake of glutamate,[152] resulting in large increases in extracellular glutamate.[148,153] This increased extracellular concentration of glutamate then becomes neurotoxic and forms the basis for the excitotoxic theory of ischemia.[154–156] There are presently known four postsynaptic receptors for the excitatory neurotransmitters, the NMDA receptor, the quisqualate (α-amino-3-hydroxy-5-methyl-4-isoxazole, AMPA) receptor, the kainate receptor[157] (all of which are inotropic receptors located in cell membranes), and the metabotropic receptor in mitochondrial membranes, which is coupled to phospholipase C.[5] There are high concentrations of NMDA receptor in those brain regions that show selective vulnerability to ischemia, layers 3,5, and 6 of the cerebral cortex, the thalamus, the striatum, the Purkinje and granule cell layers of the cerebellum, and the CA_1 region of the hippocampus. AMPA receptors occur in deep layers of cerebral cortex, the thalamus, the striatum, the molecular layer of the cerebellum, and in the pyramidal cell layer and striatum lucidum of the hippocampus. Kainate receptors have been found only in the striatum lucidum of the hippocampus. Glutamate acts on all four receptors, whereas aspartate acts only on the NMDA receptor. All three cell membrane receptors are linked to membrane cation channels. The kainate and AMPA receptors are linked to membrane channels that allow the influx of Na^+,[147] and the NMDA receptor is linked to membrane channels that allow the influx of Na^+ and Ca^{2+}.

THE NMDA RECEPTOR-ION CHANNEL COMPLEX The NMDA receptor is coupled to a membrane channel permeable to either Na^+ or Ca^{2+} that can be blocked by magnesium (Mg^{2+}) attached within the ion channel[158] (Fig. 5.7). It is theorized that Mg^{2+} ions retain water, and in this bulky state block the NMDA channel.[157] The blockade of the NMDA receptor by Mg^{2+} is voltage dependent. Zinc (Zn^+) can act as an antagonist of Mg^{2+} by attaching to the Mg^{2+} binding sites within the ion channel. Both chemical and electric signals affect the activity of the NMDA receptor-channel complex. Glutamate and aspartate excite the NMDA receptor. Glycine, usually an inhibitory transmitter, binds at a different site on the NMDA receptor to allow activation by glutamate. If glycine is not present, normal concentrations of glutamate cannot

FIGURE 5.7 *Speculative schematic diagram of the NMDA receptor-controlled ion channel complex. Glutamate binding is facilitated by glycine and antagonized by competitive antagonists. Magnesium (Mg^{2+}), zinc (Zn^{2+}), and noncompetitive antagonists block the ion channel at specific binding sites.*

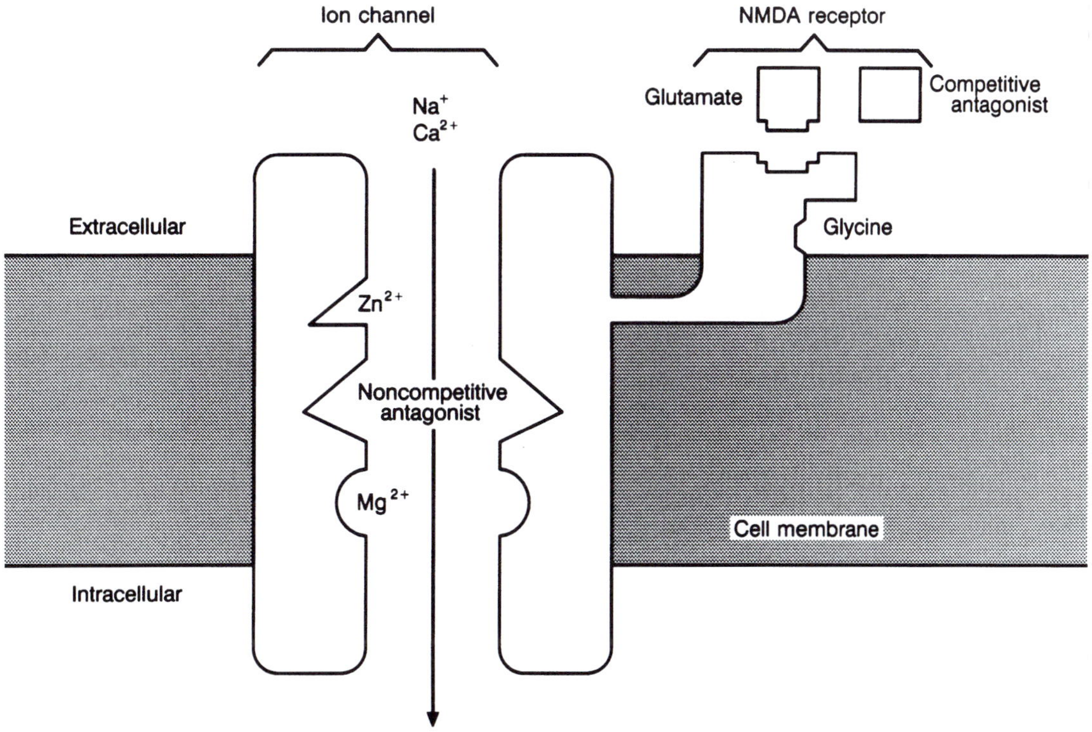

open the NMDA receptor-controlled ion channels, although greater than normal concentrations can. Depolarization of the neuron also regulates the NMDA receptor and its ion channel activity. At the normal resting membrane potential, the NMDA ion channel is closed so that glutamate binding to the receptor will induce little ion flux. Depolarization excites the NMDA receptor and dislodges the Mg^{2+} ions that block the NMDA channel when the cell is at rest. Activation of the NMDA receptor by glutamate then takes place to open the ion channel, allowing influx of Na^{+} and/or Ca^{2+} into the neuron.

Under certain pathologic conditions, including ischemia, glutamate can become a neurotoxin to produce both immediate injury and delayed neuronal death. Immediate neuronal injury occurs following severe ischemia and is due to acute cell swelling. Increased concentrations of extracellular glutamate released during ischemia activate the NMDA receptor to open the membrane ion channels allowing an influx of Na^{+}, a secondary passive influx of Cl^{-} and with it, water, to produce cell swelling.[159–162] The cell swelling will eventually cause lysis of the cell membrane and death.[162]

There is also a more slowly evolving neuronal degeneration in which neuronal injury following ischemia may not be apparent for up to 24 hours. Although Ca^{2+} can enter the cell through several routes—voltage-sensitive channels activated by membrane depolarization, nonspecific leak conductance associated with cell swelling, and reverse operation of the Na^{+}-Ca^{2+} exchange mechanism—the membrane channels controlled by NMDA receptors appear to be important for glutamate-related injury, which may involve the selectively vulnerable regions of the brain.[163] The prolonged depolarizing action of excess glutamate maintains the NMDA receptor-controlled channel in an open state, allowing an increased influx of Ca^{2+}. It is theorized that the resultant increase in intracellular Ca^{2+} starts a cascade of reactions ultimately responsible for neuronal degeneration (Fig. 5.5). Calcium entry into neuronal postsynaptic terminals can also increase the release of glutamate, thereby further propagating injury via a positive feedback loop. This late propagation, in conjunction with the intrinsically delayed nature of the calcium-dependent glutamate injury, may account for the fact that ischemic neurologic injury can require 24 to 72 hours to develop fully.[164–166]

Early observations on the excitotoxic theory of ischemia-induced neuronal damage centered around the NMDA receptor because its ion channel is highly permeable to Ca^{2+}. Glutamate via its activation of the NMDA receptor has been implicated as a mediator of neuronal damage during ischemia by the following information:

1. The distribution of excitatory neurotransmitter receptors occurs primarily in those areas of the brain that are considered to be selectively vulnerable to ischemia.[167]
2. Ischemia is associated with an increased concentration of glutamate in the extracellular space within a few minutes after cessation of blood flow.[168]

Evidence for the Mediation of Neuronal Injury by Glutamate

High concentration of glutamate receptors occurs in areas of brain selectively vulnerable to ischemia

Increased concentrations of glutamate occur during ischemia

Increased neuronal firing occurs following ischemia

Interruption of glutaminergic nerve tracts to areas of high concentration of glutamate receptors decreases ischemic injury

High concentrations of Mg^{2+} that block NMDA receptor-controlled ion channels decreases ischemic injury

Pharmacologic blockade of NMDA receptor-controlled ion channels decreases ischemic injury

Toxic intracellular calcium accumulation occurs in areas of brain selectively vulnerable to ischemia

3. There is increased neuronal firing in the hippocampus produced by excitatory amino acids for up to 24 hours following ischemia.[169]
4. The interruption of glutaminergic nerve tracts to areas of high concentration of glutamate receptors has been reported to protect against ischemic injury.[170]
5. High concentrations of Mg^{2+}, which block synaptic transmission in general and NMDA receptor-controlled ion channels specifically, decrease ischemic neuronal injury.[171,172]
6. Pharmacologic blockade of postsynaptic NMDA receptors attenuates ischemic neurologic injury.[160]
7. In the first few minutes of reperfusion, Ca^{2+} accumulates in neurons in a nonselective pattern presumably due to entry through the voltage-dependent channels and impaired outward pumping of calcium, with even a reversal of the Na^+-Ca^{2+} exchange pump.

When energy metabolism is restored, the less vulnerable neurons rapidly return to normal appearance whereas the neurons in the regions vulnerable to ischemia continue accumulation of Ca^{2+}, leading to neuronal damage. This is hypothesized to be a consequence of burst firing brought about through the activation of NMDA receptors and Ca^{2+} influx through the NMDA receptor-controlled channels.[172]

There are several types of antagonists to the NMDA receptor-ion channel complex.[173] The action of glutamate can be antagonized *competitively* by compounds that compete for the glutamate receptor binding site. Normally occurring competitive antagonists are highly polar molecules with poor BBB penetration. Competitive antagonists have been synthesized that do cross the BBB and therefore can act following systemic administration. However, because of the difficulty in making a nontoxic competitive antagonist with adequate BBB penetration that is effective in low concentrations, most biochemical research has concentrated on the noncompetitive antagonists.

Sites of Antagonism on the N-*Methyl*-D-*aspartate Receptor-Controlled Ion Channel*

Glutamate binding site (competitive)

Glycine binding site (noncompetitive)

Ion channel binding sites (noncompetitive)

- Magnesium binding site
- Zinc binding site
- Phencyclidine binding site
- Other sites (dextorphan, dextromethorphan)

Interference with secondary effects of glutamic excitatory neurotransmission

The action of glutamate can also be antagonized *noncompetitively* by compounds that bind within the ion channel, thereby impeding ion flux through the channel. These include Mg^{2+}, Zn^+, and other compounds that bind to a separate phencyclidine binding site within the channel, including dizocilipine maleate and the dissociative anesthetics, ketamine and phencyclidine, which block the NMDA receptor-associated ion channel in the open state. Dextorphan and dextromethorphan are also noncompetitive antagonists that block the ion channel in the closed state.[147] Noncompetitive antagonists are lipid soluble, easily cross the BBB, tend to concentrate in the brain, and have short half-lives. The effect of the noncompetitive antagonists cannot be overcome by increasing the concentration of glutamate, which would displace competitive antagonists. Noncompetitive NMDA antagonists have significant side effects including non-NMDA-mediated excitatory synaptic transmission, impairment of learning,[174] morphologic neuronal changes, and psychomimetic and adverse behavioral properties.[175]

NMDA receptor antagonists have been studied to determine their effect on neurologic outcome following ischemia. However, the results have been conflicting.[176,177] Improved outcome has been reported when NMDA antagonists were given after the onset of ischemia.[160,178–182]

Many of these reported improvements were based only on histologic changes emphasizing areas of known NMDA receptor concentration, the selectively vulnerable areas. Studies on the effects of NMDA antagonists in global ischemia have produced mixed results.[175,183–185] In those studies reporting improvement following complete ischemia, the noncompetitive receptor antagonist, dizocilipine maleate, was given.[183–185] This drug is known to decrease body temperature if not aggressively maintained so that decreases in brain temperature could have provided the observed neurologic protection rather than the dizocilipine maleate itself. This animal research supports the continued movement toward clinical trials of NMDA receptor antagonists in patients suffering from stroke or the multifocal brain ischemia associated with cardiopulmonary bypass.[186]

Antagonists to the glycine binding site have also been synthesized.[187] These too have been shown to prevent some neuronal injury following ischemia.[188,189] Agents that interfere with the secondary effects of excessive NMDA activation or inhibit glutamate release during ischemia are also being investigated. In the future, these compounds might prove advantageous because they do not interfere with normal NMDA-mediated neuronal transmission. Further research may demonstrate that blockade of Ca^{2+} entry at one site may be enough to provide protection from ischemic neuronal damage or it may demonstrate that a multidrug approach causing blockade of Ca^{2+} at all sites is necessary for protection.

THE AMPA RECEPTOR-ION CHANNEL COMPLEX Recent investigation has centered upon the AMPA receptor-controlled ion channel complex. The AMPA receptor gates a channel that is unselectively permeable to monovalent cations (Na^+, K^+, H^+). AMPA receptor activation can cause depolarization of the plasma membrane, allowing Na^+ influx; can cause voltage-dependent ion channels to open allowing Ca^{2+} influx, and can reverse the Na^+-Ca^{2+} exchange mechanism.

Recent research now indicates that nonglutamate receptor activation is responsible for the excessive influx of Ca^{2+} in the postischemic period. Although an NMDA antagonist blocks Ca^{2+} entry through the NMDA receptor-controlled ion complex channel, an AMPA antagonist could prevent depolarization of the cell and consequently prevent Ca^{2+} entry through NMDA receptor-controlled ion channels, voltage-sensitive ion channels and prevent the reversal of the Na^+-Ca^{2+} exchanger.[190] AMPA receptor antagonists such as 2,3-dihydroxy-6-nitro-7-sulfamoyl-benzo [*F*]quinoxaline (NBQX) readily cross the BBB and can decrease ischemic neuronal injury even when administered following ischemia. The exact intracellular mechanisms whereby AMPA receptor activation contributes to cell injury is unknown, but blockade by AMPA receptor antagonists can block glutamate release during ischemia,[191] block the increase in intracellular Ca^{2+} occurring during ischemia,[182] and prevent neuronal injury.[192] AMPA receptor antagonists appear to lack the psychostimulant and psychotomimetic effects of the NMDA receptor antagonists but do depress glucose utilization.

Present evidence suggests that selective neuronal death after cerebral ischemia does involve excitatory neurotransmitters. NMDA and/or AMPA antagonists may offer a new strategy for the treatment of ischemic brain injury. This new approach is supported by a scientific foundation and some promising results with therapy in a variety of animal models of ischemia. The identification of several different classes of drugs that can block excitation at postsynaptic receptors opens the possibility for prevention and treatment for cerebral ischemia. Further studies should identify active compounds and their possible use in preventing or ameliorating the neurologic damage produced by ischemia.

Nitric Oxide

Nitric oxide (NO) is involved in many normal physiologic functions including vasodilation, platelet aggregation and adhesion, and neurotransmission. NO is synthesized from L-arginine by the enzyme NO synthase from the oxidation of L-arginine. The tonic release of NO maintains normal vasculature in a state of vasodilation so that inhibition of NO produces vasoconstriction manifested by a decrease in blood pressure and a decrease in blood flow.[193] three types of NO synthase occur in the brain: I within neurons, II within macrophages and glia, and III within endothelial cells. Types I and III are Ca^{2+}-calmodulin-dependent enzymes that are activated by an increase in intracellular Ca^{2+} concentration. Once activated, NO synthase releases a low level of NO. During ischemia with massive Ca^{2+} influx, there is first an overproduction of NO. NO can potentiate excitatory neurotransmission by stimulating glutamate and aspartate release.[194] This excitatory neurotransmission would activate the NMDA receptor-controlled ion channels to allow further influx of Ca^{2+} resulting in further intracellular accumulation (a positive feedback mechanism). This mechanism implicates NO in the excitotoxic theory of cell damage and death following ischemia. Other potential mechanisms of NO-mediated toxicity include direct damage to proteins, DNA, and membrane lipids by the free radical form of NO although its low concentration and short half-life suggest that the NO free radical may not directly mediate neuronal damage. Rather, NO can combine with the superoxide radical to form the highly reactive free radicals, peroxynitrite and hydroxyl radical, which can cause widespread cellular damage by inducing peroxidation of lipids within cell membranes and oxidative damage to DNA and proteins. NO can also produce direct inactivation of enzymes in mitochondrial oxidative phosphorylation such that ATP is not replenished. Two feedback mechanisms do exist to limit the toxicity of NO and oppose the cascade of ischemic cell death. NO can limit influx of Ca^{2+} through NMDA receptor-controlled ion channels, thereby further inhibiting the production of NO; and NO can produce vasodilation and decrease platelet aggregation to improve the fluidity of the blood and maintain blood flow to ischemia areas (Fig. 5.8). Therefore NO has diverse physi-

FIGURE 5.8 *Schematic of proposed role of nitric oxide following cerebral ischemia. (From Dawson,[194] with permission.)*

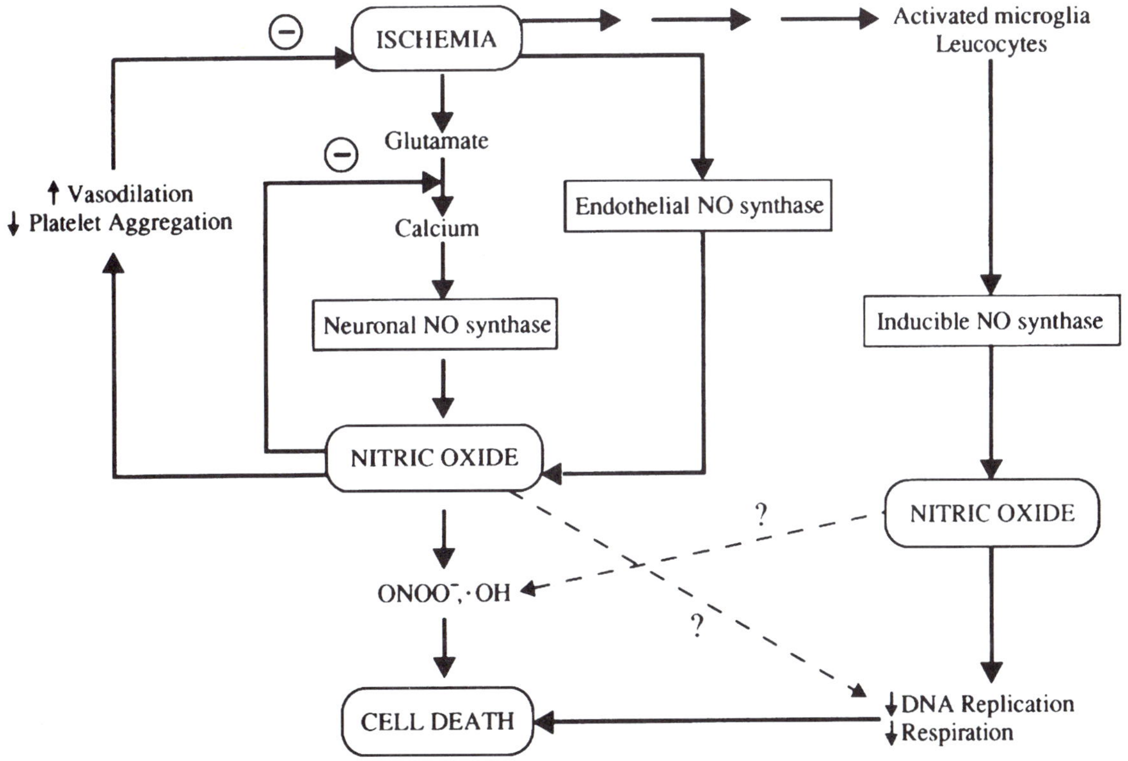

ologic actions that may both ameliorate and exacerbate cell damage and death. Much ongoing research is being done to more clearly define its role during and following ischemia.

Endogenous Neuroprotection Factors

In response to ischemia, the brain itself is capable of initiating a cascade of events in neurons and glia designed to prevent further damage. Recent research has identified several neuroprotection factors (NPFs) whose expression is increased in response to brain injury.[195] These NPFs are capable of attenuating neuronal injury initiated by ischemia through excess concentrations of excitatory amino acids and free radicals. These NPFs enhance cellular systems involved in the maintenance of Ca^{2+} homeostasis and free radical metabolism. Several compounds have been developed that can mimic the action of NPFs by activating signal transduction. Whether these compounds either alone or in combination with other protective agents can prevent neurologic damage remains to be investigated. These compounds do present a promising new approach to brain protection.

CEREBRAL PROTECTION

Protection implies improved outcome as evidenced by electrophysiologic, metabolic, or histologic indexes of recovery or, ultimately, by improved clinical neurologic recovery. Cerebral protection can be achieved by pretreatment (this is also referred to as *prevention*) in anticipation of an ischemic event such as may occur during neurosurgery or cardiac surgery that limits subsequent neuronal injury or death. Protection may also be achieved by treatment during or after ischemia in an attempt to minimize initial tissue damage and to prevent or ameliorate secondary insults resulting from the ischemia. This may be referred to as *resuscitation*.

In *focal* ischemia, protection can be accomplished by optimizing the substrate supply/demand ratio. This can be achieved by increasing blood flow to improve collateral circulation or decreasing the energy demands of the ischemic cells. Because cerebral blood vessels within an ischemic area will be maximally dilated, vasodilating agents will have little effect on improving regional CBF. An increase in rCBF to this ischemic area can be achieved only by an increase in perfusion pressure in the ischemic area. Inotropic agents can maintain or increase systemic blood pressure such that CBF in the ischemic area will passively increase. A reduction in any ischemic-induced cerebral edema that causes increased intracranial pressure (ICP) in the area may also increase cerebral perfusion pressure and rCBF. Suppression of cerebral metabolism will decrease the requirements for oxygen and substrate delivery.

In complete *global* ischemia in which there is no blood flow or metabolism, the above protective measures can have no effect. Therapy is aimed at those secondary processes thought to contribute to the ultimate neurologic damage such as cerebral edema, hypoperfusion, hypermetabolism, and cell and membrane damage. Protection from global ischemia includes delaying the development of membrane failure and inhibiting the processes leading to irreversible cell damage, such as blocking excitatory neurotransmission, blocking Ca^{2+} influx, preventing intracellular lactic acidosis, and enhancing the effect of time by slowing all reactions within the cell, thereby delaying the occurrence of the secondary consequences of ischemia. Many therapeutic agents may be protective if their administration is coordinated with endogenous cellular repair.

THERAPY

Deliberate Hypothermia

The capacity of hypothermia to protect the brain and other vital organs during periods of decreased or absent oxygen delivery is well known and used daily during cardiac surgery. It is common for total circulatory arrest to be induced in patients for up to 60 minutes at 15 to 18°C without any subsequent neurologic injury. In the 1960s profound hypothermia was a popular technique used to protect the brain from ischemia during neurosurgery when temporary cerebral ischemia was produced during the temporary clipping of an aneurysm. However, it was very difficult technically, requiring femoral-femoral bypass and heparinization. It provided excellent surgical exposure, but because of the heparinization and the low temperature, there was an increase in postoperative bleeding with subsequent neurologic deficits. Because of the complexity of the technique and the high risk/benefit ratio, the technique was largely abandoned.

The theory of hypothermic brain protection was based on the fact that hypothermia *empirically* delays those processes leading to irreversible loss of cell function and cell death. Because $CMRO_2$ was the only measurement of cellular activity at the time, it was assumed that the ability of hypothermia to protect the brain or other organs against damage from ischemia was due solely to its ability to decrease global cerebral metabolism, thereby decreasing the consumption of high-energy substrates and decreasing the accumulation of toxic metabolites. It was assumed that the lower the temperature, the lower the cellular metabolism, and therefore the longer the period of ischemia that the brain could tolerate.

Hypothermia decreases the global energy requirements of the brain by decreasing both the activation metabolism required for neuronal function and the residual metabolism necessary for the maintenance of cellular integrity. The relationship between temperature and global cerebral metabolism is expressed by the temperature coefficient Q_{10}, which is the ratio of the rates of oxygen consumption separated by 10°C.[196] However, this relationship is not linear because hypothermia affects both components of neuronal oxygen metabolism.[197] A Q_{10} of approximately 2.2 to 2.4 between the temperatures of 37 and 27°C is consistent with the Q_{10} for most biologic reactions.[196,198,199] However, between 27 and 14°C, the Q_{10} is approximately 4.5[196,198] The large increase in Q_{10} that occurs in this temperature range is accompanied by cessation of neuronal function (the EEG is progressively suppressed and eventually becomes isoelectric). Below 14°C, with the total cessation of neuronal function, the Q_{10} again approximates 2.2 to 2.4.[196] Thus, if a decrease in global cerebral metabolism were the only mechanism by which hypothemia protected the brain, knowledge of the Q_{10} would permit calculation of the duration of tolerable ischemia. This concept has been supported by past observations that at normothermia, the human brain can tolerate 5 to 8 minutes of complete global ischemia without sustaining neurologic injury, whereas at 15 to 20°C the human brain can tolerate approximately 60 minutes of ischemia (i.e., at 15 to 20°C cerebral oxygen consumption [$CMRO_2$] is approximately 1/10th the normothermic value, allowing an approximate 10-fold increase in the duration of ischemia the brain can tolerate without injury.[200]

However, recent studies have indicated that a decrease in global cerebral metabolism may not be the only mechanism by which hypothermia provides protection from ischemia. Animal studies have demonstrated that small differences in brain temperature can critically determine the extent of neuronal injury. It has been reported[201–205] that decreases of 2 to 6°C in brain temperature markedly attenuated or abolished histopathologic damage in selectively vulnerable areas of the brain following incomplete global ischemia; the lower the temperature, the less injury. These dramatic changes in histopathology occurred despite the fact that these differences in brain temperature had no significant effect on global cerebral metabolism. These same mild decreases in brain temperature have been reported to reduce significantly mortality and neurologic deficit.[206]

Only one study[207] has suggested that small 1 to 3°C differences in temperature significantly reduces anaerobic metabolism. Because this is the only evidence that small changes in brain temperature significantly alter global cerebral metabolism, other mechanisms for the observed protective effect have been proposed. These include effects on ion homeostasis, excitatory neurotransmission,[141,208] Ca^{2+} and K^{+} flux, enzyme function, free radical production or scavenging, membrane lipid peroxidation, and membrane stability including permeability of the BBB. If these protective effects of small decreases in brain temperature can be substantiated with studies of neurologic function or outcome following focal and complete global cerebral ischemia, mild hypothermia may become a very useful technique clinically. Based on the results from the animal studies, deliberate mild hypothermia has been advocated for brain protection in patients.[208] Preliminary investigations[209–212] report that mild hypothermia can reduce ICP and improve neurologic outcome in patients sustaining severe head injury. There was no increased incidence of cardiac arrhythmias, coagulopathies, or pulmonary complications in the patients undergoing hypothermia.[209] One study[213] has investigated the use of deliberate mild hypothermia in patients undergoing craniotomy. This study reported its feasibility and safety but did not study its efficacy for brain protection. Mild hypothermia was easily achieved intraoperatively, but rewarming was more difficult, although this did not delay emergence. A recent survey of neuroanesthesiologists reported that 70 percent use some form of mild hypothermia (deliberate or passive) during aneurysm clipping for brain protection. Despite the lack of randomized clinical outcome studies, the use of transient mild hypothermia (3 to 4°C) is advocated for operative procedures that may put the patient at risk of transient cerebral ischemia.

The significant side effects occurring with deep hypothermia are attenuated or avoided with mild hypothermia. The side effects of mild to moderate hypothermia include effects on the circulatory system, cardiac system, pulmonary system, neurologic function, coagulation function, metabolism, immune system, and endocrine system.[214]

Complications of Hypothermia

CARDIOVASCULAR COMPLICATIONS

- Myocardial depression
- Arrhythmias including ventricular fibrillation
- Hypotension
- Inadequate tissue perfusion
- Ischemia

COAGULATION

- Thrombocytopenia
- Fibrinolysis
- Platelet dysfunction
- Increased bleeding

METABOLISM

- Slowed metabolism of anesthetic agents
- Prolonged neuromuscular blockade
- Increased protein catabolism

SHIVERING

- Increased oxygen consumption
- Increased carbon dioxide production
- Increased cardiac output
- Aterial oxygen desaturation
- Hemodynamic instability

Proposed Mechanisms of Protection by Hypothermia

- Decrease in cerebral metabolism
- Maintenance of the integrity of membrane ion channels
- Preservation of ion homeostasis
- Decrease in excitatory neurotransmission
- Decrease in calcium flux
- Prevention of lipid peroxidation
- Maintenance of the blood-brain barrier

CIRCULATORY SYSTEM Hypothermia causes increased peripheral vascular resistance with an increase in cardiac afterload. During hypothermia, fluid leaves the intravascular space, causing an increase in hematocrit and blood viscosity. Blood viscosity increases 4 to 6 percent for every 1°C temperature decrease.[215] Hypothermia suppresses antidiuretic hormone causing diuresis. This together with shunting of peripheral blood centrally results in a further decrease in intravascular volume. Therefore the hypothermic patient will be more susceptible to hypovolemia than normothermic patients.

CARDIAC SYSTEM Hypothermia (even mild) may cause significantly greater postoperative myocardial ischemia and angina.[216] This is most likely due to shivering and the resultant increased cardiac output and to an increased level of catecholamines, producing higher myocardial oxygen demands when the hypothermia is not corrected prior to the cessation of anesthesia. For every 1°C decrease in core temperature (between 36.5 and 33.5°C), the probability of shivering is increased by 33 percent.[217] Conversely, hypothermia can decrease ventricular contractility and diastolic relaxation, thereby decreasing cardiac output. This can act synergistically with anesthetic drugs that decrease myocardial contractility. Mild hypothermia can impair the efficacy of any inotropic cardiac medications. At temperatures below 32°C, atrial fibrillation[218] may occur, and below 30°C, spontaneous ventricular fibrillation can occur, which may be very difficult to treat.[219]

PULMONARY SYSTEM Rewarming from mild hypothermia has been associated with pulmonary edema[220] and decreased oxygenation.[216]

NEUROLOGIC FUNCTION Hypothermia will prolong the latency of somatosensory and motor-evoked potentials and can prolong the latency of brainstem auditory-evoked potentials. This must be considered in the interpretation of these measurements during neurosurgery using mild hypothermia. Rewarming after mild hypothermia can increase ICP such that other therapeutic interventions may be necessary.[209]

COAGULATION Hypothermia can cause platelet sequestration and dysfunction,[221] increased fibrinolysis, and a decrease in the enzymatic activity required for clotting independent of clotting factor concentration.[222] This results in an abnormal increase in clotting parameters: prothrombin time, partial thromboplastin time, and thrombin time. Clinical laboratories routinely perform these studies at 37°C, which do not accurately measure the hypothermic clotting defect. These defects result in prolonged bleeding time and greater blood loss. During neurosurgery any coagulopathy predisposes to intracranial bleeding.[223] If induced hypothermia is to be used as a protective measure during neurosurgery, meticulous attention must be paid to hemostasis.

METABOLIC EFFECTS In addition to lowering metabolic rate, hypothermia shifts the oxyhemoglobin dissociation curve to the left, thereby reducing the amount of oxygen available to the tissues. This may contribute to a metabolic acidosis. If the minute volume is not adjusted, the lower CO_2 production during hypothermia will result in a respiratory alkalosis, which can compensate in part for the metabolic acidosis. Hypothermia affects the solubility of gases in the blood. With each 1°C decrease, pH increases by 0.015, PCO_2 decreases by 4.4 percent, and PO_2 decreases by 7.2 percent.[219] Misinterpretation of blood gas concentrations corrected to body temperature may result in a relative brain tissue acidosis, which can abolish CBF autoregulation. Hypothermia will slow the metabolism of the anesthetics and neuromuscular blocking agents such that caution should be taken when dosing with these agents. Hypothermia decreases citrate metabolism such that citrate toxicity may occur during transfusion.[224]

IMMUNOLOGIC EFFECTS Mild hypothermia decreases leukocyte mobility and phagocytosis.[225] This immunologic suppression combined with decreased peripheral blood flow can increase the risk of wound infection. This may account for the higher incidence of sepsis and pneumonia in recent trials of mild hypothermia in the treatment of closed head injury.[209,211]

Although core temperature is a rigidly guarded physiologic phenomenon,[226] mild hypothermia can be easily induced in surgical patients because anesthesia interferes with thermoregulation controlled by the hypothalamus, and produces a 2 to 4°C decrease in the vasoconstriction threshold. Intraoperative hypothermia occurs with an initial rapid decrease in core temperature caused by redistribution of body heat to the periphery followed by a slower decrease in temperature when heat loss exceeds metabolic heat production. Body temperature plateaus at 33 to 35°C when vasoconstriction decreases heat loss. Other factors include inadequate cutaneous insulation, evaporation of surgical antiseptic solutions, inhalation of dry, cold gases, administration of cold intravenous fluids; and heat loss from surgical incisions. Deliberate hypothermia to approximately 34°C can usually be achieved passively by uncovering patients in cool operating rooms and the administration of sufficient anesthesia to prevent thermoregulatory vasoconstriction.

Rewarming from mild hypothermia will decrease peripheral vascular resistance and may cause a decrease in blood pressure.[227] Rewarming after mild hypothermia should be instituted in the operating room such that the patient can be near normothermia at the time of emergence from anesthesia. The severe blood flow inhomogeneity, hypoxemia, and metabolic acidosis occurring during rewarming from deep hypothermia[228,229] do not occur following mild hypothermia. The efficacy of rewarming may be limited until thermoregulatory vasoconstriction ceases. The rate of intraoperative surface rewarming is approximately 0.7°C per hour and is inversely related to body surface area. Following rewarming, core temperature will decrease approximately 0.6°C in the next 30 minutes. However, in the next few hours the patient may actually become hyperthermic, which could have adverse effects on neurologic function.[213]

Warming devices include electrically heated humidifier circuits, fluid warmers, electrical and circulating water warming blankets, convective forced air warming blankets, and infrared heating lamps. Forced air rewarming is the fastest method of increasing body heat content and mean body temperature.[226] These devices are all associated with complications such as burns and skin irritation. Care must be taken in their use. There is a 40 percent incidence of postoperative shivering. This can increase oxygen consumption 200 to 600 percent and aggravate wound pain. Shivering can be treated by skin surface warming or the administration of meperidine (25 mg).

Risk factors should be identified in any patient at risk for neurologic injury in whom deliberate mild hypothermia is contemplated. Careful consideration of the adverse effects of mild hypothermia in each patient must be made before using the technique of mild deliberate hypothermia for protection from neurologic injury.

Risk Assessment for Patients Undergoing Deliberate Hypothermia

MINIMAL RISK

Younger patients (<60 yr)

Normal coagulation and immune status

Little intraoperative fluid shifts

MILD RISK

Predisposition to coronary artery disease

Low body surface area

Major fluid resuscitation

Older patients (>60 yr)

MODERATE RISK

Known cardiovascular disease

Coagulopathy

CONTRAINDICATIONS

Cryoglobinemia

Other cold-induced disease

Anesthetics

BARBITURATES Anesthetic agents that have been used to protect the brain from ischemia can exert their protective effects in three ways[12,55]: (1) reduction in oxygen demand, (2) increase in oxygen delivery, and (3) inhibition of deleterious pathologic intracellular processes. These categories are not mutually exclusive as any one agent may provide protection via more than one mechanism.

Barbiturates have served as the prototype for anesthetic protection against cerebral ischemia. Their primary mechanism of protection has been attributed to their ability to decrease the $CMRO_2$, thereby increasing the ratio of oxygen supply to oxygen demand. Specifically, it has been proposed that the barbiturates selectively decrease the energy expenditure required for synaptic transmission and neuronal function without affecting the energy required for basic neuronal integrity.[230,231] The reduction in cerebral oxygen consumption that parallels the reduction in neuronal function reaches a plateau when neuronal function is abolished as seen by an isoelectric EEG.[11] This decrease in $CMRO_2$ is accompanied by a parallel decrease in CBF and cerebral blood volume (CBV), which is the mechanism by which the barbiturates decrease ICP. It is also the mechanism by which barbiturates may redistribute rCBF and shunt blood from normal areas of brain to ischemic areas.[232,233] Both of these mechanisms may contribute secondarily to the protective effect of barbiturates. Other proposed mechanisms of barbiturate protection during cerebral ischemia are listed in the accompanying box.

Proposed Mechanisms of Barbiturate Protection

- Decrease in cerebral metabolic requirements
- Improvement in distribution of rCBF
- Suppression of seizures
- Supression of catecholamine-induced hyperactivity
- Anesthesia, deafferentation, immobilization
- Loss of thermoregulation
- Decrease in ICP
- Decrease in cerebral edema
- Decrease in CSF secretion
- Scavenging of free radicals
- Stabilization of membranes
- Blocking of calcium channels
- Alteration in fatty acid metabolism

Abbreviations: rCBF, regional cerebral blood flow; ICP, intracranial pressure; CSF, cerebral spinal fluid.

Before discussing the potential for cerebral protection with barbiturates (and other anesthetics), it is important to differentiate between reports concerning focal or incomplete ischemia, and those concerning complete ischemia. With the onset of complete global ischemia, brain function is abolished within 15 to 30 seconds and basal metabolism is almost immediately reduced or abolished, precluding any further metabolic suppression by anesthetics. Complete global ischemia also obviously prevents any vascular effects, such as redistribution of CBF, that are possible with regional or incomplete ischemia. By contrast, during focal ischemia wherein neuronal function is not completely abolished and the ischemic area continues to consume energy at greater than basal levels, anesthetics such as barbiturates can decrease metabolism down to basal levels and perhaps either prolong the brain's tolerance for the injury or prevent infarction altogether.[11] Because barbiturates are also capable of constricting normal vessels, they might shunt blood flow toward the ischemic area (inverse steal) and thereby provide protection.[234] This latter mechanism could not be operative during global ischemia. If barbiturate-induced brain protection is determined solely by its ability to decrease cerebral metabolic demand associated with neuronal function and/or favorably redistribute CBF, then it is not surprising that cerebral protection is not demonstrable in the event of complete ischemia, whereas a beneficial effect is demonstrable in models of focal ischemia.[235]

There are no confirmed studies demonstrating that barbiturates provide any cerebral protection after complete global ischemia in either experimental animal models of cardiac arrest or humans resuscitated from cardiac arrest.[236] Despite a flurry of interest in the 1980s, the use of barbiturates is not justified in an attempt to prevent irreversible anoxic and ischemic brain injury following cardiac arrest.[237]

In contrast is the primarily positive experimental evidence in laboratory animals that barbiturates provide protection from neurologic injury after focal cerebral ischemia.[238–243] However, the reports are contradictory and confusing because of the many variables that influenced outcome besides the barbiturate administration. The effectiveness of barbiturate protection in focal ischemia can be affected by the experimental model, species differences, the type of barbiturate, dose, timing and duration of administration, the temporary or permanent nature of the focal ischemic insult, cardiovascular and respiratory responses to barbiturates, glucose levels, brain and body temperature, and incidence of seizures.

Early studies of barbiturate protection reported that either a massive bolus dose or a smaller bolus dose followed by a continuous infusion of *pentobarbital* to suppress neuronal function and reduce cerebral energy demand,[66,244,245] redistribute or increase CBF,[232,246] and inhibit the formation of cerebral edema[247–249] provided some level of protection by decreasing neurologic injury, increasing neuronal survival time, or reducing infarct size.[240,241,243,246] Applying the results of these animal studies to evaluate the effects of barbiturates in clinical trials of intraoperative focal ischemia or stroke has been difficult because the large doses of barbiturate required for protection are associated with cardiovascular and respiratory complications.[250]

Reports of barbiturate protection for *temporary* focal ischemia are also contradictory. Postischemic treatment with high-dose pentobarbital was reported to protect from ischemic injury, the mechanism of action being reduction of cerebral edema and ICP with redistribution of rCBF.[242] Other studies reported that pentobarbital[251] or thiopental[252] failed to protect from neurologic injury.

Clinical studies describing the protective effects of thiopental are mostly anecdotal, and there is little clinical evidence for the efficacy of barbiturates in preventing or treating focal ischemia. In humans there is only one prospective randomized clinical study that has demonstrated improved neurologic function following focal ischemia suffered by patients undergoing open heart cardiac procedures using normothermic perfusion.[253] The cerebral protective effects of thiopental are specific to this patient population. It has been reported that thiopental does not reduce the number of strokes in patients undergoing coronary artery bypass grafting.[254]

Despite the relatively few studies demonstrating the efficacy of barbiturates in protecting against temporary focal ischemia, prophylactic barbiturate therapy continues to be recommended for cerebral protection when a transient ischemic episode is possible such as during carotid endarterectomy,[255–258] aneurysm procedures requiring transient occlusion of the parent artery,[259–261] extracranial to intracranial bypass procedures,[262,263] profound induced hypotension,[264] and cardiopulmonary bypass procedures requiring an open ventricle.[253] Concern that large doses of barbiturates produce cardiovascular depression and drug-induced coma delaying evaluation of neurologic function postoperatively has resulted in the recommendation of small single doses of barbiturate.[11,258,259,261–263,265] The appropriate dose of barbiturate is thought to be one that produces EEG burst suppression. Normal anesthetizing doses of thiopental (3 to 7 mg/kg) will produce EEG burst suppression. for less than 5 to 10 minutes,[252] whereas larger doses of thiopental (10 to 25 mg/kg) produce burst suppression on the EEG that lasts only 10 minutes.[256]

If a sufficient dose of thiopental is given to produce burst suppression on the EEG, the vessel can be clamped within 10 to 15 seconds.[264] Ideally the occluded vessel should be briefly opened every 5 to 10 minutes (if possible and without hemorrhage) in order for subsequent small doses of thiopental (1 to 2 mg/kg) to reach the region of ischemia. If this is not possible, a continuous infusion of thiopental (10 to 20 mg/kg/h) should be given to maintain burst suppression throughout the ischemic period.[266] The EEG should be monitored to ascertain the proper dose of thiopental needed to produce burst suppression in each patient. Blood pressure should be maintained within normal limits, with a phenylephrine infusion if necessary.

ETOMIDATE Although barbiturates have been proposed for brain protection, the high doses required to achieve and maintain an isoelectric EEG result in a prolonged duration of tracheal intubation[253] and profound hypotension requiring vasopressor support.[253,267] Etomidate has gained some favor as a neuroprotective agent because it produces less of these side effects. Etomidate is a nonbarbiturate imidazole derivative that has minimal direct cardiovascular effects[268–270] and a shorter half-life, allowing a more rapid awakening than high-dose thiopental.

Etomidate is similar to thiopental in that it produces a dose-related decrease in neuronal function with an accompanying decrease in $CMRO_2$ and CBF.[271–274] Etomidate is also a direct cerebral vasoconstrictor with the ability to significantly decrease CBF. This effect on CBF is independent of its effect on cerebral metabolism.[271] Although CBF is markedly decreased by etomidate, CO_2 reactivity remains intact.[272–274]

Proposed mechanisms by which etomidate may provide protection against ischemia include the above-mentioned decrease in $CMRO_2$ reduction in intracranial blood volume, decrease in ICP,[271,275] decrease or redistribution of CBF,[276] membrane stabilization, and inhibition of FFA liberation.[277] Several studies in animal models have shown that etomidate provides protection during incomplete global ischemia.[278–281] Postischemic administration of etomidate has no beneficial effect on recovery.[282]

Despite the advantages of producing greater cardiovascular stability and having a shorter half-life than thiopental, enthusiasm for use of etomidate has been dampened by its major side effects: myoclonic movements and suppression of adrenal cortical function. Adrenal cortical suppression by etomidate is of concern because it may attenuate a patient's ability to withstand intraoperative and postoperative stress.[283] In normal patients undergoing elective surgery, a single dose of etomidate can produce adrenal cortical suppression lasting 24 hours or more.[284,285] This effect is dose related and is more pronounced if continuous infusions are used (as required for brain protection).[286,287] There have been no reports of increased morbidity or mortality after an induction dose of etomidate and it is important to note that the initial reports of symptomatic etomidate-induced adrenal cortical suppression were in critically ill patients receiving continuous infusions of etomidate for long-term sedation.[288] Etomidate blocks 11β-hydroxylase and thereby affects the synthesis of cortisol, corticosterone, aldosterone, and 17α-hydroxyprogesterone[286,289] but not the response of the receptors. Supplemental administration of exogenous steroids should prevent the adverse effects of adrenal cortical suppression. This becomes less of an issue in most neurosurgical patients who routinely receive intravenous glucocorticoids to minimize cerebral edema and ICP.

Although a myriad of anecdotal clinical studies have reported brain protection with etomidate, no randomized controlled studies have been done. These studies need to be done to further define the ability of etomidate to act as a protective agent for intraoperative ischemia. Until then, etomidate is an unproven option to the barbiturates for brain protection.

PROPOFOL Propofol (2,6-diisopropylphenol) is an intravenous hypnotic anesthetic agent[290] used for both the induction of anesthesia[291] and for the maintenance of anesthesia[292] and has been widely used as an anesthetic for neurosurgical patients.[293] Propofol decreases neuronal activity on the EEG with an accompanying decrease in $CMRO_2$ and CBF and an increase in cerebrovascular resistance (CVR).[294–298] Because its effect on neuronal activity, $CMRO_2$, and CBF appear to be similar to those of thiopental, it has been hypothesized that propofol might provide some degree of cerebral protection against ischemia. Other proposed mechanisms of protection by propofol include an attenuation of neurotransmitter release in response to ischemia.[299]

Propofol has been reported to provide some brain protection in hypoxia,[300] and incomplete global ischemia.[301–303] In animal studies of focal cerebral ischemia, propofol does not seem to provide brain protection.[304] Nevertheless, because prompt awakening occurs following prolonged propofol infusions, propofol has become popular for brain protection during cerebrovascular surgery when the brain is at risk for focal ischemia.[305] To date this practice is unsupported by research. In addition, there have been several case reports of propofol-induced seizure activity, myoclonus, or opisthotonus.[306–308] This would be detrimental in patients recovering from neurosurgery who had sustained some degree of ischemia. Until studies in animal models and clinical studies demonstrate the efficacy of propofol for brain protection it cannot be recommended that propofol be used for this purpose.

ISOFLURANE The volatile anesthetics are also capable of decreasing neuronal activity on the EEG with an accompanying decrease in $CMRO_2$ and CBF. Isoflurane[309,310] and the newer volatile anesthetics, desflurane and sevoflurane, are capable of inducing a level of anesthesia that suppresses EEG activity without significantly adversely affecting hemodynamics. If the primary mechanism for cerebral protection during ischemia is a reduction in neuronal activity and cerebral metabolism, then one would expect that isoflurane might be protective during focal and incomplete global ischemia but not during complete global ischemia during which neuronal activity is abolished by the ischemia itself.[311,312] Animal studies have supported this concept. In models of incomplete global ischemia, isoflurane was shown to provide protection[311,313,314] but not in a model of near complete global ischemia.[315] Mechanisms of action proposed for cerebral protection by isoflurane include metabolic suppression, prevention of a cerebral hyperthermic response to ischemia,[316] suppression of sympathetic activity,[317] and a decrease in glutamate receptors preventing Ca^{2+} influx and the calcium cascade to cell death.[318] In animal studies of regional ischemia, there are conflicting results on the effect of isoflurane as a protective agent.[319–321] The protection provided by thiopental in regional cerebral ischemia may be accounted for not only by metabolic suppression, but also possibly by an advantageous redistribution of CBF secondary to the vasoconstriction produced in the nonischemic brain areas. Due to its vasodilatory properties, this latter effect is not possible with isoflurane and theoretically an opposite effect may occur.[314]

There is, however, evidence in humans that isoflurane provides some protection in regional ischemia but only when compared to the effects of other volatile anesthetics. No comparison to intravenous anesthetics has been made. In studies of patients undergoing carotid endarterectomy, the critical CBF (that blood flow below which the majority of patients developed ipsilateral EEG changes of ischemia during carotid occlusion) was significantly lower during isoflurane anesthesia[33] than during anesthesia with halothane,[31,32] enflurane,[32] or Innovar.[32] And there was a significantly lower incidence of ischemic changes on the EEG during carotid endarterectomy with isoflurane anesthesia than with either halothane or enflurane.[322] The decreased incidence of intraoperative ischemia in those patients receiving isoflurane occurred despite the fact that their preoperative neurologic risk status was greater than those patients receiving halothane or enflurane. In this clinical situation isoflurane provides better protection than other volatile anesthetics.

NITROUS OXIDE Nitrous oxide (N_2O) may affect cerebral protection. The literature is confusing concerning the effects of N_2O on CBF and $CMRO_2$ because of species variations in potency and response. The minimum alveolar concentration (MAC) of N_2O varies from 82 percent to 275 percent. This potency variation cannot be corrected by adjustment of dose so that most animal studies have used 70 percent N_2O despite this MAC variation among species. N_2O has little effect on $CMRO_2$ and CBF in the rat[323] but significantly increases CBF and $CMRO_2$ in dogs,[324,325] pigs,[326] goats,[327] and rabbits.[328] In the absence of other anesthetics N_2O significantly increases CBF and $CMRO_2$ in humans. This effect appears to be due to stimulation of sympathetic activity by N_2O.[329] Because of these species-specific effects, the literature on the effect of N_2O for brain protection is conflicting. It has been reported that N_2O alone worsens neurologic outcome[330] but that the use of other anesthetics in combination with N_2O may attenuate this effect.[331,332] Clinically, N_2O may have a detrimental effect if used alone when there is a risk of cerebral ischemia. However, this seldom occurs when other potent inhalation anesthetics or opioids are used in addition to N_2O. Many of these may modify the effect of N_2O. Both its varying potency and subsequent metabolic effect in different animal species and its effect on sympathetic activity should be considered before using N_2O as the control in animal models of cerebral ischemia and studies of brain protection.

LOCAL ANESTHETICS Lidocaine is the local anesthetic most frequently studied in determining the cerebral effects of local anesthetics. Its action blocks Na^+ channels in the cell that restricts both Na^+ influx and K^+ efflux. By blocking these ion fluxes, lidocaine may decrease the work of the cell membrane ATP-dependent ion pumps and the attendant energy requirements necessary to maintain ion homeostasis.[333] In the normal brain this would appear as a decrease in cerebral metabolism, whereas in the ischemic brain this decrease in energy requirement might provide protection from ischemia. Lidocaine significantly reduces $CMRO_2$ when administered in both subepileptogenic doses[334,335] and massive doses above the seizure threshold.[56]

It has been reported that low-dose lidocaine does provide some measure of brain protection in animal models.[336,337] Massive doses of lidocaine do not provide cerebral protection from ischemia[338] unless the circulation is supported.[56] High-dose lidocaine does have a direct toxic effect on oxidative phosphorylation.[339] Therefore, any decrease in cerebral metabolism produced by large doses of lidocaine may be due to a variety of factors both protective and toxic, including membrane stabilization, inhibition of neuronal function, and uncoupling of oxidative phosphorylation. Until more studies are done that show lidocaine to be a cerebral protective agent, it should not be used for this purpose.

Calcium Entry Blockers

The calcium entry blockers form a heterogenous group of drugs including derivatives of papaverine, dihydropyridine, and piperazine. These drugs block the influx of Ca^{2+} through the voltage-sensistive ion channels into the cells[53] and can block intracellular flux of calcium into mitochondria.[340,341] They are structurally and operationally distinct from the antagonists of excitatory neurotransmitters that also block the entry of Ca^{2+} into the cell but through the excitatory amino acid neurotransmitter receptor-controlled ion channels.

The calcium entry blockers vary in their effects on the myocardium and on the vasculature by affecting different vascular beds. The source of calcium necessary for contraction of large cerebral arteries is extracellular. This is unlike systemic arteries which use a bound intracellular pool of calcium for contraction.[342] This makes the cerebral vessels especially responsive to the calcium entry blockers. The calcium entry blockers that have been studied for brain protection have been chosen because of their preferential effect on cerebral vessels. These include flumarizine, lidoflazine, nimodipine, and nicardipine. Protection by these agents has been studied in focal ischemia and in complete global ischemia secondary to cardiac arrest. To date the only calcium entry blocker that has been shown to provide cerebral protection from ischemia clinically is nimodipine.

NIMODIPINE Nimodipine, a dihydropyridine derivative, is the calcium entry blocker most extensively studied for its protective effects against cerebral ischemia. It has been studied in animal models of focal ischemia and in patients with acute strokes or following subarachnoid hemorrhage (SAH). It has also been studied in animal models of complete cerebral ischemia and in patients surviving cardiac arrest.

Nimodipine has been most extensively studied for its role in the treatment of vasospasm following SAH. Several prospective randomized, blinded, placebo-controlled studies[343–347] on the use of nimodipine in patients following SAH reported that patients treated with nimodipine had significantly lower incidence of delayed ischemic deficits or death or had significantly better neurologic outcome than those patients given placebo. Although the number of patients in each of these studies was small, a metaanalysis of these studies clearly demonstrated that nimodipine treatment administered following SAH significantly decreased the incidence of delayed ischemic defects.[348] However, nimodipine has had no demonstrable effect on the extent and severity of vasospasm as determined by cerebral angiography. Nimodipine produces the most improvement in patients with moderate symptoms but produces little or no improvement in patients with severe symptoms.[349] The mechanism(s) of action of nimodipine in the amelioration of neurologic damage following SAH remain unclear. Nimodipine may be affecting the vasculature but does not seem to prevent vasospasm (at least as determined grossly by angiography), although it may lessen the severity of the vasospasm. It may be acting through its effects on neurons by preventing Ca^{2+} entry into the cells, Ca^{2+} sequestration by mitochondria, and the subsequent alterations in FFA metabolism and the arachidonic acid cascade. Based on the above studies, oral nimodipine, (60 mg four times a day) is now recommended for patients with mild to moderate symptoms following SAH due to aneurysm rupture.

Mechanisms of Action of Calcium Entry Blockers

VASCULATURE

Vasodilation

Prevention of vasospasm

NEURONAL TISSUE

Block calcium entry into cells

Block calcium sequestration by mitochondria

- After free fatty acid metabolism
- Alter arachidonic acid cascade

In studies of the protective effect of nimodipine in focal ischemia or stroke, nimodipine decreases infarct size and improves neurologic recovery.[350,351] In patients with acute stroke, nimodipine produced a significant improvement in regional CBF to the ischemic hemisphere, indicating that nimodipine produced an inverse (or Robin Hood) steal.[352] In two randomized blinded, placebo-controlled trials of patients with acute strokes, treatment with nimodipine orally (120 mg daily) for 1 month following the stroke resulted in significantly less mortality and significantly faster and better improvement in neurologic function.[353,354] However, nimodipine had a differential effect on recovery. Neurologic recovery was greater in those patients whose initial deficits were mild to moderate. If the initial deficits were severe, nimodipine produced no improvement.[354] These studies on CBF and neurologic outcome suggest that improvement in neurologic function is correlated with improvement in CBF to the ischemic area and its penumbra. If the ischemia is mild, nimodipine may improve CBF enough to restore normal neurologic function. If the ischemia is so severe that CBF is below the threshold for cell survival, treatment with nimodipine will have no effect. These clinical trials are promising and suggest that nimodipine may be of benefit if started within 24 hours of the onset of stroke and administered in addition to standard treatment.

Following complete cerebral ischemia, nimodipine significantly ameliorates postischemic hypoperfusion.[355–357] This flow enhancement by nimodipine is regionally heterogeneous but tends to redistribute blood flow such that areas of low flow receive a greater increase in CBF than areas of high flow, another example of a Robin Hood steal.[358] Nimodipine has also been shown to significantly improve neurologic recovery.[359] The fact that nimodipine improved both postischemic hypoperfusion and neurologic outcome supports the hypothesis that postischemic hypoperfusion does contribute to the ultimate neurologic damage occurring after complete global ischmia. A prospective randomized, blinded placebo-controlled study of patients resuscitated from cardiac arrest reported that there was no improvement in survival rate or neurologic function in those patients receiving nimodipine. However, in a subset of patients in whom advanced life support measures were delayed 10 minutes or more from the onset of cardiac arrest, treatment with nimodipine did significantly improve survival rate.[360,361]

The above studies suggest that calcium entry blockers may be able to provide limited protection of or improvement in neurologic function when given to treat cerebral ischemia. Whether the major mechanism(s) of action for this protection is an effect on the cerebral vasculature causing improvement in or redistribution of CBF or whether it is due to other subcellular neuronal effects has yet to be determined.

Steroids

Mechanisms of action of glucocorticoids proposed for cerebral protection include stabilization of membranes, reduction of cerebral edema (especially that associated with intracranial tumors), scavenging of free radicals, reduction of CSF production, and an increase in the seizure threshold.[362,363] Steroid administration significantly reduces cerebral edema associated with brain tumors.[364] However, high-dose steroid therapy provides no additional improvement in neurologic outcome when used in the management of severe head trauma.[365–368] The administration of glucocorticoids can be associated with increased blood sugar, which itself is detrimental in the setting of ischemia. Therefore the administration of glucocorticoids for the treatment of severe head injury is not indicated.

Phenytoin

Cerebral protection by phenytoin has been reported in a variety of animal models of reduced oxygen delivery, including incomplete ischemia[369] and global ischemia.[370,371] One uncontrolled clinical study reported that patients receiving phenytoin after cardiac arrest made a nearly complete recovery.[372] However, another study failed to demonstrate any protective effect of phenytoin.[373] Phenytoin decreases CBF but has no effect on cerebral metabolism;[374] it stabilizes membranes and slows the release of K^+ from ischemic neurons.[375] This may prevent constriction of vascular smooth muscle, which would decrease CBF, an increase in glial water content, and cytotoxic edema. Phenytoin has also been shown to attenuate FFA accumulation during complete global ischemia, thereby preventing the arachidonic acid cascade leading to the production of endoperoxides, prostaglandins, and free radicals and the potential detrimental effects these could have in ischemic cells.[376] Further studies are necessary to determine whether there is a clinical role for phenytoin in the treatment of cerebral ischemia.

Hyperventilation

Controlled hyperventilation producing hypocapnia is an effective short-term means of reducing ICP by decreasing CBF and CBV. CBF and CBV have a linear relationship with carbon dioxide. When $PaCO_2$ decreases, cerebral vessels vasoconstrict until the limit of vasoconstriction is reached, which occurs at a $PaCO_2$ of approximately 20 mmHg. If $PaCO_2$ decreases below 18 to 20 mmHg, ischemia may occur.[13] If hyperventilation is utilized clinically, $PaCO_2$ is kept between 20 and 30 mmHg, which produces vasoconstriction without inducing ischemia.

It is hypothesized that hyperventilation might exert a protective effect in focal cerebral ischemia by vasoconstricting normal cerebral vessels, thereby shunting blood from normal tissue to the ischemic area (Robin Hood steal).[377] Hyperventilation begun before experimental focal ischemia has been shown to decrease the incidence of cerebral infarction.[378] However, it has no effect if begun after ischemia.[379,380] Conversely, it has been reported that increased $PaCO_2$ improved CBF in areas of ischemia.[381] Because of these conflicting reports, hyperventilation is rarely used as a method for improving outcome from focal cerebral ischemia except in the presence of increased ICP.

Hypertension

Cerebral ischemia interferes with normal cerebrovacular reactivity such that autoregulation is lost. CBF then becomes pressure dependent, that is, any decrease or increase in cerebral perfusion pressure will be accompanied by a parallel change in CBF. In focal ischemia, neurologic outcome is improved, and infarct size is decreased when CBF is improved with moderately induced hypertension.[382–384] It has also been demonstrated that moderately induced hypertension in patients who have developed focal cerebral ischemia can improve CBF to the ischemic area[385,386] and improve neurologic function.[387] Cerebral vasospasm occurring as a consequence of SAH is usually accompanied by ischemia and disturbed autoregulation. Several studies have demonstrated that both CBF and abnormalities in neurologic function resulting from vasospasm can be improved by increasing arterial pressure.[388–393]

Induced hypertension may be effective in protecting the brain from ischemia only if cerebral perfusion pressure is raised before endothelial cells and the BBB have been damaged by the ischemia.[394] If hypertension is induced after these cells are injured and the BBB damaged, the raised cerebral arterial pressure may cause extravasation of blood and fluid into ischemic tissue, which would result in intracerebral hemorrhage, increased cerebral swelling, intracranial hypertension, and an exacerbation of the ischemia.[394] The efficacy of induced hypertension to treat focal ischemia will depend on a combination of factors including timing, an intact BBB, extent of impaired autoregulation in the area of ischemia, and the appropriate blood pressure elevation.

Hypervolemia

Although there is little evidence to substantiate a direct relationship between intravascular volume and CBF,[395,396] expansion of intravascular volume by colloid infusion has been commonly used to treat focal cerebral ischemia.[397,398] Colloid intravascular volume expansion together with induced hypertension have been used to improve CBF to the ischemic area and improve neurologic outcome in patients with vasospasm and focal ischemia after SAH.[390,392,399]

Hemodilution

Factors that determine the viscosity of blood include hematocrit, erythrocyte aggregation, erythrocyte flexibility, platelet aggregation, and plasma viscosity.[394] During and after cerebral ischemia blood viscosity increases as a result of low blood flow and a shift in electrolytes and water from plasma to tissue. Theoretically, hemodilution would decrease blood viscosity and improve cerebral perfusion during and after ischemia. There are three types of hemodilution depending on the amount of volume expansion. These are hypovolemic, isovolemic, and hypervolemic hemodilution.[400] Hypovolemic hemodilution is produced by phlebotomy and less fluid replacement. Isovolemic hemodilution is produced by exchanging fluid for blood. Hypervolemic hemodilution is produced by infusion of fluid (colloid or crystalloid) into the circulation. Hypervolemic hemodilution has been commonly used in patients with focal ischemia and has been shown to improve cerebral perfusion of ischemic brain and to decrease neurologic deficits.[388,389,401,402]

CLINICAL RECOMMENDATIONS

When a temporary episode of incomplete or focal ischemia is anticipated intraoperatively, as during carotid endarterectomy, aneurysm procedures requiring transient occlusion of the parent artery, extracranial to intracranial bypass procedures, profound induced hypotension, and cardiopulmonary bypass procedures requiring an open ventricle, several factors can be optimized in the perioperative period to maximize cerebral protection. These include anesthetic agent, mean arterial pressure, blood glucose level, and temperature.

During focal or incomplete cerebral ischemia, electrical activity persists and agents that reduce cerebral metabolism by decreasing neuronal activity should provide some protective effects. The prophylactic use of thiopental has been recommended for brain protection in situations of possible temporary focal or incomplete ischemia. Induced hypertension has been demonstrated to provide some degree of protection during focal ischemia if autoregulation is abolished and CBF becomes passively dependent upon cerebral perfusion pressure. It is recommended that the mean arterial blood pressure be increased by 10 to 20 percent with a phenylephrine infusion in an attempt to increase CBF. Another important consideration during the perioperative period is the blood (and hence the brain) glucose level. Because elevated glucose levels appear to aggravate the effects of cerebral ischemia, it is recommended that patients at risk for temporary focal or incomplete ischemia not receive glucose-containing solutions in the perioperative period and that blood glucose levels be routinely monitored. The administration of insulin to normalize blood glucose levels before, during, or after a potentially ischemic event has not been well studied but is a recommended practice.

There is now enough animal data demonstrating protection from cerebral ischemia by mild hypothermia that its use is recommended for patients at risk for ischemia intraoperatively. However, normothermia should be achieved once the risk of ischemia is over. Intraoperative complete global ischemia is fortunately uncommon. Currently there is little that can be done to improve neurologic outcome following complete ischemia other than prompt and aggressive resuscitation. During episodes of either complete or focal ischemia, it is important not to overlook the basics of adequate oxygenation and ventilation and cardiovascular stability.

SUMMARY

The impact of cerebral ischemia in human disease makes understanding the mechanisms by which ischemia produces irreversible cell damage of utmost importance. In the past few years there has been a flurry of research into the pathogenesis of this ischemia. Studies have indicated not only that processes occurring during ischemia contribute to cell injury, but that events occurring after restoration of the cerebral circulation are associated with secondary processes that also contribute to cell injury and ultimate neurologic damage. These and other yet to be determined mechanisms must be explored and elucidated. This will aid the clinician in making rational choices about therapy either for prevention of cerebral ischemia or for treatment to prevent irreversible cell damage once the ischemia has occurred.

References

1. Catterall WA: The molecular basis of neuronal excitability. Science 223:653, 1984
2. Raine CS: Neurocellular anatomy. p. 21. In Siegel GJ, Albers RW, Agranoff BW et al (eds): Basic Neurochemistry. Little, Brown, Boston, 1981
3. Siesjö BK: Cerebral circulation and metabolism. J Neurosurg 60:883, 1984
4. Siegel GJ, Stahl WL, Swanson PD: Ion transport.

p. 107. In Siegel GJ, Albers RW, Agranoff BW et al (eds): Basic Neurochemistry. Little, Brown, Boston, 1981
5. Siesjö BK: Calcium-mediated processes in neuronal degeneration. Ann NY Acad Sci 747:140, 1994
6. New W, Jr: Cellular mechanisms: a clinical view. p. 45. In Ream AK, Fogdall RP (eds): Acute Cardiovascular Management: Anesthesia and Intensive Care. Lippincott-Raven, Philadelphia, 1982
7. Cafe C, Torri C, Marzatico F: Cellular and molecular events of ischemic brain damage. Functional Neurol 8:121, 1993
8. Roos A, Boron WF: Intracellular pH. Physiol Rev 61:296, 1981
9. Fiskum G: Mitochondrial damage during cerebral ischemia. Ann Emerg Med 14:840, 1985
10. Astrup J: Energy-requiring cell functions in the ischemic brain. Their critical supply and possible inhibition in protective therapy. J Neurosurg 56:482, 1982
11. Michenfelder JD: The interdependency of cerebral function and metabolic effects following massive doses of thiopental in the dog. Anesthesiology 41:231, 1974
12. Messick JM, Jr, Milde LN: Brain protection. In Stoelting RK (ed): Advances in Anesthesia. Year Book Medical Publishers, Chicago, 1987
13. Siesjö BK: Utilization of substrates by brain tissues. p. 110. In: Brain Energy Metabolism. John Wiley & Sons, New York, 1978
14. Lewis LD, Ljunggren B, Norberg K, Siesjö BK: Changes in carbohydrate substrates, amino acids, and ammonia in the brain during insulin-induced hypoglycemia. J Neurochem 23:659, 1974
15. Randle PJ, Garland PB, Hales CN et al: Interactions of metabolism and the physiological role of insulin. p. 1. In Pincus Gt(ed): Recent Progress in Hormone Research. Vol. 22. Academic Press, San Diego, 1966
16. Newsholme EA, Start C: Regulation in Metabolism. p. 1. John Wiley & Sons, London, 1973
17. Rafaelson OJ: Studies on a direct effect of insulin on the central nervous system: a review. Metabolism 10:99, 1961
18. Crone C: Facilitated transfer of glucose from blood into brain tissue. J Physiol 181:103, 1965
19. Buschiazzo PM, Terrell EB, Regen DM: Sugar transport across the blood-brain barrier. Am J Physiol 219:1505, 1970
20. Gilboe DD, Andrews RL, Dardenne G: Factors affecting glucose uptake by the isolated dog brain. Am J Physiol 219:767, 1970
21. Daniel PM, Love ER, Pratt OE: Insulin and the way the brain handles glucose. J Neurochem 25:471, 1975
22. Hofer, RE, Lanier WL: The effects of insulin infusion on plasma and brain glucose in hyperglycemic diabetic rats. A comparison with placebo-treated diabetic and non-diabetic rats. Anesthesiology 75:673 1991
23. Lajtha AL, Maker HS, Clarke DD: Metabolism and transport of carbohydrates and amino acids. p. 329. In Siegel GJ, Albers RW, Agranoff BW et al (eds): Basic Neurochemistry. Little, Brown, Boston, 1981
24. Raichle ME: The pathophysiology of brain ischemia. Ann Neurol 13:2, 1983
25. Rehncrona S, Folbergrova J, Smith DS, Siesjö BK: Influence of complete and pronounced incomplete cerebral ischemia and subsequent recirculation on cortical concentrations of oxidized and reduced glutathione in the rat. J Neurochem 34:477, 1980
26. Rehncrona S, Rosen I, Siesjö BK: Excessive cellular acidosis: an important mechanism of neuronal damage in the brain. Acta Physiol Scand 110:435, 1980
27. Astrup J, Siesjö Bk, Symon L: Thresholds in cerebral ischemia—the ischemic penumbra. Stroke 12:723, 1981
28. Symon L, Pasztor E, Branston NM: The distribution and density of reduced cerebral blood flow following acute middle cerebral artery occlusion: an experimental study by the technique of hydrogen clearance in baboons. Stroke 5:355, 1974
29. Astrup J, Symon L, Branston NM, Lassen NA: Cortical evoked potential and extracellular K^+ and H^+ at critical levels of brain ischemia. Stroke 8:51, 1977
30. Heiss WD: Flow thresholds of functional and morphological damage of brain tissue. Stroke 14:329, 1983
31. Sharbrough FW, Messick JM, Jr, Sundt TM Jr: Correlation of continuous electroencephalograms with cerebral blood flow measurements during carotid endarterectomy. Stroke 4:674, 1973
32. McKay RD, Sundt TM, Michenfelder JD et al: Internal carotid artery stump pressure and cerebral blood flow during carotid endarterectomy:

modification by halothane, enflurane, and Innovar. Ansthesiology 45:390, 1976

33. Messick JM, Jr, Casement B, Sharbrough FW et al: Correlation of regional cerebral blood flow (rCBF) with EEG changes during isoflurane anesthesia for carotid endarterectomy: critical rCBF. Anesthesiology 66:344, 1987
34. Branston NM, Strong AJ, Symon L: Extracellular potassium activity, evoked potential and tissue blood flow. Relationships during progressive ischemia in baboon cerebral cortex. J Neurol Sci 32:305, 1977
35. Jones TH, Morawetz RB, Crowell RM et al: Thresholds of focal cerebral ischemia in awake monkeys. J Neurosurg 54:773, 1981
36. Hossmann KA: Post-ischemic resuscitation of the brain: Selective vulnerability versus global resistance. Prog Brain Res 63:3, 1985
37. Collins RC, Dobkin BH, Choi DW: Selective vulnerability of the brain: new insights into the pathophysiology of stroke. Ann Int Med 110:992, 1989
38. Jorgensen MB: The role of signal transduction in the delayed necrosis of the hippocampal CA1 pyramidal cells following transient ischemia. Acta Neurol Scand 143:1, 1993
39. Sims N: Energy metabolism and selective neuronal vulnerability following global cerebral ischemia. Neurochem Res 17:923, 1992
40. Cao W, Carney JM, Duchon A et al: Oxygen free radical involvement in ischemia and reperfusion injury to the brain. Neurosci Lett 88:233, 1988
41. Rehncrona S, Kagstrom E: Tissue lactic acidosis and ischemic brain damage. Am J Emerg Med 1:168, 1983
42. Bulkey GB: Free radical-mediated reperfusion injury: a selective review. Br J Cancer, suppl. VIII, 55:66, 1987
43. Ames A, Wright RL, Kowada M et al: Cerebral ischemia. II. The no-reflow phenomenon. Am J Pathol 52:437, 1968
44. Fischer EG, Ames A: Studies on mechanisms of impairment of cerebral circulation following ischemia: effect of hemodilution and perfusion pressure. Stroke 3:538, 1973
45. Arsenio-Nunes ML, Hossmann K-A, Farkas-Bargeton E: Ultrastructural and histochemical investigation of the cerebral cortex of cat during and after complete ischemia. Acta Neuropathol 26:329, 1973
46. Hossmann K-A, Hossmann V: Coagulopathy following experimental cerebral ischemia. Stroke 8:249, 1977
47. Kagstrom E, Smith M-L, Siesjö BK: Local cerebral blood flow in the recovery period following complete ischemia in the rat. J Cereb Blood Flow Metab 3:170, 1983
48. Beckstead JE, Tweed WA, Lee J, MacKeen WL: Cerebral blood flow and metabolism in man following cardiac arrest. Stroke 9:569, 1978
49. Steen PA, Newberg LA, Milde JH, Michenfelder JD: Nimodipine improves cerebral blood flow and neurologic recovery after complete cerebral ischemia in the dog. J Cereb Blood Flow Metab 3:38, 1983
50. Paschen W, Djuricic BM, Bosma H-J, Hossmann K-A: Biochemical changes during graded ischemia in gerbils. 2. Regional evaluation of cerebral blood flow and brain metabolites. J Neurol Sci 58:37, 1983
51. Hossmann K-A, Zimmermann V: Resuscitation of the monkey brain after 1 hour complete ischemia. I. Physiological and morphological observations. Brain Res 81:49, 1974
52. Vanhoutte PM: Calcium entry blockers, vascular smooth muscle, and systemic hypertension. Am J Cardiol, suppl. B 55:17, 1985
53. del Zoppo GJ: Microvascular changes during cerebral ischemia and reperfusion. Cerebrovasc Brain Metab Rev 6:47, 1994
54. Hallenbeck JM: Blood-damaged tissue interaction in experimental brain ischemia. Acta Neurochir 60:233, 1994
55. Bircher NG: Ischemic brain protection. Ann Emerg Med 14:784, 1985
56. Astrup J, Sorensen P, Rahbek Sorensen H: Inhibition of cerebral oxygen and glucose consumption in the dog by hypothermia, pentobarbital, and lidocaine. Anesthesiology 55:263, 1984
57. Hillered L, Ernster L, Siesjö BK: Influence of in vitro lactic acidosis and hypercapnia on respiratory activity of isolated rat brain mitochondria. J Cereb Blood Flow Metab 4:430, 1984
58. Hamud F, Fiskum G: Loss of maximal respiratory and Ca^{++} uptake capacities by rat brain mitochondria during cerebral ischemia. Biophys J 47:414a, 1985
59. Kagstrom E, Smith M-L, Siesjö BK: Recirculation in the rat brain following incomplete ischemia. J Cereb Blood Flow Metab 3:183, 1983
60. Lundggren B, Norberg K, Siesjö BK: Influence of tissue acidosis upon restitution of brain energy

metabolism following total ischemia. Brain Res 77:173, 1974
61. Siesjö BK: Cell damage in the brain: a speculative synthesis. J Cereb Blood Flow Metab 1:155, 1981
62. Zimmer R, Lang R: Rates of lactic acid permeation and utilization in the isolated dog brain. Am J Physiol 299:432, 1975
63. Welsh FA, Ginsberg MD, Rieder W, Budd WW: Deleterious effect of glucose pretreatment on recovery from diffuse cerebral ischemia in the cat. II. Regional metabolite level. Stroke 11:355, 1980
64. Nordstrom C-H, Rehncrona S, Siesjö BK: Effects of phenobarbital in cerebral ischemia. II. Restitution of cerebral energy state, as well as glycolytic metabolites, citric acid cycle intermediates and associated amino acids. Stroke 9:335, 1978
65. Yoshida S, Busto R, Martinez E et al: Regional brain energy metabolism after complete versus incomplete ischemia in the rat in the absence of severe lactic acidosis. J Cereb Blood Flow Metab 5:490, 1985
66. Hossmann K-A, Lechtape-Gruter H, Hossmann V: The role of cerebral blood flow for the recovery of the brain after prolonged ischemia. Z Neurol 204:281, 1973
67. Plum F: What causes infarction in ischemic brain? The Robert Wartenberg lecture. Neurology 33:222, 1983
68. Smith M-L, von Hanwehr R, Siesjö BK: Changes in extra- and intracellular pH in the brain during and following ischemia in hyperglycemic and in moderately hypoglycemic rats. J Cereb Blood Flow Metab 6:574, 1986
69. Marsh WR, Anderson RE, Sundt TM Jr: Effect of hyperglycemia on brain pH levels in areas of focal incomplete cerebral ischemia in monkeys. J Neurosurg 65:693, 1986
70. Chopp M, Frinak S, Walton DR et al: Intracellular acidosis during and after cerebral ischemia: in vivo nuclear magnetic resonance study of hyperglycemia in cats. Stroke 18:919, 1987
71. Combs DJ, Dempsey RJ, Maley M et al: Relationship between plasma glucose, brain lactate, and intracellular pH during cerebral ischemia in gerbils. Stroke 21:936, 1990
72. Pulsinelli W, Waldman S, Sigsbee B et al: Experimental hyperglycemia and diabetes mellitus worsen stroke outcome. Trans Am Neurol Assoc 105:21, 1980
73. Kraig RP, Chesler M: Astrocytic acidosis in hyperglycemia and complete ischemia. J Cereb Blood Flow Metab 10:104, 1990
74. Pulsinelli WA, Waldman S, Rawlinson D, Plum F: Moderate hyperglycemia augments ischemic brain damage: a neuropathologic study in the rat. Neurology 32:1239, 1982
75. Sieber FE, Koehler RC, Brown PR et al: Diabetic chronic hyperglycemia and cerebral pH recovery following global ischemia in dogs. Stroke 25:1449, 1994
76. Hsu SS, Meno JR, Zhou JG et al: Influence of hyperglycemia on cerebral adenosine production during ischemia and reperfusion. Am J Physiol 261:H398, 1991
77. Phillis JW, Simpson RE, Walter GA: The effect of hyperglycemia on extracellular levels of adenosine in the hypoxic rat cerebral cortex. Brain Res 524:336, 1990
78. Corradetti R, Lo Conte G, Moroni F et al: Adenosine decreases aspartate and glutamate release from rat hippocampal slices. Eur J Pharmacol 104:19, 1984
79. Cronstein BN, Rosenstein ED, Kramer SB et al: Adenosine: a physiologic modulator of superoxide anion generation by human neutrophils. Adenosine acts via an A2 receptor on human neutrophils. J Immunol 135:1366, 1985
80. Choi KT, Illievich UM, Zornow MH et al: Effect of hyperglycemia on peri-ischemic neurotransmitter levels in rabbit hippocampus. Brain Res 642:104, 1994
81. Dietrich WD, Alonso O, Busto, R: Moderate hyperglycemia worsens acute blood-brain barrier injury after forebrain ischemia in rats. Stroke 24:111, 1993
82. Ginsberg MD, Welsh FA, Budd WW: Deleterious effect of glucose pretreatment on recovery from diffuse cerebral ischemia in the cat. I. Local cerebral blood flow and glucose utilization. Stroke 11:347, 1980
83. Duckrow RB, Beard DC, Brennan RW: Regional cerebral blood flow decreased during chronic and acute hyperglycemia. Stroke 18:52, 1987
84. Harik SI, LaManna JC: Vascular perfusion and blood-brain glucose transport in acute and chronic hyperglycemia. J Neurochem 51:1924, 1988
85. Sieber FE, Traystman RJ: Special issues: glucose and the brain. Crit Care Med 20:104, 1992
86. Siemkowicz E, Hansen AJ: Clinical restitution following cerebral ischemia in hypo-, normo-,

and hyperglycemic rats. Acta Neurol Scand 58:1, 1978
87. Lanier WL, Stangland KJ, Scheithauer BW et al: The effects of dextrose infusion and head position on neurologic outcome after complete cerebral ischemia in primates: examination of a model. Anesthesiology 66:39, 1987
88. Myers RE, Yamaguchi S: Nervous system effects of cardiac arrest in monkeys. Preservation of vision. Arch Neurol 34:65, 1977
89. D'Alecy LG, Lundy EF, Barton KJ, Zelenock GB: Dextrose containing intravenous fluid impairs outcome and increases death after eight minutes of cardiac arrest and resuscitation in dogs. Surgery 100:505, 1986
90. Strong AJ, Miller SA, West IC: Protection of respiration of a crude mitochondrial preparation in cerebral ischaemia by control of blood glucose. J Neurol Neurosurg Psychiatry 48:450, 1985
91. Longstreth WT, Jr, Inui TS: High blood glucose level on hospital admission and poor neurological recovery after cardiac arrest. Ann Neurol 15:59, 1984
92. Longstreth WT, Jr, Diehr P, Inui TS: Prediction of awakening after out-of-hospital cardiac arrest. N Engl J Med 308:1378, 1983
93. Browning RG, Olson DW, Stueven HA et al: 50% dextrose: antidote or toxin? Ann Emerg Med 19:683, 1990
94. Nedergaard M: Transient focal ischemia in hyperglycemic rats is associated with increased cerebral infarction. Brain Res 408:79, 1987
95. Pulsinelli WA, Levy DE, Sigsbee B et al: Increased damage after ischemic stroke in patients with hyperglycemia with or without established diabetes mellitus. Am J Med 74:540, 1983
96. Berger L, Hakim A: The association of hyperglycemia with cerebral edema in stroke. Stroke 17:865, 1986
97. Cox NH, Lorains JW: The prognostic value of blood glucose and glycosylated haemoglobin estimation in patients with stroke. Postgrad Med J 62:7, 1986
98. DeCourten-Myers G, Myers RE, Schoolfield L: Hyperglycemia enlarges infarct size in cerebrovascular occlusion in cats. Stroke 19:623, 1988
99. Hoffman WE, Braucher E, Pelligrino DA et al: Brain lactate and neurologic outcome following incomplete ischemia in fasted, nonfasted, and glucose-loaded rats. Anesthesiology 72:1045, 1990
100. Nedergaard M, Diemer NH: Focal ischemia of the rat brain with special reference to the influence of plasma glucose concentration. Acta Neuropathol 73:131, 1987
101. Prado R, Ginsberg MD, Dietrich WD et al: Hyperglycemia increases infarct size in collaterally perfused but not end-arterial vascular territories. J Cereb Blood Flow Metab 8:186, 1988
102. Woo E, Chan YW, Yu YL et al: Admission glucose level in relation to mortality and morbidity outcome in 252 stroke patients. Stroke 19:185, 1988
103. Siesjö BK, Katsura K, Kristian T: The biochemical basis of cerebral ischemic damage. J Neurosurg Anesth 7:47, 1995
104. White BC, Wiegenstein JG, Winegar CD: Brain ischemic anoxia. Mechanisms of injury. JAMA 251:1586, 1984
105. Heistad DD: Protection of the blood-brain barrier during acute and chronic hypertension. Fed Proc 43:205, 1984
106. Cottrell JE: Possible mechanisms of pharmacological neuronal protection. J Neurosurg Anesth 7:33, 1995
107. Wolfe LS: Eicosanoids: prostaglandins, thromboxanes, leukotrienes, and other derivatives of carbon-20 unsaturated fatty acids. J Neurochem 38:1, 1982
108. Wieloch T, Siesjö BK: Ischemic brain injury: the importance of calcium, lipolytic activities, and free fatty acids. J Pathol Biol 5:269, 1982
109. Egan RW, Paxton J, Kuehl FA: Mechanism for irreversible self-deactivation of prostaglandin synthetase. J Biol Chem 257:7329, 1976
110. van den Kerckhoff W, Hossmann K-A, Hossman V: No effect of prostacyclin on blood flow, regulation of blood flow and blood coagulation following global cerebral ischemia. Stroke 14:724, 1983
111. DeWitt DS, Kong DL, Lyeth BG et al: Experimental traumatic brain injury elevates brain prostaglandin E_2 and thromboxane B_2 levels in rats. J Neurotrauma 5:303, 1988
112. Kong DL, Prough DS, Whitley JM et al: Hemorrhage and intracranial hypertension in combination increase cerebral production of thromboxane A_2. Crit Care Med 19:532, 1991
113. Rehncrona s, Westerberg E, Akesson B, Siesjö BK: Brain cortical fatty acids and phospholipids during and following complete and severe incomplete ischemia. J Neurochem 38:84, 1982
114. Dempsey RJ, Roy MW, Meyer KL, Donaldson

DL: Indomethacin-mediated improvement following middle cerebral artery occlusion in cats. J Neurosurg 62:874, 1985
115. Hallenbeck JM, Furlow TW: Prostaglandin I_2 and indomethacin prevent impairment of post-ischemic brain reperfusion in the dog. Stroke 10:629, 1979
116. Boulu RG, Plotkine M, Gueniau C et al: Effect of indomethacin in experimental cerebral ischemia. J Pathol Biol 30:278, 1982
117. Grice SC, Chappell ET, Prough DS et al: Ibuprofen improves cerebral blood flow after global cerebral ischemia in dogs. Stroke 18:787, 1987
118. Stevens MK, Yaksh TL, Hansen RB, Anderson RE: The effect of cyclo-oxygenase inhibition by zomepirac sodium on reflow, cerebral autoregulation and EEG recovery in the cat after global ischemia. J Cereb Blood Flow Metab 6:691, 1986
119. Prough DS, Kong D, Watkins WD et al: Inhibition of thromboxane A_2 production does not improve post-ischemic brain hypoperfusion in the dog. Stroke 17:1272, 1986
120. Clark IA, Cowden WB, Hunt NH: Free radical induced pathology. Med Res Rev 5:297, 1985
121. Freeman BA, Crapo JD: Biology of disease: free radicals and tissue injury. Lab Invest 47:412, 1982
122. Fuller BJ, Gower JD, Green CJ: Free radical damage and organ preservation: fact or fiction? Cryobiology 25:377, 1988
123. Floyd RA: Role of oxygen free radicals in carcinogensesis and brain ischemia. FASEB J 4:2587, 1990
124. Watson BD, Ginsberg MD: Ischemic injury in the brain: role of oxygen radical-mediated processes. Ann NY Acad Sci 559:269, 1989
125. Evans PH: Free radicals in brain metabolism and pathology. Br Med Bull 49:577, 1993
126. Hall ED: Cerebral ischaemia, free radicals and antioxidant protection. Biochem Soc Trans 21:334, 1993
127. Siesjo BK, Katsura K: Ischemic brain damage: focus on lipids and lipid mediators. Adv Exp Med Biol 318:41, 1992
128. DelMaestro RF: An approach to free radicals in medicine and biology. Acta Physiol Scand 492:153, 1980
129. White BC, Aust SD, Arforsk E, Aronson LD: Brain injury by ischemic anoxia: hypothesis extension—a tale of two ions? Ann Emerg Med 13:862, 1984
130. Cerchiari EL, Hoel TM, Safar P, Sclabassi RJ: Protective effects of combined superoxide dismutase and deferoxamine on recovery of cerebral blood flow and function after cardiac arrest in dogs. Stroke 18:869, 1987
131. Schmidley JW: Free radicals in central nervous system ischemia. Stroke 21:1086, 1990
132. Brown K, Fridovich I: Superoxide radical and superoxide dismutase: threat and defense. Acta Physiol Scand, (suppl) 492:9, 1980
133. Halliwell B, Gutteridge JMC: Oxygen free radicals and the nervous system. Trends Neurosci 8:22, 1985
134. Southorn PA, Powis G: Free radicals in medicine. I. Chemical nature and biologic reactions. Mayo Clin Proc 63:381, 1988
135. Southorn PA, Powis G: Free radicals in medicine. II. Involvement in human disease. Mayo Clin Proc 63:390, 1988
136. Siesjö BK: Brain cell death in aging and ischemia: are free radicals involved? Monogr Neurol Sci 11:1, 1984
137. Hall ED: The role of oxygen radicals in traumatic injury: clinical implications. J Emerg Med (suppl) 11:31, 1993
138. Babbs CF: Role of iron ions in the genesis of reperfusion injury following successful cardiopulmonary resuscitation: preliminary data and a biochemical hypothesis. Ann Emerg Med 14:777, 1985
139. Yamasaki Y, Kogure K: Possible contribution of free radicals and lipid peroxidations on pathogenesis of post-ischemic brain damage. Hum Cell 5:341, 1992
140. Kirsch JR, Hellfaer MA, Lange DG, Traystman RJ: Evidence for free radical mechanisms of brain injury resulting from ischemia/reperfusion-induced events. J Neurotrauma, (suppl) 9:S157, 1992
141. Traystman RJ, Kirsch JR, Koehler RC: Oxygen radical mechanisms of brain injury following ischemia and reperfusion. J Appl Physiol 71:1185, 1991
142. Hall ED, Braughler JM: Central nervous system trauma and stroke. II. Physiological and pharmacological evidence for involvement of oxygen radicals and lipid peroxidation. Free Rad Biol Med 6:303, 1989
143. Hall ED, Pazara E, Braugler JM: 21-Aminosteroid lipid peroxidation inhibitor U74006F protects against cerebral ischemia in gerbils. Stroke 19:997, 1987
144. Hall ED, Yonkers PA: Attenuation of postis-

chemic cerebral hypoperfusion by the 21-aminosteroid U47006F. Stroke 19:340, 1988
145. Yip PK, He YY, Hsu CY et al: Effect of plasma glucose on infarct size in focal cerebral ischemia-reperfusion. Neurology 41:899, 1991
146. Meldrum B: Possible therapeutic applications of antagonists of excitatory amino acid neurotransmitters. Clin Sci 68:113, 1985
147. Choi DW: Glutamate neurotoxicity and diseases of the nervous system. Neuron 1:623, 1988
148. Clark GD: Role of excitatory amino acids in brain injury caused by hypoxia-ischemia, status epilepticus, and hypoglycemia. Clin Perinatal 16:459, 1989
149. Fonnum F: Glutamate: a neurotransmitter in mammalian brain. J Neurochem 42:1, 1984
150. Hertz L: Functional interactions between neurons and astrocytes. I. Turnover and metabolism of putative amino acid transmitters. Prog Neurobiol 13:277, 1979
151. Storm-Mathisen J, Iversen L: Uptake of [3H]glutamic acid in excitatory nerve endings: light and electron microscopic observations in the hippocampal formation of the rat. Neuroscience 4:1237, 1987
152. Drejer J, Benveniste H, Diemer NH et al: Cellular origin of ischemia-induced glutamate release from brain tissue in vivo and in vitro. J Neurochem 45:145, 1985
153. Silverstein FS, Buchanan K, Johnston MV: Perinatal hypoxia-ischaemia disrupts striatal high-affinity [^{3}H] glutamate uptake into synaptosomes. J Neurochem 47:1614, 1982
154. Benveniste H: Brain microdialysis. J Neurochem 52:1667, 1989
155. Benveniste H: The excitotoxin hypothesis in relation to cerebral ischemia. Cerebrovasc Brain Metab Rev 3:1213, 1991
156. Benveniste H, Huttemeier PC: Microdialysis—theory and application. Prog Neurobiol 35:195, 1990
157. Barnes DM: NMDA receptors trigger excitement. Science 239:254, 1988
158. Albers GW, Goldberg MP, Choi DW: *N*-Methyl-D-aspartate antagonists: ready for clinical trial in brain ischemia? Ann Neurol 25:398, 1989
159. Choi DW: Ionic dependence of glutamate neurotoxicity in cortical cell culture. J Neurosci 7:369, 1987
160. Choi DW, Koh J, Peters S: Pharmacology of glutamate neurotoxicity in cortical cell culture attenuation by NMDA antagonists. J Neurosci 8:185, 1988
161. Olney JW, Price MT, Samson L et al: The role of specific ions in glutamate neurotoxicity. Neurosci Lett 65:65, 1986
162. Rothman SM: The neurotoxicity of excitatory amino acid is produced by passive chloride influx. J Neurosci 5:1483, 1985
163. Murphy SN, Thayer SA, Miller RJ: The effects of excitatory amino acids on intracellular calcium in single mouse striatal neurons in vitro. J Neurosci 7:4145, 1987
164. Kironi T: Delayed neuronal death in the gerbil hippocampus following ischemia. Brain Res 239:57, 1982
165. Petito CK, Feldmann E, Pulsinelli WA et al: Delayed hippocampal damage in humans following cardiorespiratory arrest. Neurology 37:1281, 1987
166. Pulsinelli WA, Brierly JB, Plum F: Temporal profile of neuronal damage in a model of transient forebrain ischemia. Ann Neurol 11:491, 1982
167. Collins RC: Selective vulnerability of brain: new insights from the excitatory synapse. Metab Br Dis 1:231, 1986
168. Beneviste H, Dreger J, Schousboe A, Diemer NH: Elevation of the extracellular concentrations of glutamate and aspartate in rat hippocampus during transient cerebral ischemia monitored by intracellular microdialysis. J Neurochem 43:1369, 1984
169. Suzuki R, Yamaguchi T, Li CL et al: The effects of 5-minute ischemia in Mongolian gerbils. II. Changes of spontaneous neuronal activity in cerebral cortex and CA1 sector of hippocampus. Acta Neuropathol 60:217, 1983
170. Wieloch T, Gusafsson I, Westerberg E: MK-801 does not protect against brain damage in a rat model of cerebral ischemia. Neurochem Int 12:24, 1988
171. Kass IS, Lipton P: Mechanisms involved in irreversible anoxic damage to the in vitro hippocampal slice. J Physiol 332:459, 1982
172. Rothman SM: Synaptic activity mediates death of hypoxic neurons. Science 220:536, 1983
173. Meldrum BS, Evans MC, Swan JH et al: Protection against hypoxic/ischaemic brain damage with excitatory amino acid antagonists. Med Biol 65:153, 1987
174. Collingridge GL, Bliss TV: NMDA receptors—their role in long term potentiation. Trends Neurosci 10:288, 1988

175. Albers GW: Potential therapeutic uses of *N*-methyl-D-aspartate antagonists in cerebral ischemia. Clin Neuropharmacol 13:177, 1990
176. Michenfelder JD, Lanier WL, Scheithauer BW et al: Evaluation of the glutamate antagonist dizocilipine maleate (MK-801) on neurologic outcome in a canine model of complete cerebral ischemia: correlation with hippocampal histopathology. Brain Res 481:228, 1989
177. Simon RP, Swan JH, Griffiths T et al: Blockage of *N*-methyl-D-aspartate receptors may protect against ischemic damage in the brain. Science 226:850, 1984
178. Foster AC, Gill R, Iverson LL et al: Systemic administration of MK-801 protects against ischaemia-induced hippocampal neurodegeneration in the gerbil. Br J Pharmacol 90:9P, 1987
179. McDonald JW, Silverstein FS, Johnston MV: MK-801 protects the neonatal brain from hypoxic-ischemic damage. Eur J Pharmacol 140:359, 1987
180. Simon RP, Bartkowski H, Roman R: Attenuation of infarct size by pharmacologic inhibition of excitatory amino acid neurotransmission by specific NMDA antagonist administered 15 minutes after stroke. Neurology 38:147, 1988
181. Steinberg GK, Saleh J, Kunis D: Delayed treatment with dextromethorphan and dextorphan reduces cerebral damage after transient focal ischemia. Neurosci Lett 89:193, 1988
182. Himori N, Tanaka Y, Kurasawa M et al: Dextorphan attenuates the behavioral consequences of ischemia and the biochemical cqnsequences of anoxia: possible role of N-methyl-D-aspartate receptor antagonism and ATP replenishing action in its cerebroprotecting profile. Psychopharmacology 111:152, 1993
183. Boast CA, Gerhardt SC, Pastor G et al: The *N*-methyl-D-aspartate antagonists CGS 19755 and CPP reduce ischemic brain damage in gerbils. Brain Res 442:345, 1988
184. Boast CA, Gerhardt SC, Janak P: Systemic AP7 reduces ischemic brain damage in gerbils. p. 249. In Hicks TP, Lodge D, McLennan H (eds): Excitatory Amino Acid Transmission. Alan R Liss, New York, 1987
185. Wieloch T, Lindvall O, Blomquist P et al: Evidence for amelioration of ischemic neuronal damage in hippocampal formation by lesions of the perforant path. Neurol Res 7:24, 1985
186. Albers GW, Goldeberg MP, Choi DW: Do NMDA antagonists prevent neuronal injury? Yes. Arch Neurol 49:418, 1992
187. Rothman SM, Olney JW: Glutamate and the pathophysiology of hypoxic-ischemic brain damage. Ann Neurol 19:105, 1986
188. Patel JB, Ross LE, Duncan B et al: Administration of glycine antagonists, HA-966 and 7-chlorokynurenic acid reduce ischemic brain damage in gerbils. Soc Neurosci Abstr 15:43, 1989
189. Hartley DM, Monyer H, Colamarino SA et al: 7-Chloro-kynurenate blocks NMDA receptor-mediated neurotoxicity in cortical cell cultures. Soc Neurosci Abstr 15:762, 1989
190. Gill R: The pharmacology of alpha-amino-3-hydroxy-5-methyl-4-isoxazole propionate (AMPA)/kainate antagonists and their role in cerebral ischemia. Cerebrovasc Brain Metab Rev 6:223, 1994
191. Gaspary HL, Simon RP, Graham SH: BW1003C87 and NBQX reduce glutamate release and cerebral ischemic necrosis. Eur J Pharmacol 262:197, 1994
192. Buchan AM: Do NMDA antagonists prevent neuronal injury? No. Arch Neurol 49:420, 1992
193. Macrae IM, Dawson DA, Norrie JD, McCulloch J: Inhibition of nitric oxide synthesis: effects on cerebral blood flow and glucose utilization in the rat. J Cereb Blood Flow Metab 13:985, 1993
194. Dawson DA: Nitric oxide and focal cerebral ischemia: multiplicity of actions and divers outcome. Cerebrovasc Brain Metab Rev 6:299, 1994
195. Mattson MP, Scheff SW: Endogenous neuroprotection factors and traumatic brain injury: mechanisms of action and implications for therapy. J Neurotrauma 11:3, 1994
196. Michenfelder JD, Theye RA: Hypothermia: effect on canine brain and whole body metabolism. Anesthesiology 29:1107, 1968
197. Michenfelder JD, Milde JH: The effect of profound levels of hypothermia (below 14°C) on canine cerebral metabolism. J Cereb Blood Flow Metab 12:877, 1992
198. Steen PA, Newberg LA, Milde JH, Michenfelder JD: Hypothermia and barbiturates: individual and combined effects on canine cerebral oxygen consumption. Anesthesiology 58:527, 1983
199. Michenfelder JD, Milde JH: The relationship among canine brain temperature, metabolism, and function during hypothermia. Anesthesiology 75:130, 1991
200. Lanier WL: Cerebral metabolic rate and hy-

pothermia: their relationship with ischemic neurologic injury. J Neurosurg Anesth 7:216, 1995
201. Busto R, Dietrich WD, Globus MY-T et al: Differences in intraischemic brain temperature critically determine the extent of ischemic neuronal injury. J Cereb Blood Flow Metab 7:729, 1987
202. Minamisawa H, Nordstrom CH, Smith ML et al: The influence of mild body and brain hypothermia on ischemic brain damage. J Cereb Blood Flow Metab 10:365, 1990
203. Busto R, Dietrich WD, Globus MY et al: Postischemic moderate hypothermia inhibits CA1 hippocampal ischemic neuronal injury. Neurosci Lett 101:299, 1989
204. Busto R, Globus MY, Dietrich WD et al: Effect of mild hypothermia on ischemia-induced release of neurotransmitters and free fatty acids in rat brain. Stroke 20:904, 1989
205. Warner DS, McFarlane C, Todd MM et al: Sevoflurane and halothane reduce focal ischemic brain damage in the rat: possible influence on thermoregulation. Anesthesiology 79:985, 1993
206. Clifton GL, Jiang JL, Lyeth BG et al: Marked protection by moderate hypothermia after experimental traumatic brain injury. J Cereb Blood Flow Metab 11:114, 1991
207. Berntman L, Welsh FA, Harp JR: Cerebral protective effect of low-grade hypothermia. Anesthesiology 55:495, 1981
208. Zornow MH: Inhibition of glutamate release: a possible mechanism of hypothermic neuroprotection. J Neurosurg Anesth 7:148, 1995
209. Marion DW, Obrist WD, Carlier PM et al: The use of moderate therapeutic hypothermia for patients with severe head injuries: a preliminary report. J Neurosurg 79:354, 1993
210. Shiozaki T, Sugimoto H, Taneda M et al: Effect of mild hypothermia on uncontrollable intracranial hypertension after severe head injury. J Neurosurg 79:363, 1993
211. Clifton GL, Allen S, Barrodale P et al: A phase II study of moderate hypothermia in severe brain injury. J Neurotrauma 10:263, 1993
212. Clifton GL: Systemic hypothermia in treatment of severe brain injury. J Neurosurg Anesth 7:152, 1995
213. Baker KZ, Young WL, Stone G et al: Deliberate mild intraoperative hypothermia for craniotomy. Anesthesiology 81:361, 1994
214. Schubert A: Side effects of mild hypothermia. J Neurosurg Anesth 7:139, 1995
215. Chen RYZ, Chien S: Hemodynamic functions and blood viscosity in surface hypothermia. Am J Physiol 235:H136, 1978
216. Frank SM, Beattie C, Christopherson R et al: Unintentional hypothermia is associated with postoperative myocardial ischemia. Ther Perioperative Ischemia Randomized Anesthesia Trial Study. Anesthesiology 78:468, 1993
217. Leinhart A, Fiez N, Deriaz H: Postoperative shivering: analysis of main associated factors. Ann Fr Anesth Reanim 11:488, 1992
218. Okada M: The cardiac rhythm in accidental hypothermia. J Electrocardiol 17:123, 1984
219. Reuler JB: Hypothermia: pathophysiology, clinical settings, and management. Ann Int Med 89:519, 1978
220. Morales CF, Strollo PJ: Noncardiogenic pulmonary edema associated with accidental hypothermia. Chest 103:971, 1993
221. Valeri CR, Feingold H, Cassidy G et al: Hypothermia-induced reversible platelet dysfunction. Ann Surg 205:175, 1987
222. Patt A, McCroskey BL, Moore EE: Hypothermia-induced coagulopathies in trauma. Surg Clin North Am 68:775, 1988
223. Kalfas IH, Little JR: Postoperative hemorrhage: a survey of 4992 intracranial procedures. Neurosurgery 23:343, 1991
224. Ludbrook J, Wynn V: Citrate intoxication: a clinical and experimental study. Brit Med J 2:523, 1958
225. VanOss CJ, Absolam DR, Moore LL et al: Effect of temperature on chemotaxis, phagocytic engulfment, digestion, and O_2 consumption of human polymorphonuclear leukocytes. J Reticuloendothel Soc 27:561, 1980
226. Sessler DI: Deliberate mild hypothermia. J Neurosurg Anesth 7:38, 1995
227. Sterba JA: Efficacy and safety of prehospital rewarming techniques to treat accidental hypothermia. Ann Emerg Med 20:896, 1991
228. Steen PA, Soule EH, Michenfelder JD: Detrimental effect of prolonged hypothermia in cats and monkeys with and without regional cerebral ischemia. Stroke 10:522, 1979
229. Steen PA, Milde JH, Michenfelder JD: The detrimental effects of prolonged hypothermia and rewarming in the dog. Anesthesiology 52:224, 1980
230. Michenfelder JD, Theye RA: The effects of anes-

thesia and hypothermia on canine cerebral ATP and lactate during anoxia produced by decapitation. Anesthesiology 33:430, 1970
231. Steen PA, Michenfelder JD: Mechanisms of barbiturate protection. Anesthesiology 53:183, 1980
232. Branston NM, Hope DT, Symon L: Barbiturates in focal ischemia of primate cortex: effects on blood flow distribution, evoked potential, and extracellular potassium. Stroke 10:647, 1979
233. Feustal PJ, Ingvar MC, Severinghaus JW: Cerebral oxygen availability and blood flow during middle cerebral artery occlusion: effects of pentobarbital. Stroke 12:858, 1981
234. Corkill G, Sivalingam S, Reitan JA et al: Dose dependency of the post-insult protective effect of pentobarbital in the canine experimental stroke model. Stroke 9:10, 1978
235. Michenfelder JD: Anesthesia and the Brain. p. 95. Churchill Livingstone, New York, 1988
236. Brain Resuscitation Clinical Trial I Study Group: Randomized clinical study of thiopental loading in comatose survivors of cardiac arrest. N Engl J Med 314:397, 1986
237. Yatsu FM: Cardiopulmonary-cerebral resuscitation. N Engl J Med 314:440, 1986
238. Black KL, Weidler DJ, Jallad NS et al: Delayed pentobarbital therapy of acute focal cerebral ischemia. Stroke 9:245, 1978
239. Hankinson HL, Smith AL, Nielsen SL, Hoff JT: Effect of thiopental on focal cerebral ischemia in dogs. Surg Forum 25:445, 1974.
240. Hoff JT, Smith AL, Hankinson HL, Nielsen SL: Barbiturate protection from cerebral infarction in primates. Stroke 6:28, 1975
241. Michenfelder JD, Milde JH, Sundt TM, Jr: Cerebral protection by barbiturate anesthesia use after middle cerebral artery occlusion in Java monkeys. Arch Neurol 33:345, 1976
242. Selman WR, Spetzler RF, Jackson D et al: Regional cerebral blood flow following middle cerebral artery occlusion and barbiturate therapy in baboons. J Cereb Blood Flow Metab 1:S214, 1981
243. Smith AL, Hoff JT, Nielsen SL, Larson CP: Barbiturate protection in acute focal ischemia. Stroke 5:1, 1974
244. Michenfelder JD, Milde JH: Influence of anesthetics on metabolic, functional, and pathologic responses to regional cerebral ischemia. Stroke 6:405, 1975
245. Nilsson L, Siesjö BK: The effect of phenobarbital anesthesia on blood flow and oxygen consumption in the rat brain. Acta Anesthesiol Scand, suppl. 57:18, 1975
246. Ochai C, Asano T, Takakura K et al: Mechanisms of cerebral protection by pentobarbital and nizofenone correlated with the course of local cerebral blood flow changes. Stroke 13:788, 1982
247. Lawner P, Laurent J, Simeone F et al: Attenuation of ischemic brain edema by pentobarbital after carotid ligation in the gerbil. Stroke 10:644, 1979
248. Smith A, Marque J: Anesthetics and cerebral edema. Anesthesiology 45:64, 1976
249. Simeone F, Frazer G, Lawner P: Ischemic brain edema: comparative effects of barbiturates and hypothermia. Stroke 10:8, 1979
250. Michenfelder JD, Milde JH: Cerebral protection by anaesthetics during ischemia (review). Resuscitation 4:219, 1975
251. Levy DE, Brierley JB: Delayed pentobarbital administration limits ischemic brain damage in gerbils. Ann Neurol 5:59, 1979
252. Gelb AW, Floyd R, Lok P et al: A prophylactic bolus of thiopental does not protect against prolonged focal cerebral ischemia. Can Anaesth Soc J 33:173, 1986
253. Nussmeier NA, Arlund C, Slogoff S: Neuropsychiatric complications after cardiopulmonary bypass: cerebral protection by a barbiturate. Anesthesiology 64:165, 1986
254. Zaidan JR, Klochany A, Martin WM et al: Effect of thiopental on neurologic outcome following coronary artery bypass grafting. Anesthesiology 74:406, 1991
255. Gross CE, Adams HP, Jr, Sokoll MD, Yamada MD: Use of anticoagulants, electroencephalographic monitoring and barbiturate cerebral protection in carotid endarterectomy. Neurosurgery 9:1, 1981
256. Hicks RG, Kerr DR, Horton DA: Thiopentone cerebral protection under EEG control during carotid endarterectomy. Anaesth Intensive Care 14:22, 1986
257. Spetzler RF, Martin N, Hadley MN et al: Microsurgical endarterectomy under barbiturate protection: a prospective study. J Neurosurg 65:63, 1986
258. McMeniman WJ, Fletcher JP, Little JM: Experience with barbiturate therapy for cerebral protection during carotid endarterectomy. Ann R Coll Surg Engl 66:361, 1984
259. Ditmore QM, Samson DS, Beyer CW: Traumatic

middle cerebral artery aneurysm: case report. Neurosurgery 6:293, 1980
260. Belopavlovic M, Buchthal A, Beks JWF: Barbiturates for cerebral aneurysm surgery. Acta Neurochir 76:73, 1985
261. Hoff JT, Pitts LH, Spetzler R, Wilson CB: Barbiturates for protection from cerebral ischemia in aneurysm surgery. Acta Neurol Scand, suppl. 56:158, 1977
262. Lawner PM, Simeone FA: Treatment of intraoperative middle cerebral artery occlusion with pentobarbital and extracranial-intracranial bypass. J Neurosurg 51:710, 1975
263. Spetzler RF, Selman WR, Roski RA, Bonstelle C: Cerebral revascularization during barbiturate coma in primates and humans. Surg Neurol 17:111, 1982
264. Michenfelder JD: Cerebral preservation for intraoperative focal ischemia. Clin Neurosurg 32:105, 1985
265. Moffat JA, McDougall MJ, Brunet D et al: Thiopental bolus during carotid endarterectomy—rational drug therapy? Can Anaesth Soc J 30:615, 1983
266. Barson WG: Pharmacologic therapeutic modalities: barbiturates. Crit Care Q 5:63, 1983
267. Todd MM, Drummond JC, Hoi Sang U: The hemodynamic consequences of high-dose thiopental anesthesia. Anesth Analg 64:681, 1985
268. Criado A, Masenda J, Navarro E et al: Induction of anaesthesia with etomidate: haemodynamic study of 36 patients. Br J Anaesth 52:803, 1980
269. Fragen RJ, Caldwell N, Brunner EA: Clinical use of etomidate for anesthesia induction: a preliminary report. Anesth Analg 55:730, 1976
270. Gooding JM, Weng JT, Smith RA et al: Cardiovascular and pulmonary responses following etomidate induction of anesthesia in patients with demonstrated cardiac disease. Anesth Analg 58:40, 1979
271. Milde LN, Milde JH, Michenfelder JD: Cerebral functional, metabolic, and hemodynamic effects of etomidate in dogs. Anesthesiology 63:371, 1985
272. Cold GE, Eskesen V, Eriksen H et al: CBF and $CMRO_2$ during continuous etomidate infusion supplemented with N_2O and fentanyl in patients with supratentorial cerebral tumour. A dose-response study. Acta Anaesthesiol Scand 29:490, 1985
273. Cold GE, Eskesen V, Eriksen H et al: Changes in $CMRO_2$, EEG, and concentration of etomidate in serum and brain tissue during craniotomy with continuous etomidate supplemented with N_2O and fentanyl. Acta Anaesthesiol Scand 30:159, 1986
274. Renou AM, Vernhiet J, Macrez P et al: Cerebral blood flow and metabolism during etomidate anaesthesia in man. Br J Anaesth 50:1047, 1978
275. Dearden NM, McDowall DG: Comparison of etomidate and althesin in the reduction of increased intracranial pressure after head injury. Br J Anaesth 57:361, 1985
276. Wauquier A: Brain protective properties of etomidate and flunarizine. J Cereb Blood Flow Metab, suppl. 2:S53, 1982
277. Nemoto EM, Shiu GK, Bleyaert AL: Efficacy of therapies and attenuation of brain free fatty acid liberation during global ischemia. Crit Care Med 9:397, 1981
278. Tulleken CAF, van Dieren A, Jonkman J. Kalenda Z: Clinical and experimental experience with etomidate as a brain protective agent. J Cereb Blood Flow Metab, suppl. 2:S92, 1982
279. Milde LN, Milde JH: Preservation of cerebral metabolites by etomidate during incomplete cerebral ischemia in dogs. Anesthesiology 65:272, 1986
280. Wauquier A, Ashton D, Clincke G, Niemegeers CJE: Anti-hypoxic effects of etomidate, thiopental, and methohexital. Arch Int Pharmacodyn Ther 249:330, 1981
281. Watson JC, Drummond JC, Patel PM et al: An assessment of the cerebral protective effects of etomidate in a model of incomplete forebrain ischemia in the rat. Neurosurgery 30:540 1992
282. Bohrer H, Hoyer S, Krier C: The influence of etomidate upon cerebral metabolites after complete brain ischemia in the rat. Eur J Anaesth 8:233, 1991
283. Longnecker DE: Stress free: to be or not to be. Anesthesiology 61:643, 1984
284. Fragen KJ, Shanks CA, Molteni A, Avram MJ: Effects of etomidate on hormonal responses to surgical stress. Anesthesiology 61:652, 1984
285. Zurick AM, Sigurdsson H, Koehler LS et al: Magnitude and time course of perioperative adrenal suppression with single dose etomidate in male adult cardiac surgical patients. Anesthesiology 65:A248, 1986
286. Wagner RL, White PF: Etomidate inhibits adrenocortical function in surgical patients. Anesthesiology 61:647, 1984

287. Wagner RL, White PF, Kan PB et al: Inhibition of adrenal steroidogenesis by the anesthetic etomidate. N Engl J Med 310:1415, 1984
288. Ledingham I, Finlay WEI, Watt I, McKee JI: Etomidate and adrenocortical function. Lancet 1:1434, 1983
289. Fraser R, Watt I, Gray CE et al: The effect of etomidate on adrenocortical function in dogs before and during hemorrhagic shock. Endocrinology 6:2266, 1984
290. James R, Glen JB: Synthesis, biological evaluation and preliminary structure-activity considerations of a series of alkyphenols as intravenous anaesthetic agents. J Med Chem 23:1350, 1980
291. Rogers KM, Adam HK, Dewar KMS et al: ICI 35 868, a new i.v. anaesthetic: preliminary findings in 20 patients. Br J Anaesth 52:230P, 1980
292. Galletly DC, Short TG: Total intravenous anaesthesia using propofol infusion—50 consecutive cases. Anaesth Intens Care 16:150, 1988
293. Freedman M, Levy ER: Propofol intravenous anaesthesia for neurosurgery. S Afr Med J 74:10, 1988
294. Ramani R, Todd MM, Warner DS: Dose-related changes in CBF and $CMRO_2$ during propofol infusions in rabbits. Anesthesiology 73:A702, 1990
295. Van Hemelrijck J, Fitch W, Mattheussen M et al: Effect of propofol on cerebral circulation and autoregulation in the baboon. Anesth Analg 71:49, 1990
296. Madsen JB, Guldager M, Jensen PM: CBF and $CMRO_2$ during neuroanesthesia with continuous infusion of propofol. Acta Anaesth Scand, suppl. 91, 33:143, 1989
297. Pinaud M, Lelausque JN, Fauchoux N et al: Effects of propofol on cerebral hemodynamics and metabolism in patients with head trauma. Anesthesiology 69:A569, 1988
298. Vandesteene A, Trempont V, Engelman E et al: Effect of propofol on cerebral blood flow and metabolism in man. Anaesthesia suppl. 43:42, 1988
299. Illievich UM, Zornow MH, Choi KT et al: Effects of hypothermia or anesthetics on hippocampal glutamate and glycine concentrations after repeated transient global cerebral sicehmia. Anesthesiology 80:177, 1994
300. Varner PD, Vinik HR, Funderburg C: Survival during severe hypoxia and propofol or ketamine anesthesia in mice. Anesthesiology 69:A571, 1988
301. Weir DL, Goodchild CS, Graham DZ: Propofol: effects on indices of cerebral ischemia. J Neurosurg Anes 1:284, 1989
302. Kochs E, Hoffman WE, Werner C Thomas et al: The effect of propofol on brain electrical activity, neurologic outcome, and neuronal damage following incomplete ischemia in rats. Anesthesiology 76:245, 1992
303. Milde LN, Milde JH, Michenfelder JD: The comparative cerebral protective effects of propofol, thiopental and fentanyl in a canine model of incomplete global cerebral ischemia. Anesthesiology (in press)
304. Tsai YC, Huang SJ, Lai YY et al: Propofol does not reduce infarct volume in rats undergoing permanent middle cerebral artery occlusion. Acta Anaesthesiol Sin 32:994, 1994
305. Ravussin P, deTribolet N: Total intravenous anesthesia with propofol for burst suppression in cerebral aneurysm surgery: preliminary report of 42 patients. Neurosurgery 32:236, 1993
306. Nowack WJ, Jordan R: Propofol, seizures and generalized paroxysmal fast activity in the EEG. Clin Electroencephalogr 25:110, 1994
307. Makela JP, Iivanainen M, Pieninkeroinen IP et al: Seizures associated with propofol activity. Epilepsia 34:832, 1993
308. Finley GA, MacManus B, Sampson SE et al: Delayed seizures following sedation with propofol. Can J Anaesth 40:863, 1993
309. Stockard J, Bickford R: The neurophysiology of anesthesia. Monogr Anaesthesiol 2:3, 1975
310. Newberg LA, Milde JH, Michenfelder JD: The cerebral metabolic effects of isoflurane at and above concentrations that suppress cortical electrical activity. Anesthesiology 59:23, 1983
311. Newberg LA, Michenfelder JD: Cerebral protection by isoflurane during hypoxia or ischemia. Anesthesiology 59:29, 1983
312. Drummond JCL: Brain protection during anesthesia. Anesthesiology 79:877, 1993
313. Newberg LA, Milde JH, Michenfelder JD: Systemic and cerebral effects of isoflurane-induced hypotension in dogs. Anesthesiology 60:541, 1984
314. Murr R, Schurer L, Berger S et al: Effects of isoflurane, fentanyl, or thiopental anesthesia on regional cerebral blood flow and brain surface PO_2 in the presence of a focal lesion in rabbits. Anesth Analg 77:898, 1993
315. Warner DS, Deshpande JK, Wieloch: The effect of isoflurane on neuronal necrosis following

near complete forebrain ischemia in the rat. Anesthesiology 64:19, 1986

316. Warner DS, McFarlane C, Todd MM et al: Sevoflurnae and halothane reduce focal ischemic brain damage in the rat. Possible influence on thermoregulation. Anesthesiology 79:985, 1993
317. Hoffman WE, Thomas C, Albrecht RF: The effect of halothane and isoflurane on neurologic outcome following incomplete cerebral ischemia in the rat. Anesth Analg 76:279, 1993
318. Bickler PE, Buck LT, Hansen BM: Effects of isoflurane and hypothermia on glutamate receptor-mediated calcium influx in brain slices. Anesthesiology 81:1461, 1994
319. Nehls DG, Todd MM, Spetzler RF et al: A comparison of the cerebral protective effects of isoflurane and barbiturates during temporary focal ischemia in primates. Anesthesiology 66:453, 1987
320. Milde LN, Milde JH, Lanier WL, Michenfelder JD: Comparison of the effects of isoflurane and thiopental on neurologic outcome and neuropathology following temporary focal cerebral ischemia in primates. Anesthesiology 69:905, 1988
321. Warner DS, Zhou JG, Ramani R et al: Reversible focal ischemia in the rat: effects of halothane, isoflurane, and methohexital anesthesia. J Cereb Blood Flow Metab 11:794, 1991
322. Michenfelder JD, Sundt TM, Fode N, Sharbrough FW: Isoflurane when compared to enflurane and halothane decreases the frequency of cerebral ischemia during carotid endarterectomy. Anesthesiology 67:336, 1987
323. Carlsson C, Hagerdal M, Siesjö BK: The effect of nitrous oxide on oxygen consumption and blood flow in the cerebral cortex of the rat. Acta Anaesthesiol Scand 20:91, 1976
324. Milde LN, Milde JH, Gallagher WJ: Effects of sufentanil on cerebral circulation and metabolism in dogs. Anesth Analg 70:138, 1990
325. Sakabe T, Kuramoto T, Inoue S et al: Cerebral effects of nitrous oxide in the dog. Anesthesiology 48:195, 1978
326. Manohar M: Impact of 70 percent nitrous oxide administration on regional distribution of brain blood flow in unmedicated healthy swine. J Cardiovasc Pharmacol 7:463, 1985
327. Pelligrino DA, Miletich DJ, Hoffman WE et al: Nitrous oxide markedly increases cerebral cortical metabolic rate and blood flow in the goat. Anesthesiology 60:405, 1984
328. Drummond JC, Scheller MS, Todd MM: The effect of nitrous oxide on cortical cerebral blood flow during anesthesia with halothane and isoflurane with and without morphine in the rabbit. Anesth Analg 66:1083, 1987
329. Ebert TJ, Kampine JP: Nitrous oxide augments sympathetic outflow: direct evidence from human peroneal nerve endings. Anesth Analg 69:444, 1989
330. Werner C, Hoffman WE, Thomas C et al: Ganglionic blockade improves neurologic outcome from incomplete ischemia in rats: partial reversal by exogenous catecholamines. Anesthesiology 73:923, 1990
331. Baughman VL, Hoffman WE, Thomas C et al: The interaction of nitrous oxide and isoflurane with incomplete cerebral ischemia in the rat. Anesthesiology 70:767, 1989
332. Warner DS, Zhou J, Ramani R et al: Nitrous oxide does not alter infarct volume in rats undergoing reversible middle cerebral artery occlusion. Anesthesiology 73:686, 1990
333. Astrup J, Skovsted P, Gjerris F et al: Increase in extracellular potassium in the brain during circulatory arrest. Effects of hypothermia, lidocaine, and thiopental. Anesthesiology 55:256, 1981
334. Ingvar M, Shapiro HM: Selective metabolic activation of the hippocampus during lidocaine-induced pre-seizure activity. Anesthesiology 54:33, 1981
335. Sakabe T, Maekawa T, Ishikawa T et al: The effects of lidocaine on canine cerebral metabolism and circulation related to the electroencephalogram. Anesthesiology 40:433, 1974
336. Evans DE, Catron PW, McDermott JJ et al: Effect of lidocaine after experimental cerebral ischemia induced by air embolism. J Neurosurg 70:97, 1989
337. Shokunbi MT, Gelb AW, Wu XM et al: Continuous lidocaine infusion and focal feline cerebral ischemia. Stroke 21:107, 1990
338. Shokunbi MT, Gelb AW, Peerless SJ et al: An evaluation of the effect of lidocaine in experimental focal cerebral ischemia. Stroke 17:962, 1986
339. Milde LN, Milde JH: The deterimental effect of lidocaine on cerebral metabolism measured in dogs anesthetized with isoflurane. Anesthesiology 67:180, 1987

340. Allen GS: Role of calcium antagonists in cerebral arterial spasm. Am J Cardiol 55:149B, 1985
341. Siesjö BK: Historical overview: calcium, ischemia, and death of brain cells. Ann NY Acad Sci 522:638, 1988
342. Thorens S, Haeusler G: Effects of some vasodilators on calcium translocation in intact and fractionated vascular smooth muscle. Eur J Pharmacol 54:79, 1979
343. Allen GS, Ahn HS, Preziosi TJ et al: Cerebral arterial spasm—a controlled trial of nimodipine in patients with subarachnoid hemorrhage. N Eng J Med 308:619, 1983
344. Philippon J, Grob R, Dagreou F et al: Prevention of vasospasm in subarachnoid hemorrhage. A controlled study with nimodipine. Acta Neurochir 82:110, 1986
345. Neil-Dwyer G, Mee E, Dorrance D et al: Early intervention with nimodipine in subarachnoid haemorrhage. Eur Heart J 8:41, 1987
346. Ohman J, Heiskanen O: Effect of nimodipine on the outcome of patients after aneurysmal subarachnoid haemorrhage and surgery. J Neurosurg 69:683, 1988
347. Pickard JD, Murray GD, Illingworth R et al: Effect of oral nimodipine on cerebral infraction and outcome after subarachnoid haemorrhage: British aneurysm nimodipine trial. Br Med J 298:636, 1989
348. Robinson MJ, Teasdale GM: Calcium antagonists in the management of subarachnoid haemorrhage. Cerebrovasc Brain Metab Rev 2:205, 1990
349. Petruk KC, West M, Mohr G et al: Nimodipine treatment in poor-grade aneurysm patients: results of a multicenter double-blind placebo-controlled trial. J Neurosurg 68:505, 1988
350. Meyer FB, Anderson RA, Yaksh TL, Sundt TM, Jr: Effect of nimodipine on intracellular brain pH, cortical blood flow, and EEG in experimental focal cerebral ischemia. J Neurosurg 64:617, 1986
351. Germano IM, Bartkowskilt M, Cassel ME, Pitts LH: The therapeutic value of nimodipine in experimental focal cerebral ischemia. J Neurosurg 67:81, 1987
352. Gelmers HJ: Effect of nimodipine on post-ischaemic cerebrovascular reactivity as revealed by measuring regional cerebral blood flow. Acta Neurochir 63:283, 1982
353. Gelmers HJ: The effects of nimodipine on the clinical course of patients with acute ischaemic stroke. Acta Neurol Scand 69:232, 1984
354. Gelmers HJ: Gorter K, deWeert CJ, Wiezer HJ: A controlled trial of nimodipine in acute ischemic stroke. N Engl J Med 318:203, 1988
355. Kazda S, Hoffmeister F, Garthoff B et al: Prevention of the postischemic impaired reperfusion of the brain by nimodipine. Acta Neurol Scand (suppl) 60:302, 1979
356. Steen PA, Newberg LA, Milde JH, Michenfelder JD: Cerebral blood flow and neurologic outcome when nimodipine is given after complete cerebral ischemia in the dog. J Cereb Blood Flow Metab 4:82, 1984
357. Milde LN, Milde JH, Michenfelder JD: Delayed treatment with nimodipine improves cerebral blood flow after complete cerebral ischemia in the dog. J Cereb Blood Flow Metab 6:332, 1986
358. Smith M-L, Kagstrom E, Rosen I et al: Effect of the calcium antagonist nimodipine on the delayed hypoperfusion following incomplete ischemia in the rat. J Cereb Blood Flow Metab 3:543, 1983
359. Steen PA, Gisvold SE, Milde JH et al: Nimodipine improves outcome when given after complete cerebral ischemia in primates. Anesthesiology 62:406, 1985
360. Roine RO, Kaste M, Kinnunen A, Nikki P: Safety and efficacy of nimodipine in resuscitation of patients outside hospital. Br Med J 294:20, 1987
361. Roine RO, Kaste M, Kinnunen A et al: Nimodipine after resuscitation from out-of-hospital ventricular fibrillation. A placebo-controlled, double-blind, randomized trial. JAMA 264:3171, 1990
362. Pappium HM, McCann WP: Effects of steroids on cerebral edema in cats. Arch Neurol 20:207, 1969
363. Reulen HJ: Steroids and Brain Edema. p. 65. Springer-Verlag, New York, 1972
364. Galicich JH, French LA: Use of dexamethasone in the treatment of cerebral edema resulting from brain tumors and brain surgery. Am Pract 12:169, 1961
365. Braakman R, Schouten HJA, Blaauw-van Dishoeck M et al: Megadose steroids in severe head injury. Results of a prospective double-blind clinical trial. J Neurosurg 58:326, 1983
366. Cooper PR, Moody S, Clark WK et al: Dexamethasone and severe head injury. A prospective double blind study. J Neurosurg 51:307, 1979
367. Saul TG, Ducker TB, Salcman M et al: Steroids

in severe head injury. A prospective randomized clinical trial. J Neurosurg 54:596, 1981
368. Dearden NM, Gibson JS, McDowall DG et al: Effect of high-dose dexamethasone on outcome from severe head injury. J Neurosurg 64:81, 1986
369. Cullen JA, Aldrete JA, Jankovsky L, Romos-Salas F: Protective action of phenytoin in cerebral ischemia. Anesth Analg 58:165, 1979
370. Aldrete JA, Romos-Salas F, Vankovsky L, Franatovic Y: Effect of pretreatment with thiopental and phenytoin on post ischemic brain damage in rabbits. Crit Care Med 7:466, 1979
371. Suzuki J, Abiko H, Mizoi K et al: Protective effect of phenytoin and its enhanced action by combined administration with mannitol and vitamin E in cerebral ischaemia. Acta Neurochir 88:56, 1987
372. Aldrete JA, Romos-Salas F, Mazzia VDB, Tan SL: Phenytoin for brain resuscitation after cardiac arrest: an uncontrolled clinical trial. Crit Care Med 9:474, 1981
373. Deshpande JK, Wieloch T: The role of diphenylhydantoin in the treatment of ischemic brain damage. Anesthesiology, suppl. 65:A318, 1986
374. Artru AA, Michenfelder JD: Cerebral protective, metabolic, and vascular effects of phenytoin. Stroke 11:377, 1980
375. Artru AA, Michenfelder JD: Anoxic cerebral potassium accumulation reduced by phenytoin: mechanism of cerebral protection? Anesth Analg 60:41, 1981
376. Shiu GK, Nemoto EM, Nemmer J: Dose of thiopental, pentobarbital, and phenytoin for maximal therapeutic effects in cerebral ischemia anoxia. Crit Care Med 11:452, 1983
377. Lassen NA: The luxury-perfusion syndrome and its possible relation to acute metabolic acidosis localized within the brain. Lancet 2:1113, 1966
378. Soloway M, Nadel W, Albin MS, White RJ: The effect of hyperventilation on subsequent cerebral infarction. Anesthesiology 29:975, 1968
379. Soloway M, Moriarty G, Fraser JG, White RJ: Effect of delayed hyperventilation on experimental cerebral infarction. Neurology 21:479, 1971
380. Yamaguchi T, Regli F, Waltz A: Effects of hyperventilation with and without carbon dioxide on experimental cerebral ischemia and infarction. Brain 95:123, 1972
381. Kogure K, Fujishima M, Scheinberg P, Reinmuth OM: Effects of changes in carbon dioxide pressure and arterial pressure on blood flow in ischemic regions of the brain in dogs. Circ Res 24:557, 1969
382. Hayashi S, Nehls DG, Kieck CF et al: Beneficial effects of induced hypertension on experimental stroke in awake monkeys. J Neurosurg 60:151, 1984
383. Hope DT, Branston NM, Symon L: Restoration of neurological function with induced hypertension in acute experimental cerebral ischemia. Acta Neurol Scand, suppl. 64:506, 1977
384. Waltz AG: Effect of blood pressure on blood flow in ischemic and nonischemic cerebral cortex. The phenomenon of autoregulation and luxury perfusion. Neurology 18:613, 1968
385. Aberg E, Adielsson G, Almqvist A et al: Multicenter trial of hemodilution in ischemic stroke—background and study protocol. Stroke 16:885, 1985
386. Goldberg HI, Banka RS, Reivich M: Effect on regional cerebral blood flow in ischemic stroke of vasopressor therapy. Stroke 8:6, 1977
387. Wise G, Sutter R, Burkholder J: The treatment of brain ischemia with vasopressor drugs. Stroke 3:135, 1972
388. Kassell NF, Peerless SJ, Durward QJ et al: Treatment of ischemic deficits from vasospasm with intravascular volume expansion and induced arterial hypertension. Neurosurgery 11:337, 1982
389. Brown FD, Hanlon K, Mullan S: Treatment of aneurysmal hemiplegia with dopamine and mannitol. J Neurosurg 49:525, 1978
390. Giannotta SL, McGillicuddy JE, Kindt GW: Diagnosis and treatment of postoperative cerebral vasospasm. Surg Neurol 8:286, 1977
391. Kosnik EJ, Hunt WE: Postoperative hypertension in the management of patients with intracranial arterial aneurysms. J Neurosurg 45:148, 1976
392. Montgomery EB, Jr, Grubb RL Jr, Raichle ME: Cerebral hemodynamics and metabolism in postoperative cerebral vasospasm and treatment with hypertensive therapy. Ann Neurol 9:502, 1981
393. Muizelaar JP, Becker DP: Induced hypertension for the treatment of cerebral ischemia after subarachnoid hemorrhage. Direct effect on cerebral blood flow. Surg Neurol 25:317, 1986
394. Hoff JT: Cerebral circulation. J Neurosurg 65:579, 1986
395. Little JR, Slugg RM, Latchaw JP, Jr et al: Treatment of acute focal cerebral ischemia with concentrated albumin. Neurosurgery 9:552, 1981

396. Wood JH, Snyder LL, Simeone FA: Failure of intravascular volume expansion without hemodilution to elevate cortical blood flow in region of experimental focal ischemia. J Neurosurg 56:80, 1982
397. Gilroy J, Barnhart MI, Meyer JS: Treatment of acute stroke with dextran 40. JAMA 210:293, 1969
398. Matthews WB, Oxbury JM, Grainger KM, Greenhall RC: A blind controlled trial of dextran 40 in the treatment of ischemic stroke. Brain 99:193, 1976
399. Kassell NF, Drake CG: Timing of aneurysm surgery. Neurosurgery 10:514, 1982
400. Kusunoki M, Kimura K. Nakamura M et al: Effects of hematocrit variations of cerebral blood flow and oxygen transport in ischemic cerebrovascular disease. J Cereb Blood Flow Metab 1:413, 1981
401. Grotta JC, Pettigrew LC, Allen S et al: Baseline hemodynamic state and response to hemodilution in patients with acute cerebral ischemia. Stroke 16:790, 1985
402. Wood JH, Simeone FA, Fink EA, Golden MA: Hypervolemic hemodilution in experimental focal cerebral ischemia. Elevation of cardiac output, regional cortical blood flow, and ICP after intravascular volume expansion with low molecular weight dextran. J Neurosurg 59:500, 1983

6 FLUID MANAGEMENT OF THE NEUROSURGICAL PATIENT

ROBERT S. ALPHIN

NIKOLAUS GRAVENSTEIN

Perioperative fluid management of neurosurgical patients continues to be an area of evolving refinement. It is well accepted that fluid therapy can markedly influence the clinical course of patients with an intracranial injury or mass. This influence may manifest as an effect on cerebral edema formation, cerebral perfusion pressure (CPP), and/or glucose and electrolyte homeostasis. Debate continues between neurosurgeons, trauma surgeons, and anesthesiologists as to the most appropriate fluid management for these patients. Classical teaching has suggested that perioperative fluid restriction is necessary to avoid cerebral edema and worsening of neurologic outcome.[1,2] This was based on the observation that patients who receive large volumes of crystalloid uniformly develop peripheral edema. The logical assumption that followed was that cerebral edema accompanied peripheral edema and that, therefore, such fluids were to be avoided.

Clearly, overzealous fluid administration (particularly with hypoosmolar solutions) may create osmotic and hydrostatic pressure gradients favoring the formation of cerebral edema and intracranial hypertension. Conversely, fluid restriction may create additional potentially detrimental side effects that must be considered as well. In 1967, Jelsma and Mc Queen restricted fluid intake in dogs and showed only a 1% reduction in brain water per content, per day, of fluid restriction despite an 8% decrease in body weight.[3] Applied to a normal adult, this may yield as much as a 50-ml decrease in brain water. This may be of benefit to the patient with intracranial hypertension. However, dehydration and the associated hypovolemia may result in hemodynamic instability and a decreased CPP, particularly in response to positive pressure ventilation and induction of anesthesia that outweighs any benefit of reduced brain water. Likewise, reduction in cardiac output may worsen atelectasis and increase intrapulmonary shunting.

Both hypotension and hypoxemia have been shown to worsen outcome in head-injured patients, presumably by contributing to secondary brain injury.[5,6] Indeed, even modest experimental reductions in blood pressure and oxygenation have been demonstrated to be harmful to the brain with impaired autoregulation, suggesting that maintenance of CPP is critical to preserving or improving outcome.[7–10] Aggressive fluid restriction may also compromise renal perfusion and contribute to prerenal azotemia as well as electrolyte and acid-base disturbances. Newer studies have changed clinical thinking by indicating that it is the composition, not the vol-

Goals of Fluid Management

1. Minimize cerebral edema formation while avoiding intravascular volume depletion
2. Maintain hemodynamic stability to preserve adequate cerebral perfusion pressure
3. Maintain electrolyte and glucose homeostasis
4. Reduce brain size

ume of administered fluids, that is the primary determinant in the development of cerebral edema.

Another important intraoperative consideration is brain size. The focus is hemodynamic stability and maintenance of cerebral perfusion along with avoidance of cerebral edema or, even more preferable, actual reduction of brain mass. The smaller and more pliant the brain is, the less retraction and retraction pressure is required to achieve exposure. This limits the amount of brain ischemia resulting from obtaining adequate operative exposure. The methods to best achieve these objectives continue to be actively investigated. This chapter presents a framework to guide clinical decision making with respect to fluid management in the neurosurgical patient. General goals of fluid management in neurosurgical patients should address the issues listed in the accompanying box.

GENERAL CONSIDERATIONS

It is perhaps easiest to divide perioperative fluid management into exogenous fluid administration and endogenous fluid manipulation to evaluate the effect on intracranial contents and pressure. The skull represents a rigid, closed space that contains brain tissue (± lesion), cerebrospinal fluid (CSF), and blood (Fig. 6.1). Because the encasing structures are rigid, an increase in any compartment volume without a compensatory decrease in another or others necessarily increases intracranial pressure (ICP), particularly when compensatory mechanisms (i.e., decreases in other compartments, are overwhelmed (Fig. 6.2). Of these compartments, the intracranial blood can undergo rapid volume changes in response to physiologic (e.g., $PaCO_2$ and blood pressure), pharmacologic (e.g., vasodilation and vasoconstriction), or mechanical (e.g., central venous and/or cerebral venous

FIGURE 6.1 *Schematic of CNS inside a rigid compartment. Note that 80% (dark shading) of the contents is tissue, 10% (stippled area) blood, and 10% (crosshatching) CSF.*

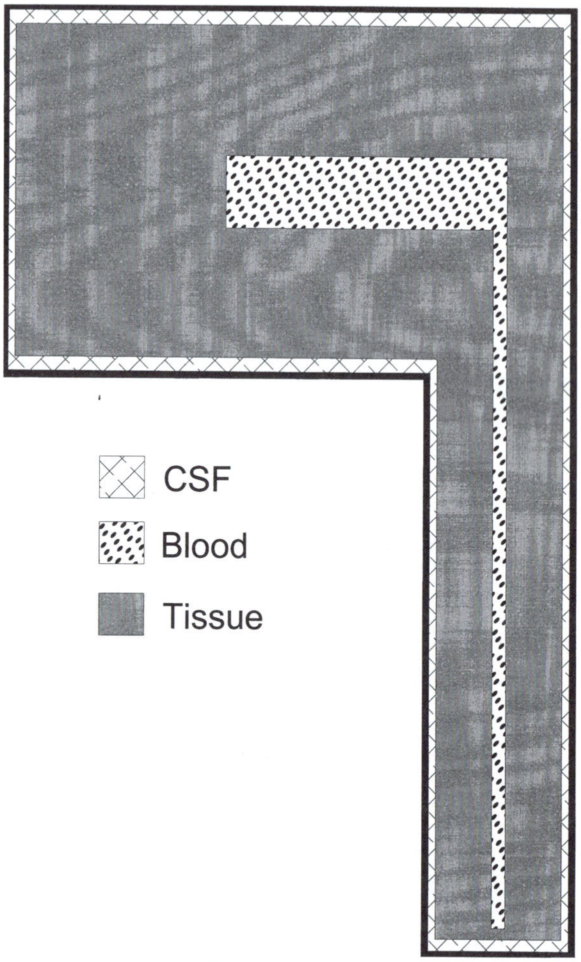

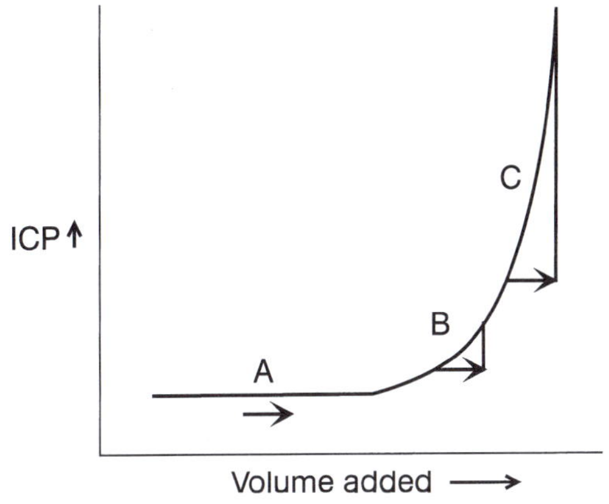

FIGURE 6.2 *Intracranial elastance curve.* A, *Normal elastance (no or minimal ICP increase with small increase in intracranial volume.* B, *Reduced elastance (small ICP increase with small increase in intracranial volume).* C, *Poor elastance (large ICP increase with small increase in intracranial volume).*

pressure [CVP]) stimuli. The CSF compartment may also undergo abrupt volume changes associated with drainage of CSF (e.g., ventriculostomy) or less acutely compensate for increased ICP by displacing CSF into the spinal subarachnoid space, slowing CSF production or increasing its resorption. Brain tissue also contributes to intracranial pressure via two mechanisms: (1) the presence of additional tissue (e.g., mass) and (2) regulation of interstitial brain water content. Because inappropriate perioperative fluid management may contribute to interstitial brain tissue water (edema) and increased ICP or, conversely, to inadequate cerebral perfusion (i.e., hypovolemia causing hypotension and brain tissue ischemia), it can influence neurologic outcome.

PHYSIOLOGY OF WATER MOVEMENT

In order to have a mental model that allows anticipation of the effects of fluid administration or manipulation, you must have an understanding of the principles governing water movement across physiologic membranes in general and in the central nervous system (CNS) in particular.

Generally speaking, water movement between intravascular and extravascular compartments is subject to the characteristics of the local capillary endothelium, the principal barrier between these compartments, as well as the osmotic, oncotic, and hydrostatic pressure gradients.

OSMOTIC AND ONCOTIC PRESSURE

Osmotic pressure is a function of the total number of osmotically active, dissolved particles (osmoles) in that solution, otherwise known as *osmolarity*. Osmolarity is the *calculated* number of osmotically active particles per liter of solution and may be determined if the molecular weight (MW) of the solute and its tendency to dissociate are known. For example, 1 g molecular weight (GMW) of glucose (MW = 180 g/mole) dissolved in 1 L of water will create a 1 osmolar solution. One gram molecular weight of sodium chloride (MW = 58.4 g/mole) dissolved in 1 L of water, however, will create a 2 osmolar solution because it dissociates into two osmotically active ions. A solution that has 1/1000 osm dissolved per liter will have an osmolarity of 1 milliosmole per liter (mosm/L). Normal serum osmolarity is approximately 285 mosm/L and may be calculated by Equation 6.1:

$$2\ \text{Na} + \text{glucose}/18 + \text{blood urea nitrogen}/2.3 \quad (6.1)$$

Confusion often arises over the use of the terms osmolarity and osmolality.[11,12,13] As stated above, osmolarity is a calculated value that assumes complete dissociation of all particles in solution. Osmolality, however, is a *measured* value of the number of osmotically active particles per kilogram of solvent (mosm/kg). It is typically determined by measuring freezing point depression and is one of the colligative properties of a solution. Although osmolality may be estimated by calculating osmolarity, it generally results in an overestimation of the true osmolality as a consequence of the incomplete dissociation of all the particles in solution. For example, normal saline (0.9% sodium chloride) has a calculated osmolarity of 308 mosm/L (154 meq Na^+ + 154 Cl^-), assuming complete dissociation of all sodium and chloride ions. However, normal saline's measured osmolality is 282 mosm/kg, because not all of the NaCl molecules remain dissociated in solutions. Therefore, osmolality is, theoretically, a better measure of a solution's osmotic pressure. Practically speaking, the terms are often used interchangeably when referring to physiologic solution, because these solutions are relatively dilute. This does not do justice to the resulting osmotic pressure differences (consider NaCl 308 mosm/L calculated vs. 282 mosm/kg measured), which, as we hope to impress upon the reader below, can have considerable impact on free water movement across the blood-brain barrier (BBB). It is prudent to inquire of your own hospital laboratory as to when the calculated value is reported typically as with a blood gas or chemistry result and when the measured one is reported.

Osmotically active particles draw water across a semipermeable membrane (e.g., capillary endothelium) from an area of low osmolality to one of high osmolality until the solute concentration is equal on both sides of the membrane. An osmolality difference generates a powerful osmotic pressure gradient for water movement, which has been calculated to be 19.3 mmHg/mosm/kg difference across the membrane. For plasma, with a normal osmolality of 285 mosm/kg, this creates an osmotic pressure of approximately 5,500 mmHg. Sodium, chloride, and other ions account for most of the plasma osmolality and thus contribute the most to osmotic pressure (See Eq. 6.1). Interestingly, and perhaps at first surprisingly, the osmotic pressure exerted by plasma proteins is relatively small (24 mmHg) when compared with total plasma osmotic pressure. The contribution of plasma proteins (e.g., albumin, globulins) to osmotic pressure is called *oncotic pressure*. Stated differently, oncotic pressure contributes just a little more than 1 mosm/kg toward total plasma osmolality.

STARLING'S LAW

Starling's law defines water movement between the intra- and extravascular spaces as the difference between hydrostatic forces favoring water removal from capillaries and the osmotic forces that draw water back into the intravascular space[13] (Eq. 6.2):

$$Qw = K_f\,A[(P_c - \pi) - \sigma(\pi_c - \pi_i)]$$

where

- Qw = net amount of water movement between intra- and extravascular spaces
- K_f = filtration coefficient of the membrane (rate of fluid filtration/min/mmHg/100 g tissue
- A = surface area of the semipermeable membrane
- P_c = capillary hydrostatic pressure
- P_i = interstitial hydrostatic pressure
- σ = reflection coefficient (ranges from O → 1, quantifies the leakiness of the membrane to solutes), like the filtration coefficient, it varies between tissue types (small in dense tissues like brain and muscle with little solute movement across the membrane, large in the more permeable tissues of the lungs, intestines, etc.)
- π_c = plasma oncotic pressure
- π_i = interstitial oncotic pressure

Capillary hydrostatic pressure, tissue hydrostatic pressure (usually negative in nonedematous tissues), and tissue oncotic pressure all act to move water from the vascular into the extravascular compartment (Fig. 6.3). Plasma oncotic pressure is the only force promoting resorption of water back into the capillaries. In most situations, the sum of these forces results in a small net outward flow from capillaries to the interstitial space. This fluid is subsequently cleared by the lymphatic system, which actively pumps it back into the circulation thereby preventing extravascular fluid accumulation or

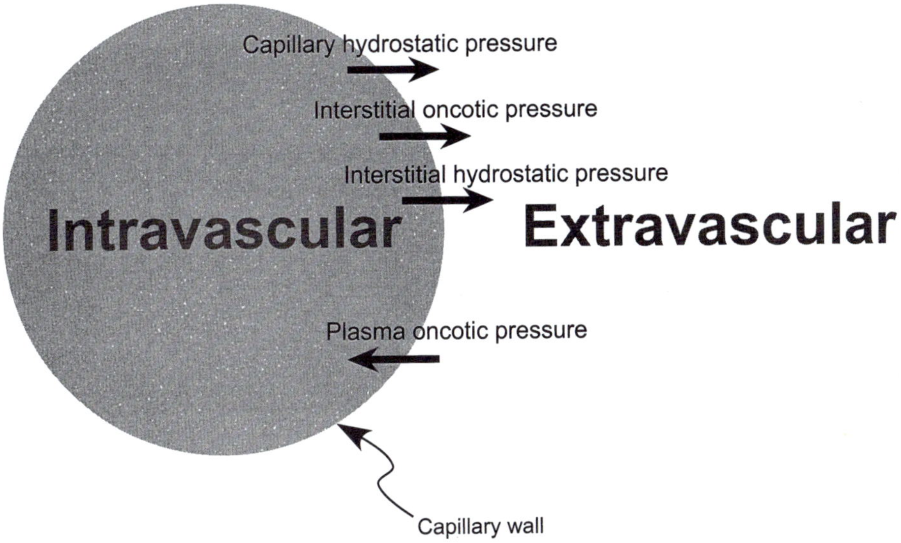

FIGURE 6.3 *Schematic of fluid movement described by Starling's law (compare to Eq. 6.2). Arrows show direction of effect on water movement.*

edema. The lymphatics are interesting in that as interstitial edema occurs they are mechanically stented open after which fluid then enters them following a hydrostatic gradient.

CAPILLARY ENDOTHELIAL BARRIER TO WATER MOVEMENT (EDEMA)

Peripheral Tissues

In most tissues of the body, the cells of the capillary endothelium are loosely connected (loose junctions) and are freely permeable to water and most dissolved particles (such as ions and glucose) (Fig. 6.4). Molecules larger than 30,000 to 40,000 daltons, such as plasma proteins, are unable to freely cross most physiologic membranes since they are larger than the typical peripheral capillary endothelial pore size of 60 to 70 Å. Therefore, in most tissues of the body, only oncotic and hydrostatic pressure gradients govern water movement, because dissolved particles are freely mobile and therefore cannot create an osmotic pressure difference. Total plasma osmolality (and hence total osmotic pressure) plays no appreciable role in water movement in peripheral tissues. Indeed, Starling's law (see Eq. 6.2) does not even account for the effect of ions, because they move freely across peripheral membranes and therefore do not and cannot create concentration gradients for water movement. The clinical impact of Starling's law is seen regularly in the operating room and intensive care unit. Patient's who undergo volume resuscitation with large volumes of crystalloid often develop generalized edema secondary to a dilutional decrease in plasma oncotic pressure and equilibration of water between intra- and extravascular compartments. Similarly, patients with severe congestive heart failure or patients in the head-down position often develop dependent edema due to increased local venous pressure and therefore higher intravascular hydrostatic pressure (see Fig. 6.3). This effect is augmented by the fact that most peripheral tissues are highly compliant (e.g., bowel, lung, skin) and have relatively low baseline interstitial hydrostatic pressure, which facilitates water accumulation.

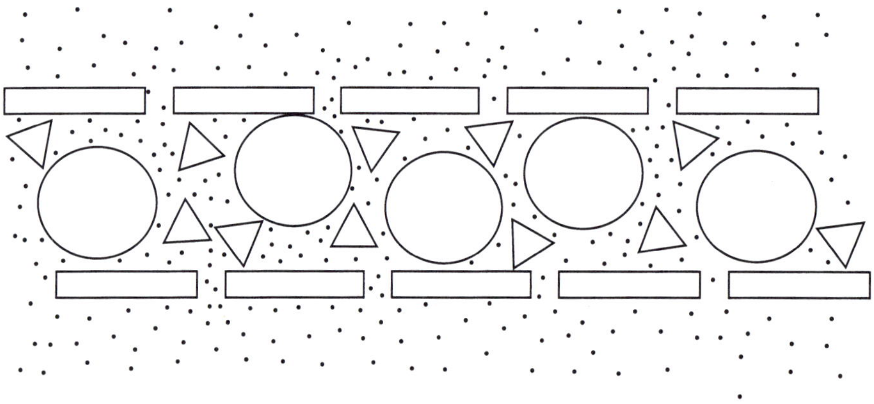

FIGURE 6.4 *Schematic of peripheral capillary. Note the loose junction (i.e., 60–70 Å space between capillary endothelial cells. Boxes, capillary endothelial cell; circles, red blood cells; triangles, particles molecular weight greater 30,000 to 40,000 daltons are too large to cross the junctions between peripheral capillary endothelial cells; stippled area, particles with size less than 70 Å (e.g., ions, glucose).*

Central Nervous System

The CNS is quite different from other tissues with respect to water movement (Fig. 6.5). In the CNS, water movement is governed by the BBB, a specialized capillary endothelium that is connected via "tight junctions".[14] In contrast to peripheral capillaries, pore size in the BBB capillaries is only one-tenth that of the periphery at 7 to 9 Å.[15] This makes the BBB impermeable not only to large molecules, but also most ions as well. Water, however, remains freely permeable along concentration gradients. Free water administration has been demonstrated to readily cause cerebral edema and increase ICP.[16,17] Because the intact BBB is impermeable to both ions and proteins and the number of ions is orders of magnitude greater than the number of plasma proteins, the oncotic contribution to water movement in the brain is necessarily quite small whereas the osmotic effect is large. This is the fundamental distinction between CNS and peripheral capillary beds. Even large reductions in plasma oncotic pressure have minimal effects on total plasma osmolality and osmotic pressure and, therefore, net water movement in the CNS. In comparison, a seemingly small reduction in plasma osmolality may drastically increase brain water content. Such effects were dramatically demonstrated as far back as 1919 by Weed and McKibben, who measured CSF pressure in cats who received hypotonic intravenous solu-

FIGURE 6.5 *Schematic of brain capillary and BBB. Note the tight connections that are really only permeable to water and not ions or small molecules (compare to Fig. 6.4) between cells. See Figure 6.4 for explanation of symbols.*

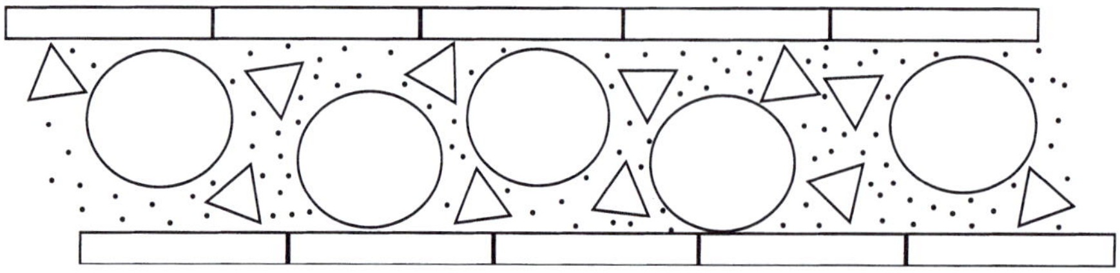

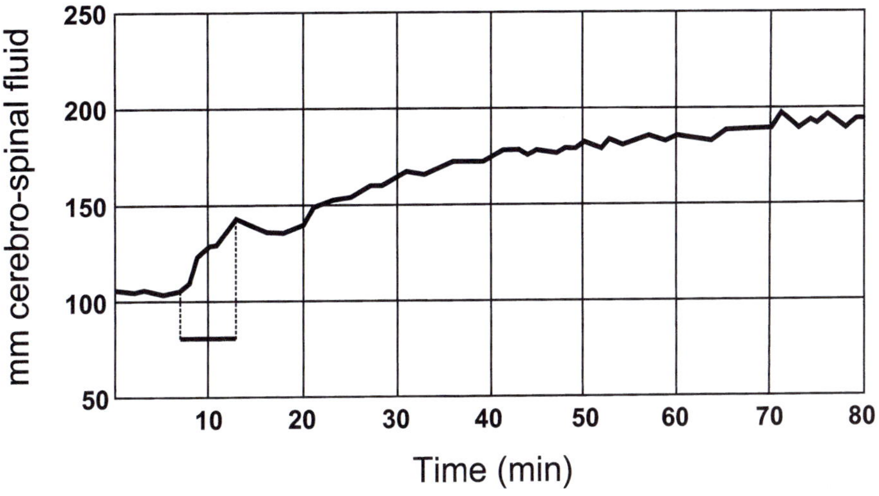

FIGURE 6.6 *Cerebrospinal fluid pressure change over time, following injection of 20 ml sterile water in a cat. (From Weed and McKibben,[19] with permission.)*

tions.[17,18] (Fig. 6.6). Indeed, it has been shown experimentally by several investigators that large reductions in plasma oncotic pressure minimally influence water movement across the BBB, whereas small changes in plasma osmolality have a significant impact on water movement and edema formation.[19,20]

Brain tissue is also quite inelastic compared to most peripheral tissues due to its dense network of glial cells. This limits efflux of water to the interstitium because tissue hydrostatic pressure rises rapidly with even very small increases in interstitial volume (e.g., cerebral edema), preventing further edema formation. Thus, normal capillary hydrostatic pressure is insufficient to produce significant cerebral edema. This is most easily appreciated when considering the small reductions in plasma oncotic pressure, which produce edema in compliant peripheral tissues but not in the inelastic brain. A reduction in plasma osmolality or a sustained large increase in cerebral venous pressure and, therefore, capillary hydrostatic pressure, however, can produce a much greater driving force for edema formation.[20,21]

To summarize, plasma osmolality and, therefore, total osmotic pressure, not oncotic or hydrostatic pressure, is the predominant force governing water movement across the BBB into brain tissue. Cerebral edema readily develops as water moves into brain tissue in the presence of decreased plasma osmolality, as seen following hypoosmolar fluid administration (Fig. 6.6) or in association with hyponatremia. Likewise, water is removed from the brain interstitium when plasma osmolality is increased with hyperosmolar agents (e.g., mannitol and hypertonic saline). Stated another way, the brain acts much more like an osmometer than an oncometer; thus, as far as the brain is concerned, small changes in plasma osmolality are much more important than even large reductions in plasma oncotic pressure.[22–26]

INJURY TO THE CNS

The previous discussion assumes the presence of an intact BBB to regulate water movement in and out of the CNS. In many patients, however, normal BBB function is lost in some regions as a consequence of trauma, subarachnoid or intercerebral hemorrhage, tumor, cerebral ischemia, or preexisting hypertension. In this situation, the permeability to all osmotically active particles may be markedly increased in that portion of the BBB that is damaged. In an area of abnormal BBB function, few, if any, osmotic or oncotic pressure gradients can be established and water movement will be insensitive to changes in plasma osmolality and/or oncotic pressure behaving much more like the periphery as shown schematically in Figure 6.4 than in the normal CNS as depicted in Figure 6.5. This leaves intravascular hydrostatic pressure as the sole driving force for water movement and edema formation in the area of injury. However, the inelastic brain tissue resists edema formation from normal hydrostatic forces at the site of injury unless the area of injury is extensive (e.g., large contusion, stroke, or tumor) or CVP is very high (overresuscitation of a trauma victim), edema at the site of injury will minimally impact upon overall intracranial pressure. If plasma osmolality is reduced, however, this permits and promotes edema formation in surrounding areas of brain with an intact BBB, potentially increasing intracranial pressure, morbidity, and mortality.[20] In addition, an increase in CVP or a decrease in cerebral venous drainage may decrease CPP and increase ICP by increasing cerebral blood volume and also contribute to brain injury and poorer outcome.[21] Conversely, an important concept is that administration of hyperosmolar solutions can decrease ICP by increasing plasma osmolality and reducing interstitial edema in areas of normal brain, compensating for edema in the injured area.[27–29] In fact, experimental evidence suggests that in the setting of brain trauma, it is changes in plasma osmolality in those regions of normal brain with an intact BBB that most influence edema formation and ICP.[30–34]

FLUID ADMINISTRATION CHOICES

The clinician is faced with a variety of choices when considering fluid administration options for a neurosurgical patient. Debate continues over the advantages of colloids as compared to crystalloids. The risks associated with blood product administration have helped define and limit their uses. A promising new therapy for use in head-injured patients is the use of hyperosmolar crystalloids. Appropriate fluid selection must be directed toward the physiologic goals of minimizing cerebral edema, preserving cerebral perfusion and optimizing cerebral oxygen delivery.

Crystalloids

Crystalloids encompass a wide range of solutions that may be categorized according to their osmolality relative to plasma. They may also be further subdivided into glucose and non–glucose-containing solutions. All maintenance and resuscitation crystalloids contain low-MW solutes less than 30,000 to 40,000 daltons (e.g., ions, +/– glucose). Accordingly, they have no oncotic pressure (Table 6.1).

HYPOOSMOLAR Hypoosmolar crystalloids (i.e. those with as osmolality less than normal plasma, 285 mosm/kg) should not be used for neurosurgical patients except for the rare patient being treated for diabetes insipidus (DI). Any solution containing 5% dextrose should be viewed as During need to abbreviate terms used only once or twice having an effective osmolality that is actually 259 mosm/kg less than that stated; as glucose (osmolality 259) is rapidly metabolized leaving behind a glucose-free fluid or in the case of 5 percent dextrose in water, plain water. Excess free water in these solutions will lower plasma osmolality and create an osmotic gradient that pulls fluid across the BBB, causing the accumulation of interstitial brain water. This is especially hazardous in patients with preexisting intracranial hypertension.

Further inspection of Table 6.1 helps explain the observations by some that lactated Ringer's (LR) may actually cause brain edema as well. This is because the osmolality (measured) versus osmolarity (calculated) is approximately 250 versus 273. When compared to a normal plasma osmolality of 285, it is apparent that LR is hypoosmolar, thus, a considerable amount of free water accompanies LR administration. In fact, each liter of LR contains roughly 10% free water (100 ml) relative to normal plasma osmolality. These ob-

TABLE 6.1 *Osmolarity and osmolality of common intravenous fluids*

FLUID	OSMOLARITY (mosm/L)	OSMOLALITY (mosm/kg)
Water	0	0
D_5W	252	259
D_5.2NS	325	321
NS	308	282
LR	273	250
D_5LR	525	524
3% Saline	1,027	921
6% Hetastarch	310	307
20% Mannitol	1,098	1,280
Plasma protein fraction	290	276
5% Albumin	290	283
Plasmalyte	294	271

Abbreviations: D_5, 5% dextrose in water; D_5.2NS, 5% dextrose in 0.2 normal saline; NS, normal saline; LR, lactated Ringer's solution; D_5LR, 5% dextrose in lactated Ringer's solution.

servations support the routine use of 282 mosm/kg normal saline in place of LR during neurosurgical procedures in which patients are likely to have elevated ICP or when larger fluid volumes are necessary to maintain hemodynamic stability.

ISOOSMOLAR Isoosmolar crystalloid solutions (normal saline, Plasmalyte, and Normosol-R) have an osmolality that more closely approximates that of plasma. This prevents the development of osmotic gradients across the intact BBB and limits cerebral edema formation. Isoosmolar crystalloids should be administered in a way that maintains euvolemia to avoid hemodynamic instability. Larger volumes of saline-containing solutions may precipitate a hyperchloremic metabolic acidosis as bicarbonate is renally excreted to maintain electrochemical neutrality. This phenomenon is usually self-limiting, resolves within 24 hours, and requires no treatment.

HYPEROSMOLAR There continues to be considerable interest in the use of hyperosmolar solutions for resuscitation of brain-injured patients. These solutions *increase* plasma osmolality, creating osmotic gradients across the intact BBB, favoring water removal from brain tissue. The concept implementing this effect is not a new one, as hyperosmolar solutions like mannitol, urea, and glycerol have been used for decades to achieve intraoperative brain relaxation and ICP reduction. Urea and glycerol, however, have fallen out of favor due to their propensity to cause rebound intracranial hypertension.[35]

Mannitol Mannitol, the most widely used osmotic agent today, is a six-carbon sugar compound (MW = 182) that is excreted unchanged in the urine. Its clinical usefulness in reducing brain bulk is due primarily to its hyperosmolality (20% solution → 1280 mosm/kg), which will dehydrate brain tissue across an intact BBB. In addition, it may further decrease ICP by reductions in cerebral blood volume[36] and rate of CSF formation.[37–39]

Like other hyperosmolar solutions, however, mannitol is ineffective in dehydrating injured brain because osmotic gradients cannot be established. Because mannitol promotes water movement only in areas of normal brain, it may be less effective in reducing ICP with more extensive brain injuries. There is also concern that if mannitol moves across the injured BBB down its own concentration gradient, it may contribute to a rebound increase in ICP.[40–44] This, fortunately, does not appear to be a common clinical phenomenon. More likely, however, is a transient increase in ICP following bolus administration of mannitol. It has been reported that mannitol may exert a biphasic effect in ICP. Initially, ICP may increase from the acute increase in intravascular volume[45] or as cerebral vasodilation occurs in response to an acute increase in plasma osmolality.[35,46] This is rapidly followed by a sustained decrease in ICP as brain tissue is dehydrated.

In fact, the clinical significance of this transient mannitol-associated rise in ICP may be overstated. Instead, the effect of mannitol on ICP may depend more on the preexisting intracranial pressure. Increases in ICP have been demonstrated following mannitol administration in animals and humans with normal baseline ICP.[45,47,48] In the setting of intracranial hypertension, however, ICP does not appear to increase further with mannitol and likely will decline immediately.[47,49,50]

Mannitol is commonly given in 0.25 to 1.0 g/kg doses as an intravenous infusion over 15 minutes. Larger doses (more than 2 g/kg) have not uniformly caused further reductions in ICP and may precipitate intravascular volume overload as well as electrolyte and acid-base disturbances.[45,51,52] Of interest are reports of higher doses of mannitol: more than 2 g/kg, providing an additional cerebral protective effect via (1) enhancing cerebral blood flow[53,54] and (2) scavenging free radicals produced during episodes of neuronal ischemia.[55–57] Higher doses of mannitol may cause pontine hemorrhage and/or myelin disruption.

Clearly, the physiologic effects of mannitol on intracranial contents are multiple and sometimes conflicting. It remains, however, a popular and clinically reliable method to lower ICP and achieve brain relaxation in neurosurgical patients.

Hyperosmolar Salt Solutions More recently, hyperosmolar saline solutions have been evaluated for use in the treatment of hypovolemic shock and control of intracranial hypertension. These solutions may also decrease CSF production[58] but, more importantly, increase plasma osmolality, subsequently drawing water intravascularly to restore circulating plasma volume and reduce ICP. Like mannitol, normal brain tissue with an intact BBB is dehydrated to compensate for edema formation in injured brain, thus reducing ICP. Many investigators report that hyperosmolar saline is more effective than isoosmolar crystalloids or colloids in restoring intravascular volume and cerebral blood flow while simultaneously decreasing ICP.[24,26,34,59–69] In addition, there is anecdotal evidence of hyperosmolar saline effectively reducing ICP after conventional mannitol and hyperventilation therapy had failed.[70]

Clinical use of hyperosmolar saline (e.g., 3% saline) is usually limited to 500 to 1,000 ml in the adult patient to avoid extreme hypernatremia. It is not uncommon to see serum sodium levels rise to the range of 150 to 160 meq/Ler. Levels higher than this may be associated with seizures and mental status changes.[71] A theoretical concern is the development of central pontine myelinolysis from the acute increase in plasma sodium. This has not been reported in patients with normal plasma sodium levels who then receive hyperosmolar saline but has usually been associated with rapid correction of chronic hyponatremia.[72,73]

An additional concern that merits investigation is the effect of longer-term hyperosmolar saline therapy (i.e., 24 to 72 hours). Prough et al. reported no improvement in intracranial pressure or cerebral blood flow in cats with cerebral percussion injury and mild hemorrhage resuscitated with 3 percent normal saline. Furthermore, many animals demonstrated a delayed rise in ICP, suggesting that 3 percent normal saline may eventually increase cerebral edema and cause rebound intracranial hypertension.[74] This may be problematic for the clinician who is caring for the neurosurgical patient in the ICU following surgery.

Outside this single report, hyperosmolar salt solutions appear to be an attractive alternative for initial volume resuscitation and ICP reduction. Early studies are promising in models with and without brain injury. We look forward to further investigations to define all potential physiologic effects.

Glucose Administration and Hyperglycemia

The administration of glucose in the perioperative period is relatively contraindicated for neurosurgical patients exceept to treat hypoglycemia. Not only may glucose solutions cotribute to plasma hypoosmolality, glucose administration and hyperglycemia have repeatedly been associated with worsened neurologic outcome.[75–78] The evidence is convincing that glucose administration, with or without hyperglycemia, contributes to worsened outcome following global cerebral ischemia. It is less clear how it may affect focal ischemia in the CNS, because both beneficial and adverse effects have been demonstrated following focal neuronal ischemia.[78–81]

The plasma glucose level for aggravation of ischemic damage has not been firmly established but may well be less than 200 mg/dl. Likewise, it is not known how well blood glucose levels correlate with those in the brain. Glucose is transported into brain cells primarily by a saturable, carrier-mediated mechanism that can be affected by blood glucose levels.[82] It is our clinical practice to administer insulin to neurosurgical patients with a blood glucose greater than 200 mg/dl, although several studies have failed to demonstrate any effect of insulin on glucose transport in brain cells.[83,84] The efficacy of insulin therapy in reducing neurologic morbidity resulting from hyperglycemia has yet to be established.

A more difficult question to answer is the mechanism by which glucose loading or hyperglycemia worsens neurologic outcome. Initial studies pointed to lactic acid production from anaerobic metabolism of glucose during ischemia as the factor aggravating postischemic brain injury.[76,85] Lactic acidosis has not conclusively been determined to be the causative mechanism; in fact, other investigators have shown a neuroprotective effect of lactate.[86,87]

Despite these controversies, the take-home message and clinical preference is clear: avoid glucose administration and hyperglycemia when there is a risk of brain or spinal cord ischemia.

Colloids

Colloidal solutions (i.e., those with an oncotic pressure similar to plasma) have traditionally been favored by neurosurgeons concerned that reduction in oncotic pressure causes cerebral edema. Now there is much evidence suggesting that brain water content is similar with and without brain injury following colloid or isoosmolar crystalloid administration.[20,26,30,33,88] Zhaung et al, recently demonstrated that colloids did not decrease cortical water content or improve ICP and cerebral oxygen delivery after 24 hours in a swine model when compared to conventional crystalloid therapy.[89] Further evaluation is needed, however, to investigate longer-term effects (e.g., occurrence of rebound cerebral edema formation) following colloid versus crystalloid therapy before conclusively stating that colloidal therapy is without clinical advantage or detriment. Based on the available data, colloids are an expensive but acceptable alternative to isoosmolar crystalloids with no apparent advantages to the recipient with respect to cerebral edema and ICP. Colloids and hypertonic crystalloids are more effective in rapidly restoring intravascular volume and hemodynamic stability during hypovolemic shock than equivalent volumes of isoosmolar solutions. Therefore, when large volume fluid resuscitation is anticipated in a neurosurgical patient, it is reasonable to consider a combination of colloids and hyperosmolar or at a minimum isoosmolar crystalloids to preserve hemodynamic stability and minimize secondary brain injury. As previously discussed, there is growing support for hyperosmolar crystalloid therapy in this setting as well.

A variety of colloidal solutions are available for use by clinicians. These include polymerized glucose solutions like dextran, hetastarch and pentastarch, plasma derivatives, (albumin, Plasmanate), and blood products. Table 6.2 lists

TABLE 6.2 *Commonly used colloidal solutions*

COLLOID	DOSE	COMMENTS
Dextran 40	2 g Dextran/kg body weight (Hyperoncotic to plasma)	1. 50% renal excretion/24 h 2. Interference with blood typing and cross-matching if infuse >20% of blood volume 3. Allergic reactions <0.03% patients (anaphylaxis)
Dextran 70	2 g Dextran/kg body weight (oncotic pressure similar to plasma)	4. May cause coagulopathy by dilutional effects or coating of blood cellular elements and endothelium
Hetastarch (Hespan)	20–30 ml/kg/24 h	1. 30% renal excretion/24 h 2. Very low incidence of allergic reaction 3. Larger doses may prolong PT/PTT, thus limiting its use in neurosurgery; dilution of clotting factors, inhibition of platelet function, decrease in factor VIII activity
Pentastarch	20–30 ml/kg/24 h	1. Lower molecular weight than hetastarch, thus more complete renal elimination (70%/24 h) 2. May have fewer adverse effects on coagulation than hetastarch
Albumin	1:1 with blood loss	1. 5% and 25% solutions available for use 2. No effects on clotting 3. No allergic reactions 4. No infection risk 5. Expensive!
Plasmanate (purified protein fraction)	1:1 with blood loss	1. Contains 80–90% albumin 2. Impurities may cause transient hypotension 3. No advantages over albumin
Fresh frozen plasma	Variable	Indicated only for replacement of clotting factors during coagulapathy, risk of hepatitis and HIV transmission
Red blood cells	Variable	Indicated only for improving oxygen-carrying capacity secondary to anemia, infectious transmission risk like FFP

Abbreviations: PT, prothrombin time; PTT, partial thromboplastin time; HIV, human immunodeficiency virus; FFP, fresh-frozen plasma.

commonly used colloidal solutions, recommended dosages, and comments pertaining to their use.

Fluid Manipulation

Fluid manipulation, the other mechanism by which fluid management occurs during the perioperative period is accomplished by decreasing the fluid volume inside the cranial cavity. We have alluded to this earlier with respect to the administration of mannitol and hyperosmolar saline. Some other methods that reduce cerebral volume include enhancing cerebral venous drainage by establishing a head neutral and elevated position as opposed to a head-turned position when this is an option. Other options include (1) hyperventilation (2% decrease in cerebral blood flow per 1 Torr decrease in $PaCO_2$), (2) cerebral vasoconstriction (e.g., barbiturate administration), (3) maintaining PaO_2, $PaCO_2$, and mean arterial pressure (MAP) within cerebral autoregulatory limits, (4) CSF drainage, (5) surgical decompression, (6) diuresis, and (7) lowering CVP.[91,92]

Osmotic diuresis with mannitol is the most commonly utilized method for reducing brain water content in the perioperative period. Furosemide, a loop diuretic, is also effective in decreasing brain water and therefore ICP as well. It is often the preferred diuretic in those patients with marginal cardiac reserve who may not tolerate the intravascular volume loading that occurs with mannitol administration. Furosemide has been shown to lower brain water content and ICP more effectively than mannitol when administered in large doses (1 mg/kg).[45] Unlike mannitol, however,it has not always consistently lowered ICP when used as a single agent.[93] When furosemide is used in combination with mannitol, a greater and more sustained decrease in ICP has been demonstrated than seen with either drug alone.[93] Roberts et al, confirmed this in an animal model and determined that the largest and most prolonged reduction in ICP was observed when furosemide was given 15 minutes after a mannitol bolus.[94] Even small doses of furosemide (5 to 20 mg) appear to augment ICP reduction by prolonging the period of increased plasma osmolality with mannitol, thus allowing for continued brain dehydration across the BBB.[94] When this technique is used, you must anticipate a more profound diuresis and the accompanying electrolyte alterations and reductions of intravascular volume that may require treatment. Although furosemide is effective in the pharmacologic treatment of cerebral edema and reduction in ICP, its use is best reserved for when mannitol alone is inadequate or in those patients in whom mannitol may be contraindicated.

ELECTROLYTE ABNORMALITIES

Electrolyte abnormalities are common in neurosurgical patients and usually affect sodium, chloride, or potassium homeostasis. Abnormalities may result directly from the associated intracranial injury and/or may be iatrogenically induced. Whatever the cause, close monitoring, especially of serum Na^+ and K^+ values, allows timely recognition and prompts treatment to prevent additional morbidity.

Sodium and Chloride

Hyponatremia may occur in association with a reduced, normal, or increased intravascular volume. Hypovolemic hyponatremia may accompany prolonged diuretic usage. Likewise, a small percentage of neurosurgical patients may develop a clinical syndrome known as *cerebral salt wasting* in which intravascular volume depletion accompanies primary natriuresis. It is important to differentiate this from the syndrome of inappropriate secretion of antidiuretic hormone in which intravascular volume status is relatively normal. Dilutional hyponatremia may also occur with administration of hypoosmolar crystalloids or with the intravascular volume overload that may accompany mannitol administration. It may also be seen in patients with significant underlying cardiac or renal dysfunction.

Determination of the underlying cause is the initial and most important step in appropriately treating hyponatremia. Severe reductions in sodium (less than 120 to 130 meq/L) may be associated with cerebral edema, seizures, or mental status changes, which can make neurologic evaluation difficult. Furthermore, overzealous correction of hyponatremia may precipitate central pontine myelinolysis; therefore, conservative sodium correction therapy is recommended: 1 to 2 meq/L/h up to 12 meq/L/day.[95]

Hypernatremia in neurosurgical patients is most commonly associated with the development of DI, particularly following pituitary surgery. The diagnosis of DI is suggested by copious dilute urine in the presence of increased plasma osmolality and sodium. It may occur intraoperatively but most often occurs in the immediate postoperative period. Treatment requires judicious administration of hypoosmolar crystalloids (e.g., 0.45% saline and DDAVP (1-desamino-8-D-arginine vasopressin) (1 to 4 μg IV/SC q 12 to 24 hours) to reestablish isoosmolality and euvolemia. Short-lived hypernatremia also accompanies the use of hyperosmolar saline and usually requires no treatment. A hyperchloremic metabolic acidosis also commonly occurs with hyperosmolar saline therapy. The pH may decrease to below 7.30 as bicarbonate is renally excreted in the presence of excess chloride ions; however, equilibrium is usually spontaneously reestablished within 24 hours. Again, no intervention is typically required unless a more significant acidosis develops as a result of other factors.

Potassium

Hypokalemia may result from renal losses of potassium following diuretic administration or from excess mineralocorticoid activity associated with steroid therapy. Similarly, plasma levels of potassium may drop while total body potassium stores remain normal during hyperventilation or insulin therapy for hyperglycemia, because potassium is shifted intracellularly. True potassium depletion may require treatment perioperatively to avoid cardiac irritability and dysrhythmias; however, our clinical experience suggests that it is generally not necessary to treat low plasma levels associated with the temporary intracellular shift of potassium.

Hyperkalemia has been associated with mannitol administration and is seemingly dose dependent. It is usually a transient phenomenon that requires no treatment unless there is significant underlying renal dysfunction. It has been reported that hyperkalemic electrocardiogram abnormalities have been observed following mannitol administration.[96]

CONCLUSIONS

To summarize, both perioperative fluid administration *and* manipulation can significantly influence cerebral water content, intracranial pressure, and cerebral perfusion. The brain appears to function most like an osmometer, responding to small changes in plasma osmolality, whereas water movement in peripheral tissues is more dependent on oncotic and hydrostatic pressure gradients. Hypoosmolality is one of the most significant etiologic factors under the control of the anesthesiologist in the development of cerebral edema. Oncotic pressure has little effect on water movement across the BBB, thus isoosmolar crystalloids, not colloids, are recommended for maintenance of intravascular volume in neurosurgical patients. We refer the reader again to Table 6.1 to be reminded which crystalloids are in actuality hypotonic.

Maintenance of euvolemia and adequate CPP are critical in avoiding secondary brain injury and additional morbidity and mortality. Glucose appears to contribute to brain injury, thus, glucose administration and hyperglycemia are to be avoided as well. Hyperosmolar therapy continues to be an important method of reducing intracranial pressure and is promising as an alternative means of volume resuscitation in the neurosurgical patient.

References

1. Shenkin HA, Bezier HS, Bouzarth WF: Restricted fluid intake. Rational management of the neurosurgical patient. J Neurosurg 45:432, 1976
2. American College of Surgeons: Advanced trauma life support course. Instructor's Manual, 1988
3. Jelsma LF, McQueen JD: Effect of experimental water restriction on brain water. J Neurosurg 26:35, 1967
4. Colley PS, Cheney FW, Butler J: Mechanism of change in pulmonary shunt flow with hemorrhage. J Appl Physiol 42:196, 1977
5. Chesnut RM, Marshall LF, Klauber MR et al: The role of secondary brain injury in determining outcome from severe head injury. J Trauma 34:216, 1993
6. Pietropaoli JA, Rogers FB, Shackford SR et al: The deleterious effects of intraoperative hypotension on outcome in patients with severe head injuries. J Trauma 33:403, 1992
7. Ishige N, Pitts LH, Pogliani L et al: Effect of hypoxia on traumatic brain injury in rats. 1. Changes in neurological function, electroencephalograms, and histopathology. Neurosurgery 20:848, 1987
8. Ishige N, Pitts LH, Berry I et al: The effects of hypovolemic hypotension on high-energy phosphate metabolism of traumatized brain in rats. J Neurosurg 68:129, 1988
9. Jenkins LW, Moszynski K, Lyeth BG et al: Increased vulnerability of the mildly traumatized rat brain to cerebral ischemia: the use of controlled secondary ischemia as a research tool to identify common or different mechanisms contributing to mechanical and ischemic brain injury. Brain Res 477:211, 1989
10. Dewitt DS, Prough DS, Taylor CL et al: Reduced cerebral blood flow, oxygen delivery, and electroencephalographic activity after traumatic brain injury and mild hemorrhage in cats. J Neurosurg 76:812, 1992
11. Deardorff DL: Osmotic strength, osmolality and osmolarity. Am J Hosp Pharm 37:504, 1980
12. Gennari FJ: Current concepts. Serum osmolality. Uses and limitations. N Engl J Med 310:102, 1984
13. Starling EH: On the absorption of fluids from the connective tissue spaces. J Physiol 19:312, 1896
14. Pollay M, Roberts PA: Blood-brain barrier: a definition of normal and altered function. Neurosurgery 6:675, 1980
15. Fenstermacher JD: Volume regulations of the central nervous system. p. 383. In Staub NC, Taylor AE (eds): Edema. Raven Press, New York, 1984
16. Dodge PR, Crawford JD, Probst JH: Studies in experimental water intoxication. Arch Neurol 3:513, 1960
17. Weed LH, McKibben PS: Experimental alteration of brain bulk. Am J Physiol 48:531, 1919
18. Weed LH, McKibben PS: Pressure changes in the cerebro-spinal fluid following intravenous injection of solutions of various concentrations. Am J Physiol 48:512, 1919
19. Tommasino C, Moore S, Todd MM: Cerebral effects of isovolemic hemodilution with crystalloid or colloid solutions. Crit Care Med 1988;16:862–8.
20. Zornow MH, Todd MM, Moore SS: The acute cerebral effects of changes in plasma osmolality and oncotic pressure. Anesthesiology 67:936, 1987
21. Cuypers J, Matakas F, Potolicchio SJ Jr: Effect of central venous pressure on brain tissue pressure and brain volume. J Neurosurg 45:89, 1976
22. Albright AL, Latchaw RE, Robinson AG: Intracranial and systemic effects of osmotic and oncotic therapy in experimental cerebral edema. J Neurosurg 60:481, 1984
23. Poole GV, Johnson JC, Prough DS et al: Cerebral hemodynamics after hemorrhagic shock: effects of the type of resuscitation fluid. Crit Care Med 14:629, 1986
24. Prough DS, Johnson JC, Poole GV et al: Effects on intracranial pressure of resuscitation from hemorrhagic shock with hypertonic saline versus lactated Ringer's solution. Crit Care Med 13:407, 1985
25. Shackford SR, Norton CH, Todd MM: Renal, cerebral, and pulmonary effects of hypertonic resuscitation in a porcine model of hemorrhagic shock. Surgery 104:553, 1988
26. Todd MM, Tommasino C, Moore S: Cerebral effects of isovolemic hemodilution with a hypertonic saline solution. J Neurosurg 63:944, 1985
27. Clasen RA, Cooke PM, Pandolfi S et al: Hypertonic urea in experimental cerebral edema. Arch Neurol 12:424, 1965
28. Pappius HM, Dayes LA: Hypertonic urea. Its effect on the distribution of water and electrolytes in normal and edematous brain tissues. Arch Neurol 13:395, 1965
29. Bell BA, Smith MA, Kean DM et al: Brain water measured by magnetic resonance imaging. Correlation with direct estimation and changes af-

ter mannitol and dexamethasone. Lancet 1:66, 1987
30. Zornow MH, Scheller MS, Todd MM, Moore SS: Acute cerebral effects of isotonic crystalloid and colloid solutions following cryogenic brain injury in the rabbit. Anesthesiology 69:180, 1988
31. Kaieda R, Todd MM, Cook LN, Warner DS: Acute effects of changing plasma osmolality and colloid oncotic pressure on the formation of brain edema after cryogenic injury. Neurosurgery 24:671, 1989
32. Kaieda R, Todd MM, Warner DS: Prolonged reductions in colloid oncotic pressure does not increase brain edema following cryogenic injury in rabbits. Anesthesiology 71:554, 1989
33. Warner DS, Boehland LA: Effects of iso-osmolal intravenous fluid therapy on postischemic brain water content in the rat. Anesthesiology 68:86, 1988
34. Zornow MH, Scheller MS, Shackford SR: Effect of a hypertonic lactated Ringer's solution on intracranial pressure and cerebral water content in a model of traumatic brain injury. J Trauma 29:484, 1989
35. Shenkin HA, Golubuff B, Haft H: Further observations on the effects of abruptly increased osmotic pressure of plasma on cerebrospinal-fluid pressure in man. J Neurosurg 22:563, 1965
36. Muizelaar JP, Wei EP, Kontos HA, Becker DP: Mannitol causes compensatory cerebral vasoconstriction and vasodilation in response to blood viscosity changes. J Neurosurg 59:822, 1983
37. Sahar A, Tsipstein E: Effects of mannitol and furosemide on the rate of formation of cerebrospinal fluid. Exp Neurol 60:584, 1978
38. Rudehill A, Gordon E, Ohman G et al: Pharmacokenetics and effects of monnitrol on hemodynamics, blood and cererospinal fluid electrolytes, and osmolality during intracranial surgery. J Neurosurg Anesthesiol 5:4, 1993
39. Donato T, Shapira Y, Artru A, Powers K: Effect of mannitol on cerebrospinal fluid dynamics and brain tissue edema. Anesth Analg 78:58, 1994
40. Rudehill A, Gordon T, Ohman G et al: Pharmacokinetics and effects of mannitol on hemodynamics, blood and cerebrospinal fluid electrolytes, and osmolality during intracranial surgery. J Neurosur Anesthesiol 5:4, 1993
41. McManus ML, Strange K: Rapid volume regulation in brain cells exposed to hypertonic saline. J Neurosurg Anesthesiol 4:300, 1992
42. McManus ML, Strange K: Rebound swelling of astroglial cells exposed to hypertonic mannitol (abstract). Anesthesiology 79:A769, 1993
43. McManus ML, Strange K: Acute volume regulation of brain cells in response to hypertonic challenge. Anesthesiology 78:1132, 1993
44. Kaufmann AM, Cardoso ER: Aggravation of vasogenic cerebral edema by multiple-dose mannitol. J Neurosurg 77:584, 1992
45. Cottrell JE, Robustelli A, Post K, Turndorf H: Furosemide- and mannitol-induced changes in intracranial pressure and serum osmolality and electrolytes. Anesthesiology 47:28, 1977
46. Coté CJ, Greenhow DE, Marshall BE: The hypotensive response to rapid intravenous administration of hypertonic solutions in man and in the rabbit. Anesthesiology 50:30, 1979
47. Abou-Madi M, Trop D, Abou-Madi N, Ravussin P: Does a bolus of mannitol initially aggravate intracranial hypertension? A study of various $PaCO_2$ tensions in dogs. Br J Anaesth 59:630, 1987
48. Zornow MH, Oh YS, Scheller MS: A comparison of the cerebral and hemodynamic effects of mannitol and hypertonic saline in a rabbit model of brain injury abstracted. Anesthesiology 69:A623, 1988
49. Ravussin P, Abou-Madi M, Archer D et al: Changes in CSF pressure after mannitol in patients with and without elevated CSF pressure. J Neurosurg 69:869, 1988.
50. Marshall LF, Smith RW, Rauscher LA, Shapiro HM: Mannitol dose requirements in brain-injured patients. J Neurosurg 48:169, 1978
51. Manninen PH, Lam AM, Gelb AW, Brown SC: The effect of high-dose mannitol on serum and urine electrolytes and osmolality in neurosurgical patients. Can J Anaesth 34:442, 1987
52. Berry AJ, Peterson ML: Hyponatremia after mannitol administration in the presence of renal failure. Anesth Analg 60:165, 1981
53. Jafar JJ, Johns LM, Mullan SF: The effect of mannitol on cerebral blood flow. J Neurosurg 59:754, 1986
54. Meyer FB, Anderson RE, Sundt TM, Yaksh TL: Treatment of experimental focal cerebral ischemia with mannitol. Assessment by intracellular brain pH, cortical blood flow, and electroencephalography. J Neurosurg 66:109, 1987
55. Suzuki J, Takahashi A, Yoshimoto T, Seki H: Use of balloon occlusion and substances to protect ischemic brain during resection of posterior fossa AVM. Case report. Stroke 63:626, 1985

56. Yoshimoto T, Sakamoto T, Watanabe T et al: Experimental cerebral infarction. Part 3: Protective effect of mannitol in thalamic infarction in dogs. Stroke 9:217, 1978
57. Little JR: Modification of acute focal ischemia by treatment with mannitol. Stroke 9:4, 1978
58. Foxworthy JC, Artru AA: Cerebrospinal fluid dynamics and brain tissue composition following intravenous infusion of hypertonic saline in anesthetized rabbits. J Neurosurg Anesth 2:256, 1990
59. Gunnar W, Jonasson O, Merlotti G et al: Head injury and hemorrhagic shock: studies of the blood-brain barrier and intracranial pressure after resuscitation with normal saline solution, 3% saline solution, and dextran-40. Surgery 103:398, 1988
60. Gunnar WP, Merlotti GJ, Barrett J, Jonasson O: Resuscitation from hemorrhagic shock. Alterations of the intracranial pressure after normal saline, 3% saline and dextran-40. Ann Surg 204:686, 1986
61. Prough DS, Johnson JC, Stump DA et al: Effects of hypertonic saline versus lactated Ringer's solution on cerebral oxygen transport during resuscitation from hemorrhagic shock. J Neurosurg 64:627, 1986
62. Prough DS, Johnson JC, Stullken EH et al: Effects on cerebral hemodynamics of resuscitation from endotoxic shock with hypertonic saline versus lactated Ringer's solution. Crit Care Med 13:1040, 1985
63. Prough DS, Whitley JM, Taylor CL et al: Regional cerebral blood flow following resuscitation from hemorrhagic shock with hypertonic saline. Influence of a subdural mass. Anesthesiology 75:319, 1991
64. Wisner DH, Schuster L, Quinn C: Hypertonic saline resuscitation of head injury: effects on cerebral water content. J Trauma 30:75, 1990
65. Schmoker JD, Zhuang J, Shackford SR: Hypertonic fluid resuscitation improves cerebral oxygen delivery and reduces intracranial pressure after hemorrhagic shock. J Trauma 31:1607, 1991
66. Ducey JP, Mozingo DW, Lamiell JM et al: A comparison of the cerebral and cardiovascular effects of complete resuscitation with isotonic and hypertonic saline, hetastarch, and whole blood following hemorrhage. J Trauma 29:1510, 1989
67. Shackford SR, Zhuang J, Schmoker J: Intravenous fluid tonicity: effect on intracranial pressure, cerebral blood flow, and cerebral oxygen delivery in focal brain injury. J Neurosurg 76:91, 1992
68. Fisher B, Thomas D, Peterson B: Hypertonic saline lowers raised intracranial pressure in children after head trauma. J Neurosurg Anesthesiol 4:4, 1992
69. Scheller MS, Zornow MH, Oh YS: A comparison of the cerebral and hemodynamic effects of mannitol and hypertonic saline in a rabbit model of acute cryogenic brain injury. J Neurosurg Anesthesiol 3:291, 1991
70. Worthley LI, Cooper DJ, Jones N: Treatment of resistant intracranial hypertension with hypertonic saline. Report of two cases. J Neurosurg 68:478, 1988
71. Sotos JF, Dodge PR, Meara P, Talbot NB: Studies in experimental hypertonicity. I. Pathogenesis of the clinical syndrome, biochemical abnormalities and cause of death. Pediatrics 26:925, 1960
72. Sterns RH, Riggs JE, Schochet SS Jr: Osmotic demyelination syndrome following correction of hyponatremia. N Eng J Med 314:1535, 1986
73. Kleinschmidt-DeMasters BK, Norenberg MD: Rapid correction of hyponatremia causes demyelination: relation to central pontine myelinolysis. Science 211:1068, 1981
74. Prough DS, DeWitt DS, Taylor CL et al: Hypertonic saline does not reduce intracranial pressure or improve cerebral blood flow after experimental head injury and hemorrhage in cats abstract. Anesthesiology 75:A544, 1991
75. Lanier WL, Stangland KJ, Scheithauer BW et al: The effect of dextrose infusion and head position on neurological outcome after complete cerebral ischemia in primates: examination of a model. Anesthesiology 66:39, 1987
76. Pulsinelli WA, Waldman S, Rawlinson D, Plum F: Moderate hyperglycemia augments ischemic brain damage: a neuropathologic study in the rat. Neurology 32:1239, 1982
77. Drummond JC, Moore SS: The influence of dextrose administration on neurologic outcome after temporary spinal cord ischemia in the rabbit. Anesthesiology 70:64, 1989
78. D'Alecy LG, Lundy EF, Barton KJ, Zelenock GB: Dextrose containing intravenous fluid impairs outcome and increases death after eight minutes of cardiac arrest and resuscitation in dogs. Surgery 100:505, 1986
79. De-courten-Meyers G, Myers RE, Schoolfield L: Hyperglycemia enlarges infarct size in cerebrovascular occlusion in cats. Stroke 19:623, 1988
80. Ginsberg MD, Prado R, Dietrich WD et al: Hyper-

glycemia reduces the extent of cerebral infarction in rats. Stroke 18:570, 1987
81. Zasslow MA, Pearl RG, Shuer LM et al: Hyperglycemia decreases acute neuronal ischemic changes after middle cerebral artery occlusion in cats. Stroke 20:519, 1989
82. Seisjö BK: Brain energy metabolism. Utilization of substrates by brain tissues. p. 110. John Wiley & Sons, New York, 1978
83. Crone C: Facilitated transfer of glucose from blood into brain tissue. J Physiol (Lond) 181:103, 1965
84. Gilboe DD, Andrews RL, Dardenne G: Factors affecting glucose uptake by the isolated dog brain. Am J Physiol 219:767, 1970
85. Welsh FA, Ginsberg MD, Rieder W, Budd WW: Deleterious effect of glucose pretreatment on recovery from diffuse cerebral ischemia in the cat. II. Regional metabolite levels. Stroke 11:355, 1980
86. Choi DW, Monyer H, Giffard RG et al: Acute brain injury, NMDA receptors, and hydrogen ions: observations in cortical cell cultures. Adv Exp Med Biol 268:501, 1990
87. Giffard RG, Monyer H, Christine CW, Choi DW: Acidosis reduces NMDA receptor activation, glutamate neurotoxicity, and oxygen-glucose deprivation neuronal injury in cortical cultures. Brain Res 506:339, 1990
88. Wisner D, Busche F, Sturm J et al: Traumatic shock and head injury: effects of fluid resuscitation on the brain. J Surg Res 46:49, 1989
89. Zhuang J. Shackford S, Schmoker JD, Pietropaoli JA Jr: Colloid infusion after brain injury: effect on intracranial pressure, cerebral blood flow, and oxygen delivery. Crit Care Med 23:140, 1995
90. Stump DC, Strauss RG, Henriksen RA et al: Effects of hydroxyethyl starch on blood coagulation, particularly factor VIII. Transfusion 25:349, 1985
91. Todd MM, Weeks JB, Warner DS: The influence of intravascular volume expansion on cerebral blood flow and blood volume in normal rats. Anesthesiology 78:945, 1993
92. Todd MM, Weeks JB, Warner DS: Microwave fixation for the determination of cerebral blood volume in rats. J Cereb Blood Flow Metab 13:328, 1993
93. Pollay M, Fullenwider C, Roberts PA, Sterens FA: Effect of mannitol and furosemide on blood-brain osmotic gradient and intracranial pressure. J Neurosurg 59:945, 1983
94. Roberts PA, Pollay M, Engles C et al: Effect on intracranial pressure of furosemide combined with varying doses and administration rates of mannitol. J Neurosurg 66:440, 1987
95. Snyder NA, Fiegal DW, Arieff AI: Hypernatremia in elderly patients. A heterogeneous, morbid, and iatrogenic entity. Ann Intern Med 107:309, 1987
96. Moreno M, Murphy C, Goldsmith C: Increase in serum potassium resulting from the administration of hypertonic mannitol and other solutions. J Lab Clin Med 73:291, 1969

7 NEURODIAGNOSTIC PROCEDURES

MARK F. TRANKINA

Although there are few indications for the use of general anesthesia in adults for diagnostic radiologic procedures, agitated adults, pediatric patients, or the mentally retarded may require either general anesthesia or heavy sedation. Occasionally, even in cooperative patients such as trauma victims, it may be prudent to use general endotracheal anesthesia for airway protection. Furthermore, intravenous sedation in some high-risk patients may be more hazardous than general anesthesia; airway control prevents carbon dioxide–induced increases in intracranial pressure (ICP) that can be seen in these patients with sedation alone.

In selecting an anesthetic technique for a specific procedure, both the anesthetic implications of the patient's disease process and the needs of the radiologist must be carefully balanced. The anesthesiologist may be confronted with a radiologic suite designed poorly for performing general anesthesia. Problems include isolated locations, lack of space, bulky radiologic apparatus, and personnel unaccustomed to the needs of anesthesia.

This chapter reviews the common neurodiagnostic procedures in relation to the requirements placed on the anesthesiologist. As anesthesiologists, we should be familiar with these procedures, the positions required, and problems encountered to facilitate communication with the radiologist. Finally, the difficulties in monitoring specifically associated with magnetic resonance imaging (MRI) are outlined.

GENERAL CONSIDERATIONS

Evaluation of a patient who is to undergo a neurodiagnostic procedure should be similar to that required for any general anesthetic because it may become necessary to change from local analgesia/sedation to a general anesthetic, sometimes under very difficult conditions. In the neurologic patient population, additional factors must be considered. The presence of cerebrovascular disease may suggest the possibility of coronary artery disease and the need for closer hemodynamic monitoring. If an intracranial mass lesion is present, signs of increased intracranial pressure should be sought. Patients with upper motor lesions (not cerebral palsy[1]), lower motor lesions, encephalitis, cerebral vascular accidents, closed head injury, severe burns, and acute trauma as well as patients after prolonged bed rest are at risk for a hyperkalemic response to succinylcholine.[2–5] Parkinson's disease does not appear to be a problem.[6] Prolonged patient immobility also raises concern about possible increased central nerious system depressant effects of anesthesia. The patient may be unable to give an adequate history due to a decreased level of consciousness, and associated systemic or serious chronic disease states may not be recognized. The possibility of a full stomach, cervical spine injury, and possible multiple organ involvement should be considered. Preparation of the patient may be inadequate because these patients often are received from wards unfamiliar with preanesthetic care.

Many neurodiagnostic procedures are invasive and may cause some discomfort, but none should absolutely require a general anesthetic because of the procedure itself. These procedures do require patient immobility for prolonged periods (i.e., cooperation for adequate studies). This often can be accomplished with compassionate encouragement and intravenous sedation. When this is not possible, increased sedation or even general anesthesia may be required. When hypercapnia is a concern or the airway is tenuous, it is prudent to protect the airway with an endotracheal tube after facilitation with general anesthesia.[7,8]

Nausea is a common complaint during radiologic procedures. Risk is potentially increased when the patient is anxious and positioning places the stomach above the head. Metoclopramide, given 2 hours before the procedure, and H_2-blockers often are efficacious.

Most radiologic suites are poorly suited for anesthesia and rarely is an anesthesiologist consulted on their design. However, equipment for monitoring, ventilation, and resuscitation must be equivalent to that used in the operating room. Electrocardiographic (ECG) monitoring is essential because dysrhythmias may be the first sign of increased pressure on the brainstem, especially in the presence of controlled ventilation. Measures to improve comfort (e.g., foam padding of extremities and bladder catheterization) tend to improve patients' acceptance of long procedures.

COMPUTED TOMOGRAPHY

Computed tomography (CT) uses a well-collimated narrow beam of x-rays that are projected through the study object from many angles of incidence in an axial plane. The transmitted photons are then detected by gamma detectors on the opposite side of the study object. A computer, using Fourier transformation, then analyzes the data including absorption values of the sample relative to its location, the location of the x-ray beam and the detectors, and produces images as cross-sectional slices or "cuts." The differences in the radiation absorption coefficient between different normal tissues as well as between normal and abnormal tissues enable the computer to separate these tissues from each other.

Since its introduction, CT has been extremely useful for intracranial pathology and has become the most widely used neuroradiologic procedure.[9] More recently, it has been used to investigate intraspinal and paraspinal pathology such as spinal neoplasms and anomalies, herniated discs, and spinal stenosis.[10–12] Conventional techniques such as cerebral pneumoencephalography and angiography are unable to produce the image quality or the almost total safety seen with CT. In addition, CT has sensitivity of greater than 100 times that of conventional x-rays. Samples of low density such as air and cerebrospinal fluid (CSF) appear as darker shades, whereas more dense tissues such as blood, bone, and intracranial calcifications are indicated by lighter shades. Brain parenchyma takes on an intermediate shading, whereas cerebral edema appears less dense than normal brain tissue.[13] Abnormalities are recognized as either differences in density from adjacent tissues or when density differences are not present, by displacement of structures such as the ventricles.[14] Enhancement of intracranial neoplasms, infarcts, vascular lesions, and abscesses is obtained by intravenous administration of water-soluble iodinated contrast material.[15]

Hazards of Computed Tomography

CT is a noninvasive procedure unless contrast material is used for enhancement. This doubles the scan time and exposes the patient to the potential problems associated with contrast material (see below). General anesthesia is rarely required with adults, and in one study, 17 percent of all patients receiving anesthesia have suffered acute head trauma.[13]

During a 30-minute scan, the patient is exposed to the amount of radiation associated with a conventional skull radiograph or 1.0 to 2.5 rads. The highest radiation field in the room is from x-ray emitter tube leakage. An anesthesiologist positioned away from the emitter tube should expect to receive a skin dose of 1 to 2 mrads/h.[16] This dose should allow safe participation in a full daily schedule.[13] Lead shields and radiation monitoring badges should be worn at all times.

Anesthetic Management

Anesthetic considerations include those discussed above as well as several others. Space is usually limited because the scanners are large and sometimes are placed in rooms not originally designed for them. Anesthetic equipment and monitoring should meet the same standards as those in the operating room. In my institution, anesthetic gases are piped in to a conventional anesthesia machine and a circle system is usually used. A Bain circuit attached to a bracket mounted system of flowmeters and vaporizers can be used to conserve space.[17] Monitoring should include ECG, blood pressure, precordial stethoscope, and pulse oximetry. CT suites are kept cool to prevent equipment malfunction, and therefore temperature must be closely monitored, especially in small children.

Adequate sedation should include the following: rapid action, controllable duration of action, safety, dependable immobilization, and ease of administration. This ideal sedative most likely does not exist, yet many attempts at mixtures or "cocktails" have been described.[17,18] Respiratory depression and even cardiac arrest have been described with these mixtures (and virtually all sedative techniques), and much of the experience is anecdotal.[19] Thompson et al.[18] described a cocktail of intramuscular (IM) atropine, meperidine, promethazine, and secobarbital supplemented with intravenous secobarbital as needed, with a failure rate of 12 percent (i.e., inadequate radiologic study) and a complication rate of 3.5 percent. An alternative is a single drug such as choral hydrate in a dose of 80 mg/kg orally, as is often used by the radiology department.[18] Other possibilities include pentobarbital 5 to 6 mg/kg IM, with a maximum dose of 200 mg given 30 minutes before the study.[17] Varner et al.[20] used IM methohexital 10 mg/kg with excellent results in infants and children (i.e., sedation in 3.3 minutes and arousability in 50 minutes). Rectal barbiturates such as methohexital 25 mg/kg can be adequate for short procedures and avoid the pain associated with intramuscular barbiturates. Burckart et al.[21] used rectal thiopental 25 to 45 mg/kg with excellent results: adequate sedation in 97 percent, mean onset time of 8 minutes, and mean duration of 2.75 hours.

At my institution, mixtures are rarely used. A common technique is titration to effect of individual drugs such as midazolam 1 mg at a time with fentanyl 1 to 2 μg/kg intravenously if the procedure is to be painful. Conscious sedation with propofol delivered by a syringe pump has also been used frequently with great success. Unconscious sedation with propofol is advocated by some authors even in pediatric patients.[22,23] Oral midazolam 0.5 to 0.8 mg/kg is frequently used in children and can facilitate the placement of an intravenous line.

Ketamine has been touted as a useful agent because it maintains a clear airway and stable hemodynamics.[24] However, ketamine increases cerebral blood flow and ICP,[25] with resultant apnea having been described.[26] In addition, airway problems and unpredictability of motion have been described.[17,27] Therefore, its use in neurodiagnostics cannot be advocated. Despite some recent research advocating ketamine for cerebral protection, I believe that it is not indicated for clinical use in these patients.

Attempts at sedation may fail and be especially dangerous when the airway becomes questionable or CO_2 retention occurs. Patients with borderline or established intracranial hypertension would not be expected to tolerate sedation alone. Detailed attention to technique and an understanding of the disease process and cerebrovascular physiology are necessary. Because the patient's head is inaccessible during the study, intubation of the trachea is prudent, regardless of the reason for general anesthesia. In addition, many centers have used the laryngeal mask airway (LMA) with great success. Given the patient's pathologic process, induction of anesthesia should follow the same criteria outlined elsewhere in this text. Induction of anesthesia can include thiopental, oxygen, and relaxant.[13] This technique allows for rapid recovery and early assessment of neurologic status. Volatile agents,[27] with or without propofo,[28] can be safely used with precautions as outlined elsewhere in the text. Controlled ventilation with moderate hyperventilation can facilitate ICP control. It is more efficient and probably safer to schedule studies requiring general anesthesia immediately before going to surgery so that all these can be achieved with the same anesthetic experience.

Examination of the posterior fossa may require extreme flexion of the neck, especially in children with severe hydrocephalus.[29] This may cause discomfort in the conscious patient, and analgesia/sedation or even general anesthesia may be required.[13] In addition, flexion may cause a kink in an endotracheal tube, compromise blood flow to the brain, or produce brainstem compression in the presence of a large infratentorial mass.[7]

PNEUMOENCEPHALOGRAPHY

This unpleasant procedure has been almost totally eliminated in the United States by CT and MRI. It may still be used in some centers without access to MRI in the diagnosis of small mass lesions in the sellar and cerebellopontine angle regions. Gaseous contrast is placed into the lumbar subarachnoid space and the patient's position manipulated, while in a special chair, to move the gas intracranially to outline the pathologic lesion. It is important to avoid increases in cerebral ventricular pressure, which may decrease air entry into the necessary regions. Complications include headache, nausea, vomiting, hypertension, hypotension, tachycardia, and bradycardia.[30] Major complications include syncope, cardiovascular collapse, air embolus, and brainstem herniation.[31] These complications can occur abruptly, and diagnosis may be difficult. If hemodynamic compromise occurs after lumbar puncture but before air injection, herniation is the probable cause. If compromise occurs soon after air injection, then embolism should be considered. In addition to the usual supportive measures, the left lateral decubitus position for air embolism and subarachnoid injection of saline for brainstem herniation should be considered.[17] Despite the fact that pneumoencephalography is one of the most uncomfortable procedures, it is usually performed by using only sedation to facilitate diagnosis of the many potential complications that would be more difficult under general anesthesia.

ANGIOGRAPHY OF THE CENTRAL NERVOUS SYSTEM

CT and MRI have reduced the use of angiography in neurodiagnosis, but it often is still used to evaluate vascular lesions such as arteriovenous malformations, carotid atherosclerosis, vasculopathy, cerebral aneurysms, and certain tumors. Arterial puncture and catheterization may produce spasm, hematomas, embolization of atherosclerotic plaques, thrombosis, intimal dissection, and compression of smaller branch vessels.[32] Other complications include transient global amnesia,[33] cortical blindness,[33] and multiple cholesterol emboli syndrome.[34] Pain and burning may be produced by the contrast medium in the vascular distribution site, although this has decreased in incidence with the introduction of newer media. Spasm may be especially dangerous in the presence of a leaking intracerebral aneurysm, in which existing spasm may be worsened. Anaphylaxis can also be seen with the use of contrast media, but this is less common after intra-arterial than intravenous injection (see section on contrast media). Contrast media can also be associated with hypotension and dysrhythmias as well as convulsions, loss of speech or sight, and paralysis.[35]

Spinal cord angiography is almost always performed by using selective injection techniques coupled with subtraction technology. Many of these patients already have spinal cord damage, and further damage to the cord by introduction of contrast media is a significant hazard. Local analgesia with sedation is most commonly used so that the patient's neurologic status can be assessed throughout the procedure. Some patients develop paroxysmal lower limb contractures during injection of the anterior spinal artery. These contractures are reported to respond to diazepam 5 mg injected directly into the angiography catheter without tissue toxicity.[36]

Cerebral angiography uses percutaneous catheterization of the femoral artery, which is well tolerated by the patient, has fewer complications than direct carotid artery puncture, and allows selective angiography. Digital subtraction techniques reduce the total volume of intra-arterial contrast and the procedural duration. Local anesthesia is commonly used for the same reasons as above. Sedation can include midazolam and/or propofol with small amounts of narcotics titrated to avoid respiratory depression.

General anesthesia, although rarely used in the United States, allows for increased patient comfort and immobility, and angiogram quality may be enhanced by mild hyperventilation (30 mmHg $PaCO_2$).[37–39] Hypocarbia slows cerebral circulation, allowing greater concentration of the contrast medium and improving clarity of the image, particularly in children. Angiographic quality in patients with brain tumor can also be enhanced by hypocarbia because it can invoke an intracerebral steal. Tumor vessels do not constrict with hypocarbia; therefore blood and contrast are shunted to the tumor, which becomes well delineated.[37] However, hyperventilation in the presence of a ruptured intracranial aneurysm has been questioned because it may increase spasm.[39] Others[40] have reported variable effects of changes in $PaCO_2$ on spastic intracerebral vessels. Clayton et al.,[4] in a randomized study, found equivalent study quality and superior hemodynamic stability with local/sedation as compared with general anesthesia. A reasonable anesthetic technique could include thiopental, muscle relaxant, volatile anesthetic agents, propofol, narcotics, and controlled ventilation. If volatile agents are used, then mild hypocarbia may be used to attenuate their cerebral vasodilatory effects, which can decrease the quality of images obtained.[37]

A recent large multicenter study (NASCET) found a 17 percent reduction in stroke 2 years after carotid endarterectomy in symptomatic patients with a stenosis greater than 70 percent.[42] This has increased the use of carotid angiography, which remains the gold standard despite the increasing sensitivity of CT/MRI angiography and ultrasound techniques. MRI tends to overestimate stenosis compared with angiography.[43] Data from the NASCET group suggests that ultrasonography should be used to screen patients before angiography.[44] Earnest et al.,[45] in a prospective study of 1,517 angiograms, found an incidence of all neurologic complications of 2.6 percent, with an overall incidence of permanent deficit of 0.33 percent and of 0.63 percent in patients studied for cerebrovascular disease. Permanent deficits tend to occur as a worsening of a preexisting deficit.[46] Incidence of ischemic events increases in the presence of systolic hypertension and after long angiographic procedures.[46]

MYELOGRAPHY

Myelography is used to define the contents of the thecal sac and any extrinsic impressions on the sac. Contrast agents are placed intrathecally, diffusing throughout the CSF. Before CT and MRI, myelography was the primary diagnostic tool for evaluation of the spinal canal contents and surrounding structures. CT following intrathecal contrast increases the specificity of CT for extradural disease, but this may soon be totally replaced by the noninvasive MRI.

Children often will need the assistance of the anesthesiologist because a completely motionless patient is required. Suggestions for anesthetic technique are as mentioned above, with the exception that ketamine may be appropriate for extradural studies because it can provide a quiet child with little airway support required. Children typically are placed in the lateral position for lumbar puncture, then supine with legs up to facilitate movement of the contrast agent throughout the subarachnoid space. During this period, the patient's head is flexed to prevent movement of the contrast through the foramen magnum. Special vigilance in regards to the airway are necessary while the head is flexed, particularly if an endotracheal tube is used.

Complications related to myelography usually are related to reactions to the use of contrast agents. Epidural hematoma, meningitis, seizures, extradural contrast injections, and postdural puncture headache have all been described after myelography. Adults with severe radiculopathy can have difficulty lying still for long scans. This can be successfully handled by adding local anesthetics to the contrast agent to achieve adequate conduction block.

MAGNETIC RESONANCE IMAGING

Purcell and Bloch described nuclear magnetic resonance (NMR) in the late 1940s, and the technique of NMR spectroscopy has been used extensively as a method of chemical analysis since that time.[2] Lauterbur suggested in 1973 that the these same techniques based on chemical shift be used for MRI. The computerized localization of data used in CT was almost directly transferable to imaging with NMR signals in the place of x-rays. This lead to the rapid development of clinically useful scanners in the late 1970s. A decade earlier, CT eliminated the need for diagnostic pneumoencephalography and echoencephalography and greatly reduced the number of cerebral angiograms, lumbar punctures, and electroencephalograms.[47] MRI has already displaced CT in many diagnostic situations and will continue to increase in popularity as cost and scanning times decrease. Magnetic resonance spectroscopy, which is used to elicit biochemical information from many different nuclei (^{1}H, ^{19}F, ^{31}P, ^{13}C), is based on the same physical principles as MRI. The number and complexity of MRI systems continue to increase, and new applications for the technology are still being developed.

MRI is based on the interaction of radio waves with nuclei (usually hydrogen, which is abundant in the body) in the presence of a strong magnetic field. The nuclei act like small bar magnets and align parallel with the field. A pulse of radio-frequency (RF) energy directed into the study sample at a frequency specific to the nuclei will knock the nuclei out of alignment. When the RF pulse is removed, the nuclei rotate back to their original position, emitting an RF signal at the same frequency. A variety of receiving antennas (coils) is used to detect the RF energy as it is released from the body.[48] The RF signals are collected with several different combinations of magnetic field gradients and projections to enable the image to be reconstructed by computer analysis using Fourier transformation in a manner similar to CT.[49]

Two time constants describe this RF signal decay. T_1 is the longitudinal relaxation time and describes the time for the vector of the spins to revert to their original orientation.[47] On T_1-weighted scans, simple fluids such as CSF or urine appear dark. These scans are useful to demonstrate anatomy and are quick to perform.[48] T_2 describes the spin-spin relaxation, which is relaxation in the transverse direction.[50] On T_2-weighted scans, CSF or urine appear bright. These scans take longer to perform but usually have a greater sensitivity to pathologic lesions.

Several types of magnets are used in MRI, but the most commonly used is the superconducting electromagnet. These magnets are made of special alloys such as niobium-titanium and kept in cyrogens such as liquid nitrogen and helium to reduce resistance to the passage of electric current. Because of this induced superconductivity, the magnet is always "on." An emergency power off switch can be used to decrease the field strength, but to completely down a magnet, it must be drained of cyrogen, which takes several hours and is potentially dangerous to personnel. This "magnet on" situation likely requires the removal of the patient from the scanning room to perform emergency procedures such as endotracheal intubation.[50,51]

Dependence of MRI on weak RF signals creates special problems for locating these units as well for monitoring the patient. During the actual scanning when the RF signal is on, the signal from the pulse oximeter will interfere with imaging. Any electric monitoring cables attached to the patient may act as antennae, carrying stray signals to the scanner and thereby reducing the quality of the image. These artifacts show up as white streaks across the image. In addition, the scanners magnetic field must be shielded from outside magnetic effects created by moving ferrous objects such as electric motors (e.g., certain types of intravenous pumps).

Hazards of MRI to the Patient

One of the many advantages of MRI is the increased safety for patients as well as providers because ionizing radiation is not used. Yet, several other potential hazards to the patient and provider exist.

The strong static magnetic field is believed to be safe even with prolonged exposure.[52] Present generation scanners use a static field in the range of 0.1 to 2.0 Tesla (T) as compared with the earth's magnetic field, which is approximately 0.05 mT. No adverse effects have been associated with fields up to 2 T, which is also the recommended maximum level. However, the static field may be hazardous for patients with implanted devices. Dislocation of intracranial aneurysm clips has been described during MRI.[53] Some of these clips are ferromagnetic and large enough to experience torque in some scanners. In recent years, many institutions have moved to nonferromagnetic materials for aneurysm clips. By contrast, most other vascular clips, such as those used in abdominal surgery or coronary bypass surgery, are not sufficiently ferromagnetic to present a problem. Patients with ferromagnetic fragments (e.g., metal shavings) in critical locations such as the eye should be excluded from MRI to prevent local tissue damage by fragment motion. Large orthopedic appliances such as total hip prostheses are not highly ferromagnetic and do not pose a risk to the patient during MRI, although they can cause image artifact.[48]

The high static magnetic field may propel loose ferromagnetic (iron, steel, nickel, or cobalt) items such as safety pins or scissors around the scanning room, placing patients and staff at risk. Older anesthesia machines should be bolted to the wall and steel gas tanks replaced with aluminum versions (Fig. 7.1). Recently, nonferromagnetic machines such as the Ohmeda Excel 210 have become available and appear to perform reliably in the MRI environment.[54] Ferromagnetic materials in this modified machine have been replaced by either aluminum or high-grade stainless steel. The unit includes an absorber system, scavenging valve, O_2 monitor, and a positive end-expiratory pressure valve in addition to the recommended safety features. My institution has used this machine with great success for some time. As field strength falls off more rapidly to the sides of the magnet, this would be the safer position for the anesthesia machine (Fig. 7.2). Analog wrist watches may be damaged, and magnetic data stored on tape, floppy disks, or credit cards may be erased.

ECG monitoring throughout the cardiac cycle is difficult due to magnetic field gradient artifacts. A time-varying filter ECG gating device has been developed to improve ECG interpretation throughout the scan.[55] Artifact can be minimized and QRS detection maximized by using leads V5 and V6.[56] ECG quality is improved by keeping electrodes close together near the center of the scanner, placing all loops of cable parallel

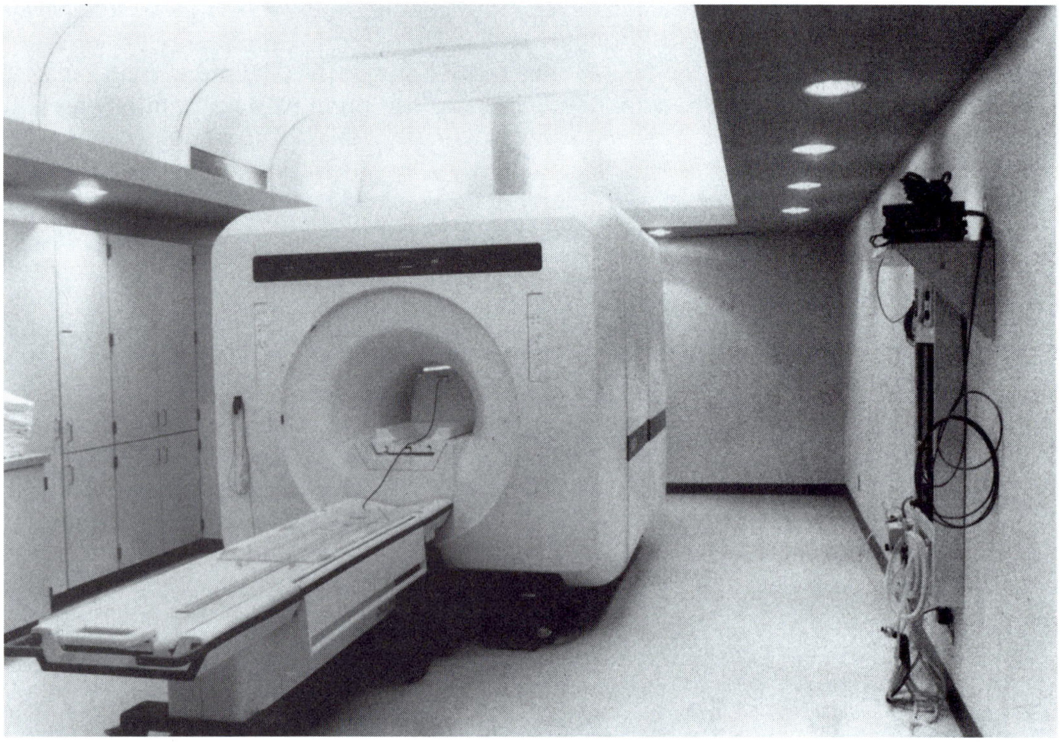

FIGURE 7.1 *MRI scanning room arrangement showing an older anesthesia machine bolted to the wall.*

to the magnetic field lines, and twisting the cable.[57] One piece electrode packs are commercially available to facilitate easy central placement. Static magnetic fields exceeding 0.1 T cause T-wave abnormalities of the ECG. These changes increase linearly up to 2 T but revert to normal when the field is removed and are not associated with changes in hemodynamics or dysrhythmias.[58] Several companies, such as Magnetic Resonance Equipment, manufacture reasonably effective monitoring units that include ECG, pulse oximetry, end-tidal CO_2, and invasive monitors. These units are easy to use, reliable, and show a waveform (Fig. 7.3), but are costly.

Patients with cardiac pacemakers should not undergo MRI. Potential problems include pacemaker inhibition or reversion to an asynchronous mode, programming changes, reed switch closure, or torque on the pacemaker generator.[59,60] It is suggested that the pacemaker service be consulted if a patient with a permanent pacemaker must undergo MRI. In addition, the rapidly changing magnetic fields that are superimposed on the main static field generate internal electrical currents. Although the current generated by MRI is low, pacemaker microcircuitry may be affected. One recent study[61] evaluated seven dual-chamber and two single-chamber systems in a 0.5 T MRI scanner in vitro. As expected, the reed switch was noted to activate followed by asynchronous stimulation once the generators were placed in the magnetic field. MRI scanning showed no influence on the stimulation function nor on the pacemaker programming. The authors' recommendations were that pacemakers should be programmed in the asynchronous mode during MRI scans to avoid inhibition and that MRI is safe with the newer-generation pacemakers. Another recent small

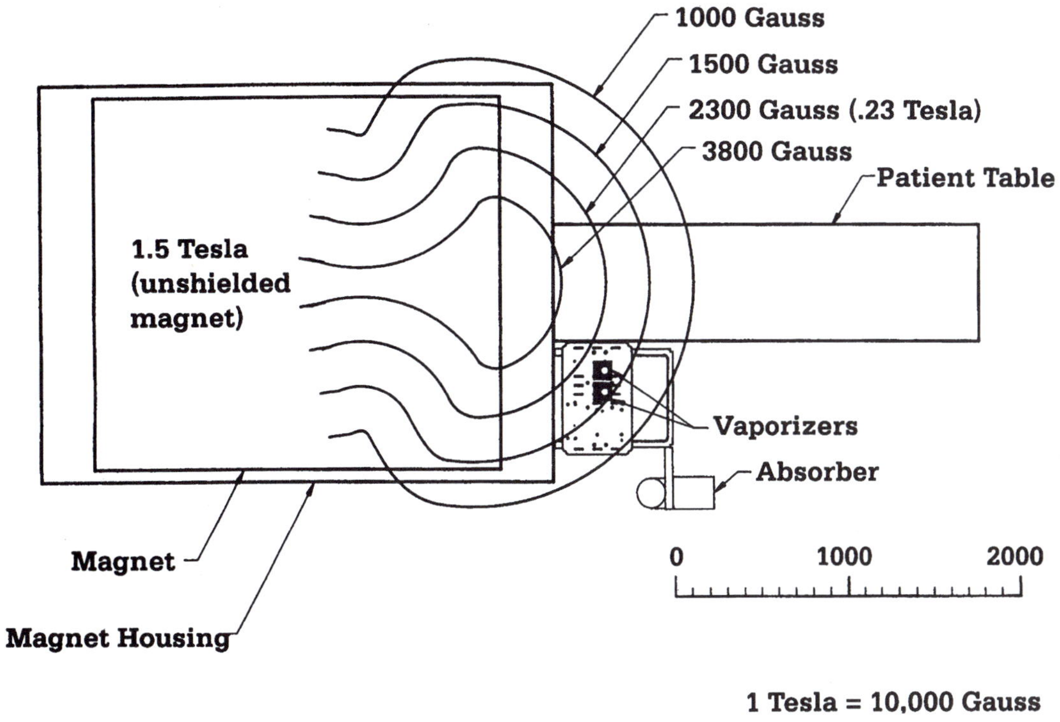

FIGURE 7.2 *Because field strength falls off more rapidly at the sides of the magnet, placement of the anesthesia machine at the side of the MRI machine is safest.*

series of five patients using pacemakers of one manufacturer (Pacesetter) suggested relative safety of these units in a 1.5 T field.[62] It is doubtful that these conclusions pertain to all pacemaker manufacturers, and further study is warranted.

Ventriculoperitoneal shunts may cause image artifact but do not preclude an MRI study. Artificial heart valves and middle ear prostheses must be considered on an individual basis, yet most do not represent a contraindication to MRI.

MRI is believed to be safe during pregnancy because many bioassays for embryologic development have shown no adverse effects from the procedure. Yet, until more experience has been gained, MRI probably should be restricted in pregnancy to critical need situations.[48] In addition, rapid repetition of changing magnetic fields may theoretically induce seizures in patients with epilepsy. To date, this complication has not been described.

Other problems for patients include claustrophobia and mechanical noise. The incidence of claustrophobia has been reported to range from 3 to 7 percent.[50] One study revealed a temporary hearing loss in 43 percent of unprotected patients.[63] This suggests that all patients, awake or anesthetized, should have ear protection if feasible.

It must be remembered that in systems that use liquid nitrogen as coolant, a major leak in that coolant system is signaled by an audible alarm. This is a true emergency that could place both the patient and anesthesiologist at risk for hypoxia because the scanning room would quickly fill with N_2. Intubated patients most likely are safe if the airway is secured and the patient is receiving supplemental O_2. However, the anesthesiologist would quickly become hypoxic.

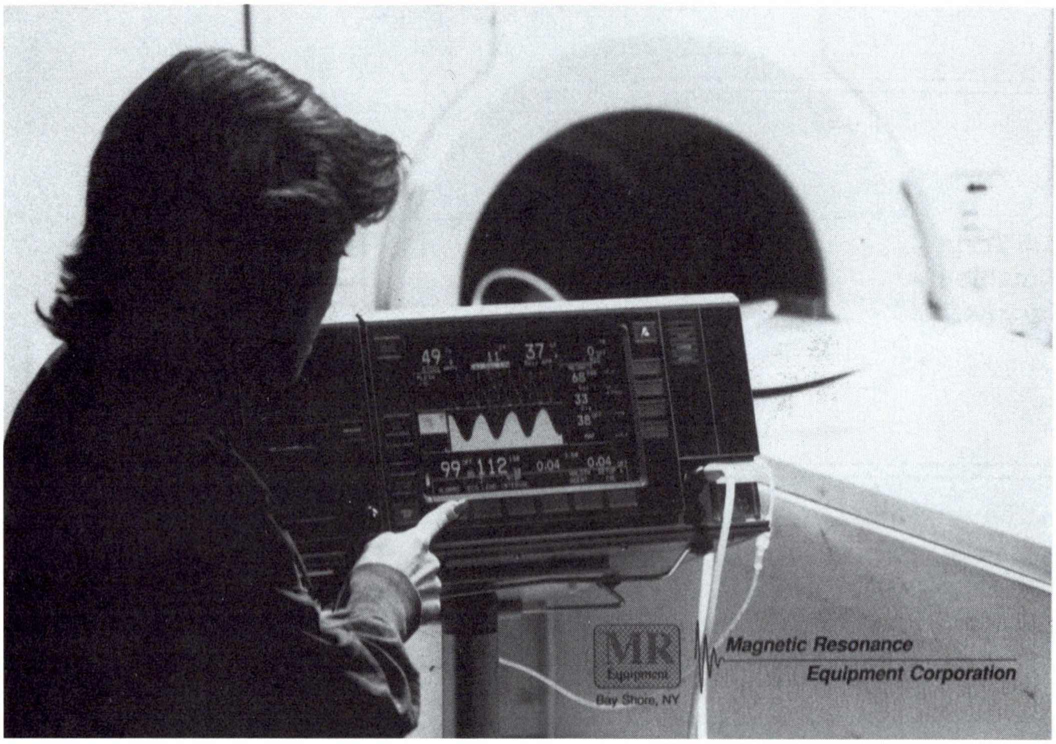

FIGURE 7.3 *Magnetic Resonance Equipment's monitoring unit, which includes ECG, pulse oximetry, end-tidal CO_2 monitor, and invasive monitors.*

An extra Mapleson system could be used to deliver O_2 to the anesthesiologist while caring for the patient during a major leak. Theoretically, the anesthesiologist would be better not breathing the gas content of the room (i.e., holding his or her breath) while reaching for his or her own supplemental O_2 system or leaving the room. Scanning rooms do have increased ventilation systems, but the efficacy of these during a leak is unproven. It is suggested in some MRI equipment manuals that a chair be thrown through the scanning room window to facilitate ventilation in the event of a major leak.

Indications for MRI

MRI offers several advantages for imaging. It can be used easily in several different planes, which allows elucidation of many anatomic regions and pathologies. There is no bone artifact, so it is possible to view soft tissues near bone as never before. Tissues vary much more in their magnetic relaxation behavior, the basis for MRI, than they do in their X-ray absorption, which is basis for CT contrast. Because of this, MRI delivers very high tissue contrast, allowing many times greater sensitivity than computed tomography[47] (Table 7.1 for comparison).

Anesthetic Management

As discussed above, monitoring can be quite difficult in the MRI environment. Patients are well hidden during most scans. The most important monitor is the anesthesiologist, who can remain in close proximity to the patient without much risk. Within the bore of the magnet, all ferro-

TABLE 7.1 *Efficacy of MRI relative to CT for the initial diagnosis of central nervous system diseases*

DISEASE	MRI	CT
Cerebrovascular		
TIA-RIND	++	±
Emboli	+++	+
Ischemic infarction	++++	+++
Intracerebral hemorrhage	+++	++++
Trauma		
Craniocerebral	++	+++
Spinal	+++	+++
Tumors		
Glioma		
Low-grade supratentorial	+++	++
High-grade supratentorial	++++	++++
Meningioma supratentorial	++	++++
Pituitary	++	++++
Sinuses and orbits	++++	+++
Brainstem	++++	+
Cervical spine	++++	±
Cervical disc disease	+++	+++
Lumbar disc disease	+++	+++
Regional cerebral blood flow	[a]	+++

[a] Research phase, of great future potential.

(Adapted from Council on Scientific Affairs,[47] with permission.)

magnetic materials should be avoided. Loops of wire can significantly degrade image detection. A brass or plastic precordial stethoscope can safely be used. As long as the dial of the sphygmomanometer is kept away from the magnet to prevent interference, oscillatory blood pressures can easily be obtained. Automated blood pressure monitors (e.g., Dinamap) may malfunction in the scanning room, frequently cause image artifact, and must be evaluated on an individual basis. Use of telemetry for ECG eliminates the need for wires, providing an adequate display in the absence of RF signals.[64] The RF signal does produce a background noise, but the QRS can usually be discerned. Capnography monitors need to be switched to high-power suction and longer tubing introduced. Data from these machines have been questioned.[50] Pulse oximetry can be used during the critical periods of patient adjustment and positioning. During the actual scanning, when the RF signal is on, most oximeters will interfere with imaging. Newer models (e.g., Biochem 1040) should interfere less with imaging. Ventilators should be of the fluidic type that are made of mostly nonmagnetic materials whose performance is unaffected by the static field, such as the Monaghan 225 SIMV volume ventilator.[65]

Actual anesthetic should be as described for CT. Any general anesthetic requires intubation of the trachea[50] or use of the LMA[66] in appropriate patients. Some authors to not advocate the use of the LMA during MRI in any situation.[67] At present, no good study exists that supports the routine use of the LMA. If used, the LMA pilot balloon should be taped out of the scanning field because it contains ferromagnetic material and will cause image artifact.

REACTIONS TO CONTRAST MEDIA

Radiographic intravenous contrast media are divided into two categories: (1) organic compounds complexed to iodine, which has high density allowing increased contrast effect, and (2) paramagnetic compounds, which are used for MRI (see below). Iodinated contrast media (ICM) are administered intravenously, intra-arterially, and intrathecally. Approximately 5 percent of radiographic examinations involving

ICM are complicated by an adverse reaction to the ICM, one-third of these reactions being severe and requiring immediate attention. Yet, despite prompt treatment, there are approximately 500 fatalities in the United States per year related to ICM examinations[68] (0.006 percent incidence of death after ICM studies[58]). Different radiographic studies have different incidences of reactions (e.g., 10.1 percent after intravenous cholangiography versus 2.3 percent with angiography involving intra-arterial injection), and the manner of ICM injection (i.e., infusion versus bolus) also influences risk. Patients allergic to seafood or shellfish and patients with asthma have a 10 to 15 percent incidence of reaction.[69] Patients with a history of allergy or atopy can increase the risk of reaction 1.5 to 10-fold compared with normals.[70,71] The risk of subsequent reactions in patients who are considered at risk by virtue of previous reactions to ICM ranges from 17 to 35 percent, yet many of these patients undergo repeat ICM examinations without signs of reaction.[71,72] Patients with cardiac disease are four to five times more likely to have reactions.[70] Fewer reactions occur when less than 20 g iodine total dose is used.[73] A recently developed class of ICM (low-osmolar contrast media) can greatly reduce reaction risk and deliver adequate contrast but costs 12 to 15 times more than traditional ICM.[74] Adverse reactions to ICM have not been reported under general anesthesia, yet anesthesiologists must be ready to assist the radiologist at any time because few studies require general anesthesia.

Types of Reactions

All patients receiving ICM undergo certain adverse reactions caused by the relative hypertonicity of the agents. These reactions are similar to those seen after the injection of any hyperosmolar solution. There is an initial brief hypertensive response followed by mild hypotension. Central venous, right ventricular, and pulmonary artery pressures increase, as does cardiac output, but systemic vascular resistance decreases.[75] A decrease in myocardial contractility and conduction abnormalities can also be seen. The ECG may reveal ischemic changes after injection of ICM, even in healthy adults and children.[76] Decreased hematocrit, increased osmolarity, and an eventual osmotic diuresis occur in almost all patients. This rapid initial increase in intravascular volume may be hazardous in patients with decreased left ventricular function. Renal or hepatic dysfunction may lead to impaired excretion of ICM. Patients with sickle cell disease must be well hydrated because the increased osmolarity can precipitate sickling in hemoglobin SS containing red blood cells, leading to a sickle cell crisis.

Some patients, however, have idiosyncratic reactions to ICM, ranging from nausea and flushing to anaphylactoid shock. The most prominent reactions seem to be related to the release of histamine and include dizziness, weakness, urticaria, pruritis, cutaneous flush, and hypotension. In a excellent comprehensive review, Goldberg[77] divided these reactions into five classes:

1. *vasomotor*, peripheral vasodilation from direct action of the ICM[78]
2. *vasovagal*, from central nervous system effects of the media[78]
3. *dermal*, erythematous and urticarial response to histamine release
4. *osmotic*, as discussed above
5. *anaphylactoid*, which involves release of histamine and other mediators

Most of these reactions will be transient and require little treatment. Yet, the potentially most harmful, anaphylactoid, is the type most likely to require the expertise of anesthesiologists. These reactions may occur within 1 minute of administration with as little as 0.1 ml ICM or may take up to 6 to 8 hours to develop. Prodromal symptoms include nausea/vomiting (seen in 20 percent of anaphylactoid reactions), hypotension/dysrhythmias (10 to 13 percent), and respiratory distress (20 percent).[79] Pharyngeal edema may progress quickly to upper airway obstruction and may severely limit ventilation.[80]

Treatment of ICM Reactions

Proper treatment of ICM reactions (Table 7.2) requires reliable intravenous access, and this should be implemented as soon as any ICM reaction is suspected. ECG and blood pressure should be monitored. The vast majority of systemic reactions will be treated by the radiologist, with most reactions requiring little more than reassurance. Guidelines for prevention and treatment of these reactions for the radiologist have recently been formulated.[81] Anaphylaxis and severe bronchospasm will require further intervention and frequently the assistance of the anesthesiologist.

Epinephrine (3 to 5 μg/kg IV) is used as a bronchodilator, to increase contractility and peripheral vascular resistance and to decrease histamine release. Aminophylline (5 mg/kg/20 min bolus followed by infusion) is also used to relax bronchiolar smooth muscle. Anticholinergics (atropine 0.5 to 2.0 mg IV) can relax bronchiolar smooth muscle somewhat, decrease secretions, and may decrease the release of histamine.[82] Antihistamines are probably of little value if unsupplemented, because specific receptors blocked by these drugs may have already been activated. Because of the low toxicity of antihistamines, many authors continue to recommend their use. Steroids are often used empirically to stabilize membranes and therefore decrease histamine release and capillary permeability. Early intervention with airway management as needed may prevent a more difficult situation later.

Prophylaxis Against ICM Reactions

Evaluation of risk with intradermal skin testing is unreliable,[69,83–85] and pretesting with an intravenous injection of a small volume of ICM is of little benefit.[75] Many studies have demonstrated the benefit of pretreating all patients who are at high risk for ICM reaction (previous reaction, allergy, atopic disease, cardiac disease).[71,86–88] The best prophylaxis seems to be a course of antihistamines and steroids started at least 18 hours before examination.[77] The routine use of H_2-antagonists has not yet been shown to be efficacious. However, many of our faculty routinely use steroids, H_1-blockers and H_2-blockers in high-risk patients.

Paramagnetic Contrast Agents

These agents are gadolinium-based and exclusively intravenous and are well tolerated, with an overall adverse reaction rate of 1 to 4 percent.[89] These agents work indirectly by shortening the T_1 and T_2 relaxation times of structures

TABLE 7.2 *Treatment of contrast media reactions*

Adrenergic agonists	Epinephrine 3–5 μg/kg IV bolus Epinephrine 1–4 μg/min IV infusion
Methylxanthines	Aminophylline 5–6 mg/kg/20 min, initial dose Aminophylline 0.5–0.9 mg/kg/hr, maintenance dose
Anticholinergics	Atropine 0.5–2.0 mg IV
Antihistamines	Diphenhydramine 25–50 mg IV
Steroids	Methylprednisolone 100–1,000 mg IV Dexamethasone 4–20 mg IV
Intravenous fluids	Normal saline (infuse to maintain normal blood pressure)

(From Goldberg,[77] with permission.)

adjacent to the site of contrast delivery.[90] Neoplasm, infection, inflammation, and ischemia/infarction can all show enhancement, which is depicted as brighter relative to surrounding structures.

Presently, the most common agent, gadopentetate, is an ionic moiety with a good safety profile. Yet, nonionic agents such as gadoteridol and gadodiamide have recently become available in an attempt to further improve on the safety profile. Animal studies suggest that nonionic agents do indeed cause less hemodynamic derangement.[91]

SUMMARY

Many of the considerations for administration of anesthesia to patients undergoing neurodiagnostic procedures are the same as those for patients with the same disease process undergoing neurosurgical procedures. Yet, anesthesia in locations remote from the operating room can be most challenging. These challenges will continue to increase in frequency and complexity in the coming years as the technologies involved persist in their evolution. The anesthesiologist must be ever vigilant and should have an understanding of the special requirements related to these technologies.

References

1. Dierdorf SF, McNiece WL, Rao CC et al: Effect of succinylcholine on plasma potassium in children with cerebral palsy. Anesthesiology 62:88, 1985
2. Cowgill DB, Mostello LA, Shapiro HM: Encephalitis and a hyperkalemic response to succinycholine. Anesthesiology 40:409, 1974
3. Cooperman LH, Strobel GE, Jr, Kennell EM: Massive hyperkalemia after administration of succinylcholine. Anesthesiology 32:161, 1970
4. Gravlee GP: Succinylcholine-induced hyperkalemia in a patient with Parkinson's disease. Anesth Analg 59:444, 1980
5. Stevenson PH, Birch AA: Succinylcholine-induced hyperkalemia in a patient with a closed head injury. Anesthesiology 51:89, 1979
6. Muzzi DA, Black S, Cucchiara RF: The lack of effect of succinylcholine on serum potassium in patients with Parkinson's disease [letter]. Anesthesiology 71:322, 1989
7. Shapiro HM, Aidinis SJ: Neurosurgical anesthesia. Surg Clin North Am 55:913, 1975
8. Smith AL: Barbiturate protection in cerebral hypoxia. Anesthesiology 47:285, 1977
9. Hounsfield GN: Computerized transverse axial scanning (tomography). 1. Description of system. Br J Radiol 46:1016, 1973
10. Di Chiro G, Schellinger D: Computed tomography of spinal cord after lumbar intrathecal introduction of metrizamide (computer-assisted myelography). Radiology 120:101, 1976
11. Di Chiro G, Doppman JL, Wener L: Computed tomography of spinal cord arteriovenous malformations. Radiology 123:351, 1977
12. Hammerschiag SB, Wolpert SM, Carter BL: Computed tomography of the spinal canal. Radiology 121:361, 1976
13. Aidinis SJ, Zimmerman RA, Shapiro HM et al: Anesthesia for brain computer tomography. Anesthesiology 44:420, 1976
14. Ambrose J: Computerized x-ray scanning of the brain. J Neurosurg 40:679, 1974
15. Lin JP: Computed tomography of the head in adults. Postgrad Med 60:113, 1976
16. Perry BJ, Bridges C: Computerized transverse axial scanning (tomography). 3. Radiation dose considerations. Br J Radiol 46:1048, 1973
17. Wolfson B, Hetrick WD: Anesthesia for neuroradiologic procedures. p. 104. In Cottrell JE, Turndorf H (eds): Anesthesia and Neurosurgery. CV Mosby St. Louis, 1986
18. Thompson JR, Schneider S, Ashwal S et al: The choice of sedation for computed tomography in children: a prospective evaluation. Radiology 143:475, 1982
19. Mitchell AA, Louik C, Lacouture P et al: Risks to children from computed tomographic scan premedication. JAMA 247:2385, 1982
20. Varner PD, Ebert JP, McKay RD et al: Methohexital sedation of children undergoing CT scan. Anesth Analg 64:643, 1985
21. Burckart GJ, White TJ, III, Siegle RL et al: Rectal thiopental versus an intramuscular cocktail for sedating children before computerized tomography. Am J Hosp Pharm 37:222, 1980
22. Vangerven M, Van Hemelrijck J, Wouters P et al: Light anaesthesia with propofol for paediatric MRI. Anaesthesia 47:706, 1992

23. Levati A, Colombo N, Arosio EM et al: Propofol anaesthesia in spontaneously breathing paediatric patients during magnetic resonance imaging. Acta Anaesthesiol Scand 40:561, 1996
24. Corssen G, Groves EH, Gomez S, Allen RJ: Ketamine: its place for neurosurgical diagnostic procedures. Anesth Analg 48:181, 1969
25. Wyte SR, Shapiro HM, Turner P, Harris AB: Ketamine-induced intracranial hypertension. Anesthesiology 36:174, 1972
26. List WF, Crumrine RS, Cascorbi HF, Weiss MH: Increased cerebrospinal fluid pressure after ketamine. Anesthesiology 36:98, 1972
27. Ferrer Brechner T, Winter J: Anesthetic considerations for cerebral computer tomography. Anesth Analg 56:344, 1977
28. Valtonen M: Anaesthesia for computerised tomography of the brain in children: a comparison of propofol and thiopentone. Acta Anaesthesiol Scand 33:170, 1989
29. Paxton R, Ambrose J: The EMI scanner. A brief review of the first 650 patients. Br J Radiol 47:530, 1974
30. Wolfson B, Siker ES, Wible LR, Dubansky J: Pneumoencephalography using neuroleptanalgesia. Anesth Analg 47:14, 1968
31. Jacoby J, Jones JR, Ziegler J: Pneumoencephalography and air embolism: simulated anesthetic death. Anaesthesia 20:336, 1959
32. Field JR, Robertson JT, DeSaussure RL: Complications of cerebral angiography in 2000 consecutive cases. J Neurosurg 19:775, 1962
33. Zagoria RJ: Iodinated contrast agents in neuroradiology. Neuroimaging Clin North Am 4:1, 1994
34. Rosansky SJ, Deschamps EG: Multiple cholesterol emboli syndrome after angiography. Am J Med Sci 288:45, 1984
35. Lundervold A, Engeset A: Recordings of EEG, ECG, EMG and intra-arterial blood pressure during cerebral angiography. Acta Radiol Diagn Stockh (suppl) 270:198, 1967
36. Doppman JL, Albertson K, Ramsey R, Saltzstein SL: Intra-arterial valium: its safety and effectiveness. Radiology 106:335, 1973
37. Dallas SH, Moxon CP: Controlled ventilation for cerebral angiography. Br J Anaesth 41:597, 1969
38. Edmonds Seal J, du Boulay G, Bostick T: The effect of intermittent positive pressure ventilation upon cerebral angiography with special reference to the quality of the films—a preliminary communication. Br J Radiol 40:957, 1967
39. Samuel JR, Grange RA, Hawkins TD: Anaesthetic technique for carotid angiography. The use of hyperventilation to improve the angiographic demonstration of intracranial tumours. Anaesthesia 23:543, 1968
40. du Boulay G, Edmonds Seal J, Bostick T: The effect of intermittent positive pressure ventilation upon the calibre of cerebral arteries in spasm following subarachnoid haemorrhage—a preliminary communication. Br J Radiol 41:46, 1968
41. Clayton DG, O'Donoghue BM, Stevens JE, Savage PE: Cardiovascular response during cerebral angiography under general and local anaesthesia. Anaesthesia 44:599, 1989
42. Beneficial effect of carotid endarterectomy in symptomatic patients with high-grade carotid stenosis. North American Symptomatic Carotid Endarterectomy Trial Collaborators. N Engl J Med 325:445, 1991
43. Vanninen RL, Manninen HI, Partanen PK et al: How should we estimate carotid stenosis using magnetic resonance angiography? Neuroradiology 38:299, 1996
44. Eliasziw M, Rankin RN, Fox AJ et al: Accuracy and prognostic consequences of ultrasonography in identifying severe carotid artery stenosis. North American Symptomatic Carotid Endarterectomy Trial (NASCET) Group. Stroke 26:1747, 1995
45. Earnest F, IV, Forbes G, Sandok BA et al: Complications of cerebral angiography: prospective assessment of risk. Am J Roentgenol 142:247, 1984
46. Dion JE, Gates PC, Fox AJ et al: Clinical events following neuroangiography: a prospective study. Stroke 18:997, 1987
47. Magnetic resonance imaging of the central nervous system. Council on Scientific Affairs. Report of the Panel on Magnetic Resonance Imaging. JAMA 259:1211, 1988
48. Larson DA, Yock DH, Yock DH, Jr. Magnetic resonance imaging–an update. Minn Med 71:95, 1988
49. Edelstein WA, Hutchison JM, Johnson G, Redpath T: Spin warp NMR imaging and applications to human whole-body imaging. Phys Med Biol 25:751, 1980
50. Nixon C, Hirsch NP, Ormerod IE, Johnson G: Nuclear magnetic resonance. Its implications for the anaesthetist. Anaesthesia 41:131, 1986
51. Geiger RS, Cascorbi HF: Anesthesia in an NMR scanner [letter]. Anesth Analg 63:622, 1984
52. Budinger TF: Nuclear magnetic resonance (NMR) in vivo studies: known thresholds for health effects. J Comput Assist Tomogr 5:800, 1981
53. New PF, Rosen BR, Brady TJ et al: Potential haz-

ards and artifacts of ferromagnetic and nonferromagnetic surgical and dental materials and devices in nuclear magnetic resonance imaging. Radiology 147:139, 1983
54. Rao CC, Krishna G, Emhardt J: Anesthesia machine for use during magnetic resonance imaging [letter]. Anesthesiology 73:1054, 1990
55. Rokey R, Wendt RE, Johnston DL: Monitoring of acutely ill patients during nuclear magnetic resonance imaging: use of a time-varying filter electrocardiographic gating device to reduce gradient artifacts. Magn Reson Med 6:240, 1988
56. Dimick RN, Hedlund LW, Herfkens RJ et al: Optimizing electrocardiograph electrode placement for cardiac-gated magnetic resonance imaging. Invest Radiol 22:17, 1987
57. Wendt RE, III, Rokey R, Vick GW, III, Johnston DL: Electrocardiographic gating and monitoring in NMR imaging. Magn Reson Imaging 6:89, 1988
58. Tenforde TS, Gaffey CT, Moyer BR, Budinger TF: Cardiovascular alterations in Macaca monkeys exposed to stationary magnetic fields: experimental observations and theoretical analysis. Bioelectromagnetics 4:19, 1983
59. Pavlicek W, Geisinger M, Castle L et al: The effects of nuclear magnetic resonance on patients with cardiac pacemakers. Radiology 147:149, 1983
60. Fetter J, Aram G, Holmes DR, Jr et al: The effects of nuclear magnetic resonance imagers on external and implantable pulse generators. Pacing Clin Electrophysiol 7:720, 1984
61. Lauck G, von Smekal A, Wolke S et al: Effects of nuclear magnetic resonance imaging on cardiac pacemakers. Pacing Clin Electrophysiol 18:1549, 1995
62. Gimbel JR, Johnson D, Levine PA, Wilkoff BL: Safe performance of magnetic resonance imaging on five patients with permanent cardiac pacemakers. Pacing Clin Electrophysiol 19:913, 1996
63. Brummett RE, Talbot JM, Charuhas P: Potential hearing loss resulting from MR imaging. Radiology 169:539, 1988
64. Roth JL, Nugent M, Gray JE et al: Patient monitoring during magnetic resonance imaging. Anesthesiology 62:80, 1985
65. Dunn V, Coffman CE, McGowan JE, Ehrhardt JC: Mechanical ventilation during magnetic resonance imaging. Magn Reson Imaging 3:169, 1985
66. Rafferty C, Burke AM, Cossar DF, Farling PA: Laryngeal mask and magnetic resonance imaging [letter]. Anaesthesia 45:590, 1990
67. Peden CJ, Menon DK, Hall AS et al: Magnetic resonance for the anaesthetist. Part II: Anaesthesia and monitoring in MR units. Anaesthesia 47:508, 1992
68. Lasser EC, Lang J, Sovak M et al: Steroids: theoretical and experimental basis for utilization in prevention of contrast media reactions. Radiology 125:1, 1977
69. Shehadi WH, Toniolo G: Adverse reactions to contrast media: a report from the Committee on Safety of Contrast Media of the International Society of Radiology. Radiology 137:299, 1980
70. Ansell G, Tweedie MC, West CR et al: The current status of reactions to intravenous contrast media. Invest Radiol 15:S32, 1980
71. Greenberger P, Patterson R, Kelly J et al: Administration of radiographic contrast media in high-risk patients. Invest Radiol 15:S40, 1980
72. Witten DM, Hirsch FD, Hartman GW: Acute reactions to urographic contrast medium: incidence, clinical characteristics and relationship to history of hypersensitivity states. Am J Roentgenol Radium Ther Nucl Med 119:832, 1973
73. Ansell G: Adverse reactions to contrast agents. Scope of problem. Invest Radiol 5:374, 1970
74. Jacobson PD, Rosenquist CJ: The introduction of low-osmolar contrast agents in radiology. Medical, economic, legal, and public policy issues. JAMA 260:1586, 1988
75. Cote CJ, Greenhow DE, Marshall BE: The hypotensive response to rapid intravenous administration of hypertonic solutions in man and in the rabbit. Anesthesiology 50:30, 1979
76. Pfister RC, Hutter AM, Jr: Cardiovascular radiology. Cardiac alterations during intravenous urography. Invest Radiol 15:S239, 1980
77. Goldberg M: Systemic reactions to intravascular contrast media. A guide for the anesthesiologist. Anesthesiology 60:46, 1984
78. Lindgren P: Hemodynamic responses to contrast media. Invest Radiol 5:424, 1970
79. Lalli AF: Contrast media reactions: data analysis and hypothesis. Radiology 134:1, 1980
80. Smith PL, Kagey Sobotka A, Bleecker ER et al: Physiologic manifestations of human anaphylaxis. J Clin Invest 66:1072, 1980
81. Cohan RH, Leder RA, Ellis JH: Treatment of adverse reactions to radiographic contrast media in adults. Radiol Clin North Am 34:1055, 1996
82. Kaliner M: Symposium on allergic lung disease. IV. Immunologic mechanisms for release of chemical mediators of anaphylaxis from human lung tissue. Can Med Assoc J 110:431, 1974

83. Yocum MW, Heller AM, Abels RI: Efficacy of intravenous pretesting and antihistamine prophylaxis in radiocontrast media—sensitive patients. J Allergy Clin Immunol 62:309, 1978
84. Arroyave CM: An in vitro assay for radiographic contrast media idiosyncrasy. Invest Radiol 15:S21, 1980
85. Fischer HW, Doust VL: An evaluation of pretesting in the problem of serious and fatal reactions to excretory urography. Radiology 103:497, 1972
86. Millbern SM, Bell SD: Prevention of anaphylaxis to contrast medium. Anesthesiology 50:56, 1979
87. Kelly JF, Patterson R, Lieberman P et al: Radiographic contrast media studies in high-risk patients. J Allergy Clin Immunol 62:181, 1978
88. Zweiman B, Mishkin MM, Hildreth EA: An approach to the performance of contrast studies in contrast material-reactive persons. Ann Intern Med 83:159, 1975
89. Byrd SE, Darling CF, Allen E: Contrast agents in neuroimaging. Neuroimaging Clin North Am 4:9, 1994
90. Saini S: Advances in contrast-enhanced MR imaging. Principles. AJR 156:236, 1991
91. Saeed M, Li HT, Wendland MF et al: Comparison of cardiovascular response to ionic and nonionic magnetic resonance susceptibility contrast agents. Invest Radiol 29:319, 1994

8 CEREBRAL ANEURYSM AND ARTERIOVENOUS MALFORMATION

SUSAN BLACK
CHERI A. SULEK
ARTHUR L. DAY

Patients presenting for intracranial cerebrovascular surgery represent a diverse population. These patients range in age from newborn to elderly and have a wide variety of signs and symptoms associated with their disease. Despite their diversity, anesthetic management of all patients with cerebrovascular disease revolves around a few basic principles: maintenance of adequate cerebral blood flow (CBF) and optimal cerebral perfusion pressure (CPP), decreasing risk for intracranial hemorrhage, minimizing risk of cerebral ischemia and preventing resultant neurologic injury, and avoidance of cerebral hyperperfusion. This chapter addresses these issues as they relate to each patient group and describes concerns unique to certain cerebrovascular diseases and their anesthetic management.

INTRACRANIAL ANEURYSMS

Pathophysiology and Management

Rupture of an intracranial aneurysm occurs in 28,000 people per year in North American and results in morbidity or mortality in approximately 18,000.[1,2] Introduction of the operating microscope and the use of microsurgery for repair of intracranial aneurysms in the 1960s resulted in the first improvement in outcome for these patients. Over the last decade additional changes in management have been introduced including early surgery, aggressive treatments for cerebral vasospasm, and further advances in surgical technique. However, morbidity and mortality following subarachnoid hemorrhage (SAH) from an intracranial aneurysm remains high.

CURRENT DIAGNOSIS, MANAGEMENT, AND OUTCOME

Natural History. The natural history following rupture of an intracranial aneurysm is grim. Nonsurgical treatment following aneurysmal SAH results in 60 to 63% mortality at 6 months to 1 year.[3,4] Asymptomatic intracranial aneurysms rupture at a rate of 1 to 2% per year. Symptomatic unruptured intracranial aneurysms rupture at a much higher rate, over 5% per year.[4] Once symptomatic aneurysms rupture, the mortality and morbidity are significant, with mortality rates as high as 88% reported.[4] Unruptured symptomatic giant intracranial aneurysms have the most ominous prognosis of the unruptured aneurysms, with mortality or severe morbidity reported in 80% of conservatively treated patients.[4]

A number of factors have been identified as risk factors for aneurysmal SAH. These are listed in the accompanying box. Increasing size is a risk factor for hemorrhage. Although studies have identified a critical diameter above which risk of rupture is higher, ranging from 4 to 10 mm, others were unable to identify a critical size below which the risk of rupture was lower.[4–10] Currently, most neurosurgeons consider any aneurysm with the possible exception of very small aneurysms (3 mm or less) as having the potential to hemorrhage. As a result, most would recommend clipping virtually any unruptured intracranial aneurysm unless the patient's medical condition is such that the risk of surgery and anesthesia is excessive.[4] The risk of SAH increases with increasing age. Most cases of SAH occur between the 4th and 6th decades.[4] The female-to-male ratio in SAH patients is 1.6:1.[1,11,12] The female predominance is stronger after age 40 to 50.[12] Hypertension is not a risk factor for development of intracranial aneurysm or the occurrence of SAH. However, once SAH occurs, hypertensive patients have a poorer prognosis.[4] Family history of aneurysmal SAH is associated with a higher incidence of intracranial aneurysm (6.7 percent).[13] In addition these aneurysms tend to hemorrhage at a younger age and smaller size, suggesting a more aggressive nature.[4,13–15] Certain systemic diseases are associated with a higher risk for intracranial aneurysm including Ehlers-Danlos syndrome, coarctation of the aorta, polycystic kidney disease, and fibromuscular dysplasia (20 to 40 percent incidence of intracranial aneurysm).[4] Substance abuse including tobacco, alcohol, and cocaine have all been reported to increase the risk for SAH.[4] Pregnancy is associated with an increased risk for rupture of intracranial aneurysms throughout the pregnancy and postpartum period, highest in the week of labor and the first several weeks postpartum.[16,17] Finally alterations in hemodynamics of the intra- and extracranial cerebral vasculature may increase the risk for development and rupture of intracranial aneurysms.[4] All types of persistent carotid-basilar anastomosis have been reported to be associated with aneurysms. Similarly, an unbalanced circle of Willis is associated with an increased risk for aneurysm. Ligation of the carotid artery has resulted in development of aneurysms of the contralateral carotid artery.[4,18] Likewise the incidence of aneurysms is increased in patients with an arteriovenous malformation (AVM). The majority of these aneurysms occur on the feeding vessels of the AVM.[19–21]

Risk Factors for an Aneurysmal Subarachnoid Hemorrhage

- Size
- Age
- Gender
- Hypertension
- Heredity
- Systemic disease
- Substance abuse
- Pregnancy
- Intracranial hemodynamic abnormalities

Diagnosis. Diagnosis of intracranial aneurysms most commonly follows SAH (in 90% of patients).[2] Signs and symptoms of SAH include severe headache, nuchal rigidity, focal neurologic deficits, and altered level of consciousness. In addition patients may develop autonomic disturbances manifested as fever, vomiting, and electrocardiographic (ECG) changes.[2] Confirmation of the diagnosis can be made with lumbar puncture or more commonly magnetic resonance imaging (MRI) or computed tomography (CT) for detection of intracerebral hemorrhage. A CT scan is positive in more than 90% of patients, especially if done soon after SAH.[2] Precise determination of location and anatomy of an intracranial aneurysm is made by angiography. Warning signs and symptoms occur in up to one-third of patients prior to major aneurysmal SAH and may be due to minor hemorrhage (sentinel bleeding) or aneurysmal enlargement. Time between warning signs and major SAH averages 2 to 3 weeks. Occurrence of a sentinel bleed, if recognized, may lead to diagnosis and aneurysm clipping with excellent outcome. However, if unrecognized, the presence of sentinel bleeding may have a negative impact on prognosis.[4]

Less commonly, aneurysms are diagnosed without hemorrhage. Symptoms related to unruptured aneurysms may be due to compression of surrounding structures or embolism of intraluminal thrombus. Finally, aneurysm may be detected on CT or MRI for unrelated symptoms.

Clinical Grade. The clinical condition of a patient with an intracranial aneurysm is most commonly described using an accepted grading system such as the Hunt-Hess modification of the Botterell classification. (Table 8.1) [22] Any discussion of outcome and treatment impact on outcome following aneurysmal SAH must take into account the presenting grade. Clinical grade on admission is the single most important determinant of outcome following SAH regardless of treatment utilized.

Outcome. The most recent large series investigating outcome following aneurysmal SAH was the International Cooperative Study on the Timing of Aneurysm Surgery published in 1990. This series included 3,521 patients. The mortality rate was 26 percent, morbidity, 16 percent and complete recovery, 58 percent. During the time period of this study, some of the current common treatment regimens, such as hypervolemic hemodilution and calcium channel blockers, were either not utilized or not used universally.[1] More recently completed smaller studies utilizing these modalities suggest there might be some improvement in outcome above that reported following the Cooperative Study.[23–26] Factors influencing outcome are listed in the accompanying box. The three most important factors influencing outcome are the neurologic status on admission, age of the patient, and presence of vasospasm on admission angiography. Figure 8.1 demonstrates the impact of clinical grade at admission on outcome.[1]

TABLE 8.1 *Hunt-Hess classification of clinical grade*

GRADE	DESCRIPTION
0	Unruptured
I	Minimal headache or nuchal rigidity
II	Moderate to severe headache, nuchal rigidity, ± cranial nerve palsy
III	Drowsiness, confusion, or mild focal deficit
IV	Stupor, hemiparesis, early decerebrate rigidity, and vegetative disturbances
V	Deep coma, decerebrate rigidity, moribund

Factors Influencing Outcome After a Subarachnoid Hemorrhage

- Admission neurologic status (level of consciousness or clinical grade)
- Age
- Vasospasm on admission angiography
- Aneurysm size (<12 mm better outcome)
- Aneurysm location (internal carotid and middle cerebral arteries better outcome)
- Hypertension (worse outcome)
- Distribution of subarachnoid clot
- Pre-existing medical conditions
- Plasma glucose levels (hyperglycemia worse outcome)

Management. The causes of morbidity and mortality following SAH are listed in Table 8.2. Vasospasm, the direct effects of the initial hemorrhage, rebleeding, and surgical complications were the leading causes of morbidity and mortality in the International Cooperative Study on the Timing of Aneurysm Surgery.[1] Current management is directed at reducing morbidity and

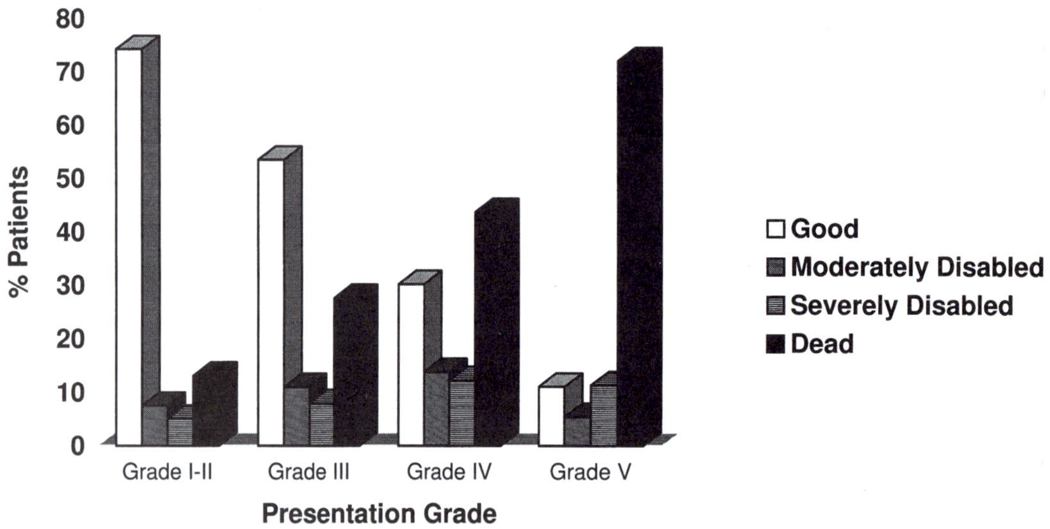

FIGURE 8.1 *Impact of admission clinical grade on outcome with the percentage of patients having each outcome at last follow-up (good, moderately disabled, severely disabled, or dead) by presenting clinical grade (From Kassell et al.,[1] with permission.)*

mortality due to these causes. In most centers SAH patients are managed aggressively with emergent diagnostic studies to allow for rapid diagnosis and institution of treatment. Following diagnosis of aneurysmal SAH, early surgery for clipping of the bleeding aneurysm, vasospasm prophylaxis, and aggressive treatment for symptomatic vasospasm is the rule in most neurosurgical centers.

TABLE 8.2 *Causes of morbidity and mortality following an SAH*

CAUSE	PERCENTAGE PATIENTS WITH MORBIDITY/ MORTALITY
Vasospasm	13.5
Direct effects of first SAH	10.6
Rebleeding	7.5
Surgical complications	4
Intracerebral hemorrhage	2
Hydrocephalus	1.7
Complications of medical therapy	0.7
Other or unknown	2.4

Abbreviation: SAH, subarachnoid hemorrhage.

CEREBRAL VASOSPASM

Incidence. Cerebral vasospasm following SAH remains the leading cause of morbidity and mortality in those patients who survive the initial event or a rebleed despite advances in early recognition, early surgical intervention, and treatment including aggressive invasive measures. Delayed ischemic neurologic deficits or symptomatic vasospasm occurs in as many as 15 to 35% of patients after SAH.[1,27,28] Angiographic vasospasm is more common than symptomatic vasospasm, occurring in 30 to 70% of patients between days 4 and 14 post-SAH.[27] Symptomatic vasospasm significantly contributes to the poor outcome of patients who initially present with a good clinical grade.

Vasospasm is characterized by abnormal arterial narrowing usually in the vascular territory of the ruptured aneurysm, but it can develop in distal vessels and rarely diffusely. The risk of cerebral vasospasm correlates well with the amount of blood in the basal subarachnoid space around the circle of Wills.[29,30] The clinical grade of the patient is not predictive of development of vasospasm and only provides a guide for timing of surgery and perhaps prognosis. Fisher et al. classified the risk of vasospasm according to the amount and distribution of subarachnoid blood detected by CT scan (Table 8.3).[30] The highest-risk patients have either a thick localized subarachnoid clot or vertical layers more than 1 mm thick (Fisher Grade III). Intraventricular or intraparenchymal clot does not predispose to the development of vasospasm.

Antifibrinolytic drugs utilized to prevent rebleeding iatrogenically increase the risk of vasospasm. Hyponatremia and hypovolemia, characteristic of cerebral salt wasting (CSW), have been associated with an increased risk of vasospasm and cerebral infarction. It was previously felt that early surgical intervention was associated with an increased likelihood of vasospasm development due to early manipulation of the cerebral vessels. There are recent studies that support early surgery and report a decreased incidence of delayed cerebral ischemia or better outcome after SAH in better-grade patients.[29,31] Early clot removal during surgery has had controversial results and has not consistently been associated with a reduction in vasospasm.[32] The trend, at least in the United States, has been toward early surgical intervention with the predominant goals of eliminating risk of rebleeding and safely allowing the aggressive treatment of vasospasm.

TABLE 8.3 *Fisher grade of SAH*

GROUP	BLOOD ON CT SCAN
I	No subarachnoid blood detected
II	Diffuse or thin vertical layer <1 mm thick
III	Localized subarachnoid clot and/or vertical layer >1 mm thick
IV	Intraventricular or intraparenchymal clot with diffuse or no SAH

Abbreviations: SAH, subarachnoid hemorrhage; CT, computed tomography.

(From Fisher et al.,[30] with permission.)

Etiology. The pathophysiology of cerebral vasospasm is not well understood but is likely complex and multifactorial (Table 8.4). The development of vasospasm clearly requires the presence of hemoglobin or its breakdown products. The time period of risk begins approximately 4 days after the initial hemorrhage as the subarachnoid clot begins to lyse. Oxyhemoglobin, the predominant and most spasmogenic breakdown product of hemoglobin, plays a key role in the initiation of vasospasm.[33–35] Other breakdown products that may be contributory include iron, hematin, and heme.[35]

Cerebral vasospasm is characterized by smooth muscle contraction but chronically there is structural and morphologic damage to the endothelium: smooth muscle necrosis, infiltration by inflammatory cells, disruption of the endothelial barrier, and fibrosis of the vessel wall.[33,36] Ultimately, free radical and inflammatory-induced endothelial injuries result in ischemia with excitatory amino acid release and finally calcium ion flux alteration with cell death.

Cerebral vasospasm may also be mediated by an imbalance between endothelin-1 and endothelium-derived relaxant factor (EDRF). Hemoglobin and oxyhemoglobin can stimulate endothelin-1 synthesis and inhibit EDRF activity.[37–39] The pathogenesis of vasospasm is complex and with elucidation of the mechanisms involved more specific treatment can be directed toward the causative agents.

Cerebral vasospasm has an insidious onset clinically presenting as confusion or decreased

TABLE 8.4 *Etiology of cerebral vasospasm following aneurysmal SAH*

AGENT	MECHANISM AND OBSERVATIONS
Oxyhemoglobin	Initiation of chain leading to vasospasm, potent vasoconstrictor, releases superoxide anion during autoxidation to methemoglobin, vasospasm produced by injection into CSF
Superoxide anion	Converted to H_2O_2 by superoxide dismutase, interacts with H_2O_2 to generate free radicals, oxidizes nitric oxide (loss of vasodilator potency)
Free radicals	Endothelial injury, lipid peroxidation in cell membranes
Lipid peroxides	Potent vasoconstrictors, CSF levels increased in vasospasm
Platelet aggregating factor	Mediator of platelet aggregation, chemoattractant-mediating inflammatory reaction
Endothelin-1	Potent vasoconstrictor, CSF levels increased after SAH, regulates vascular tone in balance with EDRF, such as nitric oxide

Abbreviations: SAH, subarachnoid hemorrhage; CSF, cerebrospinal fluid; EDRF, endothelium-derived relaxing factor.

consciousness as CBF declines, progressing to a focal neurologic deficit corresponding to the arterial territory in spasm. Symptoms depend on the degree of vasospasm, arterial territory of spasm, and adequacy of collateral circulation. Other etiologies for a change in neurologic status must be sought, including rebleeding, seizures, hydrocephalus, or metabolic disorders. Neurologic deficits can be minor or severe and reversible or permanent. If vasospasm is not ameliorated with treatment, then cerebral infarction will ensue, ultimately leading to permanent deficit or death.

The diagnosis can be made with transcranial Doppler or angiography. Transcranial Doppler can be utilized not only for diagnosis, but also for following progression of vasospasm and efficacy of treatment. In our laboratory, vasospasm is defined as a mean middle cerebral artery blood flow velocity greater than 120 cm/sec or middle cerebral artery peak blood flow velocity greater than 200 cm/sec. It is important for the physician to understand that vasospasm may be detected radiographically but can be clinically silent and is termed *symptomatic vasospasm* only when the delayed ischemic neurologic deficit corresponds to an area of vasospasm on an angiogram. Severe vasospasm is defined angiographically as a 50 percent or greater decrease in arterial diameter. Vasospasm can be detected intraoperatively by a change in somatosensory-evoked potentials (SSEP) or by surgical visualization of the vessel in spasm often with pallor of the surrounding parenchyma (Fig. 8.2).

Therapy. Treatment and prophylactic measures are listed in Table 8.5. The mainstay of treatment for established cerebral vasospasm involves the initiation of hypervolemic, hypertensive, hemodilution (HHH) therapy either postoperatively in the intensive care unit or intraoperatively. When the diagnosis is established, aggressive treatment should be initiated if the aneurysm is already clipped. In the face of an unclipped aneurysm, there is a risk of rebleeding if aggressive measures are instituted, but successful treatment has been reported in some centers.[40] Mild volume expansion with crystalloid and colloid is often instituted prophylactically in patients at high risk for vasospasm prior to aneurysm clipping in our institution. There is still considerable controversy over which aspect of HHH therapy is most important and whether CBF is elevated by increasing cardiac output or mean arterial blood pres-

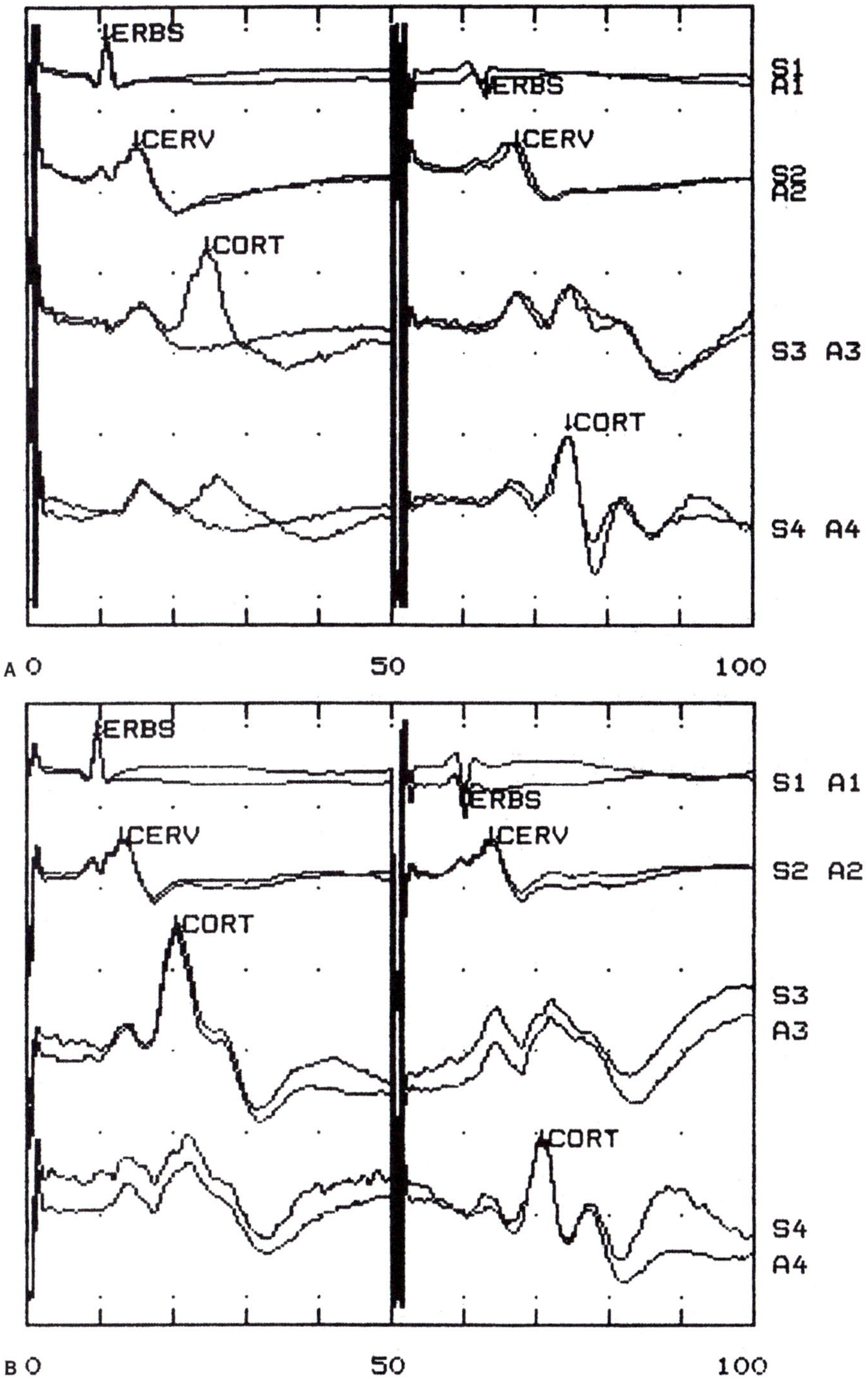

FIGURE 8.2 *Cerebral vasospasm detected by SSEP monitoring. (A) upper tracing shows baseline median nerve SSEP during surgery to clip giant right internal carotid artery aneurysm, with the lower tracing demonstrating a decrease in right cortical SSEP with development of vasospasm. T (B) Recovery of SSEP tracing after local papaverine and systemic induced hypertension.*

TABLE 8.5 *Management of cerebral vasospasm*

	Mechanism of Action
Prophylaxic Measures	
Hypervolemia	Increased CBF
Early surgery	Clot removal; allows aggressive treatment of vasospasm
TPA	Lysis of clot
Calcium channel antagonists	Prevention of calcium influx/cell death
Tirilazad	Inhibition of Fe-mediated lipid peroxidation
Aspirin (?)	Antiplatelet effect
Treatment of Established Vasospasm	
Hypervolemia	Increase CBF
Hypertension (induced)	Increase CBF
Hemodilution	Decrease blood viscosity
Angioplasty	Mechanical disruption
Papaverine	Nonspecific smooth muscle vasodilator

Abbreviations: CBF, cerebral blood flow; TPA, tissue plasminogen activator.

sure (MAP). It is known that HHH therapy can be efficacious in reversing or improving ischemic deficits. There are no large trials randomizing HHH therapy to assess efficacy of each factor alone. Of those patients who develop delayed ischemic neurologic deficits, 70 to 80 percent will achieve a good outcome with HHH therapy.[41,42]

Volume expansion is initiated with crystalloid, colloid, or packed red blood cells (only if the hematocrit is extremely low) to increase CBF either by increasing cardiac output or blood pressure. Hetastarch is not advocated by some for hypervolemic therapy as coagulopathy has been reported with its use.[43] It is prudent to place a pulmonary artery catheter prior to aggressive volume expansion in order to optimize cardiac parameters and to avoid potential complications commonly associated with this treatment. Levy and Giannotta determined the most useful cardiac parameters that could be used clinically to optimize hypervolemic therapy with pulmonary artery catheter monitoring.[44] After construction of a Starling curve with colloids in all patients, it was determined that pulmonary capillary wedge pressure (PCWP) best correlated with cardiac index, stroke volume index, and left ventricular stroke work index.[44] Since its publication, most clinicians have optimized cardiac status of the patient by following PCWP and cardiac output or index. There are new data to suggest that stroke volume index significantly correlates with end-diastolic volume index end-systolic volume index, and right ejection fraction when using a right ventricular pulmonary artery catheter (Stachniak, unpublished data). There was no correlation with PCWP and stroke volume index (Stachniak, unpublished data). In significantly ill patients being volume challenged, estimates of pressure are often inadequate, volume measurements may be more accurate and should be used instead. If cardiac output is not increased with maximized volume expansion alone, inotropic support with dobutamine or dopamine should be considered.

It has been known for many years that by increasing systemic blood pressure to hypertensive levels ischemic deficits can be alleviated by augmenting CBF and CPP through the spastic vessels or improving collateral blood flow.[41,45,46]

Autoregulation is often impaired following SAH implying that CBF is blood pressure dependent. Elevation in blood pressure may be achieved with hypervolemic therapy alone or augmented with vasopressors, such as phenylephrine or dopamine. In our institution systolic blood pressure is increased to a level of 180 mmHg or greater.

Hemodilution is generally achieved with intravascular volume expansinn with optimal hematocrit determined to be in the 30 to 32 percent range. The sole effectiveness of improving the rheological properties of the blood is questionable. Hemodilution increases CBF by decreasing viscosity of the blood. In a canine model of ischemia, a hematocrit of 30 percent was associated with the smallest infarct size.[47] Volume expansion with hemodilution seems to be more efficacious in ameliorating vasospasm than nondilutional hypervolemia.[48,49] Most neurosurgeons and critical care physicians maximize all three components of HHH therapy to optimize cardiac performance in an effort to increase CBF. HHH therapy is associated with intracranial and systemic complications. Aggressive HHH may exacerbate cerebral edema or result in hemorrhagic infarction if an infarct is present at the institution of treatment.[50] Systemic complications may include pulmonary edema, myocardial infarction, dilutional hyponatremia, or complications related to line placement.

Calcium channel antagonists, specifically nimodipine or nicardipine, are initiated in all SAH patients after admission and continued for 21 days. The role and efficacy of nimodipine have come under scrutiny recently. Nimodipine and nicardipine were originally felt to increase CBF by a cerebral vasodilatory effect related to smooth muscle relaxation; however, recent data suggest that their real role may be in the prevention of calcium influx and cell death.[31] Clinical trials utilizing nimodipine or nicardipine (even low doses) have been associated with a decreased incidence in severity of vasospasm and development of symptomatic vasospasm but overall outcome at 3 months is no different from those patients receiving a placebo.[51–53] Radiographically vasospasm is not consistently affected by calcium channel blockers. Nicardipine is not widely utilized clinically due to its cost and restricted intravenous route of administration and associated problems with systemic hypotension (with high doses), pulmonary edema, and azotemia.[51]

The 21-amino steroid tirilazad mesylate is currently being investigated in large clinical human trials worldwide. Its mechanism of action involves the inhibition of iron-mediated lipid peroxidation. The use of tirilazed in animal models attenuates chronic vasospasm after SAH.[54–56] Kassell and colleagues recently evaluated the efficacy of tirilazad mesylate in ameliorating symptomatic vasospasm and improving neurologic outcome following SAH in the first limb of the randomized, double-blind, vehicle-controlled trial of, 1023 patients.[57] The group of patients treated with 6 mg/kg/day of trilizad had a better neurologic outcome and lower mortality rate at 3 months after SAH compared to the vehicle-treated and trilizad-treated groups receiving lower total doses (0.6 mg/kg or 2 mg/kg/day). There was a trend toward a reduction in symptomatic vasospasm in the group treated with 6 mg/kg/day tirilazad that did not reach statistical significance. Women benefited from tirilazad less than their male counterparts. Currently another limb of the trial utilizing increased doses of tirilazad in women is in progress.

More aggressive, invasive measures are available if HHH therapy is ineffective or significant complications occur. Transluminal balloon angioplasty has been successfully utilized in the treatment of symptomatic vasospasm; 60 to 80 percent of patients will derive benefit with improvement in neurologic status after angioplasty.[27,58] The effectiveness of angioplasty may be secondary to disruption of structural changes in the vessel wall promoting vasospasm. Vessels may narrow again following angioplasty making it important to follow clinical status closely or perform serial transcranial Doppler studies. Angioplasty is not recommended in the presence of an unclipped aneurysm and should be initiated within 18 hours of onset of neurologic symptoms for best results.[59] Angioplasty has been employed intraoperatively for acute development of vasospasm resistant to induced hypertension and volume expansion. Risks associated with angioplasty include disruption of the aneurysm clip and dissection or rupture of the vessel wall.

Papaverine has been utilized topically intraoperatively or postoperatively as an intra-arterial injection for established vasospasm. It directly relaxes smooth muscle and is effective as long as chronic constrictive changes are not present in the vessel wall. Superselective intra-arterial injections of papaverine have been effective in attenuating vasospasm in distal or bifurcated vessels not accessible by angioplasty catheters.[60] The mechanism by which spastic vessels remain patent after papaverine use is unknown.

Several clinical trials have studied the use of intracisternal or intrathecal tissue plasminogen activator (TPA) initiated at the time of aneurysm clipping and in some studies continued postoperatively. TPA reduces the subarachnoid clot and theoretically should decrease the incidence of vasopasm. TPA has been shown to reduce the incidence of radiographic and symptomatic vasospasm.[61–63] As expected it can be associated with hemorrhagic intracranial complications.

The use of free radical scavengers, predominantly superoxide dismutase, has only be evaluated in animals. Its use for the prevention of vasospasm has yielded mixed results.[64,65] Superoxide dismutase not only scavenges free radicals by breaking down superoxide anion but also inhibits the oxidation of nitric oxide by superoxide anion. Other experimental studies have utilized platelet aggregating factor (PAF) antagonist and anti-PAF immunoglobulin, with encouraging results in rabbits.[36] The use of aspirin has not been investigated in humans except for the recent report of an observational prospective trial in patients using aspirin prior to or after SAH and documentation of the incidence of delayed cerebral ischemia.[66] Aspirin did not prevent the development of delayed cerebral ischemia but reduced the incidence of permanent neurologic deficits and cerebral infarction by CT scan in those patients with salicylates in the urine on admission.[66] Drugs with antiplatelet function may be beneficial if the bleeding risk does not outweigh their benefit.

REBLEEDING

Incidence and Outcome. In patients managed conservatively, the risk of rebleeding in the first 3 months following SAH is approximately 33%. The risk of rebleeding is highest in the first 2 weeks following the initial hemorrhage. The risk of rebleeding in the first week is 10 to 17 percent and in the second week after initial SAH 10 to 12 percent. One- third of the total rebleeds occur by the end of the first week and 50 percent by the end of 2 weeks. During the third and fourth weeks, the rate of rebleeding is 7 to 8 percent per week and during the second and third months 1.8 percent per week.[67,68] Morbidity and mortality from rebleeding are up to 50 percent, with most patients having at least a transient worsening of neurologic status. The combination of a high rate of rebleeding in the early period after aneurysmal SAH and the major risk of increased morbidity and mortality associated with rebleeding has lead to increasing enthusiasm for early surgery (within 3 days of initial hemorrhage) for aneurysm clipping.

Risk Factors. Perioperative factors felt to influence the risk for rebleeding include time since initial hemorrhage, size of aneurysm, transmural pressure, and surgical difficulties. Transmural pressure is defined as intra-aneurysmal pressure minus the pressure in the surrounding tissues. Intra-aneurysmal pressure is equal to intra-arterial pressure, and intracranial pressure, (ICP) is the pressure in the surrounding tissues. Thus, prior to clipping of the aneurysm, one important component of perioperative management is monitoring and control of systemic blood pressure. Excessive increases in blood pressure could lead to increased risk for rebleeding by increasing transmural pressure and wall tension within the aneurysmal sac. On the other hand, excessive degrees of hypotension may lead to worsening of cerebral ischemia in patients experiencing cerebral vasospasm. Perhaps the most prudent course is to attempt to determine the individual patient's usual blood pressure range and plan perioperative management to maintain blood pressure within or near the patient's "normal" blood pressure range. Likewise, impact of any intervention on ICP must be carefully considered. Unless the SAH has resulted in elevated ICP, maneuvers known to lower ICP, such as hyperventilation, are not instituted preoperatively because of concern that decreases in ICP could increase the risk for bleeding by increasing transmural pressure. However, intraoperatively, if the brain is "tight," the increased difficulty of the operative procedure could also lead to increased risk of rupture. A common approach is to avoid measures known to lower ICP preoperatively and intraoperatively until the dura is opened. Once the dura is open, ICP is no longer a component of the transmural pressure gradient. At that point, interventions to decrease brain bulk such as hyperventilation, and osmotic diuresis may be indicated to "soften" the brain and facilitate surgical exposure. Any improvement in operating conditions would likely decrease the risk for technical difficulties that could lead to intraoperative rupture.

In the past, antifibrinolytic agents were utilized to decrease the risk for rebleeding prior to surgery and clipping. These agents did lower the risk for rebleed. However, the incidence of neurologic morbidity and mortality related to cerebral vasospasm increased.[69,70] As a result, the overall results were unchanged, and these agents are no longer utilized at most neurosurgical centers.

PERIOPERATIVE COMPLICATIONS

Metabolic/Electrolyte. The most common metabolic disturbances associated with aneurysmal SAH involve the regulation of sodium and water homeostasis. Hyponatremia occurs in 9 to 33 percent of patients following SAH[71,72]; hypernatremia occurs less frequently with a reported incidence of approximately 10 percent.[73] CSW, syndrome of inappropriate secretion of antidiuretic hormone (SIADH), and diabetes insipidus (DI) are the most common syndromes associated with SAH and electrolyte disorders. Early recognition of a sodium/volume disturbance can avoid life-threatening problems and prevent further neurologic deterioration.

Hyponatremia following SAH may be attributed to the development of CSW or SIADH. Historically SIADH was the presumptive etiology of hyponatremia and natruresis in SAH patients; however, recent literature would support CSW as the most frequent syndrome resulting in hyponatremia.[74–76] Hyponatremia manifests as mental confusion, lethargy, nausea, seizures, or coma as serum levels acutely approach 120 meq/L or less. The brain can compensate for gradual development of hyponatremia with little or no associated clinical symptoms.

CSW is characterized by hyponatremia and a negative sodium balance; it is differentiated from SIADH by the presence of volume depletion. CSW and SIADH are otherwise indistinguishable by laboratory data: serum sodium less than 135 meq/L; serum osmolality greater than 280 mOsm/kg water; urine osmolality greater than serum osmolality; and urine sodium greater than 25 meq/L.[77] The diagnosis should only be made in the absence of renal, adrenal, hepatic, or thyroid disease or diuretic use.

The etiology of CSW is controversial but speculated to be due to either the release of atrial natruretic factor (ANF) or a natruretic digoxin-like substance from the central nervous system or altered neural input in the regulation of renal sodium reabsorption.[71,78] The production of ANF, a peptide hormone with potent natruretic, diuretic, and vasorelaxant properties produced by the atrial myocardium and brain, is postulated to be the primary mechanism. ANF levels are significantly elevated following SAH which may be due to hypothalamic dysfunction from vasospasm of feeding vessels or hematoma near the hypothalamic axis.[78] The significance of these elevations is not well understood, but it has been suggested that cerebral spinal fluid (CSF) ANF may play a role in CSF dynamics and regulation of ICP.[79] Interestingly not all patients with elevated ANF levels develop hyponatremia, and there is often no significant difference in levels between those patients who develop hyponatremia and those who do not.[71] The development of hyponatremia is probably not the result of elevated ANF levels alone and may require associated neural regulation or control to produce associated natruresis.

Patients with CSW are volume depleted and require treatment with fluid and sodium replacement. Fluid replacement may be achieved with crystalloid (i.e., normal saline), colloid, or packed red blood cells. Sodium replacement can be accomplished with fluids or increased dietary intake. If serum sodium levels are dangerously low or the above measures are ineffective, treatment with hypertonic saline should be instituted. Fluid restriction and diuretics, utilized in the treatment of SIADH, are dangerous, contributing to or worsening cerebral vasospasm by decreasing CPP and increasing blood viscosity in the face of hypovolemia. The correction of sodium deficits should be governed by the rapidity of decline in plasma levels, especially with chronic hyponatremia. Rapid correction of hyponatremia can lead to the development of central pontine myelinolysis. If a patient with cerebral vasospasm and hyponatremia is misdiagnosed with SIADH, fluid restriction and resultant further volume depletion will potentate cerebral ischemia, which may ultimately lead to infarction. Wijdicks et al. described 44 patients with hyponatremia following SAH of which 26 were fluid restricted and 18 maintained normal volume intake.[74] Twenty-one out of twenty-six patients with fluid restriction and 6 of 18 with normal intake developed cerebral infarction detected by CT or at autopsy. Only 19 of 90 patients with normal sodium levels had evidence of cerebral infarction. A higher mortality rate was described in those patients with cerebral infarction and hyponatremia. In most cases hyponatremia and natruresis preceded the development of cerebral ischemia or infarction.

CSW should be the leading differential in a patient with SAH and hyponatremia. Correct diagnosis is imperative to avoid inappropriate fluid restriction and exacerbation of cerebral vasospasm-induced ischemia. Fortunately the disorder is usually self-limited and resolves with time and continued fluid and sodium replacement.

The SIADH is not uncommon among neurosurgical patients but is probably an infrequent entity after aneurysmal SAH. Clinical manifestations of SIADH are similar to CSW. By laboratory data, SIADH mimics CSW, but most importantly, volume status of the patient is vastly different. SIADH is characterized by a dilutional hyponatremia secondary to excessive water reabsorption with an *increased or normal intravascular volume*. Hypothalamic or pituitary dysfunction from vasospasm or hemorrhage after SAH may account for increased antidiuretic hormone (ADH) release. It has been reported in patients with anterior cerebral, anterior communicating, and internal carotid artery aneurysms, with the highest incidence in association with anterior communicating artery aneurysms.[80,81] The onset of SIADH is variable; there is an initial rise in ADH after aneurysm rupture, but this is usually nonspecific and stress related.

The diagnosis of SIADH is made by the combination of blood and urine laboratory testing with assessment of volume status. If serum sodium levels are extremely low, use of hypertonic saline or diuretics is recommended. Fluid restriction is generally the treatment of choice if the sodium levels are not dangerously low and the patient is asymptomatic. Correction should be slow and not exceed more than a 20 meq/L increase in serum sodium levels over the first 48 hours of treatment. Chronic treatment may require fluid restriction alone or in combination with demeclocycline, furosemide, or phenytoin.[82]

Central DI has also been described following SAH and after aneurysm clipping; it has even developed as a result of mass effect from a large aneurysm. Its development has been described with anterior communicating and internal carotid artery aneurysms and associated with hypothalamic or pituitary dysfunction.[73,80] DI is characterized by hypernatremia, dilute urine output, and volume depletion.

The same mechanisms for the production of hypothalamic or pituitary dysfunction described in CSW and SIADH are operative in DI. DI may also develop secondary to mass effect especially from a giant aneurysm with similar effects as a sellar or suprasellar mass.[73] DI may even manifest intraoperatively if blood supply to the hypothalamic-pituitary axis is compromised.

Hypernatremia manifests as tremulousness, irritability, ataxia, spasticity, mental confusion, seizures, or coma as serum sodium levels acutely rise. DI is characterized by elevated serum sodium levels, urine output more than 250 to 300 ml/h, urine specific gravity less than 1.005, elevated serum osmolality, and decreased urine osmolality. The primary dysfunction is the excretion of free water as a result of low ADH levels. The diagnosis cannot be made in the presence of adrenal dysfunction. An osmotic diuresis due to mannitol or glucosuria will contribute to a high urine output but can easily be differentiated by urine specific gravity and the presence of large quantities of glucose. A water deprivation test can confirm the diagnosis of DI but is dangerous and not advocated in SAH patients.

The initial treatment of DI involves the replacement of the free water deficit by increasing oral intake or administration of hypotonic crystalloid (i.e, 5 percent clestrose in water, quarter or half normal saline). Administration of free water is not routinely recommended to avoid rapid overcorrection and administration concomitantly of dextrose that will increase urine output further and potentially worsen neurologic outcome if cerebral ischemia develops. Close monitoring of electrolytes, input/output, urine specific gravity, and daily weights is prudent. If urine output is excessive and intravenous fluid replacement is not adequate, drug treatment with arginine vasopressin (aqueous Pitressin) or desmopressin (DDAVP) is justified. Rapid correction may lead to central pontine myelinolysis. Chronic DI usually requires long-term treatment with intranasal DDAVP.

There are limited case reports of pituitary dysfunction and DI associated with cavernous and supraclinoid internal carotid artery aneurysms especially if giant.[73] Endocrine abnormalities should be investigated if the history and patient presentation are suggestive of pituitary dysfunction. The most common abnormalities involved in order of frequency are the pituitary-gonadal, pituitary-adrenal, and pituitary-thyroid axes.[73]

Respiratory. Pulmonary dysfunction is common following aneurysmal SAH and may complicate the perioperative management of these patients. Disease presentation may range from benign and self-limiting to potentially life-threatening, depending on the extent and nature of the underlying pathophysiology. Patients with SAH are at increased risk for respiratory complications due to hemodynamic events at the time of hemorrhage, frequent initial loss of consciousness, obtunded state; and prolonged bed rest or cardiac dysfunction secondary to hemorrhage.

Neurogenic pulmonary edema (NPE) is a complication of central nervous system disease frequently reported after SAH, intracranial hemorrhage, seizures, hydrocephalus, brain tumors, and severe head injury.[83,84] Its incidence has been reported to be up to 70 percent of patients at autopsy after aneurysm rupture, but most cases are probably subclinical and missed.[85]

The pathogenesis of NPE is very controversial and not well understood. There appears to be an association between elevated ICP and the development of NPE.[86] It is theorized that increased ICP resulting from severe neurologic insult produces intense sympathetic activation and catecholamine release from the hypothalamus and portions of the upper and ventrolateral medulla.[86] The etiology of pulmonary edema may be the result of elevated pulmonary microvascular pressures, a permeability abnormality, or most likely a combination of both.[83,87,88]

NPE may present acutely or have a more insidious onset several hours or days after the initial hemorrhage.[86,89] Its presentation may be fulminant and life-threatening but more commonly is subclinical or mild. Presenting symptoms depend on the severity of the pathology. NPE acutely manifests as tachypnea and dyspnea with crackles on chest examination, tachycardia, and low-grade fever. A rare presentation is fulminant disease with production of abundant pink frothy secretions, cyanosis and acute respiratory failure. Hypoxemia and intrapulmonary shunting may be evident by arterial blood gases. There is no characteristic chest x-radiographic pattern to distinguish it from other etiologies of pulmonary edema. The diagnosis is essentially one of exclusion. Aspiration of gastric contents is the primary alternate diagnosis, but the two may be difficult to distinguish initially. Usually, NPE resolves within 24 to 48 hours.[86]

Treatment of NPE is generally supportive with supplemental oxygen or continuous positive airway pressure by mask. If respiratory failure ensues, tracheal intubation, positive pressure ventilation, and institution of positive end-expiratory pressure (PEEP) is advocated. Institution of PEEP in patients with elevated ICP is safe as long as levels of PEEP are less than 10 cm water.[90] Elevations in ICP associated with low levels of PEEP are generally due to increasing dead space ventilation and not venous outflow obstruction.[90] Pulmonary artery catheter monitoring may only be helpful to rule out other etiologies of pulmonary edema. Aggressive treatment of ICP has been suggested in patients with evidence of NPE. The risk of aneurysm rebleed, related to altering the transmural pressure gradient, must be weighed with the benefit of treatment of increased ICP prior to the institution of aggressive measures. Phenytoin and adrenergic blockade only appear to be helpful in a prophylactic manner.

Aspiration of gastric contents occurs frequently after aneurysmal SAH. Patients sustaining SAH are at an increased risk of aspiration due to loss of consciousness at the time of hemorrhage or persistent obtunded state with associated blunting of airway reflexes. Aspiration may be self-limited and resolve quickly but can be complicated by the development of pneumonia depending on the pH and quantity of the aspirate. Clinical presentation is very similar to NPE, and initial treatment should be the same. The chest radiograph may be indistinguishable from pulmonary edema. If aspiration is suspected, steroids are not recommended, and antibiotics should only be instituted with documentation of pneumonia and infection. Early initiation of antibiotics may lead to overgrowth of an organism that may be resistant to conventional antibiotics. Aggressive pulmonary toilet and intubation with positive pressure ventilation may be needed if pneumonia develops and is severe.

Pulmonary embolus should always be considered in a SAH patient who suffers an acute decline in pulmonary status. Patients with SAH have been categorized as a moderate-risk group for the development of deep venous thrombosis (DVT) and pulmonary embolus.[91] The actual incidence of thromboembolism in this patient population is not well documented, but it is known that the mortality rate from pulmonary embolus is high among the general neurosurgical population. There is a large body of evidence to support the use of prophylactic measures to reduce the incidence of DVT.

The clinical presentation can be subtle and nonspecific to catastrophic with cardiovascular collapse and death. The most common presenting symptoms are dyspnea and pleuritic chest pain. A normal arterial blood gas, chest X-radiograph, and ECG do not rule out the diagnosis. The diagnosis may be made with a ventilation/perfusion lung scan, pulmonary angiography or documentation of DVT by Doppler ultrasound, impedance plethysmography, or venogram.

Prophylactic treatment should be instituted in all patients with SAH. Graduated stockings or intermittent pneumatic compression devices are advocated for all patients after SAH and should be terminated only when routine ambulation commences. Anticoagulants are contraindicated in all patients with a ruptured unclipped aneurysm or intracranial hemorrhage. They can probably be initiated with some degree of safety between postoperative weeks 1 and 6.[91] Low-molecular-weight heparin and heparinoids are the newest agents that may revolutionize DVT prophylaxis. They appear to be safer with reduced risk of bleeding and are more effective than conventional treatment. If pulmonary embolus does occur and anticoagulation is contraindicated, placement of a Greenfield filter in the inferior vena cava may be indicated to prevent further embolization.

Pulmonary edema is a common comtlication with HHH therapy instituted prophylactically in high-risk patients or for the treatment of established cerebral vasospasm. Its incidence is approximately 10 to 30 percent in the absence of coexisting cardiac dysfunction.[92,93] If pulmonary edema develops in the setting of HHH treatment for severe cerebral vasospasm, no specific therapy for the pulmonary edema except supportive ventilatory care and maintenance of oxygenation may be feasible. The morbidity and mortality associated with vasospasm are high, and aggressive treatment is often necessary to reverse neurologic deficits. If oxygenation becomes problematic, then the level of HHH therapy may need to be decreased or diuresis initiated. If HHH therapy is only prophylactic, then a mild decrease in fluid administration or cautious diuresis may be instituted.

Pulmonary edema resulting from myocardial injury should be sought in the absence of a demonstrable primary pulmonary source. The severity of hemodynamic or respiratory compromise will dictate aggressiveness of treatment. Pulmonary edema may be mild or even subclinical and only warrant supplemental oxygen. Intubation, mechanical ventilation, diuretics, and even inotropic support should be considered if severe myocardial dysfunction and hypoxemia develops. Prophylactic HHH therapy may be reduced to prevent contribution to edema formation.

ECG and Dysrhythmias Reported Following an Aneurysmal SAH

ECG CHANGES (50–70%)

Inverted T- waves
ST-T wave changes
Shortened PR interval
QT_c prolongation
Peaked P waves
U waves
Q waves

DYSRHYTHMIAS (UP TO 90%)

PVC
Ventricular tachycardia
Ventricular fibrillation
Supraventricular tachycardia
Premature atrial contraction
Atrial fibrillation
Heart block
Idioventricular rhythm
Torsades de Pointes

Abbreviations: ECG, electrocardiogram; SAH, subarachnoid hemorrhage; PVC, premature ventricular contraction.

Cardiac. ECG abnormalities are evident in 50 to 70% of patients following SAH.[94,95] However, there is still considerable debate over the clinical significance of these findings. These ECG abnormalities may mimic myocardial ischemia or infarction and may be accompanied by elevations in cardiac enzymes, complicating the patient's clinical picture. It is often challenging for the anesthesiologist, neurosurgeon, and critical care intensivists to treat these patients during the perioperative period. The clinical significance and true incidence, other than anecdotal, of these findings is unknown.

ECG abnormalities have been documented in patients with SAH, cerebrovascular accidents or infarctions, head injury, meningitis, and tumors.[96–98] The first association between ECG changes and SAH was observed in 1947.[99] For years it was postulated that these changes were the result of central nervous system influences and not representative of true myocardial injury. However, autopsy findings and recent data utilizing echocardiography (ECHO) and thallium scintigraphy have provided evidence that these ECG changes may reflect cardiac injury.

ECG abnormalities are common following SAH. In one study looking at perioperative ECG changes, the highest incidence of abnormal ECGs occurred in patients in poor clinical grade.[100] New ECG changes developed intraoperatively and postoperatively in 35 and 65 percent of patients, respectively. Only fluctuating postoperative ECG changes were associated with a worse neurologic outcome. In the majority of reports however, there are no consistent relationships between aneurysm location, poor neurologic grade, poor neurologic outcome, and cardiac dysfunction. Some evidence suggests that ECG abnormalities and cardiac dysfunction associated with SAH occurs more commonly in postmenopausal women. Arrhythmias are also common and have been reported in as many as 90 percent of SAH patients when studied by Holter monitoring.[101,102] These arrhythmias are often more frequent and severe within 48 hours of hemorrhage.[101]

Elevations in cardiac enzymes (creatine kinase and myocardial isoenzyme) may accompany ECG abnormalities in as many as 50 percent of patients after SAH but usually do not approach the levels seen with transmural infarction.[103,104] Additional evidence of cardiac injury has been documented by ECHO and thallium scintigraphy (Table 8.6).[94,95,105] Interestingly in the limited studies available, patients with myocardial dysfunction do not appear to have a higher cardiac morbidity and mortality and usually succumb to neurologic complications (primarily cerebral vasospasm).

The etiology of ECG changes, arrhythmias, and myocardial injury is likely the result of intense catecholamine release at the time of SAH. At autopsy some patients have both myocardial and hypothalamic lesions, which further supports catecholamine release resulting from hypothalamic injury as a possible mechanism for coronary vasospasm and subsequent ischemia.[106,107] The myocardial lesions at autopsy often occur in the absence of demonstrable coronary artery stenosis and are often subendocardial and diffuse, involving the left ventricle. However, not all patients with ECG abnormalities have myocardial lesions at autopsy. In experimental models, ECG changes and arrhythmias have been attenuated or prevented by C2 cordotomy, propranolol, and cocaine.[108–110] Phentolamine and propranolol have been utilized to block sympathetic response in patients following SAH to prevent the development of myocardial injury.[103,107] The hypothalamus may be the source of stimulation for catecholamine release secondary to hemorrhage, infarction, or vasospasm involving this structure at the time of SAH. Recently there has been interest generated in the role of the insular cortex as an arrhythmogenic center and possible contributor to ECG changes if damaged.[111–113] Norepinephrine lev-

TABLE 8.6 *Cardiac evaluation following an aneurysmal SAH*

STUDY	TEST	ABNORMALITY	INCIDENCE	FOLLOW-UP
Pollick et al.[94]	ECHO	Severe LV dysfunction	4/13 (all 4 had inverted T waves)	LV function improved at > 7 days
Kono et al.[105]	Angiography	LV hypokinesis, no coronary artery disease or spasm	7/7 with ST elevation	Improvement in LV function
Szabo et al.[95]	Thallium scintigraphy	Abnormal perfusion with redistribution	6/19 (all 6 had abnormal ECG, not all with abnormal ECG had abnormal thallium)	

Abbreviations: SAH, subarachnoid hemorrhage; ECHO, echocardiogram; LV, left ventricular; ECG, electrocardiogram.

els are elevated at the time of SAH, and mechanism of injury may be systemic effects or high local tissue levels.[94,107,114,115]

There are no large clinical trials documenting significance of myocardial dysfunction in this setting or increased cardiac morbidity and mortality if cardiac injury is present. As a result, the best method to treat SAH patients with evidence of cardiac injury is speculative. Further diagnostic options include ECHO, thallium scintigraphy, or cardiac catheterization. A transesophageal ECHO may be better than transthoracic ECHO to assess wall motion abnormalities, valvular function, and ejection fraction but is not practical unless the patient is in the operating room or intubated so that sedation or anesthesia can be administered to blunt the hypertensive response to probe insertion. Many patients with aneurysmal SAH will have risk factors associated with development of atherosclerotic coronary disease, making it difficult to differentiate between those patients with cardiac dysfunction secondary to SAH and those with underlying occlusive coronary artery disease. Further work-up (i.e., adenosine thallium testing) if cardiac dysfunction exists is based upon underlying risk factors and whether additional information will alter surgical timing or intervention. Cardiac catheterization is not routinely performed at our institution in the presence of a ruptured aneurysm. Results from catheterization are unlikely to alter management because coronary revascularization is not an option prior to aneurysm clipping. In a patient with suspected myocardial dysfunction secondary to SAH no further work-up beyond serial ECHOs and cardiac enzymes may be necessary. Because most neurosurgical centers believe early surgery after SAH is preferable and because there is no clear evidence of increased cardiac morbidity or mortality in patients with ECG abnormalities associated with SAH, delaying surgery to wait until wall motion abnormalities improve is not currently recommended. Diagnostic procedures should be requested only if they will allow for improved perioperative management of the patient.

Management depends on the hemodynamic stability of the patient. If hemodynamic instability is present, placement of a pulmonary artery catheter is prudent to optimize cardiac status with vasopressors, inotropic agents, or blood products. A transesophageal ECHO may be helpful in guiding the intraoperative course of the patient during aneurysm surgery. It is not known whether SAH patients should receive the same treatment as those with documented atherosclerotic coronary artery disease and ischemia. Until more is known about the outcome of these patients from a cardiac standpoint, the appropriate treatment is controversial. β-Blockade may be protective but is not always feasible, especially in those at risk for or in cerebral vasospasm receiving concomitant treatment to increase cardiac output and blood pressure. Nitroglycerin use is also controversial, because its effects on cerebral vasculature may be deterimental in the postoperative period should cerebral edema develop.

Despite the potential myocardial injury associated with an abnormal ECG at the time of SAH, the clinical significance of these findings is not well understood. In the limited data available, the patients with myocardial dysfunction die secondary to neurologic complications from the cerebral aneurysm and not cardiac-related events. Typically myocardial ischemia or infarction secondary to coronary artery disease is associated with an increased risk of cardiac complications or reinfarction, especially during anesthesia, but the long-term outcome and risk associated with anesthesia may differ in the subset of patients with SAH-related cardiac injury. It is theorized that SAH patients develop a stunned myocardium with reversible postischemic injury. In the few studies in the literature, SAH-induced wall motion abnormalities improve or normalize with time. Delays in the timing of surgical intervention and inappropriate initiation of anticoagulant therapy have been reported resulting from ECG patterns resembling ongoing ischemia or infarction. It is not known if timing of aneurysm surgery should be altered in these patients. This subset of patients may not tolerate HHH therapy that is initiated prophylactically or for the treatment of established cerebral vasospasm. At this time there is still controversy surrounding the perioperative care of these patients.

Optimal management of patients with intracranial aneurysms must take into account the pathophysiology of the disease process and should not focus solely on avoidance of any single complication or source of morbidity. It requires balancing of often conflicting concerns, the importance of which vary in each patient and at different times in the perioperative period in an individual patient. The course taken must be individualized to match the risk for each problem in a given patient at a given moment.

Perioperative Issues in Intracranial Aneurysm Patients

TIMING OF SURGERY One of the most extensively investigated aspects of management of the SAH patient is the optimal timing of surgery. During the early decades of aneurysm surgery, operative repair was generally delayed to allow for some neurologic recovery prior to operation. However, during the waiting period, many patients deteriorated from both rebleeding and vasospasm. The proposed advantages of early (0 to 3 days) versus late (more than 7 to 10 days post-SAH) surgery are listed in the accompanying box. If one of the goals of aneurysm clipping is to prevent rebleeding, early surgery would provide the greatest decrease in morbidity and mortality from rebleeding, because the rate of rebleeding is highest in the early days following SAH. It could also be argued that by eliminating the risk of rebleeding, vasospasm could be treated more aggressively should it develop. Of concern when considering early surgery is that some studies have suggested that the risk for vasospasm is greater if the brain is manipulated early after SAH. Neurosurgeons have also noted that in some patients operated on early the brain is "red and angry," increasing likelihood of a difficult exposure and potentially increased operative complications. Finally, if operative outcome alone is considered, operative results are better in patients undergoing late operations. However, these results do not take into account morbidity and mortality occurring in patients waiting for delayed procedures.

Proposed Advantages of Early Versus Late Surgery

EARLY SURGERY[a]

Eliminate risk for rebleeding

Allow aggressive vasospasm therapy

Removal of clot

LATE SURGERY[b]

Less risk for vasospasm

Better operative conditions

Lower operative morbidity/mortality

[a] Zero to three days.
[b] More than 7 to 10 days post–subarachnoid hemorrhage.

The International Cooperative Study on the Timing of Aneurysm Surgery studied 3,521 SAH patients prospectively and related overall management results on the planned surgical timing.[116] There were no differences in outcome in those patients with early surgery (0 to 3 days) versus those with late surgery (11 to 14 days post-SAH) planned. Patients operated on between days 7 and 10 fared worst. As expected, rebleeding was decreased in those patients operated on early. The risk of morbidity or mortality related to cerebral vasospasm was similar between early and late surgery. Those patients operated on in the intermediate periods had high rates of both rebleeding and vasospasm. Surgeons noted "tight brains" in nearly 50 percent of early surgery patients as compared to 20 percent of patients in the late group. However, the incidence of brain contusion, laceration, requirement for major brain resection, and intraoperative rupture was not different. These results suggest that any increase in operative difficulty did not translate to increased risk for surgical complications. Although operative results were better in the late surgery group, this was balanced by morbidity and mortality while waiting for late surgery, so that management results were the same in both early and late surgery. The authors' conclusions were that there was no difference in outcome between early and late surgery and that if effective therapy for vasospasm could be found, the advantages of early surgery would become more obvious.[1,116] Calcium channel blockers and HHH therapy were not routinely utilized in these patients. As these techniques are accepted as advantageous in patients following SAH for prevention and treatment of symptomatic cerebral vasospasm, the authors' reasoning, although not proven, may be true. In a subset of the International Cooperative Study, the results from the North American centers were evaluated. In this group, although the mortality was similar in the early and late surgery patients, the likelihood of a good recovery was increased by early surgery.[28]

Currently the most accepted management strategy is early surgery for most patients presenting in good clinical condition (grades I to III) following SAH. The optimal plan for patients presenting in poor condition (grades IV and V) is less clear. Some recent studies have suggested that early surgery and aggressive management in selected poor-grade patients may result in an improvement in outcome without an increased rate of survival in a vegetative state. In these studies poor-grade patients were selected for early surgery and aggressive management by clinical (controllable ICP and/or improvement after ventriculostomy) and CT scan (absence of evidence of irreversible brain damage) criteria. They then underwent early surgery for clipping of the aneurysm and aggressive postoperative management aimed at prevention and treatment of vasospasm and control of ICP. Good outcome was achieved in 45 to 50 percent of grade IV and V patients selected for aggressive management. Mortality was approximately 25 percent with severe disability in the remainder.[23,24]

PHARMACOLOGIC CONTROL OF BLOOD PRESSURE

Goals. The one common goal in blood pvessure management of all aneurysm patients is to avoid excessive swings in systemic pressure. Beyond that, desired blood pressure control varies with different conditions and different times in the perioperative period. Prior to clipping, hypertension may increase the risk for rupture. In patients at risk for vasospasm, hypotension may worsen neurologic deficits. Consequently, excessive lowering of blood pressure may not be indicated, even in the presence of unclipped aneurysms. Should ischemic neurologic deficits develop, induced hypertension may be indicated. This is preferably done only after securing the aneurysm but on occasion may be necessary prior to clipping.

The ideal agent to manipulate blood pressure in these patients would be have no adverse effect on CBF, would not impair cerebral autoregulation or cerebrovascular responsiveness to $PaCO_2$, would have rapid onset and offset, be titratable, and would provide cerebral protection or at least not increase risk for cerebral injury. Available hypotensive agents are listed in Table 8.7.

Sympathetic Blocking Agents. Sympathetic blocking agents have been used successfully in neurosurgical patients and have minimal impact on CBF, autoregulation, and CO_2 responsiveness.[117] Their disadvantages as a group include negative inotropic effects and varying potential to potentiate bronchospasm. They may be ideal agents to lower blood pressure when hypertension and tachycardia have developed related to stimulation, in patients with coronary artery disease where their decrease in myocardial oxygen demand is advantageous, and as supplemental agents when tachycardia has developed during use of other agents to lower blood pressure. Of these agents, esmolol, with its ultrashort half-life may be the single best agent in the perioperative period. Many advocate its use to blunt hemodynamic response to brief and intense stimulation, such as laryngoscopy and placement of the pin fixation device.

Vasodilators. Nitroprusside provides rapid and reliable decreases in blood pressure. It may well be the drug with which we have the greatest clinical experience in neuroanesthesia. However, there are significant disadvantages associ-

TABLE 8.7 *Vasoactive agents for use in neurovascular procedures*

AGENT	DOSE	ONSET (MIN)	HALF-LIFE	CBF EFFECT	ADVANTAGE	DISADVANTAGE
Esmolol	0.5–3 μg/kg bolus; 20–300 μg/kg/min	1–2	9 min	None	B-1 selective	Negative inotrope
Labetalol	5–300 mg	1–5	6 h	Minimal	Combined a and B blockade, ↓ risk of CHF and bronchospasm	Long duration, less titratable, heart block, CHF
Propanolol	0.5–6 mg	~5	2 h	Minimal		Long duration, nonselective, less titratable, CHF, bronchospasm
Sodium nitroprusside	0.5–8 μg/kg/min	1	2–3 min	Increase	Titratable, rapid, extensive clinical experience	Potential ↑ ICP, reflex tachycardia, rebound HTN, impair autoregulation, and CO_2 response, cyanide toxicity
Nitroglycerin	≥0.5 μg/kg/min	1	3–5 min	Increase	↑ Coronary blood flow	Potential ↑ ICP, methemoglobinemia
Trimethaphan	0.5–5 mg/min	1–5	10 min	Less increase	Titratable, less potential ↑ ICP	Tachyphylaxis, cycloplegia, cerebral ischemia at >CPP than SNP, NTG
Adenosine	0.06–0.35 mg/kg/h	<1	<1 min	None or decrease	Titratable, ↓ CMR	Rebound hypertension

Abbreviations: CBF, cerebral blood flow, CHF, congestive heart failure; ICP, intracranial pressure; HTN, hypertension; CPP, cerebral perfusion pressure; SNP, sodium nitroprusside; NTG, nitroglycerin; CMR, cerebral metabolism.

ated with its use, including increases in CBF with the potential for increases in ICP. This effect may be most evident when nitroprusside is used to treat hypertension in the presence of impaired cerebral autoregulation, as occurs with administration of volatile anesthetic agents.[118] In addition reflex tachycardia and rebound hypertension may develop. The rebound hypertension may be a particularly worrisome effect following AVM resection.

Nitroglycerin may also be used to lower blood pressure. Its ability to treat hypertension or induce hypotension may be less reliable than that of nitroprusside. The primary indication for nitroglycerin over nitroprusside would be use in patients with known or suspected coronary artery disease.

Ganglionic Blocking Agents. Trimethaphan is the ganglionic blocking agent most commonly utilized in neurosurgical patients. Its primary advantage is lack of significant impact on CBF or ICP in neurosurgical patients. The rapid development of tachyphylaxis and pupillary dilation have resulted in its limited use in recent years. The use of trimethophan has been largely replaced with the use of vasodilators and/or β-blockers.

SURGICAL OPTIONS Surgery offers clear and obvious benefits for the patient harboring an intracranial aneurysm, including freedom from rebleeding risks, enhanced ability to aggressively treat subarachnoid hemorrhage-induced vasospasm, and, for giant lesions, reduction of mass effect against critically important structures (i.e., optic nerve and brainstem). To maximize these advantages, the neurosurgeon must be able to safely and efficiently enter the cranial vault, perform the dissection necessary for exposure, and clip the aneurysm without undue risks of parenchymal injury, premature aneurysm rupture, or parent vessel (or perforator) compromise. Careful planning is essential to achieve these goals and requires close cooperation and communication between all members of the operating room team.

Basic Surgical Techniques. The neurosurgeon must first select an operative approach that provides an excellent trajectory to aid exposure of the desired brain region. Improper exposure and direct mechanical injury from retraction-induced contusion and ischemia can be major causes of perioperative complications, and the chosen approach should aim at key skull base regions whose radical removal provides excellent exposure with minimal need for brain retraction. The sphenoid ridge, anterior clinoid process, lateral and medial petrous apex, mastoid bone, and occipital condyle can all be refashioned extensively without causing neurologic morbidity, and skull base techniques that remove these regions should be an integral part of the modern aneurysm surgeon's armamentarium.

Once the appropriate amount of bone has been removed, the next step involves a gentle manipulation of the brain so that the desired area comes into full view. The surgical microscope (with its improved lighting, stereoscopic vision, and television camera), self-retaining brain retractors, and dedicated microinstrumentation are all essential components of this stage of the procedure. A tight brain must be relaxed prior to subarachnoid dissection to avoid significant retraction and should be anticipated preoperatively in patients with significant subarachnoid blood, hydrocephalus, or intraparenchymal or intraventricular hemorrhage. CSF drainage (through a ventriculostomy, spinal drain, or nick in the basal subarachnoid cisterns) combined with hyperosmotic solutions (i.e., mannitol) to shrink the brain parenchyma and mild hyperventilation to reduce cerebral blood volume will usually suffice. Removal of a "safe" region and amount of an intraparenchymal clot may be needed in some cases to achieve the desired state.

Trans-sylvian arachnoid attachments between the frontal and temporal lobes can then be safely separated (anterior circulation lesions) or the temporal lobe or cerebellum mobilized and gently retracted (posterior circulation aneurysms) with minimal risks of dissection-induced pial disruption. The subarachnoid dissection is continued until proximal control of the parent artery harboring the aneurysm is attained, staying on a "safe" surface of the vessel away from perforator origins and the aneurysm fundus. In most instances, the neck of the aneurysm can then be exposed and safely clipped without a need for focal or global circulatory arrest.

Some aneurysms, however, because of their large size, location, associated atheroma or thrombus, thinness of their walls, or complex shapes and branching patterns, cannot be safely clipped without high risks of parent vessel or perforator damage or premature aneurysm rupture and will require some type of circulatory arrest or diversion during the final stages of dissection and clipping. The need for these special techniques (i.e., temporary clipping, circulatory arrest, or revascularization) can often be anticipated preoperatively and obviously should be employed *before* a catastrophe arises to be maximally effective and protective.

Focal Circulatory Arrest. Exposure of the parent vessel proximal to the aneurysm's origin, thereby providing the ability to temporarily clip the artery if necessary, is a dominant principle of aneurysm surgery. Temporary proximal clipping is often all that is considered for most small or large aneurysms and is usually indicated by the intraoperative identification of a thin-walled or complex-shaped lesion or one with adherent branches in whom the last stages of the dissection risks premature aneurysm rupture. This technique usually effectively lowers the pulsatile tension on the aneurysm wall, allowing the final aspects of the dissection and clipping to be accomplished quickly, accurately, and more safely.

The need for temporary proximal parent vessel clipping combined with clipping of exiting branches (trapping) can often be anticipated preoperatively and is generally indicated for giant aneurysms or those with intraluminal thrombus or atherosclerosis in whom the aneurysm bulk must be decompressed prior to clip placement. This technique is accompanied by complete isolation of a focal part of the circulation (hence, the term *trapping*) and carries more ischemia risks than temporary proximal ligation only, particularly if perforators originate from the trapped segment.

Regardless of the type of focal circulatory arrest chosen, the patient is loaded with a cerebral protective agent (i.e., barbiturates), and the blood pressure is elevated before the temporary clip is applied. Relative mild hypothermia (33° to 35°C) may add further protection to these measures. Evoked potential monitoring is very helpful in assessing the depth of cortical suppression with the protective medicines and in guiding blood pressure maintenance levels. Except in emergency situations, the length of focal circulatory arrest should not exceed 15 to 20 minutes.

Global Circulatory Arrest. This methodology requires a concerted effort between the cardiac surgeons and the neurosurgery team, and because each patient must have a thorough preoperative cardiac evaluation, it is not a procedure to be decided upon at the last minute. General indications for circulatory arrest procedures include situations in which (1) the aneurysm size or location prevents control of the entering or proximal vessels, (2) the period of temporary occlusion is expected to be prolonged, well beyond 15 minutes, and (3) manipulation of the distended aneurysm or its associated perforators are deemed excessively hazardous. The most common lesion for which this technique is considered is the large or giant basilar apex aneurysm.

The exposure and most of the aneurysm dissection is done before the deep hypothermia and circulatory arrest are begun. Once the aneurysm is directly visualized, a decision is made whether the lesion can be clipped with brief focal arrest or will need complete circulatory hypoperfusion. Once begun, the body temperature is rapidly lowered to severely hypothermic levels (16° to 18°C). After the pump is turned off, the surgeon has a maximum of 45 to 60 minutes of reasonably safe cerebral protection, during which the aneurysm must be reconstructed and flow re-established. This protected interval can be somewhat lengthened by keeping the pump going at low flows (profound hypothermia and hypotension) but with increased coagulopathy complication risks.

By placing slightly negative pressure within the vascular system, a giant aneurysm that does not contain intraluminal thrombus will completely collapse, allowing clipping without further distortion of already overstretched perforators. These perforators must be carefully identified and marked beforehand, as they will be difficult to discriminate from arachnoid bands once the pump is stopped. This technique requires meticulous hemostasis during all stages of the procedure, as postoperative bleeding complications are common and hazardous, especially in cases with prolonged pump times or temporal lobe retraction.

Revascularization Procedures. Flow augmentation is also a very effective method to provide cerebral protection during some complex aneurysm procedures, but unfortunately, these techniques are often only considered after a catastrophe has already been set in motion. Several methods of flow augmentation procedures can be utilized, including (1) an arterial bypass between the extracranial and intracranial circulations, using the superficial temporal or occipital artery as a donor source, and a peripheral middle cerebral artery, posterior cerebral artery, superior cerebellar artery, or posterior inferior cerebellar artery branch as the recipient, (2) a similarly constructed but higher-flow venous anastomosis, using the saphenous vein to connect major arterial trunks (i.e., cervical internal or external carotid artery with a deep M-1 or M-2 middle cerebral artery segment), or (3) an internal bypass, during which adjacent intracranial arteries with different sources of blood are anastomosed together (i.e., superior cerebellar artery to posterior cerebral artery).

Like the other types of protective techniques, revascularization procedures are most effective if performed before an emergency arises. These methods are essential in situations where a segment of the parent vessel must be sacrificed in order to completely obliterate the aneurysm (i.e., dissecting, severely arteriosclerotic, or intracavernous lesions). The choice between an arterial or venous bypass is made based on the size of the available arterial donor vessel and the amount of blood volume needed to supply the isolated distal circulation territory. In general, an arterial-to-arterial bypass has superior patency rates and lower complication rates, but a superficial temporal artery may not be acutely able to provide enough blood to keep an entire middle cerebral artery circulation patent.

TEMPORARY VESSEL OCCLUSION

Indications. Temporary clipping of the parent vessel of an intracranial aneurysm is utilized to isolate the aneurysm from the systemic circulation usually during the final stages of dissection and permanent clip application to decrease risk for intraoperative rupture. It may also be utilized during repair of giant aneurysms to allow for opening of the aneurysm sac and removal of thrombus, so that the dissection can be completed and the clips properly applied. Finally temporary clips may be utilized to control hemorrhage following intraoperative rupture. Elective use of temporary clips has increased as evidence has accumulated that their use is not associated with an increased risk for ischemic neurologic injury postoperatively.

The likelihood of neurologic injury during application of temporary clips depends on the adequacy of collateral blood flow, the duration of potential ischemia, and the ability to provide cerebral protection.

Protection. When temporary clips are placed on the parent vessel, the brain supplied by that vessel is at risk for temporary focal cerebral ischemia and infarction. The degree of risk depends on the adequacy of collateral blood flow to the territory supplied by the clipped artery. It is rarely possible preoperatively to know with certainty the adequacy of the collateral blood supply. As a result many neurosurgeons and neuroanesthesiologists choose to utilize cerebral protective agents during temporary clipping. Many anesthetic agents have been touted as cerebral protective agents, including etomidate, barbiturates, and isoflurane. However, the only agent commonly available to anesthesiologists with proven cerebral protective effects during temporary focal cerebral ischemia in both animal and human studies is thiopental. The dose of thiopental for cerebral protection used in most centers is that necessary to achieve electroencephalographic (EEG) burst suppression. Ideally that is accomplished utilizing intraoperative EEG monitoring.[119] The dose range is generally a 5 to 15 mg/kg bolus followed by an infusion of 10 to 15 mg/kg/h. If intraoperative EEG monitoring is not available, empiric administration of thiopental in this dose range is likely advantageous.

Although the neuroprotective effects of thiopental in this dose range for temporary focal cerebral ischemia are proven in animal and human models, the protective effects of thiopental during intracranial aneurysm have not been studied in a randomized fashion. Nonetheless, administration of thiopental as a cerebral protective agent during application of temporary clips is a common and accepted practice in neuroanesthesiology. It is unlikely that a prospective randomized study of this practice will be conducted.

Use of etomidate for cerebral protection during aneurysm surgery has been advocated.[120] There are no studies prospectively evaluating the protective effects of etomidate in this or any other patient population. Animal studies investigating the protective effects of etomidate during temporary focal cerebral ischemia report varying neuroprotective effects. Currently the use of etomidate for cerebral protection during temporary clipping is not supported by available data.

Monitoring. It is also possible to monitor the adequacy of cerebral perfusion during temporary clipping with the use of intraoperative neurologic monitoring. This is most commonly done with SSEP. For this to be effective the pathways monitored must be supplied by the vessels at risk during the operative procedure, for example, median nerve SSEP monitoring during clipping of a middle cerebral artery aneurysm (see Ch. 4). Loss or alteration of the SSEP during application of a temporary clip indicates that blood flow is inadequate to maintain function of the neural tissue. The blood flow may or may not be adequate to prevent cell death. In our experience, if the SSEP is unaltered during temporary clipping or is depressed for shorter than 15 minutes during temporary clipping, the likelihood of a new postoperative neurologic deficit is extremely low.[121] Use of evoked potential monitoring has been of greater clinical utility during surgery for aneurysms of the anterior circulation (internal carotid artery or its branches) than posterior circulation aneurysms.[122]

Blood Pressure Management. Adequacy of collateral blood depends in part on perfusion pressure. If the brain supplied by the clipped artery is ischemic, the resistance vessels will be maximally vasodilated and blood flow will be pressure dependent. Autoregulation in that area of the brain is lost. As a result, CPPs tolerated prior to placement of the temporary clips may result in cerebral ischemia and/or infarction once the clips are placed. Once temporary clips are in place, the CPP is usually allowed to increase either by decreasing or discontinuing the administration of agents lowering systemic blood pressure or by administration of vasopressors. Routine induced hypertension is not a common practice. However, induced hypertension may be utilized empirically if it is felt that the collateral flow is likely to be marginal. It may also be initiated in response to evidence of cerebral ischemia detected via intraoperative neurologic monitoring.

INDUCED HYPOTENSION

Indications. At one time induced hypotension was used commonly during intracranial aneurysm surgery to lower transmural pressure, "softening the aneurysms sac," thereby decreasing risk of intraoperative rupture. In recent years its routine use has become uncommon. Studies have suggested that routine use of induced hypotension during aneurysm dissection and clipping does not reduce the incidence of intraoperative rupture but may increase the possibility of neurologic injury should intraoperative rupture occur and temporary clips be required to control hemorrhage.[123]

Induced hypotension may still be utilized in selected circumstances to decrease the pressure within the aneurysm sac when application of temporary clips is not appropriate. Also it may

Relative Contraindications to Induced Hypotension

- Ischemic cerebrovascular disease
- Coronary artery disease
- Hypovolemia
- Anemia
- Severe hypertension
- Extremes of age

be necessary to decrease bleeding should intraoperative rupture occur. Arterial hemorrhage from the aneurysm site can obscure the surgeons view, making it difficult or impossible to place either temporary or permanent clips properly. In this situation, the only alternative to control the bleeding is to lower systemic blood pressure, allowing the surgeon to better visualize the vessel and apply either temporary or permanent clips. Once the hemorrhage is controlled, the induced hypotension is discontinued.

Contraindications. There are few absolute contraindications to induced hypotension. The accompanying box lists relative contraindications to induced hypotension.[124,125] The potential benefits of induced hypotension must be weighed against the increased risk of induced hypotension in patients with these conditions. In patients with poorly or uncontrolled hypertension, the limits of cerebral autoregulation are shifted to higher pressures. However, induced hypotension is not contraindicated in these patients. Rather the lowest "safe" CPP is higher than the 50 mmHg (lower limit of cerebral autoregulation) for normotensive patients. Most believe that a 30% decrease in MAP from preoperative values is safe in these patients. In patients with well-controlled hypertension, the cerebral autoregulatory curve should have returned to normal values.

Complications. Complications of induced hypotension are uncommon. Table 8.8 lists reported complications and incidence when available. Complications of induced hypotension relate primarily to end-organ hypoperfusion. To minimize risks of induced hypotension, careful monitoring of adequacy of perfusion to end organs (ECG, evoked potentials, urine output), avoidance of concomitant hypovolemia or anemia further compromising oxygen delivery, and assurance of adequate ventilation and oxygenation are critical.

Agents. Any of the agents listed in Table 8.7 can be used for induced hypotension. The agents currently most commonly utilized during neurovascular procedures include nitroprusside, esmolol, and isoflurane. Isoflurane- and nitroprusside-induced hypotension to a CPP of 50 mmHg have all been shown to be associated with preservation of normal cerebral energy states (absence of cerebral ischemia).[126,127] Tri-

TABLE 8.8 *Complications of induced hypotension*

COMPLICATION	INCIDENCE (%)	COMMENT
Cerebral thrombosis or ischemia	0.1–0.2	May be higher in patients at risk for vasospasm
Coronary artery thrombosis	0.3–0.7	
Renal insufficiency	0–0.2	Decreased RBF, GFR, urine output common intraoperatively
Hepatic failure	Not reported	
Postop pulmonary dysfunction	Rare	Increased V/Q mismatching intraoperatively
Rebound hypertension		Common after SNP
Increased bleeding at operative site	0.9	Likely due to inadequate hemostasis (small vessels missed during hypotension)

Abbreviations: RBF, renal blood flow; GFR, glomerular filtration rate; SNP, sodium nitroprusside.

methaphan-induced hypotension resulted in metabolic evidence of cerebral ischemia at higher pressures than nitroprusside or isoflurane in animal models.[126,127] There is no single best agent for inducing hypotension during neurovascular procedures, and the agent can be chosen based on specific indications in certain patients (i.e., nitroglycerin in patients with coronary artery disease) or based on the anesthesiologist's experience with particular drugs.

INTENTIONAL HYPOTHERMIA

Rationale. Hypothermia has accepted cerebral protective effects. The clinical situation in which this protective effect is well recognized, and most commonly utilized is profound hypothermia and circulatory arrest for repair of complex congenital cardiac anomalies and proximal aortic aneurysms. In these patients, absence of systemic perfusion is tolerated for periods up to (and on occasion exceeding) 1 hour without evidence of neurologic injury. Profound hypothermia is utilized in these cases with temperatures in the range of 15° to 18°C.

The protective effects of hypothermia have been attributed to decreases in cerebral metabolic rate, at least in part. For many years it has been believed that the degree of cerebral protection hypothermia can provide is in proportion to the decreases in cerebral metabolic rate. This is based on the assumption that the primary mechanism for cerebral protection from hypothermia is temperature-dependent decreases in cerebral metabolic activity. In recent years multiple animal studies have demonstrated that the degree of cerebral protection afforded by mild degrees of hypothermia far exceeds the decrease in metabolic rate.[128] Thus some additional mechanism must account in part for the cerebral protection from hypothermia in addition to protection related to decreased metabolic demand.

History. In the earlier decades of aneurysm surgery, intentional hypothermia was a relatively commonly utilized technique. Most often moderate hypothermia (28° to 30°C) was utilized via active surface cooling. In addition profound hypothermia (12° to 18°C) via cardiopulmonary bypass was also utilized. However, as surgical skill improved with experience, and with routine use of the operating microscope, neurologic morbidity from intraoperative cerebral ischemia began to decrease. Significant morbidity was attributed to both moderate and profound hypothermia. Because the risks of intentional moderate or profound hypothermia began to exceed the improvement in neurologic outcome attributed to temperature-related cerebral protection, the routine use of these techniques was abandoned.[129]

Current Use. Because mild decreases in temperature (to 34° to 35°C) have demonstrated cerebral protective effects in multiple animal models, interest in intentional mild intraoperative hypothermia during neurovascular procedures has increased in recent years. Anesthesiologists have had experience managing this level of hypothermia because this level of hypothermia often occurs unintentionally in the operative period. Unintentional hypothermia is associated with known risks, including cardiac dysrhythmias and shivering, resulting in profound increases in oxygen consumption, placing patients with limited cardiac reserve at risk for perioperative cardiac morbidity. However, if body temperature remains only mildly hypothermic (above 32° to 34°C) and the patient is rewarmed prior to emergence from anesthesia, this level of hypothermia is believed to be associated with little to no morbidity and mortality. Because of these observations, intentional mild hypothermia during neurovascular procedures is practiced by many neuroanesthesiologists and neurosurgeons during procedures believed to be associated with a risk of intraoperative temporary cerebral ischemia.[130,131]

As yet there are no clinical trials proving the efficacy of intentional mild hypothermia for cerebral protection during intracranial neurovascular procedures. Likewise the optimal decrease in temperature has not been identified, nor has the ideal site for measuring temperature been determined. It appears that traditional sites for measurement of core temperature, nasopharyngeal and tympanic membranes, may overestimate brain temperature once the cranium is opened and exposed to the cooler ambient temperature of the operating theater.[132] Nonetheless the practice of intentional hypothermia prior to aneurysm clipping is gaining in popularity.

Most practice this by initiation of either active or passive cooling following induction of anesthesia. Reduction in core temperature to 33° to 35°C can often be achieved by simply uncovering the anesthetized patient during the period of surgical preparation. Additional use of cooling blankets, either with circulating water or convection blankets, will further decrease temperature if the desired degree of hypothermia is not achieved prior to completion of surgical preparation and draping. In addition fluids and gases are not warmed. Once the aneurysm is clipped and closure is begun, active warming is then initiated.

Using these practices, there are reported series in neurosurgical patients in which intentional hypothermia was utilized without complications.[130,131] These studies did not address the efficacy of the practice in improving neurologic outcome.

CARDIOPULMONARY BYPASS AND DEEP HYPOTHERMIC ARREST

Indications. The use of cardiopulmonary bypass with deep hypothermic circulatory arrest is currently reserved for the most difficult aneurysms. In general these are giant and/or complex aneurysms often of the posterior circulation. Aneurysms in which the neck is broad cannot be readily accessed or in which proximal and distal control of the parent vessels is difficult are considered for this technique. In some complex and/or large aneurysms, it may not be possible to clip the neck of the aneurysm without first opening the aneurysmal sac. This often can be achieved safely without excessive bleeding using temporary clips and barbiturate cerebral protection. However, in rare circumstances, it may not be possible to gain adequate access to the parent arteries to utilize temporary clips, or the number of vessels and the anticipated duration of temporary clipping may make traditional temporary clipping and protection likely to be inadequate. It is in these circumstances that cardiopulmonary bypass and profound hypothermia may offer an advantage.[133–135] Cardiopulmonary bypass with profound hypothermia provides cerebral protection, increasing the brain's tolerance to cerebral ischemia. In the presence of profound hypothermia, temporary clips can be utilized for time periods that might not be considered safe in the normothermic or mildly hypothermic patient. Very low bypass flows can also be utilized in the absence of temporary clips or prior to clip application to facilitate the final stages of dissection by decreasing the pressure and flow within the aneurysm and surrounding vessels. Complete circulatory arrest provides a bloodless field for permanent clipping, allowing the aneurysm to be slack. Also, during circulatory arrest the aneurysm can be opened to evacuate thrombus and identify any arterial branches arising from the aneurysm. This allows for accurate clip application in these difficult aneurysms, so that the entire aneurysm is obliterated and no critical cerebral vessels are compromised by the clips.

Techniques. Table 8.9 summarizes perioperative management. Preoperatively, patients are identified in whom the cardiopulmonary bypass to facilitate aneurysm clipping is likely to be necessary. The patient is positioned and prepared so that access to the chest and groins is possible. After initial dissection is completed, the neurosurgeon inspects the aneurysm and surrounding vessels to determine if cardiopulmonary bypass is necessary. Often, available information preoperatively suggests that cardiopulmonary bypass may be necessary. However, once the aneurysm is exposed, it is determined that the aneurysm can be clipped successfully without bypass.

Cardiopulmonary bypass may be initiated either by cannulating the femoral artery and vein (fem-fem bypass) or by cannulating the right atrium and proximal aorta (open chest bypass). The potential advantages of fem-fem bypass compared to open chest bypass are listed in

TABLE 8.9 *Management of hypothermic cardiopulmonary bypass and circulatory arrest*

TIME	ISSUES
Preoperative	Cerebrovascular anatomy Echo to rule out AI if fem-fem bypass is planned
Induction	Position patient for access to head, groin chest Position TEE to monitor LV PA catheter, pacing wires EEG and SSEP
Exposure	Neurosurgeon decides if CPB needed Initiate barbiturate infusion
Prior to CBP	Cannula placement, venous return to RA or IVC Administer heparin, check ACT Withdraw pacing wires
Initiation of bypass and cooling	Consider esmolol Monitor LV for distension Consider KCl if persistent VF Monitor EEG for burst suppression Monitor SSEP for evidence ischemia Monitor core or brain temperature
Circulatory arrest and/or trickle flow	Monitor time Maintain barbiturate infusion Monitor temperature for warming
Rewarming	Discontinue barbiturates Surgeon checks clip placement Defibrillate if necessary
Separation from CBP	Pace if necessary Monitor TEE, filling pressures to optimize cardiac performance, vasoactive drugs as necessary
Postbypass	Continue to monitor myocardial function Reverse heparin, check reversal Neurosurgeon obtains careful hemostasis Evaluate coagulation status Monitor EEG for return of activity and symmetry Monitor SSEP
Postoperative	Emergence likely delayed if used barbiturate High index suspicion for intracerebral bleed Monitor temperature, coagulation

Abbreviations: AI, aortic insufficiency; TEE, transesophageal echocardiography; LV, left ventricle; PA, pulmonary artery; EEG, electroencephalogram; SSEP, somatosensory-evoked potentials; CPB, cardiopulmonary bypass; RA, right atrium; IVC, inferior vena cava; ACT, activated clotting time; VF, ventricular fibrillation.

Table 8.10.[129,133] No studies in the neurosurgical population have been carried out comparing open chest to fem-fem bypass. Some believe in patients undergoing cardiac surgery use of fem-fem bypass is associated with increased postoperative neurologic complications. However, this is likely related to the patient population requiring fem-fem bypass for cardiac surgical procedures. Fem-fem bypass is utilized more commonly than open chest bypass for neurosurgical procedures.

Cardiopulmonary bypass requires full heparinization. It usually is initiated following craniotomy and initial dissection in preparation for aneurysm clipping. This minimizes the portion of the intracranial dissection that is carried out after heparinization. Fem-fem bypass may utilize one or both femoral veins for venous return. If possible, the venous cannula is placed into the right atrium to optimize venous return and maximize flow. The patient is then cooled to 10 to 20°C.[133–135] The rate of cooling is dependent on total bypass flow and is often slower during fem-fem bypass than open chest bypass. As the body cools, dysrhythmias predictably occur. Initially bradycardia develops. This is followed by ventricular fibrillation at 23 to 30°C, then asystole. Once the desired temperature is reached, the bypass flows may be decreased to very low flows (trickle flows 10 ml/kg/min) or the patient exsanguinated and circulatory arrest initiated. Very low flows have been advocated by many who state very low flow improves operating conditions dramatically and can be tolerated for much longer periods (several hours) than complete circulatory arrest without permanent neurologic injury. The maximal duration of tolerable circulatory arrest during profound hypothermia is not defined. It is shorter in adults than children and would be expected to be shorter in patients at risk for ischemic cerebrovascular disease. Most authors suggest 60 minutes as a maximum circulatory arrest time. Following successful aneurysm clipping, circulation is restored and rewarming begun. At 25 to 30°C sinus bradycardia or ventricular dysrhythmias usually develop.[133–135] During the rewarming period, the neurosurgeon inspects the aneurysm and surrounding vessels for bleeding and optimal clip placement. If this is satisfactory, cardiopulmonary bypass is terminated once the patient is normothermic and in sinus rhythm. Heparinization is reversed before closure of the craniotomy is begun. This allows the neurosurgeon to ensure that adequate hemostasis has been obtained. Following termination of bypass, optimal hemostasis is critical in avoiding postoperative complications that once plagued this technique.[129] This is achieved by meticulous surgical techniques as well as close monitoring of the coagulation sta-

TABLE 8.10 *Advantages and disadvantages of cardiopulmonary bypass techniques*

ADVANTAGES	DISADVANTAGES
Fem-fem Bypass	
Eliminates need for sternotomy	Lower maximal flow
Less invasive	Increased risk of cannula problems
Lower blood loss	Slower cooling and warming
	Inability to decompress heart
Open Chest Bypass	
Higher maximal flows	Increased postop pulmonary complications
More traditional	More invasive
Access to heart if problems arise	Higher operative blood loss

tus and administration of proper drugs (protamine in correct dose) and blood products (most commonly platelets).[133–135]

Special Concerns. There are a number of special concerns during cardiopulmonary bypass and hypothermic circulatory arrest, including bleeding diathesis with risk of excessive blood loss intraoperatively or postoperative intracerebral hemorrhage with devastating results. In addition, the impact of nonpulsatile flow and cooling on the cerebral blood supply, especially in patients with recent SAH, is not clearly defined. Other problems unique to fem-fem bypass must be considered. These include ventricular distension and the development of ventricular dysrhythmias.

There are multiple factors contributing to the coagulopathy that routinely is present after cardiopulmonary bypass, including decreased platelet count, platelet dysfunction, increased fibrinolytic activity, increased antithrombin activity, decreased coagulation factor levels or increased factor consumption, and inadequate heparin reversal. Although some surgeons utilize routine administration of multiple blood products and drugs to potentiate coagulation,[133] a more conservative approach would be to optimally reverse the heparin effects, monitor coagulation, and consider early administration of platelets.[133] Some centers routinely harvest 2 to 3 units of whole blood prior to initiation of bypass that are then reinfused following termination of bypass. This is an attempt to conserve the patients platelets and coagulation factors for use postbypass.

Little is known about the impact of cardiopulmonary bypass on the cerebral blood supply in patients with abnormal cerebral vasculature. This would likely be a greater concern in those patients with prior evidence of cerebrovascular ischemic disease or those suffering a recent SAH and are at risk for cerebral vasospasm. In the series reported in the literature, a majority of the patients suffering neurologic injury following these procedures were those operated upon after SAH.[134] When possible, some form of intraoperative monitoring of adequacy of cerebral perfusion would indicate if cerebral ischemia develops intraoperatively prior to the period of profound hypothermia. In our institution, we monitor these patients with SSEP for anterior circulation aneurysms. Most centers utilizing cardiopulmonary bypass to facilitate aneurysm clipping also utilize thiopental infusion to increase cerebral protection throughout the operative period. Barbiturate infusion is initiated sometime prior to cooling and titrated to maintain burst suppression by electro encephogram (EEG) monitoring. Barbiturate infusion is generally terminated following successful clipping of the aneurysm.[133–135] The efficacy of this approach is unproven. Administration of barbiturates during the period from prior to cooling to postrepair of aneurysm usually results in administration or relatively large total doses of thiopental. This most often results in a delayed emergence from anesthesia until the first or second postoperative day.

The optimal temperature for cooling is not known. Series generally report cooling to 10 to 15°C in order to ensure cerebral isoelectricity.[133–135] This is considered the endpoint for maximal cerebral protection. Likewise the ideal site for temperature measurement is not clear. Of the standard measurement sites of core temperature—esophageal, nasopharyngeal, tympanic membrane, rectal, and bladder—all have been shown to either not accurately reflect brain temperature or not reliably correlate with EEG activity during the periods of rapid temperature change during cooling.[132,133]

When fem-fem bypass is utilized, problems may arise related to the lack of direct access to the heart. These include risk for left ventricular distension. This may occur as a result of blood returning to the left atrium via the pulmonary veins (via the bronchial and pulmonary arteries). If excessive distension develops, increases in left ventricular, left atrial, and pulmonary vascular pressures may result leading to damage of these tissues. The risk for left ventricular distension during fem-fem bypass is increased in the presence of aortic insufficiency, sequestered pulmonary lobe, large bronchial arteries, and increased thebesian blood flow.[133] Transesophageal echocardiography (TEE) intraoperatively can monitor for development of left ventricular distension, which is most likely to occur during low-flow periods. If it develops, the chest can be opened and a vent placed in the left ventricle. Also the TEE may be useful during termination of cardiopulmonary bypass and in the postbypass period to access the ventricular function and cardiac volumes to optimize the patient's hemodynamic status.

An additional concern during fem-fem bypass is that as the myocardium is cooled, ventricular fibrillation will develop at some point and persist until cardiac standstill occurs at lower temperatures. During the period of ventricular fibrillation, the myocardium may be at increased risk for ischemic injury. Infusion of esmolol as cooling is begun may lower the fibrillatory threshold, the temperature at which fibrillation begins. If fibrillation develops and is persistent, some anesthesiologist recommend administering small doses of KCl (10 to 20 meq) via a central venous line to induce cardiac standstill.[133] During open chest bypass, cardioplegia may be administered to arrest the heart, or cold irrigant solution may be place around the heart to speed its cooling, thereby providing some degree of myocardial protection. During rewarming, ventricular fibrillation could again develop. External defibrillation must be available. In our institution, we also routinely utilize a pulmonary artery catheter with a port available for placing ventricular pacing wires. These wires are placed and tested prior to the initiation of bypass. Prior to bypass and circulatory arrest, the wires are withdrawn (after the position for maximal capture is noted) to prevent wire perforation of the right ventricle on bypass. At the time of weaning from cardiopulmonary bypass or in the postbypass period, the wires can be advanced and pacing initiated should bradydysrhythmias develop.

Complications.. Intracerebral hemorrhage is the most likely complication following cardiopulmonary bypass and hypothermia. In recent series it is rare following aneurysm clipping but common after use of cardiopulmonary bypass and hypothermic arrest for resection of AVMs. As a result, this technique is rarely if ever used for AVM resection. Cardiopulmonary bypass itself is not without risk of complication. These risks include myocardial injury due to incomplete myocardial protection during cooling and circulatory arrest, vessel injury at cannulation sites, and failure to wean from bypass. Although significant morbidity from cardiopulmonary bypass alone is an uncommon event, it must be considered. Finally because these patients have high-risk aneurysms, they have a higher incidence of neurologic complications postoperatively than patients with an aneurysm that can be approached using traditional techniques. This is a result of their presenting condition, not a complication of the technique itself.

Contraindications. Patients with cardiovascular disease would be expected to be at higher risk for this technique. Patients with preoperative cerebral ischemic deficits or cerebral vasospasm would be at greater risk for developing cerebral infarctions during circulatory arrest than those patients without preoperative compromise of cerebral blood supply. Use of fem-fem bypass is contraindicated in patients with aortic insufficiency, presence of patent ductus arteriosus, aortic coarctation, or aortic aneurysm because this form of bypass has a high complication rate in the presence of these conditions.[133] Most recommend routine preoperative ECHO to rule out these conditions prior to fem-fem bypass. If present, consideration must be given to open chest bypass.

Outcome. There are no controlled trials comparing outcome following clipping of these complex aneurysm with and without the use of cardiopulmonary bypass and deep hypothermic arrest. This technique is generally reserved for those cases in which the experienced neurovascular surgeon believes the likelihood of neurologic injury is high using traditional techniques. In the reported series of such patients operated on using bypass and hypothermic arrest, the results are encouraging.

Anesthetic Management of the Aneurysm Patient

PREOPERATIVE MANAGEMENT

Preoperative Evaluation. Preoperative evaluation of the patient scheduled for intracranial aneurysm repair should begin with assessment of the neurologic disorder and associated problems. The manner of presentation influences likely perioperative events. Patients presenting following SAH will have a different set of problems than those presenting with unruptured aneurysms. Following SAH, patients are at risk for development of cerebral vasospasm or rebleeding, the relative risk depending on the timing since initial hemorrhage and other prognostic findings as discussed earlier in this chapter. In addition they are at risk for the cardiac, pulmonary, and metabolic disturbances known to be associated with SAH, including ECG abnormalities with or without myocardial dysfunction, NPE, aspiration pneumonia, CSW, and DI. Although none of these complications are contraindications to surgery, their presence may further complicate intraoperative management. Patients presenting with neurologic symptoms related to local pressure effects of the aneurysm on surrounding brain tissue usually have giant aneurysms. These aneurysms often are technically more difficult for the surgeon to repair. As a result the neurosurgeon may be contemplating use of adjunct techniques, such as temporary clips and barbiturate coma or a cardiopulmonary bypass and hypothermic circulatory arrest. In patients in whom these techniques are considered, the patient's cardiopulmonary status should be evaluated preoperatively. The presence of significant cardiopulmonary disease may influence the choice of adjunct techniques. Preoperative preparation to improve cardiopulmonary status or changes in intraoperative management may be indicated in patients in whom these techniques are needed.

The preoperative neurologic exam should be noted. It is unlikely that the patient's neurologic status will improve in the immediate postoperative period. Thus the patient who is very lethargic preoperatively is not likely to be a candidate for immediate postoperative extubation. The presence of a new focal neurologic deficit on emergence is of critical importance to note. It may indicate improper clip placement, hematoma formation, or the development of vasospasm, all of which require prompt treatment if neurologic improvement is to be obtained. In order to accurately diagnose a new deficit, a thorough knowledge of the patient's preoperative neurologic status is needed.

Intracranial aneurysms most commonly present in the 5th to the 7th decades.[3,136] The anesthesiologist should anticipate the presence of disease processes common in this age range (e.g., hypertension, obesity, diabetes mellitus, atherosclerosis, and chronic pulmonary disease). The preoperative history, physical exam, and laboratory investigations should be reviewed for these illnesses.

Neurodiagnostic studies should be reviewed. The location and size of the aneurysm will be indicated on MRI and angiography. This information will determine the operative approach and need for adjunct techniques. Multiple aneurysms are present in up to 20 percent of patients.[3,137] Multiple aneurysms may be clipped at the initial operation depending on their location and operating conditions. Otherwise, the aneurysm responsible for the SAH or those considered at greatest risk for rupture will be clipped first. The presence of an unclipped aneurysm has important anesthetic implication, especially in hemodynamic management on emergence and postoperatively. The presence of vasospasm on preoperative angiography influences intraoperative fluid and hemodynamic management. Likewise the amount of and location of blood on the preoperative CT or MRI scan indicate risk for development of cerebral vasospasm. Patients with cerebral vasospasm preoperatively or at high risk for development for cerebral vasospasm may require more aggressive monitoring in order to optimize fluid and hemodynamic status either intraoperatively or postoperatively.

Preoperative electrolyte abnormalities may be present and should be corrected or at least improved preoperatively. Elevated blood glucose may be associated with worsened neurologic deficit after temporary focal cerebral ischemia,[138] and most neuroanesthesiologists would recommend correcting significant hyperglycemia preoperatively.

Most patients following aneurysmal SAH will be on nimodipine or some other calcium channel blocker for prevention of delayed ischemic neurologic deficits related to vasospasm. The use of these drugs is not associated with increased risk for intraoperative hemodynamic instability.[139] Other modalities for treatment of vasospasm may be used. Their likely impact on anesthetic management should be considered.

Premedication. Routine use of sedative premedication is not indicated in any neurosurgical patient. In patients with an altered level of consciousness, even small doses of sedative medication could result in obtundation. In addition, in patients with intracranial mass lesions, medications causing only initial mild sedation may also lead to mild hypoventilation. In the presence of limited intracranial elastance, mild increases in $PaCO_2$ can lead to significant increases in ICP with progressive decreasing level of consciousness and further hypoventilation and increasing $PaCO_2$ and ICP.

In some patients with intracranial aneurysms, preoperative level of consciousness may be normal and there may be no mass lesion. In these patients, the risk of omitting sedation may be greater. Excessive anxiety and sympathetic activation may lead to preoperative hypertension that in itself may be quite dangerous in the presence of a vascular lesion in a given patient. Clearly a thorough preoperative evaluation and visit with the patient are indicated along with appropriate choice of sedative agents and doses for the individual patient.

INDUCTION The choice of agents for induction of anesthesia should be guided by knowledge of the effects of each agent on cerebral and cardiovascular dynamics. An induction strategy should be designed to avoid excessive increases in transmural pressure and significant increases or decreases in ICP pressure or profound hypotension. The relative importance of each of these concerns varies.

The primary concern is avoidance of increases in transmural pressure, which could increase the risk for rupture of the aneurysm. Rupture of the aneurysm at the time of induction of anesthesia is associated with an extremely poor prognosis (50 to 100 percent mortality).[137,140] For this reason great care is taken to avoid increases in systemic blood pressure and decreases in ICP (transmural pressure = arterial pressure − ICP). Most of our induction agents cause decreases in CBF and ICP. However, their use is not associated with frequent aneurysm rupture. It is critical to plan the induction so that the decrease in ICP accompanying induction does not occur in concert with an increase in systemic blood pressure. Thiopental, the most commonly used induction agent in neuroanesthesia, causes a profound decrease in CBF and ICP as well as a decrease in systemic blood pressure. However, it often does not provide adequate control of the hemodynamic response to laryngoscopy and intubation. This is particularly true if a single induction dose of thiopental is combined with a nondepolarizing muscle relaxant for intubation. When thiopental or any induction agent is used, it is critical to not only ensure an adequate level of anesthesia prior to laryngoscopy, but also to ensure adequate blunting of the hemodynamic response.

Unless the aneurysm is associated with a hematoma or obstructive hydrocephalus, the ICP is usually not elevated. In most situations, then, it is simply necessary to avoid only maneuvers or drugs known to cause significant increases in intracranial volume, such as hypercarbia or hypoxia. Likewise, hyperventilation during induction should also be avoided, unless signs of elevated ICP are present. In those patients with hydrocephalus or hematoma, maneuvers to lower ICP should be instituted. However, the impact of excessive lowering of ICP on the transmural pressure gradient should be kept in mind.

Although in most patients with intracranial aneurysms, hypertension is much more feared than hypotension, in those patients with vasospasm present preoperatively, hypotension can result in cerebral ischemia and lead to equally devastating complications. It is not possible to know for certain which patients have developed vasospasm prior to the development of symptoms. A reasonable approach would be to avoid excessive decreases in MAP to below autoregulatory range in all patients and in those with known vasospasm to attempt to maintain the patient's blood pressure to within the range associated with an absence of ischemic symptoms preoperatively.

Monitoring. Determination of appropriate perioperative monitoring is based on the patient's condition, planned operative procedure, and likely immediate postoperative management. For example, in a patient with mild myocardial dysfunction and a straightforward aneurysm clipping without use of any adjunct techniques planned, the anesthesiologist might consider placing a monitor of central venous pressure but elect against it. However, if the same patient is considered to be at relatively high risk for cerebral vasospasm in the postoperative period, the decision might be made to place a central venous or pulmonary artery line. It might now provide some useful information intraoperatively as well as be of benefit postoperatively to manage hypervolemic hemodilution for the treatment of vasospasm.

Routine monitors during general anesthesia may be expected to reveal abnormalities in a significant percentage of aneurysm patients. Following SAH, ECG abnormalities are common. Hypoxemia may also develop related to aspiration pneumonia in patients that suffered a loss of consciousness or due to NPE. Monitoring of end-tidal caroon aioxide is also critical, as alterations of desired CO_2 levels occur throughout the operative course. Since mild deliberate hypothermia is becoming a common practice, at least one reliable site for temperature monitoring is crucial. Monitoring of urine output is important to access adequacy of diuresis following administration of mannitol or other diuretics to decrease brain bulk and improve surgical exposure. In addition, unexpected high urine output may signal development of DI or CSW.

In addition to the monitors considered current standard of care, patients undergoing repair of an intracranial aneurysm need a direct measure of arterial pressure. Precise control of systemic blood pressure within a relatively narrow range is necessary for optimal anesthetic and surgical management. Excessive hypertension outside the patient's normal blood pressure range must be avoided. In order to do this optimally, a direct measure of arterial pressure is required and should be placed prior to the first significant stress to the patient. The arterial line may be placed awake if adequate local anesthetic infiltration is utilized. Alternatively it may be placed following induction of anesthesia if several conditions are met:

1. Hemodynamic stability following induction of anesthesia must be likely.
2. The arterial line should be placed prior to laryngoscopy. It is imperative that the stress response to laryngoscopy be adequately blocked and monitored.
3. Adequate personnel must be available so that expert management of the airway and monitoring of the patient are possible during placement of any additional monitors.

Use of central venous or pulmonary artery pressure monitoring is not universally indicated based on the procedure alone. In our institution, one of the neuroanesthesiologists places a central venous catheter for whom in all patients use of vasoactive drugs is anticipated, whereas others utilize central lines less frequently. Factors to consider include cardiovascular status as with other preexisting conditions, likelihood of cerebral vasospasm and need for hypervolemic therapy, and anticipated use of adjunct techniques. In most instances, fluid shifts and blood loss during aneurysm repair are minor and in and of themselves do not necessitate placement of a central venous line.

Agents. In general, an anesthetic technique should be planned to allow for prompt emergence and neurologic assessment after completion of the operative procedure. Induction agents should be chosen with this in mind. Thiopental is the most commonly used agent. Additional drugs may be necessary to provide adequate blunting of the hemodynamic response to the stress of laryngoscopy. Propofol can also be utilized for induction, but given the duration of the procedure, there is little advantage to its shorter duration of action for either induction or maintenance. Narcotics may also be utilized as the primary agent or to supplement induction with other agents.

The choice of muscle relaxant for induction or maintenance is less critical than using the drug so that the patient is adequately prepared prior to laryngoscopy. This requires timing the onset of action of the muscle relaxant, administration of agents to blunt the stress response, and the stimulus itself optimally so that coughing, straining, and hypertension do not occur.

Stress Response. Hypertension associated with laryngoscopy or head pinning that follows shortly can be disastrous. These stress responses can be blunted by additional doses of the induction agent, narcotics, lidocaine, sympathetic blockers, such as esmolol, or vasodilators, most commonly, sodium nitroprusside. In most institutions, narcotic doses adequate to blunt the hemodynamic response completely to these intense stimuli are not often used in neurosurgical procedures. This is primarily due to the fact that these higher-dose narcotic techniques may not allow for the early emergence and neurologic assessment that is so often the goal in neuroanesthesiology. Drugs such as esmolol and nitroprusside are ideal for this scenario. They are titratable and have rapid onset and offset of action. Thus the pharmacokinetics of these agents are ideally matched to the time course of the intense and brief stimuli occurring at the beginning of these procedures. Laryngoscopy and head pinning are likely the greatest stimuli during the procedure. They are transient and followed by the long surgical preparation in which little stimulation occurs. If longer-acting agents are utilized to blunt the hemodynamic response during these events, problems with hypotension would likely soon develop.

MAINTENANCE The primary goals of intraoperative anesthetic management during aneurysm repair are (1) to maintain hemodynamic stability and very strict control of hemodynamic parameters, (2) optimize cerebral perfusion, (3) facilitate surgical exposure and safe aneurysm clipping, and (4) maximize tolerance for temporary cerebral ischemia should it develop. There are no perfect agents or techniques to accomplish these goals.

Agents. Successful anesthetic management has been described using the volatile anesthetic agents, narcotics, barbiturates, etomidate, propofol, and nitrous oxide. There is no clear agent of choice for these patients (Table 8.11). There are no outcome studies supporting the use of any anesthetic agent for aneurysm surgery. In a different patient population (patients with an intracranial mass), no outcome difference was found utilizing different anesthetic techniques (volatile, narcotic based, propofol).[141]

The techniques utilized most commonly are probably isoflurane as the primary agent, supplemented with narcotics, and narcotic-based techniques supplemented with low-dose isoflurane with or without nitrous oxide. There are a number of potential problems with these techniques. Both isoflurane and nitrous oxide use can lead to increased CBF and ICP should intracranial elastance be increased. In addition, both these agents depress (SSEPs) that may be utilized during aneurysm clipping. None of these agents have proven cerebral protective effects. In fact, some animal studies suggest that the use of nitrous oxide might increase the risk for cerebral infarction in the presence of temporary focal cerebral ischemia.[142] Because of this concern and the absence of any clear advantage to the use of nitrous oxide, some neuroanesthesiologists avoid its use during aneurysm surgery. Should temporary clips be utilized in-

TABLE 8.11 *Available anesthetic agents for intracranial aneurysm procedures*

AGENT	ADVANTAGES	DISADVANTAGES
Isoflurane	Least ↑ CBF, ↓ CVR of volatile agents Allows prompt emergence May be hypotensive agent Vast clinical experience	No proven cerebral protection ↑ CBF, ↓ CVR
Enflurane	Allows prompt emergence	↑ CBF, ↓ CVR Seizures No cerebral protection
Halothane	Allows prompt emergence	Greatest ↑ CBF, ↓ CVR No cerebral protection
Desflurane	Most rapid emergence	Greater ↑ CBF, ↓ CVR than isoflurane
Nitrous oxide	Allows prompt emergence	↑ CBF, ↓ CVR May worsen ischemic injury
Thiopental	Proven cerebral protection ↓ CBF, ↑ CVR, ↓ CMR	Delayed emergence if used for maintenance
Etomidate	↓ CBF, ↑ CVR, ↓ CMR	Delayed emergence if used for maintenance No clearly proven cerebral protection
Propofol	↓ CBF, ↑ CVR, ↓ CMR	No proven cerebral protection
Sufentanil	Hemodynamic stability Allows prompt emergence	No cerebral protection Controversy around CBF, CVR effects
Fentanyl	Hemodynamic stability Allows prompt emergence	No cerebral protection Controversy around CBF, CVR effects
Alfentanil	Hemodynamic stability Allows prompt emergence	No cerebral protection Controversy around CBF, CVR effects

Abbreviations: CBF, cerebral blood flow; CVR, cerebrovascular resistance; CMR, cerebral metabolism.

traoperatively (potentially creating temporary focal cerebral ischemia), an agent with proven protective effects should be added. To date the only anesthetic agent with proven cerebral protective effects in both animal models and patients is thiopental.[119] Use of thiopental infusion as the primary anesthetic agent would offer the potential for cerebral protection but does result in delayed emergence in most cases.[143]

The choice of muscle relaxant is not influenced by the procedure itself, except for the likely extended duration. Although muscle relaxation is not needed for the procedure itself, absence of muscle relaxation can result in two potential complications. Increased thoracic and abdominal muscle tone may lead to increased central venous pressure and ICP elevations in patients with intracranial elastance abnormalities. If at some point in the procedure it becomes necessary to lighten the anesthetic depth, the patient is at risk for coughing or moving. Coughing or bucking can lead to sudden and dramatic increases in ICP and worsening of surgical exposure. Moving the head in pin fixation can result in injury to the patient.

Fluids. In the past, hypovolemia was the rule for most neurosurgical patients. However, for patients undergoing aneurysm repair, normovolemia should be maintained. The risk for cerebral vasospasm and resultant neurologic deficit has been shown to be higher in the presence of hypovolemia.[144] Should induced hypotension be needed, its safety as well as ease of control is increased in normovolemic patients.

In choosing fluid to maintain normovolemia, it is the osmotic, not oncotic, pressure that is the important determinant of the impact of fluid resuscitation on ICP and cerebral edema. As a result, hypotonic fluids should be avoided and isotonic or hypertonic fluids utilized. Use of colloid solutions is of no particular benefit over crystalloids. Administration of glucose-containing solutions has been shown to worsen the neurologic deficit following temporary focal cerebral ischemia.[138,145] Perioperative fluids should be glucose free and blood glucose levels monitored. In general blood glucose levels should be maintained below 150 to 200 mg/dl. However, there is no clear outcome data in patients to support this approach.

Physiologic Parameters. In general the patient's blood pressure should be maintained within the range that is normal for the patient. Excessive decreases in blood pressure may result in cerebral ischemia should vasospasm be present. Hypertension may increase the risk for intraoperative aneurysm rupture.

Hyperventilation prior to opening the dura may lead to a decrease in ICP and increase in transmural pressure. This could in turn cause an increased risk for rupture. Normocarbia or mild hypocarbia are usually maintained prior to opening the dura. Once the dura is opened, ICP is no longer a component of the transmural pressure equation. Hyperventilation may then be initiated as directed by the need for decreasing brain bulk to facilitate surgical exposure. Routine aggressive hyperventilation is not indicated in aneurysm surgery.

TECHNIQUES TO FACILITATE SURGICAL EXPOSURE As with any other intracranial procedure, it may be necessary to implement measures to improve operative exposure. The need for these techniques will vary depending on the site and size of the aneurysm and the condition of the brain. Following SAH, some patients will have "swollen" brains in the early period following hemorrhage. The use and choice of techniques should be a joint decision between the anesthesiologist and neurosurgeon.

Should the dura be tense on removing the bone flap, the anesthesiologist should first make sure that factors leading to increased ICP are not present. These include poor positioning with obstruction of cerebral venous drainage in the neck, hypercarbia, hypoxia, high levels of volatile anesthetic especially in the absence of hyperventilation, increased muscle tone, and head-down positioning.

Sudden development of a tight brain, especially prior to exposure of the aneurysm, should alert the surgeon and anesthesiologist to the possibility of intracranial hemorrhage. If this is the case, the dissection and removal of the clot should proceed more quickly.

Hyperventilation. Hyperventilation decreases CBF by increasing cerebrovascular resistance (CVR). Maximal decreases in CBF occur at a $PaCO_2$ of 25 mmHg. Hyperventilation should not be instituted prior to opening the dura. Routine, extreme degrees of hyperventilation are not indicated. Instead, the degree of hyperventilation should be guided by the quality of the exposure and needs of the surgeon for decreasing brain bulk.

Diuretics. Both osmotic diuretics and loop diuretics are effective in lowering brain water and decreasing brain bulk. Mannitol in doses of 0.25 to 1 mg/kg is the most commonly used agent during neurosurgical procedures. The onset of mannitol effect is 15 to 30 minutes after administration.[146] Its administration should be timed so that the effect is present as the dura is opened and dissection begun. Hypovolemia and electrolyte abnormalities may develop after the use of mannitol. Usually these complications are dose dependent. However, on occasion patients administered small doses of mannitol may have a profound response. In all patients fluid status and electrolytes should be carefully monitored following mannitol administration. In patients with cardiac or renal insufficiency, use of mannitol may be associated with an increased incidence of complications, including fluid overload and congestive heart failure.

CSF Drainage. Removal of CSF either via a lumbar drain, ventriculostomy, or ventricular puncture after the dura is open is effective in decreasing intracranial content volume and facilitate surgical exposure. Excessive draining of CSF, especially prior to opening the dura, may lead to the development of subdural hematoma. If the brain becomes too slack, traction on the bridging veins may develop as the brain shrinks, leading to tearing of one of these vessels and hematoma formation.

Barbiturates. The administration of barbiturates leads to a decrease in CVR and ICP. In cases of a tight brain refractory to other maneuvers, barbiturates may be successful in decreasing brain bulk. Unless administered as an infusion, the barbiturate effect will be transient.

INTRAOPERATIVE RUPTURE

Incidence, Timing, Outcome Intraoperative rupture of intracranial aneurysms is fortunately an uncommon occurrence. The risk is felt to be related to size, location, timing since original SAH, transmural pressure gradient, and technical problems. The anesthesiologist can impact only upon the latter two factors. Anesthetic management is designed to avoid increases in transmural pressure gradient, and techniques are utilized as indicated to decrease brain bulk and thereby facilitate surgical exposure.

Should intraoperative rupture occur, its impact upon outcome is related to the timing of the rupture. Rupture of the aneurysm during induction of anesthesia and up through the early phases of the exposure is associated with a 50 to 100% mortality and 50 to 100 percent neurologic morbidity.[137,140,147] When rupture occurs prior to exposure, dramatic increases in ICP may develop, and the operative dissection and ability to carefully expose and clip the aneurysm are greatly impaired. Rupture in the later phases of dissection, after the aneurysm is exposed, carries a much lower morbidity and mortality. If rupture occurs during manipulation of the aneurysm as the dissection is nearing its completion, the operative course is much less complicated. The neurosurgeon may be able to apply temporary clips to obtain control of the bleeding and quickly complete the dissection and permanent clip application. Much of the morbidity and mortality related to intraoperative rupture has to do with vascular injury and suboptimal clip placement necessitated by the premature rupture.

Anesthetic Management. Should rupture occur during induction and up to incision, the prudent course is not clear. Both proceeding with the planned procedure and terminating the procedure to allow the situation to stabilize carry a dismal prognosis.[148]

If the operation is underway at the time of the rupture, close communication and cooperation between the anesthesiologist and neurosurgeon is the single most important factor in successful management. Should rupture occur early in the exposure, maneuvers to decrease brain bulk promptly may be needed to allow the surgeon to quickly find and evacuate the hematoma and locate and apply clips to the aneurysm or parent vessel. If rupture occurs in the later phases of dissection, the most common course is to lower systemic blood pressure, often to or occasionally below the limits of cerebral autoregulation, to decrease bleeding and facilitate location of the vessels and clip application. If temporary clips are then applied, which is the usual course, and the bleeding controlled, it may then be indicated to allow blood pressure to return to or occasionally above "normal" levels to improve collateral flow to the brain supplied by the clipped vessel. Although on occasion large volumes of blood may be lost, resulting in hemodynamic instability, the more common complication related to intraoperative rupture during the final stages of dissection is improper clip placement or cerebral ischemia related to temporary clipping.

EMERGENCE

Timing. Whenever possible, emergence and neurologic examination at the termination of the operation should be the goal of the anesthetic plan. Should the clip placement have resulted in vascular compromise and ischemia or a hematoma formed, prompt recognition and diagnosis are crucial to successful treatment and reversal of neurologic deficit. On occasion, this may not be possible due either to the patient's underlying medical condition requiring an anesthetic plan not conducive to prompt emergence, administration of large doses of barbiturates during periods of temporary clipping, or the patient's preoperative neurologic status.

Stress Response. Relatively light levels of anesthesia are necessary toward the end of the closure. This may result in hypertension and tachycardia. The stress response may be treated with vasodilators or β-blockers. This is particularly critical in patients with underlying cardiac disease or in the 20% of patients with multiple aneurysms who may have unclipped aneurysm present at the completion of the operative procedure.

ARTERIOVENOUS MALFORMATIONS

Pathophysiology and Management

CURRENT DIAGNOSIS, MANAGEMENT, AND OUTCOME AVMs are congenital lesions that consist of abnormal direct communications between small arteries and veins without intervening capillaries. The feeding arteries are abnormally dilated and may show medial hypertrophy, endothelial thickening, as well as degeneration and attenuation of the arterial wall. The nidus is composed of tortuous, thin-wall dilated vessels. Cerebral tissue within the nidus is gliotic. Draining veins are large, develop within the nidus, and follow a tortuous course to the surface of the nidus. Surrounding brain may be atrophic, presumably from chronic cerebral ischemia. Characteristics of AVMs are listed in Table 8.12.[149–155] The pathophysiology of AVMs is related to excessive blood flow through the abnormal vasculature. This may lead to intracranial hemorrhage, development of a seizure focus, or cerebral ischemia of surrounding or remote normal brain tissue. This ischemia develops as an increasing proportion of the CBF is shunted through the low-resistance AVM, resulting in inadequate blood flow to the remainder of the brain.

Historical Perspective. Although AVMs were first described in the latter half of the 19th century, it was not until the early 20th century that surgery was attempted.[150] Initial attempts at complete surgical resection were limited to relatively small lesions located in easily assessable areas remote from critical brain areas. As experience has increased, larger lesions in more remote areas have been approached surgically. In recent years, nonsurgical therapies as adjunct to surgery or in place of surgery have seen increasing use, especially in more complex lesions.

Presentation. AVMs are most commonly diagnosed during the third and forth decades of life. However, in some series, the peak incidence of diagnosis occurs prior to age 30, and in others, diagnosis occurs more frequently between age 40 and 50. In general, it is a disease of young adults. Hemorrhage and seizures are the most common presentation. Less common presentations include focal neurologic deficit, symptoms of intracerebral steal, and congestive heart failure (in neonates) (Table 8.13).[150–152,154]

At diagnosis, the AVM may be graded according to a grading system proposed by Spetzler and Martin (Table 8.14). The grading system is based on size, pattern of venous drainage, and neurological eloquence of the adjacent brain. The grading system has been demonstrated to be predictive of neurologic outcome in surgically treated lesions (Fig. 8.3).[156] Its use will be help-

TABLE 8.12 *Characteristics of AVM*

CHARACTERISTIC	INCIDENCE
Location	
Supratentorial	70–97%
Parietal	27–40%
Frontal	12–32%
Temporal	16–24%
Other	9–23%
Infratentorial	3–30%
Deep	5–18%
Size	
Small (<2–3 cm)	8–49%
Medium (2–6 cm)	40%
Large (>3–6 cm)	41–51%
Type	
Multiple unit	82%
Single unit (one artery, fistula, vein)	10%
Straight line (one artery and vein)	3%
Combined (extra and intracranial feeding arteries)	3%
Venous wall	2%
Age at presentation	Peak incidence between age 30 and 40 years
Male: female ratio	1.1:1
Feeding arteries	MCA involved in ≥50% 30–50% supplied by branches of more than one major artery (ACA, MCA, PCA)
Venous drainage	Closest venous sinus (40% superior sagittal sinus)
Intracranial aneurysm	3–10%
Location of associated aneurysm	
Major feeding artery	34%
Proximal portion system feeding AVM	25%
Remote	41%

Abbreviations: AVM, arteriovenous malformation; ACA, anterior cerebral artery; MCA, middle cerebral artery; PCA, posterior cerebral artery.

ful in comparing outcomes from various modern treatment options.

The diagnosis of AVM is confirmed by MRI, magnetic resonance angiography (MRA), and conventional cerebral angiography. MRI is superior to angiography in demonstrating the nidus and involved brain structures. However, angiography is necessary to delineate the vascular supply and conventional cerebral angiography may be superior to MRA.[157]

Natural History. Rational selection of an appropriate treatment option depends on a thorough understanding of the natural history of the disease process. Several studies have looked at long-term outcome in nonsurgically managed

TABLE 8.13 *Presenting signs of cerebral AVM*

PRESENTATION	INCIDENCE (%)
Hemorrhage	30–86
Seizure	8–46
Headache	1–34
Focal neurologic deficit	4–23
Other	6–16
Hydrocephalus	
Elevated ICP	
Bruit	
Syncope	
Confusion	
CHF	
Incidental	≤3

Abbreviations: AVM, arteriovenous malformation; ICP, intracranial pressure; CHF, congestive heart failure.

TABLE 8.14 *AVM grading system*[a]

GRADED FEATURE	POINTS ASSIGNED
Size of AVM	
Small (<3 cm)	1
Medium (3–6 cm)	2
Large (>6 cm)	3
Eloquence of adjacent brain	
Noneloquent	0
Eloquent	1
Pattern of venous drainage	
Superficial only	0
Any draining vein deep	1

[a] Grade = sum of points assigned. Grade VI is AVMs currently considered unresectable.

Abbreviation: AVM, arteriovenous malformation.

patients with intracranial AVMs. However, these data likely do not represent natural history of the disease in that patients were assigned to nonsurgical management based on some characteristic of their lesion or clinical condition.[140,152,154] The assignment to surgical and nonsurgical management has varied greatly over recent decades. In these studies, likelihood of neurologic deficit developing with the initial hemorrhage is 50 to 80 percent, with a mortality of 10 to 11 percent. The risk of rehemorrhage after initial presentation with hemorrhage is reported to be 6 to 20 percent in the first year and 2 to 4 percent per year thereafter. Mortality is noted to

FIGURE 8.3 *Operative outcome by AVM grade with the percentage of patients with each outcome (no deficit, minor deficit, major deficit, or death) with grades I to V AVMs preoperatively.*

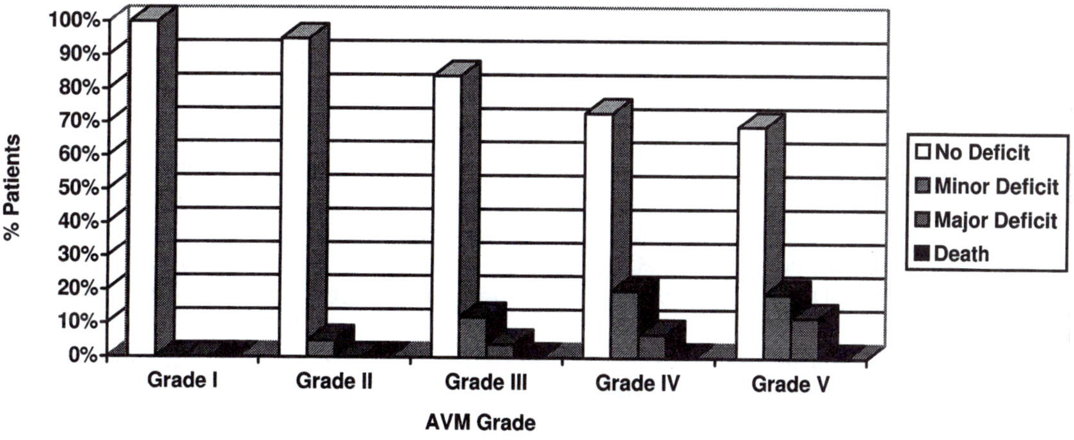

be 1 percent per year. If initial presentation is seizures, the bleeding rate is 2 to 3 percent per year. Studies do exist in which the assignment to conservative management appears to be relatively random.[151] In this patient population, the risk of hemorrhage was not related to initial presentation and was essentially constant over the first 20 years at 4 percent per year. Major morbidity occurred at a rate of 1.7 percent per year and mortality at 1 percent per year.

From these reviews, several points are fairly clear. Unlike intracranial aneurysms, the risk of subsequent hemorrhages is not dramatically higher in the very early period following initial hemorrhage. Morbidity and mortality after initial hemorrhage are high. The ultimate risk of hemorrhage subsequent to diagnosis and resultant major morbidity and mortality is also high. Given the young age at initial presentation, conservative management is likely to result in a 30 to 50 percent risk of major morbidity or mortality over the expected life span of the patient.

Considering this information, decisions regarding choice of intervention are made based on size, location of the AVM and its impact on expected operative difficulty and complications, neurologic condition of the patient, age of the patient, and general medical condition of the patient as it impacts on his or her operative risk and likely life expectancy.

Perioperative Issues

TREATMENT OPTIONS

Conservative Management. Treatment options for patients with intracranial AVMs include conservative therapy with no attempt to excise or obliterate the anomaly. As discussed, the natural history of this disease process suggests that the risk of morbidity and mortality during conservative management is significant, on the order of 2 to 3 percent per year. Medical management is considered primarily when the risk of more aggressive management is considered excessive, based either on the nature of the AVM or the patient's condition. With the introduction of intravascular obliteration techniques and radiosurgery, the indications for true conservative management for AVMs have decreased. Current options for obliteration of the AVM include surgical excision, intravascular embolization techniques, radiosurgery, or a combination of these modalities. In order to improve long-term outcome, complete resection or obliteration of the AVM is necessary. Partial resection or obliteration does not alter long-term morbidity or mortality.

Surgical Resection Standard surgical excision is the approach with the longest record of consistent use and analysis of results. It is not without risks. Operative mortality is reported between 0 and 11 percent. New neurologic deficits postoperatively occur in 5 to 15 percent of patients. Overall permanent neurologic deficits are present in 15 to 40 percent of patients treated with surgical excision of their AVM. This includes deficits present preoperatively as well as new postoperative deficits.[53,149,155,158–162] Postoperative outcome is correlated with grade of the AVM preoperatively.[156,160,163] Good outcome was obtained in 90 percent or more of patients with low-grade lesions (grades I to III), whereas major morbidity or mortality occurs in 40 to 50 percent of patients presenting with high-grade lesions.[160,163] Once total excision or obliteration of an AVM is accomplished, neurologic improvement is likely. In one series, serious neurologic deficit was found in 24 percent patients immediately postoperatively but in only 8 percent of the same patients at long-term follow-up.[160]

Newer Modalities. In recent years intravascular embolization and radiosurgery have also been used increasingly to treat AVMs. The treatment goal of intravascular embolization may be total obliteration of the lesion via embolization alone or decrease in the size and blood flow through the AVM to facilitate surgical resection or radiosurgery. Intravascular embolization is more commonly utilized as an adjunct to surgery than as a primary technique. In order to perform intravascular embolization of an AVM, it is necessary to also perform superselective angiography to identify all feeding arteries and the anatomy of adjacent normal vessels. In addition, the ability to correctly place very small catheters in the feeding arteries is critical. To access safety of embolization of a feeding vessel, provocative testing may be utilized. Once the catheter is palced in the vessel to be embolized, amobarbital is injected, and the patient is tested for development of a neurologic deficit as a result of the selective anesthesia produced by the amobarbital. As the embolization progresses, blood flow patterns may change, and retesting with amobarbital may be indicated. Use of provocative testing improves the safety of intravascular embolization techniques.

The choice of embolization agents depends on whether proximal occlusion of feeding vessels or penetration of the agent into the nidus is planned. Occlusion of proximal vessels is used primarily as a preoperative adjunct, because with time, there will be enlargement of collateral vessels and ultimate reconstitution of the nidus. The deep surgically inaccessible feeding vessels are usually chosen for embolization. For proximal occlusion, detachable balloons and platinum coils are utilized. Agents designed to penetrate into the nidus include cyanoacrylates, polyvinyl alcohol particles, ethanol, and microfibrillar collagen. These agents can be used when embolization is a preoperative adjunct or a sole therapy.[164]

Results of intravascular embolization have been reported in many relatively small series. Intravascular embolization, as a presurgical adjunct, is successful in decreasing intraoperative blood loss and making the resection technically easier. Combined surgery with preoperative embolization has been reported to result in a 70 to 90 percent complete cure rate in patients with large complex lesions. In addition, it has been successfully used to decrease risk for normal perfusion pressure breakthrough postresection by gradually decreasing blood flow to high-flow AVMs prior to complete surgical resection. Preoperative embolization may occur in one or several stages. Embolization as a sole technique has been reported to have a success rate of only 6 to 17 percent.[165] Complications from intravascular embolization include transient ischemic attacks (2 to 30 percent), with highest rates occuring with agents that penetrate into the nidus, stroke (2 to 20 percent), with the highest rates occuring with dominant hemisphere AVM embolization and when using agents penetrating into the nidus; hemorrhage (4 to 9 percent with a 30 percent mortality); gluing of the catheter to the brain with liquid adhesive agents: recanalization of occluded AVMs; and passage of embolic agents into the lung.[164]

Radiosurgery for intracraial lesions was first described in 1951. Its current use in AVM therapy is primarily in patients considered not to be surgical candidates because of the size and locaton of the lesion, condition of the patient, or patient refusal of surgery. A relatively high success rate of obliteration of the nidus and resolution of symptoms is reported in low-grade and small AVMs (50 to 75 percent). Most consider it much less efficacious in lesions over 3 cm.[165,166] Prior embolization may be utilized to decrease the size prior to radiosurgery. Obliteration of the nidus is not expected until 2 years after radiation therapy, leaving the patient at risk of hemorrhage during that period.[164]

Modern treatment of AVMs frequently involves a combination of one or more of the available options. Since the availability of intravascular embolization and radiosurgery techniques in addition to surgical excision, the managemnet outcome of AVMs has improved.[163]

NORMAL PERFUSION PRESSURE BREAKTHROUGH Normal perfusion pressure breakthrough (NPPB) is a complication that may follow surgical resection or total obliteration of an AVM via embolization. It is characterized by cerebral edema, swelling, and intracerebral hemorrhage in some patients. It occurs in 10 to 20 percent of patients following AVM obliteration.[167,168] The incidence of morbidity or mortality related to NBBP is much lower.

Etiology. The etiology of NPPB is felt to be a loss of autoregulation of CBF to CPP changes in normal brain either surrounding the AVM or remote to the AVM. This loss of autoregulation is believed to develop as a result of chronic ischemia of the normal brain. Perfusion pressure within the feeding arteries of an AVM is decreased due to the low resistance. This reduced perfusion pressure is also present in more proximal vessels of the circle of Willis. To maintain adequate CBF in the presence of lowered perfusion pressure, cerebral vasodilation occurs in the remainder of the brain, both ipsilateral and contralateral to the AVM. If the AVM is a very high-flow, low-resistance AVM, the decrease in CPP may be so great that the capacity for cerebral autoregulatory vasodilation is exhausted.[169] As a result chronic cerebral ischemia and loss of autoregulatory capacity may develop in these patients. This chronic ischemia then results in a vasomotor paralysis, so that CBF becomes pressure dependent. Once the AVM is resected and the low-resistance shunt is now absent, pressure within the cerebral arteries increases and blood flow to the remaining tissues may increase dramatically. An increase in CPP and CBF in the presence of loss of autoregulation may result in severe cerebral edema and hemorrhage.

Risk Factors. High-flow, low-resistance AVMs have the highest risk of development of NPPB. Classically these are felt to be large AVMs. These patients may also present with symptoms of focal cerebral ischemia, either cerebral dysfunction or transient ischemic attacks, and rarely complete stoke. On angiography, high flow through the AVM and delayed filling of nonfeeding arteries may be observed.[170–174]

Prevention. In recent years the incidence of NBBP has decreased. This has occurred as a result of progressive, staged embolization of feeding vessels of AVMs, especially large, high-flow AVMs. By staging the embolizations, gradual decreases in the blood flow through the anomaly, increases in resistance to AVM flow, and increases in the CPP to the surrounding cerebral tissue are seen. This allows the chronically ischemic area to adjust to smaller increases in perfusion pressure and potentially allows for a return of cerebral autoregulation.

Treatment Once NBBP develops, treatment is supportive to allow time for the cerebral vasculature to recover its autoregulatory ability. To minimize risk for intracerebral hemorrhage, blood pressure is lowered. Inadequate control of blood pressure during stimulation (emergence, transport, respiratory care) can result in life-threatening intracerebral hemorrhage. The vessels maintain reactivity to $PaCO_2$, so hyperventilation is effective in decreasing CBF and cerebral edema.[170–174] Indomethacin has been reported to be effective in some cases.[175]

Anesthetic Management

PREOPERATIVE MANAGEMENT

Timing of Surgery. Like aneurysms, once an AVM has bled, the risk of a second hemorrhage is increased. However, unlike aneurysms, the risk of rebleeding is no greater in the immediate period after the first hemorrhage.[151] As a result, urgent surgery after initial presentation of an AVM, even after hemorrhage, is rarely necessary. The exception is if the hemorrhage is causing mass effect and secondary injury. In this situation, the hematoma should be evacuated and the AVM may be resected at the same setting if it is technically possible.

Prior to surgery, the patient's neurologic condition should be optimized. If the he or she has suffered neurologic injury as a result of a hemorrhage, waiting for stabilization of neurologic condition is appropriate. In patients with large, high-flow AVMs or those with deep feeding arteries, preoperative embolization should be carried out to decrease the risk for blood loss and technical difficulties intraoperatively. These procedures usually do not require general anesthesia.

Evaluation. The patient's neurologic condition and presenting symptoms should be determined. Patients presenting with intracranial hemorrhage may have suffered a neurologic injury. Usually these patients are allowed to stabilize neurologically prior to surgery. They may have remaining fixed neurologic deficits, such as hemiplegia, that impact upon anesthetic management. Patients presenting with seizures may be on anticonvulsant medications that have drug interactions with some of the agents (i.e., nondepolarizing muscle relaxants) used intraoperatively. Symptoms of cerebral ischemia from steal phenomena should be sought. This may indicate a high-flow AVM with an increased risk of intraoperative blood loss and NPPB. Usually these patients will have received embolization preoperatively. Evidence of mass effect from large lesions should also be sought.

Diagnostic Tests. These patients will all have had preoperative angiography and MRI. From these studies size and vascularity of lesions can be determined. Lesions with deep feeding vessels may present more intraoperative difficulties with bleeding during resection. Those with surface feeding vessels or draining veins, especially with evidence of bony erosion of the skull, are of concern. During removal of the bone flap in this group of patients, pathologic vessels may be torn, and significant hemorrhage occurs before the surgeon has access to the AVM. In these cases, excellent vascular access may prove lifesaving. If the AVM is located in proximity to structures that can be monitored with intraoperative neurologic monitoring, use of monitoring modalities should be considered as well as the impact of their use on anesthetic management. The same is true for lesions with feeding arteries that also supply critical areas of the brain (i.e., middle cerebral artery feeder vessels may indicate risk of ischemia to the sensory cortex).

The anesthesiologist should also be familiar with what preoperative embolization procedures have been carried out. The degree to which the AVM has been embolized will influence the intraoperative course dramatically. The need for invasive monitoring, venous access, and use of intraoperative neurologic monitoring will depend on not only the size and location of the AVM at presentation, but also the status of the feeding vessels and draining veins after embolization is complete.

INDUCTION

Monitoring. Monitoring in patients undergoing resection of an AVM is similar to that for patients undergoing clipping of intracranial aneurysms. Because precise control of the MAP intraoperatively is necessary, arterial pressure should be monitored directly. Compared to intracranial aneurysms, risk of spontaneous hemorrhage from AVMs related to increases in systemic blood pressure is not so great. Studies have suggested that changes in blood pressure that commonly accompany induction and intubation may not be associated with risk of AVM hemorrhage. This may be due to the fact that the mean pressure within the AVM feeding arteries is often lower than systemic mean pressure.[176] Nonetheless, careful control of blood pressure is desirable. However, placement of an arterial line prior to induction and intubation, although desirable, is not so critical as it is in aneurysm patients. The ability to have continuous monitoring of systemic pressure is critical during the surgical procedure when mild induced hypotension to decrease bleeding during resection may be indicated and to aid in management should excessive bleeding occur.

The risk for large, potentially life-threatening hemorrhage is probably greater during AVM resection than during aneurysm clipping. Because of the potential for large and rapid sifts in volume status, patients with cardiac disease may benefit from monitoring of central volume status. This may be accomplished via TEE or invasive pressure monitoring of central venous pressure and/or pulmonary artery pressures. Children, especially neonates, are at risk for development of congestive heart failure from high-flow lesions and may also benefit from monitoring of cardiac filling pressures.

Depending on the location of the AVM and its feeding arteries, critical cerebral tissue may be at risk. Some of these critical areas can be evaluated via neurologic monitoring intraoperatively, for example, upper-extremity SSEPs can monitor function of the sensory cortex supplied by the middle cerebral artery if this vessel is involved in supplying the lesion. Review of the lesion, its feeding vessels, and the planned operative approach will determining the likely usefulness of intraoperative neurologic monitoring.

Agents. As with aneurysm patients, it is important to maintain stability of intracranial dynamics and systemic hemodynamics. In addition, in patients with large AVMs, intracranial elastance may be increased and the risk for elevations in ICP increased. The choice of agents for induction is less important than attention to the principles of avoiding large changes in MAP or maneuvers resulting in increases in CBF and ICP. Thiopental, etomidate, and propofol would all be appropriate agents for induction. The use of an agent such as ketamine, known to increase ICP and MAP in most patients, would rarely if ever be indicated. In most patients the choice of muscle relaxant has little impact on the neurologic status. Succinylcholine can increase ICP, less so after administration of a defasiculating dose of some nondepolarizing muscle relaxants (metocurine, curare, but not pancuronium). However, if the use of succinylcholine is indicated based on airway considerations, the risk of transient small increases in ICP is outweighed by the potential problems (aspiration, loss of the airway) that could result from avoidance of its use. The impact of induction agents on the ability to perform intraoperative neurologic monitoring should be considered. For example, large doses of benzodiazepines may impair the ability to monitor (SSEPs).

MAINTENANCE

Agents. Many anesthetic techniques, including primary volatile anesthetics, narcotic-based techniques, and balanced anesthetics, have been used with success in patients undergoing AVM resection. Sufentanil, alfentanil, and fentanyl have all been used without problems. Although some controversy remains regarding their impact on ICP, most neuroanesthesiologists feel that the agents have similar effects on intracranial dynamics and that the agents are safe for use in neurosurgical patients. Indeed, the hemodynamic stability provided by primary narcotic techniques is an advantage in this patient population. Of the volatile agents, isoflurane remains the primary agent for use in neurosurgical patients because of its limited potential to increase CBF and ICP as compared to the other available agents. Although propofol decreases ICP and CBF, which is advantageous in neurosurgical patients, the relatively long duration of these procedures make propofol a less ideal agent. If monitoring of evoked potentials is planned, levels of volatile agents and/or nitrous oxide must be limited to that which is compatible with adequate recording of evoked potentials in each patient (in general less than 1 minimum alveolar concentration).

Induced Hypotension. Induced hypotension may be useful to decrease intraoperative blood loss during the resection of the AVM. Drugs and techniques are described earlier in this chapter. If intraoperative neurologic monitoring indicates development of cerebral ischemia during vessel clipping as the AVM is resected, induced hypotension (if it is being utilized) may need to be abandoned. By allowing the blood pressure to increase, areas made ischemic by the clipping may receive increased blood flow through collateral vessels. Once the AVM is resected, but prior to closure, the surgeon may request that induced hypotension be discontinued to allow inspection of the AVM resection bed to ensure that no small vessels remain. Vessels that are not visible or bleeding during induced hypotension may begin to bleed once blood pressure returns to normal levels. Postoperative complications may be avoided if this is detected prior to closure of the dura and cranium.

Bleeding. Intraoperative hemorrhage is always a concern during repair of intracranial vascular anomalies. With aneurysm clipping, bleeding most often results in problems related to obscuring the surgeon's view of the vessels and increasing the difficulty of the procedure.

Much less often, bleeding during aneurysm clipping leads to problems related to blood loss. However, with AVMs, intraoperative bleeding leads to both increased technical difficulty for the neurosurgeon and hemodynamic compromise related to volume loss. Adequate vascular access must be obtained in these patients. Likely blood loss can be anticipated only by reviewing the angiographic and MRI data and discussion of the operative plan with the neurosurgeon. In addition to adequate venous access, appropriate amounts of blood must be available and care given in monitoring and maintaining temperature should massive blood loss occur. With increased use and success of preoperative embolization, the frequency of life-threatening hemorrhage during AVM resection has decreased. Nonetheless, the anesthesiologist must remain aware and prepared for this potential problem.

EMERGENCE Anesthetic management should be planned to allow for prompt emergence and neurologic assessment. Potential intraoperative problems, such as hemorrhage and cerebral ischemia related to clipping of feeding arteries, may lead to development of new neurologic deficits. Prompt recognition of these problems, their diagnosis, and correction are necessary if neurologic recovery is to occur. If emergence is delayed and results in delayed diagnosis of an intraoperative neurologic injury, the chance of recovery for neurologic function may be lost.

Two serious complications may develop after AVM resection: NPPB and intracranial hemorrhage into the resection bed. Each of these may be more likely to occur in the presence of uncontrolled increases in blood pressure. Very meticulous blood pressure control is indicated during completion of the procedure, emergence, and postoperatively. The appropriate desired range for blood pressure control should be determined based on the patient's preoperative blood pressure and likely risk for development of NPPB or hemorrhage. The likely risk for development of these complications depends on the size and blood flow of the AVM preoperatively and the course of the operative procedure. Discussion of management plans between the anesthesiologist and neurosurgeon caring for the patient can ensure optimal management of these patients will occur.

Bleeding into the AVM resection bed in the postoperative period can lead to serious new neurologic injury and major morbidity and mortality. The risk of this may be decreased by careful inspection of the bed after completion of the resection, intraoperative angiography after the resection to determine completeness of the resection, and careful control of blood pressure in the postoperative period. Careful and frequent neurologic exams will allow for early diagnosis and treatment should postoperative hemorrhage occur.

To achieve prompt emergence and avoid hypertension, plans must be made to manage the patient's blood pressure during emergence. These decisions must be made early in the procedure rather than as the hypertension develops. Available agents are discussed earlier in this chapter. No agent is the single best choice.

References

1. Kassell NF, Torner JC, Haley EC, Jr et al: The International Cooperative Study on the Time of Aneurysm Surgery. I. Overall management results. J Neurosurg 73:18, 1990
2. Day AL, Salcman M: Subarachnoid hemorrhage. Am Fam Practice 40:95, 1989
3. Locksley HB: Report on the Cooperative Study of Intracranial Aneurysm and Subarachnoid Hemorrhage: Section V, Part I. J Neurosurg 25:219, 1966
4. Barrow DL, Reisner A: Natural history of intracranial aneurysm and vascular malformations (Chapter 1). Clin Neurosurg 40:3, 1993
5. Crompton MR: Mechanism of growth, rupture in cerebral berry aneurysm. Br Med J [Clin Res] 1:1138, 1966
6. Freytag E: Fatal rupture of intracranial aneurysms: survey of 250 medicolegal cases. Arch Pathol 81:418, 1966
7. McCormick WF, Acosta-Rua GJ: The size of intracranial saccular aneurysm: an autopsy study. J Neurosurg 33:422, 1970

8. Wiebers DO, Whisnant JP, O'Fallen WM: The natural history of unruptured intracranial aneurysms. N Engl J Med 304:696, 1981
9. Wiebers DO, Whisnant JP, Sundt TM, Jr et al: The significance of unruptured intracranial saccular aneurysms. J Neurosurg 66:23, 1987
10. Juvela S, Matti P, Heiskanen O: Natural history of unruptured intracranial aneurysm: a long-term follow-up study. Neurosurgery 79:174, 1993
11. Pakarinen S: Incidence, aetiology, and prognosis of primary subarachnoid hemorrhage: a study based on 589 cases diagnosed in a defined urban population during a defined period. Acta Neurol Scand, suppl. 29:1, 1967
12. Weir B: Intracranial aneurysms and subarachnoid hemorrhage: an overview. p. 1308. In Wilkins RH, Rengachary SS (eds): Neurosurgery, McGraw-Hill, New York, 1991
13. Norrgard O, Angquist KA, Fodstad H et al: Intracranial aneurysms and heredity. Neurosurgery 20:236, 1987
14. Sakai N, Sakata K, Yamada H et al: Familial occurrence of intracranial aneurysms. Surg Neurol 2:2529, 1974
15. Lozano AM, Leblanc R: Familial intracranial aneurysms. J Neurosurg 66:522, 1987
16. Barno A, Freeman DW: Maternal deaths due to spontaneous subarachnoid hemorrhage. Am J Obstet Gynecol 125:384, 1976
17. Robinson JL, Hall CJ, Sedzimir CB: Subarachnoid hemorrhage in pregnancy. J Neurosurg 36:27, 1972
18. Salar G, Mingrino S: Development of intracranial saccular aneurysms: report of two cases. Neurosurgery 8:462, 1981
19. Azzam CJ: Growth of multiple peripheral high flow aneurysms of the posterior inferior cerebellar artery associate with a cerebellar arteriovenous malformation. Neurosurgery 21:934, 1987
20. Batjer HH, Suss RA, Samson D: Intracranial arteriovenous malformations associated with aneurysms. Neurosurgery 18:29, 1986
21. Sahs AL, Perret GE, Locksley HB et al (eds): Intracranial Aneurysms and Subarachnoid Hemorrhage: A Cooperative Study. JB Lippincott, Philadelphia, 1969
22. Hunt WE, Hess RM: Surgical risk as related to time of intervention in the repair of intracranial aneurysms. J Neurosurg 28:14, 1968
23. Nowak G, Schwachenwald R, Arnold H: Early management in poor grade aneurysm patients. Acta Neurol 126:33, 1994
24. Bailes JE, Spetzler RF, Hadley MN, Baldwin HZ: Management morbidity and mortality of poor-grade aneurysm patients. J Neurosurg 72:559, 1990
25. Lanzino G, Kassell NF, Germanson T et al: Plasma glucose levels and outcome after aneurysmal subarachnoid hemorrhage. J Neurosurg 79:885, 1993
26. Niskanen MM, Hernesniemi JA, Vapalaht MP, Kari A: One-year outcome in early aneurysm surgery: prediction of outcome. Acta Neurochir 123:25, 1993
27. Newell DW, Eskridge JM, Mayberg MR et al: Angioplasty for the treatment of symptomatic vasospasm following subarachnoid hemorrhage. J Neurosurg 71:654, 1989
28. Haley EC, Kassell NF, Torner JC: The International Cooperative Study on the Timing of Aneurysm Surgery: The North American experience. Stroke 23(2):205, 1992
29. Inagawa T: Effect of early operation on cerebral vasospasm. Surg Neurol 33:239, 1990
30. Fisher CM, Kistler JP, Davis JM: Relation of cerebral vasospasm to subarachnoid hemorrhage visualized by computerized tomographic scanning. Neurosurgery 6:1, 1980
31. Solomon RA, Onesti ST, Klebanoff L: Relationship between the timing of aneurysm surgery and the development of delayed cerebral ischemia. J Neurosurg 75:56, 1991
32. Inagawa T, Yamamoto M, Kamiya K: Effect of clot removal on cerebral vasospasm. J Neurosurg 72:224, 1990
33. MacDonald RL, Weir BK: Cerebral vasospasm and free radicals. Free Rad Biol Med 16:633, 1994
34. Foley PL, Takenaka K, Kassell NF, Lee KS: Cytotoxic effects of bloody cerebrospinal fluid on cerebral endothelial cells in culture. J Neurosurg 81:87, 1994
35. Otsuji T, Endo S, Hirashima Y et al: An experimental model of symptomatic vasospasm induced by oxyhemoglobin in rabbits. Stroke 25:657, 1994
36. Hirashima Y, Endo S, Otsuji T et al: Platelet-activating factor and cerebral vasospasm following subarachnoid hemorrhage. J Neurosurg 78:592, 1993
37. Baykaner MK: Evidence for the participation of vascular endothelium originated humoral fac-

tors to cerebral vasospasm. Acta Neurochir 124:135, 1993
38. Cosentino F, Katusic ZS: Does endothelin-1 play a role in the pathogenesis of cerebral vasospasm? Stroke 25:904, 1994
39. Barone FC, Globus MYT, Price WJ et al: Endothelin levels increase in rat focal and global ischemia. J Cereb Blood Flow Metab 14:337, 1994
40. Swift DM, Solomon RA: Unruptured aneurysms and postoperative volume expansion. J Neurosurg 77:908, 1992
41. Origitano TC, Wascher TM, Reichman OH, Anderson DE: Sustained increased cerebral blood flow with prophylactic hypertensive hypervolemic hemodilution ("triple-H" therapy) after subarachnoid hemorrhage. Neurosurgery 27:729, 1990
42. Kassell NF, Peerless SJ, Durward QJ et al: Treatment of ischemic deficits from vasospasm with intravascular volume expansion and induced arterial hypertension. Neurosurgery 11:337, 1982
43. Trumble ER, Muizelaar JP, Myseros JS et al: Coagulopathy with the use of hetastarch in the treatment of vasospasm. J Neurosurg 82:44, 1995
44. Levy ML, Giannotta SL: Cardiac performance indices during hypervolemic therapy for cerebral vasospasm. J Neurosurg 75:27, 1991
45. Farhat SM, Schneider RC: Observations on the effect of systemic blood pressure on intracranial circulation in patients with cerebrovascular insufficiency. J Neurosurg 27:441, 1967
46. Kosnik EJ, Hunt WE: Postoperative hypertension in the management of patients with intracranial arterial aneurysms. J Neurosurg 45:148, 1976
47. Lee SH, Heros RC, Mullan JC, Korosue K: Optimum degree of hemodilution for brain protection in a canine model of focal cerebral ischemia. J Neurosurg 80:469, 1994
48. Wood JH, Simeone FA, Kron RE, Snyder LL: Experimental hypervolemic hemodilution: physiological correlations of cortical blood flow, cardiac output, and intracranial pressure with fresh blood viscosity and plasma volume. Neurosurgery 14:709, 1984
49. Wood JH, Snyder LL, Simeone FA: Failure of intravascular volume expansion without hemodilution to elevate cortical blood flow in region of experimental focal ischemia. J Neurosurg 56:80, 1982
50. Shimoda M, Oda S, Tsugane R, Sato O: Intracranial complications of hypervolemic therapy in patients with a delayed ischemic deficit attributed to vasospasm. J Neurosurg 78:423, 1993
51. Haley EC, Kassell NF, Torner JC: A randomized controlled trial of high-dose intravenous nicardipine in aneurysmal subarachnoid hemorrhage. J Neurosurg 78:537, 1993
52. Mercier P, Alhayek G, Rizk T et al: Are the calcium antagonists really useful in cerebral aneurysmal surgery? A retrospective study. Neurosurgery 34:30, 1994
53. Ohman J, Servo A, Heiskanen O: Long-term effects of nimodipine on cerebral infarcts and outcome after aneurysmal subarachnoid hemorrhage and surgery. J Neurosurg 74:8, 1991
54. Zuccarello M, Marsch JT, Schmitt G et al: Effect of the 21-aminosteroid U-74006F on cerebral vasospasm following subarachnoid hemorrhage. J Neurosurg 71:98, 1989
55. Matsui T, Asano T: Effects of new 21-aminosteroid tirilazad mesylate (U74006F) on chronic cerebral vasospasm in a "two-hemorrhage" model of beagle dogs. Neurosurgery 34:1035, 1994
56. Kanamaru K, Weir BKA, Findlay JM et al: M, Macdonald RL. A dosage study of the effect of the 21-aminosteroid U74006F on chronic cerebral vasospasm in a primate model. Neurosurgery 27:29, 1990
57. Kassell NF, Haley EC, Apperson-Hansen C et al: Randomized, double-blind, vehicle-controlled trial of tirilazad mesylate in patients with aneurysmal subarachnoid hemorrhage: a cooperative study in Europe, Australia, and New Zealand. J Neurosurg 84:221, 1996
58. Higashida RT, Halbach VV, Tsai FY et al: Interventional neurovascular techniques for cerebral revascularization in the treatment of stroke. Am J Radiol 163:793, 1994
59. Le Roux PD, Newell DW, Eskridge J et al: Severe symptomatic vasospasm: the role of immediate postoperative angioplasty. J Neurosurg 80:224, 1994
60. Kaku Y, Yonekawa Y, Tsukahara T, Kazekawa K: Superselective intra-arterial infusion of papaverine for the treatment of cerebral vasospasm after subarachnoid hemorrhage. J Neurosurg 77:842, 1992
61. Mizoi K, Yoshimoto T, Fujiwara S et al: Prevention of vasospasm by clot removal and intrathecal bolus injection of tissue-type plasminogen

activator: preliminary report. Neurosurgery 28:807, 1991
62. Mizoi K, Yoshimoto T, Takahashi A et al: Prospective study on the prevention of cerebral vasospasm by intrathecal fibrinolytic therapy with tissue-type plasminogen activator. J Neurosurg 78:430, 1993
63. Zabramski JM, Spetzler RF, Lee KS et al: Phase I trial of tissue plasminogen activator for the prevention of vasospasm in patients with aneurysmal subarachnoid hemorrhage. J Neurosurg 75:189, 1991
64. Shishido T, Suzuki R, Qian L, Hirakawa K: The role of superoxide anions in the pathogenesis of cerebral vasospasm. Stroke 25:864, 1994
65. Kajita Y, Suzuki Y, Oyama H et al: Combined effect of L-arginine and superoxide dismutase on the spastic basilar artery after subarachnoid hemorrhage in dogs. J Neurosurg 80:476, 1994
66. Juvela S: Aspirin and delayed cerebral ischemia after aneurysmal subarachnoid hemorrhage. J Neurosurg 82:945, 1995
67. Locksley HB: Report on the Cooperative Study of Intracranial Aneurysms and Subarachnoid Hemorrhage: Section V, Part II. Natural history of subarachnoid hemorrhage: intracranial aneurysms and arteriovenous malformations. J Neurosurg 25:321, 1966
68. Whisnant JP, Phillips LH, Sundt TM: Aneurysmal subarachnoid hemorrhage: timing of surgery and mortality. Mayo Clin Proc 57:471, 1982
69. Adams HP: Early management of the patient with recent aneurysmal subarachnoid hemorrhage. Stroke 17:1068, 1986
70. Kassell NF, Torner JC, Adams HP: Antifibrinolytic therapy in the acute period following aneurysmal subarachnoid hemorrhage. J Neurosurg 61:225, 1984
71. Diringer M, Ladenson PW, Stern BJ et al: Plasma atrial natriuretic factor and subarachnoid hemorrhage. Stroke 19:1119, 1988
72. Kroll M, Juhler M, Lindholm J: Hyponatremia in acute brain disease. J Int Med 232:291, 1992
73. Fernandez-Real JM, Fernandez-Castaner M, Villabona C et al: Giant intrasellar aneurysm presenting with panhypopituitarism and subarachnoid hemorrhage: case report and literature review. Clin Invest 72:302, 1994
74. Wijdicks EFM, Vermeulen M, Hijdra A, van Gijn J: Hyponatremia and cerebral infarction in patients with ruptured intracranial aneurysms: is fluid restriction harmful? Ann Neurol 17:137, 1985
75. Maroon JC, Nelson PB: Hypovolemia in patients with subarachnoid hemorrhage: therapeutic implications. Neurosurgery 4:223, 1979
76. Nelson PB, Seif SM, Maroon JC, Robinson AG: Hyponatremia in intracranial disease: perhaps not the syndrome of inappropriate secretion of antidiuretic hormone (SIADH). J Neurosurg 55:938, 1981
77. Weinand ME, O'Boynick PL, Goetz KL: A study of serum antidiuretic hormone and atrial natriuretic peptide levels in a series of patients with intracranial disease and hyponatremia. Neurosurgery 25:781, 1989
78. Rosenfeld JV, Barnett GH, Sila CA et al: The effect of subarachnoid hemorrhage on blood and CSF atrial natriuretic factor. J Neurosurg 71:32, 1989
79. Doczi T, Joo F, Vecsernyes M, Bodosi M: Increased concentration of atrial natriuretic factor in the cerebrospinal fluid of patients with aneurysmal subarachnoid hemorrhage and raised intracranial pressure. Neurosurgery 23:16, 1988
80. Landolt AM, Yasargil MG, Krayenbuhl H: Disturbances of the serum electrolytes after surgery of intracranial arterial aneurysms. J Neurosurg 37:210, 1972
81. Doczi T, Bende J, Huszka E, Kiss J: Syndrome of inappropriate secretion of antidiuretic hormone after subarachnoid hemorrhage. Neurosurgery 9:394, 1981
82. Andreoli TE: Disorders of fluid volume, electrolyte and acid-base balance. p. 515. In Wyngaarden JB, Smith LH (eds): Cecil Textbook of Medicine. 17th Ed. W Saunders, Philadelphia, 1985
83. Touho H, Karasawa J, Shishido H et al: Neurogenic pulmonary edema in the acute stage of hemorrhagic cerebrovascular disease. Neurosurgery 25:762, 1989
84. Fein IA, Rackow EC: Neurogenic pulmonary edema. Chest 81:318, 1982
85. Weir BK: Pulmonary edema following fatal aneurysm rupture. J Neurosurg 49:502, 1978
86. Colice GL, Matthay MA, Bass E, Matthay RA: Clinical commentary: neurogenic pulmonary edema. Am Rev Respir Dis 130:941, 1984
87. Minnear FL, Kite C, Hill LA, Van der Zee H: Endothelial injury and pulmonary congestion char-

acterize neurogenic pulmonary edema in rabbits. J Appl Physiol 63:335, 1987
88. Maron MB: A canine model of neurogenic pulmonary edema. J Appl Physiol 59:1019, 1985
89. Pender ES, Pollack CV: Neurogenic pulmonary edema: case reports and review. J Emerg Med 10:45, 1992
90. Cooper KR, Boswell PA, Choi SC: Safe use of PEEP in patients with severe head injury. J Neurosurg 63:552, 1985
91. Hamilton MG, Hull RD, Pineo GF: Venous thromboembolism in neurosurgery and neurology patients: a review. Neurosurgery 34:280, 1994
92. Medlock MD, Dulebohn SC, Elwood PW: Prophylactic hypervolemia without calcium channel blockers in early aneurysm surgery. Neurosurgery 30:12, 1992
93. Archer DP, Shaw DA, Leblanc RL, Tranmer BI: Hemodynamic considerations in the management of patients with subarachnoid hemorrhage. Can J Anaesth 38:454, 1991
94. Pollick C, Cujec B, Parker S, Tator C: Left ventricular wall motion abnormalities in subarachnoid hemorrhage: an echocardiographic study. J Am Coll Cardiol 12:600, 1988
95. Szabo MD, Crosby G, Hurford WE, Strauss HW: Myocardial perfusion following acute subarachnoid hemorrhage in patients with an abnormal electrocardiogram. Anesth Analg 76:253, 1993
96. Kreus KE, Kemila SJ, Takala JK: Electrocardiographic changes in cerebrovascular accidents. Acta Med Scand 185:327, 1969
97. Hersch C: Electrocardiographic changes in subarachnoid haemorrhage, meningitis, and intracranial space-occupying lesions. Br Heart J 26:785, 1964
98. Koskelo P, Punsar S, Sipila W: Subendocardial haemorrhage and ECG changes in intracranial bleeding. Br Med J 1:1479, 1964
99. Byer E, Ashman R, Toth LA: Electrocardiograms with large, upright T waves and long Q-T intervals. Am Heart J 33:796, 1947
100. Manninen PH, Gelb AW, Lam AM et al: Perioperative monitoring of the electrocardiogram during cerebral aneurysm surgery. J Neurosurg Anesth 2:16, 1990
101. Di Pasquale G, Pinelli G, Andreoli A et al: Holter detection of cardiac arrhythmias in intracranial subarachnoid hemorrhage. Am J Cardiol 59:596, 1987
102. Andreoli A, Di Pasquale G, Pinelli G et al: Subarachnoid hemorrhage: frequency and severity of cardiac arrhythmias: a survey of 70 cases studied in the acute phase. Stroke 18:558, 1987
103. Neil-Dwyer G, Cruickshank J, Stratton C: Betablockers, plasma total creatine kinase and creatine kinase myocardial isoenzyme, and the prognosis of subarachnoid hemorrhage. Surg Neurol 25:163, 1986
104. Fabinyi G, Hunt D, McKinley L: Myocardial Creatine kinase isoenzyme in serum after subarachnoid hemorrhage. J Neurol Neurosurg Psych 40:818, 1977
105. Kono T, Morita H, Kuroiwa T et al: Left ventricular wall motion abnormalities in patients with subarachnoid hemorrhage: neurogenic stunned myocardium. J Am Coll Cardiol 24:636, 1994
106. Doshi R, Neil-Dwyer G: A clinicopathological study of patients following a subarachnoid hemorrhage. J Neurosurg 52:295, 1980
107. Neil-Dwyer G, Walter P, Cruickshank JM et al: Effect of propranolol and phentolamine on myocardial necrosis after subarachnoid hemorrhage. Br Med J 2:990, 1978
108. Melville KI, Blum B, Shister HE, Silver MD: Cardiac ischemic changes and arrhythmias induced by hypothalamic stimulation. Am J Cardiol 12:781, 1963
109. Estanol BV, Loyo MV, Mateos JH et al: Cardiac arrhythmias in experimental subarachnoid hemorrhage. Stroke 8:440, 1977
110. Offerhaus L, Van Gool J: Electrocardiographic changes and tissue catecholamines in experimental subarachnoid haemorrhage. Cardiovas Res 3:433, 1969
111. Svigelj V, Grad A, Tekavcic I, Kiauta T: Cardiac arrhythmia associated with reversible damage to insula in a patient with subarachnoid hemorrhage. Stroke 25:1053, 1994
112. Oppenheimer SM, Cechetto DF, Hachinski VC: Cerebrogenic cardiac arrhythmias: cerebral electrocardiographic influences and their role in sudden death. Arch Neurol 47:513, 1990
113. Oppenheimer SM, Gelb A, Girvin JP Hachinski VC: Cardiovascular effects of human insular cortex stimulation. Neurol 42:1727, 1992
114. Benedict CR, Loach AB: Clinical significance of plasma adrenaline and noradrenaline concentrations in patients with subarachnoid haemorrhage. J Neurol Neurosurg Psych 41:113, 1978
115. Grad A, Kiauta T, Osredkar J: Effect of elevated plasma norepinephrine on electrocardiographic

changes in subarachnoid hemorrhage. Stroke 22:746, 1991
116. Kassell NF, Torner JC, Jane JA et al: The International Cooperative Study on the Timing of Aneurysm Surgery. 2. Surgical results. J Neurosurg 73:37, 1990
117. Muzzi DA, Black S, Losasso TJ, Cucchiara RF: Labetalol and esmolol in the control of hypertension after intracranial surgery. Anesth Analg 70:68, 1990
118. Michenfelder, JD, Milde JH: The interaction of sodium nitroprusside, hypotension, and isoflurane in determining cerebral vasculature effects. Anesthesiology 69:870, 1988
119. Nussmeier NA, Arlund C, Slogoff S: Neuropsychiatric complication after cardiopulmonary bypass: cerebral protection by a barbiturates. Anesthesiology 64(2):165, 1986
120. Samson D, Batjer HH, Bowman G et al: A clinical study of the parameters and effects of temporary arterial occlusion in the management of intracranial aneurysm. Neurosugery 34:22, 1994
121. Freedman WA, Chadwick GM, Verhoeven JS et al: Monitoring of somatosensory evoked potentials during surgery of middle cerebral artery aneurysms. Neurosurgery 29(1):98, 1991
122. Freedman WA, Kaplan BL, Day AL et al: Evoked potential monitoring during aneurysm operation: observations after fifty cases. Neurosurgery 20:92, 1987
123. Abe K: Vasodilators during cerebral aneurysm surgery (review article). Can J Anaesth 40:775, 1993
124. Lam AM: Induced hypotension. Can Anaesth Soc J 31:556, 1984
125. Little DM: Induced hypotension during anesthesia and surgery. Anesthesiology 16:320, 1955
126. Newberg LA, Milde JH, Michenfelder JD: Systemic and cerebral effects of isoflurane-induced hypotension in dogs. Anesthesiology 60:541, 1984
127. Michenfelder JD, Theye RA: Canine systemic and cerebral effects of hypotension induced by hemorrhage, trimethaphan, halothane, or nitroprusside. Anesthesiology 46:188, 1977
128. Minamisawa H, Smith ML, Siesjo BK: The effect of mild hyperthermia and hypothermia on brain damage following 5, 10, and 15 minutes of forebrain ischemia. Ann Neurosurg 28:26, 1990
129. Michenfelder JD: Cerebral preservation for intraoperative focal ischemia. Clin Neurosurg 32:105, 1986
130. Baker KZ, Young WL, Stone JG et al: Deliberate mild intraoperative hypothermia for craniotomy. Anesthesiology 81:361, 1994
131. Clifton GL, Christensen ML: Use of moderate hypothermia during elective craniotomy. J Tex Med 88:66, 1992
132. Black S, Sulek CA, Mahla ME, Cucchiara RF: Comparison of brain temperature with tempanic membrane and esophageal temperatures in neurosurgical patients. J Neurosurg Anesth 6:310, 1994
133. Chaney MA: Profound hypothermic circulatory arrest for noncardiac surgery via the closed-chest technique. Anesth Analg 76:892, 1993
134. Ausman JI, Malik GM, Tomecek FJ et al: Hypothermic circulatory arrest and the management of giant and large cerebral aneurysms. Surg Neurol 40:289, 1993
135. Williams MD, Rainer WG, Fieger HG, Jr et al: Cardiopulmonary bypass, profound hypothermia, and circulatory arrest for neurosurgery. Ann Thorac Surg 52:1069, 1991
136. Bonita R, Thomson S: Subarachnoid hemorrhage: epidemiology, diagnosis, management, and outcome. Stroke 16:591, 1985
137. Sundt TM, Kobayashi S, Fode NC, Whisnant JP: Results and complications of surgical management of 809 intracranial aneurysms in 722 cases: related and unrelated to grade of patient, type of aneurysm, and of surgery. J Neurosurg 56:753, 1982
138. Lanier WL, Stangland KJ, Scheithauer BW et al: The effects of dextrose infusion and head position on neurologic outcome after complete cerebral ischemia in primates: examination of a model. Anesthesiology 66:39, 1987
139. Stullken EH, Johnston WE, Prough DS et al: Implications of nimodipine prophylaxis of cerebral vasospasm on anesthetic management during intracranial aneurysm clipping. J Neurosurg 62:200, 1985
140. Schramm J, Cedzich C: Outcome and management of intraoperative aneurysm rupture. Surg Neurol 40:26, 1993
141. Todd MM, Warner DS, Sokoll MD et al: a prospective comparative trial of three anesthetics for elective supratentorial craniotomy: propofol/fentanyl, isoflurane/nitrous oxide, and fentanyl/nitrous oxide. Anesthesiology 78:1005, 1993
142. Baughman VL, Hoffman WE, Thomas C et al: The interaction of nitrous oxide and isoflurane

with incomplete cerebral ischemia in the rat. Anesthesiology 70:767, 1989
143. Grundy BL, Pashayan AG, Mahla ME: Three balanced anesthetic techniques for neuroanesthesia: infusion of thiopental sodium with sufentanil or fentanyl compared with inhalation of isoflurane. J Clin Anesth 4:372, 1992
144. Drake CG: Management of cerebral aneurysm. Stroke 12:273, 1981
145. Pulsinelli WA, Levy DE, Sigsbee B et al: Increased damage after ischemic stroke in patients with hyperglycemia with or without established diabetes mellitus. Am J Med 74:540, 1983
146. Fearnside MR, Adams CP: The treatment of raised intracranial pressure following aneurysm surgery. J Neurol Neurosurg Psychiatry 43:957, 1980
147. Batijer H, Samson D: Intraoperative aneurysmal rupture: incidence, outcome, and suggestions for surgical management. Neurosurgery 18:701, 1986
148. Tsementzis SA, Hitchcock ER: Outcome from "rescue clipping" of ruptured intracranial aneurysms during induction anaesthesia and endotracheal intubation. J Neurol- Neurosurg Psychiatry 48:160, 1985
149. Parkinson D, Bachers G: Arteriovenous malformations: summary of 100 consecutive supratentorial cases. J Neurosurg 53:285, 1980
150. Perret G, Nishioka H: Report on the cooperative study of intracranial aneurysms and subarachnoid hemorrhage. VI. Arteriovenous malformations. J Neurosurg 25:467, 1966
151. Ondra SL, Troupp H, George ED, Schwab K: The natural history of symptomatic arteriovenous malformations of the brain: a 24-year follow-up assessment. J Neurosurg 73:387, 1990
152. Graf CJ, Perret GE, Torner JC: Bleeding from cerebral arteriovenous malformation as part of their natural history. J Neurosurg 58:331, 1983
153. Guidetti B, Delitala A: Intracranial arteriovenous malformations: conservative and surgical treatment. J Neurosurg 53:149, 1980
154. Wilkins RH: Natural history of intracranial vascular malformations: a review. Neurosurgery 16:421, 1985
155. Stein BM, Wolpert SM: Arteriovenous malformations of the brain. II. Current concepts and treatment. Arch Neurol 37:69, 1980
156. Spetzler RF, Martin NA: A proposed grading system for arteriovenous malformations. J Neurosurg 65:476, 1986
157. Nussel F, Wegmuller H, Huber P: Comparison of magnetic resonance angiography, magnetic resonance imaging and conventional angiography in cerebral arteriovenous malformation. Neuroradiology 33:56, 1991
158. Heros RC, Tu YK: Is surgical therapy needed for unruptured arteriovenous malformations? Neurology 37:279, 1987
159. Abad JM, Alvarez F, Manrique M et al: Cerebral arteriovenous malformations: comparative results of surgical vs conservative treatment in 112 cases. J Neurosurg Sci 27:203, 1983
160. Heros RC, Korosue K, Diebold PM: Surgical excision of cerebral arteriovenous malformations: late results. Neurosurgery 26:570, 1990
161. Spetzler RF, Martin NA, Carter LP et al: Surgical management of large AVM's by staged embolization and operative excision. J Neurosurg 67:17, 1987
162. Deruty R, Mottolese C, Soustiel JF, Pelissou-Guyotat-I: Association of cerebral arteriovenous malformation and cerebral aneurysm: diagnosis and management. Acta Neurochir (Wien) 107:133, 1990
163. Deruty R, Pelissou-Guyotat I, Mottolese C et al: Amat D: The combined management of cerebral arteriovenous malformation: experience with 100 cases and review of the literature. Acta Neurochir (Wien) 123:101, 1993
164. Barnwell SL, Dowd CF, Higashida RT et al: Therapy for cerebral arteriovenous malformations. p. 1225. In Apuzzo MLJ (ed): brain surgery: Complication Avoidance and Management. Vol. 3. Churchill Livingstone, New York, 1993
165. Seifert V, Stolke D, Mehdorn HM, Hoffman B: Clinical and radiological evaluation of long term results of stereotactic proton beam radiosurgery in patients with cerebral arteriovenous malformations. J Neurosurg 81:683, 1994
166. Yamamoto M, Jimbo M, Kobayashi M et al: Long-term results of radiosurgery for arteriovenous malformation: neurodiagnostic imaging and histological studies of angiographically confirmed nidus obliteration. Surg Neurol 37:219, 1992
167. Young WL, Kafer A, Prohovnik I et al: Pressure autoregulation is intact after arteriovenous malformation resection. Neurosurgery 32:491, 1993
168. Young WL, Prohovnik I, Ornstein E et al: Monitoring of intraoperative cerebral hemodynamics

before and after arteriovenous malformation resection. Anesth Analg 67:1011, 1988
169. Diehl RR, Henkins H, Nahser HC et al: Blood flow velocity and vasomotor reactivity in patients with arteriovenous malformations: a transcranial Doppler study. Stroke 25:1574, 1994
170. Day AL, Friedman WA, Sypert GW, Mickle JP: Successful treatment of the normal perfusion pressure breakthrough syndrome. Neurosurgery 625, 1982
171. Spetzler RF, Wilson CB, Weinstein P et al: Normal perfusion pressure breakthrough theory. Clin Neurosurg 25:651, 1978
172. Nornes H, Grip A: Hemodynamic aspects of cerebral arteriovenous malformations. J Neurosurg 53:456, 1980
173. Morgan MK, Johnson I, Besser M, Baines D: Cerebral arteriovenous malformations, steal and the hypertensive breakthrough threshold: an experimental study in rats. J Neurosurg 66:563, 1987
174. Costantino A, Vinters HV: A pathologic correlate of the "steal" phenomenon in a patient with cerebral arteriovenous malformation. Stroke 17:103, 1986
175. Hansen PA, Knudson F, Jacobsen M et al: Indomethacin in controlling normal perfusion pressure "breakthrough" in a case of large cerebral arteriovenous malformation. J Neurosurg Anesthesiol 7:117, 1995
176. Young WL, Pile-Spellman J: Anesthetic considerations for interventional neuroradiology. Anesthesiology 80:427, 1994

9 EXTRACRANIAL VASCULAR DISEASE

MICHAEL E. MAHLA

MARK F. TRANKINA

EXTRACRANIAL VASCULAR SURGERY IN PERSPECTIVE

Carotid endarterectomy (CEA) remains one of the most commonly performed noncardiac vascular surgery procedures in the United States. Its frequency has been reduced somewhat in recent years because of a concern that carotid artery surgery was over used and provided little significant stroke risk reduction, particularly in asymptomatic patients. In 1988, a panel of experts published their findings after reviewing more than 1,500 CEAs from both academic and private settings during the preceding 5 years.[1] They found that only one-third of all the CEAs reviewed were performed for what they considered appropriate reasons. One-third were performed for debatable reasons, and one-third of the operations were inappropriate. The authors published their findings, and this article among others had a profound effect on the number of CEAs performed. Simultaneously with this review, several large international trials were begun to answer the question of whether medical or surgical treatment is more appropriate for patients with symptomatic and asymptomatic carotid narrowing of varying degrees. Results from both the North American and European symptomatic CEA trials showed that a subset of symptomatic patients with critical carotid stenosis (greater than 70 percent luminal narrowing) clearly has a better outcome with surgical therapy.[2,3] Symptomatic patients with lesser degrees of stenosis are still being randomized to medical and surgical treatment groups, and no definitive results are yet available. Several smaller trials involving a comparison of medical versus surgical therapy in patients with asymptomatic carotid stenosis failed to demonstrate a difference in the incidence of stroke after carotid surgery in patients with less than 90 percent stenosis.[4–6] However, these trials were not large enough to detect small but significant differences in outcome.

Recently, the larger multicenter asymptomatic carotid atherosclerosis study (ACAS) reported interim results of a subgroup of patients with more than 60 percent luminal narrowing.[7] There was an absolute 5-year stroke reduction of 5.8 percent in the surgical group, with a relative risk reduction of 55 percent.

Thus, CEA is now indicated when the procedure can be performed with acceptable surgical and medical risk in the following patients:

Symptomatic (transient ischemic attack [TIA], reversible ischemic neurologic deficit [RIND], or nondisabling stroke within 3 months before surgery) patients with more than 70 percent stenosis in the carotid artery supplying the symptomatic cerebral hemisphere Asymptomatic patients with greater than 60 percent luminal narrowing of either internal carotid artery

Acceptable surgical mortality rates are less than 1 percent, and stroke-related morbidity is less than 3 percent for patients who have had a TIA; surgical mortality and stroke-related morbidity are less than 2 percent for patients with asymptomatic carotid stenosis. All the studies comparing medical and surgical therapy were based on this or a similar complication rate.[1,2,6]

These studies appear to have had a major impact on clinical practice. At our institution, the number of CEAs performed declined steeply during the late 1980s. Since the data involving patients with severe stenoses from the North American and European symptomatic CEA trials were released, there has been a modest increase in the number of CEAs performed. Compared with 10 years ago, however, patients presenting for carotid artery surgery now, on the average, have more cerebral symptoms and a greater degree and number of cerebrovascular stenoses. The number of patients undergoing CEA who are asymptomatic preoperatively has not yet increased dramatically.

PREOPERATIVE EVALUATION

Patients undergoing CEA have a relatively high risk of perioperative complications involving primarily the central nervous system (CNS) and the cardiovascular system (CVS). With the acceptable stroke-related morbidity rate of 2 to 3 percent and reported myocardial infarction (MI) rate of up to 5 percent, careful preoperative evaluation of both of these systems is warranted to identify those areas in which risk reduction is possible.

Central Nervous System

Evaluation of the CNS involves primarily three areas: the cerebral circulation, other risk factors for perioperative stroke, and the patient's current level of neurologic function.

CEREBRAL CIRCULATION Carotid artery disease may cause cerebral symptoms by two mechanisms—embolism or hemodynamic insufficiency. Embolic disease presents with the classic TIA or RIND. An arterial embolus from a carotid arteriosclerotic plaque lodges in the distal cerebral circulation, producing a localized neurologic deficit that clears when the embolus breaks up. In a TIA, breakup occurs quickly, and symptoms associated with a TIA resolve within a few minutes (Fig. 9.1). The embolus breaks up more slowly during a RIND, and symptoms, although eventually clearing completely, may take up to 24 hours to resolve.

Hemodynamic disease may also present as a TIA or RIND. A critical narrowing of the lumen of the carotid artery potentially may reduce cerebral blood flow (CBF) by decreasing cerebral perfusion pressure (mean arterial pressure minus intracranial pressure or central venous

FIGURE 9.1 *Most patients with symptoms referred to carotid artery stenosis have transient ischemic attacks caused by small emboli from the carotid artery that lodge in the distal cerebral circulation and subsequently break up.*

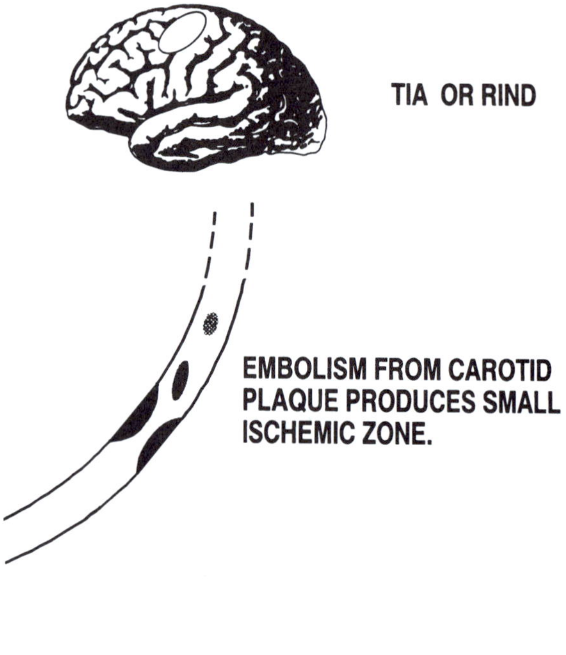

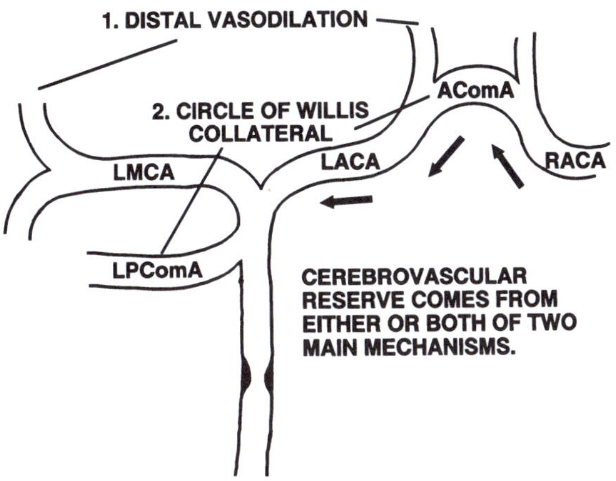

FIGURE 9.2 *Mechanisms of cerebrovascular reserve: when the ipsilateral carotid artery narrows, flow may be increased by either relying on circle of Willis collateral or on distal cerebral vasodilation.*

pressure, whichever is higher). Normally, however, cerebrovascular reserve prevents significant drops in CBF. Patients with carotid artery narrowing can maintain CBF via cerebrovascular reserve in two ways (Fig. 9.2). Blood may be supplied by collateral blood flow from the circle of Willis via either the anterior communicating artery or the posterior communicating artery. Alternatively, or in addition, the cerebral microcirculation distal to the carotid obstruction may dilate, thereby decreasing outflow resistance and preserving blood flow. Patients who develop TIA or RIND by a hemodynamic mechanism have totally exhausted their cerebrovascular reserve. As long as cerebral perfusion pressure is above a certain critical level, the patient is asymptomatic. Symptoms are produced when perfusion pressure falls below a critical level. In a patient without critical carotid stenosis, autoregulation-mediated vasodilation would compensate for any usual fall in blood pressure and maintain CBF. In the patient with critical carotid stenosis and exhausted cerebrovascular reserve, autoregulation-mediated vasodilation cannot compensate because maximal vasodilation has already occurred (Fig. 9.3). Decreases in perfusion pressure thus result in symptoms. Embolic and hemodynamic disease may occur simultaneously, and either of these presentations may be accompanied by a history of completed stroke.

When evaluating patients for CEA, the preoperative angiogram, including the opposite carotid and the vertebral circulation, should be evaluated carefully. If possible, the function of the circle of Willis should also be known. Symptomatic patients with exhausted cerebrovascular reserve may have critical reductions in CBF with decreases in perfusion pressure even within the range of cerebral autoregulation. These patients should have even transient drops in blood pressure vigorously treated during surgery, especially if no form of neurologic monitoring is used. Symptomatic patients without significant (greater than 70 percent) luminal narrowing or patients with significant narrowing but good collateral circulation are likely experiencing embolic events. These patients may tolerate lower blood pressures during surgery.

Knowledge of which patients will likely require aggressive management of hypotension from a CNS standpoint would be extremely useful, because hemodynamic interventions to increase blood pressure may increase the risk of myocardial ischemia and MI in these patients who frequently also have significant ischemic

FIGURE 9.3 *Exhausted cerebrovascular reserve: the patient without any further cerebrovascular reserve will become symptomatic when blood pressure falls (e.g., on arising rapidly from a chair or bed).*

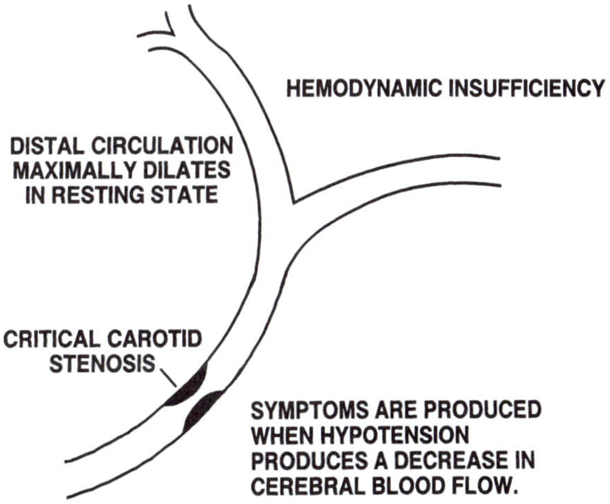

cardiovascular disease. Some recent studies have suggested that it may be possible to delineate preoperatively which patients with critical luminal narrowing have the least cerebrovascular reserve and are at highest risk for cerebral ischemia or stroke.[8–11] From this information, it might also be possible to infer which patients need vigorous treatment for even mild hypotension. Preoperative cerebrovascular reserve can be tested using laboratory tests of CBF including inhaled 60 percent xenon followed by computed tomography scanning, single photon emission computed tomography, positron emission tomography, or transcranial Doppler (TCD). A baseline blood flow study is performed. The patient is then given a cerebral vasodilator, such as inhaled carbon dioxide or intravenous acetazolamide, and the blood flow study is repeated. If the patient is unable to increase flow to a region of the brain, maximal cerebral vasodilation has already occurred in that area. Blood flow to such a region of the brain may actually *decrease* because the vessels that supply blood to normal areas of the brain are still able to vasodilate in response to the cerebral vasodilator. This vasodilation of normal vessels will "steal" blood from the area where maximal dilation has already occurred. If the asymptomatic patient shows an area of brain without cerebrovascular reserve, surgery may be indicated to increase carotid flow. If the symptomatic patient shows absent cerebrovascular reserve, he or she may be in imminent danger of hemodynamic stroke and may need urgent surgery. If the symptomatic patient can increase blood flow to all areas of the brain, the patient is not maximally using reserve resources and is likely experiencing embolic rather than hemodynamic events. If surgery is planned for this type of patient, transient or prolonged reduction in blood pressure that may occur during surgery may be better tolerated (from a cerebral standpoint). These studies suggest a method to evaluate which patients undergoing surgery are at highest risk for hypotension-related cerebral ischemia. Much more work is needed, however, before these expensive tests become routine or a standard of care, especially because one recent study failed to show that patients with preoperative evidence of decreased or absent cerebrovascular reserve had an increased likelihood of intraoperative cerebral ischemia.[12]

OTHER RISK FACTORS FOR PERIOPERATIVE STROKE Several other types of patients have increased risk for perioperative ischemia and stroke.[13] These include patients with recent stroke, intracranial luminal narrowing, significant contralateral carotid narrowing or vertebral narrowing, and contralateral carotid occlusion and a history of stroke. Studies have also suggested that postoperative hypertension is associated with a higher risk of perioperative stroke.[14,15] Poorly controlled hypertension preoperatively is associated with a higher incidence of both intraoperative and postoperative blood pressure instability. Logic would dictate that preoperative control of blood pressure could reduce the incidence of postoperative hypertension, which in turn could reduce the incidence of postoperative stroke. Although this conclusion is logical, it has not been systematically studied and is entirely unsupported by data.

LEVEL OF NEUROLOGIC FUNCTION The patient's preoperative level of neurologic function is important for several reasons. Immediate reexploration of the carotid artery may, in some circumstances, be indicated when the patient wakes up with a neurologic deficit that was not present before surgery. Reexploration is not appropriate if the deficit was present preoperatively. Preexisting deficits may actually worsen transiently after general anesthesia without any surgical cause. The abnormal brain presumably recovers function after anesthesia more slowly than normal brain. This slow recovery is manifested by transient loss of function. This phenomenon is well known to anesthesiologists who regularly anesthetize patients with prior stroke. However, postanesthesia worsening of preexisting neurologic deficits has not been scientifically studied, and the normal time course of such an exacerbation is not known. Anesthetic-induced worsening of neurologic deficit should, therefore, be a diagnosis of exclusion. Finally, the presence of a preoperative neurologic deficit may increase the risk of hyperkalemia associated with the use of succinylcholine to facilitate intubation during induction.

Cardiovascular System

Cardiovascular complications continue to be a clinically significant source of morbidity and mortality in high-risk patients undergoing CEA.[17] Despite the improved outcome of modern perioperative care, the advancing age of the U.S. population is leading to an increased percentage of patients with serious cardiac disease who present for surgery. Perioperative CVS dynamics appear to play a central role in the evolution of myocardial ischemia and adverse cardiac outcome.[18–20] It appears likely that the combination of severe coronary artery disease CAD and perioperative hemodynamic instability that is common during CEA, is partly responsible for the prevalence of myocardial ischemia in these patients.[21] Unfortunately, the mechanisms causing perioperative myocardial ischemia and its related outcomes are poorly understood.[22]

A strong relationship exists between peripheral vascular disease and significant cardiovascular disease.[23] Hypertension is present in about 80 percent of patients undergoing CEA.[24] The prevalence of severe CAD in patients with known peripheral vascular disease ranges from 37 to 78 percent.[25] Hertzer et al.[26] in a prospective study of 506 patients with neurologic symptoms or bruits, showed that greater than 26 percent of patients with extracranial cerebrovascular disease have severe correctable CAD. Severe, surgically correctable coronary artery disease was documented in 37 percent of patients in this series suspected to have CAD by history, compared with 16 percent of those who were not. Severe inoperable coronary disease was present in 9.8 and 1.5 percent of these respective subsets. Severe inoperable disease was especially common (14 percent) among diabetics patients; only 7 percent of these patients had normal coronary arteries. In another prospective study, Chimowitz et al.[27] recently examined cardiac outcome of patients with asymptomatic carotid stenosis presenting for CEA as part of a Veterans Administration study. About 45 percent of patients in this series had a history of CAD (angina, previous coronary artery bypass grafting [CABG] MI by history or electrocardiogram) [ECG]. A follow-up period of 48 months revealed that 43 percent of patients with CAD and 33 percent without a history of CAD had cardiac ischemic events. In patients without a history of CAD, the first cardiac event was MI or sudden death in 56 percent. In this negative history group, factors that were independently associated with cardiac events included diabetes, peripheral vascular disease, and intracranial occlusive disease. Thus, it seems that patients even without known CAD but with other risk factors should be considered high risk for adverse cardiac sequelae.

Urbinati et al.[28] evaluated the role of silent CAD in patients with symptomatic high-grade carotid stenosis. Silent CAD (abnormal testing with no history, symptoms or resting ECG signs of CAD) was found in 25 percent of patients by exercise ECG and thallium myocardial scintigraphy. Although silent CAD did not affect perioperative outcome during a 5.4-year follow-up period, cardiac ischemic events occurred in 29 percent of patients with silent CAD as compared with 1.2 percent without CAD. Gersh et al.[25] suggest that all patients with peripheral vascular disease should be considered to be at lifelong risk for adverse cardiac events and should undergo appropriate clinical and laboratory evaluation followed by the appropriate treatment.

Hypertension should be well controlled medically before surgery if possible. Asiddao et al.[24] demonstrated that postoperative hypertension and transient neurologic deficits are more frequent in patients with inadequate preoperative control of blood pressure (greater than 170/95) as compared with adequate control or normotension. This must be balanced against the risk of potential focal cerebral ischemia if the blood pressure is too aggressively treated preoperatively. Other studies[29] have shown that poor preoperative control also leads to wider swings of blood pressure during the intraoperative period, which potentially could lead to cardiovascular morbidity.

The strong association between carotid and CAD, as well as the high associated adverse cardiac event rate, warrants careful preoperative assessment. The clinician is faced with a complex strata of algorithms and confusing/conflicting data in the environment of cost-containment/litigation. The decision-making process varies greatly in different centers, and often the preoperative workup is the first cardiac evaluation of the patient. Ten years ago, the pathway was easy because little was known about the subject. Several factors, though, have led to an explosion of information in recent years, leading to difficulty in practical application for the busy

Clinical Predictors of Increased Perioperative Cardiovascular Risk (MI, Congestive Heart Failure, Death)

MAJOR PREDICTORS

Unstable coronary syndromes

Recent myocardial infarction[a] with evidence of important ischemic risk by clinical symptoms or noninvasive study

Unstable or severe[b] angina (Canadian class III or IV)[c]

Decompensated congestive heart failure

Significant arrhythmias

High-grade atrioventricular block

Symptomatic ventricular arrhythmias in the presence of underlying heart disease

Supraventricular arrhythmias with uncontrolled ventricular rate

Severe valvular disease

INTERMEDIATE PREDICTORS

Mild angina pectoris (Canadian class I or II)[c]

Previous MI by history or pathologic Q waves

Compensated or previous congestive heart failure

Diabetes mellitus

MINOR PREDICTORS

Advanced age

Abnormal ECG (left ventricular hypertrophy, left bundle-branch block, ST-T segment abnormalities)

Rhythm other than sinus (e.g., atrial fibrillation)

Low functional capacity (e.g., inability to climb one flight of stairs with a bag of groceries)

History of stroke

Uncontrolled systemic hypertension

[a] American College of Cardiology defines "recent myocardial infarction" as greater than 7 days but 30 days or less.
[b] May include "stable" angina in patients who are unusually sedentary.
[c] Campeau L. Grading of angina pectoris. Circulation 54:522, 1976.
(Adapted from Fleisher and Eagle,[23] with permission.)

Cardiac Risk Stratification for Noncardiac Surgical Procedure[a]

HIGH RISK (REPORTED CARDIAC RISK OFTEN MORE THAN 5 PERCENT)

Emergent major operations, particularly in the elderly

Aortic and other major vascular surgery

Peripheral vascular surgery

Anticipated prolonged surgical procedures associated with large fluid shifts or blood loss

INTERMEDIATE RISK (REPORTED CARDIAC RISK GENERALLY LESS THAN 5 PERCENT)

Carotid endarterectomy

Head and neck surgery

Intraperitoneal and intrathoracic surgery

Orthopaedic surgery

Prostate surgery

LOW RISK (REPORTED CARDIAC RISK GENERALLY LESS THAN 1 PERCENT)[b]

Endoscopic procedure

Superficial procedure

Cataract removal

Breast surgery

[a] Risk is combined incidence of cardiac death and nonfatal MI.
[b] Patients in this group do not generally require further preoperative cardiac testing.
(Adapted from Fleisher and Eagle,[23] with permission.)

clinician. Fortunately, this increasingly complex situation was noted, and recently the American College of Cardiology/American Heart Association Task Force published its practice guidelines for evaluation of these patients.[30] These guidelines were prepared with the help of an anesthesiologist expert in the field, are intended to simplify the process, and will be updated on a regular basis. They proposed an algorithm based on six steps, the first of which is to evaluate the urgency of surgery. Unstable coronary syndromes should be identified and appropriate treatment implemented. The need for further testing depends on the interaction of the clinical risk factors, surgery risk (e.g., CABG), and functional capacity. CABG should be considered if it is likely to improve long-term survival. In other words, the guidelines state that coronary revascularization indications are identical in the preoperative period and the nonsurgical setting. Prudence suggests that all clinicians involved with these patients become familiar with these guidelines because they most certainly will be used by our medical colleagues and members of the law community. It is estimated that more than $1 billion is spent annually on cardiac testing before vascular surgery.[23]

Active congestive heart failure has been associated with increased perioperative morbidity.[31] Stabilization of left ventricular function is prudent, and the cause should be elicited. This leads to rational selection of perioperative monitors. Unstable angina is also associated with increased risk.[31] The associated hypercoagulable state and increased catecholamine levels that are seen during the perioperative period may exacerbate the underlying process in unstable angina.[23]

Several studies have suggested that exercise capacity is an important factor.[32] Yet, exercise stress testing is rarely indicated preoperatively in patients who have excellent capacity during normal life. Preoperative cardiac testing is often suggested in patients who cannot exercise (e.g., claudication). The planned anesthetic may be of significantly greater stress than that encountered during daily life. Pharmacologic testing has been advocated in these patients. Boucher et al.[33] studied a moderate risk group of 48 peripheral vascular patients with dipyridamole thallium imaging. They reported eight ischemic cardiac events in 16 patients who had redistribution and no events in patients with normal scans. This led to increased enthusiasm and attempts to apply these tests to all patients.

Eagle et al.[34] evaluated the implications of prior risk factors in determining the value of preoperative testing. Two hundred consecutive vascular surgery patients were studied retrospectively. Patients without clinical risk factors

(ECG Q waves, angina, diabetes mellitus, age older than 70 years, medicated ventricular ectopic activity) had only a 3 percent incidence of perioperative morbidity, and noninvasive testing could not further stratify risk. Patients with three or more risk factors had a morbidity rate of 50 percent, and noninvasive testing also did not help stratify risk. Preoperative dipyridamole thallium scanning was helpful in the moderate-risk group (one or two risk factors). This concept was further validated by L'Italien et al.[35] Two recent studies have shown the reduced value of noninvasive testing when all patients are studied in a consecutive fashion.[36,37] In essence, the low prevalence of cardiac events limits the ability to predict which patients require preoperative intervention.[22]

Other advocated tests include dobutamine stress echocardiography, Holter monitoring for silent ischemia, and angiography. Stress echocardiography has been shown to have excellent negative and positive predictive values in several large series and appears to be best used in moderate-risk patients.[38,39] Holter monitoring predicted poor outcome in several series, but it does not further stratify risk on the basis of ischemic quantity.[40,41] Transthoracic echocardiography was recently studied by the Mangano group as a preoperative tool and was found to offer little in stratifying cardiac risk.[42] Angiography, which has high costs and some risk itself, should be reserved for patients with many clinical markers or a highly positive stress test in whom coronary revascularization is being considered.[23]

Clinical studies have demonstrated that cardiac outcome after CEA often is not adequately predicted by the standard criteria of history, physical findings, and rest ECG.[43] Based on the Task Force algorithm,[30] patients without major but with intermediate predictors of clinical risk and moderate or better functional activity can proceed with CEA with little chance of perioperative death or MI. Similarly, if two or more intermediate predictors are present along with poor functional capacity, further noninvasive testing should be performed before CEA. Noninvasive test results may lead to a recommendation to proceed with surgery because the risk of coronary intervention may approach or even exceed the risk of the proposed CEA. The decision to proceed with preoperative coronary angiography and myocardial revascularization should be based primarily on indications independent of the vascular procedure as stated in the task force guidelines. Patients with high-risk or unstable coronary artery disease may benefit from preoperative coronary revascularization in regard to long-term prognosis, although this hypothesis remains unproven. In all patients, careful monitoring during and after operation is essential.

MONITORING DURING CAROTID SURGERY

As with the preoperative evaluation, most monitoring during CEA is directed at the CVS and neurologic systems.

Cardiovascular Monitoring

Cardiovascular monitoring during surgery is generally determined by the nature of the operation and the patient's preoperative medical condition. Carotid surgery itself presents little cardiovascular risk with regard to fluid shifts or bleeding, but considerable changes in heart rate or blood pressure may occur during and after manipulation of the carotid artery and baroreceptor. The patient's preoperative cardiovascular status may necessitate extensive intraoperative monitoring to assess either ventricular function, the balance between myocardial oxygen supply and demand, or both. Monitors that have been used for this purpose include the ECG with continuous ST-segment analysis, invasive arterial blood pressure monitoring, pulmonary artery pressure monitoring, and transesophageal echocardiography. There are no clear-cut outcome studies documenting the efficacy of these monitors in detecting and preventing cardiovascular complications, and choice of monitors must be determined by the clinical needs of

Monitors of the Nervous System during Carotid Surgery

MONITORS OF BLOOD FLOW

Transcranial Doppler blood flow velocity

Radioactive (^{133}Xenon) washout

Jugular venous PO_2 and cerebral oximetry

MONITORS OF FUNCTION

Neurologic examination: continuous; local or regional technique

Electroencephalogram (EEG): scalp recordings (unprocessed, processed); direct cortical recordings

Evoked potentials: somatosensory; Cortical, scalp recordings

the patient in combination with the expertise and experience of the anesthesiologist.

Central Nervous System Monitoring

Monitoring of the CNS examines the balance between cerebral oxygen supply and demand. In our opinion, some form of CNS monitoring should be performed in any CEA. Monitors used for such purposes are listed in the accompanying box.

THE AWAKE PATIENT The awake patient gives direct access to multiple levels of neurologic function. There are no costs associated with either equipment or monitoring employees, and superficially, interpretation seems simple. However, unless the surgeon is quick and gentle, the patient may not tolerate surgery without significant sedation. Sedation decreases the specificity of the monitor because decreases in sensorium may be caused either by drugs, CNS ischemia, or both. Finally, cerebral ischemia is not always immediately reversible and may be exacerbated by poor control of oxygenation and ventilation. Because access to the airway is limited by the patient's position and surgical drapes, quick control of the airway to optimize oxygenation and ventilation during a period of cerebral ischemia is not easy and may be impossible. Because most studies quote a conversion rate to general anesthesia (for unspecified reasons) of between 5 and 15 percent,[44–47] the unprotected airway is a significant problem in the awake patient undergoing CEA. In addition, if some other form of monitoring (e.g., electroencephalogram [EEG]) is not also used, conversion to general anesthesia will leave the patient's nervous system unmonitored.

THE ELECTROENCEPHALOGRAM The EEG is a plot of the spontaneous electrical activity generated by the cerebral cortex. The surface-recorded EEG represents the summation of excitatory and inhibitory postsynaptic potentials produced by the pyramidal cells in the cerebral cortex. Generation of the spontaneous EEG requires approximately 50 percent of the oxygen used by the brain. The remainder of the oxygen is used for maintenance of cell viability (Fig. 9.4). If the oxygen supply to the brain becomes limited by either reduced blood flow or hypoxemia, the brain will use all available oxygen re-

FIGURE 9.4 *Roughly 50 percent of the oxygen demand of the brain is used to generate the spontaneous EEG. The remainder is used for maintenance of cellular integrity (ionic gradients, etc.).*

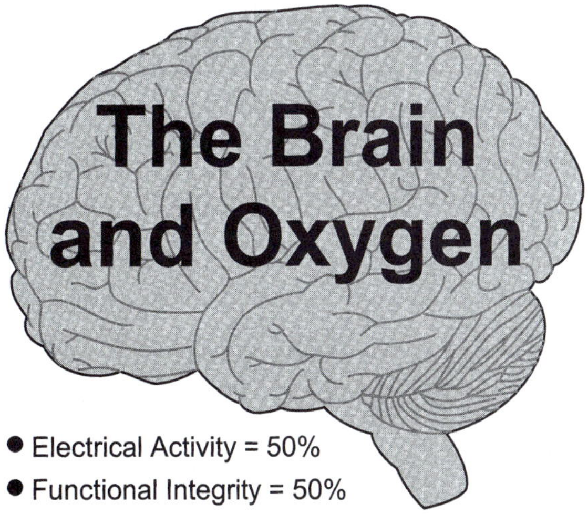

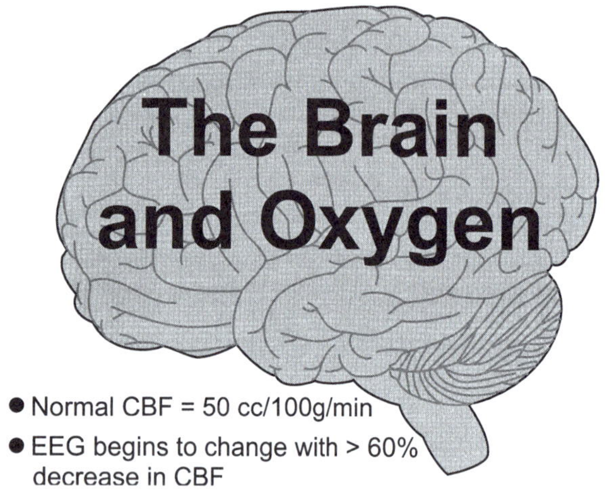

FIGURE 9.5 *Relationship of EEG to reduction in cerebral blood flow.*

sources for maintenance of cell viability. Electrical activity fails.

The EEG has been shown conclusively to reflect the balance between cerebral oxygen supply and oxygen demand during carotid surgery.[48,49] As cerebral blood flow falls below 20 ml.100 g^{-1}.min^{-1}, frequency of the EEG activity slows (Fig. 9.5). As ischemia worsens, the EEG voltage also decreases, with the EEG ultimately becoming isoelectric at a blood flow of approximately 10 ml.100 g^{-1}.min^{-1}. These threshold blood flow values for EEG change appear to be somewhat lower when isoflurane is used as the maintenance anesthetic, even in relatively low concentrations in combination with nitrous oxide and narcotics.[49] The EEG will become isoelectric *before* irreversible damage to the cortex occurs. However, just as the ischemic interval on ECG correlates to postoperative MI after coronary bypass surgery, increasing duration of severe EEG changes increases the likelihood of stroke after CEA.

The most extensive experience with intraoperative EEG during CEA has been obtained at the Mayo Clinic by using 16-channel strip-chart recording.[48] Such an application of EEG requires a technician both to set up the monitor and to interpret the large amount of data generated. At that institution in a series of what is now more than 5,000 patients, there has never been a case of a patient awakening at the conclusion of surgery with a neurologic deficit that was not detected by EEG.

When such technical assistance is not available, simpler processed EEG monitors using two or four channels can provide information that is easy to follow over time and to interpret with only moderate loss of the ability to detect ischemia.[50,51] Most processed EEG machines convert the plot of voltage versus time (Fig. 9.6) to a plot of frequency and power versus time. The processed EEG can be displayed so that the anesthesiologist performing the anesthetic can easily monitor the EEG data as well as other vital signs. EEG display methods include compressed spectral array, density spectral array, pie graphs, and others (see Fig. 4.4).

The optimum number of channels that should be used for monitoring the EEG has not been determined, however. Increasing the number of channels increases both the cost of the instrument and of the personnel required to operate the instrument. Each scalp electrode can only detect EEG activity within a few centimeters of its location. Decreasing the number of channels thus decreases the amount of cerebral cortex that is monitored. Electrodes can be strategically placed, however. The watershed distributions of the middle and anterior cerebral arteries are most likely at highest risk for ischemia caused by hypotension, placement of carotid cross-clamp, or embolism. Electrodes placed over these watershed distributions would thus be most likely to pick up an important decrease in blood flow. Indeed, a recent study[52] has shown that compared with 16-channel EEG monitoring, there is no significant loss in the sensitivity of the EEG for detecting ischemia if four channels are used with electrodes placed in this fashion.

All these processed EEG monitors will process and display both real physiologic signals and noise. It is not always apparent from the processed data display which data represent real brain activity. For example, ECG activity detected on the scalp will appear as delta EEG ac-

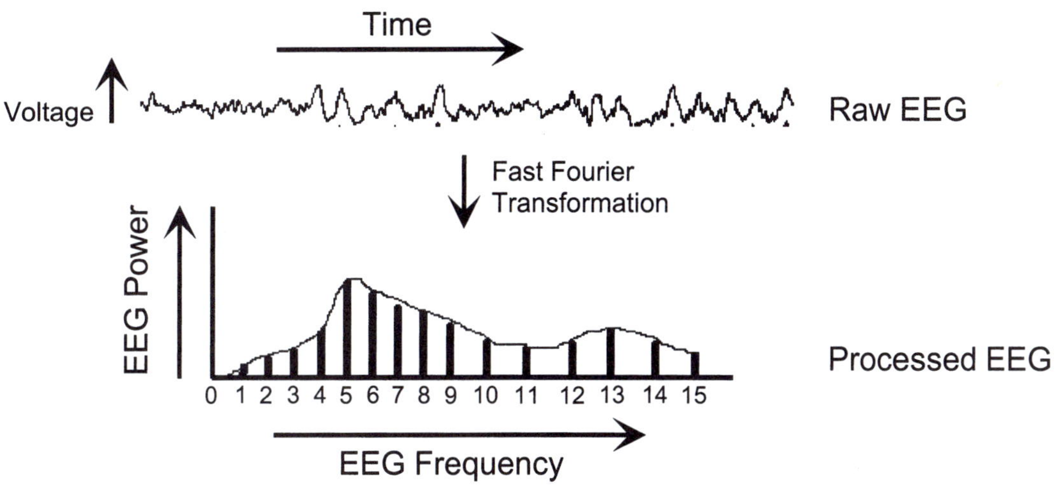

FIGURE 9.6 *Processed EEG monitors usually convert the standard plot of voltage versus time to frequency and power versus time.*

tivity. Therefore, all processed EEG monitors must have the ability to display unprocessed raw EEG to confirm that the signals monitored are real brain activity.

These monitors do not require extensive training to operate or interpret and can be readily mastered by any practicing anesthesiologist. Several cautionary notes are needed, however. First, changes in anesthetic technique may produce global EEG changes that are indistinguishable from global mild or severe ischemia. For example, there is no way to distinguish between a flat EEG produced by severe global ischemia and a flat EEG produced by a large dose of thiopental. Therefore, anesthetic technique must be tightly controlled, particularly when monitoring for mild ischemia. Secondly, anesthesiologists who are planning to begin EEG monitoring in the operating room should spend time with a neurologist at their hospital of employment or preferably with personnel at a center where intraoperative monitoring is already performed. This training will enable the anesthesiologist to recognize real EEG signals as opposed to artifact and to learn the "typical" EEG changes associated with anesthetic drugs and with changes in anesthetic depth.

SOMATOSENSORY EVOKED POTENTIALS

Somatosensory evoked potentials (SSEPs) differ from spontaneous EEG in that electrical activity in the brain is evoked by the application of an electric shock to a peripheral nerve (usually the median or posterior tibial nerve). This evoked activity is much smaller than the spontaneous EEG and is produced only by a relatively small area of cortex (the somatosensory cortex). SSEPs require stimulating devices, a recording device, and a computer to allow signal averaging necessary to record such a small signal. This type of monitoring is continuous and could be performed by an anesthesiologist not responsible for conducting the anesthetic. However, it is better performed by a technologist. The SSEP waveform is simpler in appearance than the EEG and is described in terms of latency and amplitude (see Fig. 4.9). The latency of the response is the amount of time that it takes from the application of the stimulus to the peak of the recorded response. Because the waveform is simpler, changes in SSEP may be easier to interpret than changes in EEG. An increase in cortical response latency of greater than 1 ms and a decrease in cortical response amplitude of greater than 50 percent are thought to be indicative of ischemia.

However, there are conflicting data as to whether the SSEP is as sensitive as the EEG to reductions in CBF during carotid surgery,[53,54] and in the laboratory, the SSEP appears to be less sensitive.[55] Because of the technical requirements and uncertainty regarding sensitivity, the SSEP has not attained great popularity for monitoring during CEAs. It does, however, possess one major advantage. When barbiturates are given for cerebral protection, the EEG becomes isoelectric and cannot be used to detect ischemia during that period. The SSEP, however, is only moderately depressed and still readily recordable during barbiturate cerebral protection.[56] In our clinical experience, the SSEP is effective for monitoring during carotid vascular surgery.

TRANSCRANIAL DOPPLER ULTRASOUND

The TCD is a device that found use in the operating room as a monitor of CBF during the 1980s. It uses the Doppler shift of sound waves reflected off moving red blood cells to measure blood flow velocity in the basal cerebral arteries (most commonly, the middle cerebral artery) (see Fig. 4.22). The waveform produced resembles an arterial pulse waveform and is easily quantified (see Fig. 4.23) into systolic, mean, and diastolic flow velocities and pulsatility index. Pulsatility index is a calculated parameter that was originally thought to correlate very well with cerebrovascular resistance.[57] More recently, however, a study has suggested that the correlation may not be so straightforward.[58]

When interpreting TCD values, an assumption is made that changes in blood flow velocity in cerebral arteries reflects changes in cortical CBF. As long as blood flow velocity is maintained, CBF is presumed to be adequate. Reductions in blood flow velocity below a critical value would reflect critical reductions in blood flow that could produce ischemia. This assumption would only be true so long as the measurement angle of the Doppler probe is nearly constant and the diameter of the conducting cerebral arteries does not change.

Unfortunately, this monitor has not been adequately validated in a large series of intraoperative cases against either established monitors of CBF, such as the EEG, or against direct cortical CBF measurements. One early study showed no significant correlation between measured CBF and middle cerebral artery blood flow velocity.[59] Several more recent series involving relatively small numbers of patients have, however, suggested that TCD is useful. Two recent articles documented an increase in perioperative neurologic morbidity if more than 10 particulate embolic events were detected during surgery[60,61] (see Fig. 9.7). Other studies have suggested that TCD detection of emboli occurs commonly without concomitant changes in the EEG.[62,63] Finally, several studies have used TCD successfully to predict which patients are at risk for postoperative hyperperfusion syndrome (see later). Increases in the mean flow velocity of more than 175 percent or in the pulsatility index of more than 100 percent predicted the development of hyperperfusion-related postoperative symptoms.[64,65] Finally, although one large multi-institutional study of TCD during 1,500 CEAs did not formally compare TCD with other methods of assessing the adequacy of CBF, the investigators did find an excellent correlation, however, between prolonged reduction in blood flow and postoperative stroke.[66] Of more interest, however, was their finding that the use of a shunt in patients without significant reduction in CBF velocity increased the risk of stroke six times, suggesting that routine shunting is not benign.

The major uses of TCD have been described primarily during the cross-clamping period. The period of carotid cross-clamping is only a relatively small portion of the time that the patient with carotid disease is at risk for ischemia, and most strokes occur at other times during surgery or postoperatively. Little data are available about the nature and degree of acceptable TCD changes during the remainder of the operation. Normal variations in blood flow velocities in patients without cerebrovascular disease appear to be large and not necessarily associated with definable events (Pushayan AG; Mahla ME; unpublished data). Technically satisfactory recordings cannot be obtained in some patients

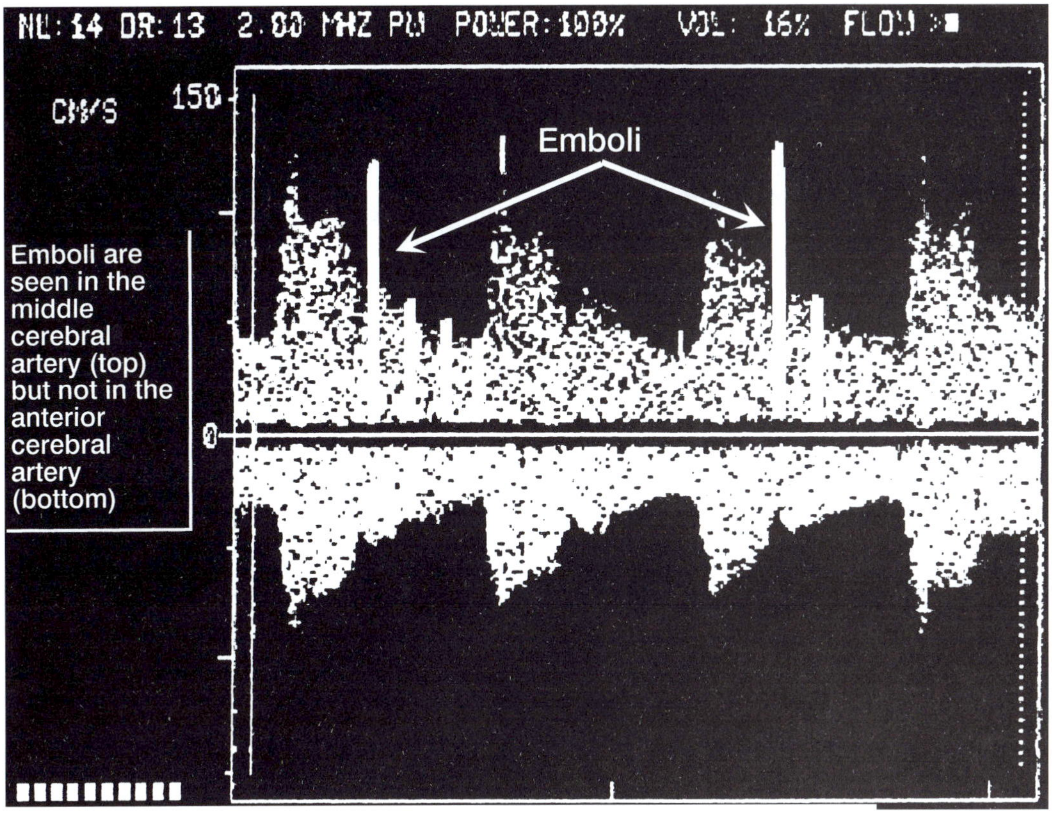

FIGURE 9.7 *Transcranial Doppler waveform demonstrating cerebral microemboli.*

(particularly elderly women), rendering TCD measurement useless in these individuals.

TCD is very attractive because it is easy to use and continuous. Manufacturers have developed new hardware and software that have changed the device from a diagnostic tool to a monitor. TCD clearly is of benefit in the laboratory evaluation of patients with cerebrovascular disease. Much further laboratory and clinical work is needed, however, before this device can be used universally in place of other monitoring techniques during carotid surgery. This monitor appears to be valuable as an adjunct to electrophysiologic monitoring and may be extremely useful in detecting particulate or air embolism to cerebral circulation that allows immediate surgical intervention to prevent further embolization.

REGIONAL CEREBRAL BLOOD FLOW

Regional CBF may be directly measured intraoperatively. CBF can be measured with an array of detectors placed over the head that detect radioactivity associated with either intravenous or intracarotid injection of radioactive xenon. The radioactivity washout pattern is directly dependent on CBF. Although this measurement may be repeated multiple times during surgery, it is not a continuous measurement and is usually performed only just before and after carotid cross-clamping. CBF measurements supplement, but are not a substitute for, a continuous monitor of cerebral function. Because these measurements require radioactive xenon as well as sophisticated computer analysis, they are unlikely to become widely popular or the standard of care in the near future.

CEREBRAL OXIMETRY A new continuous indirect measurement of regional CBF uses near-infrared transmission spectroscopy. This now commercially available instrument uses a single probe secured to the scalp with adhesive. (Multichannel instruments are not yet available). In transmission spectroscopy, infrared light is passed through the skull and measures the venous oxygen saturation in the very superficial portion of the cortex beneath the probe (see Fig. 4.26). Preliminary studies exposing animals to severe levels of hypoxemia show that cerebral hemoglobin oxygen saturation detected by this device falls before EEG changes occur.[67] In addition, several studies in humans document cerebral oximetry's ability to detect falls in brain hemoglobin oxygen saturation.[68–70] One study, however, showed a substantial contribution of the extracranial circulation to the measured value.[71] Thus, a major problem with this monitoring device involves what it is actually measuring. Although this monitor looks very promising, studies are only preliminary. As with the TCD, there are no *large* clinical studies comparing this monitor to established monitors of CBF such as EEG or radioactive xenon washout. This monitor must be considered experimental but potentially useful at this time.

INTERNAL CAROTID ARTERY STUMP PRESSURE Internal carotid artery stump pressure is defined as the pressure remaining in the carotid artery distal to the cross-clamp. A stump pressure of more than 50 mmHg has been hypothesized to represent adequate collateral circulation via the circle of Willis or the external carotid circulation. Unfortunately, stump pressure does not correlate to measured regional CBF or EEG changes when this hypothesis is tested clinically.[72–75] Also, in patients anesthetized with regional anesthesia, stump pressures do not correlate reliably to the development (or lack of development) of neurologic symptoms after application of the carotid cross-clamp. In our opinion, although many surgeons continue to use this method, there are no data to support the continued use of this technique to monitor adequacy of CBF.

The Bottom Line

Some form of neurologic monitoring during CEA is needed in today's practice. A published consensus statement from a multidisciplinary group concludes that EEG, evoked potentials, or an awake patient currently meet the standard of care for neurologic monitoring during CEA.[76] Although several of the other modalities appear promising, they either are not continuous (regional CBF) or lack sufficient clinical trials to conclude that they clearly are as effective as other established monitoring methods (TCD, cerebral oximetry).

ANESTHETIC TECHNIQUES DURING CAROTID SURGERY

Premedication of the patient undergoing CEA may help prevent preinduction hypertension, tachycardia, and potential myocardial ischemia associated with preoperative anxiety. However, use of premedication may increase the incidence of postoperative somnolence, which would be difficult to distinguish from cerebral ischemia or infarction. Long-acting premedication, particularly the benzodiazepines, should thus be avoided. Shorter-acting benzodiazepines and narcotics may be useful. Their effects on CNS monitoring should, however, be considered before their use. All regularly scheduled cardiovascular drugs should usually be given.

Regional/Local Anesthesia

The patient undergoing CEA with regional anesthesia may be satisfactorily blocked with a deep and superficial cervical plexus block or with a single injection high in the interscalen groove (at the C4 level). Simple local infiltration (field block) has also been widely reported as an effective technique. These techniques allow continuous neurologic examination during surgery. In addition, excellent hemodynamic stability associated with regional anesthesia seems to result in a very low incidence of perioperative MI.[44,45,47,77–79] Indeed, several studies have shown significantly improved hemodynamic stability when compared with patients undergoing CEA under general anesthesia.[46,80–82] This observation has led some to consider regional anesthesia the technique of choice for CEA. Unfortunately, few of these studies are prospective, randomized, controlled studies, and none involve very large numbers. However, in the opinion of one of the authors (M.E.M.) based on considerable personal experience, it is very likely that during CEA the requirement for vasoactive drugs for control of blood pressure either intraoperatively or postoperatively is lower with regional or local anesthesia.

Regional anesthesia has several disadvantages, however. First, the operative experience may be unpleasant for the patient, particularly if the operation is long and the surgeon is not gentle. This patient may require significant sedation with benzodiazepines, narcotics, or both. Such sedation produces a decrease in the level of consciousness, which may be confused with or, in fact, mask cerebral ischemia while the patient sleeps. Second, if the patient experiences CNS ischemia that does not promptly reverse, oxygenation and ventilation are not necessarily well controlled, and cerebral ischemia may worsen if the patient becomes systemically hypoxemic or hypercapnic. Reported incidence of conversion to general anesthesia ranges from 5 to 15 percent.

General Anesthesia

Considerations for the patient undergoing CEA with general anesthesia fall into three main areas: (1) anesthetic technique used, (2) how hemodynamics are controlled, and (3) control of carbon dioxide and glucose. There is no evidence based on outcome data that favors the use of one anesthetic technique for CEA over another. There is considerable controversy about whether isoflurane may protect the brain from ischemia and therefore be the agent of choice for CEA. On the promising side, data from the Mayo Clinic showed that EEG changes suggestive of ischemia occur at a much lower CBF with isoflurane (8 ml.100 g^{-1}.min^{-1}) than with halothane or enflurane (18 ml.100 g^{-1}.min^{-1}).[49] On the negative side, data from primates subjected to regional cerebral ischemia showed that animals pretreated with isoflurane had no protection from regional cerebral ischemia whereas animals pretreated with thiopental showed significant protection. Outcome in primates receiving isoflurane for protection was actually worse than control animals who were given no agents for protection at all.[83]

There is also controversy about whether patients should be given a bolus of thiopental before carotid cross-clamping to protect the brain from ischemia. Barbiturates have been demonstrated in both animals and humans to provide protection from focal cerebral ischemia if given before the insult. The mechanism for this protection is not clear. Barbiturates when given in a dosage sufficient to abolish all EEG electrical activity will reduce the cerebral metabolic rate by nearly 50 percent. Originally, investigators thought that this metabolic rate reduction was responsible for cerebral protection. More recently, however, other investigators have found that neither etomidate[84] nor isoflurane,[83] both of which reduce cerebral metabolic rate, are able to provide significant protection from focal ischemia. Indeed, these drugs may actually worsen outcome.[83,84]

Although protective treatment with thiopental seems logical, there is no outcome evidence that barbiturate pretreatment reduces either the incidence or severity of perioperative stroke during CEA. Second, most strokes do not occur during the period of carotid cross-clamping, but rather are caused by particulate embolism either before or after carotid repair. Finally, thiopental treatment will render the EEG isoelectric for a period of time. During that time, EEG is useless for detecting cerebral ischemia that could be treated by elevation of blood pressure, shunting, or both. In our opinion, there is some rationale to giving a bolus of thiopental to a patient with multiple critical stenotic lesions in whom temporary shunting would be dangerous or impossible. If test cross-clamping immediately results in severe EEG slowing and loss of power, cross-clamping should be released. After restoration of flow, thiopental may be given before reclamping the artery for definitive repair. We do not recommend use of bolus thiopental for cerebral protection except in that circumstance.

Carotid artery surgery is often associated with wide swings in blood pressure. It has been traditionally thought that such blood pressure swings were caused by transient surgically induced dysfunction of the carotid baroreceptors, but there may be other mechanisms involved. Some surgeons claim that injection of local anesthetic around the baroreceptor is effective in controlling blood pressure changes. However, a prospective randomized studies of injection of the carotid sinus nerve as a method of controlling blood pressure during and after CEA failed to demonstrate any benefit.[85] In fact, the incidence of perioperative hypertension was actually increased.

Clinicians have evolved two main methods of treating and preventing these changes in blood pressure. Blood pressure may be controlled by changes in anesthetic drug level or with hemodynamic agents such as phenylephrine, ephedrine, esmolol, nitroprusside, or nitroglycerine. A recent study suggested that control of hypotensive episodes by withdrawal of anesthetic is associated with a lower incidence of ventricular wall motion abnormalities suggestive of myocardial ischemia. Control of hypotension with titrated phenylephrine was associated with a greater incidence and severity of wall motion abnormalities.[86] These data suggest that control of hemodynamics by adjusting anesthetic agent concentration is preferred. However, frequent adjustments of anesthetic agent needed for control of hemodynamics may be associated with EEG changes that could increase the difficulty associated with interpretation of the EEG. In another recent study of 171 CEAs, phenylephrine was given only during persistent, EEG-diagnosed ischemia that did not respond to shunting, release of cross-clamp, or other means of increasing blood pressure within 2 minutes.[87] The incidence of MI was quite low (1.2 percent, nonfatal) and not increased in the patients given phenylephrine. We recommend this approach, which seems logical and avoids drug-induced alterations in the EEG.

In addition to blood pressure, other parameters must also be controlled. Because carbon dioxide is a potent cerebral vasodilator, changes in arterial carbon dioxide are associated with changes in CBF. Increases in the partial pressure of arterial carbon dioxide ($PaCO_2$) will cause cerebral vasodilation. In areas of ischemic brain, blood vessels are already maximally vasodilated. Increases in $PaCO_2$ can only dilate vessels in nonischemic brain. Dilation of these vessels may steal blood from areas of the brain where maximal dilation has already occurred. Decreases in $PaCO_2$ cause cerebral vasoconstriction and theoretically could increase blood flow to ischemic areas by decreasing flow to normal areas. This phenomenon has not been shown to occur reliably, however, and there is some laboratory evidence that hypocapnia may aggravate the effects of ischemia on cerebral metabolism.[88] Therefore, during CEA, $PaCO_2$ should be kept at preoperative levels and should not be adjusted unless cerebral function is monitored with EEG during the adjustment to document the effect.[89]

Another parameter under the control of the anesthesiologist is the glucose level. In animal studies, the brain has been shown to be more susceptible to ischemic injury when the animal is given glucose before and during the insult period.[90–92] Patients with poorly controlled blood sugar presenting with stroke may have a worse neurologic outcome,[93–95] but some investigators think that the hyperglycemia seen in these patients may reflect the stress of a more severe stroke.[96] Although no outcome studies have proved this hypothesis, these data would suggest that withholding perioperative glucose and close monitoring of glucose levels in all patients would be prudent during CEA because there is a risk for cerebral ischemia.

Cerebral Hyperperfusion Syndrome

Blood pressure swings often continue for several days into the postoperative period and may require continued use of vasoactive drugs. Patients with severe stenoses of carotid vessels are at particular risk for postoperative hypertension. Because of the stenosis-induced reduction in cerebral perfusion pressure, parts of the intracerebral circulation in these patients can no longer autoregulate and will be maximally vasodilated preoperatively to preserve CBF. With restoration of cerebral perfusion pressure after CEA, the brain experiences greatly increased CBF. Because the involved brain could not autoregulate preoperatively, increased blood flow after CEA cannot be reduced to normal values. Cerebral edema and possible intracranial hemorrhage may ensue.[97] These patients must have very careful postendarterectomy control of hypertension to prevent this catastrophic syndrome. Patients who experience intracranial hemorrhage have a very high mortality rate. Recent studies have suggested that TCD ultrasound monitoring may be used to detect those patients who are at particular risk for this syndrome and allow prophylactic pharmacologic reduction of blood pressure to safe levels.[64,65]

The Issue of Cost

Several recent studies have either proved or suggested that patients undergoing CEA may do so much less expensively.[98–100] In fact, at our own institution a retrospective comparison was made of 60 patients who underwent CEA with 30 patients receiving each anesthetic technique. The demographic data on the two groups were not statistically different in any area. The hospital cost (not patient charges) for patients undergoing CEA in the regional anesthesia group was less than 50 percent of the cost for the patients who had general anesthesia (Harward, unpublished data) (Fig. 9.8A and B). Considering hospital DRG reimbursement for CEA, this savings means the difference between a $500 loss (general anesthesia) and a $5,500 profit. Nearly all this cost savings came from two areas: intensive care unit (ICU) care and time in the hospital. None of the patients who had regional anesthesia required postoperative intensive care and all went home the morning after surgery. Virtually all the patients in the general anesthesia group went to the ICU postoperatively and stayed in the hospital slightly more than 3 days. It is not clear why either the ICU or the longer hospital stay was necessary, except that both have been common practice for many years. Studies performed in other institutions have suggested that this practice may, indeed, not be necessary in most cases.[98–100]

Several questions must be answered before these cost data become compelling. First, what is the mechanism of the greater hemodynamic stability? Does regional anesthesia itself provide protection from hemodynamic instability or does general anesthesia cause the instability? If regional anesthesia provides protection, then a combined technique may be the technique of choice because it controls the airway in case of

FIGURE 9.8 *Cost of carotid artery surgery. (A) General versus regional anesthesia—hospital cost versus reimbursement. (B) Most of the difference in hospital cost relates to length of stay and ICU care.*

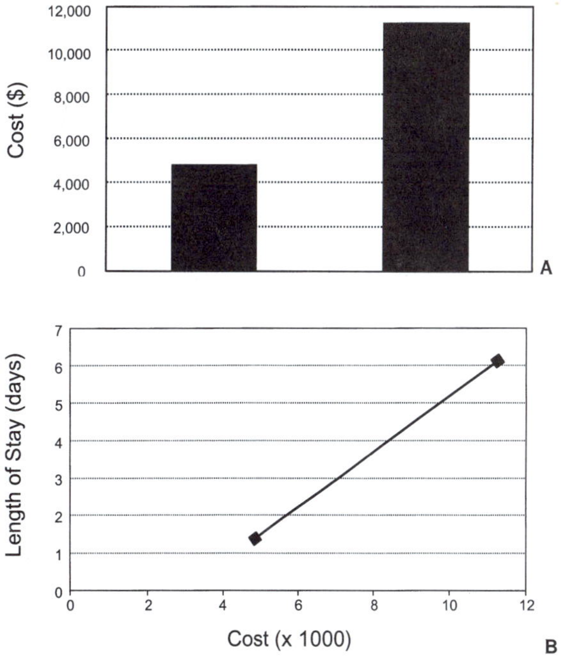

cerebral ischemia, eliminates the need for patient cooperation, and still provides the hemodynamic stability that will allow a shorter hospital stay. Second, when is it safe to send patients home after CEA? The vast majority, but clearly not all strokes, occur within 24 hours of surgery. Cardiovascular events are actually more common on the third than the first postoperative day. Much of the total cost savings for a year will be lost if a devastating complication occurs at home that could have been detected and treated earlier with a presumably better outcome were the patient still in the hospital. Certainly, those studies that have been published suggest that is safe to send patients home early after CEA, but the numbers reported in the literature are still too small to make this a standard of care. Clearly, the insurance industry will and has seized on this data and will pressure the clinical community to use regional anesthesia and send patients home early. It is thus *very* important for us as a clinical community to answer these two questions.

EXTRACRANIAL-INTRACRANIAL BYPASS OPERATIONS

The extracranial-intracranial (EC-IC) bypass operation used to be performed much more frequently than it currently is. This operation was used for symptomatic patients with intracranial narrowing of the carotid artery. In the EC-IC bypass, most commonly the superficial temporal artery is anastomosed with a distal branch of the middle cerebral artery through a small craniotomy. This anastomosis increases flow (albeit in reverse) in the distribution of the middle and anterior cerebral arteries ipsilateral to the operation. Other extracranial and intracranial arteries may also be used, but these are the most commonly used. A prospective, randomized trial published in the mid-1980s,[101,102] however, demonstrated that this operation together with aggressive reduction of medical risk factors was no more effective than aggressive medical therapy alone in preventing subsequent stroke or in reducing the severity of strokes. This study provoked considerable controversy, especially related to the way that the patients were randomized to medical and surgical treatment groups. Some reviewers thought that the highest-risk patients were assigned nonrandomly to receive surgical treatment, thus biasing the study and rendering its conclusions invalid. Despite the fact that this study is not widely accepted in the academic community, EC-IC bypass is not commonly performed now and is reserved only for patients in whom aggressive medical therapy has failed to stop symptoms.

The EC-IC bypass operation also has other uses that are accepted. The most common use of this operation is to preserve cerebral circulation in the case of patients with giant intracranial aneurysms that cannot be clipped in the usual fashion. For example, a patient with a giant internal carotid artery aneurysm that cannot be clipped (e.g., extending into the cavernous sinus and involving the portion of the carotid artery encased in the skull), ligation of the internal carotid artery in the neck with clipping of the internal carotid artery distal to the aneurysm will trap the aneurysm and cut of its blood supply. However, the patient may then suffer from inadequate flow to the anterior and middle cerebral arteries on that side. If a trial occlusion of the internal carotid artery conducted in the angiography suite produces neurologic symptoms, an EC-IC bypass may be performed before trapping the aneurysm to preserve CBF after the aneurysm is trapped.

Anesthetic Considerations

In patients with intracranial occlusive disease, anesthetic considerations are identical with those discussed previously for CEA. These patients also have significant cardiovascular disease and will require the same types of monitoring for both the CNS and CVS. The only significant difference between the operations involves the more routine use of barbiturate cerebral protection during the EC-IC bypass operation. Because a distal branch of a major cerebral vessel must be occluded temporarily to allow the anastomosis between it and the extracranial vessel, barbiturates may be given to produce EEG electrical silence. SSEP monitoring may then be used to assess adequacy of middle cerebral artery and anterior cerebral artery blood flow. The more proximal the branch of the cerebral vessel used for the anastomosis, the more likely the surgeon is to request barbiturate protection. When anticipating the use of barbiturate protection, the patient's left ventricular function must be carefully evaluated and appropriate monitoring (e.g., transesophageal echocardiography or pulmonary artery catheter) established if there is significant compromise. If the patient has normal ventricular function, the primary effect of high-dose barbiturate therapy will be to reduce preload (venodilation). An infusion of phenylephrine is usually sufficient to treat the resulting hypotension. If the patient has compromised left ventricular function, inotropic support will likely be needed.

INTERVENTIONAL NEURORADIOLOGY

Neuroradiologists are taking an increasing role in the treatment of patients with carotid disease. Balloon angioplasty and stent placement are being performed at an increasing rate to treat both lesions that are not surgically accessible and those that would normally be treated by surgery.[103–105] The anesthetic technique for these procedures has not yet been well defined. Some centers use monitored anesthesia care and depend on ability to assess the neurologic function of the awake patient as the monitor of the adequacy of the cerebral circulation. Other centers prefer general anesthesia because it better controls patient movement and allows prompt administration of barbiturates in the case of damage to the arterial circulation (dissection, embolization, rupture) that may require immediate surgical intervention. If general anesthesia is used, all the neurologic and cardiovascular monitoring considerations discussed for CEA apply to interventional neuroradiology as well. The anesthetic considerations are also similar because these patients, of course, have the same cardiovascular diseases.

CONCLUSIONS

CEA as a surgical procedure is being better defined with respect to its indications. This redefinition *may* result in an increased number of operations performed. Anesthesiologists, because of their expertise in monitoring and cardiovascular physiology, can take a leading role in intraoperative monitoring and treatment of the CNS and CVS that are at significant risk during this operation. These areas have the greatest potential for improving overall morbidity and mortality in this challenging operation.

References

1. Winslow CM, Solomon DH, Chassin MR et al: The appropriateness of carotid endarterectomy. N Engl J Med 318:721, 1988
2. North American Symptomatic Carotid Endarterectomy Trial Collaborators: Beneficial effect of carotid endarterectomy in symptomatic patients with high-grade carotid stenosis. N Engl J Med 325:445, 1991
3. European Carotid Surgery Trialists Collaborative Group: MRC European carotid surgery trial: interim results for symptomatic patients with severe (70–99%) or with mild (0–29%) carotid stenosis. Lancet 337:1235, 1991
4. The Casanova Study Group: Carotid surgery versus medical therapy in asymptomatic carotid stenosis. Stroke 22:1229, 1991
5. Hobson RW, Weiss DG, Fields WS et al: Efficacy of carotid endarterectomy for asymptomatic carotid stenosis. The Veterans Affairs Cooperative Study Group. N Engl J Med 328:221, 1993
6. Mayo Asymptomatic Carotid Endarterectomy Study Group: Results of a randomized controlled trial of carotid endarterectomy for asymptomatic carotid stenosis. Mayo Clin Proc 67:513, 1992
7. Brott T, Toole JF: Medical compared with surgical treatment of asymptomatic carotid artery stenosis. Ann Intern Med 123:720, 1995
8. Miller JD, Smith RR, Holaday HR: Carbon diox-

ide reactivity in the evaluation of cerebral ischemia. Neurosurgery 30:518, 1992
9. Cikrit DF, Burt RW, Dalsing MC et al: Acetazolamide enhanced single photon emission computed tomography (SPECT) evaluation of cerebral perfusion before and after carotid endarterectomy. J Vasc Surg 15:747, 1992
10. Steiger HJ, Aaslid R, Stoos R: Dynamic computed tomographic imaging of regional cerebral blood flow and blood volume. A clinical pilot study. Stroke 24:591, 1993
11. Piepgras A, Schmiedek P, Leinsinger G et al: A simple test to assess cerebrovascular reserve capacity using transcranial Doppler sonography and acetazolamide. Stroke 21:1306, 1990
12. Thiel A, Zickmann B, Stertmann WA et al: Cerebrovascular carbon dioxide reactivity in carotid artery disease. Relation to intraoperative cerebral monitoring results in 100 carotid endarterectomies. Anesthesiology 82:655, 1995
13. Sieber FE, Toung TJ, Diringer MN et al: Preoperative risks predict neurologic outcome of carotid endarterectomy related stroke. Neurosurgery 30:847, 1992
14. Asiddao CB, Donegan JH, Whitesell RC, Kalbfleisch JH: Factors associated with perioperative complications during carotid endarterectomy. Anesth Analg 61:631, 1982
15. Archie JP Jr. The relationship of early hypertension following carotid endarterectomy to intraoperative cerebral ischemia. Ann Vasc Surg 2:108, 1988
16. Prys-Roberts C, Meloche R, Foex P: Studies of anaesthesia in relation to hypertension. I. Cardiovascular responses of treated and untreated patients. Br J Anaesth 43:122, 1971
17. Rihal CS, Gersh BJ, Whisnant JP et al: Influence of coronary heart disease on morbidity and mortality after carotid endarterectomy: a population-based study in Olmsted County, Minnesota (1970–1988) [published erratum appears in J Am Coll Cardiol 20:1304, 1992]. J Am Coll Cardiol 19:1254, 1992
18. Mangano DT, Browner WS, Hollenberg M et al: Association of perioperative myocardial ischemia with cardiac morbidity and mortality in men undergoing noncardiac surgery. The Study of Perioperative Ischemia Research Group [see comments]. N Engl J Med 323:1781, 1990
19. Mangano DT, Hollenberg M, Fegert G et al: Perioperative myocardial ischemia in patients undergoing noncardiac surgery—I: Incidence and severity during the 4 day perioperative period. The Study of Perioperative Ischemia (SPI) Research Group. J Am Coll Cardiol 17:843, 1991
20. McCann RL, Clements FM: Silent myocardial ischemia in patients undergoing peripheral vascular surgery: incidence and association with perioperative cardiac morbidity and mortality. J Vasc Surg 9:583, 1989
21. Landesberg G, Erel J, Anner H et al: Perioperative myocardial ischemia in carotid endarterectomy under cervical plexus block and prophylactic nitroglycerin infusion [see comments]. J Cardiothorac Vasc Anesth 7:259, 1993
22. Bodenheimer MM: Noncardiac surgery in the cardiac patient: what is the question? [see comments]. Ann Intern Med 124:763, 1996
23. Fleisher LA, Eagle KA: Screening for cardiac disease in patients having noncardiac surgery [comment]. Ann Intern Med 124:767, 1996
24. Asiddao CB, Donegan JH, Whitesell RC, Kalbfleisch JH: Factors associated with perioperative complications during carotid endarterectomy. Anesth Analg 61:631, 1982
25. Gersh BJ, Rihal CS, Rooke TW, Ballard DJ: Evaluation and management of patients with both peripheral vascular and coronary artery disease. J Am Coll Cardiol 18:203, 1991
26. Hertzer NR, Beven EG, Young JR et al: Coronary artery disease in peripheral vascular patients. A classification of 1000 coronary angiograms and results of surgical management. Ann Surg 199:223, 1984
27. Chimowitz MI, Weiss DG, Cohen SL et al: Cardiac prognosis of patients with carotid stenosis and no history of coronary artery disease. Veterans Affairs Cooperative Study Group 167. Stroke 25:759, 1994
28. Urbinati S, Di Pasquale G, Andreoli A et al: Frequency and prognostic significance of silent coronary artery disease in patients with cerebral ischemia undergoing carotid endarterectomy [see comments]. Am J Cardiol 69:1166, 1992
29. Prys Roberts C, Greene LT, Meloche R, Foex P: Studies of anaesthesia in relation to hypertension. II. Haemodynamic consequences of induction and endotracheal intubation. Br J Anaesth 43:531, 1971
30. Eagle KA, Brundage BH, Chaitman BR et al: Guidelines for perioperative cardiovascular evaluation for noncardiac surgery. Report of the American College of Cardiology/American Heart Association Task Force on Practice Guidelines. Committee on Perioperative Cardiovascular

Evaluation for Noncardiac Surgery. Circulation 93:1278, 1996
31. Goldman L: Assessment of the patient with known or suspected ischaemic heart disease for noncardiac surgery. Br J Anaesth 61:38, 1988
32. McPhail N, Calvin JE, Shariatmadar A et al: The use of preoperative exercise testing to predict cardiac complications after arterial reconstruction. J Vasc Surg 7:60, 1988
33. Boucher CA, Brewster DC, Darling RC et al: Determination of cardiac risk by dipyridamole-thallium imaging before peripheral vascular surgery. N Engl J Med 312:389, 1985
34. Eagle KA, Coley CM, Newell JB et al: Combining clinical and thallium data optimizes preoperative assessment of cardiac risk before major vascular surgery. Ann Intern Med 110:859, 1989
35. L'Italien GJ, Paul SD, Hendel RC et al: Development and validation of a Bayesian model for perioperative cardiac risk assessment in a cohort of 1,081 vascular surgical candidates [see comments]. J Am Coll Cardiol 27:779, 1996
36. Mangano DT, London MJ, Tubau JF et al: Dipyridamole thallium-201 scintigraphy as a preoperative screening test. A reexamination of its predictive potential. Study of Perioperative Ischemia Research Group [see comments]. Circulation 84:493, 1991
37. Baron JF, Mundler O, Bertrand M et al: Dipyridamole-thallium scintigraphy and gated radionuclide angiography to assess cardiac risk before abdominal aortic surgery [see comments]. N Engl J Med 330:663, 1994
38. Poldermans D, Fioretti PM, Forster T et al: Dobutamine stress echocardiography for assessment of perioperative cardiac risk in patients undergoing major vascular surgery [see comments]. Circulation 87:1506, 1993
39. Poldermans D, Arnese M, Fioretti PM et al: Improved cardiac risk stratification in major vascular surgery with dobutamine-atropine stress echocardiography. J Am Coll Cardiol 26:648, 1995
40. Raby KE, Goldman L, Creager MA et al: Correlation between preoperative ischemia and major cardiac events after peripheral vascular surgery [see comments]. N Engl J Med 321:1296, 1989
41. Fleisher LA, Rosenbaum SH, Nelson AH et al: Preoperative dipyridamole thallium imaging and ambulatory electrocardiographic monitoring as a predictor of perioperative cardiac events and long-term outcome [see comments]. Anesthesiology 83:906, 1995
42. Halm EA, Browner WS, Tubau JF et al: Echocardiography for assessing cardiac risk in patients having noncardiac surgery. Study of Perioperative Ischemia Research Group. Ann Intern Med 125:433, 1996
43. Calvin JE, Kieser TM, Walley VM et al: Cardiac mortality and morbidity after vascular surgery. Can J Surg 29:93, 1986
44. Shah DM, Darling RC, Chang BB et al: Carotid endarterectomy in awake patients: its safety, acceptability, and outcome. J Vasc Surg 19:1015, 1994
45. Donato AT, Hill SL: Carotid arterial surgery using local anesthesia: a private practice retrospective study. Am Surg 58:446, 1992
46. Forssell C, Takolander R, Bergqvist D et al: Local versus general anaesthesia in carotid surgery. A prospective, randomised study. Eur J Vasc Surg 3:503, 1989
47. Hafner CD, Evans WE: Carotid endarterectomy with local anesthesia: results and advantages. J Vasc Surg 7:232, 1988
48. Sundt TM Jr, Sharbrough FW, Piepgras DG et al: Correlation of cerebral blood flow and electroencephalographic changes during carotid endarterectomy. Mayo Clin Proc 56:533, 1981
49. Messick JM Jr, Casement B, Sharbrough FW et al: Correlation of regional cerebral blood flow (rCBF) with EEG changes during isoflurane anesthesia for carotid endarterectomy: critical rCBF. Anesthesiology 66:344, 1987
50. Spackman TN, Faust RJ, Cucchiara RF et al: A comparison of a periodic analysis of the EEG with standard EEG and cerebral blood flow for the detection of ischemia. Anesthesiology 66:229, 1987
51. Kearse LA, Brown EN, McPeck K: Somatosensory evoked potentials sensitivity relative to electroencephalography for cerebral ischemia during carotid endarterectomy. Stroke 23:498, 1992
52. Craft RM, Losasso TJ, Perkins WJ et al: EEG monitoring for cerebral ischemia during carotid endarterectomy (CEA): how much is enough? abstracted Neurosurg Anesth 6:301, 1994
53. Kearse LA, Brown EN, McPeck K: Somatosensory evoked potentials sensitivity relative to electroencephalography for cerebral ischemia during carotid endarterectomy. Stroke 23:498, 1992
54. Lam AM, Manninen PH, Ferguson GG et al: Monitoring electrophysiologic function during carotid endarterectomy: a comparison of somatosensory evoked potentials and conventional

electroencephalogram. Anesthesiology 75:15, 1991
55. Branston NM, Ladds A, Symon L, Wang AD: Comparison of the effects of ischaemia on early components of the somatosensory evoked potential in brainstem, thalamus, and cerebral cortex. J Cereb Blood Flow Metab 4:68, 1984
56. Drummond JC, Todd MM, U HS: The effect of high dose sodium thiopental on brain stem auditory and median nerve somatosensory evoked responses in humans. Anesthesiology 63:249, 1985
57. Aaslid R, Markwalder TM, Nornes H: Noninvasive transcranial Doppler ultrasound recording of flow velocity in basal cerebral arteries. J Neurosurg 57:769, 1982
58. Czosnyka M, Richards HK, Whitehouse HE, Pickard JD: Relationship between transcranial Doppler-determined pulsatility index and cerebrovascular resistance: an experimental study. J Neurosurg 84:79, 1996
59. Halsey JH, McDowell HA, Gelman S: Transcranial Doppler and rCBF compared in carotid endarterectomy. Stroke 17:1206, 1986
60. Gaunt ME, Brown L, Hartshorne T et al: Unstable carotid plaques: preoperative identification and association with intraoperative embolisation detected by transcranial Doppler. Eur J Vasc Endovasc Surg 11:78, 1996
61. Ackerstaff RG, Jansen C, Moll FL et al: The significance of microemboli detection by means of transcranial Doppler ultrasonography monitoring in carotid endarterectomy. J Vasc Surg 21:963, 1995
62. Jansen C, Moll FL, Vermeulen FE et al: Continuous transcranial Doppler ultrasonography and electroencephalography during carotid endarterectomy: a multimodal monitoring system to detect intraoperative ischemia. Ann Vasc Surg 7:95, 1993
63. Jansen C, Vriens EM, Eikelboom BC et al: Carotid endarterectomy with transcranial Doppler and electroencephalographic monitoring. A prospective study in 130 operations. Stroke 24:665, 1993
64. Jansen C, Sprengers AM, Moll FL et al: Prediction of intracerebral haemorrhage after carotid endarterectomy by clinical criteria and intraoperative transcranial Doppler monitoring. Eur J Vasc Surg 8:303, 1994
65. Jorgensen LG, Schroeder TV: Defective cerebrovascular autoregulation after carotid endarterectomy. Eur J Vasc Surg 7:370, 1993
66. Halsey JHJ: Risks and benefits of shunting in carotid endarterectomy. The International Transcranial Doppler Collaborators. Stroke 23:1583, 1992
67. Rampil IJ, Litt L, Mayevsky A: Correlated, simultaneous, multiple-wavelength optical monitoring in vivo of localized cerebrocortical NADH and brain microvessel hemoglobin oxygen saturation. J Clin Monit 8:216, 1992
68. McCormick PW, Stewart M, Goetting MG et al: Noninvasive cerebral optical spectroscopy for monitoring cerebral oxygen delivery and hemodynamics. Crit Care Med 19:89, 1991
69. McCormick PW, Stewart M, Lewis G et al: Intracerebral penetration of infrared light (technical note). J Neurosurg 76:315, 1992
70. Slavin KV, Dujovny M, Ausman JI et al: Clinical experience with transcranial cerebral oximetry. Surg Neurol 42:531, 1994
71. Germon TJ, Kane NM, Manara AR, Nelson RJ: Near-infrared spectroscopy in adults: effects of extracranial ischaemia and intracranial hypoxia on estimation of cerebral oxygenation. Br J Anaesth 73:503, 1994
72. Okudaira Y, Arai H, Sato K: Cerebral blood flow alteration by acetazolamide during carotid balloon occlusion: parameters reflecting cerebral perfusion pressure in the acetazolamide test. Stroke 27:617, 1996
73. Archie JP Jr, Feldtman RW: Determinants of cerebral perfusion pressure during carotid endarterectomy. Arch Surg 117:319, 1982
74. Rowed DW, Vilaghy MI: Intraoperative regional cerebral blood flow during carotid endarterectomy. Can J Neurol Sci 8:235, 1981
75. McKay RD, Sundt TM, Michenfelder JD et al: Internal carotid artery stump pressure and cerebral blood flow during carotid endarterectomy: modification by halothane, enflurane, and innovar. Anesthesiology 45:390, 1976
76. Nuwer MR, Daube J, Fischer C et al: Neuromonitoring during surgery. Report of an IFCN Committee [see comments]. Electroencephalogr Clin Neurophysiol 87:263, 1993
77. Collier PE: Are one-day admissions for carotid endarterectomy feasible? Am J Surg 170:140, 1995
78. Kraiss LW, Kilberg L, Critch S, Johansen KJ: Short-stay carotid endarterectomy is safe and cost-effective. Am J Surg 169:512, 1995
79. Lee KS, Davis CH Jr, McWhorter JM: Low morbidity and mortality of carotid endarterectomy performed with regional anesthesia. J Neurosurg 69:483, 1988

80. Allen BT, Anderson CB, Rubin BG et al: The influence of anesthetic technique on perioperative complications after carotid endarterectomy. J Vasc Surg 19:834, 1994
81. Zuccarello M, Yeh HS, Tew JM: Morbidity and mortality of carotid endarterectomy under local anesthesia: a retrospective study. Neurosurgery 23:445, 1988
82. Luosto R, Ketonen P, Mattila S et al: Local anaesthesia in carotid surgery. A prospective study of 111 endarterectomies in 100 patients. Scand J Thorac Cardiovasc Surg 18:133, 1984
83. Nehls DG, Todd MM, Spetzler RF et al: A comparison of the cerebral protective effects of isoflurane and barbiturates during temporary focal ischemia in primates. Anesthesiology 66:453, 1987
84. Drummond JC, Cole DJ, Patel PM, Reynolds LW: Focal cerebral ischemia during anesthesia with etomidate, isoflurane, or thiopental: a comparison of the extent of cerebral injury. Neurosurgery 37:742, 1995
85. Elliot BM, Collins GJ Jr, Youkey JR et al: Intraoperative local anesthetic injection of the carotid sinus nerve. A prospective randomized study. Am J Surg 152:695, 1986
86. Smith JS, Roizen MF, Cahalan MK et al: Does anesthetic technique make a difference? Augmentation of systolic blood pressure during carotid endarterectomy: effects of phenylephrine versus light general anesthesia and of isoflurane versus halothane on the incidence of myocardial ischemia. Anesthesiology 69:846, 1988
87. Modica PA, Tempelhoff R, Rich KM et al: Computerized electroencephalographic monitoring and selective shunting: influence on intraoperative administration of phenylephrine and myocardial infarction after general anesthesia for carotid endarterectomy. Neurosurgery 30:842, 1992
88. Michenfelder JD, Sundt TM Jr: The effect of P_aCO_2 on the metabolism of ischemic brain in squirrel monkeys. Anesthesiology 38:445, 1973
89. Artru AA, Merriman HG: Hypocapnia added to hypertension to reverse EEG changes during carotid endarterectomy. Anesthesiology 70:1016, 1989
90. Lanier WL, Stangland KJ, Scheithauer BW et al: The effects of dextrose infusion and head position on neurologic outcome after complete cerebral ischemia in primates: examination of a model. Anesthesiology 66:39, 1987
91. Sieber FE, Traystman RJ: Special issues: glucose and the brain. Crit Care Med 20:104, 1992
92. Wass CT, Lanier WL: Glucose modulation of ischemic brain injury: review and clinical recommendations. Mayo Clin Proc 71:801, 1996
93. deFalco FA, Sepe-Visconti O, Fucci G, Caruso G: Correlation between hyperglycemia and cerebral infarct size in patients with stroke. A clinical and X-ray computed tomography study in 104 patients. Schweiz Arch Neurol Psychiatr 144:233, 1993
94. Broderick JP, Hagen T, Brott T, Tomsick T: Hyperglycemia and hemorrhagic transformation of cerebral infarcts. Stroke 26:484, 1995
95. Candelise L, Landi G, Orazio EN, Boccardi E: Prognostic significance of hyperglycemia in acute stroke. Arch Neurol 42:661, 1985
96. Woo J, Lam CW, Kay R et al: The influence of hyperglycemia and diabetes mellitus on immediate and 3-month morbidity and mortality after acute stroke. Arch Neurol 47:1174, 1990
97. Reigel MM, Hollier LH, Sundt TM Jr et al: Cerebral hyperperfusion syndrome: a cause of neurologic dysfunction after carotid endarterectomy. J Vasc Surg 5:628, 1987
98. Morasch MD, Hirko MK, Hirasa T et al: Intensive care after carotid endarterectomy: a prospective evaluation. J Am Coll Surg 183:387, 1996
99. Musser DJ, Calligaro KD, Dougherty MJ et al: Safety and cost-efficiency of 24-hour hospitalization for carotid endarterectomy. Am Vasc Surg 10:143, 1996
100. Luna G, Adye B: Cost-effective carotid endarterectomy. Am J Surg 169:516, 1995
101. The International Cooperative Study of Extracranial/Intracranial Arterial Anastomosis (EC/IC Bypass Study): methodology and entry characteristics. The EC/IC Bypass Study group. Stroke 16:397, 1985
102. Hornig CR, Dorndorf W, Busse O: Extracranial-intracranial anastomosis in the prevention of stroke. Results of the International EC-IC Bypass Study. Dtsch Med Wochenschr 111:243, 1986
103. Motarjeme A: Percutaneous transluminal angioplasty of supra-aortic vessels. J Endovasc Surg 3:171, 1996
104. Roubin GS, Yadav S, Iyer SS, Vitek J: Carotid stent-supported angioplasty: a neurovascular intervention to prevent stroke. Am J Cardiol 78:8, 1996
105. Higashida RT, Halbach VV, Tsai FY et al: Interventional neurovascular techniques for cerebral revascularization in the treatment of stroke. Am J Roentgenol 163:793, 1994

10 TUMOR SURGERY

SUSAN BLACK

ROY F. CUCCHIARA

BASIC PRINCIPLES

The scientific foundation of the anesthetic management of intracranial tumor patients has been discussed in depth in the first five chapters of this text. This brief review considers those concepts that are clinically applicable to the discussions in this chapter.

Intracranial Pressure

The individual volumes within the cranial vault (cerebral tissue, cerebral blood, and cerebrospinal fluid [CSF]) may be altered and produce a change in the other volumes or a change in intracranial pressure (ICP). This is important because anesthetic agents and techniques can produce acute changes in one or more of these volumes and thus in ICP. Intracranial hypertension manifested either clinically or by midline shift on computed tomographic (CT) scan suggests extra care in selecting anesthetic techniques, since ICP compensatory mechanisms have been exhausted and intracranial elastance is likely severely compromised. Clinically, the important concerns in the patient with elevated ICP are to avoid (1) further increases in ICP to a degree that would cause herniation of the brain or cerebral ischemia by reducing cerebral perfusion pressure (CPP) or (2) sudden reduction in ICP and an increase in CPP that might lead to cerebral hemorrhage, for example, as in aneurysm patients (see Ch. 8).

Control of ICP during induction and maintenance of neurosurgical anesthesia is important. Some recommend placing devices to measure ICP awake and while anesthesia is induced to prevent unknown alterations. On the other hand, we have specific drugs that decrease ICP available to us for induction. There are no data available to show that routine use of such monitored or unmonitored techniques is associated with any difference in outcome. It is probably currently a safe practice to use induction techniques in neurosurgery that do not include monitoring ICP, as suggested by the wide use of such techniques without apparent clinical ill effects or brain swelling when the dura is opened.

Cerebral blood flow (CBF) can be acutely modified by anesthetics, arterial blood gas tensions, and cerebral metabolic rate (CMR). All these can be manipulated clinically to help achieve our goals. The use of drugs for cerebral protection in tumor patients generally relates to control of ICP rather than ischemia. However, areas under a retractor or in a traumatized tumor bed may become ischemic. The use of cerebral protective agents or techniques as therapy for that type of ischemia is unsubstantiated and is a secondary consideration in agent selection.

ANESTHETIC MANAGEMENT OF THE TUMOR PATIENT

Supratentorial Tumors

CHOICE OF ANESTHETIC Most, but not all, anesthetics can be used safely in patients with cerebral lesions. There are specific effects of the agents that may require certain ancillary techniques in their administration to ensure appropriate pharmacologic and physiologic responses. The effects of the agent on ICP, CPP, CBF, CMR, promptness of return of consciousness, drug-related protection from cerebral ischemia or edema, blood pressure control, and compatibility with neurophysiologic monitoring techniques are important considerations.

Most craniotomy surgery in the United States today is probably performed following a thiopental induction of anesthesia with intubation of the trachea after a nondepolarizing relaxant. Maintenance of anesthesia is commonly accomplished with a combination of a volatile agent (usually isoflurane) and narcotic such as fentanyl, sufentanil, or alfentanil in various combinations during hypocarbia to $PaCO_2$ levels of 28 to 33 mmHg. Some institutions use propofol instead of a volatile agent. The use of nitrous oxide varies among neuroanesthesiologists.

The complex interrelationships of the anesthetics and their effects on cerebral hemodynamics and ICP are described in Chapter 3. With the use of volatile agents, an increase in ICP is an expected pharmacologic result if these drugs are used to produce deeper levels of anesthesia with normocarbia. However, this is rarely done in neoplastic neurosurgery. Most commonly, minimum alveolar concentration less than 1.0 minimum alveolar concentration (MAC) of a volatile agent is combined with moderate hyperventilation to provide an adequate level of anesthesia and to avoid increases in ICP. The greatest reduction in cerebral vascular resistance and the greatest increase in ICP is produced by halothane. In humans, this can be blunted or even eliminated by establishing hypocarbia before administration of the agent.[1] Isoflurane also reduces cerebral vascular resistance and increases ICP at normocarbia, but this response can be blocked by simultaneous introduction of hyperventilation in tumor patients.[2] Desflurane administration also results in decreases in cerebrovascular resistance and increases in CBF and ICP that at 1 MAC exceed those of isoflurane. However, at 0.5 MAC similar ICP effects may well be seen with desflurane and isoflurane.[3,4] Isoflurane remains the most commonly utilized volatile agent in neurosurgical patients. It has been suggested that patients with a midline shift on CT scan are more likely to show an elevation in ICP during isoflurane anesthesia, but the clinical applicability of the data is not striking.[5] On balance, human studies suggest that isoflurane is a safe anesthetic drug when used with hyperventilation for intracranial tumor surgery.[6]

Intravenous anesthetics (e.g., thiopental, fentanyl) decrease cerebral oxygen consumption ($CMRO_2$) and CBF together. This allows a reduction in ICP to be accomplished by modification of the vascular compartment. Thiopental safely produces a profound linked reduction in $CMRO_2$ and CBF to near half of the awake values.[7] The dramatic reduction in ICP that can be achieved with this drug clinically is secondary to these cerebral effects. Over the decades there has been a waxing and waning of enthusiasm for thiopental as an induction and maintenance agent in neurosurgical anesthesia. It is still our preferred induction agent in cerebral tumor patients. The effectiveness of thiopental as a cerebral protective drug should probably be viewed as applicable to the experimental conditions for which protection is most solidly demonstrated, that is, temporary focal cerebral ischemia by vascular occlusion techniques. Cerebral protection produced by lowering ICP in cerebral tumor patients is a distinctly different, although useful, concept. Etomidate decreases $CMRO_2$ with a lesser reduction in CBF and is a useful induction agent for special situations of hemodynamic instability.[8] It is known to produce myoclonus and possible seizure activity. Propofol also causes decreases in $CMRO_2$, CBF, and ICP.[9] Concern has been raised that in some circumstances the decrease in mean arterial pressure exceeds the decrease in ICP, resulting in lowering of CPP to pressures below the autoregulatory range in some patients.[10–12] None the less, propofol has been used safely for induction and maintenance of anesthesia in neurosurgical patients. We do not feel that it offers any real advantage for induction of open craniotomy patients. It may be used at the end of the case when isoflurane is being washed out to allow rapid emergence.

Although some early studies suggested that there were differences in the cerebral effects of fentanyl, sufentanil, and alfentanil, the majority of the studies suggest that these agents have similar effects.[13–15] Some studies in both animals and humans suggest that high doses of any of these agents can lead to increases in ICP that may be transient. The clinical implication of these results in unclear. These agents have all been utilized extensively in neurosurgical patients without ill effects.[15] These narcotics are useful in neurosurgical anesthesia because they afford maintenance of stable heart rate and blood pressure during surgical stimulus without delaying emergence or causing clinically significant adverse cerebral hemodynamic effects.

CHOICE OF MUSCLE RELAXANTS

Muscle relaxant use can probably affect the conduct of a neuroanesthetic as much as the primary agent. Succinylcholine (SCh) as yet appears unequaled in achieving total rapid paralysis for the rapid sequence intubation of the trachea. There is still controversy regarding SCh-induced increases in ICP.[16,17] However such increases are probably clinically insignificant except perhaps in the most extreme cases of intracranial hypertension. Although some recommend avoiding SCh in all patients with intracranial mass lesions, other neuroanesthesiologists continue to utilize the agent in selected patients in whom rapid onset and/or offset of muscle relaxation is critical. Since complete flaccidity is required to avoid coughing and straining during intubation of the trachea and thus avoid ICP increases, it is reasonable to use a nerve stimulator during induction and intubation in these cases. Use of short and intermediate-duration nondepolarizing muscle relaxants has been recommend by some.[18,19] Mivacurium has the shortest duration of action but a relatively slower onset of action (2 to 3 minutes).[20] Its use as a replacement for SCh for rapid sequence induction is limited by its longer onset time. A larger dose to achieve a more rapid onset time is complicated by histamine release.[21] Rocuronium in doses of 0.6 to 0.9 mg/kg has been reported to provide rapid (60 seconds) intubating conditions.[22] It may provide an alternative to SCh for rapid paralysis if the intermediate duration of action is not contraindicated. Agents such as vecuronium and rocuronium have shorter duration of action and less hemodynamic effects (vagolytic) than pancuronium.[23] Lack of cardiovascular side effects as compared to pancuronium makes these agents popular. However, the increased cost of using these agents throughout a long neurosurgical procedure must be considered.

Hemiplegia from cerebral ischemia or from cerebral tumor is associated with differences in response to nondepolarizing muscle relaxants on the two sides of the body. The affected extremities are resistant to neuromuscular blockade by nondepolarizing muscle relaxants.[24,25] In most operating room arrangements, the face and endotracheal tube are turned toward the anesthetist so that the operative field is uppermost. This places the extremities contralateral to the tumor in a position that allows easy monitoring of neuromuscular transmission. But that arm is likely to be more resistant to nondepolarizing muscle relaxants than the rest of the body, thus leading us to use a relative overdose of drug, making timely reversal difficult or impossible. However, it ensures that the patient will not move intraoperatively, because we are providing neuromuscular blockade of the most resistant muscles. SCh is associated with a significant complication in the hemiplegic patient, that of hyperkalemia.[26] The time of sensitivity is not well defined, but cases are reported from 1 week to 6 months after onset of hemiplegia.

INTRAOPERATIVE FLUIDS The patient's overall fluid and electrolyte status and specific electrolyte imbalances preoperatively and shifts in these parameters likely to occur intraoperatively guide the choice of intravenous fluids for tumor patients. Most elective patients do not seem to require the replacement of overnight fluid deficit. However, angiographic dye used in cerebral studies is osmotically active, and substantial intravascular fluid volume can be lost acutely as a result of diuresis.

An important factor in fluid administration is the integrity of the blood-brain barrier (BBB). For practical purposes, the surgical effort necessary to remove cerebral tumors always has the potential to leave the tissue immediately surrounding the resection with a damaged BBB from the trauma of resection or retractor ischemia. It is generally thought that limiting fluid administration to what is necessary to maintain hemodynamic stability helps prevent brain edema. Perhaps the converse is more applicable, that is, large volumes of fluid administered to the patient with an injured BBB contribute to cerebral edema. It is clinically unwise to allow significant intravascular hypovolemia to occur for fear of exacerbation of cerebral edema. Over the last decade the acceptable intraoperative volume administration has been liberalized somewhat.

There has been much controversy and research into the appropriate fluid types for use in neurosurgical patients. This issue is discussed in depth in Chapter 6. It appears that osmotic pressure rather than oncotic pressure of administered fluids is the determining factor in production of cerebral edema after fluid administration.[27,28] Hypotonic fluids should be avoided. Isotonic crystalloid and colloid have similar effects on cerebral edema and ICP. Hypertonic crystalloid causes the least cerebral edema or increase in ICP following fluid resuscitation.[29] Total volume of administered hypertonic saline should be guided by serum sodium determination and is usually limited to 500 to 1,000 ml in adults. If colloid administration is chosen among available agents, some concern has been raised regarding the potential for coagulopathy following hetastarch administration.[30] As long as total volume of hetastarch is limited to 1,000 ml in adults, this does not appear to be a clinical problem except possibly in patients with very vascular lesions.[31] Glucose administration has been demonstrated to increase the risk of neurologic injury following cerebral ischemia.[32–34] The most common regimen for fluid administration is non-glucose-containing isotonic fluids in volumes adequate to maintain hemodynamic stability. If volume depletion develops due to blood loss or diuretic administration, 3% saline for resuscitation is the likely best choice prior to transfusion.

CONTROL OF ICP DURING INDUCTION Many things occur sequentially during induction. Timing is important. Approaches that seem generally similar may produce very different patient responses because of timing and duration of pharmacologic intervention to balance stimulation. One popular technique is preinduction voluntary hyperventilation. Although hyperventilation decreases ICP, the application of a face mask to some awake brain tumor patients has been shown to transiently elevate ICP, perhaps due to anxiety. We do not know whether we can predict which response will occur in a given

Control of Intracranial Pressure on Induction

- Narcotic
- Nondepolarizing muscle relaxant
- Hyperventilation, ensure high SaO_2
- Blunt stress of intubation
  - Deepen anesthetic
    - Narcotic
    - Thiopental
    - Lidocaine
  - β-Blockade (short acting)
- Prompt intubation

patient. This potential problem must be balanced against the increased risk of hypoxia and elevate ICP should problems develop with the airway and preoxygenation was omitted. In addition, anxiety-induced increases in ICP may not be critical because thiopental dramatically decreases ICP in doses commonly used for induction. It is this effect on ICP that makes thiopental such a valuable induction agent in tumor patients. In addition, it is very rapid in producing unconsciousness, it is well tolerated by most patients, and it is a drug that everyone in anesthesia is familiar with and feels comfortable in using. However, it is short acting.

One of the most common mismatches in timing relative to ICP control is the use of thiopental and nondepolarizing muscle relaxants. Techniques that use this approach are valuable and are to be recommended. However, total loss of train-of-four response is sought to avoid an elevation of ICP due to coughing during intubation. Depending on the drug selected and the dose, this level of relaxation may take 3 minutes to achieve, during which time the CNS effects of the thiopental are decreasing, the patient's anesthetic level is lightening, CBF is coming up toward control, and the reduction in ICP is being reversed. Intubation at this point will likely result in elevation of blood pressure and a probable increase in ICP. Thus, the proper selection of drugs may not give the anticipated results. Additional thiopental just before intubation will blunt those responses. It may also be helpful to supplement the induction drugs with a narcotic or a β- blocker. β-Blockade will prevent hypertension with high perfusion pressures that allow breakthrough in autoregulation.

Some are concerned with the use of nitrous oxide because of studies suggesting that nitrous oxide causes an increase in $CMRO_2$, CBF, and thus ICP. It is true that nitrous oxide studies show these effects. These are not really clinically very worrisome because the effect of nitrous oxide on CBF is easily blunted by the concomitant use of thiopental or hyperventilation during induction. Even when using nitrous oxide as part of an inhalation induction, it is usual to start an intravenous line as soon as possible and administer thiopental to achieve a reduction in ICP.

Blood pressure control during induction may be important when there is loss of autoregulation in areas of pathology. Because flow is pressure dependent in areas without autoregulation and ICP is related to CBF via cerebral blood volume and we do not know which, if any, areas have lost autoregulation, it seems clinically prudent to control blood pressure to levels that the patient sustained awake. Blunting the hemodynamic response to intubation can be achieved with additional thiopental, narcotic, lidocaine, esmolol, or sodium nitroprusside.

INTRAOPERATIVE MANAGEMENT OF TIGHT BRAIN Intracranial hypertension can result in the extrusion of brain tissue when craniotomy is performed. The first sign of difficulty is usually noted by the neurosurgeon as the craniotomy flap is removed and the dura is bulging and tense. The term *tight brain* gives no clue as to etiology or course of treatment. Some observations can help assess the severity and intractability of the situation. If the dura is tense and bulging only at the lower portion of the craniectomy, palpation may reveal that the brain tissue is easily displaced upward and that the superior dura is tense only from being pushed out at the lower level. Surgical exposure may be slightly compromised in this situation, and some maneuvers may improve the situation. If the dura is tense at all edges of the craniectomy and palpation reveals fairly immobile brain beneath, surgical exposure may be severely compromised. Maneuvers may help the situation but are unlikely to bring the brain profile to the bone edge. A large dural incision will result in brain extrusion with trapping at the edges and little room to achieve exposure.

A small dural incision allows the surgeon some control of the brain while seeking to obtain exposure. Although the usual cause of such extreme tenseness of the dura is not amenable to anesthetic maneuvers, it is important to rule out correctable problems. The usual cause is intracranial hypertension because of the tumor

Therapeutic Maneuvers to Improve Tight Brain

Position, venous return
PCO_2, PO_2
Anesthetic agent, nitrous oxide
Thiopental
Mucle relaxants
Diuretics
Spinal fluid drainage
Steroids (not helpful acutely)
Pneumocephalus

mass itself. As resection is performed, the dural opening can be enlarged and the offending mass will be removed, eventually leaving a cavity where previously there was bulging brain. An ominous cause of such swelling is occult acute bleeding into the tumor. Vital signs give a clue to this. Hypertension may develop without apparent cause and appears unusually resistant to increasing anesthetic depth. Heart rate may initially rise but then slows. This response is somewhat masked by the complexity of pharmacologic and surgical interventions superimposed during anesthesia. Timing is also important. If the brain begins to vigorously bulge where it was slack before, intracerebral hemorrhage must be strongly suspected. It is helpful to the surgeon to be informed of the subtle vital sign changes suggesting this etiology, because the surgeon will need to proceed more rapidly and boldly with decompression. Because of the relationship of CPP to ICP and blood pressure, it may be unwise to try to reduce blood pressure before decompression despite the probability of bleeding.

With the use of the operating microscope, the surgeon may adjust the position of the table for best exposure without realizing that the patient is slowly being placed horizontally or head down. Readjusting the operating table to allow the head to be slightly elevated can dramatically improve the situation. Venous drainage may be compromised by extreme head positions and go unnoticed until the dura is exposed. Repositioning the alignment of head and chin to the body may be necessary.

Because it is a powerful cerebral vasodilator, an increase in $PaCO_2$ may cause a dramatic increase in ICP. Hypoxic cerebral vasodilation may produce the same effect. Reassurance that hypocarbia is achieved and hypoxia is absent can be obtained by arterial blood gas determinations supported by pulse oximetry and capnography.

Despite the overall evidence of safety of volatile anesthetics, it seems prudent to discontinue such drugs and utilize an opioid in the presence of tight brain. There may be no causal connection between volatile drugs and brain size, but changing to an opioid anesthetic eliminates any such possibility. Nitrous oxide may increase CBF, but its effect is likely to be less pronounced and easily altered by thiopental or opioids and hyperventilation. Nonetheless, discontinuation of nitrous oxide eliminates any concern of its being a causative agent for the problem. Acute administration of a sleep dose of thiopental can be expected to reduce ICP. Lack of any visible response of the brain to thiopental suggests a serious situation. In theory, sequential changes in anesthetics can help identify the agent responsible, although rarely is this helpful clinically. It is usually more practical to make several changes at once to effect a reduction in intracranial mass as quickly as possible.

Patients receiving antiseizure medications may have a shortened response to nondepolarizing muscle relaxants.[35] Return of abdominal and thoracic muscle tone during light anesthesia can raise central venous pressure and, as a result, cerebral venous pressure, thus, the presumed origin of the saying that "curare relaxes the brain." Evaluation of the level of neuromuscular blockade is an important subtle step in seeking a cause for tight brain.

Osmotic diuretics have long been shown to be effective in reducing brain size in normal brain tissue by drawing water from the interstitial tissue. In patients with intact autoregulation, mannitol results in no change in CBF and a decrease of ICP by 27 percent at 25 minutes. However, in patients with impaired autoregulation, the CBF increases by 5 percent, and there is less decrease in ICP (18 percent) at 25 minutes.[36] Furosemide in fairly large doses (e.g., 80 mg) reduces ICP, but its mechanism of action is not entirely clear.[37]

Drainage of CSF is a rapid and effective method of reducing intracranial bulk directly. Generally effective methods include subarachnoid needle and catheter techniques. Rarely, pneumocephalus may be present from some previous diagnostic test and can increase with the use of nitrous oxide.

MONITORING FOR SUPRATENTORIAL BRAIN TUMOR Routine monitoring should be employed as for any other case of this magnitude. Specific ancillary techniques useful in these cases can alter the monitoring requirements. Hypocarbia is a part of all neuroanesthetic techniques to facilitate surgical exposure and can be evaluated with capnography or mass spectrometry together with arterial blood gases. The use of a central venous catheter and direct arterial blood pressure measurement are not essential although its low risk and usefulness lead us to use the latter technique for most craniotomy procedures. Meningioma and metastatic tumors to the brain tend to bleed, suggesting monitoring that provides detailed information on hemodynamic parameters. Procedures that have a likelihood of exposing a cerebral venous sinus to the atmosphere (e.g., a tumor invading the sinus) suggest special monitoring for venous air embolism (VAE) for early detection. A right heart catheter may be lifesaving in the event of massive air embolism through an open dural sinus. ICP monitoring is popular in some centers, especially during anesthetic induction and emergence. To be useful during induction, the monitor must be placed in the awake patient. Induction agents and techniques can then be titrated to produce the desired level of ICP and anesthesia.[38]

Infratentorial Tumor

Infratentorial tumors require a change in body and head position from supine and head forward to provide surgical access to the posterior fossa. For some lesions, this can be achieved with the patient supine and with the head turned dramatically to the side. For others, the park bench, prone, or sitting position provides the desired surgical exposure.

The sitting position is said to offer some surgical advantages. Surgeons might weigh these advantages differently, but most would agree that ease of surgical exposure, the amount of blood pooling in the operative field, and the operative position of the surgeon are different among the sitting, lateral, supine, and prone positions. Some anesthesiologists believe that access to the endotracheal tube, the reduction of facial swelling, and the ability to observe facial nerve function are notable advantages of the sitting position in anesthetic management. The two most common procedures performed in the sitting position are cervical laminectomy and posterior fossa exploration. Hazards to the patient in the sitting position include VAE, hypotension, vital sign changes due to brainstem manipulation, specific cranial nerve stimulation airway obstruction, and position-related brainstem ischemia. These are not unique to the sitting position and may occur in other positions as

Practical Reasons for Selective Use of Sitting Position

- Better surgical exposure
  - Less tissue retraction and damage
  - Less bleeding
  - Less cranial nerve damage
  - More complete resection of the lesion
  - Ready access to airway, chest, and extremities
- Modern monitoring gives early warning of
  - Air embolism
  - Brainstem compromise
- Serious problems due to air embolism are uncommon

well. Our management should be directed at the prevention, early detection, and treatment of these problems.

There is much concern about the use of the sitting position, some even suggesting that it is malpractice to use this position for today's surgery. These intimidating statements may have some basis in fact but, in general, do not consider what has become a large body of information about the safety of the sitting position.

SAFETY There are several large published series of sitting cases that have a remarkably similar and favorable safety record.[39–42] The practice at our institution reflects the practice in the United States in general. The sitting position is being used less, and more posterior fossa procedures are being performed in horizontal positions. The use of the sitting position is becoming a conscious selection rather than automatic for any posterior fossa lesion. There is risk and benefit in each position, and these must be weighed in the overall care of the patient.

An outcome study puts the problem into perspective and is consistent with other studies.[42] A total of 579 posterior fossa craniectomies (333 sitting and 246 horizontal) performed concurrently at the Mayo Clinic between 1981 and 1984 were reviewed retrospectively. Intraoperatively, the incidence of hypotension was not different between groups either from induction of anesthesia to incision or from incision to closure. About 20 percent of the patients in both groups became hypotensive during each of these periods. All responded to vasopressors and/or fluids. The incidence of VAE in patients monitored with the Doppler was significantly greater in the sitting patients (45 percent) than in the horizontal patients (12 percent). An important significant difference was found in the need for blood transfusion between the two groups, confirming the traditional surgical impression that upright patients bleed less. More than 2 units of blood were required in 13 percent of the horizontal patients and in only 3 percent of the upright patients. Average blood volume transfused was also lower in the sitting patients. Postoperatively, no differences were found in cardiac or respiratory complications. The perioperative myocardial infarction rate was less than 1 percent overall and not different between groups. Respiratory complications were found in 2.5 percent and were not different between groups nor from other studies.[39]

Thus the data do not support the general selection of either the sitting or horizontal positions based on outcome. There are certain risks and advantages to each, and selection of position should be made with those in mind. In our opinion, there are some conditions that seem prudent to consider as relative contraindications to the sitting position. However, there are few objective data to support our approach. If a shunt tube is in place from the cerebral ventricular system to the right atrium, air may enter the end of the shunt as CSF drains out and be pulled into the heart. The noncollapsible tubing acts as a noncollapsible vein to allow air to pass unimpeded into the heart. This is not a potential problem with a ventriculoperitoneal shunt, since the air would have no venous access. We recommend that a patient having a ventriculoatrial shunt in place should have the shunt tied off before having an intracranial procedure per-

Relative Contraindications to Operative Sitting Position

- Ventriculoatrial shunt in place and open
- Cerebral ischemia upright awake
- Left atrial pressure (PCWP) $<$ right atrial pressure
- Platypnea-orthodeoxia
- Preoperative demonstration of patient foramen ovale or right-to-shunt
- ? Cardiac instability
    - Chest compression and resuscitation not really better in prone or lateral position
- ? Age extremes

Abbreviation: PCWP, pulmonary capillary wedge pressure.

formed in the sitting position. There are some patients who suffer cerebral ischemia whenever they assume the upright position. Their cardiovascular and cerebral vascular systems may both be implicated in this situation. These patients may present for an extracranial intracranial bypass procedure for the posterior cerebral circulation. Some surgeons believe the sitting position gives the best exposure for this procedure. We believe that we cannot be sure that we will maintain cerebral circulation in this circumstance, because we must not only put the patient upright, but also administer an anesthetic. It seems a reasonable balance of risk and benefit to do such a patient in a horizontal position.

There has been a suggestion that if the left atrial pressure (as measured by pulmonary artery occlusion pressure) is less than the right atrial pressure in the sitting position, the patient should be operated on horizontally because of increased risk of paradoxical embolism.[43] This is based on the following two important assumptions: (1) that the left atrial pressure will be greater than the right atrial pressure in the horizontal position and (2) that the atrial pressure gradient and its direction is a prognostic indicator of whether VAE will become paradoxical air embolism. Laboratory work suggests that these assumptions may not be applicable. In a pig model with an iatrogenic atrial septal defect, the relationship of atrial pressures (which side was greater) before air embolism was unrelated to the occurrence of paradoxical air embolism.[44] Thus, we believe that decisions regarding the use of the sitting position based on estimates of the preoperative atrial pressure gradients are not well founded. There are some patients who have a potential right-to-left shunt demonstrated preoperatively. There is an unusual cardiovascular illness in which the atrial gradients apparently reverse when the patient assumes the upright position.[45] In platypnea-orthodeoxia the patient is well oxygenated in the supine position but becomes desaturated in the upright position because of unsaturated blood passing from right to left at the atrial level. There are other patients in whom a patent foramen ovale is demonstrated preoperatively during a cardiac work-up. Still others may have a known right-to-left shunt. It seems that these patients might be at greater risk for paradoxical air embolism should VAE occur, and therefore, it seems prudent to avoid using the sitting position for them.

Some suggest that patients with cardiac instability or at extremes of age should not be placed in a sitting based on a possible need to resuscitate intraoperatively. We believe that it is really no easier to provide chest compression in the prone or lateral position than in the sitting position; they are equally undesirable. The rare occurrence of the need to resuscitate probably does not justify giving up whatever surgical advantage is thought to be gained by using the sitting position. Thus, these last considerations are not really relative contraindications.

MONITORING FOR INFRATENTORIAL BRAIN TUMOR In collating the data from many studies, the sitting position seems relatively safe, provided adequate monitoring is used.

The Central Nervous System. Nervous system monitoring techniques for patients in the sitting position are directed not only at minimizing the hazards of the position but also at providing positive information to the surgeon, particularly during posterior fossa exploration. The same central nervous system monitoring is required for a given infratentorial procedure regardless of surgical position. The response of the vital signs to brainstem manipulation and the response of the cranial nerves to stimulation can provide pathophysiologic data that the surgeon can utilize in real time during dissection (Table 10.1).

The electrocardiograph (ECG) is an effective monitor of brainstem compression. Spontaneous respiration has been advocated as a means of detecting transgression of the respiratory centers during posterior fossa exploration. However, large series indicate that monitoring of the ECG provides adequate warming of brainstem compromise during light anesthesia while using mechanical ventilation to maintain reduced $PaCO_2$ levels.[46] Brainstem auditory-evoked responses and somatosensory-evoked

TABLE 10.1 *Cranial nerve stimulation during posterior fossa surgery*

CRANIAL NERVE OR AREA	CLASSIC ACTIVITY DESCRIPTION WITH PHYSICAL SIGNS	ELECTRONIC DEVICE
V	Motor	
	Jaw jerk	EMG
	Sensory	
	Hypertension	Arterial line
	Bradycardia	ECG
VII	Facial twitch	EMG
X	Hypotension	Arterial line
	Bradycardia	ECG
XI	Shoulder jerk	EMG
Pons	Brainstem compression	BAEP, SSEP
	Ectopic cardiac foci	ECG
	Hypertension/hypotension	Arterial line
	Tachycardia/bradycardia	ECG
	Gasp, irregular respirations	Respirator trigger

Abbreviations: EMG, electromyography; ECG, electrocardiogram; BAEP, brainstem auditory evoked potential; SSEP, somatosensory-evoked potential.

potentials (SSEPs) can provide an electrophsiologic monitor for detection of early brainstem compromise. Stimulation of cranial nerve VII results in a facial twitch that is visible in the seated patient. EMG over the distribution of cranial nerve VII can aid in detecting stimulation when the face is not accessible to palpation or visual assessment. Facial nerve monitoring with EMG has resulted in improved VII nerve function in patients undergoing acoustic neuroma resection.[47]

Cerebral Profusion Pressure. Blood pressure and pulse rate are monitors of several interrelated systems and factors. Some operations performed in the sitting position tend to be of a type that might result in sudden and extreme changes in pulse rate and blood pressure either because of the surgery or VAE. Intra-arterial blood pressure measurements will yield instantaneous information, particularly in regard to CPP. This is most easily accomplished when the strain gauge is zeroed to the base of the skull. This can be done by using the routine zero at the heart level with the patient supine and placing the strain gauge at the level of the external auditory meatus once the patient is placed in the sitting position.

VENOUS AIR EMBOLISM

Diagnosis. Monitoring for VAE can be approached from several aspects. Monitors include a precordial Doppler, a right heart catheter, capnograph or mass spectrometer, esophageal stethoscope, transcutaneous oxygen, and transesophageal echocardiography. The most sensitive of these are the transesophageal echocardiography and Doppler, followed by expired nitrogen (EtN_2), end-tidal carbon dioxide ($EtCO_2$), transcutaneous oxygen, right heart catheter, and (least sensitive) the esophageal stethoscope. None of these monitors is totally reliable. We believe it is generally necessary to use at least three

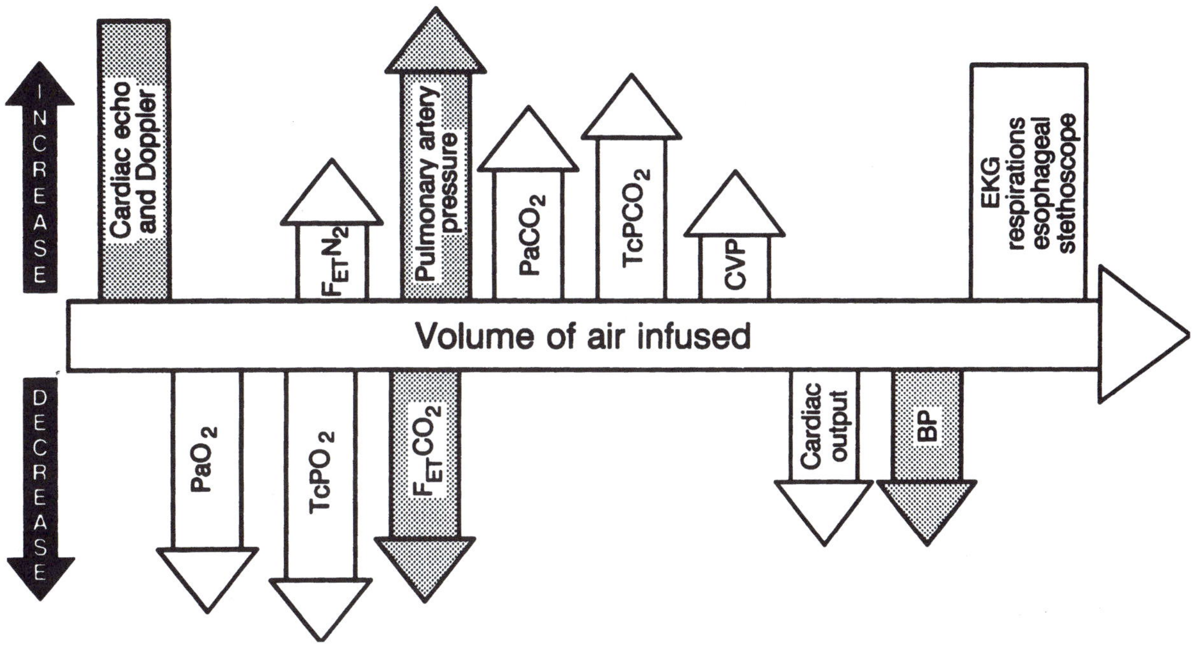

FIGURE 10.1 *Changes in detection parameters for VAE with increasing air volume. Data are aggregated from human and animal studies under a wide variety of circumstances. (From Cucchiara et al.,[92] with permission.)*

of these to ensure that VAE can detected (Fig. 10.1).

The risk of VAE is not eliminated by putting the patient horizontal, but it is reduced. A 12 percent incidence of Doppler-detected air occurs in supine infratentorial craniectomy cases.[42] Once VAE has occurred, about 20 percent of those patients will have hypotension regardless of their position. Except in the unusual situation of massive VAE, these episodes can be expected to respond promptly to vasopressor therapy.

The precordial Doppler is advocated as the basic monitoring device for the reduction of complications due to VAE. It is reasonably priced, relatively easy to use, noninvasive, and very sensitive; its position over the right heart can be verified by rapid injection of saline into the central venous circulation; and its sounds can be heard by both surgeon and anesthesiologist. Proper positioning of the precordial Doppler is relatively simple in the sitting position. However, in the prone and park bench or three-quarter positions, it can be more difficult. Our experience suggests the Doppler should be placed after the patient is positioned and care exercised that excessive pressure is not placed on the probe. Proper position can be confirmed by injection of agitated saline into a central venous catheter or large-bore peripheral intravenous line and listening for the characteristic Doppler signal. Its sensitivity has led some to criticize its use as indicating insignificant air before hemodynamic consequences ensue. Protagonists argue that such sensitivity is precisely the early warning needed to identify the occurrence of VAE and stop its entry surgically.

The use of the right heart catheter has evolved and improved such that air can frequently be aspirated when detected on Doppler. But what are the real functions of the right heart catheter?[48] Rapid injection of agitated saline through it can help confirm that the Doppler is properly placed over the right heart. The aspiration of air confirms or establishes the diagnosis of VAE. The

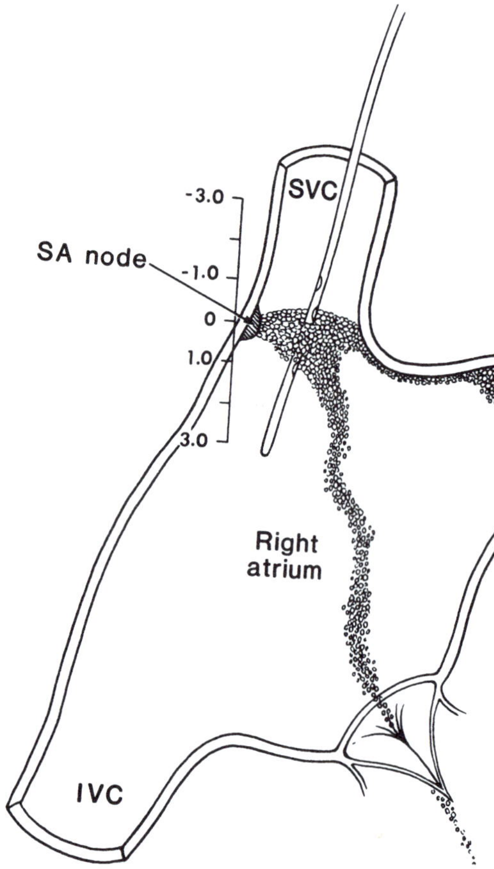

FIGURE 10.2 *In patients with VAE the air tends to localize at the atrial-SVC junction, moving through the tricuspid valve or into upright portions of the atrium. The multiorifice catheter placement most likely to aspirate air is shown. The ECG tracing from the catheter in this position is described in Figure 10.3 Conceptualization of localization of air embolism in the upright heart is based on a human cardiac model and human echocardiographic findings. SA, sinoatrial; IVC, inferior vena cava. (From Cucchiara et al.,[92] with permission.)*

role of the catheter in the treatment of VAE is more anecdotal and less solidly founded. The aspiration of air from the right atrium during VAE is occasionally lifesaving, but such occasions are very rare situations of massive VAE. Whether the routine aspiration of smaller or medium quantities of air from the heart can prevent paradoxical air embolism or cardiopulmonary complications is not known. Right atrial multiorifice catheters allow a larger amount of air to be aspirated than single-orifice catheter. Proper placement of the right atrial catheter in the high right atrium by ECG control can increase its effectiveness by placing it where the air tends to collect (Fig. 10.2).[49] A common question related to patients at risk for VAE is does concern for potential VAE and use of a precordial Doppler imply that a right atrial catheter should be used. The right atrial catheter is of limited therapeutic value, and there are a number of other treatment modalities, most importantly eliminating the source of VAE. Our practice is to weigh the likely risk for VAE in the given procedure and position against any risk associated with placing the catheter.

The right heart catheter may be positioned by ECG control, radiographs, or pressure recordings. Although it is not clear, it is likely that the ECG trace from a multiorifice catheter comes from the proximal hole, usually 2 cm from the tip.[50,51] Thus the tracing sought is a little different with these catheters. The standard concept if

FIGURE 10.3 *The intracardiac ECG from each position. With a single-orifice catheter, tracing 4 indicates midright atrial position. Because the ECG trace originates from the proximal orifice of a multiorifice catheter and the placement as shown in Figure 10.2 is desirable, tracing 2 should be sought. (From Cucchiara et al.,[50] with permission.)*

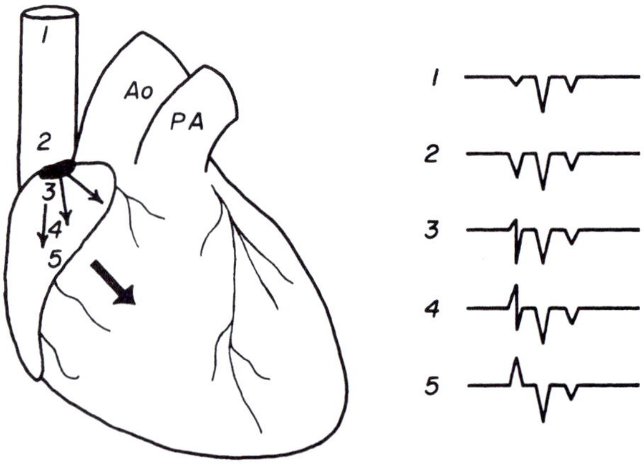

a progressively more negative P wave as the catheter is advanced still applies, but the proximal orifice should be placed in the superior vena cava (SVC), allowing the portion of the catheter that has the holes to float at the SVC-high right atrial level (Fig. 10.2). The P wave should be large and negative, with no positive component (Fig. 10.3). This indicates that the proximal orifice is not in the atrium. In practice, one can usually obtain an increasingly negative P wave that finally develops a small positive deflection and then withdraw slightly to an all-negative P wave. Care must be taken when the arm is returned to the side, because the catheter will likely migrate a little more centrally and may need to be withdrawn slightly.[52]

The use of the pulmonary artery (PA) catheter for the aspiration of VAE has generally been unsatisfactory because of the small lumen size and slow speed of blood return. However, other information can be obtained from the PA catheter. The entry of air into the pulmonary circulation causes the PA pressures to rise. One can utilize this information to evaluate when VAE has cleared the pulmonary circulation. If PA pressure rises during VAE and the Doppler clears, a return of PA pressure to previous levels suggests that the air obstructing the pulmonary circulation has been moved more distally and probably excreted through the lungs.[43]

Capnography and mass spectrometry demonstrate a decrease in $EtCO_2$ during VAE with intermediate sensitivity. One can expect to see changes in $EtCO_2$ after Doppler changes occur but before hemodynamic changes occur. When enough air is entrained to cause hemodynamic

FIGURE 10.4 *Paradoxical air as noted by transesophageal echocardiography (A) Normal. (B) Air in right atrium. (C) Air in left atrium, right atrium nearly opacified. (D) More air in left and right atrium. (From Cucchiara et al.,[54] with permission.)*

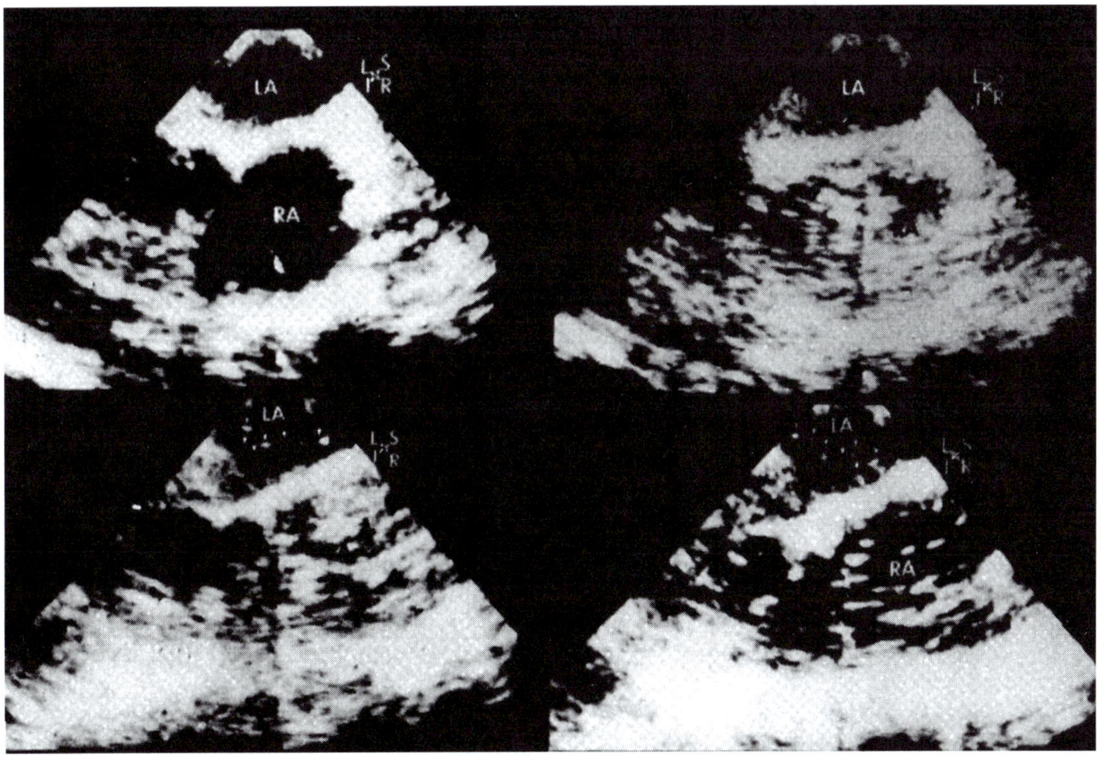

A B C D

changes, the $EtCO_2$ will usually drop within a few breaths of the Doppler change. Sensitive mass spectrometry can show increases in FeN_2 as the VAE is excreted through the lung. Transcutaneous PO_2 is also of intermediate sensitivity but has more practical and technical problems, making its use in the operating room somewhat less popular.[53]

Transesophageal echocardiography is a very sensitive monitor for VAE and allows us to visualize air in the cardiac chambers themselves. This gives us the unique opportunity to identify the occurrence of left heart air (Fig. 10.4).[54] The only other clinical way to identify paradoxical air embolism during neurosurgery is for the surgeon to visualize air in the small arteries of the brain or spinal cord. This suggests that it is already late because the air is already in the vessels to the brain in large enough amounts to be readily seen.

Treatment of VAE. The team approach is critical in achieving a reduction in complications from VAE. The anesthesiologist can make the diagnosis from the devices discussed above. The surgeon often makes the diagnosis at the same time, because it can be seen that the opened vein is entraining air rather than bleeding. The role of the anesthesiologist is to support the cardiovascular system so that ischemic injury can be avoided; the role of the surgeon is to stop the influx of air at the surgical site. We can help identify the problem area in the surgical field by several maneuvers. The surgeon can flood the field with saline to submerge the area of air entry. The application of jugular pressure at the anterior neck for about 15 seconds will frequently raise the venous pressure in the wound enough so that the vessel will back-bleed. We suggest two cautions in applying this pressure. You must attempt to feel the carotid pulsation so that it is not occluded as well. Prolonged simultaneous occlusion of the jugular veins may raise cerebral venous pressure sufficiently to cause the brain to bulge from the wound. If nitrous oxide is being administered, it should be discontinued immediately on detection of VAE. The discontinuation of nitrous oxide will slow the increase in size of the aspirated bubbles and hasten their reabsorption. The use of vasopressors and volume for preload may increase cardiac output and thereby aid in moving the air through the heart to the peripheral pulmonary circulation.

An additional use of transesophageal echocardiography is diagnosis of patent foramen ovale. Most episodes of paradoxical embolism occur via a patent foramen ovale.[55] Twenty-seven percent of people with no history of cardiac disease have a patent foramen ovale and therefore would be at risk for paradoxical air embolism during VAE.[56] In some series, echocardiography is effective in detecting patent foramen ovale.[57,58] Unfortunately in our experience as well as that of several other centers, preoperative echocardiography detects a much lower incidence of patent foramen ovale than expected.[59,60] When preoperative echocardiography or intraoperative transesophageal echocardiography (TEE) detects a patent foramen ovale, that patient is at risk for developing paradoxical air embolism. However, when echocardiography fails to detect a patent foramen ovale, the risk of paradoxical air embolism may still exist.

The use of positive end-expiratory pressure (PEEP) in these circumstances is controversial. The application of PEEP to decrease the incidence of VAE or identify the site of air entry has been advocated.[61–66] However, studies examining the effectiveness of clinically applicable levels of PEEP suggest that these levels of PEEP may be ineffective in significantly increasing central venous pressure or intracranial venous pressure and therefore may not influence the occurrence of VAE.[67,68] Concern has also been expressed that the application of PEEP may result in an increased risk for the development of paradoxical air embolism during VAE in the presence of a patent foramen ovale by increasing right atrial pressure relative to left atrial pressure.[69,70] In a study evaluating the effect of patterns of ventilation on the occurrence of paradoxical air embolism in animals with a surgically created atrial septal defect, the application of PEEP did not increase the incidence of paradoxical air embolism developing. However, with the release of PEEP an increase in right-to-left passage of air emboli occurred.[44] This can be explained by PEEP decreasing venous return to the right heart and with the release of PEEP the venous return to the right heart increasing so that for a brief period it exceeds that of the left heart. Finally, the adverse hemodynamic effects of PEEP in patients in the sitting position must be considered.[70]

The mechanics of elevation of cerebral venous pressure are not as simple as was previously thought. It appears that cerebral venous flow is carried in both collapsible (jugular veins) and noncollapsible (vertebral venous sinuses) vessels. When venous sinus pressure is highly negative, cerebral venous drainage is carried primarily through noncollapsible vessels that are protected from the neck compression. Neck compression is most effective when venous drainage is through the collapsible channels. That occurs when the venous sinus pressure is only slightly negative or positive. PEEP increased venous sinus pressure when it was very negative only if cardiac output was maintained.[67] The use of PEEP thus remains controversial, but it is our opinion, based on current literature, that the potential risks of PEEP outweigh its potential benefits.

ANESTHETIC CONSIDERATIONS There are several viable choices in agent selection for posterior fossa craniotomies, and each has its advantages and disadvantages. Some of the disadvantages can be minimized by skillful administration. Volatile anesthetics agents may be used as the primary agent. They provide smooth, easily controlled anesthetic depth, and the anesthetic depth can be measured using mass spectrometry. Little cardiovascular depression is encountered in the low concentrations required, and a predictable awakening can be accomplished at the end of the case.

The supplemental use of nitrous oxide is an area of controversy, particularly in these cases, because of the risk of VAE. When VAE occurs in the presence of nitrous oxide, the bubbles will increase in size as the N_2O diffuses into the bubble faster than the nitrogen can diffuse out. Some have suggested that nitrous oxide should be deleted in sitting cases because of this risk. Some have suggested that nitrous oxide offers an advantage in patients at risk for VAE. By diffusing into small bubbles and increasing their size, nitrous oxide could increase the sensitivity of monitors for VAE allowing for earlier detection. Some believe that more volatile agent must be used when nitrous oxide is deleted, making it a little more difficult to end a posterior fossa case without the added analgesia provided by nitrous oxide. Animal data comparing monitor sensitivity as well as hemodynamic changes during VAE with and without nitrous oxide revealed that use of nitrous oxide did not alter sensitivity of the most sensitive monitors, Doppler and TEE, while it increased the sensitivity of the less sensitive monitors. Hemodynamic effects of a given volume of VAE were unchanged by the administration of nitrous oxide if the nitrous oxide was discontinued once VAE was detected, as is the common clinical practice.[71] In a prospective randomized study of patients undergoing neurosurgical procedures in the sitting position, use of nitrous oxide did not alter incidence of VAE, hemodynamic changes associated with VAE, or time of emergence.[72] Based on these studies, the decision for use of nitrous oxide can be based on other considerations as long as the patient is monitored for VAE. If a patient undergoing a procedure with a known risk for VAE is not monitored with precordial Doppler or TEE, nitrous oxide use could increase the risk for complications should VAE occur. If the episode of VAE is not detected, the continued administration of nitrous oxide would lead to increased size of the embolism and potentially serious hemodynamic compromise.

Narcotic-based anesthetics, using low to moderate doses, supplemented with volatile agents and/or nitrous oxide, are often used and are compatable with intraoperative hemodynamic stability as well as prompt emergence at completion of the operative procedure. These cases can be done with a high-dose narcotic technique, but in general, it is difficult to have the patient actively responding at the end of surgery with this technique.[73] The significance of apnea may be confusing because it may be due to the surgery or to the opioid. Continued intubation of the trachea may be necessary to support ventilation of the lungs. Most neurosurgeons want to see the patient awake at the end of the case in the operating room to assess their work and to be sure that a catastrophic event requiring reopening has not occurred. An anesthetic technique that permits this is desirable.

With the advent of SSEPs and intraoperative EMG, our use of long-acting muscle relaxants is compromised. Muscle relaxants do not interfere with SSEP monitoring of a cervical laminectomy, for example, but when cranial nerve motor function (cranial nerve VII, for example) is being tested, we are limited in practice to muscle relaxants for intubation of the trachea and closure only. This poses additional risks, because it is most undesirable to have an open craniotomy patient suddenly strain on the endotracheal tube or move. We have avoided that situation previously by using long-acting nondepolarizing muscle relaxants. As more motor monitoring comes into practice, our use of muscle relaxants will be more limited. The anesthetic plan must incorporate consideration of these aspects of the procedure. Thus our overall anesthetic muscle relaxant technique must be altered to ensure, as best we can, that the patient will not move and that the monitoring can be used at critical times.

POSTOPERATIVE CONSIDERATIONS

The most serious immediate postoperative complication following posterior fossa craniectomy is apnea. It is very important to be able to define anesthetic-related apnea at the end of the case, because apnea resulting from surgical complications, especially hematoma, may require immediate reoperation. For that reason, is desirable to return the $PaCO_2$ to near the normal and to verify that only the smallest concentrations of anesthetic drugs are present, muscle relaxants are reversed, temperature is near normal, and any opioid effects are dissipated. The anesthetic technique should be managed with those goals in mind.

Posterior fossa craniectomy patients are subject to cranial nerve injuries that have implications for the anesthesiologists.[74] Whenever the lower cranial nerves are disturbed, traumatized, or even severed during the procedure, the anesthesiologist should be notified. If cranial nerve V is injured, sensation to the cornea will be impaired, and an eye patch should be used. The most dangerous cranial nerve injuries are to the sensory and motor nerves to the pharynx and larynx. If cranial nerves IX, X, or XII is injured, the patient is at increased risk of aspiration pneumonitis and hypoxia. The pathophysiology seems to involve inability to handle secretions either because the patient is not aware that these are in the pharynx and does not swallow them or because motor coordination of the pharyngeal muscles is impaired so that swallowing is ineffective. Sometimes the vocal cords are paretic and unable to effectively close the glottis to secretions. The process of aspiration of their own secretions is an insidious one in these patients. We have the clinical impression that they become hypoxic some hours after emerging from anesthesia. If the lower cranial nerves are significantly compromised, the patient's trachea is probably best left intubated at least overnight and probably for several days. We prefer to see the patients swallow on the endotracheal tube before extubation of the trachea to assure ourselves that at least pharyngeal sensation is present. Depending on the anesthetic technique used, this is not always possible, but observation of the event when it occurs can give you a little more confidence in removing the endotracheal tube.

Pneumocephalus occurs regularly in posterior fossa patients, but symptomatic tension pneumocephalus is uncommon. When it occurs, it requires immediate decompression. There is controversy surrounding the use of nitrous oxide and its relationship to the frequency and severity of tension pneumocephalus.[75,76]

Postoperative macroglossia resulting in airway obstruction requiring emergent tracheostomy following neurosurgical procedures in the sitting position has been reported.[77,78] It is believed to be due to obstruction of lingual venous drainage by pressure from the endotracheal tube in the flexed position. We have observed mild tongue edema following posterior fossa procedures in the three-quarter prone position that has not resulted in airway compromise.

Transsphenoidal Surgery

The pituitary gland is anatomically and functionally separated into the anterior pituitary (adenohypophysis) and posterior pituitary (neurohypophysis). Excision of adenomas of the anterior pituitary represents the vast majority of transsphenoidal operations performed, but understanding of total glandular function is necessary, as even selective removal of anterior pituitary microadenomas may often lead to posterior pituitary dysfunction. Normal anterior pituitary function is influenced both by hypothalamic releasing and inhibiting factors and by feedback from endocrine organ hormones. The posterior pituitary is responsible for storage and release of the hormones, antidiuretic hormone (ADH) and oxytocin, which are synthesized in the hypothalamus and transported to the posterior pituitary as granules in neurosecretory axons. The hormones released by the pituitary gland are listed in the accompanying box.

Pituitary Hormone Products

ANTERIOR PITUITARY

Growth hormone
Prolactin
Corticotropin
β-Lipotropin
Follicle-stimulating hormone
Luteinizing hormone
Thyrotropin

POSTERIOR PITUITARY

Antidiuretic hormone
Oxytocin

Clinical presentation of pituitary tumors is generally manifested as pressure effects secondary to tumor growth with impingement on adjacent intracranial structures or as altered endocrine function.[79,80] Pressure effects may result in headaches, cranial nerve palsies, and visual disturbances secondary to optic tract involvement. In addition, pituitary endocrine deficiency may occur secondary to compression of normal gland. Functioning pituitary adenomas may cause hypersecretion of anterior pituitary hormones, resulting in a variety of clinical syndromes. The hormones most commonly involved are prolactin, growth hormone (GH), adrenocorticotropin (ACTH), with adenomas secreting thyroid-stimulating hormone, follicle-stimulating hormone, or luteinizing hormone being rare. Prolactinomas represent the most common hyperfunctioning adenoma, followed by GH and ACTH adenomas. Hyperprolactinemia may produce the amenorrhea-galactorrhea syndrome in females and impaired libido and potency in males. Hypersecretion of GH prepuberty may lead to gigantism, whereas postpuberty, the result is acromegaly. ACTH adenomas result in the increased adrenal cortisol production of Cushing's disease. Endocrine hypofunction secondary to pressure effects on normal pituitary can be reflected as panhypopituitarism necessitating hormone replacement preoperatively. Hyposecretion of ADH secondary to pressure effects on the posterior pituitary may produce diabetes insipidus, which manifests as impairment of urine concentrating ability and overall inability to maintain body water balance, resulting in hyperosmolarity and hypovolemia.

Anesthetic Considerations

Preoperative assessment of the patient scheduled for transsphenoidal surgery necessitates an evaluation with emphasis on physiologic changes related to endocrine dysfunction. Glucose tolerance may be disturbed secondary to endocrine dysfunction, and patients should be evaluated for possible hyperglycemia. Adequacy of ADH reserve of the posterior pituitary may be determined by measuring urine concentrating ability after water deprivation.[80] Knowledge of baseline function is important, as operative manipulations may alter pituitary function, even if a small adenoma is microscopically removed. This necessitates perioperative provision of glucocorticoids and awareness of the potential postoperative development of diabetes insipidus.[81] In addition to the endocrine evaluation, the radiologic features of the tumor should be reviewed to ascertain whether pathology is limited to the sella turcica or involves suprasellar extension. Special consideration must be given to the patient presenting with Cushing's disease or acromegaly. The patient with Cushing's disease is susceptible to hypertension, hyperglycemia, hyperkalemia, skeletal muscle weakness, and increased intravascular fluid volume.[82] The acromegalic may have hypertension, hyperglycemia, and skeletal muscle weakness, as well as skeletal, soft tissue, and connective tissue abnormalities that may manifest as neuropathies, organomegaly, and alterations in airway anatomy that may make tracheal intubation difficult and may predispose to sleep apnea.[83] Airway changes include prognathism; macroglossia; pharyngeal, tonsillar, and epiglottic soft-tissue hypertrophy; vocal cord fixation; and laryngeal stenosis.[84,85] Careful preoperative assessment of the airway in the patient with acromegaly may help to anticipate difficult airway management. This may involve difficulty with obtaining good mask fit and ventilating the patient, visualizing the larynx, and advancing an endotracheal tube.[86] These investigators suggest that patients with preoperatively ascertained glottic abnormalities or those with soft-tissue abnormalities and glottic abnormalities should be considered for elective tracheostomy preoperatively. Others suggest that tracheostomy is rarely necessary in these patients, even with advanced acromegalic changes. Fiberoptic laryngoscopy and intubation of the trachea should be initially considered in acromegalic patients in whom airway management difficulties are anticipated.[87,88]

The transsphenoidal approach for microsurgical excision of pituitary adenomas is generally performed under general anesthesia, and principles for management of patients with intracranial lesions should be observed if there is associated suprasellar extension and potential increased ICP. Patient monitoring routinely includes directly (usually) or indirectly measured arterial pressure, ECG, temperature, esophageal stethoscope auscultation, and urine output. Right atrial-central venous pressure monitoring and precordial Doppler ultrasonic air detection have been suggested by some to diagnose and treat potential VAE in operations performed with a 40° head-up lift,[89] whereas others suggest that the monitoring may be omitted as head-up tilt is limited to less than 5° to 15°.[90] Induction of general anesthesia can generally be accomplished with intravenous thiopental and a nondepolarizing muscle relaxant to facilitate endotracheal intubation. SCh may be utilized, especially if a shorter duration of relaxation is desired in cases when difficult airway management is anticipated. The acromegalic airway might be such a case. The transsphenoidal approach to the pituitary usually involves nasal septal and sublabial incisions, thus necessitating oral endotracheal intubation, with the endotracheal tube and esophageal stethoscope secured to the corner of the mouth opposite to the side where the surgeons are operating (Fig. 10.5). The mouth and posterior pharynx may be packed with moist cotton gauze to prevent bleeding into the esophagus and glottic regions and thus prevent postoperative vomiting of blood. Anesthetic maintenance can be achieved with either an opioid-nitrous oxide or inhalation technique. Selection of anesthetic agents must consider the potential hypertensive and arrhythmogenic effects of epinephrine and cocaine used in submucosally injected local anesthetic mixtures by the surgeons,[81] with halothane most likely to sensitize toward these effects.

When there is suprasellar extension of the tumor, subarachnoid air may be injected to allow the tumor outline to be visualized on intraoperative fluoroscopy. The elevation of ICP produced by the air may help to deliver the tumor down-

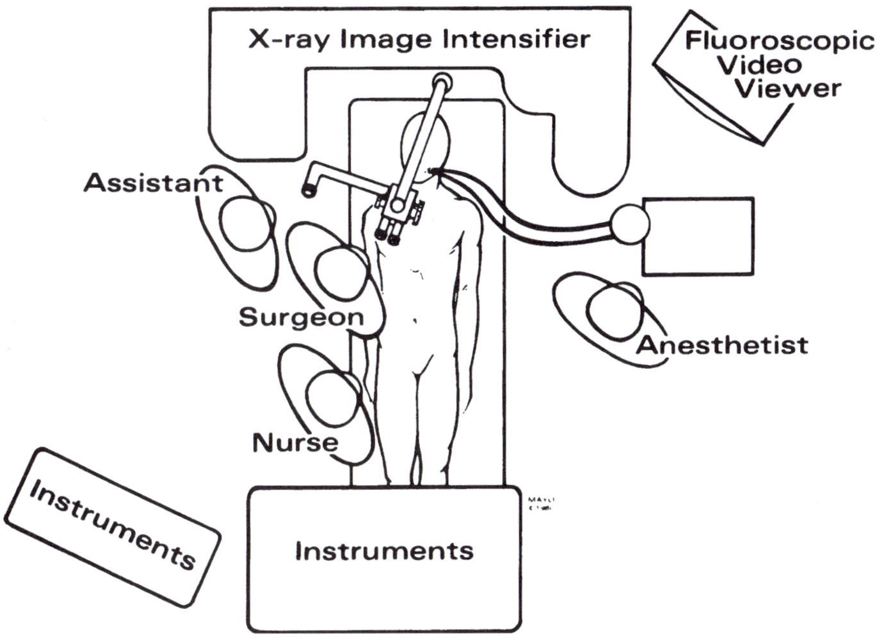

FIGURE 10.5 *Typical operating room arrangement for transsphenoidal pituitary surgery. (From Messick et al.,[90] by permission of Mayo Foundation.)*

ward into the surgeon's field. Inhaled nitrous oxide will increase the volume of the injected air rapidly There are several possible approaches to this ancillary technique, none of which has been shown to be clearly superior. You may continue the nitrous oxide and inject smaller volumes of air (e.g., 5 ml), realizing that it will expand as it reaches the cranium. One may discontinue the nitrous oxide and inject subarachnoid air (e.g., 10 ml), or one may draw the gas mixture from the inspired line and inject it. We do not utilize this third option if volatile agents are in use. The air is injected through a lumbar subarachnoid needle or catheter. As long as CSF can be aspirated from the lumbar drainage system you can help the surgeon by controlling the degree of downward push on the tumor (related to increased ICP) by removing CSF. Thus, if the air volume proves to be too large as seen from the surgeon's view of the tumor, removal of CSF can optimize the intracranial fluid dynamics. Occasionally, air will be injected but not seen on head fluoroscopy. There may be two reasons for this: (1) the lumbar drain is not subarachnoid (this can be ruled out by withdrawing CSF before and after air injection and (2) the drain is too caudad, and the air is passing cauded in the subarachnoid space rather than cephalad.

One must bear in mind the potential for operative complications. The sella turcica is bordered laterally by the cavernous sinus, which, in addition to venous structures, contains the intracavernous portion of the internal carotid artery and cranial nerves IV, V and VI. Operative manipulation in the region of the cavernous sinus can thus result in (1) hemorrhage from the carotid artery or arterial spasm secondary to arterial manipulation, (2) venous hemorrhage and potential entrainment of air into the venous system if head-up tilt is excessive, and (3) cranial nerve weakness secondary to trauma or stretching.[91] Injury to the carotid artery during transsphenoidal surgery is a catastrophic event with high mortality. Control of bleeding is extremely difficult, if not impossible. Visual complications secondary to damage to the optic nerve or chiasm may occur as well as hypothalamic damage and intracranial hemorrhage. Appearance of new visual field deficits postoperative should raise concern of possible intracranial hematoma at the operative site. Other complications include postoperative alterations in endocrine function, including the development of diabetes insipidus, which may manifest as a hypotonic polyuria and necessitates frequent reassessment of fluid status. If diabetes insipidus develops, fluid replacement should include maintenance fluids plus an amount sufficient to cover urinary losses. In addition, exogenous vasopressin may need to administered. This may be accomplished via intranasal administration of desmopressin once nasal packing is removed.[92]

References

1. Adams RS, Gronert GA, Sundt TM, Michenfelder JD: Halothane, hypocapnia, and cerebrospinal fluid pressure in neurosurgery. Anesthesiology 37:510, 1972
2. Adams RW, Cucchiara RF, Gronert GA et al: Isoflurane and cerebrospinal fluid pressure in neurosurgical patients. Anesthesiology 54:97, 1981
3. Muzzi DA, Losasso TJ, Dietz NM et al: The effect of desflurane and isoflurane on cerebrospinal fluid pressure in humans with supratentorial mass lesions. Anesthesiology 76:720, 1992
4. Muzzi DA, Daltner C, Losasso T et al: The effect of desflurane and isoflurane on cerebrospinal fluid pressure in patients with supratentorial mass lesions (abstract). Anesthesiology 75:A167, 1991
5. Grosslight K, Foster R, Colohan AR, Bedford RF: Isoflurane for neuroanesthesia: risk factors for increases in intracranial pressure. Anesthesiology 63:533, 1985
6. Madsen JB, Cold GE, Hansen ES, Bardrum B: The effect of isoflurane on cerebral blood flow and metabolism in humans during craniotomy for small supratentorial cerebral tumors. Anesthesiology 66:332, 1987
7. Cucchiara RF, Michenfelder JD: The effect of interruption of the reticular activating system on metabolism in canine cerebral hemispheres before and after thiopental. Anesthesiology 39:3, 1973
8. Milde LN, Milde JH, Michenfelder JD: Cerebral functional metabolic, and hemodynamic effects of etomidate in dog. Anesthesiology 63:371, 1985
9. Vandesteene A, Trempont V, Engelman E et al: Effect of propofol on cerebral blood flow and metabolism in man. Anaesthesia 43S:42, 1988
10. Pinaud M, Lelausque JN, Chetanneau A et al: Effects of propofol on cerebral hemodynamics and metabolism in patients with brain trauma. Anesthesiology 73:404, 1990
11. Ravussin P, Guinard JP, Ralley F, Thorin D: Effect of propofol on cerebrospinal fluid pressure and cerebral perfusion pressure in patients undergoing craniotomy. Anaethesia 43S:37, 1988
12. Herregods L, Verbeke J, Rolly G, Colardyn F: Effect if propofol on elevated intracranial pressure: Preliminary result. Anaesthesia 43S:107, 1988
13. Albanese J, Durbec O, Viviand X et al: Sufentanil increases intracranial pressure in patients with head trauma. Anesthesiology 7:493, 1993
14. Sperry RJ, Bailey PL, Reichman MV et al: Fentanyl and sufentanil increase intracranial pressure in head trauma patients. Anesthesiology 77:416, 1992
15. From RP, Warner DS, Todd MM, Sokoll MD: Anesthesia for craniotomy: a double-blind comparison of alfentanil, fentanyl, and sufentanil. Anesthesiology 73:896, 1990
16. Marsh ML, Dunlop BJ, Shapiro HM et al: Succinylcholine-intracranial pressure effects in neurosurgical patients. Anesth Analg 59:550, 1980
17. Minton MD, Stirt JA, Bedford RF: Increased intracranial pressure from succinylcholine: modification by prior nondepolarizing blockade. Anesthesiology 65:165, 1986
18. Minton MD, Stirt JA, Bedford RF, Haworth C: Intracranial pressure after atracurium in neurosurgical patients. Anesth Analg 64:113, 1985
19. Unni VK, Gray WJ, Young WB: Effects of atracurium on intracranial pressure in man. Anaesthesia 41:1047, 1986
20. Hwang KH, Kim SC, Kim SY et al: Neuromuscular and hemodynamic effects of mivacurium and succinylcholine in adult patients during nitrous oxide-propofol-fentanyl anesthesia. J Korean Med Sci 8:374, 1993
21. Loan PB, Elliott P, Mirakhur RK et al: Comparison of the hemodynamic effects of mivacurium and atracurium during fentanyl anaesthesia. Br J Anaesth 74: 330, 1995
22. De Mey JC, Debrock M, Rolly G: Evaluation of the onset and intubation conditions of rocuro-

nium bromide. Eur J Anaesthesiol, suppl. 9:37, 1994
23. Bevan DR: Newer neuromuscular blocking agents. Pharmacol Toxicol 74:3, 1994
24. Graham D: Monitoring neuromuscular block may be unreliable in patients with upper motor neuron lesions. Anesthesiology 52:74, 1980
25. Brown JC, Charlton JE: Study of sensitivity to curare in certain neurological disorders using a regional technique. J Neurol Neurosurg Psychiatry 38:34, 1975
26. Cooperman LH, Strobel GE, Kennell EM: Massive hyperkalemia after administration of succinylcholine. Anesthesiology 32:161, 1970
27. Zornow MH, Todd MM, Moore SS: The acute cerebral effects of changes in plasma osmolality and oncotic pressure. Anesthesiology 67:936, 1987
28. Zornow MH, Scheller MS, Todd MM, Moore SS: Acute cerebral effects of isotonic crystalloid and colloid solutions following cryogenic brain injury in the rabbit. Anesthesiology 69:180, 1988
29. Ducey JP, Mozingo DW, Lamiell JM et al: A comparison of the cerebral and cardiovascular effects of complete resuscitation with isotonic and hypertonic saline, hetastarch, and whole blood following hemorrhage. J Trauma 29:1510, 1989
30. Cully MD, Larson CP, Silverburg GD: Hetastarch coagulopathy in a neurosurgical patients. Anesthesiology 66:706, 1987
31. Engel AK, Losasso TJ, Weglinski MR, Muzzi DA: Does intraoperative use of hydroxyethyl starch (hespan) increase the risk of perioperative intracranial hemorrhage (ICH) in patients undergoing intracranial surgery (abstract). Anesthesiology 79:A223, 1993
32. Lanier WL, Stangland KJ, Scheithauer BW et al: The effects of dextrose infusion and head position on neurologic outcome after complete cerebral ischemia in primates: examination of a model. Anesthesiology 66:38, 1987
33. Pulsinelli WA, Levy DE, Sigsbee B et al: Increased damage after ischemic stroke in patients with hyperglycemia with or without established diabetes mellitus. Am J Med 74:540, 1983
34. Longstreth WI, Inui TS: High blood glucose level on hospital admission and poor neurological recovery after cardiac arrest. Ann Neurol 15:59, 1984
35. Messick JM, Maass L, Faust RJ, Cucchiara RF: Duration of pancuronium neuromuscular blockade in patients taking anticonvulsant medication (abstract). Anesth Analg 61:203, 1982
36. Muizelaar JP, Lutz HA, Becker DP: Effect of mannitol on ICP and CBF and correlation with pressure autoregulation in severely head-injured patients. J Neurosurg 61:700, 1984
37. Samson D, Beyer CW: Furosemide in the intraoperative reduction of intracranial pressure in the patient with subarachnoid hemorrhage. Neurosurgery 10:167, 1982
38. Bedford R, Colley P: Intracranial tumors, p. 135. In Matjasko J, Katz J (eds): Clinical Controversies in Neuroanesthesia and Neurosurgery. Grune & Stratton, Orlando, FL, 1986.
39. Standefer M, Bay JW, Trusso DO: The sitting position in neurosurgery: A retrospective analysis of 488 cases. Neurosurgery 14:649, 1984
40. Matjasko J, Petrozza P, Cohen M, Steinberg P: Anesthesia and surgery in the seated position: Analysis of 554 cases. Neurosurgery 17:695, 1985
41. Young ML, Smith DS, Murtagh F et al: Comparison of surgical and anesthetic complications in neurosurgical patients experiencing venous air embolism in the sitting position. Neurosurgery 18:157, 1986
42. Black S, Ockert DB, Oliver WC, Cucchiara RF: Comparison of outcome following posterior fossa craniectomy done in either a sitting or horizontal position. Anesthesiology 69:49, 1988
43. Perkins-Pearson NAK, Marshall WK, Bedford RF: Atrial pressures in the seated position: implication for paradoxical air embolism. Anesthesiology 57:493, 1982
44. Black S, Cucchiara RF, Nishimura RA, Michenfelder JD: Parameters affecting occurrence of paradoxical air embolism. Anesthesiology 71:235, 1989
45. Seward JB, Hayes DL, Smith HC et al: Platypnea-orthodeoxia: clinical profile, diagnostic workup, management and report of seven cases. Mayo Clin Proc 59:221, 1984
46. Michenfelder JD, Gronert GA, Rehder K: Neuroanesthesia. Anesthesiology 30:65, 1969
47. Ebersold MJ, Harner SG, Beatty CW et al: Current results of the retrosigmoid approach to acoustic neurinoma. J Neurosurg 76:901, 1992
48. Michenfelder JD: Central venous catheters in the management of air embolism: whether as well as where. Anesthesiology 55:339, 1981
49. Bunegin L, Albin M, Helsel P et al: Positioning the

right atrial catheter: a model for reappraisal. Anesthesiology 55:343, 1981
50. Cucchiara RF, Messick JM, Gronert GA, Michenfelder JD: Time required and success rate of percutaneous right atrial catheterization: description of a technique. Can Anaesth Soc J 27:572, 1980
51. Artru AA, Colley PS: The site of origin of the intravascular electrocardiogram recorded from multiorificed intravascular catheters. Anesthesiology 69:44, 1988
52. Lee D, Kuhn J, Shaffer M, Weintraub H: Migration of tips of central venous catheters in seated patients. Anesth Analg 63:949, 1984
53. Glenski JA, Cucchiara RF: Transcutaneous O_2 and CO_2 monitoring of neurosurgical patients: detection of air embolism. Anesthesiology 64:546, 1986
54. Cucchiara RF, Nugent M, Seward JB, Mesick JM: Air embolism in upright neurosurgical patients: Detection and localization by 2-D transesophageal echocardiography. Anesthesiology 60:353, 1984
55. Gazzaniga AB, Dalen JE: Paradoxical embolism: Its pathophysiology and clinical recognition. Ann Surg 171:137, 1970
56. Hagen PT, Scholz DG, Edwards WD: Incidence and size of patent foramen ovale during the first 10 decades of life: An autopsy study of 965 normal hearts. Mayo Clin Proc 59:17, 1984
57. Lynch JJ, Schuchard GH, Gross CM, Wann LS: Prevalence of right-to-left atrial shunting in a healthy population: Detection by Valsalva maneuver contrast echocardiography. Am J Cardiol 53:1478, 1984
58. Dubourg O, Bourdarias JP, Farcot JC et al: Contrast echocardiography visualization of cough-induced right to left shunt through a patient foramen ovale. J Am Coll Cardiol 4:587, 1984
59. Lechat PH, Mas JL, Lascault G et al: Prevalence of patient foramen ovale in patients with stroke. N Engl J Med 318:1148, 1988
60. Kronik G, Mosslacher H: Positive contrast echocardiography in patients with patent foramen ovale and normal right heart hemodynamics. Am J Cardiol 49:1806, 1982
61. Voorhies RM, Fraser RAR, Poznak AV: Prevention of air embolism with positive end expiratory pressure. Neurosurgery 12:503, 1983
62. Hewer AJH, Logue V: Methods of increasing the safety of neuroanesthesia in the sitting position. Anaesthesia 17:476, 1962
63. Lee DS, Lichtmann MW, Weintraub HD: Effect of PEEP on air embolism during sitting neurosurgical procedures. Anesth Analg 60:262, 1981
64. Muravchick S, DeLisser E, Welch F: The use of PEEP to identify source of cardiopulmonary air embolism. Anesthesiology 49:294, 1978
65. Albin MS: The paradox of paradoxic air embolism-PEEP, Valsalva, and patent foramen ovale. Should the sitting position be abandoned? Anesthesiology 61:222, 1984
66. Albin MS, Carroll RG, Maroon JC: Clinical considerations concerning detection of venous air embolism. Neurosurgery 3:380, 1978
67. Toung T, Ngeow YK, Long DL et al: Comparison of the effects of positive end-expiratory pressure and jugular venous compression on canine cerebral venous pressure. Anesthesiology 61:169, 1984
68. Grady MS, Bedford RF, Park TS: Changes in superior sagittal sinus pressure in children during head elevation, jugular venous compression, and PEEP. J Neurosurg 65:199, 1986
69. Cucchiara RF, Seward JB, Nishimura RA et al: Identification of patent foramen ovale during sitting position craniotomy by transesophageal echocardiography with positive airway pressure. Anesthesiology 63:107, 1985
70. Perkins NAK, Bedford RF: Hemodynamic consequences of PEEP in seated neurological patients-implications for paradoxical air embolism. Anesth Analg 63:429, 1984
71. Losasso TJ, Black S, Muzzi DA et al: Detection and hemodynamic consequences of venous air embolism: does nitrous oxide made a difference. Anesthesiology 77:148, 1992
72. Losasso TJ, Muzzi DA, Dietz NM, Cucchiara RF: Fifty percent nitrous oxide does not increase the risk of venous air embolism in neurosurgical patients operated upon in the sitting position. Anesthesiology 77:21, 1992
73. Shupak RC, Harp JR: Comparison between high-dose sufentanil-oxygen and high-dose fentanyl-oxygen for neuroanesthesia. Br J Anaesth 57:375, 1985
74. Artru AA, Cucchiara RF, Messick JM: Cardiorespiratory and cranial nerve sequelae of surgical procedures involving the posterior fossa. Anesthesiology 52:83, 1980
75. Skahen S, Shapiro HM, Drummond JC et al: Nitrous oxide withdrawal reduces intracranial pressure in the presence of pneumocephalus. Anesthesiology 65:92, 1986
76. Artru AA: Breathing nitrous oxide during closure

of the dura and cranium is not indicated. Anesthesiology 66:719, 1987
77. Ellis SC, Bryan-Brown CW, Hyderally H: Massive swelling of the head and neck. Anesthesiology 42:102, 1975
78. McAllister RG: Macroglossia—a positional complication. Anesthesiology 40:199, 1974
79. Randall RV: Clinical presentation of pituitary adenomas. p. 15. In Laws ER, Randall RV, Kern EB, Abboud CF (eds): Management of Pituitary Adenomas and Related Lesions with Emphasis on Transsphenoidal Surgery. Appleton-Century-Crofts, East Norwalk, CT, 1982
80. Tindall GF, McLanahan CS: Hyperfunctional pituitary tumors: pre- and postoperative management considerations. Clin Neurosurg 27:48, 1980
81. Messick JM, Laws ER, Abboud CF: Anesthesia for transsphenoidal surgery of the hypophyseal region. Anesth Analg 57:206, 1978
82. Tasch MD: Endocrine diseases. p. 437. In Stoelting RK, Dierdorf SF (eds): Anesthesia and Co-Existing Disease. Churchill Livingstone, New York, 1983
83. Cadieux RJ, Kales A, Santen RJ et al: Endoscopic findings in sleep apnea associated with acromegaly. J Clin Endocrinol Metab 55:18, 1982
84. Hassan SZ, Matz GJ, Lawrence AM, Collins PA: Laryngeal stenosis in acromegaly: A possible cause of airway difficulties associated with anesthesia. Anesth Analg 55:57, 1976
85. Kitahata LM: Airway difficulties associated with anesthesia in acromegaly. Br J Anaesth 43:1187, 1971
86. Southwick JP, Katz J: Unusual airway difficulty in the acromegalic patient-indications for tracheostomy. Anesthesiology 51:72, 1979
87. Ovassapian A, Doka JC, Romsa DE: Acromegaly—use of a fiberoptic laryngoscopy to avoid tracheostomy. Anesthesiology 54:429, 1981
88. Messick JM, Cucchiara RF, Faust RJ: Airway management in patients with acromegaly. Anesthesiology 56:157, 1982
89. Newfield P, Albin MS, Chestnut JC, Maroon J: Air embolism during transphenoidal pituitary operations. Neurosurgery 2:39, 1978
90. Messick JM, Faust RJ, Cucchiara RF: Anesthesia for transsphenoidal microsurgery. p. 253. In Laws ER, Randall RV, Kern EB, Abboud CF (eds): Management of Pituitary Adenomas and Related Lesions with Emphasis on Transsphenoidal Surgery. Appleton-Century-Crofts, East Norwalk, CT, 1982
91. Laws ER, Kern EB: Complications of transsphenoidal surgery. p. 329. In Laws ER, Randall RV, Kern EB, Abboud CF (eds): Management of Pituitary Adenomas and Related Lesions with Emphasis on Transsphenoidal Surgery. Appleton-Century-Crofts, East Norwalk, CT, 1982
92. Cucchiara RF, Black S, Steinkeler JA: Anesthesia for intracranial procedures. p. 849. In Barash PG, Cullen BF, Stoelting RK (eds): Clinigal Anesthesia. JB Lippincott, Philadelphia, 1989

11 EPILEPSY SURGERY

STEVEN N. ROPER

ROBERT S. ALPHIN

The patient who undergoes surgical treatment for epilepsy presents special considerations for all members of the operative team. Epilepsy is the chronic tendency for recurrent seizures, and it effects 6.25 of 1,000 individuals in the United States. Most of these patients will be well controlled on medications; however, about 30 percent of these cases are refractory to medical therapy. There are an estimated 100,000 individuals with intractable epilepsy in the United States who may be candidates for surgical treatment with 5,000 new cases presenting each year.[2] Epilepsy surgery dates back to a report of three cases that was presented by Sir Victor Horsley in 1886.[3] It has evolved over the years to be a highly effective and safe treatment modality in well-selected patients. In 1992, the Second Palm Desert International Conference on the Surgical Treatment of Epilepsies received participants from 118 epilepsy surgery centers throughout the world and obtained outcome data on 6,009 surgical patients treated between 1986 and 1990. The first conference, held in 1986, had 53 participating centers, and outcome data were obtained on 3,446 patients (representing the centers' surgical experience up to 1985).[2] These figures document the growing, worldwide recognition of epilepsy surgery as an effective and underused treatment for intractable epilepsy.

Seizures may be classified broadly as partial (with focal origin) or generalized (with diffuse, bilateral onset). The generalized seizures include generalized tonic-clonic seizures and absence seizures and tend to respond well to medical management. The partial epilepsies are more likely to be refractory to medical therapy. Current classification systems of the partial epilepsies attempt to organize them according to region of onset and etiologies that include idiopathic (no underlying cause other than possible hereditary predisposition), symptomatic (caused by a disorder of the central nervous system), and cryptogenic (presumed to be symptomatic but the etiology is currently unknown).[4]

From the surgical perspective, the epilepsies can be broadly defined by pathologic substrate and location. Lesional epilepsy has been used to describe epilepsy that occurs because of a focal structural abnormality that is demonstrable by current clinical imaging studies. Foreign tissue lesions, such as tumors and vascular malformations, comprise most of these cases.[5] Other common lesions include focal areas of abnormal cortical development such as glioneuronal hamartomas, focal cortical dysplasia, and the tubers associated with tuberous sclerosis.[6] Epileptogenic lesions can also result from destructive processes such as trauma, infarction, and infection. Mesial temporal lobe epilepsy has a strong association with hippocampal sclerosis,[7] and in these cases, seizure onset occurs in the temporal structures medial to the collateral sulcus. Nonlesional neocortical epilepsy arises in neocortex and does not have a consistent pathologic correlate. It remains the most poorly understood of the surgically treated epilepsies. Even these very general classifications become inadequate in certain situations.

In the temporal lobe, for instance, foreign tissue lesions can occur simultaneously with hippocampal sclerosis, and the implications of this "dual pathology" for surgical treatment have yet to be completely understood.[8–10]

The primary treatment for epilepsy is the use of antiepileptic drugs. Surgery is contemplated when the patient's epilepsy has proved to be intractable to medical therapy. Epilepsy is considered intractable when there are persistent disabling seizures despite maximal, tolerable medical treatment including the most current, effective anticonvulsants. In general, the goal of epilepsy surgery is to remove a focal area of epileptogenesis where all the patient's seizures originate when this occurs in an area that will not produce unacceptable neurologic deficits. Extensive testing is required to define this area and document its physiologic function. Some of this testing extends to the operative suite, and this can present special considerations for the anesthetist. Intraoperative electrocorticography (ECoG) is performed to record the interictal activity of the exposed brain. In these cases, the effect of anesthetics on electroencephalogram (EEG) activity becomes extremely important. In some cases, there is a need to define eloquent cortical regions such as the primary language areas or the primary motor or somatosensory areas via stimulation mapping in an awake patient so that special sedating techniques are required. This chapter describes the workup, surgical procedures, and anesthetic techniques involved in the surgical treatment of intractable epilepsy.

SURGICAL CONSIDERATIONS

Diagnostic Workup

The management of a patient that is being considered for epilepsy surgery can be organized into three phases. The information obtained during each phase will determine the next step toward surgical therapy, or it may determine that further surgical workup is not indicated.

Phase I consists of information gathering by noninvasive tests. This includes a thorough history and physical examination, documentation of current and previous adequate attempts at medical management, review of interictal EEG, structural and functional brain imaging studies, neuropsychological testing, and scalp/sphenoidal EEG telemetry to record seizure onset. One major goal of the initial studies is to document that intractable epilepsy is present and to determine if there is strong evidence for a unifocal onset. In some cases, noninvasive EEG telemetry alone will provide strong evidence for seizure onset in a particular area. In a growing number of patients, the combined information from noninvasive EEG telemetry and sophisticated imaging studies will provide sufficient information to recommend therapeutic surgery without further investigation with intracranial electrodes. This most commonly occurs in epilepsy that is associated with foreign tissue lesions and mesial temporal lobe epilepsy that is associated with hippocampal sclerosis. Although specific protocols and relative weighting of tests may vary between centers, most surgical programs require a focal ictal onset on noninvasive EEG and another independent test that implicates the same area with no conflicting results from any other noninvasive tests to recommend surgical resection without prior investigation with intracranial electrodes. This is not always true for epilepsy associated with foreign tissue lesions in which good results have been obtained with removal of only the lesions or the lesions and adjacent cortex and in which ictal onset by both noninvasive and invasive EEG can be misleading.[11] At the end of phase I, the patient may be found to be inappropriate for further surgical workup, in need of intracranial investigation, or appropriate for surgery without further extraoperative EEG-based testing.

In patients in whom temporal lobectomy is being considered, it is important to confirm the lateralization of language function and that the contralateral hemisphere can support major memory function. This is accomplished with the Wada test. The goal of the Wada test is to temporarily anesthetize each temporal lobe using a fast-acting barbiturate while testing for language and memory functions. This is generally accomplished through intracarotid injection of sodium amobarbital.[12] Patients are asked to memorize objects before injection and while the barbiturates are active. They are also asked to perform naming tasks. Motor strength is assessed to document that the barbiturates have produced the appropriate effects on the hemisphere. An obvious criticism of the intracarotid test for evaluating memory function is that the hippocampi are supplied primarily by the posterior cerebral artery. Depending on the relative flow from the internal carotid artery through the posterior communicating artery, there may be little to no injection of barbiturates into the posterior cerebral artery through this approach. In addition, the global effects of anesthetizing the entire distribution of the internal carotid artery may produce a change in alertness to the point at which poor performance on the memory tests may be a nonspecific finding. By using an approach through the vertebrobasilar arterial system, the posterior cerebral arteries can be cannulated individually and infused with barbiturates by experienced angiographers to test the memory functions of the hippocampi (the superselective Wada test). Despite these problems, the intracarotid Wada test has proved to be effective in assessing language and memory function in most cases.[13] The policy at the University of Florida is that all patients who may be recommended for a temporal lobe resection undergo intracarotid Wada testing before phase II or, if no phase II is planned, before surgical resection (phase III). If there are equivocal results on memory testing during the intracarotid Wada test, the patient returns at a later date for superselective Wada testing using posterior cerebral artery injections before surgery.

Because noninvasive EEG can be misleading regarding the site of seizure onset in 18 to 30 percent of patients with partial seizures,[14,15] more accurate methods for determining this area are sometimes needed. Phase II consists of monitoring electroclinical activity through invasively implanted, intracranial electrodes. The two most common types of intracranial electrodes are depth electrodes, which are placed within the brain parenchyma, and subdural electrodes, which are placed over the cortical surface. Depth electrodes are most commonly used to record from the amygdala and hippocampus on both sides in patients in whom mesial temporal lobe epilepsy has been established but lateralization is in question. Subdural electrodes can be arranged in single rows (strips) or matrices of various sizes (grids). They are generally used for recording from neocortical surfaces but can also record mesial temporal activity if placed over the parahippocampal gyrus. Subdural electrodes are used to define the boundaries of epileptogenic areas as well as to perform extraoperative stimulation mapping to localize cortical function. If phase II studies define an area of epileptogenesis that can be resected without an unacceptable functional deficit, surgical resection is recommended. Because subdural grids require a craniotomy for placement and removal and the electrodes serve to define the spatial limits of the resection, the surgical resection is performed at the time of electrode removal. Depth electrodes and subdural strips are placed through burr holes and may be removed at bedside or in a minor second surgery. For this reason, patients who have had depth electrodes placed often recover from phase II at home before returning for the craniotomy for resection.

Surgical Procedures

ELECTRODE IMPLANTATION The indications for intracranial electrode placement were discussed in the previous section. Depth electrodes are placed using stereotactic guidance. The mesial temporal structures can be approached either from the side (through the lateral temporal lobe) or from posteriorly (traversing the occipital lobe). Stereotactic systems can be broadly classified as orthogonal or arc-based. At this time, many systems still require

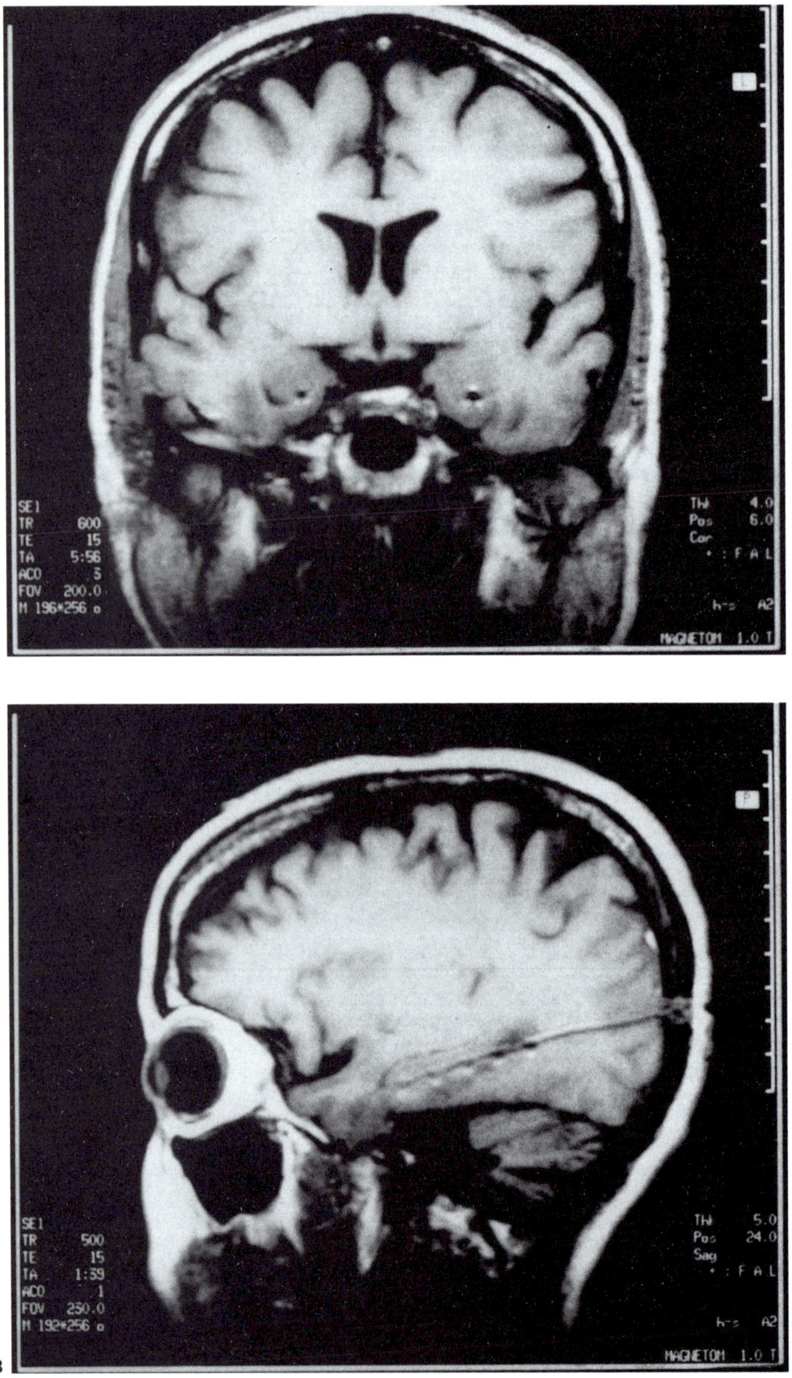

A

B

FIGURE 11.1 *T_1-weighted magnetic resonance images of a patient with bilateral depth electrodes in place. The coronal image (A) shows the most anterior contacts within both amygdalae. The sagittal image (B) shows one depth electrode traversing the long axis of the hippocampus.*

that an external frame be placed on the head in a fixed position for preoperative imaging studies and implantation of the electrodes, but the development of frameless stereotaxy is rapidly obviating the need for cumbersome and uncomfortable external frames. The typical stereotactic surgery begins at the patient's bedside with placement of the stereotactic frame under local anesthesia. Appropriate imaging studies are then performed so that the targets, entry point, and possible intervening vascular structures can be accounted for when planning the electrode trajectory. The patients are then taken to the operative suite. Depth electrodes may be placed under local anesthesia. At the University of Florida, bitemporal depth electrodes are placed from an occipital approach[16] in conjunction with bilateral subtemporal and orbitofrontal subdural strip electrodes (Fig. 11.1).[17] Because the strip electrodes require additional bilateral frontotemporal skin incisions, these procedures are carried out under general anesthesia. The surgical procedures for implantation of subdural electrodes vary, depending on the region that needs to be sampled.[18] Subdural strip electrodes can be placed through burr holes, but grids require a craniotomy (Fig. 11.2).

ANTERIOR TEMPORAL LOBECTOMY AND OTHER TEMPORAL RESECTIONS

Anterior temporal lobectomy is the most commonly performed procedure for the treatment of epilepsy. It has been modified and refined over the years to reflect an increased understanding of the role of mesial temporal structures in most cases of temporal lobe epilepsy as well as differences in how interictal and ictal EEG data are interpreted and weighed. The standard anterior temporal lobectomy removes a portion of the temporal lobe that is relatively constant between patients. This includes anterior temporal neocortex, parahippocampal gyrus, the uncus, the lateral portion of the amygdala, and the hippocampus. The amount of anterior temporal neocortex removed is 4 to 5 cm (as measured from the temporal pole over the middle temporal gyrus) in the dominant hemisphere and 5 to 6 cm in the nondominant hemisphere. The amount of hippocampus removed varies slightly between centers but usually includes 3 cm along the longitudinal axis. Spencer's modification of the standard anterior temporal lobectomy limits the neocortical resection to 3 cm from the temporal pole and carries the hippocampal resection back to the level of the superior colliculi[19] (Fig. 11.3). More recent procedures such as amygdalohippocampectomy attempt to limit the resection to the mesial temporal structures. Because the hippocampus lies within the inferomedial wall of the temporal horn, it may be approached through the sylvian fissure,[20] the middle temporal gyrus,[21] or a subtemporal approach.[21] Tailored anterior temporal lobectomies vary the amount of resected tissue based on physiologic data. These may include ictal and interictal data acquired extraoperatively through subdural electrodes or intraoperative interictal data. When intraoperative data are used to determine the extent of resection, dominant temporal lobectomies are generally performed awake with stimulation mapping of the posterior temporal speech area because the topography of interictal spiking may suggest a more posterior temporal resection than is known to be safe and because the exact location of this eloquent area varies between patients.[23]

Temporal lobe resections have a high success rate, with 68 percent of patients experiencing complete abolition of seizures and an additional 24 percent with significant improvement in seizures at 1-year follow-up.[24] The side effects of dominant temporal lobectomy include visual field defects in the contralateral superior quadrant and impaired ability to memorize lists of words and some word-finding difficulties in normal conversation. Nondominant resections may produce visual field defects, but cognitive deficits are not apparent. With complete abolition of seizures, neuropsychologic testing may show improvements in some patients.

LESIONECTOMY

Lesionectomy refers to a surgical resection for intractable epilepsy that is caused by a documented structural lesion. De-

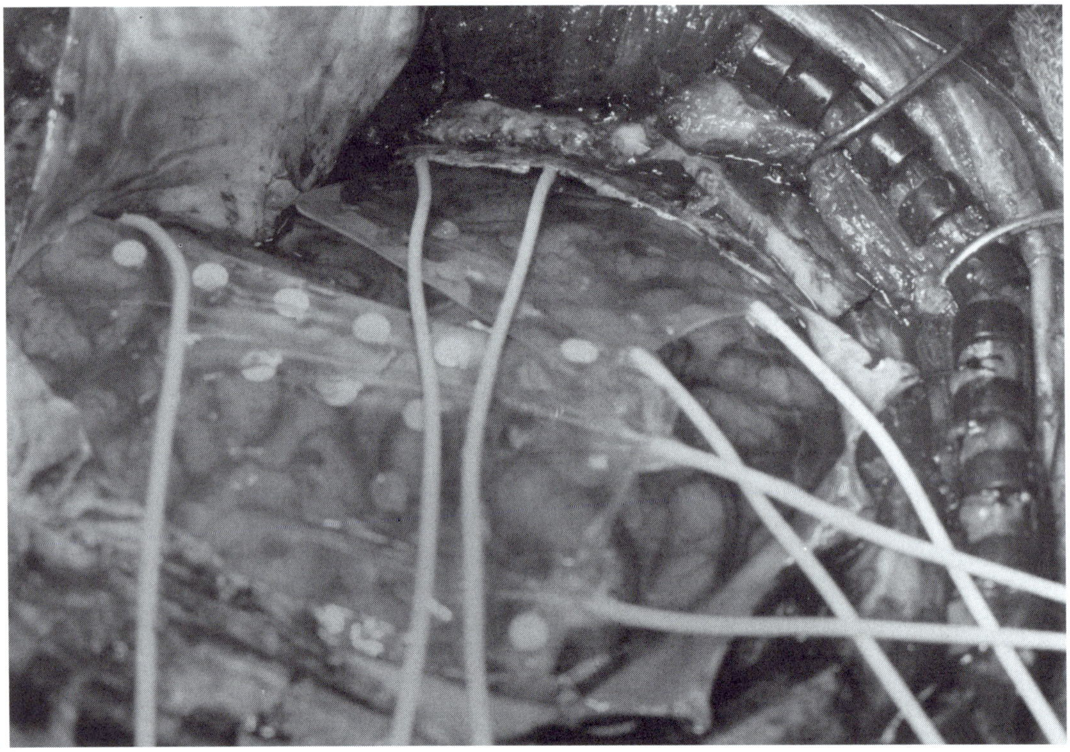

A

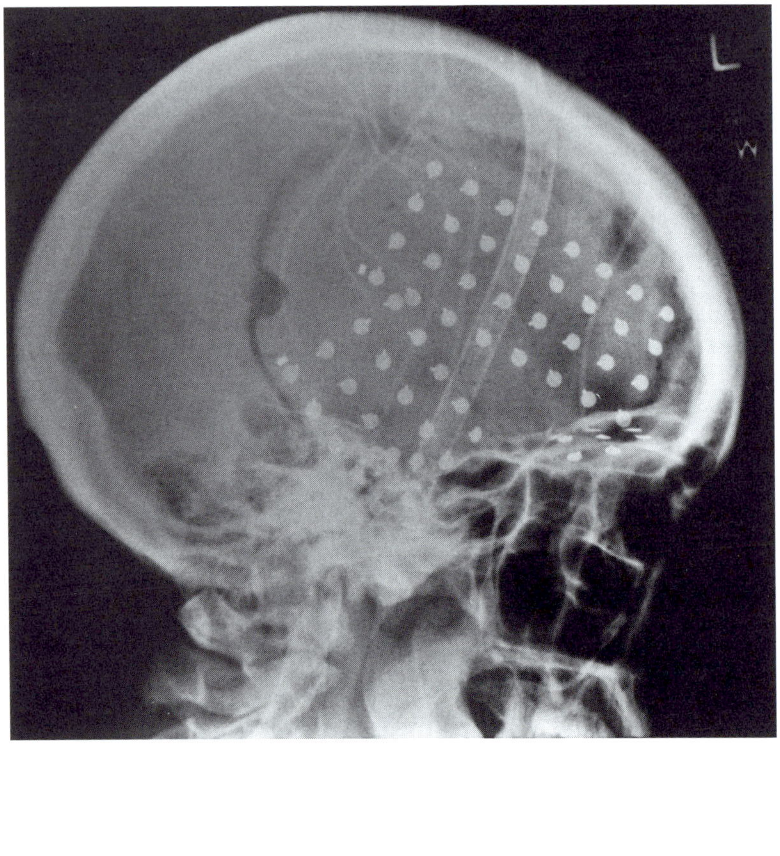

B

FIGURE 11.2 *An intraoperative photograph (A) demonstrates the implantation of subdural grid and strip electrodes. Grids are seen over the lateral surfaces of the right frontal and temporal lobes (anterior is to left and superior is at the bottom of the image). The postoperative, lateral skull radiograph (B) shows two subdural grids covering the lateral surface of the frontal and temporal lobes. (Figure continues.)*

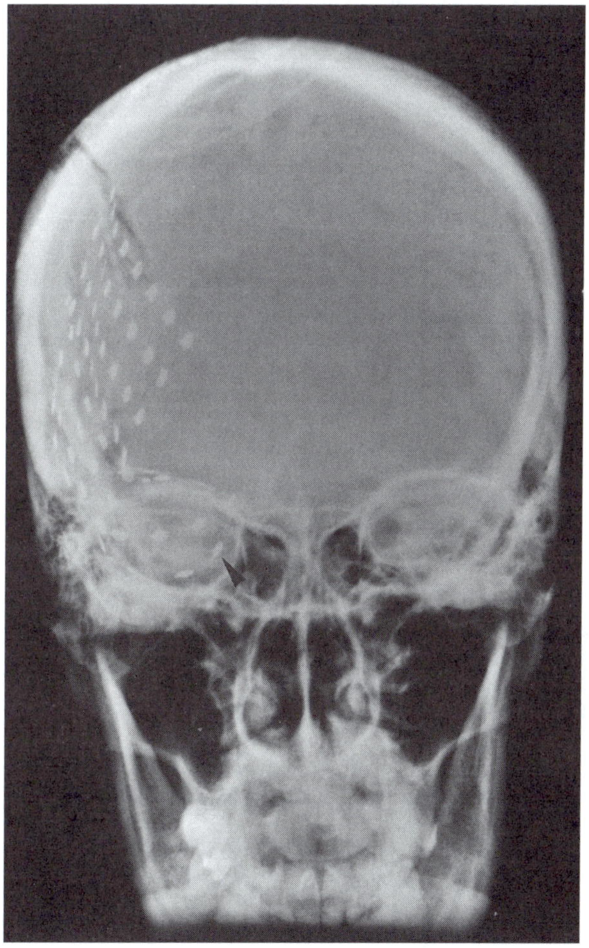
C

FIGURE 11.2 *(Continued) The anterior-posterior skull radiograph (C) shows two subdural strip electrodes extending over the inferior surface of the right temporal lobe to reach the region of the parahippocampal gyrus (arrowhead).*

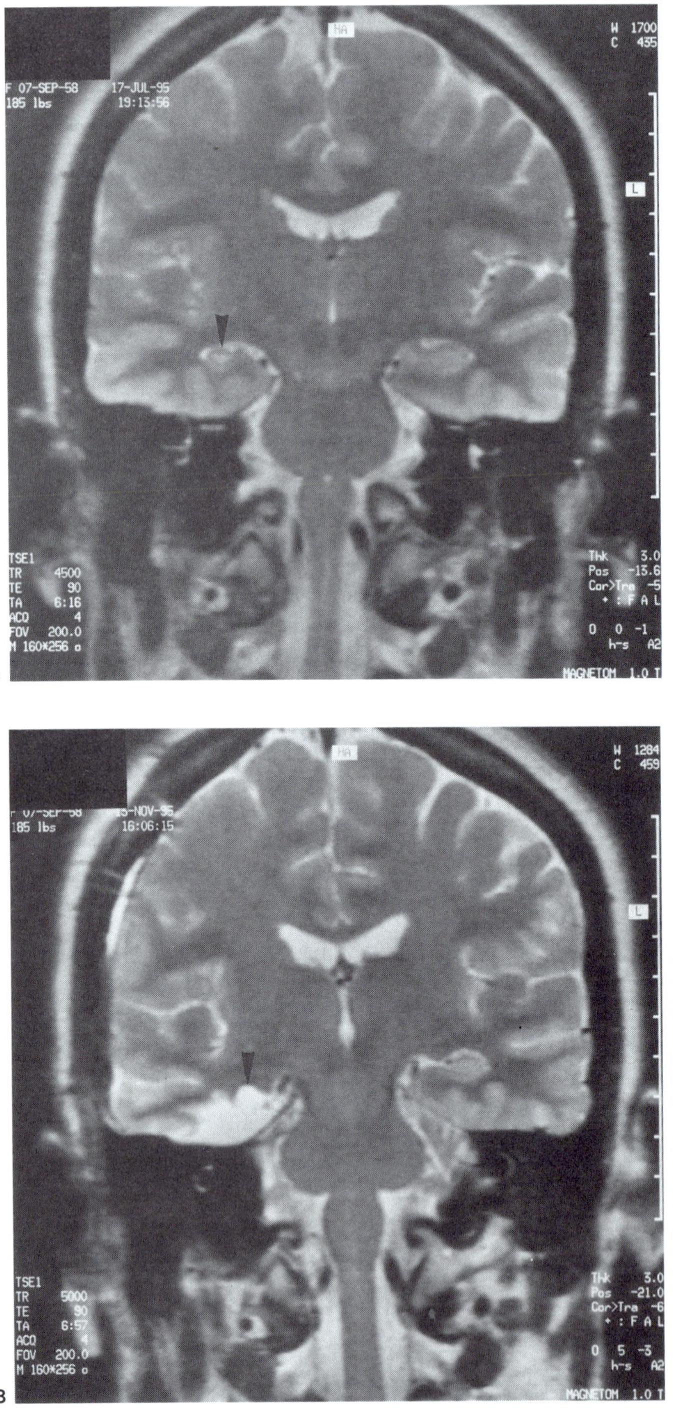

A

B

FIGURE 11.3 *Coronal, T_2-weighted magnetic resonance images of a patient with mesial temporal lobe epilepsy. The preoperative image (A) shows that the right hippocampus (arrowhead) is small and has a high T_2 signal when compared with the left one. These findings are indicative of hippocampal sclerosis. The postoperative image (B) shows the resection cavity in the location of the hippocampus and parahippocampal gyrus (arrowhead) with sparing of the lateral temporal lobe. Pathologic examination of the resected hippocampus confirmed the diagnosis of hippocampal sclerosis.*

bate still exists on whether it is sufficient to remove the lesion alone or whether additional cortex adjacent to the lesion should be resected as well to provide the best chance at seizure control, and resolution of this question is beyond the scope of this chapter (for discussion, see ref. 25). If additional cortex is to be removed, the limits of resection may be defined extraoperatively through subdural electrodes or intraoperatively using interictal data. If the lesion is near an eloquent cortical region, awake craniotomy and stimulation mapping may be necessary when intraoperative ECoG is being used to define the limits of the resection. The approaches and exposures for these resections are dictated by the location of the lesion.

EXTRATEMPORAL RESECTIONS Cortical resections for intractable seizures that extend beyond the limits of the temporal lobe are termed extratemporal resections or topectomies. If lesionectomies are removed from this group, it represents the greatest challenge to the epilepsy surgery team and holds the greatest room for improvement in surgical outcome. The area of epileptogenesis is usually defined by physiologic data acquired extraoperatively through subdural electrodes. This area may overlap with eloquent cortical regions and further limit surgical options (see below, Multiple Subpial Transection). As in lesionectomies, the surgical approaches and exposures vary according to the location of the area of epileptogenesis.

HEMISPHERECTOMY Hemispherectomy represents the epilepsy surgery with the most inclusive resections, the most stringent criteria for consideration, and the best surgical outcomes. It is performed in cases in which the area of epileptogenesis extends throughout an entire hemisphere and in which there is a preexisting hemiparesis or in which the natural history of the underlying process makes eventual hemiparesis or hemiplegia a certainty. These conditions are most frequently found in children. Underlying pathologies include Rasmussen's encephalitis, perinatal infarction of the middle cerebral artery, Sturge-Weber syndrome, and hemimegalencephaly. Although the patients have preexisting hemiparesis, increased neurologic deficits are rare because most cases have had a nonfunctional or poorly functional hemisphere since the pre- or perinatal period (when the presumed insult actually occurred) and brain maturation has occurred while relying on the "good" hemisphere. Rasmussen's encephalitis with onset in late childhood or adolescence is a notable and unfortunate exception to this rule. The remarkable capacity for reorganization of cortical function that exists up to 6 to 8 years of age also allows for compensation of neurologic deficits that may occur after hemispherectomy (e.g., children can still develop functional speech after left hemispherectomy). Unavoidable deficits after hemispherectomy include significantly impaired fine motor control in the opposite hand and some degree of contralateral, homonymous visual field defect and may represent the limits of the brain's capacity to transfer function to the opposite hemisphere.

Hemispherectomy was originally described as a complete removal of the cortical structures of one cerebral hemisphere.[26] This anatomic hemispherectomy involves a large hemicraniotomy for exposure. The hemisphere is then devascularized by clipping and transecting the anterior, middle, and posterior cerebral arteries. The hemisphere is then removed down to the level of the basal ganglia. Although seizure control rates were very good, follow-up reports on early anatomic hemispherectomies described a late deterioration in up to 25 percent of patients.[27] The complications were thought to be related to the large subdural space that was created by the hemispherectomy and predisposed to recurrent episodes of bleeding from subdural membrances. The pathologic changes in the remaining brain structures were termed superficial cerebral hemosiderosis. The effects of this process were quite severe and could result in death. To avoid this complication, Dr. Theodore Rasmussen at the Montreal Neurological Institute devised the functional hemispherectomy based on the observation that large multilobar brain resections did not produce the same late complications if a substantial amount of cortex remained in place. The functional hemispherectomy removes the central cortex and the temporal lobe. The anterior frontal and occipital lobes are left in place with their vascular supply intact but are functionally isolated from the rest of the brain by transecting the corpus callosum and the descending fiber tracts. Follow-up studies on this procedure have not shown the occurrence of late chronic hemosiderosis but have maintained seizure control rates of 86 percent.[28] More recent modifications of the procedure further limit the cortical resection while performing an extensive disconnection from within the lateral ventricle.[29]

CORPUS CALLOSOTOMY Corpus callosotomy is the only epilepsy surgery that is, by definition, palliative. The goal of the procedure is to alter the propagation of the seizure activity through the corpus callosum and, consequently, reduce the severity of the clinical manifestation of the seizure. It is most effective in the treatment of drop attacks.[30] Other seizure types can respond to corpus callosotomy, but surgical outcome rates are reduced as compared with drop attacks and vary between centers.[31–33] Drop attacks are a type of seizure that begin very rapidly and cause an alteration in postural control such that the patient will fall to the ground if not supported. They are the most physically damaging of any seizure type and will often, over time, result in a series of broken bones and other injuries. Daily management of these patients is extremely difficult for the family because of the constant threat of physical injury coupled with the fact that they often suffer some degree of mental retardation. The postural changes during drop attacks are usually atonic, but they can also be tonic or a combination of the two. These seizures are almost always seen in the context of multiple seizure types with multifocal or diffuse abnormalities on EEG. They occur commonly in children with Lennox Gastaut syndrome (which consists of multiple seizure types, mental retardation, and a 2.5 to 3-Hz spike and -wave pattern on EEG) but often persist as patients mature and outgrow the specific definitions of this syndrome.

Corpus callosotomy is performed through a right frontal craniotomy with exposure of the corpus callosum through the interhemispheric fissure. The corpus callosum is then divided in the midline. The division extends from the level of the anterior commissure (the anterior commissure is left intact) through the rostrum, genu, and body of the corpus callosum and may or may not include the splenium. The procedure may be performed as a one-stage or complete callosotomy, which includes the splenium, or as an anterior callosotomy, which divides about two-thirds of the callosum and spares the posterior body and splenium. The anterior callosotomy is recommended with the understanding that a second operation to divide the remaining posterior structures may be needed if the response to the anterior callostomy is suboptimal or transient. The rationale behind the staged approach arises from the fact that seizure control rates are better with complete callosotomy,[33] but the risk of neurologic side effects is higher with this procedure. In patients who are so severely impaired that a disconnection syndrome would not make a significant impact on their quality of life, complete callosotomy may be recommended as the initial procedure to optimize seizure outcome.

MULTIPLE SUBPIAL TRANSECTION The multiple subpial transection (MST) procedure was designed by Dr. Frank Morrell to address the difficult problem that arises when the area of epileptogenesis resides within eloquent neocortex such as the primary motor, somatosensory, or language areas. MST is based on two fundamental observations. The first is that epileptiform activity requires a critical volume of neocortex to occur,[34] and when the horizontal connections in the neocortex are interrupted at certain intervals, interictal spikes and seizures are prevented. The second is that, because of the vertical modular structure of many neocortical areas, horizontal connections within the cortex can be interrupted while preserving the major functions of the area as long as the ascending and descending connections remain intact.[35] The procedure consists of making parallel subpial cuts through the thickness of the cortex at 5 mm intervals. A small hooked instrument is passed through a needle hole in the pia to disrupt the horizontal connections within the cortex but preserve the pia and blood vessels on the cortical surface, all ascending and descending connections, and the subcortical U-fibers. MST, as described by Ford et al.,[36] relies heavily in intraoperative ECoG both in defining the area of epileptogenesis and in determining the physiologic endpoint of the procedure, which is cessation of interictal spiking. Because of this, they advocate brevital infusion in these cases to enhance interictal spiking throughout the surgery.[36] The MST literature is small when compared with the other procedures listed in this chapter, but MST either alone or in combination with an adjacent resection has produced significant improvement in seizures in 55 to 83 percent of patients.[37–39] It has been used in primary motor cortex, primary sensory cortex, and the posterior temporal speech area with preservation of function,[37] although temporary postoperative deficits can occur.

ANESTHETIC CONSIDERATIONS

The anesthesiologist plays an important role in the perioperative management of the epileptic patient. The potent physiologic effects of anticonvulsants and their potential interaction with anesthetic drugs must be considered for all epileptic patients undergoing any surgical procedure. In these patients, a primary objective for the anesthesiologist is to provide an anesthetic technique that will prevent or limit perioperative seizures. Further planning and understanding are necessary, however, to properly care for the subset of patients who undergo surgical treatment for their seizures. It is imperative to communicate early and effectively with the neurosurgeon and neurologist to establish an appropriate anesthetic plan. Thus, in medical centers where this type of surgery is routinely performed, protocols are often developed to standardize anesthetic techniques for these patients.

The anesthesiologist's responsibilities include provision of optimal operative conditions and patient safety while allowing for possible intraoperative neurophysiologic monitoring. Depending on the specific situation, this may require providing an anesthetic with anticonvulsant properties or, conversely, enhancing seizure activity with anesthetic drugs during intraoperative ECoG. For select patients, it may also require skillful monitored anesthesia care and conscious sedation for an awake craniotomy to allow intraoperative evaluation of eloquent (e.g., language, memory) cortical functions. Therefore, goals for the anesthesiologist should include the following:

1. careful preoperative patient evaluation, with particular emphasis on coexisting medical conditions, neurologic evaluation (including etiology, type and frequency of seizure activity), and anticonvulsant therapy
2. anticipation and understanding of operative and neurophysiologic monitoring plans
3. understanding of the proconvulsant and anticonvulsant effects of anesthetic drugs and their effects on EEG monitoring
4. patient education and preparation for the proposed surgical and anesthetic procedures (i.e., the potential for awake procedures, intraoperative awareness and/or discomfort, and potential complications)

PREOPERATIVE ISSUES

Anesthetic Considerations for Radiologic Evaluation

Often, anesthesiologists initially encounter epilepsy patients during evaluation for seizure surgery. Most patients undergo a variety of radiologic evaluations ranging from computed tomographs scans, magnetic resonance imaging scans, and cerebral angiography to more advanced cortical function tests such as positron emission tomography scans and Wada testing. Usually, these procedures do not require the presence of an anesthesiologist. However, with some patients (e.g., children, adults with claustrophobia, anxiety, or significant other medical problems), an anesthesiologist may be consulted to provide monitored anesthesia care, conscious sedation, or even general anesthesia to ensure patient safety and optimal test results. It is rare for EEG monitoring to be performed during these procedures; therefore anesthetic drugs with anticonvulsant properties may be used to ensure patient cooperation and immobility.

A variety of anesthetic techniques and drugs may be used, tailored to the individual patient as well as expertise of the anesthesiologist. Short-acting benzodiazepines and narcotics are acceptable for providing conscious sedation; alternatively, a propofol infusion (30 to 120 μg/kg/min) may be used to provide rapid onset and offset of sedation. It is best to avoid anesthetics (e.g., methohexital), which may trigger seizure activity and compromise patient safety and test results. Patient monitoring during conscious sedation or general anesthesia for these radiologic procedures must also take into consideration other medical conditions of the patient and should be the same as that routinely used in the operating suite. Wada testing for eloquent cortex is described under the previous Diagnostic Workup section.

Preoperative management for patients undergoing epilepsy surgery is similar to other neurosurgical patients with some additional considerations. Essentially, all these patients will be on one or more antiepileptic drugs, and each one has some impact on the anesthetist. Increasing valproate levels have been correlated with reduction in platelet counts, increase in bleeding times, and reduction in platelet aggregation,[40] and valproate has been associated with von Willebrand disease type I in children.[41] Published reports and surgeons vary on their assessment of the importance of this effect for operative hemostasis.[42] At the University of Florida, we taper patients off valproic acid several days before surgery if they are undergoing depth or subdural electrode implantation but not for open resective surgeries in which hemostasis can be confirmed before closure.

All patients are started on dexamethasone 10 mg 6 h on the evening before any of the surgeries listed in this chapter and maintained on steroids throughout the perioperative period. Before subdural grid implantation, patients are given the opportunity to donate autologous cryoprecipitate along with packed red blood cells (PRBCs all surgical patients are given the opportunity to donate PRBCs). The cryoprecipitate is used to make fibrin glue, which is placed over the exposed dura at the end of the surgery to decrease the chances of postoperative ceretrspinal fluid fistula.

Anesthetic Considerations for Intracranial Electrode Placement and Testing

Intracranial electrode placement and testing are sometimes required to localize epileptogenic foci and areas of eloquent cortical function. As described earlier, these may be a combination of depth electrodes as well as epidural or subdural grids and strip electrodes, depending on the area of cortex to be evaluated. These electrodes are most commonly placed during general anesthesia to avoid patient discomfort, although depth electrodes alone may be placed under local anesthesia using stereotactic guidance. Children and uncooperative adults, however, may require general anesthesia before placement of the stereotactic frame.

For those patients requiring general anesthesia, it is important to determine whether intraoperative ECoG will be performed at the time of electrode insertion before planning an anesthetic. If ECoG is planned during surgery, care must be taken to avoid drugs with anticonvulsant properties, which may diminish ECoG information. At the University of Florida, we have standardized our technique as follows. Preoperatively, anticonvulsant medication is continued at the discretion of the neurosurgeon. Anxiolytic premedication with a benzodiazepine is not administered. Standard intraoperative patient monitors include automated sphygmomanometry, electrocardiographic telemetry, pulse oximetry, capnography, temperature, and a precordial or esophageal stethoscope. A central venous line is generally not necessary, nor is an arterial line, unless the patient is undergoing a craniotomy. Fiberoptic awake intubation is usually used. We have had no problems intubating with the stereotactic frame in place, provided the anterior portion of the ring does not sit inferior to the nose. Induction of general anesthesia is accomplished with either propofol or thiopental, along with a nondepolarizing muscle relaxant and narcotic (fentanyl 5 to 10 $\mu g \cdot kg^{-1} \cdot hr^{-1}$ sufentanil 0.5 to 1.0 $\mu g \cdot kg^{-1} \cdot hr^{-1}$). Anesthesia is maintained with low-dose isoflurane (ET_{iso} less than 1 percent), 70 percent N_2O, continued muscle relaxation, and a narcotic infusion (fentanyl 2 to 5 $\mu g \cdot kg^{-1} \cdot hr^{-1}$ or sufentanil 0.2 to 0.8 $\mu g \cdot kg^{-1} \cdot hr^{-1}$). Once cranial bonework has begun (i.e., burr holes or craniotomy bone flap), isoflurane is discontinued until ECoG is completed, at which time it may be restarted during surgical resection (if performed at this time) and closure. The neurosurgeon may ask the anesthesiologist to help elicit epileptogenic foci intraoperatively by inducing hyperventilation or administering methohexital (0.25 to 0.5. kg^{-1}. hr^{-1}). In patients with seizure foci adjacent to the motor cortex, muscle relaxants may need to be discontinued or reversed intraoperatively to evaluate motor response to cortical stimulation. The antiepileptic drug valproic acid may inhibit platelet function, and its effect should be considered if unexpected bleeding occurs.

It is important to recognize that anesthetic requirements may be greatly increased in patients on chronic anticonvulsant therapy. Thus, more frequent dosing of muscle relaxants and higher narcotic infusion rates are often necessary to maintain adequate operative conditions. Likewise, it is necessary to discuss preoperatively with the patient the possibility of intraoperative awareness because anesthesia levels are decreased during ECoG.

Often, surgical resection is not performed at the time of electrode placement, and ECoG is deferred until the postoperative period. Any number of anesthetic techniques may then be used safely and effectively during electrode placement. In these situations, electrodes are placed, as described earlier, during general anesthesia; however, the electrodes remain in place postoperatively. This allows for ECoG and neurologic evaluation to take place while the patient is awake, in the absence of anesthetic drugs that may inhibit seizure activity. This technique is particularly useful in defining the relationship of seizure foci to cortical speech and memory areas. Once testing is completed, the patient may then return to the operating room for electrode removal and surgical resection. Alternatively, surgical resection may be deferred and electrodes may be removed during a minor surgical procedure or under aseptic bedside conditions. If the foci are determined to be operable, the patient returns after several weeks for elective surgical resection. Whether ECoG is performed intra-or postoperatively, the anesthesiologist should plan for the patient to emerge quickly and smoothly from general anesthesia and be extubated at the end of surgery so that a thorough postoperative neurologic evaluation may be performed.

Complications during electrode implantation and removal occur infrequently. Surgical bleeding is usually minimal, although intracranial hematomas have resulted from stereotactic depth electrode insertion. Hemodynamic instability is uncommon in the absence of other medical conditions, and intracranial elastance is typically normal. Rarely, patients will present with cerebral swelling and increased intracranial pressure, making electrode implantation difficult or impossible.

INTRAOPERATIVE ISSUES

Anesthetic Considerations for Surgical Resection

Once the decision has been made to proceed with the surgical resection of an epileptogenic focus, additional planning and discussion is necessary between the anesthesiologist, neurosurgeon, and patient to facilitate an optimal surgical outcome. Patients may be placed into one of three categories: (1) those who present for resection after phase I testing; (2) those who undergo surgical resection at the time of electrode deplantation; and (3) those patients in whom electrodes have been previously removed. Depending on the patient's previous surgical experiences and understanding of the planned procedure, significant patient education and preparation may be necessary, especially if an awake procedure with intraoperative neurologic evaluation is planned. Thus, a close relationship between the patient and anesthesiologist is helpful.

Several issues must be addressed by the anesthesiologist at this point:

1. What is the planned surgical procedure?
2. Will intraoperative ECoG be necessary?
3. Will an awake procedure with neurologic testing be required?

Once these factors are known, the anesthesiologist can complete the preoperative evaluation. Again, the patient's baseline neurologic status, anticonvulsant therapy, and coexisting medical conditions that may be affected by the planned surgery and anesthesia should be reviewed. Laboratory data should include anticonvulsant blood levels, if available, as well as hematologic and liver function studies to detect complications of anticonvulsant therapy. Anticonvulsants are again given preoperatively at the discretion of the neurosurgeon or neurologist. All patients should be treated with an antiemetic and antacid (sodium citrate or H_2-blocker), especially those undergoing awake procedures. Benzodiazepines are not administered preoperatively to avoid difficulty with EEG interpretation or emergence from anesthesia postoperatively. Small doses of narcotics or droperidol given intravenously may be useful in the immediate preoperative period for children and anxious adults. Intraoperative monitoring is similar to that described previously for patients undergoing electrode insertion. Arterial catheters are routinely placed in all patients undergoing a craniotomy to assist with blood pressure and ventilatory management. Central venous access is generally not necessary unless dictated by other medical problems, anticipated large blood loss, or poor peripheral venous access.

Anesthetic Techniques

The choice of an anesthetic technique for surgical resection of an epileptogenic focus depends primarily on the needs of the neurosurgeon and neurophysiologic monitoring teams. The optimal anesthetic technique during seizure surgery remains controversial. Most seizure surgery today is performed under general anesthesia, although there is no conclusive evidence (i.e., prospective, controlled studies) that demonstrates improved outcomes with either general anesthesia or conscious sedation. There are risks and benefits inherent to both techniques; thus, the physical and psychological condition of the patient as well as the skill of the surgeon and anesthesiologist must also be considered when planning an anesthetic.

Anesthetic goals should include (1) hemodynamic stability to maintain normal cerebral perfusion pressure; (2) avoidance of cerebral swelling and edema to minimize ischemia and facilitate surgical exposure; and (3) maintenance of normal fluid, electrolyte, and glucose homeostasis.

GENERAL ANESTHESIA General anesthetic techniques provide several advantages during seizure surgery. Patient cooperation and immobility are assured; furthermore, physiologic variables such as ($PaCO_2$), blood pressure, and intracranial pressure are more easily controlled to optimize operative conditions. However, neurophysiologic monitoring may be more difficult; language and memory evaluation is sacrificed, and ECoG may be diminished in some patients or with certain anesthetic agents. Because most volatile anesthetic agents cause

EEG suppression, their usefulness during seizure surgery is limited. When ECoG is planned during surgical resection, an N_2O narcotic technique with neuromuscular blockade is recommended, as described earlier for electrode implantation. The patient should be informed preoperatively that lighter anesthesia levels may be necessary during ECoG, increasing the likelihood of awareness during surgery. Inadequate analgesia is unlikely, however, if intraoperative narcotics are used.

Numerous other general anesthesia techniques have been described for use during seizure surgery. Ford et al.[36] advocate a combination of local anesthetic infiltration with general anesthesia by intravenous methohexital infusion. This technique uses the EEG activating ability of methohexital. Alternatively, Abou-Madi et al.[43] describe a technique that provides patient immobility, yet allows evaluation of the motor cortex during general anesthesia. Anesthesia is maintained with a combination of N_2O, fentanyl, and atracurium. Before ECoG, N_2O and atracurium are discontinued. Once neuromuscular function has returned, a blood pressure cuff is inflated above systolic pressure on the contralateral arm to the cortical testing area. Atracurium is readministered for muscle relaxation; however, the motor cortex can be identified by monitoring the unparalyzed arm during cortical stimulation.

Another useful drug during seizure surgery is droperidol. Commonly used during conscious sedation, droperidol is also effective for general anesthesia in combination with fentanyl and N_2O (Mahla, personal communication). It is administered in a dose of 0.1 $mg{\cdot}kg^{-1}$ intravenously over 20 minutes during induction of general anesthesia. Subsequent anesthesia is maintained with a narcotic infusion, 70 percent N_2O and neuromuscular blockade. This technique is not recommended for surgical procedures less than 4 hours in length to avoid a prolonged emergence or postoperative somnolence.

At times, despite a carefully planned anesthetic technique, ECoG recording may be inadequate. In such situations, it may be necessary to facility EEG activity with proconvulsant drugs. Methohexital, in small doses (less than 0.5 mg/kg), reliably activates the EEG in patients with temporal lobe epilepsy.[44] Likewise, ketamine[45,46] and etomidate[47,48] may also produce EEG activation. Enflurane, a seldom-used volatile anesthetic, may trigger seizure activity at higher concentrations as well.[49]

AWAKE CRANIOTOMY With refinement in neurophysiologic monitoring techniques, awake craniotomies are necessary only in a small percentage of patients, those in whom a seizure focus may be suppressed during general anesthesia or may be adjacent to an area of eloquent cortical function. Under these circumstances, an awake craniotomy may be the best or only option to identify the seizure focus and minimize brain injury.

When an awake craniotomy using local anesthesia and conscious sedation is indicated, appropriate preoperative screening is necessary to select those patients who will likely tolerate the procedure. It is important to discuss all details of the planned surgery with the patient and family. Points to be emphasized include

1. prolonged surgical procedure (often greater than 4 hours)
2. awkward body positioning with an absolute need for minimal patient movement
3. potential for significant patient discomfort (including pain, recall, nausea, and vomiting)
4. need for patient cooperation to evaluate language, memory, and motor skills
5. potential for emergent intubation and general anesthesia should the patient become uncooperative or persistent seizure activity, airway compromise, or hemodynamic instability occur

Only those patients with the ability to clearly understand risks and benefits and who in the opinion of the neurosurgeon and neuroanesthesiologist will cooperate during surgery should be considered as candidates for an awake craniotomy. Thus, children and mentally impaired adults are often not candidates for this type of surgery. Likewise, an awake craniotomy carries significantly increased risks in patients in whom airway management is predicted or known to be difficult because emergent intubation may become necessary with the patient in a suboptimal position.

Numerous techniques for conscious sedation and monitored anesthesia care have been described.[50–54] In all cases, appropriate patient positioning and surgical draping are necessary to allow for patient comfort, airway access, and prevention of peripheral nerve injuries. Standard intraoperative patient monitoring is indicated, including invasive arterial blood pressure monitoring. Oxygen administration and capnography may be accomplished via a nasal cannula.

Traditionally, techniques using intravenous narcotics and neuroleptic drugs (e.g., droperidol) have been successful for conscious sedation during awake craniotomy. Fentanyl and droperidol have been commonly used and may be administered by bolus or infusion techniques.[52,53] Fentanyl (0.5 to 0.75 $\mu g \cdot kg^{-1}$) and droperidol (up to 0.15 $mg \cdot kg^{-1}$ in divided doses) are effective in minimizing the discomfort associated with scalp infiltration and surgical exposure. It is important for the anesthesiologist to recognize the most painful parts of the procedure (scalp infiltration, surgical exposure, and closure) and titrate the anesthetic accordingly. Intraoperative ECoG and surgical resection are typically not painful. Most patients tolerate the procedure with continued reassurance and mild sedation. Occasionally, a patient will require additional small doses of narcotics (which may be titrated to a respiratory rate of 12 to 14/min) or even temporary unconsciousness with small doses of methohexital.

More recently, propofol has proved effective during awake craniotomy.[55,56] A background infusion of 50 to 150 $\mu g \cdot kg^{-1} \cdot min^{-1}$ with intermittent boluses of 0.5 to 1 $mg \cdot kg^{-1}$ provides excellent sedation; however, analgesia must be provided with supplemental narcotics or scalp infiltration of local anesthetic.

Problems arising intraoperatively during awake craniotomy have been described.[50] In addition to the potential for airway compromise during conscious sedation, other problems that have been reported include seizures with convulsions, nausea and vomiting, brain swelling, and patient somnolence or agitation. Once surgical resection and ECoG are completed, anesthetic depth may be increased for added patient comfort, or if necessary, general anesthesia can be induced. At the end of surgery, rapid patient awakening is necessary for accurate neurologic evaluation. Coughing and hypertension should be minimized to potentially reduce the risk of intracranial bleeding.

Anticonvulsant and Proconvulsant Properties of Anesthetics

Inherent to the appropriate management of patients undergoing seizure surgery is an understanding of the effects of anesthetic drugs on seizure activity. The medical literature on this subject is extensive and at times confusing because some anesthetics may exhibit both pro- and anticonvulsant properties, depending on the drug dose and the physiologic conditions under which it was administered. Modica et al.[57,58] have thoroughly reviewed this topic. What follows is a synopsis of the most clinically relevant pro- and anticonvulsant characteristics of anesthetics for the practicing anesthesiologist.

INHALATIONAL ANESTHETICS Generally, the volatile anesthetics are potent anticonvulsants that often interfere with intraoperative EEG monitoring. Refractory status epilepticus has been successfully terminated with general inhalational anesthesia.[59]

Halothane. Halothane is an effective anticonvulsant.[60] Although there are anecdotal reports of seizures with halothane anesthesia,[61,62] halothane, when used alone, has not shown proconvulsant activity.[63]

Isoflurane. Isoflurane exhibits potent anticonvulsant activity in animal studies.[64–66] It also has successfully terminated refractory status epilepticus.[59,67,68] Furthermore, it has been shown to suppress epileptogenic foci during intraoperative ECoG. Burst suppression typically occurs at greater than 2 MAC isoflurane.

Enflurane. Although enflurane is used less frequently today since the development of newer anesthetics, it possesses proconvulsant characteristics that may be beneficial during seizure surgery. Epileptiform activity has been demonstrated in both normal patients[69–71] and patients with temporal lobe epilepsy[49,72,74] under enflurane anesthesia. Its ability to produce seizures appears to be concentration- and $PaCO_2$-dependent.[74] As $PaCO_2$ is decreased from 40 torr, EEG spiking activity increases with an inspired enflurane concentration of 2.5 to 3.0 percent.[74] Burchiel et al.[75] further demonstrated that the minimum epileptogenic enflurane concentration was approximately 1 percent lower with a 20 torr reduction in $PaCO_2$ and 1 percent higher when $PaCO_2$ was increased 20 torr. There are also scattered reports of enflurane exhibiting anticonvulsant activity[76–78]; however, its proconvulsant effects are most recognized.

Desflurane and Sevoflurane. To our knowledge, neither sevoflurane or desflurane have been demonstrated to reproducibly cause or suppress seizure activity. They most likely exhibit anticonvulsant characteristics, as sevoflurane has been shown to progressively decrease EEG activity with increasing concentrations, with burst suppression occurring at 2 MAC sevoflurane.[79] Likewise, EEG activity diminishes to an isoelectric state as desflurane concentrations are increased to 2 MAC. Spiking activity has recurred, however, with concentrations greater than 2 MAC.[80] Further investigation is needed to evaluate the usefulness of these drugs during epilepsy surgery.

Nitrous Oxide. Although N_2O has anecdotally been associated with seizures,[61,81] it has not been documented to produce EEG seizure activity in patients with and without preexisting seizure disorders.[82] Furthermore, it does not appear to have clinically relevant anticonvulsant properties in humans, thus making it particularly useful in epilepsy surgery.

INTRAVENOUS ANESTHETICS

Opioids. Opioids have demonstrated both EEG suppression and activation in a variety of animal models under varying physiologic conditions. The clinical relevance of these effects in humans, however, remains controversial. There are reports of convulsive activity in humans after opioid administration, although none have been confirmed by EEG.[83–85] Several additional studies using scalp EEG monitoring have failed to demonstrate EEG activation during clinical seizure activity.[86–88] Opioids may however, produce limbic system epileptiform activity in patients with epilepsy,[89,90] although the significance of this is not well established. Generally, opioids exhibit minimal pro- or anticonvulsant activity and are, therefore, widely used during anesthesia for seizure surgery.

Barbiturates. In therapeutic anesthetic doses, barbiturates exhibit potent anticonvulsant properties. Furthermore, neither EEG or clinical seizure activity have been documented after barbiturate administration in nonepileptic patients. However, in patients with seizure disorders, it is well known that methohexital, in low doses, produces epileptiform EEG activity.[91] Thus, in doses of less than 1 mg/kg, methohexital is often effective in activating previously silent seizure foci during epilepsy surgery.[91]

Etomidate. Etomidate exhibits both pro- and anticonvulsant properties.[60,92,93] Administration of etomidate has been associated with both EEG-documented seizures and myotonic activity unrelated to seizure activity.[93–95] Like methohexital, it has been useful in activating seizure foci during epilepsy surgery.[47,48,92] In addition, it also may augment intraoperative somatosensory evoked potentials.[96,97] Etomidate has also demonstrated anticonvulsant activity in humans by terminating status epilepticus.[98,99]

Benzodiazepines. Benzodiazepines are potent anticonvulsants without any known proconvulsant activity in humans. Because of their ability to stop clinical and EEG seizure activity, they are typically avoided during epilepsy surgery to prevent suppression of epileptogenic foci. After surgery resection and ECoG are completed, however, a short-acting benzodiazepine (e.g., midazolam) may be useful to deepen anesthesia and enhance amnesia.

Ketamine. Ketamine is generally avoided during elective intracranial procedures because it may increase cerebral metabolic rate. With regard to cortical electrical activity, ketamine exhibits pro- and anticonvulsant activity. It is well documented that ketamine can activate seizure foci in patients with epilepsy.[45,100] However, EEG seizure activity has not been reported in normal patients. Myotonic movement has been noted but has not been associated with EEG seizure documentation.[101,102] It is hypothesized that these movements may be associated with subcortical seizure activity,[103,104] although this has not yet been documented in nonepileptic humans.

Propofol. There are anecdotal reports of propofol causing seizures in humans.[105–107] Subsequent investigation, however, indicates that propofol, when used as a single anesthetic agent, does not induce any electrical seizure activity in epileptic patients.[108] Furthermore, residual propofol levels have not been found to be proconvulsant after prolonged infusion periods.[109] Propofol has been shown to abolish seizures during status epilepticus, indicating anticonvulsant properties.[110] Additional investigation is warranted to confirm its effect on the EEG and use during seizure surgery.

Droperidol. Droperidol is frequently used during anesthesia for seizure surgery. When given in combination with fentanyl, it has not been shown to initiate or suppress epileptiform activity.[64]

References

1. Engel J: Seizures and Epilepsy. FA Davis, Philadelphia, 1989
2. Engel J, Shewmon DA: Who should be considered a surgical candidate? p. 23. In Engel J (ed): Surgical Treatment of the Epilepsies. 2nd Ed. Raven Press, New York, 1993
3. Horsley V: Brain surgery. BMJ 2:670, 1886
4. Commission on Classification and Terminology of the International League against Epilepsy: Proposal for revised classification of epilepsies and epileptic syndromes. Epilepsia 30:389, 1989
5. Wolf HK, Wiestler OD: Surgical pathology of chronic epileptic seizure disorders. Brain Pathol 3:371, 1993
6. Wolf HK, Wellmer J, Muller MB et al: Glioneuronal malformative lesions and dysembryoplastic neuroepithelial tumors in patients with chronic pharmacoresistant epilepsies. J Neuropathol Exp Neurol 54:245, 1995
7. Falconer MA, Serafetinides EA, Corsellis JAN: Etiology and pathogenesis of temporal lobe epilepsy. Arch Neurol 10:233, 1964
8. Fried I, Kim JH, Spencer DD: Hippocampal pathology in patients with intractable seizures and temporal lobe masses. J Neurosurg 76:735, 1992
9. Levesque MF, Nakasato N, Vinters HV, Babb TL: Surgical treatment of limbic epilepsy associated with extrahippocampal lesions: the problem of dual pathology. J Neurosurg 75:364, 1991
10. Nakasato N, Levesque MF, Babb TL: Seizure outcome following standard temporal lobectomy: correlation with hippocampal neuron loss and extrahippocampal pathology. J Neurosurg 77:194, 1992
11. Williamson PD, Boon PA, Thadani VM, et al: Parietal lobe epilepsy: diagnostic considerations and results of surgery. Ann Neurol 31:193, 1992
12. Wada J, Rasmussen T: Intracarotid injection of sodium amytal for the lateralization of cerebral speech dominance: experimental and clinical observations. J Neurosurg 17:266, 1960
13. Rausch R, Silfvenius H, Wieser HG et al: Intraarterial amobarbital procedures. p. 341. In Engel J (ed): Surgical Treatment of the Epilepsies. 2nd Ed. Raven Press, New York, 1993
14. Risinger MW, Engel J, Van Ness PC et al: Ictal localization of temporal lobe seizures with scalp/sphenoidal recordings. Neurology 39:1288, 1989

15. Spencer SS, Spencer DD, Williamson PD, Mattson RH: The localizing value of depth electroencephalography in 32 patients with refractory epilepsy. Ann Neurol 12:248, 1982
16. McCarthy G, Spencer DD, Riker RJ: The stereotaxic placement of depth electrodes in epilepsy. p. 385. In Luders HO (ed): Epilepsy Surgery. Raven Press, New York, 1991
17. Blatt DR, Roper SN, Friedman WA: Invasive monitoring of limbic epilepsy using stereotactic depth and subdural strip electrodes: surgical technique. Surg Neurol (in press)
18. Roper SN: Implantation of grid and strip electrodes. Techniques Neurosurg 1:5, 1995
19. Spencer DD, Spencer SS, Mattson RH et al: Access to the posterior medial temporal lobe structures in the surgical treatment of temporal lobe epilepsy. Neurosurgery 15:667, 1984
20. Yasargil MG, Teddy PJ, Roth P: Selective amygdalo-hippocampectomy: operative anatomy and surgical technique. p. 93. In Symon L et al. (eds): Advances and Technical Standards in Neurosurgery. Vol. 12. Springer-Verlag, New York, 1985
21. Cendes F, Dubeau F, Olivier A et al: Increased neocortical spiking and surgical outcome after selective amygdalo-hippocampectomy. Epilepsy Res 16:195, 1993
22. Hori T, Tabuchi S, Kurosaki M et al: Subtemporal amygdalohippocampectomy for treating medically intractable temporal lobe epilepsy. Neurosurgery 33:50, 1993
23. Ojemann GA, Ojemann J, Lettich E, Berger M: Cortical language localization in left, dominant hemisphere. J Neurosurg 71:316, 1989
24. Engel J, Van Ness PC, Rasmussen TB, Ojemann LM: Outcome with respect to epileptic seizures. p. 609. In Engel J (ed): Surgical Treatment of the Epilepsies. 2nd Ed. Raven Press, New York, 1993
25. Fried I, Cascino GD: Lesional surgery. p. 501. In Engel J (ed): Surgical Treatment of the Epilepsies. 2nd Ed. Raven Press, New York, 1993
26. Krynauw R: Infantile hemiplegia treated by removing one cerebral hemisphere. J Neurol Neurosurg Psychiatry 3:243, 1950
27. Oppenheimer DR, Griffith HB: Persistent intracranial bleeding as a complication of hemispherectomy. J Neurol Neurosurg Psychiatry 29:229, 1966
28. Tinuper P, Andermann F, Villemure JG et al: Functional hemispherectomy for treatment of epilepsy associated with hemiplegia: rationale, indications, results, and comparison with callosotomy. Ann Neurol 24:27, 1988
29. Schramm J, Behrens E, Entzian W: Hemispherical deafferentation: an alternative to functional hemispherectomy. Neurosurgery 36:509, 1995
30. Oguni H, Olivier A, Andermann F, Comair J: Anterior callosotomy in the treatment of medically intractable epilepsies: a study of 43 patients with a mean follow-up of 39 months. Ann Neurol 30:357, 1991
31. Fuiks KS, Wyler AT, Hermann BP, Somes G: Seizure outcome from anterior and complete corpus callosotomy. J Neurosurg 74:573, 1991
32. Gates JR, Rosenfeld WE, Maxwell RE, Lyons RE: Response of multiple seizure types to corpus callosum section. Epilepsia 28:28, 1987
33. Spencer SS, Spencer DD, Williamson PD et al: Corpus callosotomy for epilepsy. I. Seizure effects. Neurology 38:19, 1988
34. Lueders H, Bustamante LA, Zablow L, Goldensohn ES: The independence of closely spaced discrete experimental spike foci. Neurology 31:846, 1981
35. Sperry RW: Cerebral regulation of motor coordination following multiple transection of sensorimotor cortex. J Neurophysiol 10:275, 1947
36. Ford EW, Morrell F, Whisler WW: Methohexital anesthesia in the surgical treatment of uncontrollable epilepsy. Anesth Analg 61:997, 1982
37. Morrell F, Whisler WW, Bleck TP: Multiple subpial transection: a new approach to the surgical treatment of focal epilepsy. J Neurosurg 70:231, 1989
38. Sawhney IMS, Robertson IJA, Polkey CE et al: Multiple subpial transection: a review of 21 cases. J Neurol Neurosurg Psychiatry 58:344, 1995
39. Wyler AT, Wilkus RJ, Rostad SW, Vossler DG: Multiple subpial transections for partial seizures in sensorimotor cortex. Neurosurgery 37:1122, 1995
40. Gidal B, Spencer N, Maly M et al: Valproate-mediated disturbances of hemostasis: relationship to dose and plasma concentrations. Neurology 44:1418, 1994
41. Kreuz W, Linde R, Funk M et al: Valproate therapy induces von Willebrand disease type I. Epilepsia 33:178, 1992
42. Ward MW, Barbaro NM, Laxer KD, Rampil IJ: Preoperative valproate administration does not increase blood loss during temporal lobectomy. Epilepsia 37:98, 1996

43. Abou-Madi J, Trop D, Lenis S et al: Selective neuromuscular blockade for intraoperative electrocorticography. Appl Neurophysiol 50:386, 1987
44. Rockoff MA, Goudsouzian NG: Seizures induced by methohexital. Anesthesiology 54:333, 1981
45. Ferrer-Allado T, Brechner VL, Dymand A et al: Ketamine-induced electroconvulsive phenomena in the human limbic and thalamic regions. Anesthesiology 38:333, 1973
46. Corssen G, Little SC, Tavakoli M: Ketamine and epilepsy. Anesth Analg 53:319, 1974
47. Gancher S, Laxen KD, Krieger W: Activation of epileptogenic activity by etomidate. Anesthesiology 61:616, 1984
48. Ebrahim ZY, Deboer GE, Luders H et al: Effect of etomidate on the electroencephalogram of patients with epilepsy. Anesth Analg 65:1004, 1986
49. Flemming DC, Fitzpatrick J, Fariello RG et al: Diagnostic activation of epileptogenic foci by enflurane. Anesthesiology 52:431, 1980
50. Archer DP, McKenna JM, Morin L et al: Conscious-sedation analgesia during craniotomy for intractable epilepsy: a review of 354 consecutive cases. Can J Anaesth 35:338, 1988
51. Girvin JP: Resection of intracranial lesions unders local anesthesia. Int Anesth Clin 24:133, 1986
52. Manninen P, Contreras J: Anesthetic consideration for craniotomy in awake patients. Int Anesth Clin 24:157, 1986
53. Trop D: Conscious-sedation analgesia during the neurosurgical treatment of epilepsies—practice at the Montreal Neurological Institute. Int Anesth Clin 24:175, 1986
54. Welling EC, Donegan J: Neuroleptanalgesia using alfentanil for awake craniotomy. Anesth Analg 68:57, 1989
55. Kearns CF, Sinclair F, Manninen PH: A comparison of propofol and midazolam for awake craniotomy, abstracted. J Neurosug Anesth 7:306, 1995
56. Drummond JC, Iragui-Modoz VJ, Alksne CJ et al: Masking of epileptiform activity by propofol during seizure surgery. Anesthesiology 76:652, 1992
57. Modica PA, Templehoff R, White PF: Pro- and anticonvulsant effects of anesthetics (part I). Anesth Analg 70:303, 1990
58. Modica PA, Templehoff R, White PF: Pro-and anticonvulsant effects of anesthetics (part II). Anesth Analg 70:433, 1990
59. Kofke WA, Young RS, Davis P et al: Isoflurane for refractory status epilepticus: a clinical series. Anesthesiology 71:653, 1989
60. Opitz A, Marschall R, Degan R et al: General anesthesia in patients with epilepsy and status epilepticus. Adv Neurol 34:531, 1983
61. Krenn J, Porges P, Steinbereithner K: Case of anesthesia convulsions under nitrous oxide-halothane anesthesia. Anaesthesist 16:83, 1967
62. Smith PA, McDonald TR, Jones CS: Convulsions associated with halothane anaesthesia. Anaesthesia 21:229, 1966
63. Opitz A, Marschall M, Degan R et al: General anesthesia in patients with epilepsy and status epilepticus. p. 531. In Delgado-Escueta AV, Wasterlain CG, Treiman DM et al (eds): Status Epilepticus: Mechanisms of Brain Damage and Treatment Raven, New York, 1983
64. Koblin DD, Eger EI, Johnson BH et al: Are convulsant gases also anesthetics? Anesth Analg 60:464, 1981
65. Kofke WA, Ropper A, Young RSK et al: Isoflurane for status epilepticus. Neurology, 37, suppl. 1:103, 1987
66. Kofke WA, Towfighi J, O'Connell BK et al: Neuropathological effects of anesthetics used to stop status epilepticus in rats. Anesthesiol Rev 15:27, 1987
67. Meeke, RI, Sorfer BE, Gelb AW: Isoflurane for the measurement of status epilepticus. DICP 23:579, 1989
68. Ropper AH, Kofke WA, Bromfield EB et al: Comparison of isoflurane, halothane and nitrous oxide in status epilepticus (letter). Ann Neurol 19:98, 1986
69. Lebowitz MH, Blitt CD, Dillon JB: Clinical investigation of compound 347 (Ethrane). Anesth Analg 49:1, 1970
70. Bart AJ, Homi J, Linde HW: Changes in power spectra of electroencephalograms during anesthesia with fluroxene, methoxyflurane and ethrane. Anesth Analg 50:53, 1971
71. Wollman H, Smith AL, Hoffman JC: Cerebral blood flow and oxygen consumption in man during electroencephalographic seizure patterns induced by anesthesia with ethrane. Fed Proc 28:356, 1969
72. Niejadlik K, Galindo A: Electrocorticographic seizure activity during enflurane anesthesia. Anesth Analg 54:722, 1975
73. Fariello RG: Epilpetogenic properties of enflurane and their clinical interpretation. Electroenceophalgr Clin Neurophysiol 48:595, 1980

74. Lebowitz MH, Blitt CD, Dillon JB: Enflurane-induced central nervous system excitation and its relation to carbon dioxide tension. Anesth Analg 51:355, 1972
75. Burchiel KJ, Stockard JJ, Myers RR et al: Metabolic and electrophysiologic mechanisms in the initiation and termination of enflurane-induced seizures in man and cats. Electroencephalogr Clin Neurophysiol 38:555, 1975
76. Opitz A, Oberwetter WD: Enflurane or halothane anesthesia for patients with cerebral convulsive disorders? Acta Anesthesiol Scand, 71, suppl.:43, 1979
77. Gallagher TJ, Galindo A, Richey ET: Inhibition of seizure activity during enflurane anesthesia. Anesth Analg 57:130, 1978
78. Oshima E, Urabe N, Shingu K, Mori K: Anticonvulsant actions of enflurane on epilepsy models in cats. Anesthesiology 63:29, 1985
79. Scheller MS, Takeishi A, Drummond JC et al: The effects of sevoflurane on cerebral blood flow, cerebral metabolic rate for oxygen, intracranial pressure, and the electroencephalogram are similar to those of isoflurane in the rabbit. Anesthesiology 68:548, 1988
80. Lutz LJ, Milde JH, Milde, LN: The cerebral functional, metabolic, and hemodynamic effects of desflurane in dogs. Anesthesiology 73:125, 1990
81. Steen PA, Michenfelder J: Neurotoxicity of anesthetics. Anesthesiology 50:437, 1979
82. Yamamura T, Fukuda M, Takeya H et al: Fast oscillatory EEG activity induced by analgesic concentrations of nitrous oxide in man. Anesth Analg 60:283, 1981
83. Baraka A, Haroun S: Grand mal seizures following fentanyl-lidocaine (letter). Anesthesiology 62:206, 1985
84. Koren G, Butt W, Pape K et al: Morphine-induced seizures in new-born infants. Vet Hurn Toxicol 27:519, 1985
85. Molbegott LP, Flashburg MH, Karasic HL et al: Probable seizures after sufentanil. Anesth Analg 66:91, 1987
86. Bowdle TA: Myoclonus following sufentanil without EEG seizure activity. Anesthesiology 67:593, 1987
87. Scott JC, Sarnquist FH: Seizure-like movements during a fentanyl infusion with absence of seizure activity in a simultaneous EEG recording. Anesthesiology 62:812, 1985
88. Smith NT, Benthuysen JL, Bickford RG et al: Seizures during opioid anesthetic induction—are they opioid-induced rigidity? Anesthesiology 71:852, 1989
89. Cascino GD, Sharbrough FW, Elson LS et al: Intraoperative alfentanil hydrochloride in temporal lobe epilepsy: correlation with MRI-based volume studies, abstracted. Epilepsia 33:85, 1992
90. Templehoff R, Modica PA, Bernardo KL et al: Fentanyl-induced electrocorticographic seizures in patients with complex partial epilepsy. J Neurosurg 77:2, 1992
91. Gumpert J, Paul R: Activation of the electroencephalogram with intravenous brietal (methohexitone): the findings in 100 cases. J Neurol Neurosurg Psychiatry 34:646, 1971
92. Krieger W, Cooperman J, Laxer KD: Seizures with etomidate anesthesia (letter). Anesth Analg 64:1226, 1985
93. Laughlin TP, Newbert LA: Prolonged myoclonus after etomidate anesthesia. Anesth Analg 64:80, 1985
94. Ghoneim MM, Yamada T: Etomidate: a clinical and electroencephalographic comparison with thiopental. Anesth Analg 56:479, 1977
95. Doenicke A, Loffler B, Kugler J et al: Plasma concentration and EEG after various regimens of etomidate. Br J Anaesth 54:393, 1982
96. McPherson RW, Sell B, Traystman RJ: Effects of thiopental, fentanyl and etomidate on upper extremity somatosensory evoked potentials in humans. Anesthesiology 65:584, 1986
97. Sloan TB, Ronai AK, Toleikis JR et al: Improvement of intraoperative somatosensory evoked potentials by etomidate. Anesth Analg 67:582, 1988
98. Hoffman P, Schockenhoff B: Etomidate as an anticonvulsant agent. Anaesthesist 33:142, 1984
99. Pichlmayr I, Lips U, Kunkel H: Special considerations in patients with seizure disorders. p. 167. In Pichlmayr I, Lips U, Kunkel H (eds): The Electroencephalogram in Anesthesia. Springer-Verlag, Berlin, 1984
100. Bennett DR, Madsen JA, Jordan WS et al: Ketamine anesthesia in brain-damaged epileptics: electroencephalographic and clinical observations. Neurology 23:449, 1973
101. Thompson GE: Ketamine-induced convulsions (letter). Anesthesiology 37:662, 1972
102. Schwartz MS, Virden S, Scott DF: Effects of ketamine on the electroencephalograph. Anaesthesia 29:135, 1974
103. Mori K, Kawamata M, Mitani H et al: A neuro-

physiologc study of ketamine in the cat. Anesthesiology 35:373, 1971
104. Kayma Y, Iwama K: The EEG, evoked potentials and single unit activity during ketamine anesthesia in cats. Anesthesiology 36:316, 1972
105. Bredhal C: Seizures and opistotonus after propofol anesthesia. A possible connection. Ugeskr Laeger 52:748, 1990
106. Paech MJ, Storey JM: Propofol and seizures (letter). Anaesth Intensive Care 18:585, 1990
107. Thomas JS, Boheimer NO: An isolated grand mal seizure 5 days after propofol anaesthesia (letter). Anaesthesia 46:508, 1991
108. Cheng MA, Tempelhoff R, Theard MA et al: Propofol alone at high dose in adult epileptic patients: electrocorticographic results, abstracted. J Neurosurg Anesth 7:305, 1995
109. McFarlane C, Hong SY, Todd MM et al: The effects of residual propofol on seizure threshold, abstracted. J Neurosurg Anesth 7:306, 1995
110. Wood PR, Brown GPR, Pugh S: Propofol infusion for the treatment of status epilepticus (letter). Lancet 1:480, 1990

12 CERVICAL SPINE IN ANESTHESIA: EVALUATION AND APPROACH

MICHAEL E. MAHLA

Many patients undergoing neurosurgical procedures have disease, either acquired or congenital, of the cervical spine. Acquired disease may be either degenerative or traumatic. Regardless of the type of cervical spine disease, the anesthesiologist should use an organized, logical approach to the evaluation of the cervical spine. This evaluation will help the clinician decide how best to secure the airway and position the patient at the beginning of the operation and avoid creating or further aggravating preexisting neurologic injury.

There are two main areas for consideration: (1) implications of signs and symptoms of cervical spine disease, and (2) the function of the cervical spine bony structures, ligaments, and joints. Signs and symptoms of cervical spine disease are produced by compression of nervous system structures (nerve roots or spinal cord), abnormal mobility (either increased or decreased) of the cervical spine, or both. These signs and symptoms may have significant implications for the anesthesiologist. Compression or damage to neural structures could be aggravated by intubation or, more likely, positioning. Loss of function has implications for ease of intubation. The greater the loss of function, the more difficult ideal intubation conditions will be to achieve.

SIGNS AND SYMPTOMS

Signs and symptoms of cervical spine disease are produced by compression of neural structures or abnormal function of the bones, joints, and ligaments of the cervical spine. The most striking symptoms are produced by compression of or damage to neural structures.

Cervical Radiculopathy

Radiculopathy is defined as those signs and symptoms that are produced by nerve root compression. Cervical spine nerve root compression is generally produced by herniation of a cervical intervertebral disc, bony compression from either a degenerative osteophyte, or from displacement or stretching of a nerve root produced by trauma. Figure 12.1 shows the most common mechanisms of nerve root compression. Nerve root compression is frequently a dynamic process. Flexion, extension, and rotation of the head and neck may change the degree of nerve root compression. When evaluating the patient with cervical radiculopathy, it is important to assess this dynamic component. Assuming the patient has full range of motion of the

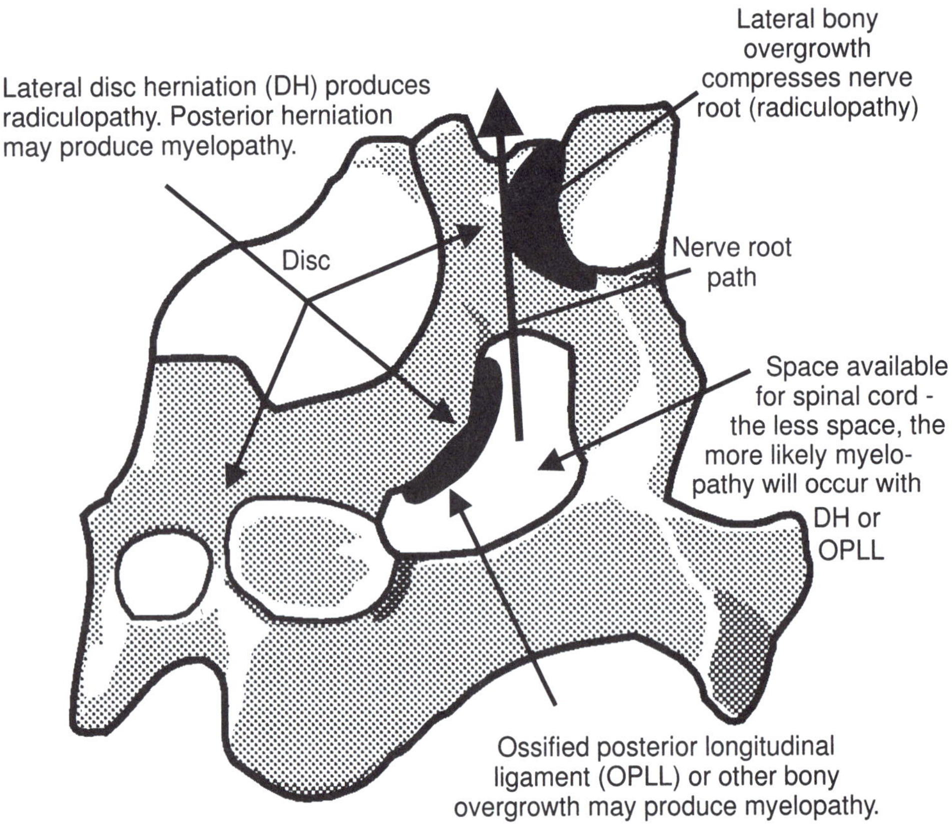

FIGURE 12.1 *Schematic of common mechanisms of cervical nerve root compression*

TABLE 12.1 *Signs and symptoms of cervical radiculopathy*

NERVE ROOT	SENSORY SYMPTOMS	MOTOR SIGNS	REFLEXES
C2	Occipital neuralgia, headache, position-related	None	Normal
C3	Dermatomal (neck) pain	None	Normal
C4	Dermatomal (neck) pain	None	Normal
C5	Deltoid pain	Deltoid weakness	Normal
C6	Pain distal to the elbow and sensory loss over thumb and index finger	Biceps weakness	Decreased biceps
C7	Pain distal to the elbow and sensory loss over index or ring finger. May have normal sensory examination because of overlapping C-6 and C-8 roots	Triceps, wrist extensor weakness	Decreased triceps
C8	Pain distal to the elbow and sensory loss over ulnar side of hand	Triceps, intrinsic hand muscles	Decrease triceps
T1	Sensory loss over ulnar side of hand	Intrinsic hand muscles	Normal

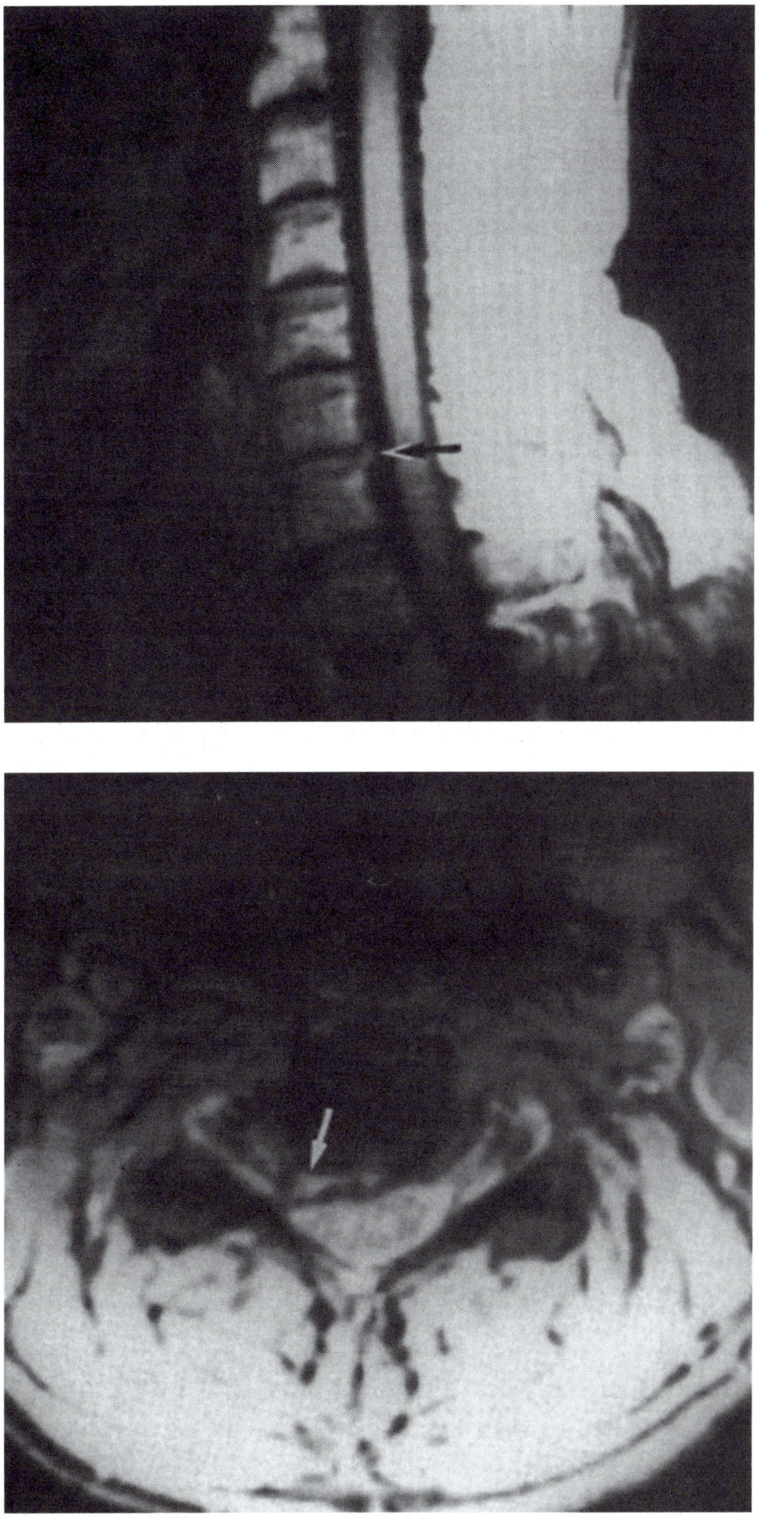

A

B

FIGURE 12.2 *Sagittal and cross-section MRI study from a patient with cervical radiculopathy. Note compression of cervical nerve root (arrow) and lack of compression of the spinal cord itself.*

TABLE 12.2 *Signs and symptoms of cervical myelopathy*

LEVEL OF COMPRESSION	SENSORY FINDINGS	MOTOR FINDINGS	REFLEXES
Above C4	Variable *bilateral sensory loss below level of compression*[a]	*Bilateral* upper and *lower extremity weakness, ataxia*	*Globally increased*
C4–T1	Variable, *bilateral* pain in upper extremities, *loss of sensation below level of compression*	*Bilateral* upper and *lower extremity weakness and ataxia below compression*	Normal above compression, decreased at level of compression, *increased below compression*

[a] Findings shown in italic script are key factors that *may* help distinguish nerve root compression from spinal cord compression.

cervical spine, if there is no change in the patient's symptoms with changes in head and neck position, then there is no significant dynamic component to the compression, and positioning considerations are much less important. If the motion of the cervical spine is limited by loss of function or pain, then for maximum safety, motion of the cervical spine after induction of anesthesia should be limited to the degree of motion possible before induction of anesthesia. Table 12.1 shows those signs and symptoms that may be found in patients with pure cervical radiculopathy. Figure 12.2 shows several views from magnetic resonance imaging (MRI) in a patient with cervical radiculopathy. Notice that the spinal cord itself is ***not*** compressed.

Cervical Myelopathy

Signs and symptoms associated with cervical myelopathy are produced by compression of the spinal cord itself at the cervical levels. Myelopathy may occur alone or (more commonly) be associated with radiculopathy. Table 12.2 describes symptoms of cervical myelopathy. Those features that distinguish myelopathy from radiculopathy are shown in italic print. It is important to assess whether there is a dynamic component to the myelopathy as well. If signs and symptoms do not change with a sustained change in the patient's position, then aggravation of spinal cord compression by motions produced by intubation or by surgical positioning may be less likely. Figure 12.3 shows an MRI in a patient with symptomatic cervical myelopathy. Note that the thecal sac and spinal cord itself are severely compromised by degenerative changes in the cervical spine of this patient with rheumatoid arthritis.

CERVICAL SPINE FUNCTION

Normal Function of the Cervical Spine[1]

FLEXION: EXTENSION There is normally a total range of motion of from 60 to 75 degrees that is roughly evenly distributed throughout the cervical spine. The greatest mobility is at the atlanto-occipital junction, with the next greatest between C5 and C7. This mobility at these joints accounts for the high incidence of degenerative changes at these levels.

TRANSLATION Normal anterior-posterior motion (translation) is limited to 2 to 3 mm at all levels. In the upper cervical spine, transverse at-

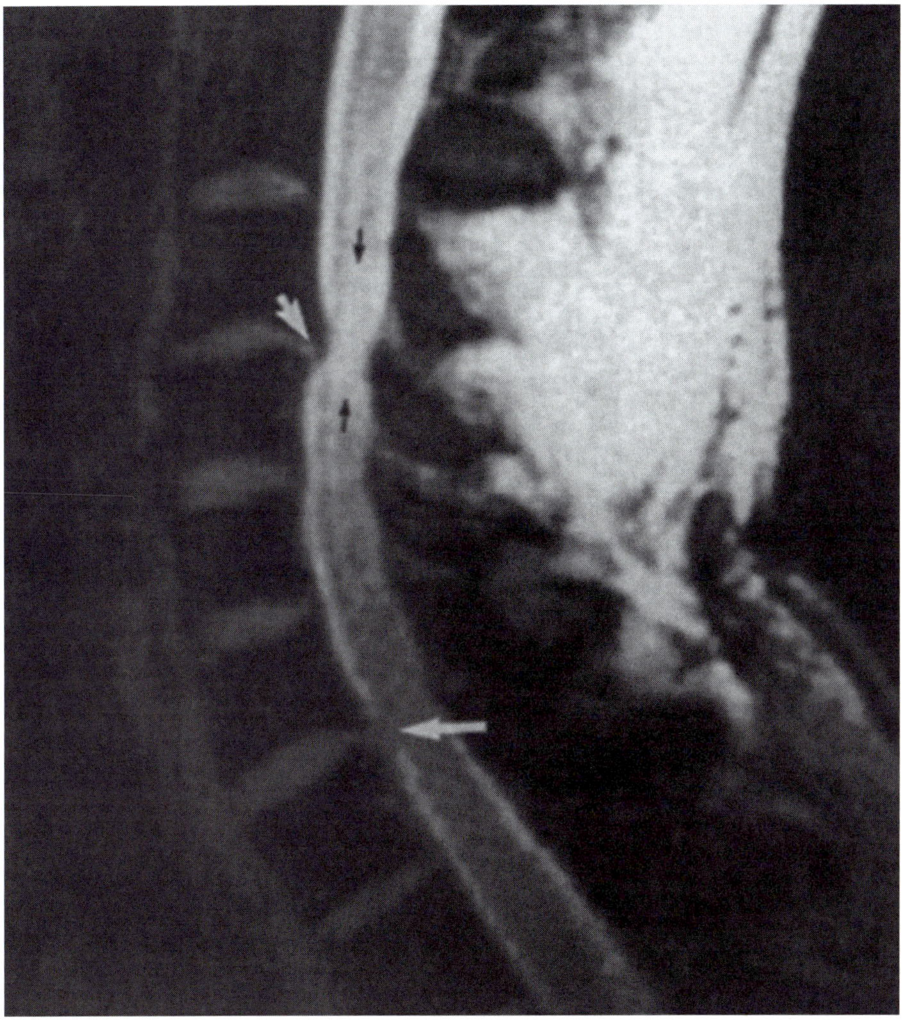

FIGURE 12.3 *Sagittal MRI view of the cervical spine in a patient with cervical myelopathy. Note marked compression of the thecal sac and spinal cord itself.*

lantal ligament holding the dens to the arch of C-1 limits this motion (Fig. 12.4A). Elsewhere, translation is limited by ligaments, facet orientation, and the disc annulus (Fig. 12.4B).

ROTATION/LATERAL BENDING Rotation and lateral bending are most important at C1–2 but also occur at lower levels. There is normally 50 degrees of rotation at C1–2. From C-2 to 5, C-10 to 12 degrees of lateral bending can occur at each level, which decreases to 4 to 8 degrees below C6.

STABILITY The cervical spine is normally well equipped to prevent motions beyond those described above, and therefore most patients will never experience damage to neural structures. The stabilizing function of the spine can be divided into anterior, middle, and posterior components[2] (Fig. 12.5). The anterior compo-

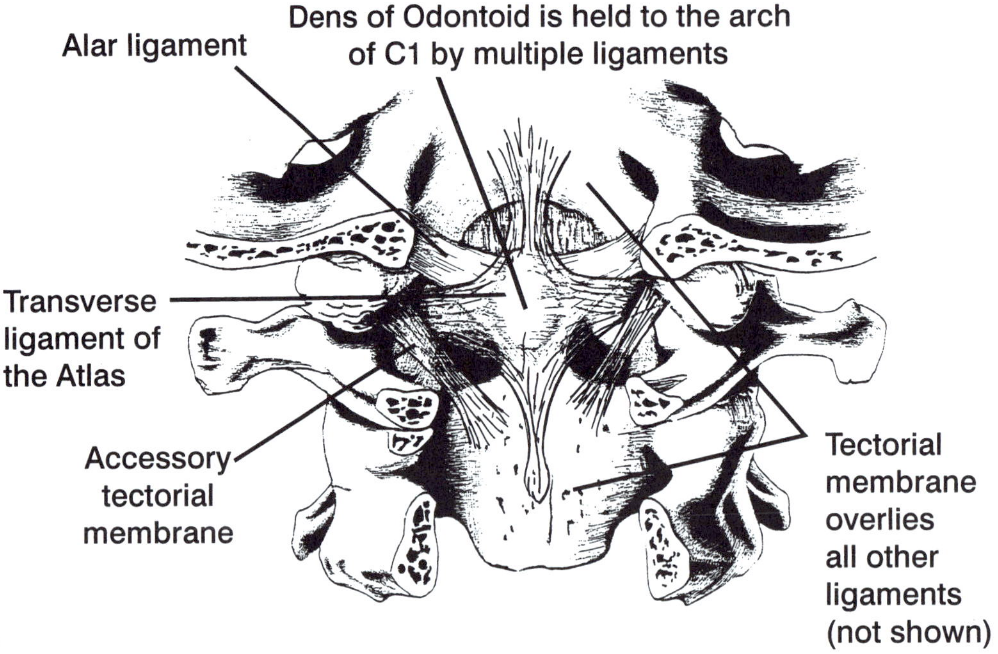

A

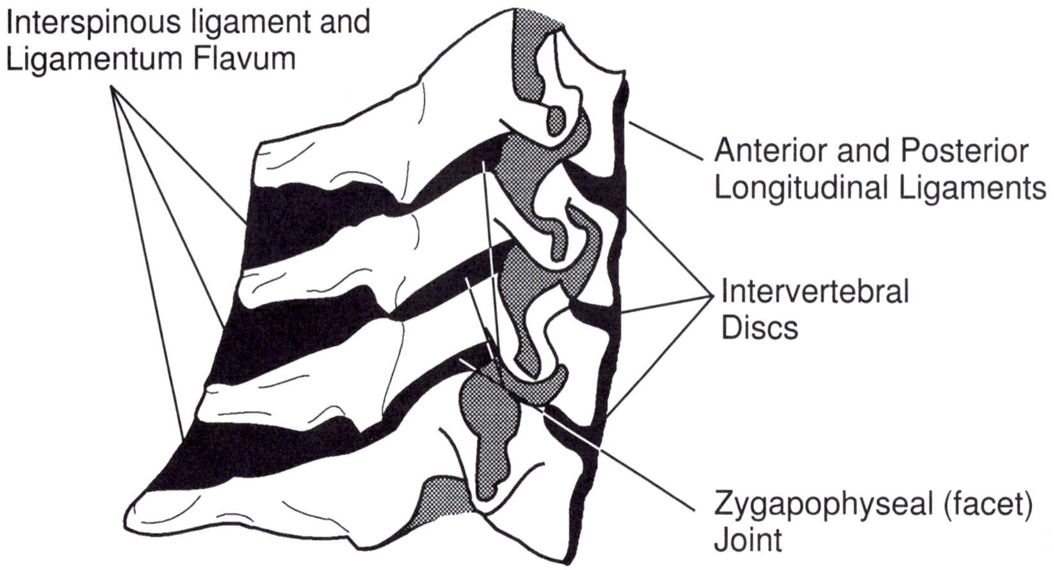

B

FIGURE 12.4 *(A) Structures preventing abnormal translation at the C1–2 level. (B) Structures preventing abnormal translation at lower cervical levels. (Fig. B adapted from Netter,*[25] *with permission.)*

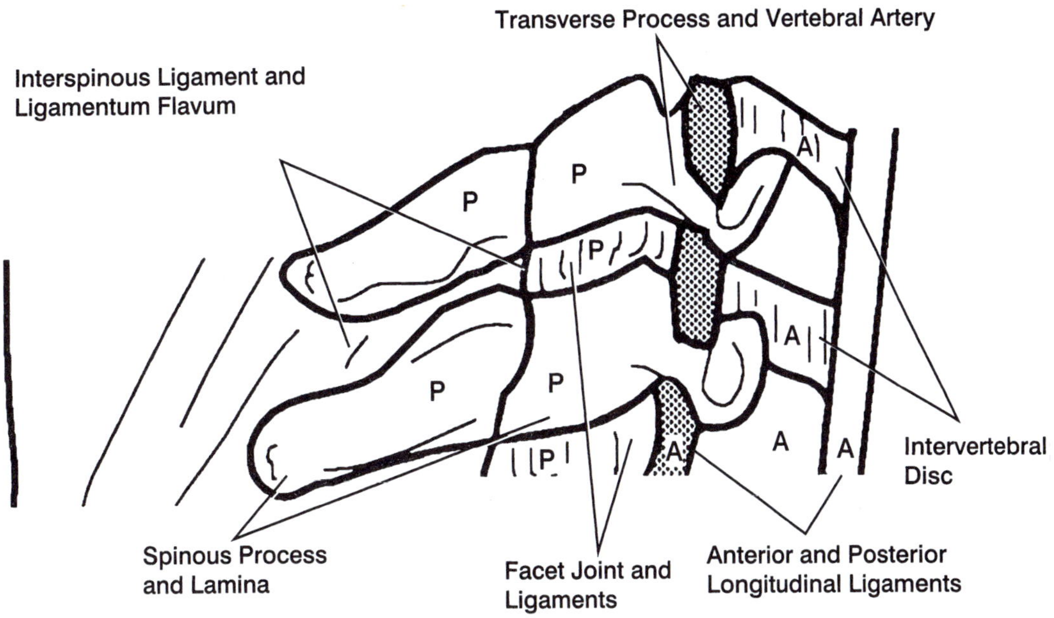

FIGURE 12.5 *Cervical spine stability is ensured by both anterior (A) and posterior (P) elements. Instability generally does not occur unless both anterior and posterior elements are disrupted.*

nent consists of the anterior longitudinal ligament and the anterior two-thirds of the vertebral body. The middle component consists of the posterior one-third of the vertebral body, the annulus fibrosis, and the posterior longitudinal ligament. The posterior component consists of the facet joints and capsules and the posterior bony covering of the canal (pedicles, laminae, and spinous processes) connected by the interspinous and supraspinous ligaments. Failure of the stabilization function (i.e., an unstable neck) will usually only occur with disruption of at least two of the three stabilizing components.

Evaluation of upper cervical spine stability includes consideration of the bony structures of the atlas and axis and complex ligamentous structures. The ligaments can be divided into inner and outer groups. The inner group consists of the paired alar ligaments, the apical ligament, the cruciform ligament, and the tectorial membrane. The outer group consists of the articular capsules, the anterior and posterior atlanto-occipital membranes, and the ligamentum nuchae[3] (Fig. 12.4). Studies have concluded that injury from excessive flexion is prevented by skeletal contact between the odontoid and the anterior arch of C1 and the foramen magnum.[4] Hyperextension injury and vertical impaction injuries at C1–2 are prevented by the tectorial membrane. Excessive lateral bending is prevented by the alar ligaments. The most important structures controlling stability of the upper cervical spine are thought to be the tectorial membrane and the alar ligament.[4] In the lower cervical spine, several studies have shown the important role of the anterior and posterior longitudinal ligaments.[5–7]

However, in the final analysis, the diagnosis of cervical spine stability is really a clinical one. If a cervical spine after injury is to be considered stable before induction of anesthesia, two things must be true. First, normal physiologic stresses and movements of the cervical spine will not produce abnormal movement or deformity. Second, there can be no compression or injury to central neural elements. Thus, for example, a patient with a compression fracture of the fifth cervical vertebral body with intact posterior elements and ligaments and a normal neurologic examination has a stable cervical spine. If, however, the compression fracture has resulted in bony disruption with compression of the spinal cord, even small, normally harmless degrees of movement may result in damage to the spinal cord, and the same skeletal injury to the cervical spine cannot be considered stable. Consultation with neurosurgical colleagues should help you decide whether the injury is stable, but the above guidelines should be helpful if consultative help is not immediately available.

ABNORMAL CERVICAL SPINE

Step 1: History and Physical Examination

Any evaluation of the cervical spine begins with the history and physical examination. Signs and symptoms that suggest cervical radiculopathy are listed in Table 12.1. There should be no lower extremity or bowel/bladder symptoms or physical findings in the patient with cervical radiculopathy. The hallmarks of cervical nerve root compression are

- sensory loss and pain associated with one or more dermatomal distributions, usually but not always unilateral
- innervated muscle weakness
- decreased reflexes in the involved muscle groups

Nerve root compression is usually unilateral but occasionally may be bilateral.

Signs and symptoms that suggest cervical myelopathy are shown in Table 12.2. Many of the signs and symptoms of myelopathy are similar to those found in radiculopathy, particularly at the level of the pathology. For example, spinal cord compression at the C6 level will frequently produce C6 radicular symptoms. Lower extremity and bowel/bladder symptoms and findings are found only in cervical myelopathy. Reflexes other than at or above the level of spinal cord compression are disinhibited by compression of the spinal cord and will be abnormally brisk. Pathologic reflexes such as the Babinski or Hoffman reflexes may also be present. Hallmarks of cervical myelopathy are

- bilateral involvement
- loss of sensation and motor function, either partial or complete, at multiple levels at and below the level of spinal cord compression
- disinhibited, increased reflexes below the level of spinal cord compression with pathologic reflexes seen

Stability of the lesion, either traumatic, degenerative, or congenital, will be determined, as described above, by an examination of the anterior and posterior components of stability.

Step 2: Clinical Significance of Cervical Spine Disease and Implications for Anesthetic Management

For the practicing anesthesiologist confronted with a patient with cervical spine abnormalities, presence of radiculopathy, myelopathy, or changes in function may necessitate substantial changes in anesthetic management.

CERVICAL RADICULOPATHY Peripheral nerves are relatively resistant to damage caused by transient compression alone. An example of this resistance is illustrated by long segment neural compression produced by tourniquets. This type of compression rarely produces sustained loss of neural function. Damage with sustained loss of function is much more likely with severe nerve stretching alone or when compression is associated with stretching of the nerve.

Compression can clearly produce symptoms (e.g., compression by an osteophyte or by a herniated disc) that can be quite severe. However, with either surgical or nonsurgical therapy, prompt correction of the compression frequently results in restoration of function to normal or near-normal levels. Such good results may not occur with axonotmetic or neurotmetic stretch injuries that result in axonal and/or neural disruption, respectively. These more severe stretch injuries of cervical nerves, however, are not normally associated with the movements caused by intubation. Thus, one could probably safely conclude that radicular compression produced either by intubation or positioning is not likely to produce permanent loss of neurologic function, although transient loss of function may well occur if the compression is prolonged, for example, by positioning. Good positioning practice should, however, prevent any prolonged loss of function.

In the patient with a prominent dynamic component to radiculopathy that produces a marked change in function with a change in position (a ***very*** rare finding in my clinical experience), the most conservative approach would be to treat this patient similarly to the patient with myelopathy and assess function by performing a neurologic examination after positioning (see below). However, most patients with cervical radiculopathy do not have a dramatic change in neurologic function after a change in neck position and may be safely intubated and positioned after induction of general anesthesia.

CERVICAL MYELOPATHY The number one consideration for patients with cervical myelopathy is maintenance of spinal cord perfusion. Although perfusion to the noninvolved areas of the spinal cord is probably normal, spinal cord compression at the level of the lesion producing myelopathy may substantially limit perfusion in that zone. Perfusion pressure in this case is limited to the mean arterial pressure minus the spinal cord compression pressure. Neurologic injury secondary to failure to maintain adequate spinal cord perfusion pressure is a real phenomenon and may, in fact, be one of the more common causes of unexplained worsening of neurologic function postoperatively in the patient with preexisting myelopathy. I am personally aware of two cases in which intraoperative hypotension produced severe aggravation of preexisting myelopathy, and there are case reports in the literature as well.[8]

Worsening of perfusion may occur by one of two important mechanisms: decreases in mean arterial pressure, or increases in spinal cord compression pressure. Hypotension can be a serious problem in these patients, and mean arterial pressure should be kept, if possible, at or above baseline values at all times during the case. Induced hypotension for reduction of blood loss should not be considered at all in patients with myelopathy unless continuous spinal cord monitoring is available. Even then, the risk-benefit ratio may be unfavorable. Inadvertent decreases in blood pressure should be promptly treated. It is unknown and likely variable from patient to patient how long decreased blood pressure can be tolerated by the compressed spinal cord.

Increases in spinal cord compression pressure may be caused by changes in head position associated with intubation and, more important, positioning. In patients with a stable cervical spine, changes in spinal cord compression associated with intubation are unlikely to be harmful, primarily secondary to their very transient nature. During a normal (i.e., nondifficult) intubation with a Macintosh- or Miller-type blade, there is measurable extension at all cervical spine levels, but it is most prominent at the occipitoatlantal (6.8 degree) and atlantoaxial (4.7 degree) joints.[9] This degree of movement is far less than their maximal capacity for movement that would be seen in an awake patient. This degree of motion may be reduced by using the Bullard laryngoscope,[10] a fiberoptic approach, or a blind nasal intubation. Even in the worse case (i.e., direct laryngoscopy), extension returns promptly to near baseline after removal of the laryngoscope. In any event, the degree of motion appears, from recent studies, to be far less than previously reported in patients with good airways undergoing technically easy laryngoscopy, particularly if stabilization maneuvers are used.[9] Intubation in patients with cervical myelopathy, normal airways, and stable cervical spine is unlikely to cause further damage to the spinal cord. Patients in whom laryngoscopy is difficult likely experience greater degrees of motion, and this statement may not apply.

Positioning may, however, introduce much more serious considerations. Positioning the patient other than supine with the head in a neutral position may cause an increase in the spinal cord compression pressure that is sustained. The cervical spinal canal is similar in many respects to the intracranial vault. The spinal cord is surrounded on all sides by a bony casing. In a patient with cervical myelopathy and accompanying spinal stenosis, there is little room for the spinal cord to maneuver. Spinal cord swelling associated with injury may produce the same conditions in patients with a normal spinal canal. Increased flexion or extension of even a few degrees may substantially increase or decrease the compression pressure on the spinal cord if the elastance of the compartment is poor. Preoperative somatosensory evoked potentials recorded in patients with long segment cervical stenosis frequently deteriorated with changes in neck position (both flexion and extension) after a relatively short period of time.[11] I have also experienced several cases in which any degree of cervical flexion at all was associated with a prompt loss of evoked potentials that was reversed with correction of head position. Thus, my approach to patients with cervical myelopathy uses awake intubation and positioning when spinal cord monitoring is not planned. Local airway analgesia is obtained using either topical analgesia or neural blockade of the superior laryngeal or glossopharyngeal nerves followed by transtracheal injection of lidocaine.[12] After intubation and positioning, allowing time for position-related neurologic problems to develop (usually about 15 to 20 minutes), a neurologic examination is performed and compared with baseline. If there are no changes, anesthesia is induced and blood pressure maintained at or above baseline values.

ABNORMAL CERVICAL SPINE FUNCTION Up until this point, we have been considering anesthetic implications of abnormalities of neurologic function produced by cervical spine disease. There are also abnormalities of cervical spine function that produce either significant loss of mobility or abnormally increased mobility that do not cause any neurologic abnormalities. Cervical spine disease that severely limits cervical spine mobility causing potential airway difficulties is generally obvious to the anesthesiologist and will be discovered in the routine preoperative evaluation of the airway. Instability, however, may not be obvious, particularly when it is asymptomatic and not associated with trauma that would result in diagnostic cervical spine radiographs (i.e., flexion/extension lateral cervical spine views). A cervical spine is considered unstable when any of the motions described above in the section on normal cervical spine function exceed normal values. The most important "instability" is associated with translation, because this type of motion can cause direct bony trauma to the spinal cord. Two to three millimeters of translation (anterior-posterior motion) is normal at all cervical levels. Any greater amount of translation is considered abnormal and unstable. There is little controversy or doubt that awake intubation and positioning is an appropriate method of airway management in the patient with cervical spine trauma resulting in instability of the cervical spine. This technique will allow the anesthesiologist to assess spinal cord function continuously and allow the patient to give immediate feedback about any manipulations associated with securing the airway or positioning that produce pain. However, as noted above, there are no data to support the contention that neurologic injury is increased in patients who are managed with asleep intubation and positioning.[13–15] When other factors such as lack of patient cooperation or understanding would make awake intubation and positioning difficult, induction of general anesthesia before intubation is clearly a safe option in the vast majority of cases. Methods of cervical spine immobilization, however, clearly affect the ability of the anesthetist to secure the airway. The presence of a cervical collar clearly increases the incidence of a grade III or IV laryngoscopic view.[16] Several authors have recommended passive immobilization with or without in-line traction as the preferred method of intubation in these cases.[13,17,18] Both of these methods have been shown to decrease movement with laryngoscopy and intubation in the patient with a normal cervical spine. Interestingly, one study demonstrated that laryngoscopy and intubation were associated with significantly less cervical spine motion (1.51 mm) than mask ventilation (2.93 mm).[19]

Patients with asymptomatic instability will usually go unrecognized, because preoperative cervical spine radiographs are generally reserved for those patients with symptomatic cervical spine disease. A few types of patients, however, have a very high incidence of asymptomatic instability and should probably be evaluated preoperatively with cervical flexion and extension radiographs. The accompanying box shows those patients who have a high incidence of unsuspected cervical spine instability. Patients with rheumatoid arthritis have a particularly high incidence of significant cervical spine instability. In a recent retrospective review of patients with rheumatoid arthritis at my institution undergoing all types of surgery except cervical operations, 38 percent of all patients without any symptoms of cervical spine disease had significant instability of the cervical spine at one or more levels, some of which were severe.[20] Figure 12.6 shows an MRI obtained from one asymptomatic patient. This patient's abnormality was thought to be so severe that the patient underwent a transoral resection of the odontoid with occipitocervical fusion instead of the planned orthopaedic hand procedure. It is thus clear from this and other studies[21–23] that the incidence of cervical spine instability in patients with rheumatoid arthritis is high, even in asymptomatic patients. Many of these patients undergo surgery (mostly orthopedic) without any special precautions for airway management or positioning and do not suffer any untoward sequelae. There are several case reports, however, documenting unexpected perioperative deaths in patients with rheumatoid arthritis, and in one of these, postmortem examination revealed that the odontoid process in an unstable C1–2 joint had caused a brainstem contusion and hemorrhage.[24]

I thus recommend that when possible, patients at increased risk for instability of the cervical spine should have flexion and extension cervical spine radiographs within 1 year of surgery. Patients who show significant (greater than 4 mm) translation at any level should be given serious consideration for awake intubation and positioning, particularly if the surgery is to be conducted in any position other than supine, head neutral. It is unknown how much translation or other motion will occur during intubation in patients with these types of instabilities, particularly under the influence of muscle relaxants. The most conservative approach would be to keep these patients awake during intubation and positioning so that all the patients' normal musculoskeletal tone is still present and no greater motion than those the patients experience on a daily basis will occur. This approach, although practiced by many clinicians, is not standard of care at this time, and most patients will do well with laryngoscopy, intubation, and positioning after induction of general anesthesia. In fact, several retrospective studies have failed to demonstrate an increased incidence of neurologic injury in patients with cervical instability after trauma associated with intubation and positioning under general anesthesia.[13–15] Much of what we do in anesthesia monitoring, however, is designed to detect and prevent rare complications. Why should we have a different

> ***Disease States Associated with Relatively Common Asymptomatic Cervical Spine Instability***
>
> Rheumatoid arthritis
>
> Down's syndrome (trisomy 21)
>
> Klippel-Feil abnormality

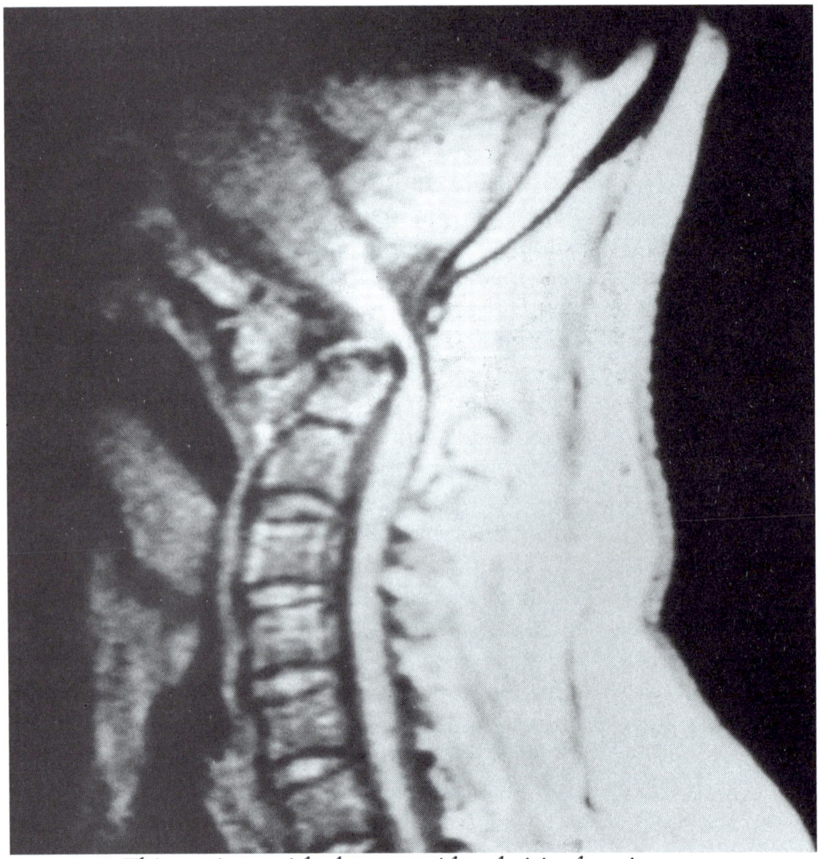

FIGURE 12.6 *This patient with rheumatoid arthritis showing severe compression of the cervical spinal cord at and just below the level of the foramen magnum was asymptomatic.*

approach for the patient with asymptomatic cervical spine instability?

SUMMARY

In conclusion, when evaluating the cervical spine, the anesthesiologist should use an organized approach that carefully documents the presence or absence of radiculopathy, myelopathy, or abnormal function of the ligaments and joints. These abnormalities have implications for anesthetic management of intubation, positioning, and blood pressure control, and a detailed understanding of the pathophysiology of cervical spine disease will help the anesthesiologist minimize the likelihood of further damage to cervical spinal cord function.

References

1. Maiman DJ, Yoganandan N, Pintar F, Hollowell J: Biomechanics of the spine. p. 2229. In Youmans JR (ed): Neurologic Surgery. 4th Ed. WB Saunders, Philadelphia, 1996
2. Denis F: The three column spine and its significance in the classification of acute thoracolumbar spine injuries. Spine 8:817, 1983
3. Fielding JW, Burstein AH, Frankel VH: The nuchal ligament. Spine 1:3, 1976
4. Werne S: Studies in spontaneous atlas dislocation. Acta Orthop Scand Suppl 23:1, 1957

5. Bailey RW: Observations of cervical intervertebral disc lesions in fractures and dislocations. J Bone Joint Surg 461, 1963
6. Bedbrook GM: Compression, flexion, and extension injuries of the cervical spine with tetraplegia. In: Proceedings of the Veterans Administration Spinal Cord Injury Conference 19:6, 1973
7. Bedbrook GM: Closed injuries of the cervical spine and spinal cord extension-rotation injuries. p. 58. In: Proceedings of the Veterans Administration Spinal Cord Injury Conference 19:58, 1973
8. Grundy BL, Nash CL Jr, Brown RH: Arterial pressure manipulation alters spinal cord function during correction of scoliosis. Anesthesiology 54:249, 1981
9. Sawin PD, Todd MM, Traynelis VC et al: Cervical spine motion with direct laryngoscopy and orotracheal intubation. Anesthesiology 85:26, 1996
10. Hastings RH, Vigil AC, Hanna R et al: Cervical spine movement during laryngoscopy with the Bullard, Macintosh, and Miller laryngoscopes. Anesthesiology 82:859, 1995
11. Kraus R, Christophis P: Functional studies of the spinal cord in chronic stenosing diseases of the cervical spine using somatosensory evoked potentials. Zentralbl Neurochir 55:96, 1994
12. Crowley WJ, Mahla ME: Awake intubation with nerve blocks and transtracheal injection of lidocaine: a 10-year experience, abstracted. Anesthesiology 79:A218, 1993
13. Suderman VS, Crosby ET, Lui A: Elective oral tracheal intubation in cervical spine-injured adults. Can J Anaesth 38:785, 1991
14. Doolan LA, O'Brien JF: Safe intubation in cervical spine injury. Anaesth Intensive Care 13:319, 1985
15. Criswell JC, Parr MJA, Nolan JP: Forum: emergency airway management in patients with cervical spine injuries. Anesthesia 49:900, 1994
16. Pennant JH, Pace NA, Gajraj NM: Role of the laryngeal mask airway in the immobile cervical spine. J Clin Anesth 5:226, 1993
17. Wood PR, Lawler PGP: Managing the airway in cervical spine injury. A review of the Advanced Trauma Life Support protocol. Anesthesia 47:792, 1992
18. Hastings RH, Marks JD: Airway management for trauma patients with potentials cervical spine injuries. Anesth Analg 73:471, 1991
19. Hauswald M, Sklar DP, Tandberg D, Garcia JF: Cervical spine movement during upper airway management: cinefluoroscopic appraisal in human cadavers. Am J Emerg Med 9:535, 1991
20. Totten JA, Mahla ME: Incidence of unsuspected cervical spine instability in asymptomatic patients with rheumatoid arthritis undergoing surgery, abstracted. Anesthesiology 77:A199, 1997
21. Cabot A, Becker A: The cervical spine in rheumatoid arthritis. Clin Orthop 131:130, 1978
22. Pellici PM, Ranawat CS, Tsairis P, Bryan WJ: A prospective study of the progression of rheumatoid arthritis of the cervical spine. J Bone Joint Surg 63A:342, 1981
23. Halla JT, Hardin JG, Vitek J, Alarcon GS: Involvement of the cervical spine in rheumatoid arthritis. Arthritis Rheum 32:652, 1989
24. Yaszemski MJ, Shepler TR: Sudden death from cord compression associated with atlantoaxial instability in rheumatoid arthritis. A case report. Spine 15:338, 1990
25. Netter FH: Atlas of Human Anatomy. Ciba-Geigy, 1989

13 VERTEBRAL COLUMN AND SPINAL CORD SURGERY

MICHAEL E. MAHLA

TERESE T. HORLOCKER

Surgery to the spine and spinal cord comprises a large percentage of neurosurgical procedures. This chapter is organized by procedure and reviews common and newly developed spine operations. An emphasis is placed on preoperative, intraoperative, and postoperative considerations that will help the clinician:

- understand what each operation involves
- understand how certain specific disease processes may alter anesthetic considerations for each operation
- preserve spinal cord blood flow to ensure a good neurologic outcome

SPINAL CORD BLOOD FLOW AND AUTOREGULATION

The vascular supply of the spinal cord is quite complex in both its origin and pattern of flow in and around the cord. There are substantial individual anatomic variations as well. Surgical manipulation and instrumentation, direct trauma, and anesthetic agents and techniques may all affect spinal cord blood flow and autoregulation. As during craniotomies, it is important to apply the principles of neuronal protection during spinal cord and vertebral column surgery to prevent spinal cord ischemia and preserve function.

Blood Supply

The spinal cord is supplied with arterial blood by one anterior and two posterolateral vessels that run the length of the cord. These vessels are supplied from segmental radicular arteries that enter the vertebral foramina and reach the spinal cord along with the nerve roots. Individual variation exists in the number of radicular arteries, their origin, and their route to the spinal cord.

ANTERIOR SPINAL ARTERY The anterior spinal artery (ASA) is formed by a branch of each vertebral artery that arises near its junction with the basilar artery. These two branches then join to form the single ASA, which then descends in the median fissure of the spinal cord (Fig. 13.1). A series of six to eight anterior radicular arteries from the vertebral, thyrocervical, costocervical, intercostal, and iliac vessels supply the ASA at intervals (variable from patient to patient) along the length of the spinal cord. The cervical and lumbar cord receive most of this blood supply. The largest of these radicular arteries is the radicularis magna (artery of

Adamkiewicz), which supplies the ASA in the thoracolumbar region of the spinal cord. Its origin is between T9 and T12 in 60 percent, between T5 and T8 in 14 percent, and below L1 in 26 percent of cases.[1] The artery of Adamkiewicz is commonly responsible for one-quarter to one-half of the total blood supply of the spinal cord.

In the upper and midcervical portions of the cord, the flow in the ASA is in the caudad direction. Because of the great variations in radicular supply, the direction of flow in the ASA is uncertain in other areas. The relatively large distances between the radicular vessels in the thoracic region place multiple "watershed" areas of the cord at risk for ischemia, particularly in the midthoracic (between artery of Adamkiewicz and cervical supply) and lumbar regions. Without radicular supplementation, the ASAs and posterior spinal arteries (PSAs) are sufficient only for the upper cervical cord. ASA ischemia results in loss of motor function and pain and temperature sensation because the anterior two-thirds of the cord is supplied by the ASA. Dorsal column functions are spared if PSAs are intact.

POSTERIOR SPINAL ARTERIES The paired PSAs arise from the vertebral arteries or the posterior inferior cerebellar arteries and descend along the posterolateral aspect of the cord. Compared with the ASA, the PSAs receive contributions from many more radicular arteries (25 to 40). The PSAs supply only the posterior one-third of the cord. Because they are widely anastomosed with each other and with radicular branches, injury to one of them will not necessarily result in any spinal cord ischemia.

Blood flow to the spinal cord is approximately 40 percent of cerebral blood flow, with the cervical and lumbosacral regions receiving twice that of the thoracic area.[2] Spinal cord blood flow autoregulates and responds to chemical factors similarly to cerebral blood flow.[2,3] Spinal cord blood flow is constant between spinal cord perfusion pressures of 60 to 150 mmHg. Outside this range, flow is pressure-dependent.[4] Ischemia may occur if spinal cord perfusion pres-

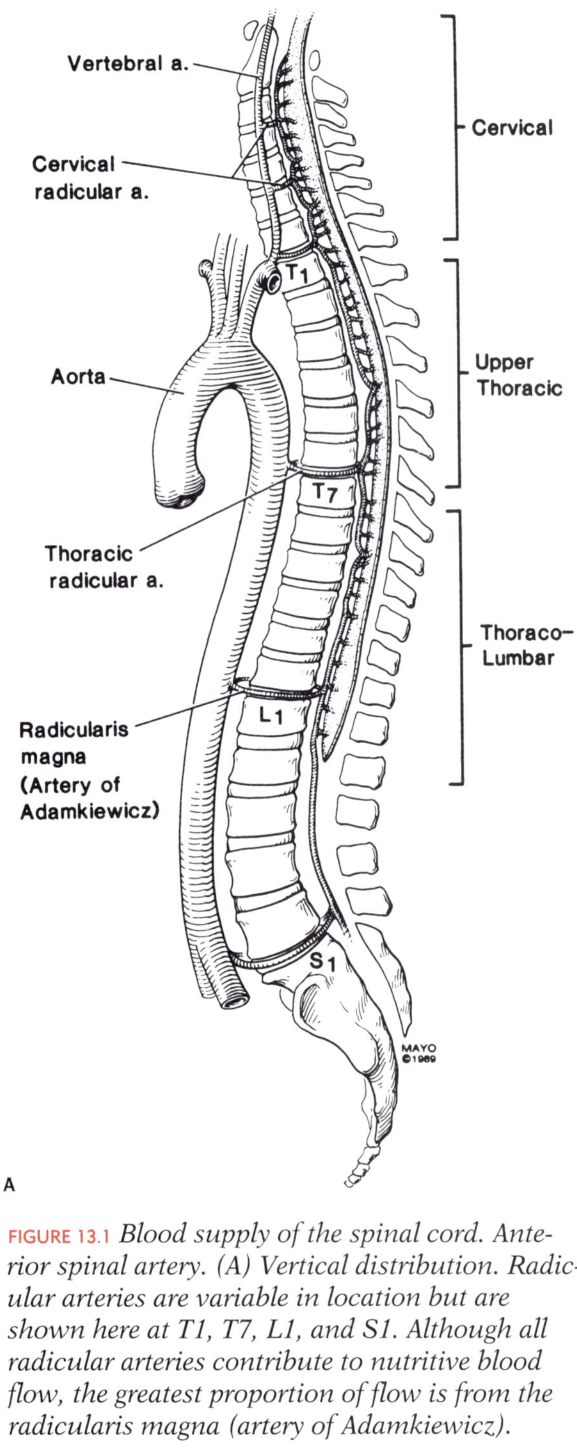

FIGURE 13.1 *Blood supply of the spinal cord. Anterior spinal artery. (A) Vertical distribution. Radicular arteries are variable in location but are shown here at T1, T7, L1, and S1. Although all radicular arteries contribute to nutritive blood flow, the greatest proportion of flow is from the radicularis magna (artery of Adamkiewicz).*

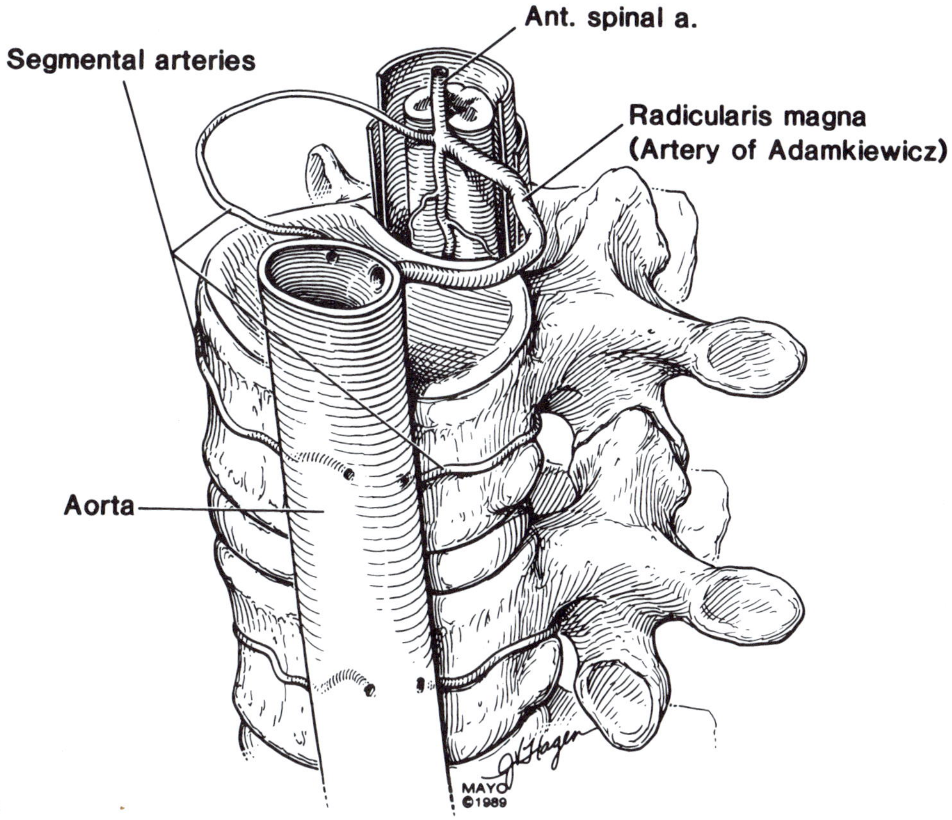

B

FIGURE 13.1 *Continued. (B) Segmental blood supply at the level of the radicularis magna, which is between T9 and T12 in 60 percent of cases. (By permission of Mayo-Clinic).*

sure falls below autoregulatory limits. Spinal cord blood flow responds to arterial oxygen and carbon dioxide tensions in the same manner as cerebral blood flow.[5] Hypocapnia decreases flow, whereas hypercapnia and hypoxia result in vasodilation and increased flow. As during intracranial surgery, autoregulation may be affected by patient pathology, trauma, surgery, and anesthetics. Maintenance of spinal cord perfusion pressure during surgery on the spine or spinal cord is every bit as important as maintaining cerebral perfusion pressure during intracranial surgery.

The spinal cord is encased in a bony enclosure that in many ways may be compared with the cranium. For example, a posteriorly directed intervertebral disc herniation pushes tissue into the spinal canal. Because the canal cannot expand, the spinal cord may be compressed. Spinal cord perfusion pressure at that level is then equal to the mean arterial pressure (MAP) minus the pressure exerted by the herniated disc. Thus, with significant spinal cord compression, even mild hypotension may cause spinal cord ischemia/infarction at the level of the compression. Maintenance of blood pressure at or above levels where the patient demonstrated function in the awake state is therefore very important in patients who have spinal cord compression from any cause.

VERTEBRAL COLUMN PROCEDURES

Surgery on the vertebral column is most commonly performed for degenerative disease, congenital abnormalities, or trauma. Spinal stenosis, spondylosis, and spondylolithesis are all forms of degenerative vertebral column disease. It is not unusual for more than one of these degenerative changes in the spine to occur concomitantly, leading to a more rapid progression of neurologic symptoms and the need for surgical intervention.

Spinal stenosis may be best defined as an inadequate space for the neural contents of the spinal canal and most commonly occurs in the lumbar spine. Patients with baseline narrowing of the spinal canal are more susceptible to the effects of trauma and aging than individuals with more available reserve space. In these patients, a major neurologic deficit may occur with only a minor injury. Fracture dislocation, disc extrusion, hyperextension (which allows nerve roots to relax and thicken and at the same time decreases space within the spinal canal), and facet hypertrophy all contribute to neural compression and ischemia. The typical presentation of uncomplicated spinal stenosis includes a long history of low back pain and dysesthesias exacerbated by walking. Symptoms disappear with sitting or lying down. Activity is usually discontinued before the development of weakness because of pain and numbness. Many patients, then, do not complain of motor deficits and only rarely show a specific sensory deficit on examination. However, in 30 percent of patients, spinal stenosis is complicated by a herniated disc. In these patients, loss of motor function, sensation, and/or reflexes may be evident.[6] Changes in the anteroposterior (AP) diameter of the spinal canal and compression of neural structures are best identified by a combination of computed tomography (CT) or magnetic resonance imaging (MRI) scan and myelography. Stenosis is rarely encountered at the L5–S1 interspace and is more frequently seen at L3–4 and L4–5 levels. Multilevel stenosis is a common finding.[7] The aim of surgery is decompression to increase available space for neural structures. Laminectomies are performed at the levels identified by myelography preoperatively. Usually two or more levels require decompression. Frequently, no stabilization or instrumentation of the spine is required for spinal stenosis initially. However, depending on how much lateral decompression near the facet joints is necessary, subsequent instability may result that will require fusion.

When spinal stenosis presents in the cervical spine, presentation may be similar to the lumbar spine but involve primarily the upper extremities and neck itself. More serious, however, is the patient who presents with spinal cord compression and myelopathy. Symptoms may then involve the upper extremities, lower extremities, bowel, and bladder and be so disabling as to render the patient unable to walk unassisted. Decompression in the cervical spine may be performed posteriorly via laminectomy or anteriorly via discectomy and corpectomy.

Degenerative disc disease, or spondylosis, results from progressive dessication of the nucleus pulposus. A fracture of the anulus fibrosus allows nuclear herniation. Reactive osteophytes and continued spondylosis result in neurologic sequelae when either the spinal cord or nerve root is compromised.[8] The initial pain accompanying a herniated disc is due to stretching of the posterior longitudinal ligament of the spine, associated nerve root compression, muscle spasm, and facet inflammation. Untreated radiculopathy may progress to numbness, weakness, and hyporeflexia in the corresponding nerve root distribution. Disc herniation usually occurs laterally, compressing nerve roots as they leave the canal. Most commonly, the C5–6 and C6–7 discs in the cervical area and L4–5 and L5–S1 discs in the lumbar area are affected. The ratio of lumbar to cervical disc disease is 6:1.[9] More than one-half of patients report a history of trauma preceding onset of symptoms even though the basic etiology is a degenerative process. Myelography is useful in supporting physical findings. The typical radiographic appearance is a filling defect corresponding to the involved interspace, with lack of definition of the root pouches. Initial treatment is immobilization and bedrest. Surgery is considered only if conservative measures are ineffective. Signs of spinal cord compression with or without root symptoms and deteriorating neurologic function (e.g., development of foot drop, leg weakness, or bowel/bladder incontinence) are indications for urgent surgery without giving conservative treatment a chance to work.

Spondylolisthesis is defined as a slipping forward of one vertebra on the vertebra beneath. Degenerative spondylolisthesis is caused by long-standing intersegmental instability. The facets and annulus fibrosis at the level of slip show severe degeneration. Although this disease does occur in the cervical spine, it is most common in the lumbar spine. The L4 interspace is involved six to nine times more often than any other level, with the L3 and L5 interspaces following in that order. [10] The incidence increases with age and occurs four times more frequently in women. The initial complaint is back pain or back and leg pain. Many patients experience pain on walking but characteristically find relief by laying down—the classic symptoms of spinal stenosis. A comparison of supine and standing lateral radiographs will allow assessment of the instability and slip present, which is exacerbated by an erect posture. Treatment depends on symptoms. If spinal stenosis accompanies spondylolisthesis, the space available for nervous system structures is further reduced, the patient will most likely be symptomatic, and surgical treatment will probably be necessary. Posterior fusion with iliac crest bone graft is the most common surgical procedure for spondylolisthesis. Reduction of the slippage with instrumentation of the listhetic vertebra may be required with symptomatic slips of greater than 50 percent.[11]

Spinal trauma can occur at any level but is most common in the lumbar (thoracolumbar junction) and the middle to lower cervical spine, which are the most mobile regions of the spinal column and are not relatively protected by the rigid chest wall and rib cage. Trauma often produces the same type of bony changes as degenerative changes. However, these changes occur much faster and give the nervous structures no time to adapt. The patient is thus more likely to be symptomatic and require surgery. In addition, trauma may cause fractures and acute ligamentous disruption that may result in serious instability, which in turn may produce further damage to nerve roots or the spinal cord if proper care is not taken.

Evaluation of the airway and approach to the cervical spine are discussed in detail in Chapter 12, and considerations discussed there apply as well to the patient with cervical spine trauma. These same considerations for cervical instability (i.e., awake positioning) may apply for spine injuries that have resulted in cord/nerve root compromise and instability in the thoracic and lumbar regions as well. Thoracic injuries are rarely unstable. There may be damage to nerve roots and spinal cord, but positioning of the patient will not usually cause further damage. The relatively rigid rib cage/thorax generally stabilizes thoracic injuries. There are exceptions to this, and neurosurgical colleagues should be consulted when there is any question of instability. Lumbar injuries are much more commonly unstable. If there is already neurologic injury or if movement of the patient into the prone position for surgery could potentially create more neural damage, some experts recommend awake positioning or a wake-up test after positioning to make certain that placing the patient into position has not created injury. Alternatively, some form of neurologic monitoring such as somatosensory (SSEP) or motor evoked potentials (MEP) may be used before and after positioning to make certain that function is preserved. Both forms of monitoring are feasible after induction of anesthesia (Ch. 4). Prompt correction of positioning that has caused new neurologic abnormalities detected early by one of these methods is more likely to restore function than if a position-related injury is undetected for an entire operation.

Spinal cord injury itself deserves special attention. In the acutely injured patient, several important factors must be considered. First, spinal cord injuries are often accompanied by other serious injuries that need consideration as well. Serious injuries involving the musculoskeletal system (18 percent), head (16 percent), lung (10.5 percent), abdomen (2.5 percent), and cardiovascular system (1.5 percent) accompany spinal cord injury.[12] Second, there are data that outcome after spinal cord injury can be improved by prompt administration of a high dose of methylprednisone (30-mg/kg loading dose followed by an infusion of 5.5 mg/kg/hr for 24 hours).[12] Although the actual amount of improvement in ultimate function gained by the administration of high-dose steroids is not dramatic, it is clinically significant. Most experts recommend administration of the above steroid regimen only if it can be instituted within 8 hours of the spinal cord injury.

Finally, spinal cord injury in both the acute and chronic time period can produce dramatic hemodynamic changes that profoundly alter anesthetic management. In the period surrounding an acute spinal cord injury, spinal cord function at and below the level of the lesion ceases ("spinal shock"). There is no motor, sensory, reflex, or sympathetic nervous system function. If the spinal cord injury level is high enough (generally above T6), loss of sympathetic nervous system function can produce significant hypotension, which can further aggravate spinal cord injury. Injuries at or above T4 may produce bradycardia as well (loss of cardioaccelerator function). This spinal shock syndrome may persist for some time after the injury (weeks). Its end is heralded by the return of reflexes below the level of the lesion.

Maintenance of a systolic blood pressure of at least 90 mmHg and an adequate cardiac output has been shown to prevent secondary injury to the spinal cord.[13] Although there is little controversy about the need to maintain blood pressure at a level sufficient for spinal cord perfusion, there is considerable controversy about how to do that. Most recommend the use of a pulmonary artery catheter to manage hemodynamics.[14] Because there is a well-known association between spinal cord injury and serious respiratory complications,[15] some experts recommend only judicious use of fluids in these patients to minimize extravascular lung water. Others, however, note that cardiac function is sometimes impaired in patients with spinal cord injury and that elevation of pulmonary wedge pressure readings to 18 mmHg with fluids resulted in restoration of acceptable blood pressure with better cardiac output than when inotropic agents with vasoconstrictor properties were used to elevate blood pressure.[16]

Patients with acute spine injuries are not always surgical candidates. Patients with a patent spinal canal in whom there is no instability or fractures are generally not operative candidates. If, however, there is instability but no extrinsic pressure on the spinal cord that could compromise spinal cord perfusion, surgery is generally performed after medical stabilization in an intensive care unit. Patients with evidence of spinal cord compression where traction either cannot (thoracic/lumbar) or fails (cervical) to relieve this compression are taken to the operating room within 24 hours of injury. Surgery is performed to relieve the pressure on the spinal cord and restore stability (see below for description of operations).[17] In these cases, surgery is performed to prevent further neurologic injury even though the patient may still have significant cardiorespiratory instability.

Patients with chronic spinal cord injury above the level of T6 may also show hemodynamic abnormalities in the form of autonomic hyperreflexia in response to a noxious stimulus. This syndrome is characterized by severe hypertension, bradycardia, and vasodilation (flushing) above the level of injury. Normally, when a neurologically intact patient experiences an injury or a noxious stimulus (e.g., a cut on the leg), there is intense reflex vasoconstriction in the area surrounding the injury. This vasoconstriction is prevented from generalizing to other areas of the leg and the other leg by inhibitory control of the sympathetic system. Spinal cord injury, however, damages or destroys this inhibitory control. Any injury or noxious stimulus (cut, full bladder, full rectum) may result in intense, generalized vasoconstriction below the level of the lesion. If the spinal cord lesion is high enough, there is not enough vascular territory remaining for vasodilation above the level of the lesion to compensate. As a result, hypertension and reflex bradycardia may result. This hypertension may be so severe as to require treatment with vasoactive drugs.

Patients undergoing surgery with a spinal cord injury at T6 or above should be considered at risk for this syndrome. The syndrome will *not* occur in the period of spinal shock. One method that we have found helpful in determining if a patient is at risk for autonomic hyperreflexia is to look for a history of spasticity and to attempt to elicit spasticity on clinical examination. If the patient has a known history of spasticity, then disinhibited spinal cord function is present and the patient is at risk for autonomic hyperreflexia. If the patient does not have a history of spasticity but testing reflexes produces sustained motor responses, the patient is also likely at risk.

If the syndrome develops intraoperatively, management with deepening the anesthetic (blocks afferent limb of reflex causing hypertension and may cause vasodilation), vasodilators (nitroprusside, nitroglycerine, hydralazine, others), or both will be needed. A preoperative spinal anesthetic sufficient to provide a level as high as the spinal cord injury will totally prevent this syndrome. Both the afferent and efferent limb of the reflex that produces hypertension are blocked.

SPECIFIC SPINAL COLUMN AND SPINAL CORD PROCEDURES

Cervical Spine

ANTERIOR PROCEDURES Before the early 1950s, virtually all surgery on the cervical spine was performed via a posterior approach. In 1955, Robinson and Smith[18] performed an anterior stabilization of the cervical spine. Three years later, Cloward described the use of the anterior approach for the removal of cervical discs compressing nerve roots or the spinal cord. Since then, anterior approaches have become much more popular. In fact, in many institutions including the University of Florida, most cervical spine surgery is conducted from an anterior approach.

Anterior Cervical Discectomy and Fusion The most common indication for anterior cervical procedures is a soft intervertebral disc herniation. This anterior approach may also used for repair of cervical spondylosis (degenerative bony overgrowth with compression of neural structures), repair of trauma to the vertebral body, and resection of bony or metastatic tumors involving the vertebral body (see below).

The approach to the spine is fairly straightforward. A small transverse incision is made on the right side (usually) at the level of the planned procedure. A left-sided approach may also be used and is associated with a lower incidence of recurrent laryngeal nerve injury. The left-sided approach is, however, harder for the right-handed surgeon. The surgeon will then develop a plane between the trachea and esophagus medially and the carotid artery laterally. The trachea and esophagus are retracted medially, and the carotid and associated structures are retracted laterally, exposing the spinal column. This retraction risks damaging the recurrent laryngeal nerve and compromising common carotid blood flow (Fig. 13.2). Lower vertebrae (T1–3) may also be approached anteriorly but require splitting of the manubrium for access.

Preoperative evaluation is routine except for evaluation of the cervical spine. It is very important to characterize the type of neurologic problem produced by the herniated cervical disc (Ch. 12). Cervical disc herniation may produce nerve root compression (radiculopathy), spinal cord compression (myelopathy), or both. Patients with spinal cord compression are at higher risk for reduced perfusion to the spinal cord at the level of the disc herniation. Even mild hypotension may not be tolerated, and intra-arterial monitoring of blood pressure may be helpful in

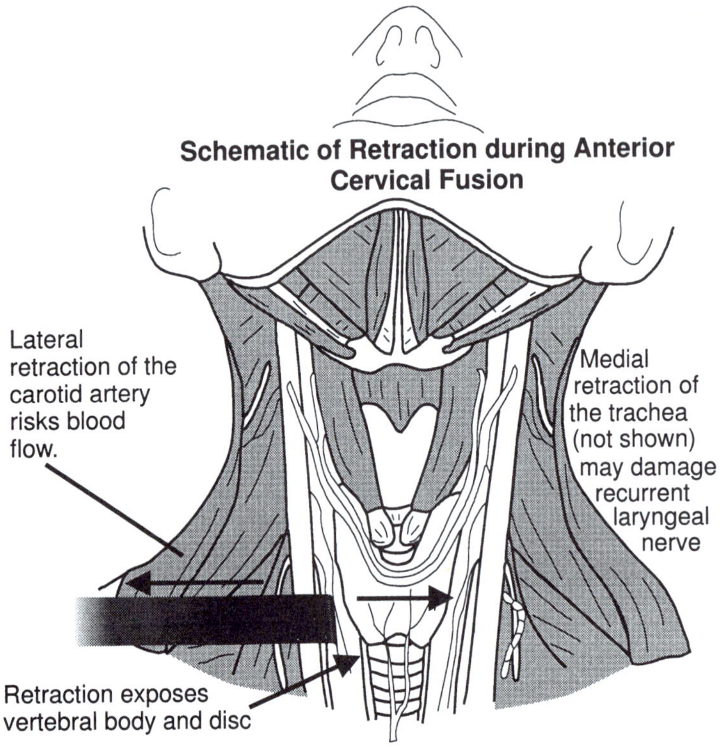

FIGURE 13.2 *In the anterior approach, damage to the recurrent laryngeal nerve or compromised common carotid artery blood flow may occur after placement of retraction to expose the cervical spine.*

managing blood pressure, particularly in patients at higher medical risk.

Intraoperatively, improper positioning may actually increase spinal cord compression. Awake intubation and positioning *may* be indicated to avoid this problem (Chapter 12). The patient is positioned supine with the head turned slightly away from the side of the incision. A chin strap is commonly placed to facilitate cervical traction (Fig. 13.3), which may be either continuous or intermittent. If continuous retraction is used, extra care must be taken to prevent the ropes from cutting into the skin of the face and ears or compressing the facial nerve. When using the strap system to put additional traction on during surgery (e.g., to facilitate placement of a bone graft), extubation may result if the strap slips off the chin. The arms are tucked to the patient's side. Padding should be placed at the elbows to avoid compression of the ulnar nerve in the olecranon fossa. The arms may need to be pulled in a caudad direction during surgery to facilitate fluoroscopic visualization of the lower cervical spine. Intravenous and arterial catheters placed in this region should be carefully secured to avoid dislodgment. Because these patients frequently have lumbar disease as well, padding should be placed under the knees to produce slight knee flexion. This flexion helps relax the sciatic nerve, reduces lumbar curvature, and will likely result in a more comfortable patient postoperatively. The surgeons are frequently standing directly against the arms of the patient and may move against the blood pressure cuff, producing incorrect readings or sometimes complete failure to measure blood pressure. The automated blood pressure cuff may be placed on the calf to avoid surgeon-induced motion artifact.

Incision and approach to the spine with retraction on the trachea/esophagus and carotid are made as described above. Compromise of the carotid artery (see above) may be detected by the anesthesiologist if the superficial temporal pulse on the operative side is located and marked before retractor placement. Loss of the superficial temporal pulse indicates common carotid compression and the need for retractor readjustment. This problem is uncommon, and one of us (M.E.M.) has observed this only three times in 10 years. The disc is then removed with the assistance of the operating microscope. After the disc is removed, the surgeon may or may not elect to perform some sort of stabilization procedure. Usually when just a disc with or without a small portion of bone is removed, placement of a bone graft is not needed. With time, the disc space collapses and spontaneous bony fusion occurs. Many surgeons prefer, however, to place an autologous (iliac crest) or homologous bone graft in the intervertebral space to facilitate a bony fusion at that level. Instrumentation is rarely needed. If more than just the disc must be removed (i.e., vertebral body), instrumentation may be required as well (see below).

Discectomy and fusion are not usually associated with large blood loss, but epidural venous bleeding may be troublesome, particularly in patients with concomitant cervical spinal stenosis. Vascular access with two large-bore intravenous lives should suffice in nearly all cases. This incision is not particularly painful, but the procedure itself may be extremely stimulating at several points during the case. Retraction of the trachea is a strong stimulus and may require deep planes of anesthesia to avoid coughing, but the patient becomes accustomed to this retraction as the case progresses and anesthesia may usually be lightened. Periosteal dissection and decompression of a nerve root are also extremely stimulating parts of this procedure.

An important anesthetic goal is to prevent excessive coughing at the conclusion of the operation. Coughing and bucking may dislodge the bone plug, which can then compromise the airway or the esophagus. This complication will require reoperation, and initial management of the airway may be very difficult. After an uncomplicated discectomy and fusion, the patient is nearly always extubated on the operating room table. Factors that would suggest caution in extubating the patient include multiple-level operation (more than two levels), major blood loss requiring large amounts of intravenous fluids, difficult tracheal retraction, and a difficult initial intubation. These factors would all tend

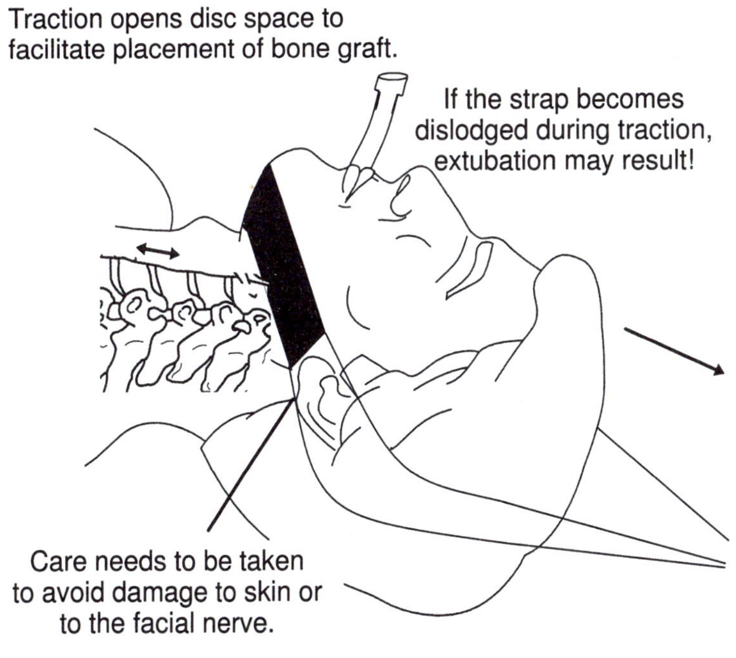

FIGURE 13.3 *Placement of a chin strap facilitates application of cervical traction, which may be needed to open up a disc space or to enable placement of a bone graft after discectomy.*

to cause postoperative tracheal/airway edema. Operations at high (i.e., C2–3) or C3–4) levels are the most likely to produce glottic edema, but significant problem are unlikely unless those factors listed above also apply.

Virtually any anesthetic technique may be used, provided the above goals are met. Some surgeons request that the patient remain unparalyzed so that they can detect patient movement associated with trespass on a nerve root or the spinal cord. This requirement will likely necessitate the use of higher doses of a narcotic and potent inhalation agent to prevent coughing associated with tracheal retraction. This may cause difficulty in patients with myelopathy who should have their blood pressure maintained at all times at or above preoperative levels where they were documented to have good neurologic function. Deep levels of anesthesia required to prevent movement may also produce hypotension. In these cases, surgical compromise is necessary and some relaxation should be used. Some form of spinal cord monitoring (Ch. 4) may be helpful during surgery, particularly in cases in which the spinal cord is compressed by osteophytes or especially by an ossified posterior longitudinal ligament, but spinal cord monitoring is clearly not a standard of care for a simple anterior cervical discectomy and fusion in the nonmyelopathic patient.

Postoperative recovery is rapid, and discharge on the first postoperative day is common, particularly if iliac crest bone grafting was not done. The patient's cervical spine will be immobilized for a period of time in a hard cervical collar to facilitate fusion. The patient's voice should be evaluated for evidence of recurrent laryngeal nerve damage. Usually, this complication is benign and does not result in airway obstruction. Spontaneous resolution in a few days to 6 weeks is the rule.

Cervical Corpectomy With Stabilization Cervical spondylosis causing compression of nerve roots or the spinal cord is treated more aggressively. Depending on the degree of disease, the procedure may vary from removal of compressive osteophytes with part of the vertebral body to a multilevel corpectomy with removal of an ossified posterior longitudinal ligament. Multiple-level vertebrectomies require reconstruction, usually with a bone graft that is held in place by a plate secured to the vertebrae above and below the levels of resection.

Preoperative and intraoperative considerations and management are identical to that described for anterior cervical discectomies above. Patients requiring a multiple-level cervical corpectomy are more likely to have cervical myelopathy with its associated blood pressure and positioning considerations than patients requiring a single-level discectomy. Blood loss is likely to be higher than for a simple discectomy, and at least two large-bore intravenous lives are a requirement. Intra-arterial blood pressure monitoring will be helpful for patients with myelopathy or medical risk factors.

The decision whether to extubate on the operating room table is more problematic for these patients. Generally, fluid requirements and duration and degree of retraction are higher in this operation. Most patients who have undergone a single-level corpectomy may be extubated safely on the operating table. The likelihood of airway problems increases with the number of vertebral bodies removed and the amount of intravenous fluid and retraction needed. Patients undergoing a three-level or more vertebrectomy should be left intubated in a head-up position and sedated overnight to allow airway edema to subside. The cuff may be let down in the morning to see if the patient can breathe around the endotracheal tube. If the patient successfully breathes around the tube, extubation is likely to be safe. If there is any question about the safety of extubation, placement of a tube changer with a port for administration of oxygen may increase the safety of extubation and the ease of reintubation if needed. Patients who have undergone a two-level corpectomy may or may not be suitable for extubation. Patients with more difficult airways at baseline or who had significant blood loss during surgery (more than 2 units) should be left intubated overnight in a head-up position and extubated the next day as described above.

Corpectomy may also be required for metastatic cancer to the cervical spine. Metastatic tumor to the cervical spine may cause symptoms of radiculopathy, myelopathy, or both. Operative intervention is necessary to prevent permanent significant loss of function in the cancer patient who would otherwise survive for a significant period of time. This intervention is palliative, for the most part, and designed to relieve nerve root or spinal cord compression. Decompressive surgery may be performed from either an anterior (corpectomy) or posterior (laminectomy) approach. Posterior approaches will generally avoid much of the tumor mass and may be just as effective in decompressing the spinal cord. When the anterior approach is indicated, anesthetic considerations for the preoperative and intraoperative management of these patients are similar to those described above. In addition, considerations imposed by the primary cancer (e.g., loss of lung function with lung cancer) must be considered. Finally, the possibility of massive, very difficult-to-control blood loss must be considered and appropriate intravenous access placed. If significant bleeding is encountered during corpectomy for malignant disease, it usually cannot be well controlled until the operation is complete.

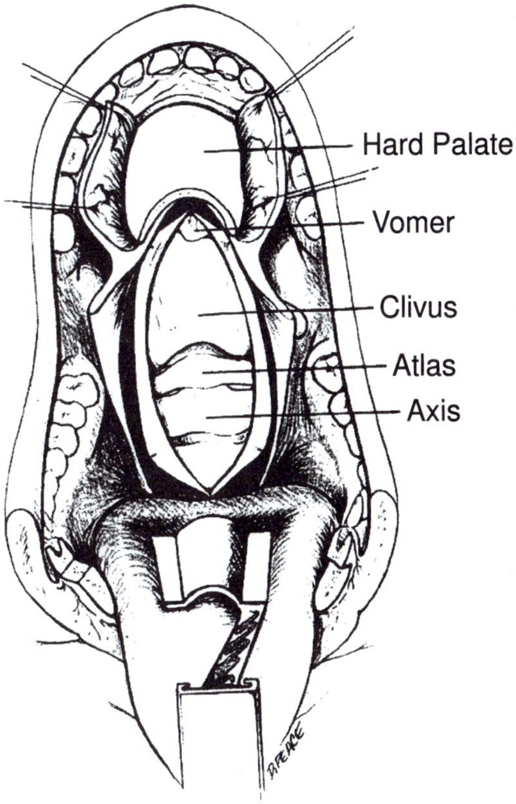

FIGURE 13.4 *Transoral approach to odontoid resection is possible because of the relation of the odontoid process to the posterior pharynx.*

Transoral Resection of the Odontoid Anterior approaches to cervical spine pathology above the level of C3 are also possible but must be approached transorally. The most common pathology requiring surgery at this high level is C1–2 instability. This instability may be congenital, traumatic, or degenerative. Symptoms are produced from either bony motion around the high cervical nerve roots, producing headache and pain, or by spinal cord compression from the odontoid process, producing myelopathy. The odontoid process is located directly behind the posterior pharyngeal wall (Fig. 13.4). Resection of the odontoid followed by an occipitocervical fusion cures the spinal cord compression and the instability causing the nerve root symptoms.

This operation is most commonly performed on patients with rheumatoid arthritis, and preoperative evaluation should focus on this disease. In patients without rheumatoid arthritis, preoperative evaluation is routine except for the cervical spine (Ch. 12). Intravenous access should consist of at least two large-bore intravenous lines because both epidural veins and the vertebral arteries themselves may be injured during this operation (Fig. 13.5). An arterial line is helpful in patients with myelopathy or in higher-risk medical patients. An oral right atrial enlargement tube or similar tube is necessary during this operation. The tube is secured out of the way with retraction similar to that used during tonsillectomies. Nasal intubation cannot be used because the endotracheal tube would directly obscure much of the surgical field. Early experience with this operation suggested that initial tracheostomy was desirable to allow ideal

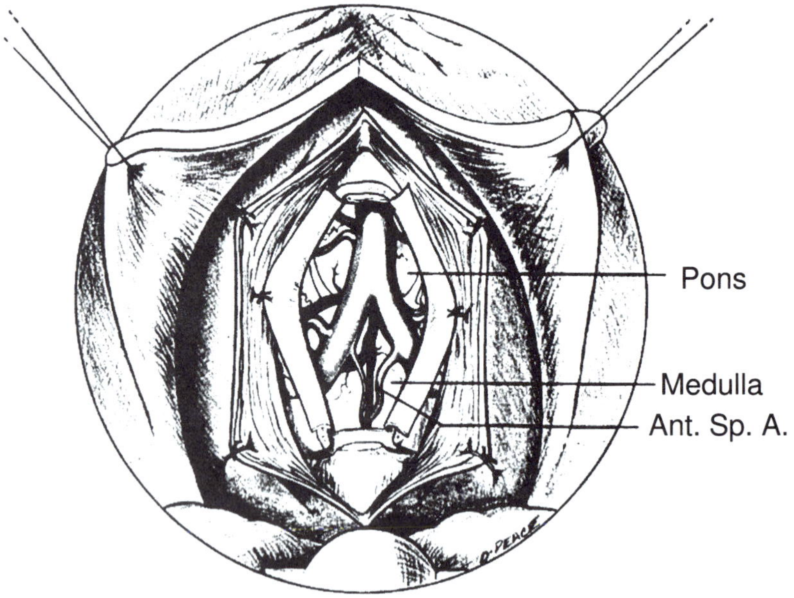

FIGURE 13.5 *Note the proximity of the vertebral arteries to the approach path for transoral resection.*

exposure and postoperative wound healing. However, later data indicate that tracheostomy, with its own set of risks/complications, is not usually needed. Patients are left intubated for several days to allow swelling in the posterior pharynx to subside. In addition, if a posterior fusion is not performed at the time of the transoral odontoid resection, the patient may be left intubated until this second operation is completed, usually several days later. Now that this operation is being more commonly performed, operative times have been reduced, and it is often feasible to do both the anterior and posterior procedure on the same day. Removal of the odontoid with its surrounding ligaments leaves the upper cervical spine very unstable. After completion of the odontoid resection, the patient is carefully turned prone. A fusion from the occiput to the first three cervical vertebrae is performed, which restores upper cervical spine stability.

At the completion of surgery, the patient is allowed to awaken enough to assess neurologic function and then sedated again to facilitate tolerance of the endotracheal tube. The patient is usually left intubated for several days to allow swelling to subside and then may be extubated as described above for patients undergoing corpectomy.

POSTERIOR PROCEDURES The most common procedures conducted from the posterior approach include decompression laminectomy (e.g., for spinal stenosis, Arnold-Chiari malformation, metastatic tumor), laminectomy for removal of intramedullary or extramedullary tumors, cervical fusions for stabilization, and nerve root procedures such as decompressions (foraminotomies) and rhizotomies. Although all anterior procedures are conducted in the same position (supine), posterior procedures may be conducted in the sitting position, prone position, or three-quarter-prone position.

Preoperative evaluation is routine except for that directed at the patient's neurologic problem and the cervical spine. The cervical spine should be evaluated as described in Chapter 12. The method of intubation and positioning will be determined by this evaluation and the patient's neurologic disease process. As with anterior approaches to surgery, patients with problems involving only the nerve roots may generally be intubated and positioned after induction of general anesthesia. Patients with instability that risks damage to the spinal cord and patients with myelopathy secondary to spinal cord compression may need to be intubated and positioned awake. This process, however, is more complicated when the surgery is conducted in the prone or sitting position. The patient is first intubated in the supine position. We will generally induce a brief period of general anesthesia by using propofol or thiopental to allow the placement of the head pinion. In the case in which the patient is already in a halo stabilization device or when use of the horseshoe head rest is planned, this step is unnecessary. After the patient awakens, either the patient moves into the prone or sitting positions or is moved into these positions. The head and neck are placed into the desired position, and the patient's neurologic function is tested. In addition, the patient is asked if there is any pain associated with the position. Once lack of pain and unchanged neurologic function is documented, general anesthesia may be induced.

Other preoperative considerations involve either the patient's preexisting neurologic function or the surgery itself. Patients with preexisting radiculopathy or myelopathy associated with muscle weakness may be at risk for hyperkalemia associated with the use of succinylcholine. The greater the amount of muscle mass involved with weakness, the greater the risk of hyperkalemia. The minimum amount of muscle/muscle groups involved that can produce hyperkalemia is unknown, and succinylcholine should only be used when the advantages to using this drug are clear (e.g., need for short duration of action, need for rapid onset, potential inability to intubate the patient).

The type and degree of hemodynamic monitoring may also be influenced by the patient's preexisting neurologic function. Patients with myelopathy either secondary to trauma or to degenerative disease may suffer worsening of spinal cord function if blood pressure is allowed to fall below baseline for any length of time. Use of an arterial line to measure blood pressure on a beat-to-beat basis will be helpful in these cases.

The surgical indication, planned procedure, and position used may also alter anesthetic planning. Procedures associated with significant blood loss may benefit from intra-arterial and central venous pressure (CVP) monitoring. Also, procedures planned for the sitting position should have intra-arterial pressure monitoring and CVP access for aspiration of air (see below).

Spinal cord monitoring may be used with many posterior cervical procedures. Monitoring is likely to be used for any procedure in which instrumentation may damage the spinal cord or nerve root (particularly sublaminar wiring) or when the surgical procedure itself risks the spinal cord or nerve roots (e.g., laminectomy for removal of tumor). Alteration of the anesthetic technique may be needed to facilitate SSEP or MEP monitoring.

The use of the sitting position for cervical laminectomy is still prevalent in some practices, but many have abandoned it for the prone or three-quarters prone position. The sitting position with its advantages and disadvantages is discussed in detail in Chapter 10. It is especially important to note that although the incidence of venous air embolism (VAE) in sitting posterior fossa cases is 40 percent, the incidence is only 5 to 25 percent in sitting cervical spine procedures. This decreased incidence may reduce the need for a CVP catheter. If attempted placement of a right atrial catheter in the sitting cervical patients is unsuccessful, it is reasonable to proceed with the case. The use of capnography, mass spectrometry, and precordial Doppler should be routine monitoring for such cases as they are noninvasive yet effective in detecting VAE. VAE does, in fact, occur during cervical laminectomies performed in any position because the wound is always above cardiac level regardless of the position of the patient. Incidences of VAE (defined by aspiration of air through a CVP catheter) in patients undergoing neurosurgical procedures in the sitting, supine, prone, and lateral positions are 25, 18, 10, and 8 percent, respectively.[19–21] These data would suggest that monitoring for air embolism should be routine during any cervical laminectomy. Positioning of the precordial Doppler may be difficult or impossible in the prone or three-quarters prone position, however.

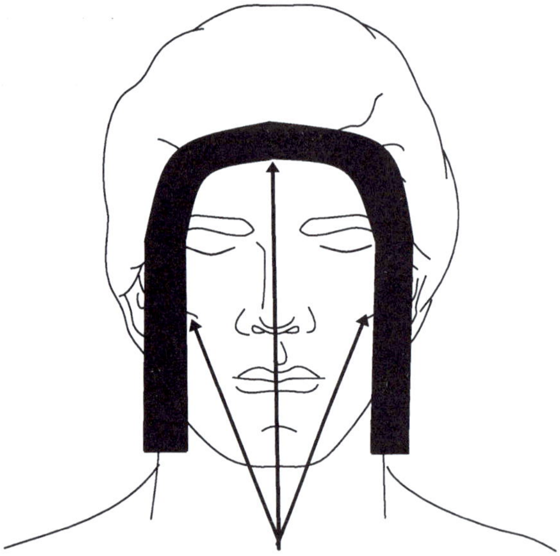

FIGURE 13.6 *Horseshoe head rest. note that proper positioning of the face places the eyes between the arms of the horseshoe. Pressure points are on the forhead and malar eminences. Eyes are free of any pressure.*

Posterior cervical spine procedures are usually conducted with the head fixed in a pinion or equivalent (e.g., halo immobilization adapted to a Mayfield head holder). The pinion provides maximal three point stabilization for the head and does not create any pressure points at all. The eyes are free of any pressure. The major disadvantage to the pinion is that if the patient attempts to move the head while fixed in a pinion, that may result in damage to the spine and serious skin lacerations. The patient needs to be kept anesthetized and paralyzed (if the operative procedure allows for muscle relaxation) until the pinion is removed after surgery. The only real alternative to the head pinion for posterior cervical spine surgery is the so-called horseshoe head rest. The horseshoe is molded to the patient's face, allowing the eyes and nose to rest between the arms of the horseshoe (Fig. 13.6). During prolonged surgery, serious pressure injury may occur to the forehead associated with the use of this device. In addition, if the patient moves during surgery, the eyes may no longer be free of any pressure and damage to vision may result.

Positioning the patient in the sitting position is described in detail in Chapter 10 and is not reviewed here. In the prone position, the patient lies on chest rolls that are sized to allow the patient's abdomen to hang free between the rolls. Keeping the abdomen suspended will minimize effects of the prone position on pulmonary function and reduce venous bleeding. The legs should be flexed at the knee with the thighs and calves padded to prevent excess pressure on the knee. The feet should be dorsiflexed slightly to prevent stretching of the anterior tibial nerve.

There are many variants of the three-quarters prone position. At the University of Florida, we use a "bean bag" positioning appliance to facilitate positioning. The patient's head is first placed in a pinion as described above. The patient is then turned into position as shown in Figure 13.7. The dependent leg is kept straight, and the superior leg is flexed 90 degrees at the knee. The body is allowed to fall forward until the desired head position can be achieved without significant rotation. An axillary roll is placed under the bean bag itself rather than under the patient. This roll allows the dependent arm to hang free and prevents compression of the brachial plexus against the head of the humerus. This method of placing the axillary roll diffuses the pressure of the roll and has not, thus far, been associated with any skin pressure injuries. There is also a risk of brachial plexus injury to the nondependent arm. This injury is likely caused by lateral bending of the neck against the dependent shoulder and taping the nondependent shoulder to improve exposure. This combination produces significant stretching of the plexus. This injury should be prevented by positioning the head and superior shoulder in such a fashion that there is no significant resting tension in the trapezius or sternocleidomastoid muscles.

Any anesthetic technique and monitoring methods may be used for posterior cervical procedures provided that the above considerations are taken into account. Drugs and techniques used for induction and intubation will be

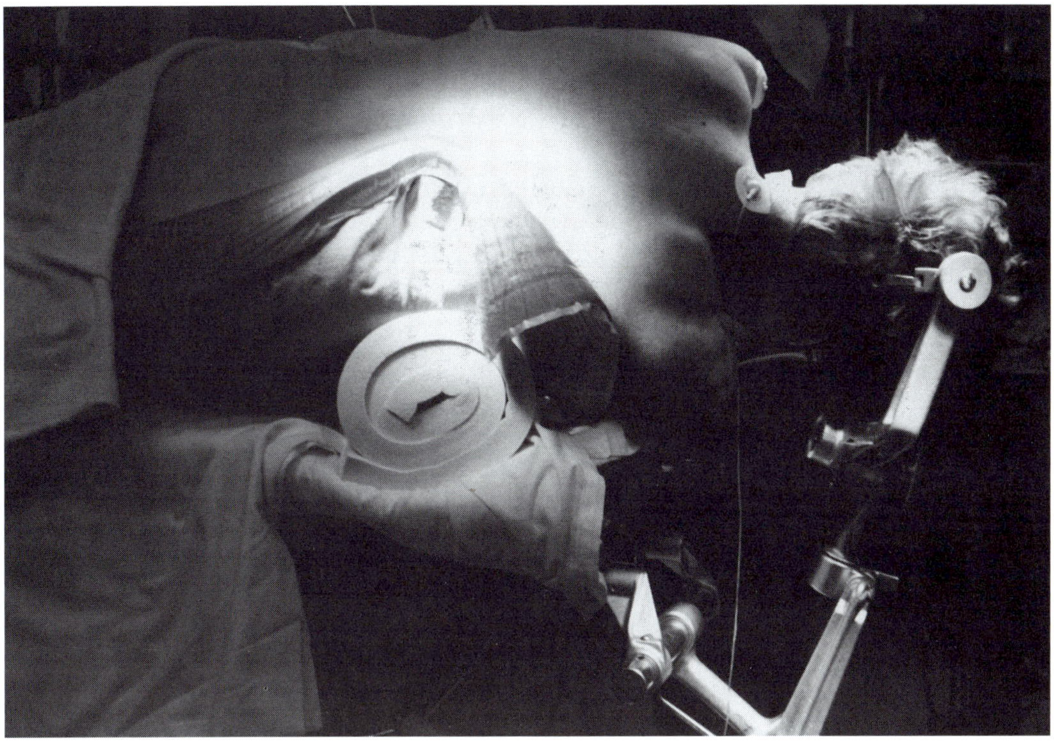

FIGURE 13.7 *Three-quarters prone position. Note the use of the bean bag appliance prevents excessive pressure of the axillary roll on the chest wall.*

determined by the need for awake intubation and positioning and whether the patient has any preexisting muscle weakness. Maintenance techniques will be influenced by whether evoked potential or electromyography (EMG) monitoring is used during surgery. Prompt awakening at the conclusion of surgery is important for assessment of neurologic function. Even if extubation is not planned, the patient should still be awakened if possible to assess neurologic function. Otherwise, complications that if detected promptly may be reversible would be missed until loss of neurologic function would be permanent.

The decision to extubate or not may be somewhat difficult and involve many factors. The main areas for consideration are neurologic function, length of case and position, amount of blood loss/intravenous fluid during surgery, and difficulty of intubation. If loss of neurologic function from the patient's pathology resulted in preoperative respiratory insufficiency, extubation is unwise in all cases. Pulmonary function will not improve during surgery, and a patient who could only marginally maintain acceptable respiratory function preoperatively will likely fail postoperatively. Patients with normal pulmonary function preoperatively should be assessed routinely (i.e., tidal volume, vital capacity, muscle strength) at the end of surgery for extubation criteria. These criteria will detect the rare patient in whom intraoperative neurologic injury will likely result in postoperative respiratory insufficiency. The one type of operation in which this problem may be more common is the resection of an intramedullary spinal cord/lower medulla tumor. These patients should be very carefully assessed for respiratory and upper extremity muscle strength and respiratory drive before extubation.

Prolonged surgery in the prone or three-quarters prone position, particularly when there is neck flexion, may result in swelling of some or all airway structures. The size of the tongue is readily assessed and may reflect swelling in the remainder of the airway. Patients with significant tongue swelling should probably not be extubated until the swelling has receded. These patients should be placed in a head-up position to allow swelling to subside during the night after surgery. Most of these patients may be extubated safely, provided they meet all other criteria, on the morning after surgery. Patients in whom there is concern may either be left intubated or extubated over a tube changer that has a port to provide oxygen supplementation. Similar airway swelling may occur after surgery in the sitting position (particularly when there is excessive neck flexion), but in our experience, airway edema after surgery in this position is much less common. In no case should a standard oral airway be used when neck flexion is planned. The superior surface of the oral airway will be pushed against the hard and soft palate by neck flexion and may result in palatal necrosis. Either a soft bite block or a plastic endotracheal tube sleeve should be used in place of the oral airway to prevent the patient from biting down on the endotracheal tube.

In cases in which there is significant blood loss requiring large amounts of intravenous fluids (more than 5 L fluid in a 70-kg or larger adult), airway edema may occur after surgery. The tongue may again be a window on the remainder of the airway. If the tongue does not show significant edema, extubation is probably safe, provided that the patient meets all other criteria. Further information may be gained from deflating the endotracheal tube cuff and occluding the endotracheal tube. If the patient is able to breathe around the endotracheal tube, significant airway edema is unlikely. As described above, patients with significant airway edema may be left intubated in a head-up position to allow edema to subside and extubated the following morning.

Finally, patients who experienced a difficult intubation should be extubated only when they are wide awake, meet all standard criteria, and are unlikely to have significant airway edema. Such patients should be treated more conservatively than patients who were intubated easily.

Thoracic and Lumbar Spine

As with cervical spine procedures, access to the thoracic and lumbar spine may be achieved from both anterior (really anterolateral) and posterior approaches. Some types of pathology require both approaches. Because there are so many indications for these operations, this chapter concentrates on the operative procedures and their associated anesthetic considerations. Anterior and posterior procedures are treated separately, although the clinician should be aware that an individual patient may require both approaches, sometimes even on the same day. Because the disease scoliosis presents so many anesthetic challenges and serves as a good general example of thoracic and lumbar spine surgery, it will be treated entirely separately and in much more detail than other thoracic and lumbar pathology with their associated operations. Thoracic spine procedures can be associated with considerable surgical trauma and morbidity, and great effort has been expended to develop more noninvasive surgical approaches to thoracic and lumbar pathology that will allow for more rapid patient recovery and less hospital time. These newer procedures are discussed along with the more traditional procedures.

SURGICAL APPROACH TO THE PATIENT WITH SCOLIOSIS Scoliosis is a deformity of the spine resulting in lateral curvature and rotation of the vertebrae and also deformity of the rib cage (Fig. 13.8). On the concave side of the curve, the discs and vertebral bodies become wedge-shaped, the posterior angles of the ribs are shallow, and the vertebrae and spinous processes rotate toward the concavity. On the convex side of the curvature, the ribs are pulled back, making the posterior angle more acute. Thoracic and lumbar regions are the most frequent sites of the primary curvature.[22]

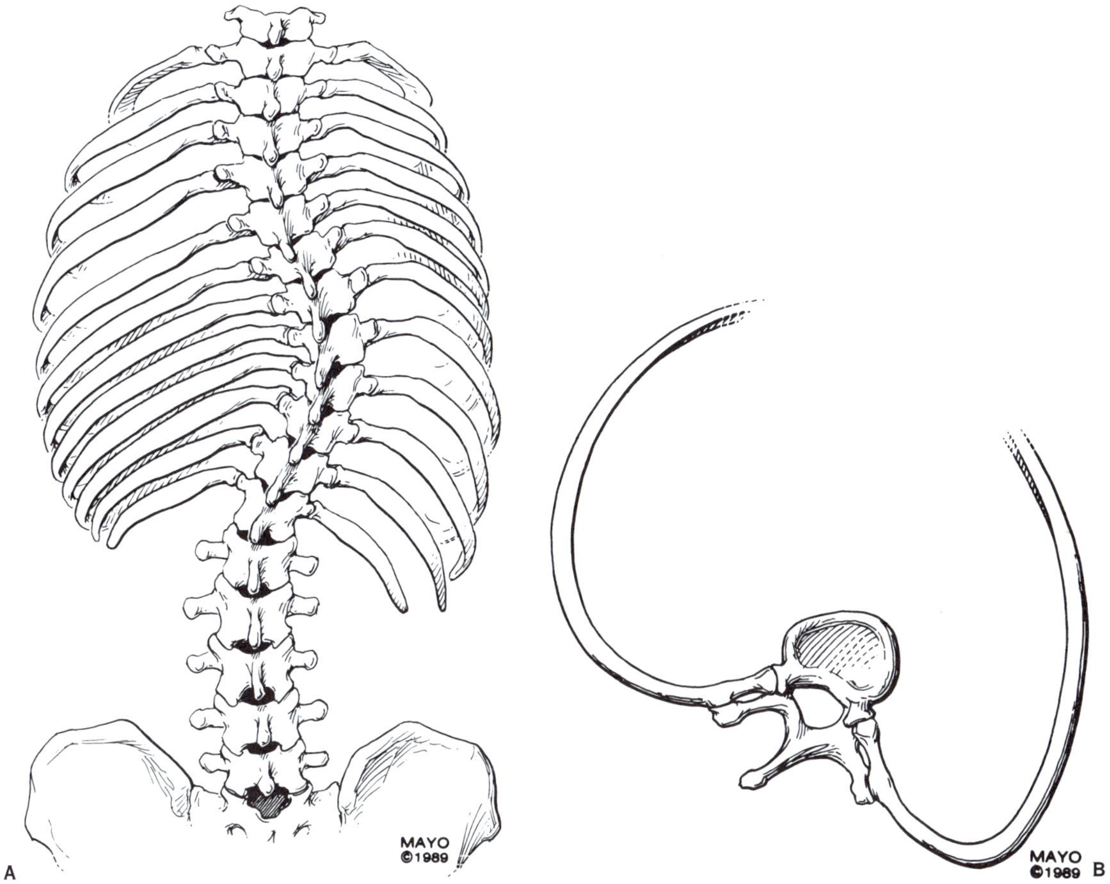

FIGURE 13.8 *(A & B): Deformity of the vertebrae and rib cage in scoliosis. Primary curvature occurs most frequently in the thoracic and lumbar regions. The vertebral bodies are wedge-shaped, and the posterior angles of the ribs are shallow on the side of concavity. On the convex side, the rib angles are more acute. (By permission of Mayo Clinic.)*

Patients with scoliosis may also develop kyphosis, or posterior rotation of the spine. Kyphoscoliosis is rare and is usually a congenital abnormality. These patients may require kyphectomy and anterior fusion in addition to posterior fusion to achieve spinal stability.[23]

The severity of the scoliosis is defined by the angle of scoliosis or Cobb angle (Fig. 13.9). The larger the angle, the more severe the scoliosis. It is generally agreed that nonoperative treatment such as application of a Milwaukee brace should be used in patients with a small curvature and in children who have not achieved skeletal maturity. Surgical correction is performed for deformities with a Cobb angle greater than 50°.[24] Improved methods of internal fixation have resulted in a trend toward earlier surgery.[25]

Classification of Scoliosis In 1973, the Scoliosis Research Society identified multiple etiologies in the development of scoliosis[26] (Table 13.1). As a result of the eradication of poliomyelitis, the incidence of scoliosis predominantly reflects the incidence of idiopathic scoliosis, which represents 75 to 90 percent of cases. The incidence is 4 per 1,000 girls and 0.3 per

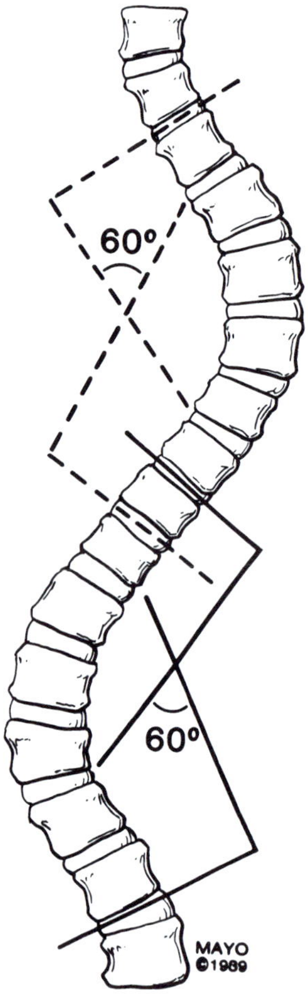

FIGURE 13.9 *Angle of scoliosis or Cobb angle. Lines are drawn parallel to the vertebral bodies at the lowest and highest borders of the curve. Perpendicular lines are drawn to these lines, and the angles are measured at the point of intersection. The angle of curvature consists of the cephalad and caudad angles. (From Mayo Clinic and foundation, with permission.)*

1,000 boys, with an overall incidence of 1.8 per 1,000.[27] The remaining 10 to 25 percent of cases are associated with neuromuscular diseases, congenital abnormalities including congenital heart disease, trauma, and mesenchymal disorders. A diagnosis of scoliosis in a patient should therefore include a family history and physical examination, with particular attention to the respiratory, cardiac, and neuromuscular systems.

IDIOPATHIC SCOLIOSIS. Idiopathic scoliosis is the most common type of scoliosis and has three well-defined periods of onset: infantile (0 to 4 years), juvenile (4 to 9 years), and adolescent (10 years to maturity). It is generally thought that the higher the curve and the earlier the onset, the worse the prognosis; however, 50 percent of cases of infantile scoliosis resolve spontaneously.

Infantile scoliosis can be classified as resolving or progressive. Male infants more frequently have progressive curves and a higher incidence of kyphosis. In one survey of 14 patients, the mean angle of scoliosis was 130 degrees, and three patients died of cardiac or respiratory failure.[28] Resolving infantile scoliosis does not usually increase beyond 30 degrees and seldom requires treatment.[26]

Adolescent idiopathic scoliosis is most common. Ninety percent of patients are girls, and 90 percent of the curves are right-sided and thoracic in origin.[29] Typically, seven to ten vertebrae are involved, and curve progression occurs rapidly. At skeletal maturity, two-thirds of patients will have a Cobb angle greater than 70 degrees and will require surgical correction. Curve progression may continue even after skeletal maturity. The average increase in the curve is 30 degrees.

Idiopathic scoliosis appears to be genetically inherited in adolescent scoliosis with an autosomal dominant mode of inheritance with reduced penetrance. The pattern has not been defined in infantile scoliosis. Although most patients with idiopathic scoliosis have no other associated anomalies, 7 percent of patients also had mental retardation, congenital heart defects, and other limb defects.[27]

SCOLIOSIS ASSOCIATED WITH NEUROMUSCULAR DISEASE. Neuropathic and myopathic scolioses are spinal curvatures caused by disease or anomalous function or development of nervous tissue or muscle. Poliomyelitis was once the leading cause of neuromuscular scoliosis. Degeneration of anterior horn cells in the spinal cord results in muscle weakness. Involvement of respiratory muscles leads to decreased force of inspiration and expiration, im-

TABLE 13.1 *Classification of spinal deformities*

I. Idiopathic
    A. Infantile (3 years of age or younger)
        1. Resolving
        2. Progressive
    B. Juvenile (4–9 years of age)
    C. Adolescent (10 years of age or older)
II. Neuromuscular
    A. Neuropathic
        1. Upper motor neuron lesion
            a. Cerebral palsy
            b. Spinocerebellar disease
                (1) Friedrich's
                (2) Charcot-Marie-Tooth
                (3) Roussy-Lévy
            c. Syringomyelia
            d. Spinal cord tumor
            e. Spinal cord trauma
            f. Other
        2. Lower motor neuron lesion
            a. Poliomyelitis
            b. Other viral myelitis
            c. Traumatic
            d. Spinal muscular atrophy
                (1) Werdnig-Hoffmann
                (2) Kugelberg-Welander
            e. Myelomeningocele (paralytic)
        3. Dysautonomia (Riley-Day)
        4. Other
    B. Myopathic
        1. Arthrogryposis
        2. Muscular dystrophy
            a. Duchenne (pseudohypertrophic)
            b. Limb-girdle
            c. Facioscapulohumeral
        3. Fiber-type disproportion
        4. Congenital hypotonia
        5. Myotonia dystrophica
        6. Other
III. Congenital
    A. Congenital scoliosis
        1. Failure of formation
            a. Wedge
            b. Hemivertebra
        2. Failure of segmentation
            a. Unilateral bar
            b. Bilateral ("fusion")
        3. Mixed
    B. Congenital kyphosis
        1. Failure of formation
        2. Failure of segmentation
        3. Mixed
    C. Congenital lordosis
    D. Associated with neural tissue defect
        1. Myelomeningocele
        2. Meningocele
        3. Spinal dysraphism
            a. Diastematomyelia
            b. Other
IV. Neurofibromatosis
V. Mesenchymal
    A. Marfan's disease
    B. Homocystinuria
    C. Ehlers-Danlos disease
VI. Traumatic
    A. Fracture of dislocation (nonparalytic)
    B. Postirradiation
    C. Postlaminectomy
    D. Other
VII. Soft tissue contractures
    A. Burn
    B. Other
VIII. Osteochondrodystrophies
    A. Achondroplasia
    B. Spondyloepiphyseal dysplasia
    C. Diastrophic dwarfism
    D. Mucopolysaccharidosis
IX. Scheuermann's disease
X. Infection
    A. Tuberculosis
    B. Bacterial
    C. Fungal
    D. Parasitic
    E. Other
XL. Tumor
    A. Benign
    B. Malignant
XII. Rheumatoid disease
    A. Juvenile rheumatoid
    B. Adult rheumatoid
    C. Marie-Strümpell
XIII. Metabolic
    A. Rickets
    B. Juvenile osteoporosis
    C. Osteogenesis imperfecta
XIV. Related to lumbosacral area
    A. Spondylolisthesis
    B. Spondylolysis
    C. Other congenital anomaly
    D. Other
XV. Thoracogenic
    A. Postempyema
    B. Post-thoracoplasty
    C. Post-thoracotomy
    D. Other
XVI. Hysterical
XVII. Functional
    A. Postural
    B. Secondary to short leg
    C. Other

paired cough, and atelectasis. Bulbar involvement impairs swallowing, predisposing the patient to aspiration and pneumonia. These patients often need aggressive preoperative pulmonary therapy. Residual effects of muscle relaxants and narcotics may cause respiratory failure postoperatively because of the limited respiratory reserve.

Patients with myelomeningocele undergoing scoliosis repair require careful positioning to avoid vertebral fractures. These patients have a high incidence of kyphosis and often require kyphectomy, including ligation of the nonfunctioning spinal cord. Ligation of the cord can lead to increases in intracranial pressure as well as the effects of sympathectomy due to cord transection. Patients with an intraventricular shunt must have shunt patency confirmed preoperatively. Profuse blood loss may occur due to scar tissue from previous repair as well as the proximity of the epidural plexus.

Neurofibromatosis, or Von Recklinghausen's disease, consists of irregular pigmented areas in the skin (café-au-lait spots) and multiple neurofibromas. There is a large spectrum of neuroskeletal abnormalities in patients with von Recklinghausen's disease. Skeletal deformities including bone cysts and scoliosis are found in 30 to 50 percent of patients. Neurofibromas arise within nerve trunks and may be located anywhere on or in the body. Most neurofibromas are asymptomatic; however, when they occur in fixed nonexpandable spaces, they may cause neural ischemia. The most clinically significant neurofibromas are those that occur in the intervertebral canal, where they may compress spinal roots, or the spinal cord or the posterior fossa, where they may compromise the acoustic nerve or medulla. There is an association between neurofibromatosis and meningiomas or gliomas. In addition, 1 percent of these patients will develop pheochromocytomas.

Cerebral palsy is a nonprogressive central motor deficit resulting from hypoxic events occurring in the prenatal or perinatal periods. Physical and intellectual disabilities are variable and may make communication difficult, resulting in poor patient cooperation. The accompanying spastic diplegia or quadriplegia may cause scoliosis, particularly in nonambulatory patients. Patients with more severe forms may have a pseudobulbar palsy, which predisposes to swallowing difficulties and aspiration. Spasticity and rigidity lead to abnormal limb positions and contractures that interfere with positioning and placement of monitoring lines.

Friedreich's ataxia is a progressive disease of the spinal cord and cerebellum that can be associated with scoliosis. Onset is usually in late childhood, and survival beyond early adult life is rare. Involvement of the spinocerebellar pathways, pyramidal tract, peripheral nerves, and dorsal columns results in gait disturbance, tremor, impairment of position sense, and in some patients, optic atrophy. Degeneration and necrosis of cardiac muscle fibers may also occur. Progressive muscle weakness involves the respiratory muscles and leads to respiratory failure.

Muscular dystrophy is the general designation of a group of chronic progressive disorders of skeletal musculature leading to weakness, atrophy, contracture, and disability. Most of these disorders are hereditary. Duchenne muscular dystrophy is an X-linked trait and is the most common form of muscular dystrophy. Patients are usually asymptomatic until 3 to 5 years of age, by which time enough muscle mass has been lost to impair function. The presenting signs typically include difficulty ascending stairs or rising from the floor, reflecting involvement of the proximal muscles in the lower extremities. By 9 years of age, 45 percent of patients are unable to ambulate independently, leading to the development of scoliosis. Death occurs before age 20 in 75 percent of patients due to respiratory or cardiac failure.[30] Pulmonary complications frequently occur in the advanced stages of muscular dystrophy. Respiratory muscle weakness with resultant alveolar hypoventilation, atelectasis, and decreased ability to clear secretions predisposes these patients to cor pulmonale, aspiration, and pneumonia. Postoperatively, they require aggressive pulmonary therapy to mobilize and remove secretions and prevent respiratory infections.

Cardiac involvement is present in more than

80 percent of patients with Duchenne muscular dystrophy. These children may have electrocardiographic (ECG) evidence of the disease when clinically asymptomatic because of their restricted activity level. The most common ECG findings of cardiomyopathy are tall precordial R waves, deep precordial Q waves, bundle branch block, PR interval prolongation, and ST segment elevation or depression. Cardiac arrhythmias may be precipitated by changes in vagal or sympathetic tone, inhalation agents, hypercapnia, or succinylcholine.[31]

Succinylcholine is contraindicated in patients with Duchenne or other muscular dystrophy.[32] The increase in muscle membrane permeability may lead to acute hyperkalemia and cardiac arrest after administration of succinylcholine. In addition, a sustained contraction in response to succinylcholine may produce difficulty in ventilation and intubation and extensive rhabdomyolysis. Subsequent myoglobinuria, an indicator of muscle trauma from prolonged contraction, may cause acute tubular necrosis and renal failure.

Patients with muscular dystrophy may be at increased risk for developing malignant hyperthermia.[33] Although an elevated resting creatine phosphokinase is often present in these patients, it is not a reliable predictive factor for malignant hyperthermia. A nontriggering anesthetic is recommended for these patients, including avoidance of depolarizing muscle relaxants and potent volatile agents. They should be observed for clinical evidence of malignant hyperthermia (e.g., hypercapnia, tachycardia, respiratory and metabolic acidosis, ventricular dysrhythmias, and an increase in body temperature). Should malignant hyperthermia be suspected, any volatile anesthetic agents should be discontinued and appropriate supportive measures initiated. Intravenous dantrolene should be administered.

In addition to the possible complications from administration of succinylcholine, these patients are also sensitive to the residual effects of nondepolarizing muscle relaxants. Paradoxically, when physical inactivity causes significant disuse atrophy of normal muscle groups, there can be resistance to nondepolarizing agents from the increased number of embryonic receptors present at the neuromuscular junction. Because of these uncertainties, a nerve stimulator should be used to guide doses of nondepolarizing muscle relaxants.

Respiratory Function in the Patient With Scoliosis (Idiopathic) Scoliosis has profound effects on the respiratory and cardiovascular systems (Fig. 13.10). In patients with untreated scoliosis, death usually occurs by age 45. Cor pulmonale or respiratory failure accounts for 60 percent of deaths.

The abnormal chest wall and mechanical disadvantage of intercostal muscles result in a restrictive pattern of pulmonary disease, which is manifested by decreases in total lung capacity and vital capacity. In one group of patients, the vital capacity was reduced to 60 percent of predicted, whereas the total lung capacity and functional residual capacity were 70 percent and 80 percent of predicted, respectively. The lung volumes and total compliance of the respiratory system are inversely related to the angle of curvature.[34] Patients with idiopathic scoliosis rarely show respiratory impairment with curves less than 65 degrees. However, curves of less than 30 degrees may be associated with severe respiratory compromise in patients with neuromuscular-associated scoliosis.[35] Tachypnea and small tidal volumes reduce the work of breathing but increase dead space ventilation and alveolar hypoventilation.[36] Alveolar development will be arrested if marked scoliosis is present before age 8.[34]

Vital capacity appears to be a reliable prognostic indicator of perioperative respiratory reserve. If vital capacity exceeds 70 percent of predicted, respiratory reserve should be adequate. Postoperative ventilation will most likely be required for patients with a vital capacity less than 40 percent of predicted.[23] Although the long-term effect of scoliosis repair is to halt the decline in respiratory function, pulmonary function acutely deteriorates immediately postoperatively. Vital capacity decreases by 40 percent and the alveolar-arterial oxygen gradient

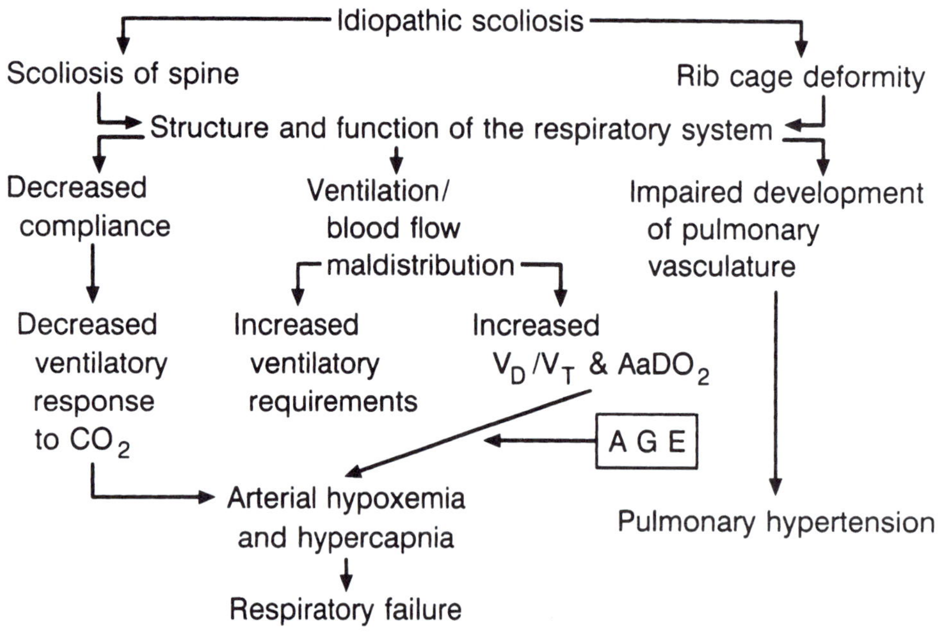

FIGURE 13.10 *Factors in idiopathic scoliosis that contribute to respiratory function abnormalities and failure. (From Kafer,[109] with permission).*

increases by 50 percent.[37] These changes may require 7 to 10 days to resolve. Significant improvement in respiratory function is unlikely and rarely exceeds a 10 percent increase in vital capacity 1 year postoperatively.[23] Occasionally, surgical correction may result in a permanent decrease in pulmonary function.[38]

The primary abnormality in gas exchange is ventilation/perfusion maldistribution, which contributes to hypoxemia. The most common arterial blood gas abnormality is a reduced oxygen tension (PaO_2) with a normal carbon dioxide tension ($PaCO_2$).[34] Deterioration of the mechanical properties of the lung results in further ventilation/perfusion maldistribution, increased ventilatory requirements, and eventually respiratory failure. Hypercapnia develops with increasing age as compensatory mechanisms fail. Prolonged hypoxia, hypercapnia, and pulmonary vascular constriction may result in irreversible pulmonary vascular changes and pulmonary hypertension.

In summary, the thoracic cage and vertebral deformities of scoliosis lead to reduced lung volumes, ventilation/perfusion abnormalities, reduced chest wall compliance, and increased pulmonary vascular resistance. The hypoxemia resulting from these functional abnormalities causes increased ventilatory requirements. Initially, these compensatory mechanisms are adequate, but the progression of skeletal deformities and age-associated deterioration in arterial blood gases eventually lead to hypercapnia, respiratory failure, and ultimately death.

Respiratory Function in Scoliosis Associated With Neuromuscular Disease In general, the prognosis of scoliosis caused by neuromuscular disease is worse than that of idiopathic scoliosis. The respiratory function of these patients is compromised not only by the skeletal abnormalities of scoliosis but also by abnormalities of the central respiratory control system, impairment of protective airway mechanisms, and loss of respiratory muscle function from denervation or myopathy. These patients frequently need postoperative ventilatory support.

Weakness of respiratory musculature produces a further decrease in total lung capacity and vital capacity and functional residual capacity. Reduction of inspiratory and expiratory forces leads to ineffective cough, atelectasis, and pneumonia. Involvement of the pharyngeal and laryngeal musculature may result in poor airway control mechanisms and aspiration. Bilateral diaphragmatic paralysis is associated with a reduction in vital capacity to 30 to 65 percent of predicted in the upright position and 15 to 30 percent of predicted in the supine position.[22]

Central nervous system involvement may cause an impaired ventilatory response to CO_2, impaired automatic control of ventilation, and infrequent sighs. Patients may also exhibit an increased sensitivity to muscle relaxants and narcotics and need to be observed carefully for signs of respiratory insufficiency.

Cardiovascular Function in Patients With Scoliosis Thoracic scoliosis may result in cardiac failure. At autopsy, these patients exhibit right ventricular hypertrophy and hypertensive pulmonary vascular changes. The skeletal deformities contribute to the elevated pulmonary vascular resistance in several ways. The rib cage compression of the lung impairs normal development of the pulmonary vascular bed and also causes alveolar collapse. This forces blood to flow through extra-alveolar vessels, which have increased resistance. Prolonged alveolar hypoxia due to hypoventilation and ventilation-perfusion mismatch eventually causes irreversible vasoconstriction and pulmonary hypertension.

Increases in right heart pressures and cor pulmonale are not only features of untreated progressive scoliosis. In a recent echocardiographic study of asymptomatic adolescents with idiopathic scoliosis, Primiano et al.[39] noted increases in pulmonary vascular resistance that were independent of severity of scoliosis. These results suggest that cardiopulmonary abnormalities develop parallel to, rather than in response to, the structural changes. ECG evidence of pulmonary hypertension and right atrial enlargement (P wave greater than 2.5 mm; R greater than S in V_1 and V_2) is late in appearance and unreliable. An echocardiogram appears to be a more sensitive preoperative screen than the ECG if findings or physical examination is suspicious. Echocardiography should also be performed in all patients with an apical murmur to determine the presence of mitral valve prolapse, which is present in 25 percent of patients with idiopathic scoliosis.

Children with congenital heart disease have an increased incidence of scoliosis. Scoliosis is especially associated with coarctation and cyanotic heart disease, suggesting a common embryonic insult. The high incidence of mitral valve prolapse in patients with scoliosis may signify a generalized soft tissue collagen defect.[40] Children with congenital cardiac anomalies may have complex patterns of blood flow that require special anesthetic considerations to maintain oxygenation and cardiac output. Even after definitive repair, residual cardiac disease may be present, and shunting may occur if hemodynamic and acid-base stability is not maintained. Patients with congenital cardiac disease and mitral valve prolapse are at increased risk for infective endocarditis and should receive antibiotic prophylaxis perioperatively.

Preoperative Assessment The primary aim of preoperative evaluation of patients with scoliosis is to detect the presence and extent of cardiac or pulmonary compromise. Respiratory reserve is assessed by exercise tolerance, vital capacity, and arterial blood gases. Despite the additional functional abnormalities in patients with coexisting neuromuscular disease (e.g., loss of abdominal muscle function and impairment of cough) the preoperative respiratory evaluation is the same as for any other respiratory disease. A history of exercise intolerance, hypercapnia, or respiratory failure indicates poor respiratory reserve and increases the likelihood of postoperative assisted ventilation. Polycythemia suggests the presence of chronic hypoxia. Pulmonary function testing should include measurement of the vital capacity (seated and supine), forced expiratory volume, and total lung capacity. Although the vital capacity is a reliable prognostic indicator of respiratory flow reserve, it does not assess brainstem regulation of respiration and the potential for postoperative respiratory insufficiency. The chest radiograph and physical examination will diagnose acute treatable pulmonary processes. Patients with severe pulmonary disease may require hospital admission preoperatively for chest physiotherapy, bronchodilators, and treatment of respiratory infections. A history of cardiac failure or a click murmur heard on examination should be further evaluated with an echocardiogram. Further cardiac studies are performed as indicated to optimize cardiovascular status preoperatively.

A brief neurologic examination is also performed at the time of the preoperative evaluation. At this time, it is important to discuss the wake-up test with the patient, emphasizing the role of the "wake-up" in diagnosing and minimizing neurologic sequelae. The patient is also reassured that little pain will be felt and that it will not be an unpleasant experience. Finally, cervical mobility and upper airway anatomy are evaluated to discover any potential airway or positioning difficulties and the need for fiberoptic intubation.

Patients should also be encouraged to participate in preoperative autologous blood donation. Collection is typically initiated 4 weeks preoperatively, allowing 4 to 7 days between donations. Usually four or more units of blood can be collected over this period of time and stored as a liquid at 4°C. A donation period greater than 4 weeks can be used for patients with greater transfusion requirements (e.g., a combined AP fusion) or for those whose cardiac status or hemoglobin level would not tolerate short intervals between blood donations. Blood collected over a more prolonged period must be stored as frozen red blood cells until surgery. Because frozen red blood cells must be transfused within 24 hours of thawing, it is important to thaw only those units that will be needed intraoperatively.

Autologous blood donation may not be feasible in young children, patients in poor overall medical condition, or those who weigh less than 100 lb. In these situations, directed donors may be available from the family members who have a blood type compatible with the patient. Directed donation units are screened for hepatitis and human immunodeficiency virus in the same manner as other homologous blood. The use of directed donation units has increased because of patient demand; however, these units have not proved to have a lower infectious risk than that of the general donor population.

Surgical Approach and Positioning

POSTERIOR APPROACH. Posterior spinal fusion is the most commonly used procedure to halt progression of spinal curvature when conservative measures have failed. Instrumentation developed by Harrington in the 1960s provides internal distraction and stability; however, prolonged casting for 6 to 18 months after surgery may be required to achieve spinal fusion.[41] Luque[42] introduced segmental spinal instrumentation, a technique that distributes correctional forces throughout the instrumented area of the spine by wiring each vertebrae in the scoliotic curve. This results in better correction of the curvature, reduced bone and implant failure, and earlier mobilization (often eliminating the need for postoperative casts or other orthopedic appliances).[43] However, the increased instrumentation associated with sublaminar segmental wire placement produces longer operative times, increased blood loss, and perhaps a higher incidence of neurologic sequelae (5 to 7 percent) compared with conventional Harrington instrumentation (1 to 2 percent). Modifications of surgical technique and experience have steadily decreased this complication.[44] The introduction of a hook or screw and rod construct by Cotrel and Dubousset (CD system) in 1984 allowed for multilevel corrective forces on the rods while reducing the risk of spinal cord injury associated with sublaminar wiring.[45] The incidence of major neurologic deficits after CD instrumentation is only 0.2 percent. Further development of the principles of CD instrumentation resulted in the ISOLA and TSRH systems and pedicle screw fixation. These systems allow more spinal flexibility and stability and improve fusion rates compared with conventional (Harrington and Luque) devices.[46] After instrumentation is completed, bone chips from the posterior iliac crest or elsewhere are placed longitudinally over the prepared site of fusion.

Optimal positioning during spine surgery is influenced by the necessity of providing good operating conditions (including a bloodless operating field) with the minimal complications. Because bleeding into the surgical incision is a significant concern, a variety of specifically designed operating tables has been constructed to decrease pressure on the abdomen. Typically, the patient is supported by chest rolls or other supports to leave the abdomen free. This allows diaphragmatic excursions and reduces paravertebral venous congestion and epidural bleeding. The Tower table, Jackson table, and Relton-Hall frame are examples of pedestal-type systems that support the patient's weight at the chest and iliac crest.

In correct prone positioning for thoracolumbar spine surgery, the head is turned to the side or positioned midline on a foam/gel head rest, the neck is slightly flexed, and the arms are anteriorly flexed and abducted to reduce tension on the brachial plexus (Fig. 13.11). If only one arm is abducted, the head should be laterally rotated toward the abducted arm to prevent stretch injury to the brachial plexus. Placement of extra padding beneath the elbow may protect the ulnar nerve from compression injury. Alternatively, both arms may be tucked alongside the patient's body. However, care must be taken to ensure usual anatomic position and also patency of indwelling arterial and venous catheters.

Because rotation of the neck in patients with cervical spondylosis may alter cerebrovertebral circulation and compromise the spinal cord, patients should be evaluated for neck pain or neurologic symptoms with neck rotation preoperatively.[47] Breasts should be positioned medial to the chest rolls to avoid pressure injury. The nipples are especially sensitive to this type of injury. The dependent ear and eye should be checked frequently during surgery to avoid injury and ischemia. Pressure on the globe can result in retinal damage, especially in patients with glaucoma. Eyes should be taped closed to avoid corneal abrasion, which occurs in the dependent eye with a frequency of 0.17 percent.[48] Use of the ophthalmic lubricants has no documented effect on the incidence of corneal abrasion. Necrosis of the dependent ear cartilage may occur if the pinna is doubled back on itself.

ANTERIOR APPROACH. The anterior approach for correction of kyphosis and scoliosis has gained

FIGURE 13.11 *Prone position. The head is turned with the dependent ear and eye protected from pressure. Chest rolls are in place, the arms are brought forward without hyperextension, and the knees are flexed. (By permission of Mayo Clinic.)*

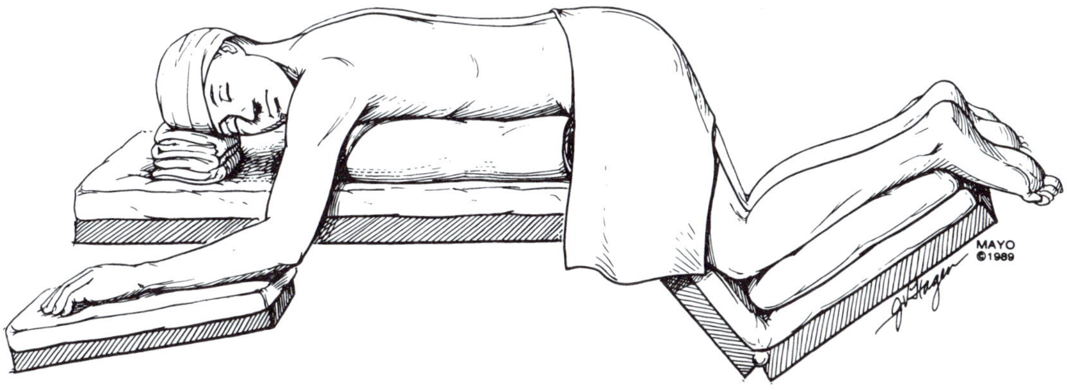

popularity over the past 10 years. Anteriorly placed instrumentation such as the Dwyer screw and cable apparatus is used when posterior elements of the spine are deficient or when there is a significant degree of lordosis requiring correction. This technique offers the advantage of a limited fusion area, a compression fusion, and less blood loss compared with the Harrington apparatus. A major disadvantage to the Dwyer apparatus is the risk of damage to the spinal cord during vertebral body screw placement, particularly in the thoracic spine, because of the relatively small size of the vertebral bodies and the large number of segmental spinal arteries that require ligation.[29] Fusion is usually accomplished with bank bone rather than an autologous source.

The anterior approach to the spine is achieved with the patient in the lateral position, usually with the convexity of the curve uppermost, although some surgeons always prefer to approach the thoracolumbar region from the left regardless of the convexity to avoid the liver and the inferior vena cava.[29] The vertebrae in the lumbar region can be exposed by a single flank incision, whereas those in the lower thoracic and lumbar area may be visualized by removing the tenth rib and dividing the diaphragm to enter the abdominal cavity. This incision will allow exposure from T9 to the pelvis. Removal of the sixth rib in addition to the tenth will increase upper thoracic exposure.[49] Wound closure requires pleural repair and reattachment of the diaphragm. The thoracoabdominal approach for anterior fusion may be associated with more postoperative respiratory insufficiency than conventional posterior fusion due to lung and diaphragmatic manipulation during scoliosis correction. Use of a double lumen endotracheal tube with collapse of the lung on the operative side will reduce the amount of lung retraction needed for exposure of the spine and decrease operative time, particularly if the operative site is above T_8. Surgery below T_8 is less likely to be aided significantly by double lumen tube placement.

COMBINED ANTERIOR AND POSTERIOR FUSION. Patients with unstable spines or those with severe primary curvatures may require both anterior and posterior instrumentation and/or fusion. Frequently, the anterior procedure is accomplished first and is followed by secondary posterior instrumentation and fusion 1 to 2 weeks later. This approach allows slightly greater distractive forces to be applied posteriorly, with less risk of damage to the spinal cord because the spine has been partially stabilized and corrected by the initial anterior procedure.[49] Anterior fusion followed by immediate posterior fusion is occasionally performed when the area to be fused is small and the primary curvature is below the diaphragm and when the patient is not at high medical risk for the procedure.

Anesthetic Management Anesthetic considerations in orthopedic surgery for scoliosis include management of a patient in the prone position, hypothermia secondary to a long procedure with an extensive exposed area, and replacement of blood and fluid losses, which may be extensive. Recently, attention has been focused on the maintenance of spinal cord integrity, the prevention and treatment of VAE, and reduction of blood loss through hypotensive anesthetic techniques.

Usual monitors include ECG, blood pressure cuff, pulse oximeter, core temperature probe, and esophageal stethoscope for monitoring breath and heart sounds. An indwelling urinary catheter is used to monitor urine output, and a nasogastric tube is placed to decompress the stomach until resolution of perioperative ileus. A capnograph is useful for assessing adequacy of ventilation as well as detecting air embolus and malignant hyperthermia. Two large-bore intravenous catheters are placed. The radial artery is cannulated for direct blood pressure measurement and assessment of blood gases. A CVP catheter is helpful in evaluating blood and fluid management and can be used to aspirate air should VAE occur. Patients with evidence of pulmonary hypertension or severe coexistent cardiovascular or pulmonary disease may require a pulmonary artery catheter, measurement of pulmonary artery and wedge pressures, and determination of serial cardiac outputs. Because the surgical wound is higher than the heart, a precordial Doppler may be used to detect VAE.

Minimal premedication is administered if the wake-up test will be used. Anesthesia is induced with thiopental (5 mg/kg), fentanyl (2 μg/kg), and pancuronium (0.1 mg/kg) unless intubation difficulties are anticipated. In some cases, fiberoptic intubation is required.

After induction and establishment of vascular access are completed, the patient is positioned for surgery. The prone position is used for the posterior approach. Pressure points should be carefully padded. A special orthopedic frame can be used to free the chest and abdomen. Increased thoracic pressure hinders effective ventilation, and elevated abdominal pressure causes engorgement of the vertebral venous plexus and excessive bleeding. Double lumen endotracheal tubes (if above T8) and lateral or semilateral positioning are used when the spine is approached anteriorly. Exposed body surfaces are wrapped or a Bair hugger (a forced-air warming device) is applied to minimize heat loss. Other methods to maintain normothermia include humidifying inhaled gases and heating intravenous fluids.

A nitrous oxide–narcotic–muscle relaxant technique supplemented as necessary by volatile anesthetics is most commonly used for maintenance of anesthesia. The use of low concentrations of inhalational anesthetics will help maintain normotension, reduce total narcotic requirements, and still allow satisfactory interpretation of SSEPs. Narcotics may be administered by either bolus or continuous infusion. A loading dose of fentanyl 2.5 μg/kg followed by an infusion of 1.5 to 2.5 μg/kg/hr or intermittent boluses of 50 to 100 μg every 20 to 30 minutes will usually provide adequate analgesia. Alternatively, an initial dose of morphine 250 μg/kg may be injected followed by 5 to 10-mg boluses every 30 to 40 minutes or a continuous infusion of 150 to 250 μg/kg/h. Continuous infusion may reduce total narcotic requirement by more than 50 percent and results in a smoother and more rapidly achievable wake-up test.[50] Excessive narcotic administration, which is more likely to occur with the intermittent bolus technique, may lead to prolonged ventilatory support and delay in postoperative neurologic evaluation. An additional advantage of the continuous narcotic infusion technique is the elimination of bolus-induced variations in SSEPs, making it easier to interpret SSEP changes that occur during surgical manipulation. Neuromuscular blockade is monitored with a nerve stimulator, preferably at the wrist. Electrodes placed for EMG monitoring can also be used to monitor twitch height. Supplemental doses of muscle relaxants are given based on twitch monitoring to prevent overdosage and enable reversal during the wake-up test.

Blood Loss Most blood losses in spinal instrumentation and fusion occur with decortication, are proportional to the number of vertebral levels decorticated, and usually necessitates perioperative transfusions. Complications associated with homologous blood transfusions include acquired immunodeficiency syndrome, hepatitis, transfusion reactions, and isoimmunization. The use of autologous blood reduces these risks; the use of preoperative autologous donations has been previously discussed. Blood loss and transfusion requirements may also be reduced through the use of positioning, intraoperative blood salvage, induced hypotension, and intraoperative hemodilution, although reported results are inconsistent.[50–53]

Patient positioning should minimize epidural venous engorgement by freeing the abdomen. Positive end-expiratory pressure is avoided to promote venous return. Subcutaneous infiltration of 1:500,000 epinephrine before skin incision may also decrease blood loss. Preoperative donation of autologous blood or infusion of a large volume of crystalloid before surgical incision to reduce the hematocrit to 25 to 28 percent decreases blood viscosity and enhances organ blood flow. Normovolemic hemodilution combined with induced hypotension and autotransfusion can decrease or eliminate the need for homologous transfusion.[52]

Moderate induced hypotension (reduction of systolic 20 mmHg from baseline or lowering MAP to 65 mmHg in the normotensive patient) has been shown to decrease blood loss, reduce transfusion requirements by 50 percent, and shorten operating times.[52,54] However, induced hypotension is not without risk and has also been reported to cause cord ischemia and neurologic deficit.[55,56] Factors associated with increased risk of spinal cord damage include preoperative hypertension, hypocapnia, intraoperative MAP less than 60 mmHg, rapid decrease in blood pressure, and anemia.[57] Patients with severe deformity, congenital scoliosis, or kyphosis may have an abnormal pattern of spinal cord blood supply, which is more easily compromised during surgical distraction or compression. The purported benefits of deliberate hypotension must be weighed against the potential risk of acute neurologic complications.

The various agents used to induce hypotension in scoliosis surgery include trimethaphan, nitroglycerine, sodium nitroprusside, halothane, enflurane, and isoflurane.[58] The volatile agents provide anesthesia as well as hypotension. Enflurane and isoflurane have less myocardial depressant effects, decrease systemic vascular resistance to a greater extent, and are less arrhythmogenic than halothane.[59] However, all volatile anesthetics produce a dose-dependent deterioration of SSEP waveforms. Sodium nitroprusside produces a reliable decrease in blood pressure and at least initially increases spinal cord blood flow but may be associated with tolerance, tachyphylaxis, toxicity, and rebound hypertension.[60] Nitroglycerin maintains or increases spinal cord blood flow but may be ineffective in achieving target blood pressure.[59,61] Pretreatment with a β-blocker, calcium channel blocker, or an angiotensin-converting enzyme inhibitor can prevent rebound hypertension and reflex tachycardia and reduce dose requirements and toxicity for intravenous hypotensive agents.[62–64]

Hypotension should be induced before surgical incision to prevent hemodilution and excess fluid administration. Blood pressure is slowly decreased to achieve a MAP of 60 to 70 mmHg or systolic blood pressure 20 to 30 mmHg less than preoperative systolic values.[52,58] On completion of the surgical procedure, blood pressure is allowed to gradually recover to prevent reactionary hemorrhage.

Spinal Cord Monitoring Paraplegia is one of the most feared complications of spinal surgery. In a series of 33,250 patients compiled by the Scoliosis Research Society for 1971 to 1979, the incidence of neurologic injuries was 1.2 percent, with partial or complete paraplegia occurring in one-half of these.[65] Only a few spinal cord injuries are the result of direct surgical trauma. Most neurologic damage is believed to be due to distraction of the spinal cord by instrumentation with disruption of arterial blood supply. Patients with severe deformity, congenital scoliosis, kyphosis (especially), or preoperative neurologic deficit are at increased risk for spinal cord injury during scoliosis surgery. When patients awaken paraplegic, neurologic recovery is unlikely; however, immediate removal of instrumentation will improve prognosis. It is therefore essential that any intraoperative compromise of spinal cord function be detected as early as possible and reversed immediately. The two methods developed to accomplish this are the wake-up test and neurophysiologic monitoring.

The wake-up test, first described by Vauzelle et al.,[66] consists of the intraoperative awakening of patients after completion of spinal instrumentation. The patients are informed of this procedure preoperatively and reassured that they will feel minimal pain and will be quickly reanesthetized after they have moved their hands and feet. Ideally, the surgeon should notify the anesthesiologist 30 to 45 minutes in advance so that bolus of muscle relaxant and narcotic can be avoided immediately before awakening the patient. During this period, the volatile anesthetic is discontinued, and the patient is allowed to gradually awaken. Narcotic infusion may be continued until 5 minutes before wake-up.[50] Awakening is accomplished by withdrawing the nitrous oxide and ventilating the patient by hand. Sealing the wound with wet packs has also been advocated to minimize the occurrence of VAE with spontaneous deep inspiration.[65] No attempt is made to fully reverse muscle relaxation, ideally leaving the patient partially paralyzed but able to make limited but detectable movements of the hands and feet. The patient is addressed by first name and is asked to move both hands and, after a positive response, both feet. Patients will usually respond within 5 minutes.[50,65,67] If the patient moves neither hands nor feet, naloxone is administered in 20-μg increments until proper patient response. Narcotic antagonists are rarely required with continuous narcotic infusion; however, narcotics given as boluses frequently require reversal at time of awakening.[50] If there is satisfactory movement of the hands but not the feet, nitrous oxide is reinstituted, the distraction on the rod is released one notch, and the wake-up test repeated. If movement still does not occur, other causes of paraplegia such as hematoma must be considered. Increasing the blood pressure and blood volume may be attempted to increase spinal cord perfusion. Throughout the test, the patient is continuously reassured, and on satisfactory completion of the test, administration of nitrous oxide is resumed and diazepam 0.15 mg/kg administered. Surgical manipulation should recommence only when the patient no longer responds to commands. Recall of the event occurs in 0 to 20 percent of patients and is only rarely viewed as unpleasant.[50,65]

To date, there has been one reported case[67a] and one case experienced by one of us (M.E.M.) in which the patient awakened with a neurologic deficit that was not predicted by the intraoperative wake-up test. In the latter case, changes in intraoperative SSEPs occurring at an unexpected time during surgery provoked the wake-up test which failed to detect a neurologic deficit. This patient was paraplegic postoperatively. Diaz and Lackhart[68] also reported a case involving a 16-year-old boy with presumed idiopathic scoliosis who had a negative wake-up test intraoperatively and normal motor function immediately postoperatively. The patient developed a flaccid quadriplegia over the next 12 hours from a previously undiagnosed syrinx, which had been extended by the scoliosis correction. These two cases cannot be truly called a false-negative wake-up test because the patient was neurologically intact at the time of the test. Subsequent deterioration of neural function cannot be detected by a test that assesses function only at the time it is applied. However, in the vast majority of cases, intraoperative awakening does predict postoperative function and has proved very valuable in the early recognition of neurologic deficits in patients undergoing surgical correction of scoliosis. This technique does not require complex electrical equipment or technical expertise for interpretation. Certain hazards of the wake-up test do exist and include recall, pain, air embolism, rod dislocation, and accidental extubation or removal of intravenous and arterial lines. In addition, the wake-up test requires patient cooperation and may be difficult to perform on young children or mentally challenged individuals.

An adjunct or alternative to the wake-up test is neurophysiologic monitoring including SSEPs, MEPs, and EMG. Monitoring of SSEPs and EMG during spinal surgery is well established.

Acute alterations in SSEP amplitude or latency signify spinal cord compromise and may be the result of direct trauma, ischemia, compression, or hematoma. A deepening of the anesthetic can also cause similar changes and must be ruled out as the source. Monitoring of the cervical response, which is resistant to changes in anesthetic technique, should help with this problem. Should changes occur, it is recommended that surgery stop, blood pressure be returned to normal or 20 percent above normal, and volatile agents decreased or discontinued.[55] Arterial blood gases may be drawn to rule out a metabolic derangement. If the waveform does not return to normal, the surgeon should release distraction on the cord. A wake-up test may be performed to corroborate SSEP changes that do not make clinical sense or occur at unexpected times. If the changes occur at a time when distraction is applied, the wake-up test is not needed. To date, no studies comparing the sensitivity of intraoperative wake-up with SSEP monitoring have been conducted. No intraoperative monitor has ever been shown to be 100 percent reliable, and SSEP monitoring is no exception. Postoperative paraplegia has been reported during spine surgery when SSEP waveforms were preserved intraoperatively (see Ch. 4).

Other Considerations

VENOUS AIR EMBOLISM. Several catastrophic events may occur during spine surgery. The large amount of exposed bone and the elevated location of the surgical incision relative to the cardiac level predispose to VAE. The actual incidence of VAE in major spine surgery is unknown, in part because complete monitoring for VAE, including a precordial Doppler, is not routinely performed in these patients. Only two cases of massive VAE during spine fusion had been described before 1991.[70,71] At that time, Albin et al.[72] presented three cases of VAE (two of which were fatal) that occurred in the prone position during simple lumbar laminectomy. Subsequent cases suggest that the incidence of VAE during spine surgery is increasing.[73,74] The presenting sign is often unexplained hypotension. A decrease in end-tidal carbon dioxide and an increase in end-tidal nitrogen may be noted on mass spectrometry. Aspiration of the CVP catheter inconsistently reveals air, although 15 ml of air was aspirated on one occasion.

The recent increase in reported cases of VAE during spine surgery may reflect the increased use of orthopaedic frames such as the Tower table, four-poster frame, and Wilson frame. These devices free the patient's abdomen from compression in the prone position and help to reduce engorgement of the venous plexuses and hence decrease bleeding. The resultant decrease in caval pressure increases the gravitational gradient and places the patient at risk for VAE. Hypovolemia may further enhance the risk of VAE. The anesthesiologist, therefore, should be aware of the possibilities of VAE because prompt diagnosis and treatment will increase patient survival. Mass spectrometry or capnography is a noninvasive and sensitive monitor and should be part of routine monitoring during these cases. In the presence of chest rolls or bolsters, a Doppler probe may be cushioned with foam rubber and taped in place. Optimal CVP catheter position for aspiration of VAE in these patients remains controversial. In the prone head-down position, the ideal location may be at the inferior vena cava–right atrial junction. Should VAE be suspected, the wound should be packed with saline, nitrous oxide discontinued, and vasopressors administered. Massive embolism may necessitate turning the patient supine and initiating cardiopulmonary resuscitation.

VASCULAR TRAUMA. Another rare complication during spine surgery is trauma to the aorta, vena cava, or iliac vessels. Unexplained hypotension or signs of hypovolemia without obvious blood loss should alert the anesthesiologist to this possibility.[75] In addition, hemothorax or pneumothorax manifested by hypoxia or a change in pulmonary compliance may occur during procedures involving the thoracic spine.

ISCHEMIC OPTIC NEUROPATHY. Postoperative blindness, particularly after cardiopulmonary bypass, is well established in the ophthalmology literature. In several large series, the incidence varies from 0.1 to 1 percent.[76] Previous reports of altered vision after spinal surgery in the prone position have been attributed to excessive pressure applied to the globe from improper positioning, resulting in occlusion of the central retinal artery.[77] Until recently, infarction of the optic nerve (ischemic optic neuropathy) had not been reported as a complication of major spinal surgery. However, five cases of ischemic optic neuropathy after spinal fusion or multilevel laminectomy have been reported since 1994.[78,79] All patients complained of visual loss in one or both eyes that had been diagnosed within days of spine surgery. The amount of vision loss ranged from decreased visual acuity or visual field defect to no light perception. Although visual acuity usually improved with time, field defects persisted.

Patient age ranged from 13 to 65 years, and all had undergone prolonged spine surgery, during which the blood pressure was deliberately maintained between 85 and 100 mmHg systolic and 45 to 65 mmHg diastolic. The lowest recorded intraoperative hemoglobin levels ranged from 7.1 to 11.7 g/dl. Arteriosclerotic risk factors such as hypertension, diabetes, and coronary artery disease were present in three cases. However, intraoperative anemia (which was not corrected because of the presumed infectious risk of homologous transfusion) and deliberate hypotension were present in all patients. This combination of risk factors was the most significant contributor to postoperative vision loss.

The clinical characteristics of ischemic optic

neuropathy after spine surgery is similar to those reported after other surgical procedures (cardiopulmonary bypass, radical neck dissection, pulmonary resection), complicated by hypotension or anemia.[79] The recent reporting of ischemic optic neuropathy after major spine surgery may be a result of changes in transfusion practice. Current guidelines for transfusion of red blood cells suggested by the American Association of Blood Banks and the National Institutes of Health are hemoglobin levels of 8 g/dl and 7 g/dl, respectively. However, these cases suggest that although anemia alone may not result in ischemic optic neuropathy, an episode of hypotension in an already anemic patient may predispose the patient to postoperative blindness, and the decision to withhold transfusion in the presence of deliberate hypotension must be given careful consideration in this patient population.

Postoperative Care Most posterior spinal fusion patients can be extubated immediately after the operation if preoperative vital capacity values were acceptable. Residual narcotic or muscle relaxant may lead to hypoventilation or apnea, especially in patients with an associated neuromuscular disease. Postoperative pneumothorax may be present. Aggressive postoperative pulmonary care, including incentive spirometry, is necessary to avoid atelectasis and pneumonia.

Continued hemorrhage is another concern in the postoperative period. Careful monitoring of systemic and central venous pressures, urine output, and wound drainage is essential. Neurologic status must also be monitored closely for deterioration.

Postoperative pain management is discussed in detail in Chapter 20. However, the site and magnitude of the surgical procedure necessitate aggressive management of postoperative analgesia in patients undergoing major spine surgery. Adequate analgesia facilitates aggressive respiratory care and early ambulation, important factors in decreasing patient morbidity and improving perioperative outcome. Historically, postoperative pain has been managed with intramuscular and, more recently, intravenous opioids. Intravenous opioids may be delivered as a continuous infusion or as intermittent boluses. Continuous infusions do not account for alterations in pain intensity (e.g., dressing changes or ambulation), whereas intermittent boluses may be administered at inadequate doses, at protracted intervals, resulting in break-through pain. However, patients receiving continuous opioid infusions should be carefully monitored for respiratory depression. Because these patients are typically monitored in an intensive care setting, a continuous opioid infusion with patient-controlled intermittent opioid boluses is an ideal method of delivering postoperative analgesia.

Opioids may also be administered intrathecally or epidurally. Preservative-free morphine may be injected intrathecally, under direct vision, by the surgeon. Ross et al.[80] reported superior analgesia and reduced hospital stays in lumbar spine surgical patients who received 0.25 mg or 0.5 mg intrathecal morphine, compared with a control group that received parenteral opioids.

A continuous epidural infusion is another technique for delivering analgesia after spine surgery. Epidural opioids (and local anesthetics) may be infused through an indwelling catheter placed in the epidural space before surgical closure. Joshi et al.[81] compared epidural fentanyl infusion (2 μg/ml, 4 to 10 ml/hr) with patient-controlled intravenous morphine in the management of postoperative pain after lumbar laminectomy. The continuous epidural infusion of fentanyl provided superior analgesia with less somnolence compared with intravenous patient-controlled morphine.[81] Epidural analgesia has several advantages compared with intrathecal administration: the dura is not breached and the presence of an indwelling catheter allows continuous, titratable, and prolonged pain relief.

In summary, anesthetic management of scoliotic patients involves a thorough preoperative evaluation of the patient's cardiac, pulmonary, and neurologic function. Intraoperative attention to temperature control, blood loss, positioning, and spinal cord integrity is essential. Continued attention to pulmonary status, neurologic function, blood loss, and pain management define postoperative concerns.

ANTERIOR THORACIC AND LUMBAR PROCEDURES Both the thoracic and lumbar spine may be approached anteriorly. The most common indications for anterior approaches are discectomy and corpectomy. As noted above, during scoliosis surgery, an anterior approach to discectomy and release of ligaments may allow greater correction in patients with severe curves and (especially) kyphosis.

Preoperative evaluation should be directed at two major areas. First, the patient's pulmonary function should be carefully evaluated. Patients without history or physical findings consistent with lung disease and a normal exercise tolerance need not be evaluated further. Patients with poor exercise tolerance and/or a significant history of lung disease should be evaluated in the same fashion as a patient undergoing a thoracic or upper abdominal procedure. The anterior approach to the thoracic spine may be associated with significant lung retraction or require the use of a double lumen tube. In a patient with poor lung reserve, this may result in significant pulmonary morbidity postoperatively and require prolonged intubation. If possible, the posterior or lateral extracavitary approach (see below), which is less traumatic to the lung, should be used in these cases.

Depending on the pathology, the spine may be approached via either a right or left thoracotomy. For higher lesions, a right thoracotomy is most common, whereas for lower thoracic and lumbar lesions, a left thoracotomy is most commonly used. The patient is positioned in the lateral decubitus position with an upper thoracic roll placed to prevent dependent brachial plexus stretching. The head is positioned in a neutral position, taking special care to avoid lateral bending of the cervical spine. Lateral bending of the neck, particularly toward the dependent shoulder, may result in stretching of the nondependent brachial plexus, especially if the shoulders are taped to facilitate positioning. A double lumen endotracheal tube is extremely helpful to minimize retraction on the lung if the lesion is located above T10. For lesions in the lower thoracic (below T10) and lumbar spine, the patient is positioned as for a nephrectomy, and a retroperitoneal approach to the spine is used.

Anterior Discectomy Most thoracic disc herniations are managed conservatively. However, in the case in which the patient develops myelopathy, progressive neurologic deterioration is common[82] and surgery is indicated. Intractable radicular pain is also a relative indication for surgery. An anterior approach is indicated for disc herniations below T_4 directly anterior or anterolateral to the spinal cord. A traditional posterior transpedicular approach is effective for lateral herniations. The use of a double lumen tube will substantially facilitate surgical exposure if the disc herniation is above T9. An intra-arterial catheter is helpful for blood gas sampling. Otherwise, invasive monitoring is generally not indicated. These operations are not commonly associated with significant blood loss, and extubation is the rule, except in patients with significant pulmonary disease or when significant intravenous fluids are needed for blood loss. Removal of a thoracic disc does not usually produce instability, and posterior stabilization is rarely necessary.

Anterior Corpectomy When the vertebral body itself or osteophytes must be removed to relieve nerve root or spinal cord compression (caused either by degenerative or metastatic disease or by trauma), corpectomy is indicated. Corpectomy is not possible from a simple posterior approach, and prior to the development of the lateral extracavitary approach, corpectomy was always approached via thoracotomy or via a flank incision (in the case of lumbar vertebrae). Considerations are identical to those for disc removal, except that blood loss may be more significant, particularly in the case of metastatic malignant disease. In these cases, massive blood loss is possible, and major intravenous access is mandatory. We generally use at least two 14-gauge peripheral intravenous lines and a 7- to 9-Fr introducer placed in a central or peripheral (generally antecubital). Removal of the vertebral body *will* most often cause instability of the thoracic or lumbar spine, and posterior stabilization using one of the methods described in the section on scoliosis will be required either in the same surgical setting or subsequently. Because surgical trauma is very significant, even patients with normal lungs may not be able to be extubated immediately postoperatively.

LATERAL EXTRACAVITARY PROCEDURES As discussed above, significant anterior procedures such as corpectomy, multilevel discectomies, or procedures in the lumbar region usually require subsequent posterior stabilization. This stabilization may be done on the same day or at a later time. If the stabilization is done on the same day, the patient's position must be changed from lateral to prone. As with any position change, care must be taken to prevent dislodgment of lines or the endotracheal tube. In addition, if a double lumen tube was used, movement of the patient to the prone position could be associated with trauma to the carina. In addition, ventilation of the patient (particularly an obese patient) in the prone position may be difficult with a double lumen tube. If there has not been significant blood loss or intravenous fluid administration during the first part of the operation, one of us (M.E.M.) recommends changing the endotracheal tube to a large-diameter single lumen tube to facilitate ventilation of the prone patient. If the stabilization is done at a later time, the patient must be kept immobile to prevent neurologic injury. This immobilization may be associated with complications such as pneumonia, deep venous thrombophlebitis, or pulmonary embolus. Thus, an approach that would enable the entire operation to be done in one sitting without changing the patient's position would be distinctly advantageous.

The lateral extracavitary approach involves the exposure and resection of the proximal portion of at least two consecutive ribs around the level of the pathology (Fig. 13.12, arrow). The lung is retracted away from the spine, giving excellent exposure to the operative side of the spine including the entire vertebral body and the space anterior to the vertebral body (Fig. 13.12). Only mild-to-moderate retraction is needed, and the surgery is possible with a single lumen tube and conventional ventilation. One of us (M.E.M.) has tried several alternative approaches to ventilation including a double lumen tube with one-lung ventilation, a bronchial blocker with one-lung ventilation, and jet ventilation. In an unpublished study at the University of Florida, use of jet ventilation was associated with the least pulmonary morbidity as judged by length of time to extubation after surgery. The study involved only a few patients, however (Fessler RF and Pashayan AG: unpublished data). Jet ventilation has the advantage that it uses an endotracheal tube that may be left in place postoperatively as needed and used with conventional positive pressure ventilation. Once jet ventilation has begun, the lung on the operative side may be gently retracted and does not move significantly or impair the surgeon's exposure. With jet ventilation, it is very difficult to deliver an adequate inhalation anesthetic dose, and total intravenous anesthesia is preferable. One of us (M.E.M.) finds total intravenous anesthesia using propofol (100 to 150 μg/kg/min) and sufentanil (0.1 to 0.2 μg/kg/hr) to be very effective for this purpose.

To illustrate the advantages of this technique, resection of a tumor of the vertebral body will be used as an example. After resection of the rib and retraction of the lung, the tumor involving the vertebral body is readily seen (Fig. 13.13). After resection of the tumor, the cavity with surrounding anterior and posterior longitudinal ligaments is seen (Fig. 13.14). Anterior stabilization with pins and methylmethacrylate is then performed (Fig. 13.15), followed by posterior stabilization (Fig. 13.16), all through the same incision in the same operation. This procedure may also be used in the lumbar spine. When this technique can be used, it provides reduced operative time and less surgical trauma for the patient.

Preoperative anesthetic considerations are identical to those for anterior thoracic and lumbar procedures. Although experience with this procedure is insufficient to prove this statement,

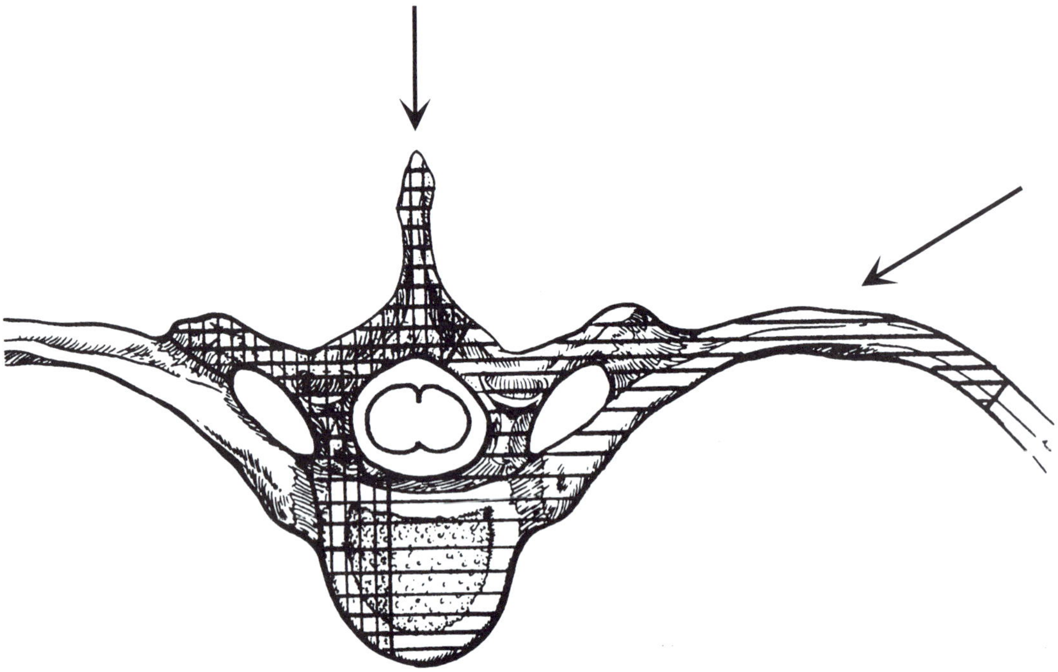

FIGURE 13.12 *Lateral extracavitary approach. The proximal portion of at least two adjacent ribs (arrow) is resected. The lung is then retracted giving excellent exposure to the vertebral body as well as the remainder of the vertebra (shaded areas). (From Fessler et al.,[110] with permission.)*

it is very likely that patients with significant pulmonary disease will tolerate this procedure better than anterior followed by posterior spinal fusions. Major intravenous access is necessary, especially in patients with malignant tumors. Intra-arterial monitoring facilitates blood gas analysis and the use of induced hypotension, when appropriate. Extubation is based on usual criteria and is more likely to be successful than following a combined anteroposterior approach.

POSTERIOR PROCEDURES Lower thoracic and lumbar microdiscectomies are the most commonly performed spine operations. The patient is placed in the prone position on chest rolls or, more commonly, the Wilson frame or equivalent. A small incision is made and the spine exposed. Through a small hemilaminotomy, the disc is approached and excised through a microoperative approach. The operations is not associated with significant blood loss, and operative trauma is usually minimal. One exception to this should be known to all anesthesiologists. It is possible for the surgeon to violate major intra-abdominal vessels if the anterior longitudinal ligament is penetrated during removal of the disc. The surgeon may not be aware of the bleeding because the ligament may immediately seal itself, and all bleeding would be into the retroperitoneal space. At lower levels, the iliac vessels are most commonly involved, but at higher levels (low thoracic, high lumbar), the aorta itself may be compromised. Treatment is immediately laparotomy and repair of the lacerated artery/vein. If the diagnosis is not considered promptly, prognosis is very poor, with most patients dying on the operating table. This diagnosis should always be considered when unexpected profound hypotension occurs during lower thoracic/lumbar disc surgery.[83–85]

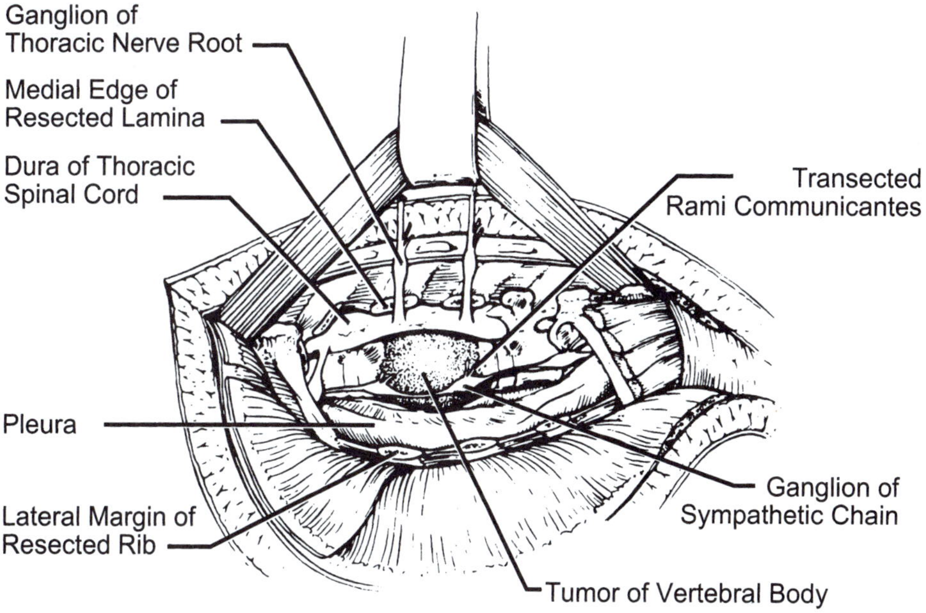

FIGURE 13.13 *Lateral extracavitary approach. After lung retraction, note excellent view of the vertebral body and associated tumor. (From Fessler et al.,*[110] *with permission.)*

FIGURE 13.14 *Lateral extracavitary approach. The tumor is now resected, giving a full view of the spinal cord and anterior and posterior longitudinal ligaments. (From Fossler et al.,*[110] *with permission.)*

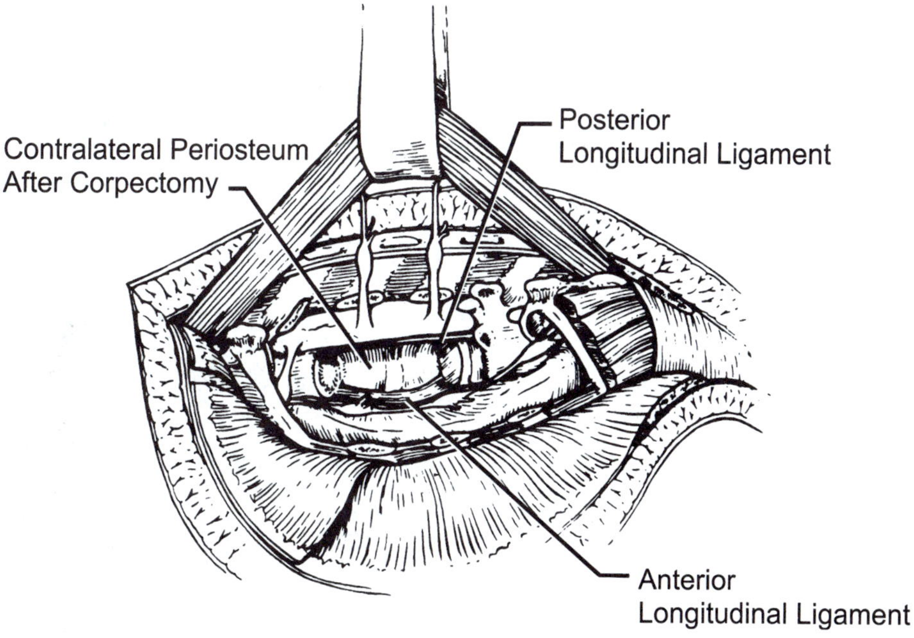

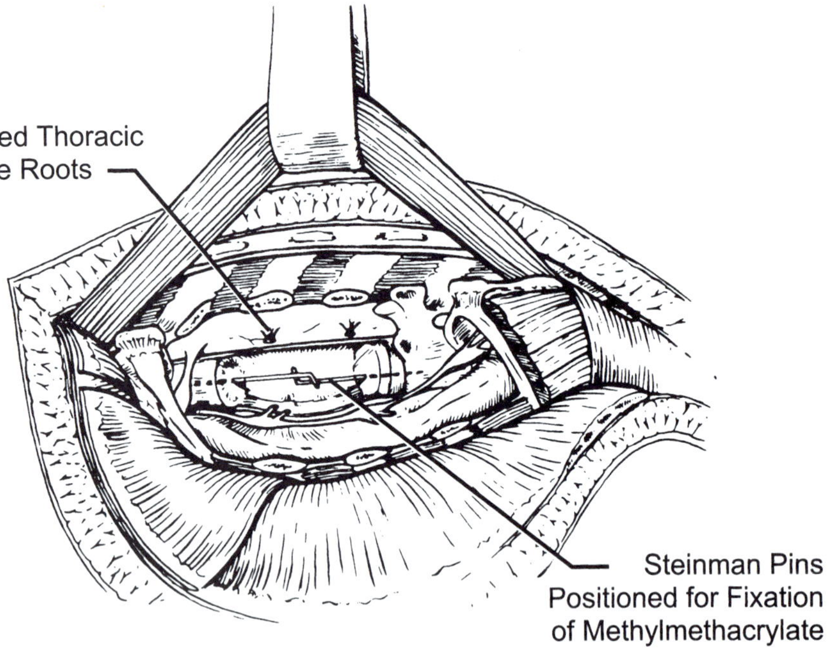

FIGURE 13.15 *Lateral extracavitary approach. Anterior stabilization may then be easily accomplished by using pins and methylmethacrylate. (From Fegler et al.,[110] with permission.)*

FIGURE 13.16 *Lateral extracavitary approach. Posterior stabilization is then performed through the same incision, all without a position change. (From Fessler et al.,[110] with permission.)*

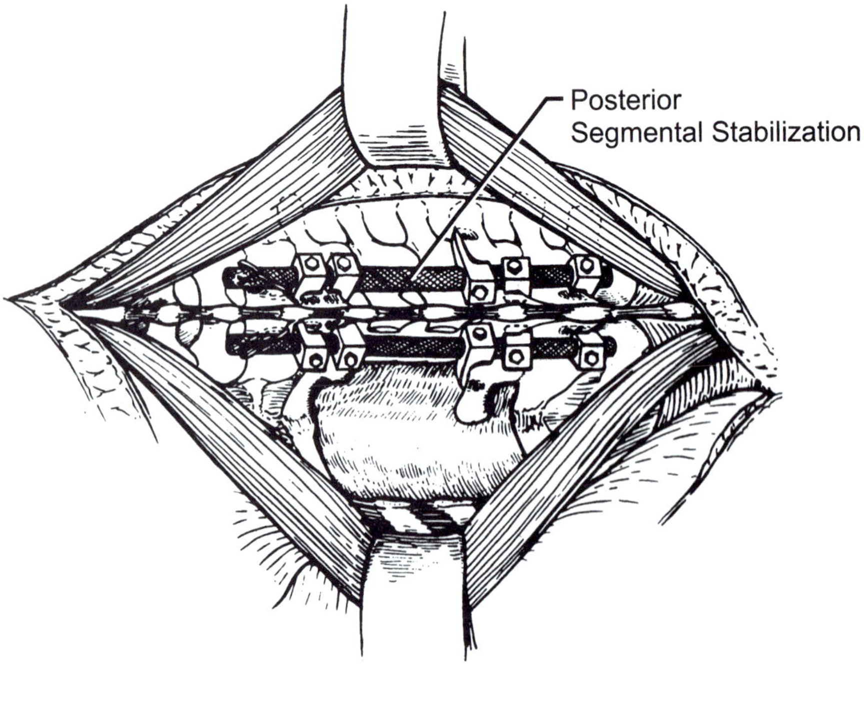

Either general or regional anesthesia can be safely administered for lower thoracic and lumbar surgery. Some anesthesiologists and surgeons prefer the use of spinal anesthesia; typically, a hypobaric solution is used. If the myelogram is performed just before surgery, the spinal anesthetic may be administered through the same needle after the contrast medium is removed. Advocates of regional anesthesia maintain that this type of anesthesia reduces blood loss and improves operating conditions by shrinking epidural veins. If a regional technique is used, a local anesthetic of sufficient duration must be selected. Should surgery last longer than the regional block, direct reinfection of the anesthetic into the subarachnoid space via the surgical incision (or above/below it) is possible. Most spine surgery, however, is performed under general endotracheal anesthesia. General anesthesia is preferred for essentially all thoracic and cervical procedures because of the high spinal level that would be required with a regional technique. In addition, general anesthesia ensures a secured airway, is associated with greater patient acceptance, and can be used for lengthy operations. Succinylcholine should be avoided if there are progressive neurologic deficits because of the possible hyperkalemic response. Some surgeons prefer that muscle relaxants be avoided altogether after induction because they think that muscle relaxants would prevent patient movement in response to trauma to nerve roots. In that case, any of the shorter duration relaxants such as atracurium, vecuronium, rocuronium, or mivacurium could be used as a single dose at induction and allowed to wear off.

"NONINVASIVE" SPINAL SURGERY Surgery on the spine, particularly for degenerative disease, is commonly associated with a significant hospital stay and prolonged recovery at home after hospitalization. As in other surgical disciplines, there has been a concerted effort to develop techniques that are less invasive, cause less postoperative pain, and still provide the desired postoperative result (usually the relief of pain and improvement of muscle strength). Several of these techniques that have special anesthetic considerations are reviewed here.

Percutaneous endoscopic discectomy has gained some popularity over the past decade. There are two main "varieties" of percutaneous discectomy. The first involves the removal of the herniated nucleus pulposus with various types of instruments, both manual and automated, under endoscopic control (similar to arthroscopic surgery). The second method involves use of a single automated instrument to remove the nucleus pulposus from the center of the disc space (under fluoroscopic control, not direct vision). There are no data to prove that these techniques are better than conventional surgery. Most reports are anecdotal, and there are no adequate prospective randomized studies. It is also clear that some of the surgeons using percutaneous techniques are applying careful selection criteria for their patients. One study considered only 13 of 326 patients suitable for percutaneous surgery.[86] Nonetheless, in appropriately selected patients, success rate appears to be high, recovery rapid, and patient satisfaction excellent.[87–90]

Initially, nearly all these procedures were conducted under local anesthesia with intravenous sedation. The surgeons were very concerned that damage to nerve roots could occur during these procedures. If the patients were under general anesthesia, associated paresthesias could not be detected, and unsuspected damage could occur. Little scientific work has been done to prove or disprove that idea. One study randomly assigned 92 patients undergoing automated percutaneous discectomy to receive either general anesthesia or local anesthesia supplemented with intravenous sedation.[91] In this small group of patients, nerve injury was not increased in the general anesthesia group. Because nerve injury is relatively uncommon, this study does not, however, have the statistical power to prove that general anesthesia is as safe as local anesthesia with respect to detection and prevention of nerve injury. We, however, greatly prefer either general or spinal anesthesia for these procedures. Most of the patients that have undergone percutaneous discectomy at our institution have had a low tolerance for any sort of pain and were not good candidates for intravenous sedation. To remain still, most patients required close to "unconscious" sedation in the prone position. Patient selection is obviously key in these cases.

The next noninvasive technique may supplant anterior thoracic and lumbar procedures (discussed above) in certain instances. A standard thoracoscope or laparoscope is placed through a small percutaneous incision, giving access to the thoracic and lumbar spines, respectively. There is a small body of literature reporting the use of these instruments for procedures ranging from simple discectomy to vertebrectomy for trauma or pathologic fractures at levels from T3 down to the lumbar spine. Morbidity reported in these small series appears to be favorable when compared with open thoractomy techniques with respect to length of time requiring a chest tube, time in the intensive care unit, and total hospitalization.[92–94]

Anesthetic considerations for these operations are essentially identical to other thoracoscopic procedures, with the added potential for significant blood loss, depending on the indication for the operation. The operation is performed with the patient in a lateral decubitus position (thoracic procedures) or in a semilateral position (lumbar procedures). The ability to provide one-lung ventilation for the thoracic-level procedures is essential because thoracoscopic techniques do not allow adequate retraction of lung tissue to provide visualization of the spine. Double lumen endotracheal tube intubation is thus necessary. One of us (M.E.M.) has not found bronchial blockers to be helpful because it is often necessary to provide apneic oxygenation or a small amount of continuous positive airway pressure (CPAP) to the nonventilated lung to improve oxygenation. These methods are not possible with a bronchial blocker or equivalent. Lumbar procedures do not need special ventilation techniques.

If the operation is performed for a simple discectomy or corpectomy for degenerative disease or trauma, two large-bore intravenous catheters and intra-arterial monitoring for sampling arterial blood gases suffice. If a multilevel corpectomy or corpectomy for metastatic malignancy is planned, then a large introducer placed in a peripheral or central vein may be helpful in the event that massive, difficult to control, blood loss occurs. CVP monitoring may also be helpful for monitoring volume status.

After completion of the surgical procedure, the lung should be carefully and completely reexpanded. In the case in which one-lung ventilation has lasted for longer than 3 hours, pulmonary edema may occur with reexpansion of the lung. Although there is no clear limit in the literature to duration of one-lung ventilation, consideration should be given to changing the endotracheal tube to a single lumen tube at the conclusion of surgery and providing postoperative ventilatory support with CPAP for several hours until it is clear that pulmonary complications are unlikely. One study involving more chronically collapsed lungs that are then reexpanded suggests that pulmonary edema will occur within 1 hour in most patients if it is going to occur at all.[95] Patients with a shorter duration of one-lung ventilation should be able to be extubated at the conclusion of surgery without a problem. In cases in which blood loss and fluid requirements are significant, the dependent lung may also become edematous. In these cases, the patient should remain intubated until weaning from the ventilator as documented by arterial blood gases is successful.

Epidural and Spinal Anesthesia After Major Spinal Surgery

Previous spinal surgery has been considered to represent a relative contraindication to the use of regional anesthesia. Many of these patients experience chronic back pain and are reluctant to undergo epidural or spinal anesthesia, fearing exacerbation of their preexisting back complaints. Several postoperative anatomic changes make needle or catheter placement more difficult and complicated after major spinal surgery. Degenerative changes such as spondylolisthesis occur in the spine below the level of fusion, increasing the potential for spinal cord ischemia and neurologic complications with regional anesthesia. In a study of 48 patients with chronic low back pain after spinal fusion, 8 showed significant spinal stenosis on CT scan and required surgical decompression.[96] The ligamentum flavum may be injured during surgery, resulting in adhesions within or obliteration of the epidural space. Spread of epidural local anesthetic may be affected by adhesions, producing an incomplete or "patchy" block. Obliteration of the epidural space may increase the incidence of dural puncture and make subsequent epidural blood patch placement impossible. Finally, needle placement in an area of the spine that has undergone bone grafting and fusion is not possible with either midline or lateral approaches; needle insertion can be accomplished only at unfused segments.

The guidelines for epidural anesthesia after spinal surgery are unclear. Daley et al.[97] reviewed the charts of 18 patients with previous Harrington rod instrumentation who underwent 21 attempts at epidural anesthesia for obstetric analgesia. Continuous lumbar epidural anesthesia was successfully established in 20 of 21 attempts; however, only ten were performed easily on the first attempt. The remaining 11 patients required excessive amounts of local anesthetics and/or complained of a patchy block. There was no correlation between the level of surgery and the ease of insertion or quality of epidural anesthesia. There were no complications except for low back pain in 2 patients with multiple attempts at catheter placement. Crosby and Halpern[98] studied 9 parturients with previous Harrington rod instrumentation who underwent epidural anesthesia for analgesia during labor and delivery. Five of the nine catheters were successfully placed on the first attempt. Four of the 9 were complicated and involved multiple attempts before successful insertion, traumatic catheter placement requiring a second insertion, inadequate epidural analgesia with subsequent dural puncture on a repeated attempt, or an inability to locate the epidural space despite attempts at two levels. Seven of the 9 patients obtained satisfactory analgesia. There were no adverse sequelae related to the epidural insertion. Hubbert[99] described attempted epidural anesthesia in 17 patients with Harrington rod instrumentation. Four of 5 patients with fusions terminating above L3-4 had successful epidural placement. However, in 12 patients with fusions extending to L5–S1 interspace,[6] attempts were unsuccessful,[5] required multiple attempts, and 1 patient had a dural puncture after multiple attempts before success at epidural placement. A false loss of resistance was reported to have occurred frequently. Howard[100] reported a case in which a 31-year-old woman with Harrington rod instrumentation to L3 received an epidural at the L4-5 level for induction of labor. Bupivacaine 0.125 percent was administered as a 5-ml bolus with subsequent infusion at 10 ml/hr. Forty minutes later, the patient had a sensory level of C3. The authors suspected subdural catheterization. No studies have reported on the complications and quality of spinal anesthesia in patients with previous spinal surgery. However, one would suspect that although needle placement may be more difficult or traumatic in these patients, the spread of local anesthetic within the subarachnoid space and quality of block would not be affected. A spinal anesthetic may be more desirable after spinal surgery because the technique is not dependent on a subjective loss of resistance but instead has a definite endpoint—the presence of cerebrospinal fluid (CSF). In addition, a smaller needle may produce less trauma and reduce the incidence of postoperative low back pain.

In summary, epidural anesthesia may be successfully performed in patients with previous spinal surgery; however, successful catheter placement will be possible on the first attempt in only 50 percent of patients even with an experienced anesthesiologist. Although adequate epidural anesthesia is eventually produced in 40 to 95 percent of patients, there appears to be a higher incidence of traumatic needle placement, inadvertent dural puncture, and unsuccessful epidural needle or catheter placement, especially if spinal fusion extends to L5–S1.[97–99] Spinal anesthesia may produce a more reliable block and cause less trauma than epidural anesthesia. Several cases of successful spinal anesthesia after inadequate epidural blockade in patients with prior correction of scoliosis have been reported.[101,102] The presence of postoperative spinal stenosis or other degenerative changes in the spine and/or preexisting neurologic symptoms may preclude the use of regional anesthesia in these patients because the block will be technically very difficult, and proper spread of the local anesthetic may never occur despite large doses.

SPINAL CORD PROCEDURES

Syringomyelia

Syringomyelia is often a slowly progressive process involving the nervous system with an onset at age 30 and a life expectancy to late middle age. Men and women are equally affected. The syrinx is an abnormal CSF-filled cavity that occupies the central part of the spinal cord, frequently in the cervical region, and that may extend upward to the medulla and downward to the thoracic segments. Pathophysiologic mechanisms remain unclear, but syringomyelia can be divided into five groups[103]: (1) communicating syringomyelia, which is most likely a result of protracted and traumatic birth injury; (2) syringomyelia associated with spinal tumors; (3) post-traumatic syringomyelia, affecting 1 to 2 percent of patients with spinal cord injury, most commonly at the thoracolumbar level[104]; (4) syringomyelia after arachnoiditis; and (5) an idiopathic form that may be accompanied by tonsillar ectopia.[105]

Presentation is variable. Sensory changes involving loss of pain and temperature in a capelike distribution with sparing of proprioception sense, vibration, and touch are typical. Motor symptoms, initially located ipsilateral to the pain and temperature deficits, consist of muscular atrophy and weakness along with absence of deep tendon reflexes. Autonomic involvement, although less common, may be manifested by Horner syndrome, resting tachycardia, orthostatic hypotension, and bowel or bladder dysfunction. Cranial nerve involvement such as vocal cord paralysis, lingual atrophy, nystagmus, and diplopia have also been described.[104]

Surgery is the only therapeutic means of halting progression or improving symptoms. Several different procedures have been advocated including posterior fossa decompression, laminectomy with syringostomy, ventriculoatrial or peritoneal shunting, and shunting of the syrinx to the subarachnoid space, pleural cavity, or peritoneum.[105] Hemilaminectomy is performed in the sitting, prone, or three-quarters prone position, usually at the widest part of the syrinx (thinnest portion of the spinal cord). Posterolateral myelotomy is made in the dorsal root entry zone, and a Silastic wick is placed to maintain patency.

Anesthetic management of syringomyelia depends on many factors. If there are associated vertebral column deformities, ventilation-perfusion abnormalities and decreased lung function may be present, and preoperative pulmonary testing is warranted.

Any increase in intracranial pressure caused by sneezing, coughing, or vomiting can alter intrasyrinx tension and theoretically result in extension of the cavity. Muscle relaxants must be administered with care. Patients with significant myelopathy may have a hyperkalemic response to depolarizing muscle relaxants and exhibit increased sensitivity to nondepolarizing agents. Thus, succinylcholine is to be avoided, and a nerve stimulator placed on an unaffected extremity should be used to assess degree of blockade when nondepolarizing muscle relaxants are used. Blood pressure control is also very important. In the patient with a syrinx, the spinal cord is compressed from within the cord itself, much as the brain is compressed in the patient with significant hydrocephalus. Thus, spinal cord perfusion pressure is the MAP minus the pressure within the syrinx. Maintenance of at least normotension is very important to prevent spinal cord ischemia. We do not allow blood pressure to fall more than 10 percent below levels at which the patient has spinal cord function in the awake state.

Autonomic dysfunction leads to special anesthetic considerations. Cardiac and peripheral vasculature responses to hypovolemia, blood loss, and increase in intrathoracic pressure (Valsalva) may be present.[106] Opiates are preferable for maintenance because the volatile agents would further depress the autonomic system.[107] Impaired autonomic tone may also result in hypothermia.

Postoperatively, the patient may still require airway management. Chronic aspiration may result in pneumonia. Some patients with depressed gag reflex or vocal cord paralysis preoperatively will recover after decompression whereas others may require tracheostomy for airway protection.

Intra- and Extradural Spinal Tumors

Spinal cord tumors may be classified as intramedullary (within the parenchyma of the spinal cord) or extramedullary (outside the parenchyma of the spinal cord). The extramedullary type of tumor comprises the largest portion of spinal neoplasms and may be either intradural or extradural. The most common types of extramedullary tumors include Schwannomas and meningiomas. Schwannomas may occur at any level of the spinal cord and are usually not highly vascular. They may be both intradural and extradural and extend out the neural foramen into the surrounding tissue. Resection of these tumors may thus be complex. Meningiomas are mainly intradural and occur mainly in the thoracic and high cervical (near foramen magnum) regions. These tumors may be more vascular.

Astrocytomas and ependymomas comprise the vast majority of intramedullary tumors. Most of these tumors are benign, but some astrocytomas in adults may be malignant. Hemangioblastomas account for about 5 percent of intramedullary tumor[108] and deserve special mention because they are frequently highly vascular lesions and are commonly associated with von Hippel-Lindau disease.

Preoperative evaluation of the patient with a spinal cord tumor follows the same principles as described above for surgery on the spinal column. Patients with tumors in the upper cervical spine may have compromised respiratory function preoperatively. Respiratory function will rarely improve and usually deteriorates postoperatively. Thus, it is important to document the degree of compromise with a careful analysis of exercise tolerance (difficult to assess if the patient is clinically weak in the arms and legs) and pulmonary function testing. A careful motor examination should be performed. Succinylcholine should probably not be used if there is any muscle weakness present. In addition, if muscle relaxation is planned during surgery, monitoring of neuromuscular blockade will be difficult if an uninvolved extremity is not available. Up-regulation of the neuromuscular receptor sites in patients with significant myelopathy will make the patient appear to be resistant to nondepolarizing relaxant agents. At the University of Florida, muscle relaxation is generally avoided if possible after induction of anesthesia. The surgeons will thus be able to detect motor movement in response to trespass on a nerve root or the spinal cord.

Positioning, as well as induction and maintenance of anesthesia, follows the principles outlined above for spinal column and operations to shunt spinal syrinxes. As in the patient with a syrinx or with spinal cord compression from a bony cause described above, maintenance of blood pressure is very important. Both the spinal cord and the tumor reside within the rigid "box" of the spinal column. If the tumor is large enough or has grown rapidly, the spinal cord may be severely compressed. Its perfusion pressure is then the MAP minus the pressure inside the spinal canal. Evoked potential monitoring may also be used, and anesthetic technique may need to be altered in these cases to accommodate monitoring, particularly in the patient with an abnormal neurologic examination preoperatively. Extubation is usually feasible except in the case of surgery in the upper cervical spine. In these cases, we generally leave the patient intubated until weaning and pulmonary testing parameters document that extubation will likely be successful. The spinal cord may develop significant edema after resection of a tumor, and this fact should be kept in mind when deciding to extubate a patient after removal of an upper cervical spinal cord tumor. Initial good respiratory function may deteriorate in the first 24 hours, and careful monitoring in an intensive care unit environment is needed even if the patient is extubated after surgery.

CONCLUSIONS

Spinal surgery comprises a significant portion of neurosurgical practice. Neuroanesthesiologists have traditionally focused most of their attention on the patient with intracranial pathology. We are only now coming to realize that all the principles regarding positioning, blood pressure management, and management of ventilation that we have applied for many years to patients with intracranial pathology are equally important in the patient with spinal column or spinal cord disease. It is hoped that realization of that fact will enable the clinician to provide anesthetic care that will maximize the chances for a good neurologic and clinical outcome.

References

1. Messick JM, Newberg LA, Nugent M, Faust RJ: Principles of neuroanesthesia for the nonneurosurgical patient with CNS pathophysiology. Anesth Analg 64:143, 1985
2. Marcus ML, Heistad DD, Ehrhardt JC, Abboud FM: Regulation of total and regional spinal cord blood flow. Circ Res 41:128, 1977
3. Hickey R, Albin MS, Bunegin B, Gelineau J: Autoregulation of spinal cord blood flow: is the cord a microcosm of the brain? Stroke 17:1183, 1986
4. Griffiths IR: Spinal cord blood flow in dogs: the effect of blood pressure. J Neurol Neurosurg Psychiatry 36:914, 1973
5. Griffiths IR: Spinal cord flow in dogs. 2. The effect of the blood gases. J Neurol Neurosurg Psychiatry 36:42, 1973
6. Ruge D: Spondylosis. p. 315. In Ruge D, Wiltse LL (eds): Spinal Disorders Diagnosis and Treatment. Lea & Febiger, Philadelphia, 1977
7. Epstein NE, Epstein JA: Lumbar spinal stenosis. p. 149. In Camins MB, O'Leary PF (eds): The Lumbar Spine. Raven Press, New York, 1987
8. Hudson A, Berry H, Mayfield F: Chronic injuries of peripheral nerves by entrapment. p. 2430. In Youmans FR (ed): Neurological Surgery, A Comprehensive Guide to the Diagnosis and Management of Neurosurgical Problems. Vol. 4. WB Saunders, Philadelphia, 1982
9. Murphey F, Simmons JCH, Brunson B: Ruptures cervical discs 1939–1972. Clin Neurosurg 20:9, 1973
10. Wiltse LL: Spondylolisthesis and its treatment; fusion with and without reduction. p. 193. In Ruge D, Wiltse LL (eds): Spinal Disorders Diagnosis and Treatment. Lea & Febiger, Philadelphia, 1977
11. Neuwirth MG: Spondylolysis and spondylolithesis in children and adults. p. 251. In Camins MB, O'Leary PF (eds): The Lumbar Spine. Raven Press, New York, 1987
12. Bracken MB, Shepard MJ, Collins WF et al: A randomized, controlled trial of methyl-prednisolone or naloxone in the treatment of acute spinal cord injury. N Engl J Med 322:1405, 1990
13. Levi L, Wolf A, Belzberg H: Hemodynamic parameters in patients with acute cervical cord trauma: description, intervention and prediction of outcome. Neurosurgery 33:1007, 1993
14. Albin MS: Acute cervical spinal injury. Crit Care Clin 1:267, 1985
15. Jackson AB, Groomes TE: Incidence of respiratory complications following spinal cord injury. Arch Phys Med Rehabil 75:270, 1994
16. Mackenzie CF, Shin B, Krishnaprasad D et al: Assessment of cardiac and respiratory function during surgery on patients with acute quadriplegia. J Neurosurg 62:843, 1985
17. Green BA, David C, Falcone S et al: Spinal cord injuries in adults. p. 1969. In Youmans R (ed): Neurological Surgery. 4th Ed. WB Saunders, Philadelphia, 1996
18. Robinson RA, Smith GW: Anterolateral cervical disc removal and interbody fusion for cervical disc syndrome. Bull Johns Hopkins Hosp 96:223, 1955
19. Cucchiara RF: Safety of the sitting position. Anesthesiology 61:790, 1984

20. Young ML, Smith DS, Murtagh F et al: Comparison of surgical and anesthetic complications in neurosurgical patients experiencing venous air embolism in the sitting position. Neurosurgery 18:157, 1986
21. Albin MS, Chang JL, Babinski M et al: Intracardiac catheters in neurosurgical anesthesia. Anesthesiology 50:67, 1979
22. Kafer ER: Respiratory and cardiovascular functions in scoliosis and the principles of anesthesia management. Anesthesiology 52:339, 1980
23. Gibbons PA, Lee IS: Scoliosis and anesthesia. Int Anesthesiol Clin 23:149, 1985
24. Youngman PME, Edgar MA: Posterior spinal fusion and instrumentation in the treatment of adolescent idiopathic scoliosis. Ann R Coll Surg Engl 67:313, 1985
25. McMaster MJ: Management of scoliosis. J R Soc Med 75:685, 1982
26. Goldstein LA, Waugh TR: Classification and terminology of scoliosis. Clin Orthop 93:10, 1973
27. Wynne-Davies R: Familial (idiopathic) scoliosis: a family survey. J Bone Joint Surg [Br] 50:24, 1968
28. Scott JC, Morgan TH: The natural history and prognosis for infantile idiopathic scoliosis. J Bone Joint Surg [Br] 37:400, 1955
29. Waugh TR, Riseborough E: Scoliosis. p. 177. In Ruge D, Wiltse LL (eds); Spinal Disorders Diagnosis and Treatment. Lea & Febiger, Philadelphia, 1977
30. Siegel IM: Diagnosis, management, and orthopaedic treatment of muscular dystrophy. Instr Course Lect 30:3, 1981
31. Seay AR, Ziter FA, Thompson JA: Cardiac arrest during induction of anesthesia in Duchenne muscular dystrophy. J Pediatr 93:88, 1978
32. Gronert GA, Theye RA: Pathophysiology of hyperkalemia induced by succinylcholine. Anesthesiology 43:89, 1975
33. Cobham IG, Davis HS: Anesthesia for muscular dystrophy patients. Anesth Analg 43:22, 1964
34. Kafer ER: Idiopathic scoliosis: mechanical properties of the respiratory system and ventilatory response to carbon dioxide. J Clin Invest 55:1153, 1975
35. Smyth RJ, Chapman KR, Wright TA et al: Pulmonary function in adolescents with mild idiopathic scoliosis. Thorax 39:901, 1984
36. Kafer ER: Idiopathic scoliosis: gas exchange and the age-dependence of arterial blood gases. J Clin Invest 58:825, 1976
37. Lin HY, Nash CL, Herndon CH, Anderson NB: The effect of corrective surgery on pulmonary function in scoliosis. J Bone Joint Surg [Am] 56:1173, 1974
38. Bayder A, Swank SM, Stiles CM, Sassoon CSH: Respiratory mechanics in anesthetized young patients with scoliosis kyphoscoliosis: immediate and delayed effects of corrective spinal surgery. Chest 97:1157, 1990
39. Primiano FP, Nussbaum E, Hirschfeld SS et al: Early echocardiographic and pulmonary function findings in idiopathic scoliosis J Pediatr Orthop 3:475, 1983
40. Hirschfeld SS, Rudner C, Nash, CL et al: The incidence of mitral valve prolapse in adolescent scoliosis and thoracic hypokyphosis. Pediatrics 40:451, 1982
41. Harrington PR: Treatment of scoliosis. Correction and internal fixation by spine instrumentation. J Bone Joint Surg [Am] 44:591, 1962
42. Luque ER: Segmental spinal instrumentation for correction of scoliosis. Clin Orthop 163:192, 1982
43. Thompson GH, Wilber RG, Shaffer JW et al: Segmental spinal instrumentation in idiopathic scoliosis. A preliminary report. Spine 10:623, 1985
44. MacEwen GD, Bunnell WP, Sviram K: Acute neurologic complications in the treatment of scoliosis. J Bone Joint Surg [Am] 57:404, 1975
45. Flores E, Rengachary SS, Hitchon PW: ISOLA instrumentation. p. 218. Hitchon PW, Traynelis VC, Rengachary SS (eds): Techniques in Spinal Fusion and Stabilization. Thieme Medical Publishers, New York, 1995
46. Hitchon PW, Follett KA: Transpedicular screw fixation of the thoracic and lumbar spine. p. 240. In Hitchon PW, Traynelis VC, Rengachary SS (eds): spine. Techniques in Spinal Fusion and Stabilization. Thiem Medical Publishers, New York, 1995
47. Schmidek H, Smith D: Anterior cervical disc excision in cervical spondylosis. p. 1327. In Schmidek H (ed): Operative Neurosurgical Techniques: Indications, Methods, and Results. Vol. 2. Harcourt Brace Jovanovich, New York, 1988
48. Cucchiara RF, Black S: Corneal abrasion during anesthesia and surgery. Anesthesiology 69:978, 1988
49. Jenkins DHR, Weeks RD, Yau ACMC, Du RR: Thoracolumbar approach T_{10}-L_1 (anterior and

anterolateral) for single-body or limited interbody fusions. p. 35. In: Manual of Spinal Surgery. Butterworths, Boston, 1981
50. Pathak KS, Brown RH, Nash CL, Cascorbi HF: Continuous opioid infusion for scoliosis fusion surgery. Anesth Analg 62:841, 1983
51. Lennon RL, Hosking MP, Gray JR et al: The effects of intraoperative blood salvage and induced hypotension on transfusion requirements during spinal surgical procedures. Mayo Clin Proc 62:1090, 1987
52. Mandel RJ, Brown MD, McCollough NC et al: Hypotensive anesthesia and autotransfusion in spinal surgery. Clin Orthop 154:27, 1981
53. Brodsky JW, Dickson JH, Erwin WD, Rossi CD: Hypotensive anesthesia for scoliosis surgery in Jehovah's Witnesses. Spine 16:304, 1991
54. McNeil JW, DeWald RL, Kuo KN et al: Controlled hypotensive anesthesia in scoliosis surgery. J Bone Joint Surg [Am] 56:1167, 1974
55. Grundy BL, Nash CL, Brown RH: Arterial pressure manipulation alters spinal cord function during correction of scoliosis. Anesthesiology 34:249, 1981
56. Grundy BL, Nash CL, Brown RH: Deliberate hypotension for spinal fusion: prospective randomized study with evoked potential monitoring. Can Anaesth Soc J 29:452, 1982
57. Lindop MJ: Complications and morbidity of controlled hypotension. Br J Anaesth 47:799, 1975
58. Patel NJ, Patel BS, Paskin S, Laufer S: Induced moderate hypotensive anesthesia for spinal fusion and Harrington-rod instrumentation. J Bone Joint Surg [Am] 67:1384, 1985
59. Yaster M, Simmons RS, Tole VT et al: A comparison of nitroglycerin and nitroprusside for inducing hypotension in children: a double blind study. Anesthesiology 65:174, 1986
60. Fahmy NR, Mossad B, Milad M: Spinal cord blood flow during induced hypotension: comparison of nitroprusside and trimethaphan. Anesthesiology 53:87, 1980
61. Spargo PM, Tait AR, Knight PR et al: Effect of nitroglycerin induced hypotension on canine spinal cord blood flows. Br J Anaesth 59:640, 1987
62. Porter SS, Asher M, Fox DK: Comparison of intravenous nitroprusside, nitroprusside-captopril, and nitroglycerin for deliberate hypotension during posterior spine fusion in adults. J Clin Anesth 1:87, 1988
63. Bernard JM, Passuti N, Pinaud M: Long-term hypotensive technique with nicardipine and nitroprusside during isoflurane anesthesia for spinal surgery. Anesth Analg 75:179, 1992
64. Bernard JM, Moren J, Demeure D et al: Diltiazem reduces the dose requirement for nitroprusside-induced hypotension. Anesth Analg 77:318, 1993
65. Dorgan JC, Abbott TR, Bentley G: Intraoperative awakening to monitor spinal cord function during scoliosis surgery. J Bone Joint Surg [Br] 66:716, 1984
66. Vauzelle C, Stagnara P, Jouvinroux P: Functional monitoring of spinal cord activity during spinal surgery. Clin Orthop 93:173, 1973
67. Jones ET, Matthews LS, Hensinger RN: The wake-up technique as a dual protector of spinal cord function during spine fusion. Clin Orthop 168:113, 1982
67a. Ben DB, Taylor PD, Haller GS: Posterior spinal fusion complicated by posterior column injury. A case report of a false-negative wake-up test. Spine 12:540, 1987
68. Diaz JH, Lockhart CH: Postoperative quadriplegia after spinal fusion for scoliosis with intraoperative awakening. Anesth Analg 66:1039, 1987
69. Ginsburg HH, Shetter AG, Raudzens PA: Postoperative paraplegia with preserved intraoperative somatosensory evoked potentials. J Neurosurg 63:296, 1985
70. Lang SA, Duncan PG, Dupius PR: Fatal air embolism in an adolescent with Duchenne muscular dystrophy during Harrington instrumentation. Anesth Analg 69:132, 1989
71. Frankel AS, Holzman RS: Air embolism during posterior spinal fusion. Can J Anaesth 35:511, 1988
72. Albin MS, Ritter RR, Pruett CE, Kalff K: Venous air embolism during lumbar laminectomy in the prone position: report of three cases. Anesth Analg 73:346, 1991
73. Horlocker TT, Wedel DJ, Cucchiara RF: Venous air embolism during spinal instrumentation and fusion in the prone position. Anesth Analg 75:152, 1992
74. Tempelhoff R, Williams EL, Vollmer DG: Is the "kneeling" prone position as dangerous as the sitting position for the development of venous air embolism? Anesth Analg 75:467, 1992
75. Thiagarajah S: Anesthetic management of spinal surgery. p. 587. In Frost EAM (ed): Anesthesiology Clinics of North America. Vol. 5. WB Saunders, Philadelphia, 1987

76. Williams EL, Hart WM, Tempelhoff R: Postoperative ischemic optic neuropathy. Anesth Analg 80:101, 1995
77. Wolfe SW, Lospinuso MF, Burke SW: Unilateral blindness as a complication of patient positioning for spinal surgery. Spine 17:600, 1992
78. Brown RH, Schauble JF, Miller NR: Anemia and hyptension as contributors to perioperative loss of vision. Anesthesiology 80:222, 1994
79. Katz DM, Trobe JD, Cornblath WT, Kline LB: Ischemic optic neuropathy after lumbar spine surgery. Arch Ophthalmol 112:925, 1994
80. Ross DA, Drasner K, Weinstein PR et al: Use of intrathecally administered morphine in the treatment of postoperative pain after lumbar spine surgery: a prospective, double-blind, placebo-controlled study. Neurosurgery 28:700, 1991
81. Joshi GP, McCarroll SM, O'Rourke K: Postoperative analgesia after lumbar laminectomy: epidural fentanyl infusion versus patient-controlled intravenous morphine. Anesth Analg 80:511, 1995
82. Fessler RG, Mack CA: Benign extradural lesions of the dorsal spine. p. 2320. In Youmans JR (ed): Neurological Surgery. 4th Ed. WB Saunders, Philadelphia, 1996
83. Bass J, Lach J, Fegelman RH: Vascular injuries during lumbar laminectomy. Am Surg 46:649, 1980
84. Shevlin WA, Luessenhop AJ, Fox JL, McCullough DC: Perforation of the anterior annulus during lumbar discectomy. Case report. J Neurosurg 38:514, 1973
85. Kiev J, Dupont JR, Kerstein MD: Injury of a medial sacral vessel during lumbar laminectomy. Ann Vasc Surg 10:63, 1996
86. Kleinpeter G, Markowitsch MM, Bock F: Percutaneous endoscopic discectomy: minimally invasive, but perhaps only minimally useful? Surg Neurol 43:534, 1995
87. Maroon JC, Onik G, Vidovich DV: Percutaneous discectomy for lumbar disc herniation. Neurosurg Clin North Am 4:125, 1993
88. Sortland O, Kleppe H, Aandahl M, Blikra G: Percutaneous lumbar discectomy. Technique and clinical result. Acta Radiol 37:85, 1996
89. Shapiro S: Long-term follow up of 57 patients undergoing automated percutaneous discectomy. J Neurosurg 83:31, 1995
90. Sakou T, Masuda A, Yone K, Nakagawa M: Percutaneous discectomy in athletes. Spine 18:2218, 1993
91. Bokesch PM, Huffnagle FT, Macauley C: Local versus general anesthesia for lumbar percutaneous discectomy. J Neurosurg Anesthesiol 5:81, 1993
92. McAfee PC, Regan JR, Fedder IL et al: Anterior thoracic corpectomy for spinal cord decompression performed endoscopically. Surg Laparosc Endosc 5:339, 1995
93. McAfee PC, Regan JR, Zdeblick T et al: The incidence of complications in endoscopic anterior thoracolumbar spinal reconstructive surgery. A prospective multicenter study comprising the first 100 consecutive cases. Spine 20:1624, 1995
94. Regan JJ, Mack MJ, Picett GD: A technical report on video-assisted thoracoscopy in thoracic spinal surgery. Preliminary description. Spine 20:831, 1995
95. Tarver RD, Broderick LS, Conces DJ: Reexpansion pulmonary edema. J Thorac Imaging 11:198, 1996
96. Laasonen EM, Soini J: Low-back pain after lumbar fusion: surgical and computed tomographic analysis. Spine 14:210, 1989
97. Daley MD, Morningstar BA, Rolbin SH et al: Epidural anesthesia for obstetrics after spinal surgery. Reg Anesth 15:280, 1990
98. Crosby ET, Halpern SH: Obstetric epidural anaesthesia in patients with Harrington instrumentation. Can J Anaesth 36:693, 1989
99. Hubbert CH: Epidural anesthesia in patients with spinal fusion. Anesth Analg 64:843, 1985
100. Howard R: Subdural catheterization and opiate administration in a patient with Harrington rods. Can J Anaesth 37:712, 1990
101. Pascoe JF, Jennings GS, Marx GF: Successful spinal anesthesia after inadequate epidural block in a parturient with prior surgical correction of scoliosis. Reg Anesth 18:191, 1993
102. Silva TSS, Popat MT: Combined spinal-epidural anesthesia in parturient with Harrington rods. Reg Anesth 19:360, 1994
103. Barnett HJM, Fox A, Vinuela F, Peerless SJ: Delayed metrizamide CT observations in syringomyelia. Ann Neurol 8:116, 1980
104. Padilla CR: Syringomyelia after spinal cord injury. Am Fam Physician 26:145, 1982
105. Barbaro NM, Wilson CB, Gutin PH, Edwards MSB: Surgical treatment of syringomyelia: favorable results with syringoperitoneal shunting. J Neurosurg 61:531, 1984
106. Ishak VA, McLone D, Seleny FL: Intraoperative autonomic dysfunction associated with Arnold-Chiari malformation. Childs Brain 7:146, 1980

107. Roelofse JA, Skipton EA, Nell AC: Anaesthesia for caesarean section in a patient with syringomyelia. S Afr Med J 65:736, 1984
108. Neumann NPH, Eggert HR, Weigel K et al: Hemangioblastomas of the central nervous system: a 10-year study with special reference to von Hippel-Lindau syndrome. J Neurosurg 70:24, 1989
109. Kafer ER: Respiratory and cardiovascular functions in scoliosis. Bull Eur Physiopathol Respir 13:299, 1977
110. Feggler RG, Nictze NN, MacMillan MM, Peace D: Latiral paraescapular extrapleural approach to the upper thoracic spine. J Neurosurg 75:349, 1991

14 NEUROMUSCULAR DISORDERS AND MUSCLE RELAXANTS

RORY S. JAFFE
GERALD A. GRONERT
NEAL W. FLEMING
JOSEPH F. ANTOGNINI

Many neurologic and muscular disorders alter patients' responses to muscle relaxants. Most of these alterations are due to a change within skeletal muscle or the neuromuscular junction. Altered responses include (1) sensitivity or resistance to relaxants, (2) hyperkalemia, (3) rhabdomyolysis with myoglobinuria, (4) muscle contracture, (5) accelerated muscle metabolism, and (6) increased intracranial pressure. This chapter will review normal responses to muscle relaxants, altered responses and their etiology, and considerations in various disease states: central and peripheral neurological disorders and myopathies. There is an excellent two-volume monograph that provides comprehensive information on myopathies.[1]

NORMAL RESPONSES

Nondepolarizing Relaxants

Nondepolarizing neuromuscular blocking drugs have two predominant sites of action. The primary action, originally demonstrated by Claude Bernard,[2] is direct competition with acetylcholine for the receptor on the postjunctional skeletal muscle cell membrane. As the relaxant molecules occupy a progressively greater percentage of receptors, there is a progressive decrease in the force of muscle contraction. At 95% receptor occupancy, intubation is feasible without the need for deep anesthesia or other modifying factors that facilitate intubation. At this point, a single twitch response will be virtually abolished.

The second action of the nondepolarizing relaxants is hypothesized to result from competitive interaction with acetylcholine at prejunctional receptors and is manifested clinically by fade: a decremental response to repetitive stimulation. Acetylcholine receptors on the prejunctional nerve terminal appear to be part of a positive feedback mechanism.[3,4] Activation of presynaptic receptors causes movement of acetylcholine from the storage pool to the readily releasable store within the distal nerve terminal. This maintains acetylcholine availability during high demand as with continued high-frequency stimulation. Blockade of these prejunctional receptors by a nondepolarizing relaxant occurs with relatively small doses. Some drugs act solely on the postjunctional membrane (e.g., α-bungarotoxin) and produce a decrease in twitch amplitude with no evidence of fade. This pattern has also been reported in a patient with peripheral polyneuropathy given curare.[5] However, most clinically used nondepolarizing relaxants have a dose-dependent combination of pre- and postjunctional effects.

Detection of fade produced by muscle relaxants is used for clinical monitoring. Train-of-four (four impulses at 2 Hz), tetanic stimuli, or sustained patient effort all repetitively stimulate the nerve and produce fade during partial paralysis. When approximately 30 to 50% of the receptors are occupied, only a high-frequency stimulus such as 100 Hz tetanus will demonstrate a diminished response.[6] When about 70 to 80% of the receptors are occupied, the patient will have difficulty holding his head off the pillow for 5 seconds or maintaining a strong grip.[7] Thus, the response to more frequent stimuli is blocked at lesser doses of relaxants and that to less frequent stimuli is blocked only at greater doses.

Some nondepolarizing muscle relaxants produce histamine release with associated hypotension and, occasionally, bronchospasm. Histamine-related side effects occur more frequently with curare, metocurine, atracurium, mivacurium, and, rarely, large doses of vecuronium.[8] These side effects are related primarily to dose and speed of administration.[9] The combined use of H_1 and H_2 antagonists will prevent or ameliorate many of the histamine-related side effects, for example, even with administration of very large doses of atracurium, 1.5 mg/kg.[9,10]

Depolarizing Relaxants

Postjunctional receptors on muscle fibers are chemically sensitive to the cholinergic agonists, responding with graded depolarization due to the cationic fluxes of potassium, sodium, and calcium. This graded depolarization alters the permeability of the adjacent electrically sensitive skeletal muscle cell membrane, which responds with an all-or-none action potential after reaching its electrical threshold. Thus, during a normal contraction, acetylcholine released from the nerve terminal chemically depolarizes the chemically sensitive membrane of the receptor site. This chemically induced depolarization activates the electrically sensitive ion channels of the cell membrane adjacent to the receptor sites. These local currents propagate across the surface membrane and into the transverse tubules.

Depolarizing relaxants such as succinylcholine initially activate muscle fibers in a manner similar to that of acetylcholine.[11,12] They initially produce depolarization of the receptor site, but the response is prolonged, producing a marked increase in the threshold of the adjacent electrically sensitive skeletal muscle membrane. This process is called *accommodation* or *cathodal depression* and results in insensitivity to acetylcholine and muscle paralysis: the so-called phase I block. With diffusion of succinylcholine away from the receptor, repolarization of the chemically sensitive membrane occurs and muscle function returns. However, with continued exposure to succinylcholine, desensitization of the motor end-plate gradually develops. Desensitization is defined as a diminished response (e.g., membrane depolarization) to equivalent doses of agonist. This is clinically apparent as a phase II block when the block from a depolarizing relaxant develops features similar to the block of nondepolarizing relaxants: fade, posttetanic facilitation, and so on. Acetylcholine released from nerve terminals does not cause desensitization, probably because of the discrete areas of depolarization induced by the quanta of acetylcholine. These quanta produce disks of depolarization across the end-plate that are self-limited and separate from each other. Each recovers quickly and independently and the lack of coalescence appears to prevent the development of desensitization (saturated disc theory).[13] Because the usual doses of succinylcholine are relatively huge, most or all the receptor sites depolarize and the areas of depolarization coalesce. This may be, in part, why desensitization is associated with succinylcholine.

Non–End-Plate Relaxants

Dantrolene is currently the only member of this group used clinically. It is not a practical everyday relaxant, but it does have certain valuable applications. It is lipophilic and difficult to dissolve in aqueous solutions unless the pH is 9.5 to 10. Even then it is relatively insoluble: 0.3 to 0.5 mg/ml. A salting-out effect may occur if water for solution contains other ions or molecules, although mannitol is included for isotonicity. Its uses include treatment of malignant hyperthermia, neuroleptic malignant syndrome, tetanus, heat stroke, and any situation in which muscle rigidity or temperature is difficult to control. An advantage over other relaxants is that the patient need not require endotracheal intubation.[14] Being lipophilic, dantrolene enters cells, in contrast to the other relaxants that are water soluble. It apparently acts by blocking calcium release from the sarcoplasmic reticulum, without altering reuptake. It will not paralyze, even in large doses, as it depresses twitch more than tetanus.[15] Patients will feel weak with larger doses. Neostigmine may transiently increase motor strength.[16,17] Dantrolene interacts adversely with calcium antagonists, resulting in cardiac depression, hyperkalemia, and complete skeletal muscle paralysis.[18–22]

ALTERED RESPONSES AND THEIR ETIOLOGY

Regulation of Acetylcholine Receptors

Chronic decreased release of acetylcholine or blockade of acetylcholine receptors causes up-regulation: greater numbers of acetylcholine receptors. Up-regulation may be mild or marked, depending on the condition. For example, certain anticonvulsants (dilantin, carbamazepine), although acutely potentiating nondepolarizing muscle relaxants, cause mild acetylcholine receptor up-regulation at the neuromuscular junction during chronic therapy.[23] Resistance to nondepolarizing muscle relaxants is related to spread of receptor sites in the perijunctional area, decreased muscle cholinesterase activity, and terminal nerve sprouting.[24] Significant hyperkalemia is not seen with mild up regulation. In situations of marked up regulation (e.g., denervation, spinal cord injury, stroke, and burns), acetylcholine receptors are spread over a large portion of the affected muscle, and resistance to nondepolarizing muscle relaxants occurs. These extrajunctional receptors appear to bind nondepolarizing muscle relaxants poorly.[25] Due to the larger number of acetylcholine receptors, many more ion channels open with succinylcholine, which can cause hyperkalemia and possibly cardiac arrest (Fig. 14.1). Down-regulation, or decreased numbers of functioning acetylcholine receptors, may occur with myasthenia gravis or exercise, leading to sensitivity to nondepolarizing muscle relaxants and resistance to succinylcholine.[26]

Nondepolarizing Relaxants

SENSITIVITY Sensitivity may occur in situations in which there is a deficiency of functional acetylcholine receptors at the neuromuscular junction (down-regulation), e.g., myasthenia gravis.[27,28] Chronic conditioning exercise can produce sensitivity,[29] presumably due, at least in part, to fewer junctional acetylcholine receptors. Sensitivity with myopathies presumably occurs either because of diminished numbers of acetylcholine receptors or because of a weak and poorly functioning contractile system.

Chronic potassium depletion[30] as well as many drugs potentiate the effect of nondepolarizing muscle relaxants; the drugs with the best evidence for this effect in humans include antibiotics (aminoglycosides, polymixin), corticosteroids (acute administration), furosemide (low dose), calcium channel blockers, and anticonvulsants (acutely) (Table 14.1).

The pharmacodynamics of vecuronium are unaltered by mild hypothermia.[31] Hypothermia may augment the effect of some relaxants[32] due to decreased metabolism and decreased muscle blood flow, which retards clearance from muscle. Atracurium lasts longer during hypothermia presumably due to temperature dependence of inactivation.[33]

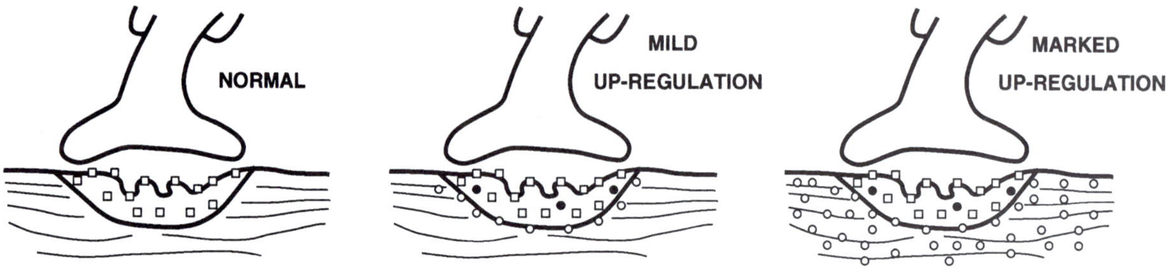

FIGURE 14.1 *Mature acetylcholine receptors are denoted by the squares, immature receptors by the unfilled circles, and unconfirmed immature receptors by the filled circles. Mild up-regulation (e.g., chronic anticonvulsant therapy) occurs as receptors increase perijunctionally; this leads to resistance to nondepolarizing muscle relaxants. The actual minimal increase is insufficient to cause hyperkalemia after succinylcholine. With marked up-regulation (e.g., burns), new receptors are diffusely spread throughout the muscle membrane; those in the perijunctional region cause resistance to nondepolarizing muscle relaxants, whereas the overall increase leads to hyperkalemia following succinylcholine. (Adapted from Melton et al.,[23] with permission.)*

RESISTANCE Increased acetylcholine receptor number produces resistance to nondepolarizing muscle relaxants. Due to up-regulation, resistance develops within a week of thermal trauma,[34–36] within 4 to 7 days following upper motor neuron lesions such as stroke or cord section[37,38] and in conjunction with disuse atrophy.[24,39,40]

If disuse is restricted to one limb, resistance can also occur in nonrestricted muscles in the absence of measurable atrophy, presumably based upon volitional "disuse" also.[30] This apparent paradox has also been noted in patients with upper motor neuron lesions.[41]

Some drugs used in neurosurgical patients produce resistance to nondepolarizing relaxants, including corticosteroids (chronic administration), furosemide (high dose), and chronic use of hydantoin derivatives (Table 14.1).[42,43]

INCREASED INTRACRANIAL PRESSURE Some nondepolarizing muscle relaxants release histamine, a cerebral vasodilator that increases cerebral blood flow and intracranial pressure in the absence of central nervous system pathology.[44,45] Normal doses of *d*-tubocurarine, but not atracurium, vecuronium, or pancuronium, apparently produce enough histamine to elevate cerebral blood flow and intracranial pressure in patients with normal intracranial compliance.[46] Histamine-induced hypotension can also decrease cerebral perfusion pressure.

PROLONGED ACTION The nondepolarizing relaxants are water soluble; their effect is dissipated by redistribution throughout the extracellular fluid, renal excretion, and liver metabolism. Atracurium and mivacurium have other routes of inactivation. Several situations may slow elimination and result in prolonged action. These include renal and hepatic insufficiency, drug overdose, shock, and hypothermia. In the latter two situations, restoration of muscle blood flow through either resuscitation or warming generally corrects the basic problem. Relative overdosage of the relaxant will also result in prolonged action. In a patient sensitive to muscle relaxants, this can occur with a small dose.

Depolarizing Relaxants

HYPERKALEMIA Hyperkalemia occurs with the administration of succinylcholine due to acetylcholine receptor up-regulation featured in several disorders[26,47,48]: lower motor neuron lesions or denervation,[49–51] upper motor neuron lesions (stroke, cord section) involving muscle weakness or spasticity,[49] thermal trauma,[52,53] chronic abdominal infection,[54,55] and direct muscle damage.[56–60] Mild up-regulation of acetylcholine receptors, as occurs in disuse atrophy, results in a modest increase in potassium efflux after succinylcholine.[48,61] Severe responses appear due to the spread of receptor sites over large areas of the skeletal muscle membrane with an accompanying increased efflux of potassium.[8,48,49,62] Although their ion conductance is slightly reduced, these extrajunctional receptors also remain open much longer when stimulated by succinylcholine.[63] Sensitivity to succinylcholine may also be due to the lack of muscle cholinesterase around these new receptors. The large increase in potassium efflux results in systemic hyperkalemia, which can precipitate cardiac arrest.

Hyperkalemia may also occur with acute rhabdomyolysis; this probably is from cell breakdown with potassium release. β-Adrenergic blockade may augment hyperkalemia resulting from potassium release, but the effect does not appear to be marked.[64,65] Verapamil does not affect the hyperkalemic response to succinylcholine.[66]

Hyperkalemia after succinylcholine has also been rarely reported in patients in hemorrhagic shock. Based on animal studies, the mechanism appears to be underlying shock-induced hyperkalemia exacerbated by the normal increase in circulating potassium after succinylcholine.[67]

TABLE 14.1 *Drugs that alter neuromuscular blockade by nondepolarizing agents*

	Potentiation
Anesthetics	Ketamine[a]
	Local anesthetics
	Propanidid
	Volatile general anesthetics
Antiarrhythmic drugs	Calcium channel blockers
	Procainamide
	Quinidine
Antibiotics	Aminoglycosides
	Clindamycin
	Lincomycin
	Polymixins
Miscellaneous	Corticosteroids (acute administration)
	Furosemide (low dose)
	Hydantoin derivatives (acute, <10 days)
	Magnesium
	Trimethaphan
Muscle relaxants	Dantrolene
	Nondepolarizers (synergy)
	Succinylcholine (phase II block)
	Antagonism
Miscellaneous	4-Aminopyridine
	Anticholinesterases
	Corticosteroids (chronic administration)
	Furosemide (high dose)
	Hydantoin derivatives (chronic, >10 days)
	Theophylline

[a] Potentiates *d*-tubocurarine but not pancuronium.
(Modified from Viby-Mogenson et al.,[53] with permission.)

INCREASED INTRACRANIAL PRESSURE This effect was first noted in 1959.[68] Succinylcholine, as it depolarizes myofibers, activates muscle spindles. The volley of afferent activity activates the electroencephalogram[69] thus increasing cerebral blood flow and cerebral spinal fluid pressure.[68,70] This activation can be blocked by paralysis with a nondepolarizing muscle relaxant.[71]

TRISMUS OR MUSCLE RIGIDITY In several situations, succinylcholine produces a contracture in skeletal muscle. This includes myotonia,[72–75] denervation,[48,49,76–78] malignant hyperthermia,[79] and instances of unknown etiology. This contracture can be benign and nonthreatening, as happens in myotonia, in which the contracture persists for 5 minutes or so, but is not associated with other major effects.[73,80] (See further discussion under Myotonia.) In denervation, the muscle contracture is associated with an extensive release of potassium and an associated increase in muscle oxygen consumption.[49] In malignant hyperthermia, total body effects may be pronounced due to increased metabolism, heat production, and acidosis.[79]

The significance of succinylcholine-induced trismus in the presence of adequate limb relaxation is controversial. Based on muscle biopsy contracture responses in these patients, trismus has been regarded as an indicator of malignant hyperthermia about 50% of the time.[81] However, two retrospective reports demonstrate a 1% incidence of trismus in children given halothane and succinylcholine,[82,83] a frequency incompatible with the incidence of clinical malignant hyperthermia. Further, none of these children developed signs of clinical malignant hyperthermia. Additional findings support the conclusion that normal masseter muscle may have slow tonic fibers that can develop contractures.[84,85] Finally, potent volatile agents such as halothane or enflurane predispose toward muscle contracture, after succinylcholine, both in vitro[86] and in vivo.[87,88] Thus, there is a spectrum of masseter muscle responses to succinylcholine (Fig. 14.2).

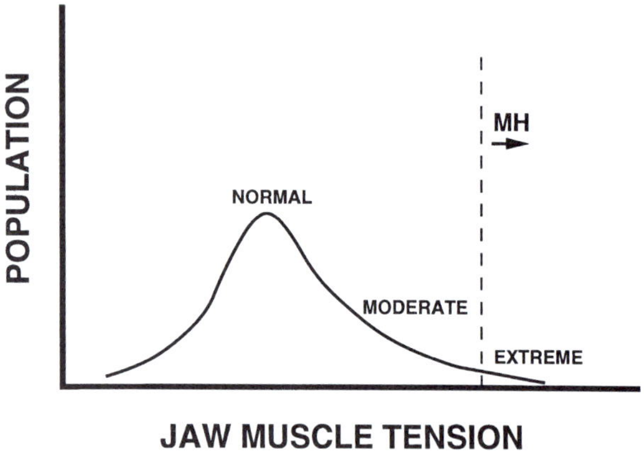

FIGURE 14.2 *There is a spectrum of responses to succinylcholine. Many normal patients will have a slight to moderate increase in jaw tension following succinylcholine. A few patients will have a marked increase in jaw tension, while rare patients will have "jaws of steel." These latter patients are more likely to have malignant hyperthermia, particularly if they also have rigidity of other muscles. It is unclear where to draw the line separating nonmalignant hyperthermia from malignant hyperthermia patients.*

There are two opposing clinical opinions regarding trismus. Some recommend that the anesthetic should be halted if possible and the procedure canceled,[89] whereas others recommend that with the use of appropriate monitoring and availability of satisfactory therapeutic modalities anesthesia and surgery may proceed.[90] The decision to proceed in part depends on the degree of rigidity, for example, postponement of surgery in cases of "jaws of steel" or total body rigidity. Should anything untoward occur, treatment for malignant hyperthermia should begin and the procedure canceled or finished as soon as possible. The single area of agreement is that these patients should ultimately undergo malignant hyperthermia testing (muscle contracture responses to halothane or caffeine). With muscle biopsy evaluation of malignant hyperthermia susceptibility in these patients, we will, with time, understand the relevance of trismus.

MALIGNANT HYPERTHERMIA In susceptible individuals, succinylcholine results in a dramatic increase in oxygen consumption and lactate production.[91,92] Used by itself, succinylcholine provokes a brief episode that may not become fulminant.[91–93] If the dose is repeated[92] or associated with the use of potent volatile anesthetic agents,[79] malignant hyperthermia is likely to become fulminant (see the subsection of Muscle, Malignant Hyperthermia).

RHABDOMYOLYSIS In normal individuals, succinylcholine usually increases blood creatine phosphokinase (CK) values[94] and provokes a modest release of myoglobin from skeletal muscle.[95–98] This is more marked when succinylcholine is used in association with potent volatile agents, such as halothane, and is less marked following pretreatment by a small dose of a nondepolarizer or when anesthesia involves a nitrous-narcotic-barbiturate technique. In some patients, the release of myoglobin may be severe, leading to extensive rhabdomyolysis, port wine urine, and the threat of renal failure.[99–101] This breakdown sometimes involves concomitant acute hyperkalemia. Rhabdomyolysis may occur in otherwise normal people or with malignant hyperthermia or certain dystrophies. With rhabdomyolysis, myoglobin release into the blood precedes the increase in CK by several hours[102] so the myoglobin rise can be completely missed.

PROLONGED ACTION Unlike nondepolarizing relaxants, it is unusual for the duration of action of succinylcholine to be significantly altered by diseases or drug interactions. The action of succinylcholine is prolonged in patients with huge overdoses, cholinesterase deficiencies, or pregnancy. Whether cimetidine prolongs blockade is controversial,[103,104] but if it does, it is not due to effects upon cholinesterase.[105]

Non-End-Plate Relaxants

There is little information concerning alteration of dantrolene's effect by disease. One patient with myasthenia gravis initially showed resistance to twitch depression by dantrolene.[106] Dantrolene produces more weakness in those susceptible to malignant hyperthermia than in normal people.[107] Alteration of clearance and metabolism may occur if there is hepatic dysfunction or shocklike states. Patients with myopathies or clinical weakness may be very sensitive to dantrolene.

EVIDENCE IN DISEASE STATES

Central Nervous System Tumors and Increased Intracranial Pressure

In 1959, Halldin and Wåhlin showed that succinylcholine increases intraspinal fluid pressure in anesthetized normal human volunteers.[68] This finding was confirmed in patients at risk for elevated intracranial pressure by McLeskey et al. in 1974.[108] Succinylcholine activates muscle spindles thereby stimulating the central nervous system; this in turn increases cerebral blood flow.[71,109,110] Whether this effect is clinically relevant is unclear. Succinylcholine has been used to prevent an increase in intracranial pressure during endotracheal suctioning,[111] but these patients had diffuse brain injuries and may not have had decreased intracranial compliance. A recent study in patients with intracranial pathology demonstrated no appreciable effect of succinylcholine on intracranial pressure.[112] If activation of muscle spindles is inhibited by prior complete nondepolarizing blockade, succinylcholine does not stimulate muscle spindles and thus does not increase intracranial pressure.[113] Administration of a smaller dose of a nondepolarizing relaxant before succinylcholine, however, produces conflicting results.[108,114] Without complete blockade of postsynaptic receptors on muscle spindles, it is possible that enough muscle spindle activation will occur to increase intracranial pressure. Many clinicians believe that an anesthetic induction involving a cerebral vasoconstrictor (e.g., thiopental), hyperventilation, and pretreatment with a nondepolarizing muscle relaxant will sufficiently attenuate increases in intracranial pressure due to succinylcholine.

Some nondepolarizing muscle relaxants release enough histamine to increase intracranial pressure. *d*-Tubocurarine, 0.6 mg/kg, increased intracranial pressure.[46] Atracurium had no effect on patients with space-occupying lesions.[115] Apparently, under the conditions of the study, atracurium's histamine release was inconsequential. Histamine release varies directly with dose and speed of administration, and the effect is attenuated by giving smaller doses at a slower rate.[9] Vecuronium generally does not alter intracranial pressure[116] but occasionally releases histamine,[8] it transiently inhibits histamine metabolism and can augment the effect of histamine released by another agent.[117,118]

Upper Motor Neuron Lesions

Upper motor neuron lesions produce sensitivity to succinylcholine and cause hyperkalemia presumably due to receptor proliferation (up-regulation).[26,48] In those disorders involving sensitivity to succinylcholine due to up-regulation, resistance to nondepolarizing relaxants should occur. This is amply demonstrated.[37,38,41,119,120] The hyperkalemic response is clinically important if a significant amount of muscle is involved; thus a monoplegia probably would not result in significant systemic hyperkalemia, whereas the paraplegic or hemiplegic patient has a marked risk.[51,121,122]

The initial flaccidity noted during the period of spinal shock or immediately after a stroke reflects neuronal inactivity, functionally like a lower motor neuron lesion.[123] In this situation, there is a rapid development of extrajunctional receptors, and the hyperkalemic response occurs within 4 days. However, experimentally, this spread is modest, similar to that in disuse atrophy, even though the hyperkalemic response, when quantitated, resembles that of denervation.[48] Also, the hyperkalemic response persists longer than spinal shock.[121,124] The duration of the hyperkalemic response to succinylcholine after an upper motor neuron lesion occurs is unknown. Succinylcholine was extensively used in the 1950s and early 1960s in patients with chronic cord lesions when succinylcholine-induced hyperkalemia was not yet recognized. There were no reports of cardiac arrest in these patients. The later reports describing cardiac arrest in patients with upper motor neuron lesions were related to lesions of more recent onset (i.e., several months). Presently, it cannot be stated for certain the duration of time for which the patient with an upper motor neuron lesion is at risk for hyperkalemia. Animal data[124] suggest that this may be limited, but although most evidence in humans suggests that this lasts about 1 year, one article reports abnormal responses up to 7 years after the lesion.[125] The authors' bias is that the absence of resistance to nondepolarizing relaxants would portend a normal response to succinylcholine. Resistance to nondepolarizing relaxants can persist for many years, longer than sensitivity to succinylcholine.[38] This resistance can be seen in either spastic or flaccid weak limbs; normal unaffected limbs (or muscles) should be used for the nerve stimulator.[37] Unaffected limbs can show a lesser degree of resistance,[41] perhaps due to disuse. When spasticity persists without any weakness, sensitivity to nondepolarizing relaxants can occur,[126] like that seen with exercise.[29]

There are many central nervous system disorders that will produce upper-motor neuron lesions and susceptibility to hyperkalemia after succinylcholine: trauma,[127,128] Huntington's chorea, stroke, tetanus,[129] spinal cord lesions,[51,121] encephalitis,[130] and multiple sclerosis involving motor nuclei.[119,125,131] If there is motor involvement—flaccidity, spasticity, or hyper-reflexia — these patients have become sensitive to succinylcholine by the fourth day after onset, and hyperkalemia will result with its use. Pretreatment will not protect against cardiac arrest in this situation,[128] and succinylcholine must be avoided in these patients.[51,132]

Closed head injuries producing coma without noticeable motor involvement have also resulted in significant hyperkalemia with succinylcholine.[127,128] Hyperkalemia after succinylcholine in patients with cerebral aneurysms and no neurologic deficit has been noted,[133] but this finding is contradicted by a more recent study.[134] The etiology of hyperkalemia in central nervous system disorders lacking overt motor neuron lesions is unclear.

Parkinson's disease, even when poorly controlled, does not appear to be a risk factor for significant hyperkalemia,[135] although there is one case reported of hyperkalemia some time after a prolonged succinylcholine infusion in a complex patient.[136] Patients with cerebral palsy or myelomeningocele demonstrate a normal response to succinylcholine and are not at risk for succinylcholine-induced hyperkalemia, perhaps because there is no recent change in motor innervation and abnormal myofibrils have degenerated.[137,138] Patients with multiple sclerosis without motor involvement may receive succinylcholine without hazard. If there has been recent onset of motor involvement in a patient with fluctuating multiple sclerosis, the risk of succinylcholine-induced hyperkalemia recurs.[125,131]

Tetanus patients can exhibit normal sensitivity to nondepolarizing relaxants,[139] and their tetany can be managed with nondepolarizing relaxants[140] or dantrolene.[14,141] With dantrolene, intubation may not be required.

Peripheral Nerve Lesions and Lower Motor Neuron Lesions

These involve destruction of the anterior horn cell or its peripheral motor nerve. Disorders include poliomyelitis, the postpolio syndrome,[142] polyneuropathy,[47] Guillain-Barré, and direct denervation.[76] In these situations, there is an extensive spread of receptor sites in extrajunctional areas. By the fourth day following onset, the involved muscle shows a marked efflux of potassium following the use of succinylcholine[49–51] as well as muscle contracture.[49,76,78] The hyperkalemic response persists until there is return of function or complete muscle atrophy. In Guillain-Barré and polio, hyperkalemia may occur after return of function (see below). Resistance to nondepolarizing relaxants is difficult to document because of the lack of function of the motor nerve.

Convalescent Guillain-Barré patients still have extensive involvement of their skeletal musculature in this denervation phenomenon. Succinylcholine may produce pronounced hyperkalemia.[143] This cannot be circumvented through use of smaller doses, because this is indeed a supersensitivity phenomenon in which doses of succinylcholine that are inadequate to paralyze normal muscle still result in pronounced hyperkalemia.[49]

The postpolio patient can have ongoing denervation, as the surviving motor neurons that have extensively arborized to those muscle fibers denervated in the initial disease now themselves prematurely senesce.[142] Gradually progressive denervation may cause few symptoms as the patient accommodates to the subtle changes. These patients present a continuing risk for succinylcholine-induced hyperkalemia.

Acquired neuromyotonia (Isaacs syndrome, armadillo syndrome) is an unusual lower motor neuron disease characterized by myokymia (muscle twitching), stiffness, and decreased tendon reflexes. The defect appears to be in the distal nerve, producing repetitive discharges. Curare produces complete relaxation,but regional nerve blockade does not.[144] These patients may be resistant to nondepolarizing muscle relaxants.[145]

Even though neurofibromatosis may cause lower motor neuron lesions, there have been several case reports of unexplained sensitivity to nondepolarizing muscle relaxants.[146–148] In one carefully studied patient without apparent peripheral neuropathy, the response to both succinylcholine and atracurium was normal.[149] These authors speculate that increased sensitivity, when it occurs, is due to elevated levels of nerve growth factor seen in some of these patients.

Charcot-Marie-Tooth disease is a hereditary disorder consisting of demyelinating peripheral neuropathy with muscle atrophy.[150] It is the most common inherited neuromuscular disease. Nondepolarizing muscle relaxants have a varying effect on Charcot-Marie-Tooth patients. The denervationlike process might lead to resistance. However, severe muscular atrophy might severely impair affected muscles' function with lower than usual degrees of blockade. Small doses and close monitoring is the most appropriate course. Despite the denervation that occurs with this disease, succinylcholine appears safe,[150] probably because these denervated muscles are severely atrophied. However, it is prudent to avoid succinylcholine in a patient with a recent acute exacerbation.

Mixed Upper and Lower Motor Neuron Lesions

Amyotrophic lateral sclerosis involves degeneration of lower motor neurons, brainstem motor nuclei, and descending pathways from upper motor neurons.[151] This combination of upper and lower motor neuron lesions results in signs of both spasticity and fasiculations. Ongoing motor unit denervation places the patient at risk for succinylcholine-induced hyperkalemia. The remaining motor neurons arborize to innervate the orphaned muscle cells, but the restored innervation apparently has a reduced margin of safety, resulting in increased sensitivity to nondepolarizing muscle relaxants, similar to that seen in myasthenia gravis.[151]

Friedreich's ataxia also involves both upper and lower motor neurons. As with amyotrophic lateral sclerosis, succinylcholine is contraindicated. Three reports feature normal sensitivity to vecuronium[152] and atracurium[153] and undue sensitivity to curare.[154]

Neuromuscular Junction

MYASTHENIA GRAVIS Approximately 5 people in every 100,000 have myasthenia gravis. In these patients, increasing effort produces increasing weakness. Muscles innervated by cranial nerves and the proximal limb musculature usually are most seriously involved. The severity of the disease varies widely among individuals, over time in the same patient, and even between muscle groups in the same patient. Myasthenia gravis is an autoimmune phenomenon in which there are deficient numbers of functioning acetylcholine receptors on the postjunctional membrane.[28,155] As a result, there can be extraordinary sensitivity to nondepolarizing relaxants. Further, the use of anticholinesterases to increase strength may place the patient in a situation in which there is an excessive acetylcholine effect similar to the phase II desensitization block seen with succinylcholine. This is called a *cholinergic crisis*.

Anticholinesterase medications are frequently withdrawn or tapered the night before an anesthetic (e.g., two-thirds the normal dose the evening before the anesthetic and none thereafter[156]) to avoid precipitating a cholinergic crisis. If anticholinesterase agents need to be continued or reinstituted, the intravenous dose is approximately 1/30th the oral dose, and the intramuscular dose is approximately 1/20th the oral dose. Before assuming that weakness is due to insufficient anticholinesterase medication, cautious testing with small doses of edrophonium (initially 2 mg IV, then 8 mg IV if no response) is warranted.[157] If muscle strength increases with edrophonium, the patient should benefit from further anticholinesterase medication. Otherwise the patient is probably overtreated.

Intubation may be facilitated when necessary with succinylcholine. Pretreatment with a small dose of nondepolarizing relaxant is potentially hazardous. These patients appear to be two to three-fold resistant to succinylcholine, but the effective dose of 95% of the patients (ED_{95}) (calculated from a limited number of patients) still is probably less than 1.0 mg/kg.[158] Onset of block with succinylcholine might be prolonged, but with 1.0 mg/kg IV, full blockade ensues.[159] A larger dose may hasten onset of block, but this has not been studied. Recovery might also be prolonged and is marked by the appearance of a nondepolarizing block, which may last for 1½ hours. This is related to the degree of cholinesterase inhibition due to anticholinesterase therapy.[160]

Nondepolarizing muscle relaxants may be avoided by utilizing the relaxant effects of the potent inhalational agents in combination with the patient's pre-existent muscle weakness.[159,161] If nondepolarizing relaxants are used, careful administration of small increments of an intermediate or short-acting agent (e.g., atracurium, cis-atracurium, rocuronium, vecuronium, or mivacurium) monitored by a nerve stimulator is safest.[156,162,163] The effective dose varies from less than 10% of normal[164] to near normal,[165] on average 40% of normal.[166] The duration of the mivacurium blockade appears slightly prolonged due to anticholinesterase drugs.[167] An anticholinesterase may be administered for antagonism but cautiously to avoid cholinergic crisis. With atracurium or mivacurium, antagonists may be unnecessary if complete spontaneous recovery is allowed to occur, as recovery time of either is reasonably short.[163,165,168] In the future, shorter-duration nondepolarizing muscle relaxants may simplify the management of these patients. Although monitoring of the neuromuscular blockade is vital, a single muscle (e.g., adductor pollicis) may not accurately reflect the status of the bulbar and respiratory muscles due to different degrees of myasthenic involvement. The ability of the patient to breathe (e.g., peak negative inspiratory pressure) and maintain his/her airway must be independently assessed before extubation and resumption of spontaneous ventilation.

Because the margin of safety of neuromuscular transmission decreases with loss of postsynaptic receptors, some drugs not classified as muscle relaxants but that alter neuromuscular transmission can increase muscle weakness in these patients. These include aminoglycosides, polymixins, quinine, quinidine, and β-adrenergic blockers.[28]

LAMBERT-EATON MYASTHENIC SYNDROME

The Lambert-Eaton myasthenic syndrome classically occurs in patients with high-grade pulmonary malignancies, although it is now recognized that the non-neoplastic form of the syndrome can occur in association with other autoimmune diseases.[169] These patients have weakness predominantly in the lower extremities and the proximal musculature, with increased fatiguability of most muscles of the body. Strength is reduced in rested muscles but increases briefly during the beginning of maximum voluntary contraction. This is related to the unique electromyography (EMG) findings of growth during stimulation. Thus, after rest, there is marked facilitation during activity, and this distinguishes it from the fade and weakness observed in myasthenia. The physiologic lesion appears to be a reduced release of quanta from the nerve terminal by the nerve impulse. These patients are generally not helped by anticholinesterase drugs and may have a normal response to succinylcholine. They may be very sensitive to the effect of nondepolarizing muscle relaxants, even in apparently unaffected muscle groups.[126]

BOTULISM, MAGNESIUM TOXICITY

Botulinum poisoning and magnesium intoxication reduce the release of transmitter quanta by each nerve impulse, mimicking the clinical and EMG features of the Lambert-Eaton syndrome.[169] It would be expected in these situations that the number and quality of postjunctional receptors may be unaltered and that there should be a normal response to succinylcholine and perhaps sensitivity to nondepolarizing relaxants, as with the Lambert-Eaton syndrome. However, in one study, magnesium reduced the effect of succinylcholine.[170] Because these patients are decidedly weak, little relaxation may be required, and if needed at all, a very small dose of a short-duration muscle relaxant may suffice.

THE INTENSIVE CARE UNIT PATIENT

Befitting the complexity of intensive care unit (ICU) patients, various neuromuscular syndromes may arise. Several appear related to prolonged nondepolarizing muscle relaxant use.

By inhibiting acetylcholine receptors, nondepolarizing muscle relaxants produce a state akin to denervation. If lack of acetylcholine receptor stimulation produces the receptor proliferation seen in denervation, you would expect to see the same with chronic blockade. Proliferation should cause resistance to nondepolarizing muscle relaxants. Dodson et al. indeed found both proliferation and resistance in these patients as well as a correlation between receptor number and muscle relaxant dose.[171] This proliferation may also explain the sporadic reports of hyperkalemia with succinylcholine in intensive care unit ICU patients.

A second phenomenon is steroid myopathy. These patients have elevated creatine kinase (CK) concentrations as well as myopathic changes in muscle biopsy specimens. There is the suggestion that neuromuscular blockers may accentuate the syndrome,[172] either because of structural similarity of the steroid-based nondepolarizing muscle relaxants[173] or from the accelerating effect that denervation (effected by neuromuscular blockade) has on the development of steroid myopathy.[174,175]

Prolonged paralysis following muscle relaxants may have several different causes. Besides the above-mentioned denervation changes and steroid myopathy, ICU patients may develop polyneuropathy of critical illness.[171,173] Also, with renal or hepatic dysfunction, the muscle relaxants or their less active metabolites may accumulate. Whatever the cause, monitoring the effects of neuromuscular blockade with a nerve stimulator will allow tracking neuromuscular function (at least in the stimulated muscle groups).

Muscle

Myopathies are not uncommon in the general population, and many are inherited. Most result from a single point mutation, so there is a high probability of recurrence within families.[122] Adequate understanding and treatment require an accurate diagnosis because the typical findings are nonspecific and variable. The progressive muscular dystrophies are heterogeneous, and their classification depends on the pattern of inheritance in the specific family, the severity, the muscle groups typically involved, and the age at onset. Myopathies that involve diminished numbers of functioning end-plate receptors or contractile bundles may produced increased sensitivity to the action of muscle relaxants in general.

OCCULT MYOPATHY Patients with an occult or undiscovered myopathy (frequently Duchenne dystrophy) may develop sudden and unexpected abnormal responses during anesthesia, usually but not always[101] in association with the use of succinylcholine. The manifestations of these responses can be abrupt and devastating, and totally unanticipated mortality is not uncommon. These responses include rhabdomyolysis, hyperkalemia, and cardiac arrest.[97,100,101,176–178] Due to the X-linked transmission of the more common dystrophies, these events predominantly occur in young boys, typically younger than 7 years old.

A series of such incidents precipitated a controversial label change for succinylcholine.[179] This has since been changed to a boxed warning. Because this risk is so small, many pediatric anesthesiologists continue to use succinylcholine in elective surgery. If cardiac arrest occurs after succinylcholine, hyperkalemia must be considered. All efforts should be expended to resuscitate the patient, including use of calcium and, in rare instances, cardiopulmonary bypass.[180]

DUCHENNES AND OTHER DYSTROPHIES Duchenne and Becker dystrophies are caused by quantitative and qualitative alterations in a single myofibril surface membrane protein, dystrophin.[181] This leads to the fundamental disorder, a severe myopathy usually detectable at birth and associated with elevated levels of CK. The Duchenne type is associated with an absence of dystrophin and Becker dystrophy is related to an abnormal dystrophin.[181] These and other similar myopathies are highly variable in part because the associated gene is large and with its many base pairs can lead to numerous mutations.

Despite a report citing a lack of problems in Duchenne patients under anesthesia,[182] several risks have been documented. The increase in permeability that is reflected by the elevated CK values makes these patients more subject to acute rhabdomyolysis after succinylcholine.[99,183] Hyperkalemic cardiac arrest after succinylcholine can occur with or without rhabdomyolysis.[184] In addition, the Duchenne patient frequently has an associated cardiomyopathy. Anesthetic depression can therefore lead to sudden cardiac arrest with difficult resuscitation.[178,185] Due to leaky muscle cell membranes, abnormal calcium fluxes may produce hypermetabolism. Thus, anesthetic problems with Duchenne dystrophy may include hypermetabolism, rhabdomyolysis, hyperkalemia, and sudden and unexpected cardiac arrest. These patients must not be given succinylcholine. The safety of potent inhalational anesthetics is disputed. Some would give volatile anesthetics, while others would not. If there is significant disuse atrophy of normal muscle due to inactivity imposed by affected myopathic muscle, there can be resistance to nondepolarizing relaxants.[24,39,186] Because of these uncertainties, the clinician should use a nerve stimulator to guide doses of nondepolarizing relaxants. The alternative is to avoid relaxants completely and intubate during depression by other agents.

Fascioscapulohumeral dystrophy is a rare syndrome distinct from the Becker and Duchenne varieties; its incidence is 1 in 100,000 and it has autosomal dominant inheritance, whereas the Becker and Duchenne are X-linked recessive. Disability is usually not severe, and cardiac involvement is not associated.[187] One patient had normal sensitivity to a bolus of atracurium but unusually fast recovery time.[188]

MYOTONIA AND PARAMYOTONIA Myotonias are disorders in which muscle relaxation is delayed after effort. Myotonic dystrophy, by far the most common form, refers to myotonic patients with significant histologic dystrophic findings, weakness, and muscular hypoplasia.[189] The other forms of myotonia are not progressive and include paramyotonia: very rare, with prolonged contracture and weakness with cold exposure; and myotonia congenita: onset early in life, prominent contractures, some muscular hypertrophy, and little weakness. We have not seen reports concerning paramyotonia. Succinylcholine produces a transient contracture in patients with myotonic dystrophy or myotonia congenita.[72–75] These contractures are not clinically associated with hyperkalemia or malignant hyperthermia as established partly from human data and from study of the myotonic goat.[190] Although recent muscle biopsy contracture data are consistent with susceptibility to malignant hyperthermia,[191,192] the association is not well supported by clinical reports (see Malignant Hyperthermia). Prolonged infusion of succinylcholine (not recommended) can produce relaxation.[75] Dantrolene has been inadequate for relaxation in myotonia,[193] probably because the multiple depolarizations overwhelm the relatively weak blockade by dantrolene, which reduces the response to a single stimulus more than to repetitive stimuli.[15] Nondepolarizing relaxants are safe in these patients; some do not appear to have undue sensitivity,[194–196] whereas others may.[197] Neostigmine may exacerbate weakness instead of reversing relaxant effects,[198] and short-duration relaxants without neostigmine reversal may be preferred.[194,199] These patients (especially those with myotonia congenita and paramyotonia) may be receiving antimyotonic drugs, including quinine and procainamide, which potentiate neuromuscular blockade with nondepolarizing agents, or phenytoin, which antagonizes blockade (Table 14.1).[42,43]

INFLAMMATORY MYOPATHIES This is a heterogeneous group of disorders, including polymyositis, dermatomyositis, and myositis ossificans progressiva, resulting from a variety of causes—parasitic, viral, inclusion bodies, infections, and immunologic alterations.[200] EMG features of inflammatory myopathies include decreased numbers of muscle fibers in a motor unit and increased percentage of polyphasic motor unit potentials. There is progressive weakness, and the anesthetic and muscle relaxant must be planned with regard to the degree of disability. Improvement in the clinical course is generally associated with increased muscle strength. With marked muscle weakness, relaxants may not be required. It is always important to estimate relaxant effects using a nerve stimulator. Because this group of disorders involves direct inflammation of muscle, it appears unlikely that hyperkalemia would be a problem with succinylcholine. Three reports concern relaxants: one observed prolonged paralysis with vecuronium,[201] and two noted normal responses with nondepolarizing relaxants.[202,203]

FAMILIAL PERIODIC PARALYSIS This is a syndrome of multiple etiologies, transmitted by autosomal dominant inheritance, featuring varying changes in serum potassium during the paralytic attack—hypokalemia, normokalemia, or hyperkalemia. Each form of periodic paralysis produces electrical inexcitability of the muscle fiber surface membrane other than at the end plate.[204] There is hypopolarization of the muscle fiber surface membrane during paralysis. Propagation of the action potential then fails because either the resting membrane potential is so small that the sodium channel is inactivated or the sodium channel is abnormally sensitive to inactivation by even minor membrane depolarization. It is unlikely that a patient would be anesthetized during an acute attack when weakness is profound. Motor weakness may persist between attacks from either destruction of muscle tissue or subclinical chronic hypopolarization ("abortive attacks").[205] If potassium levels remain normal, anesthetic agents and depolarizing and nondepolarizing relaxants are well tolerated.[206–209] Should a patient with an acute attack require anesthesia, the anesthesiologist should remember that the muscle bundles of affected muscles are inexcitable to either direct or indirect electrical stimulation during the attacks. Thus, the associated muscles are flaccid and would not require muscle relaxants. Other unaffected muscles within the body could be most easily managed by use of suitable doses of nondepolarizing relaxants.

THERMAL TRAUMA Muscle responses are altered in burned patients because of known and unknown factors altering the pharmacodynamics of the acetylcholine receptors. The final common pathway, however, is up-regulation of acetylcholine receptors.[26] Some factors have been identified: there may be denervation of some muscle beneath the burn wound. The prolonged period of convalescence imposes whole-body disuse atrophy, which is associated with mild increases in serum potassium after succinylcholine[61] and with relaxant resistance.[24,34–36,39] Careful analysis by Martyn has demonstrated that the changes due to disuse are insufficient to explain the overall altered responses to muscle relaxants.[34] There also may be a circulating plasma factor that in part confers resistance. Data from rats show increased numbers of diaphragmatic acetylcholine receptors[210] as well as proliferation of receptors in unburned limbs.[211]

Patients with thermal trauma develop a hyperkalemic response to succinylcholine by approximately 7 to 10 days postburn.[52,53] This is related to the size of the burn, but the altered response can be seen in patients with burns as small as 15% second degree. This hyperkalemic response persists until the wound is covered, and the patient is healing well and gaining weight. This period is approximately 2 months in most burn patients. Because of up-regulation, there is about a two- to threefold resistance to nondepolarizing relaxants, starting within a week of the burn.[35,36,212] This resistance to nondepolarizing relaxants is felt to wane about or after the time the hyperkalemic response disappears but can be observed up to a year following recovery from the burn.[213]

IMMOBILIZATION DISUSE ATROPHY Up-regulation occurs with disuse atrophy, associated with a modest hyperkalemic response to succinylcholine, based upon a modest spread of receptor sites in association with disuse.[61] Disuse atrophy does not generally involve the entire body, and it is therefore not regularly associated with serious and severe hyperkalemia after succinylcholine. Calculations suggest that disuse would result in an increase in arterial serum potassium of 2 to 3 mEq/L after succinylcholine only if the muscle disuse affected virtually all the skeletal muscle of the body. Clinical reports appear to demonstrate this.[214,215] Muscle disuse is associated with resistance to nondepolarizing relaxants, which is two- to threefold in a mock clinical (non–steady-state) situation[39] and eightfold in the same dog model when plasma relaxant concentrations were in near equilibrium with receptor sites.[24] Thus the patient who has disuse atrophy will have resistance to nondepolarizing relaxants in the affected limb or muscle. Neuromuscular monitoring should involve the normal muscles of that patient.

INFECTION Prolonged intra-abdominal infection, such as a subhepatic or subdiaphragmatic abscess, appears to alter relaxant responses much the same as thermal trauma.[54,55] Disuse may be a factor in this. About 7 to 10 days following onset, a hyperkalemic response develops, and the duration is related to successful convalescence, with healing and weight gain. Again, because of up-regulation, there should be associated resistance to nondepolarizing relaxants, but supporting data are lacking.

MUSCLE TRAUMA Even minor muscle trauma, for example, a degenerating nerve laid across the muscle surface, results in the development of extrajunctional receptor sites and an increase in sensitivity to cholinergic agonists.[57,58] This response can be as pronounced as with a lower motor neuron lesion. Therefore, in someone with direct muscle trauma or a muscle crush injury, a hyperkalemic response to succinylcholine, not present immediately after injury, appears within 4 days.[56,59,60] This will persist until excision or healing of the affected part. If the degree of muscle involved by the trauma is extensive, then succinylcholine is contraindicated. This may also occur after radiation[216] or ischemic atherosclerosis.[217] We suspect that resistance to nondepolarizing relaxants also occurs in this situation but have no supporting data.

METABOLIC MYOPATHIES

Malignant Hyperthermia. Potent inhalational anesthetic agents trigger this rare genetic subclinical myopathy to produce hypermetabolism and systemic acidosis. The youngest person apparently developing malignant hyperthermia was an unborn baby, whose normal mother received triggering agents for a caesarean section.[218] The baby was born with rigidity and other signs of malignant hyperthermia, presumably paternally inherited. Nondepolarizing relaxants do not trigger this syndrome, despite clinical reports incriminating curare[219] and pancuronium.[220] The latter was correctly criticized.[221] However, curare has a weak depolarizing effect: two laboratory reports indicate that curare produces a contracture in denervated muscle.[222,223] A porcine experiment cited pancuronium as a trigger, but it was given during halothane anesthesia.[224] Overall, clinical evidence supports the safety of nondepolarizing relaxants in malignant hyperthermia. The unique intracellular muscle relaxant dantrolene is specific for treating malignant hyperthermia and can be used to relax contractures or rigidity related to malignant hyperthermia or other disorders that feature contractures or severe rigidity.

Malignant hyperthermia is known to be associated with several myopathies: King Denborough syndrome[225–227] and central core disease.[228,229] In susceptible pigs, the ryanodine receptor gene on chromosome 6 is altered. In humans, this gene is on chromosome 19. A number of different ryanodine receptor mutations have been found in affected families, but in most families the gene defect is unidentified. Other potential causative mutations include abnormalities in the dihydropyridine receptor, lipase and IP_3. One patient with a chromosomal anomaly, Wolf-Hirschhorn syndrome, apparently developed malignant hyperthermia.[230] Malignant hyperthermia has also been controversially suggested as associated with other disorders. The difficulty is interpretation of a positive caffeine-halothane contracture response from a muscle biopsy in a person with no personal or family history of malignant hyperthermia.[231] Positive biopsy responses are probably not unique to malignant hyperthermia, but how should questions such as these be decided? For the neuroleptic malignant syndrome, some contracture evidence suggests an association,[232] some does not[233,234]; clinical results do not.[235] Heiman-Patterson et al. reported positive malignant hyperthermia biopsies in 10 of 25 consecutive patients being evaluated for neuromuscular disorders.[192] Two had unusual anesthesia events. Considering these data, these authors now include myotonia as malignant hyperthermia related. Yet support for this position is weak (see Myotonia and Paramyotonia).

Neuroleptic Malignant Syndrome. Neuroleptic malignant syndrome, characterized by hyperthermia, parkinsonism, rigidity, autonomic disturbances (e.g. tachycardia, diaphoresis, and blood pressure lability), dystonia, and rhabdomyolysis, occurs in some patients after initiation of neuroleptic therapy.[232,236] It can occur up to 2 months after a new agent is started and can persist for over 1 month.[236] It can also occur soon after an anesthetic in which an antiemetic neuroleptic is given.[237] Due to the resemblance of this syndrome to malignant hyperthermia, some speculate that this disease is caused by a similar or the same myofibrillar metabolic defect as malignant hyperthermia. Studies examining muscle biopsies have yielded conflicting results.[232–234] No cases of coexistent neuroleptic malignant syndrome and malignant hyperthermia have been reported, and patients with neuroleptic malignant syndrome have been treated by electroconvulsive therapy (and repetitive succinylcholine administration) without triggering malignant hyperthermia.[235,238] Note, however, that succinylcholine given during a time of rhabdomyolysis and bed rest did cause serious hyperkalemia in one patient.[239] Neuroleptic malignant syndrome may be the result of rapid decrease in dopaminergic transmission.[236] Not only does administration of neuroleptics (which are dopamine antagonists) induce the syndrome, but so does the *withdrawal* of dopaminergic drugs, such as levodopa.[240] Therapy with dopamine agonists like bromocriptine appears effective, as does the administration of dantrolene.[236] The effectiveness of dantrolene appears to be related to its reduction of muscle tone and metabolism, thereby diminishing heat production, fever, and acid-base problems.

Glycogen Storage Diseases. These can be mistaken for or associated with malignant hyperthermia; the differentiation may be difficult.[241–243] Glycogen storage diseases usually involve a compensatory metabolic acidosis because of lack of substrate. This metabolic acidosis should be identified in the preoperative period so that you are not confounded by a sudden and unexpected blood gas result. Glycogen storage diseases can be associated with malignant hyperthermia and the syndrome can be dramatically fulminant: Simmons et al. describe a 5-year-old boy whose malignant hyperthermia episode recurred repeatedly, requiring dantrolene, 16 mg/kg.[243]

Mitochondrial Myopathies. Abnormalities of mitochondrial metabolism are uncommon.[244] There are at least 25 different disease entities already identified involving defects in either mitochondrial substrate transport, substrate utilization, the respiratory chain, or energy conservation and transduction. They can be associated with hypermetabolism, for example, a threefold increase in basal oxygen consumption. These patients frequently have progressive muscular weakness and may have cardiomyopathy. They may be associated with progressive external ophthalmoplegia. Anesthetic considerations include those statements made about myopathies in general regarding overall muscle weakness or muscle atrophy (see the section Muscle).

Myoadenylate Deaminase. This is the most common of the known enzyme defects of skeletal muscle. Patients develop signs in early adulthood or middle age. They become aware of postexertional fatigue or weakness along with soreness or cramping. They never become paralyzed but their performance level diminishes. CK is mildly elevated, occasionally above 1,000. This appears to be an inherited genetic disorder involving a permanent enzyme deficit in all skeletal muscles. The enzyme is generally activated under hypoxic conditions, and therefore the patient can be tested for this with an ischemic forearm fatigue protocol. The increase in ammonia as a percentage of the increase in lactate following fatiguing ischemic exercise constitutes the criterion for diagnosis. Unequivocal diagnosis requires histoenzymatic staining of a muscle biopsy, which demonstrates the absence of adenosine monophosphate deaminase. You would not expect problems with muscle relaxants, although muscle biopsy results suggest that malignant hyperthermia may be involved.[245] This interesting theory is unsupported.

SUMMARY

Because muscle relaxants affect neuromuscular transmission, it is inevitable that there will be interactions between muscle relaxants and neuromuscular disease. The depolarizing muscle relaxant succinylcholine causes many problems in this setting. Potentially lethal hyperkalemia can be produced by succinylcholine for many months after the onset of motor neuron dysfunction, burn, infection, or muscle trauma and is always a hazard in patients with certain myopathies, especially Duchenne muscular dystrophy. It can also produce varying degrees of rhabdomyolysis and associated hyperkalemia. Succinylcholine produces trismus and can produce contracture in patients with myotonia or susceptibility to malignant hyperthermia. Succinylcholine depolarizes muscle spindles, resulting in central nervous system activation that can increase intracranial pressure. Yet succinylcholine is advantageous in some patients without these diseases because it has the fastest onset and shortest duration of all available muscle relaxants. Succinylcholine may eventually be replaced if ultrashort-acting nondepolarizing relaxants are developed.

Some nondepolarizing muscle relaxants increase intracranial pressure or decrease cerebral perfusion pressure by releasing histamine or inhibiting its metabolism. The effect may be reduced by choosing an agent with less histamine effect, administering the agent slowly, or pretreating with H_1 and H_2 blocking drugs. Clinically, only curare is known to significantly affect cerebral blood flow.

Many neuromuscular diseases affect the sensitivity to nondepolarizing relaxants. Sensitivity may vary from muscle to muscle and day to day. Commonly used drugs, including calcium channel blockers, corticosteroids, furosemide, hydantoins, volatile anesthetics, and many antibiotics also alter sensitivity. Unwanted excessive or insufficient effect can be avoided by monitoring a properly representative muscle with a nerve stimulator and judiciously administering incremental doses of muscle relaxant. Where undue sensitivity might occur, a shorter-acting drug will reduce the risk of prolonged action. Shorter-acting drugs can also minimize the need for anticholinesterase antagonism of neuromuscular blockade and reduce the problem with anticholinesterase administration in such diseases as the myotonias and myasthenia gravis. Future ultrashort-acting nondepolarizing relaxants will simplify the treatment of a patient sensitive to this class of drugs.

References

1. Engel AG, Franzini-Armstrong C, (eds). Myology: Basic and Clinical. 2nd Ed. McGraw-Hill, New York, 1994
2. Lee JA: Claude Bernard (1813–1878). Anaesthesia 33:741, 1978
3. Bowman WC: Block by depolarization (editorial). Acta Anaesthesiol Scand 38:529, 1994
4. Standaert FG: They won't go away! (editorial). Acta Anaesthesiol Scand 38:533, 1994
5. Azar I, Turndorf H: An unusual response to *d*-tubocurarine in a case of severe peripheral polyneuropathy. Anesthesiology 46:371, 1977
6. Waud BE, Waud DR: The relation between tetanic fade and receptor occlusion in the presence of competitive neuromuscular block. Anesthesiology 35:456, 1971
7. Pavlin EG: Clinical tests of recovery from neuromuscular blocking agents. Anesthesiol Clin North Am 11:379, 1993
8. Cannon JE, Fahey MR, Moss J, Miller RD: Large doses of vecuronium and plasma histamine concentrations. Can J Anaesth 35:350, 1988
9. Basta SJ: Modulation of histamine release by neuromuscular-blocking drugs. Curr Opin Anaesthesiol 5:572, 1992
10. Hosking MP, Lennon RL, Gronert GA: Combined H_1 and H_2 receptor blockade attenuates the cardiovascular effects of high-dose

atracurium for rapid sequence endotracheal intubation. Anesth Analg 67:1089, 1988
11. Burns BD, Paton WDM: Depolarization of the motor end-plate by decamethonium and acetylcholine. J Physiol (Lond) 115:41, 1951
12. Waud DR: The nature of "depolarization block." Anesthesiology 29:1014, 1968
13. Matthews-Bellinger J, Salpeter MM: Distribution of acetylcholine receptors at frog neuromuscular junctions with a discussion of some physiological implications. J Physiol (Lond) 279:197, 1978
14. Tidyman M, Prichard JG, Deamer RL, Mac N: Adjunctive use of dantrolene in severe tetanus. Anesth Analg 64:538, 1985
15. Krarup C: The effect of dantrolene on the enhancement and diminution of tension evoked by staircase and by tetanus in rat muscle. J Physiol (Lond) 311:389, 1981
16. Flewellen EH, Nelson TE, Bee DE: Effect of dantrolene on neuromuscular block by *d*-tubocurarine and subsequent antagonism by neostigmine in the rabbit. Anesthesiology 52:126, 1980
17. Lee C, Durant NN, Au E, Katz RL: Reversal of dantrolene sodium-induced depression of skeletal muscle in the cat. Anesthesiology 54:61–65, 1981
18. Lynch C III, Durbin CG, Jr, Fisher NA et al: Effects of dantrolene and verapamil on atrioventricular conduction and cardiovascular performance in dogs. Anesth Analg 65:252, 1986
19. Rubin AS, Zablocki AD: Hyperkalemia, verapamil, and dantrolene. Anesthesiology 66:246, 1987
20. Saltzman LS, Kates RA, Corke BC et al: Hyperkalemia and cardiovascular collapse after verapamil and dantrolene administration in swine. Anesth Analg 63:473, 1984
21. San Juan AC, Jr, Wong KC, Port JD: Hyperkalemia after dantrolene and verapamil-dantrolene administration in dogs. Anesth Analg 67:759, 1988
22. Yoganathan T, Casthely PA, Lamprou M: Dantrolene-induced hyperkalemia in a patient treated with diltiazem and metoprolol. J Cardiothorac Anesth 2:363, 1988
23. Melton AT, Antognini JF, Gronert GA: Prolonged duration of succinylcholine in patients receiving anticonvulsants: evidence for mild up-regulation of acetylcholine receptors? Can J Anaesth 40:939, 1993
24. Gronert GA, Matteo RS, Perkins S: Canine gastrocnemius disuse atrophy: resistance to paralysis by dimethyl tubocurarine. J Appl Physiol 57:1502, 1984
25. Sarvey JM, Albuquerque EX, Eldefrawi AT, Elderfrawi M: Effects of α-bungarotoxin and reversible cholinergic ligands on normal and denervated mammalian skeletal muscle. Membr Biochem 1:131, 1978
26. Martyn JAJ, White DA, Gronert GA et al: Up-and-down regulation of skeletal muscle acetylcholine receptors. Effects on neuromuscular blockers. Anesthesiology 76:822, 1992
27. Buzello W, Noeldge G, Krieg N, Brobmann GF: Vecuronium for muscle relaxation in patients with myasthenia gravis. Anesthesiology 64:507, 1986
28. Engel AG: Acquired autoimmune myasthenia gravis. p. 1769. In Engel AG, Franzini-Armstrong C (eds): Myology: Basic and Clinical. 2nd Ed. McGraw-Hill, New York, 1994
29. Gronert GA, White DA, Shafer SL, Matteo RS: Exercise produces sensitivity to metocurine. Anesthesiology 70:973, 1989
30. Waud BE, Amaki Y, Waud DR: Disuse and *d*-tubocurarine sensitivity in isolated muscles. Anesth Analg 64:1178, 1985
31. Heier T, Caldwell JE, Sharma ML et al: Mild intraoperative hypothermia does not change the pharmacodynamics (concentration-effect relationship) of vecuronium in humans. Anesth Analg 78:973, 1994
32. Buzello W, Schluermann D, Pollmaecher T, Spillner G: Unequal effects of cardiopulmonary bypass-induced hypothermia on neuromuscular blockade from constant infusion of alcuronium, d-tubocurarine, pancuronium, and vecuronium. Anesthesiology 66:842, 1987
33. Diefenbach C, Abel M, Buzello W: Greater neuromuscular blocking potency of atracurium during hypothermic than during normothermic cardiopulmonary bypass. Anesth Analg 75:675, 1992
34. Martyn J: Clinical pharmacology and drug therapy in the burned patient. Anesthesiology 65:67, 1986
35. Martyn JAJ, Matteo RS, Greenblatt DJ et al: Pharmacokinetics of *d*-tubocurarine in patients with thermal injury. Anesth Analg 61:241, 1982
36. Martyn JAJ, Szyfelbein SK, Ali HH et al: Increased d-tubocurarine requirement following major thermal injury. Anesthesiology 52:352, 1980

37. Graham DH: Monitoring neuromuscular block may be unreliable in patients with upper-motor-neuron lesions. Anesthesiology 52:74, 1980
38. Moorthy SS, Hilgenberg JC: Resistance to non-depolarizing muscle relaxants in paretic upper extremities of patients with residual hemiplegia. Anesth Analg 59:624, 1980
39. Gronert GA: Disuse atrophy with resistance to pancuronium. Anesthesiology 55:547, 1981
40. Waud BE, Waud DR: Tubocurarine sensitivity of the diaphragm after limb immobilization. Anesth Analg 65:493, 1986
41. Shayevitz JR, Matteo RS: Decreased sensitivity to metocurine in patients with upper motoneuron disease. Anesth Analg 64:767, 1985
42. Ornstein E, Matteo RS, Young WL, Diaz J: Resistance to metocurine-induced neuromuscular blockade in patients receiving phenytoin. Anesthesiology 63:294, 1985
43. Ornstein E, Matteo RS, Schwartz AE et al: The effect of phenytoin on the magnitude and duration of neuromuscular block following atracurium or vecuronium. Anesthesiology 67:191, 1987
44. Forbes HS, Wolff HG, Cobb S: The cerebral circulation. X. The action of histamine. Am J Physiol 89:266, 1929
45. Malkinson TJ, Cooper KE, Veale WL: Induced changes in intracranial pressure in the anesthetized rat and rabbit. Brain Res Bull 15:321, 1985
46. Tarkkanen L, Laitinen L, Johansson G: Effects of *d*-tubocurarine on intracranial pressure and thalamic electrical impedance. Anesthesiology 40:247, 1974
47. Azar I: The response of patients with neuromuscular disorders to muscle relaxants: a review. Anesthesiology 61:173, 1984
48. Gronert GA, Theye RA: Pathophysiology of hyperkalemia induced by succinylcholine. Anesthesiology 43:89, 1975
49. Gronert GA, Lambert EH, Theye RA: The response of denervated skeletal muscle to succinylcholine. Anesthesiology 39:13, 1973
50. John DA, Tobey RE, Homer LD, Rice CL: Onset of succinylcholine-induced hyperkalemia following denervation. Anesthesiology 45:294, 1976
51. Tobey RE, Jacobsen PM, Kahle CT et al: The serum potassium response to muscle relaxants in neural injury. Anesthesiology 37:332, 1972
52. Schaner PJ, Brown RL, Kirksey TD et al: Succinylcholine-induced hyperkalemia in burned patients. 1. Anesth Analg 48:764, 1969
53. Viby-Mogensen J, Hanel HK, Hansen E, Graae J: Serum cholinesterase activity in burned patients. II. Anaesthesia, suxamethonium and hyperkalaemia. Acta Anaesthesiol Scand 19:169, 1975
54. Khan TZ, Khan RM: Changes in serum potassium following succinylcholine in patients with infections. Anesth Analg 62:327, 1983
55. Kohlschütter B, Baur H, Roth F: Suxamethonium-induced hyperkalaemia in patients with severe intra-abdominal infections. Br J Anaesth 48:557, 1976
56. Birch AA, Jr, Mitchell GD, Playford GA, Lang CA: Changes in serum potassium response to succinylcholine following trauma. JAMA 210:490, 1969
57. Cangiano A, Magherini PC, Pasino E et al: Interaction of inactivity and nerve breakdown products in the origin of acute denervation changes in rat skeletal muscle. J Physiol (Lond) 355:345, 1984
58. Jones R, Vrbová G. Two factors responsible for the development of denervation hypersensitivity. J Physiol (Lond) 236:517, 1974
59. Kopriva C, Ratliff J, Fletcher JR et al: Serum potassium changes after succinylcholine in patients with acute massive muscle trauma. Anesthesiology 34:246, 1971
60. Mazze RI, Escue HM, Houston JB: Hyperkalemia and cardiovascular collapse following administration of succinylcholine to the traumatized patient. Anesthesiology 31:540, 1969
61. Gronert GA, Theye RA: Effect of succinylcholine on skeletal muscle with immobilization atrophy. Anesthesiology 40:268, 1974
62. Axelsson J, Thesleff S: A study of supersensitivity in denervated mammalian skeletal muscle. J Physiol (Lond) 149:178, 1957
63. Neher E, Sakmann B: Noise analysis of drug induced voltage clamp currents in denervated frog muscle fibres. J Physiol (Lond) 258:705, 1976
64. Maryniak JK, Henderson AM, Woodall NM et al: Beta-adrenoceptor blockade and suxamethonium-induced rise in plasma potassium. Anaesthesia 42:71, 1987
65. McCammon RL, Stoelting RK: Exaggerated increase in serum potassium following succinylcholine in dogs with beta blockade. Anesthesiology 61:723, 1984
66. Roth JL, Nugent M, Gronert GA: Verapamil does

not alter succinylcholine-induced increases in serum potassium during halothane anesthesia in normal dogs. Anesth Analg 64:1202, 1985
67. Antognini JF, Gronert GA: Succinylcholine causes profound hyperkalemia in hemorrhagic, acidotic rabbits. Anesth Analg 77:585, 1993
68. Halldin M, Wåhlin Å: Effect of succinylcholine on the intraspinal fluid pressure. Acta Anaesthesiol Scand 3:155, 1959
69. Mori K, Iwabuchi K, Fujita M: The effects of depolarizing muscle relaxants on the electroencephalogram and the circulation during halothane anaesthesia in man. Br J Anaesth 45:604, 1973
70. Lanier WL, Milde JH, Michenfelder JD: Cerebral stimulation following succinylcholine in dogs. Anesthesiology 64:551, 1986
71. Granit R, Skoglund S, Thesleff S: Activation of muscle spindles by succinylcholine and decamethonium. The effects of curare. Acta Physiol Scand 28:134, 1953
72. Mitchell MM, Ali HH, Savarese JJ: Myotonia and neuromuscular blocking agents. Anesthesiology 49:44, 1978
73. Örndahl G: Myotonic human musculature: stimulation with depolarizing agents. II. A clinicopharmacological study. Acta Med Scand 172:753, 1962
74. Paterson IS: Generalized myotonia following suxamethonium. A case report. Br J Anaesth 34:340, 1962
75. Thiel RE: The myotonic response to suxamethonium. Br J Anaesth 39:815, 1967
76. Brim VD: Denervation supersensitivity: the response to depolarizing muscle relaxants. Br J Anaesth 45:222, 1973
77. Cannon WB. A law of denervation. Am J Med Sci 198:737, 1939
78. Lee C, Yang E, Katz RL: Focal contracture following injection of succinylcholine in patients with peripheral nerve injury. Can Anaesth Soc J 24:475, 1977
79. Gronert GA, Milde JH, Theye RA: Porcine malignant hyperthermia induced by halothane and succinylcholine: failure of treatment with procaine or procainamide. Anesthesiology 44:124, 1976
80. Cody JR: Muscle rigidity following administration of succinylcholine. Anesthesiology 29:159, 1968
81. Ellis FR, Halsall PJ: Suxamethonium spasm. A differential diagnostic conundrum. Br J Anaesth 56:381, 1984
82. Carroll JB: Increased incidence of masseter spasm in children with strabismus anesthetized with halothane and succinylcholine. Anesthesiology 67:559, 1987
83. Schwartz L, Rockoff MA, Koka BV: Masseter spasm with anesthesia: incidence and implications. Anesthesiology 61:772, 1984
84. Butler-Browne GS, Eriksson P-O, Laurent C, Thornell L-E: Adult human masseter muscle fibers express myosin isozymes characteristic of development. Muscle Nerve 11:610, 1988
85. Morgan DL, Proske U: Vertebrate slow muscle: its structure, pattern of innervation, and mechanical properties. Physiol Rev 64:103, 1984
86. Fletcher JE, Rosenberg H. *In vitro* interaction between halothane and succinylcholine in human skeletal muscle: implications for malignant hyperthermia and masseter muscle rigidity. Anesthesiology 63:190, 1985
87. van der Spek AFL, Fang WB, Ashton-Miller JA et al: The effects of succinylcholine on mouth opening. Anesthesiology 67:459, 1987
88. van der Spek AFL, Fang WB, Ashton-Miller JA et al: Increased masticatory muscle stiffness during limb muscle flaccidity associated with succinylcholine administration. Anesthesiology 69:11, 1988
89. Rosenberg H: Trismus is not trivial. Anesthesiology 67:453, 1987
90. Gronert GA: Management of patients in whom trismus occurs following succinylcholine. Anesthesiology 68:653, 1988
91. Gronert GA, Theye RA: Suxamethonium-induced porcine malignant hyperthermia. Br J Anaesth 48:513, 1976
92. Lucke JN, Hall GM, Lister D: Porcine malignant hyperthermia. I. Metabolic and physiological changes. Br J Anaesth 48:297, 1976
93. Nelson TE, Jones EW, Bedell DM: Porcine malignant hyperthermia: a study on the triggering effects of succinylcholine. Anesth Analg 52:908, 1973
94. Charak DS, Dhar CL: Suxamethonium-induced changes in serum creatine phosphokinase. Br J Anaesth 53:955, 1981
95. Bernhardt D, Horder MH: CK Isoenzyme bei anaesthesie-induzierter Myoglobinurie (AIM). Anaesthesist 30:131, 1981
96. Brustowicz RM, Moncorge C, Koka BV: Metabolic responses to tourniquet release in children. Anesthesiology 67:792, 1987
97. Delphin E, Jackson D, Rothstein P: Use of suc-

cinylcholine during elective pediatric anesthesia should be reevaluated. Anesth Analg 66:1190, 1987
98. Plötz J, Braun J: Serummyoglobin nach Wiederholungsgaben von Succinylcholin und der Einfluss von Dantrolen. Klinische Untersuchungen bei Kindern in Halothannarkose. Anaesthesist 34:513, 1985
99. McKishnie JD, Muir JM, Girvan DP: Anaesthesia induced rhabdomyolysis—a case report. Can Anaesth Soc J 30:295, 1983
100. Moore WE, Watson RL, Summary JJ: Massive myoglobinuria precipitated by halothane and succinylcholine in a member of a family with elevation of serum creatine phosphokinase. Anesth Analg 55:680, 1976
101. Rubiano R, Chang J-L, Carroll J et al: Acute rhabdomyolysis following halothane anesthesia without succinylcholine. Anesthesiology 67:856, 1987
102. Florence JM, Fox PT, Planer GJ, Brooke MH: Activity, creatine kinase, and myoglobin in Duchenne muscular dystrophy: a clue to etiology? Neurology 35:758, 1985
103. Kambam JR, Dymond R, Krestow M: Effect of cimetidine on duration of action of succinylcholine. Anesth Analg 66:191, 1987
104. Stirt JA, Sperry RJ, DiFazio CA: Cimetidine and succinylcholine: potential interaction and effect on neuromuscular blockade in man. Anesthesiology 69:607, 1988
105. Cook DR, Stiller RL, Chakravorti S, Mannenhira T: Cimetidine does not inhibit plasma cholinesterase activity. Anesth Analg 67:375, 1988
106. Mora CT, Eisenkraft JB, Papatestas AE: Intravenous dantrolene in a patient with myasthenia gravis. Anesthesiology 64:371, 1986
107. Wedel DJ, Quinlan JG, Iaizzo PA: Clinical effects of intravenously administered dantrolene. Mayo Clin Proc 70:241, 1995
108. McLeskey CH, Cullen BF, Kennedy RD, Galindo A: Control of cerebral perfusion pressure during induction of anesthesia in high-risk neurosurgical patients. Anesth Analg 53:985, 1974
109. Brinling JC, Smith CM: A characterization of the stimulation of mammalian muscle spindles by succinylcholine. J Pharmacol Exp Ther 129:56, 1960
110. Cottrell JE, Hartung J, Giffin JP, Shwiry B: Intracranial and hemodynamic changes after succinylcholine administration in cats. Anesth Analg 62:1006, 1983
111. White PF, Schlobohm RM, Pitts LH, Lindauer JM: A randomized study of drugs for preventing increases in intracranial pressure during endotracheal suctioning. Anesthesiology 57:242, 1982
112. Kovarik WD, Mayberg TS, Lam AM et al: Succinylcholine does not change intracranial pressure, cerebral blood flow velocity, or the electroencephalogram in patients with neurologic injury. Anesth Analg 78:469, 1994
113. Minton MD, Grosslight K, Stirt JA, Bedford RF: Increases in intracranial pressure from succinylcholine: prevention by prior nondepolarizing blockade. Anesthesiology 65:165, 1986
114. Stirt JA, Grosslight KR, Bedford RF, Vollmer D: "Defasciculation" with metocurine prevents succinylcholine-induced increases in intracranial pressure. Anesthesiology 67:50, 1987
115. Rosa G, Orfei P, Sanfilippo M, et al: The effects of atracurium besylate (Tracrium) on intracranial pressure and cerebral perfusion pressure. Anesth Analg 65:381, 1986
116. Rosa G, Sanfilippo M, Vilardi V et al: Effects of vecuronium bromide on intracranial pressure and cerebral perfusion pressure. A preliminary report. Br J Anaesth 58:437, 1986
117. Futo J, Kupferberg JP, Moss J et al: Vecuronium inhibits histamine N-methyltransferase. Anesthesiology 69:92, 1988
118. Futo J, Kupferberg JP, Moss J: Inhibition of histamine *N*-methyltransferase (HNMT) *in vitro* by neuromuscular relaxants. Biochem Pharmacol 39:415, 1990
119. Brett RS, Schmidt JH, Gage JS et al: Measurement of acetylcholine receptor concentration in skeletal muscle from a patient with multiple sclerosis and resistance to atracurium. Anesthesiology 66:837, 1987
120. Iwasaki H, Namiki A, Omote K et al: Response differences of paretic and healthy extremities to pancuronium and neostigmine in hemiplegic patients. Anesth Analg 64:864, 1985
121. Stone WA, Beach TP, Hamelberg W: Succinylcholine—danger in the spinal-cord-injured patient. Anesthesiology 32:168, 1970
122. Thompson MW: The genetic transmission of muscle diseases. p. 1072. In Engel AG, Franzini-Armstrong C, (eds): Myology: Basic and Clinical. 2nd Ed. McGraw-Hill, New York: 1994
123. Krueger KC, Waylonis GW: Hemiplegia: lower

motor neuron electromyographic findings. Arch Phys Med Rehabil 54:360, 1973
124. Stone WA, Beach TP, Hamelberg W: Succinylcholine-induced hyperkalemia in dogs with transected sciatic nerves or spinal cords. Anesthesiology 32:515, 1970
125. Cooperman LH: Succinylcholine-induced hyperkalemia in neuromuscular disease. JAMA 213:1867, 1970
126. Brown JC, Charlton JE: Study of sensitivity to curare in certain neurological disorders using a regional technique. J Neurol Neurosurg Psychiatry 38:34, 1975
127. Frankville DD, Drummond JC: Hyperkalemia after succinylcholine administrtion in a patient with closed head injury without paresis. Anesthesiology 67:264, 1987
128. Stevenson PH, Birch AA: Succinylcholine-induced hyperkalemia in a patient with a closed head injury. Anesthesiology 51:89, 1979
129. Roth F, Wüthrich H. The clinical importance of hyperkalaemia following suxamethonium administration. Br J Anaesth 41:311, 1969
130. Cowgill DB, Mostello LA, Shapiro HM: Encephalitis and a hyperkalemic response to succinycholine. Anesthesiology 40:409, 1974
131. Walker DE, Barry JM, Hodges CV: Succinylcholine-induced ventricular fibrillation in the paralyzed urology patient. J Urol 113:111, 1975
132. Carter JG, Sokoll MD, Gergis SD: Effect of spinal cord transection on neuromuscular function in the rat. Anesthesiology 55:542, 1981
133. Iwatsuki N, Kuroda N, Amaha K, Iwatsuki K: Succinylcholine-induced hyperkalemia in patients with ruptured cerebral aneurysms. Anesthesiology 53:64, 1980
134. Manninen PH, Mahendran B, Gelb AW, Merchant RN: Succinylcholine does not increase serum potassium levels in patients with acutely ruptured cerebral aneurysms. Anesth Analg 70:172, 1990
135. Muzzi DA, Black S, Cucchiara RF: The lack of effect of succinylcholine on serum potassium in patients with Parkinson's disease (letter). Anesthesiology 71:322, 1989
136. Gravlee GP: Succinylcholine-induced hyperkalemia in a patient with Parkinson's disease. Anesth Analg 59:444, 1980
137. Dierdorf SF, McNiece WL, Rao CC et al: Effect of succinylcholine on plasma potassium in children with cerebral palsy. Anesthesiology 62:88, 1985
138. Dierdorf SF, McNiece WL, Rao CC et al: Failure of succinylcholine to alter plasma potassium in children with myelomeningocoele. Anesthesiology 64:272, 1986
139. Duvaldestin P, Gibert C, Henzel D et al: Pancuronium blood level monitoring in patients with tetanus. Intensive Care Med 5:111, 1979
140. Kerr J: Current topics in tetanus. Intensive Care Med 5:105, 1979
141. Aguilar Bernal OR, Bender MA, Lacy ME: Efficacy of dantrolene sodium in management of tetanus in children. J R Soc Med 79:277, 1986
142. Dalakas MC, Elder G, Hallett M et al: A long-term follow-up study of patients with post-poliomyelitis neuromuscular symptoms. N Engl J Med 314:959, 1986
143. Feldman JM: Cardiac arrest after succinylcholine administration in a pregnant patient recovered from Guillain-Barre syndrome. Anesthesiology 72:942, 1990
144. Jackson DL, Satya-Murti S, Davis L, Drachman DB: Isaacs syndrome with laryngeal involvement: an unusual presentation of myokymia. Neurology 29:1612, 1979
145. Sinha S, Newsom-Davis J, Mills K et al: Autoimmune aetiology for acquired neuromyotonia (Isaacs' syndrome). Lancet 338:75, 1991
146. Baraka A: Myasthenic response to muscle relaxants in von Recklinghausen's disease. Br J Anaesth 46:701, 1974
147. Magbagbeola JA: Abnormal responses to muscle relaxants in a patient with Von Recklinghausen's disease (multiple neurofibromatosis). Br J Anaesth 42:710, 1970
148. Manser J: Abnormal responses in von Recklinghausen's disease. Br J Anaesth 42:183, 1970
149. Naguib M, Al-Rajeh SM, Abdulatif M, Ababtin WA: The response of a patient with von Recklinghausen's disease to succinylcholine and atracurium. Middle East J Anesthesiol 9:429, 1988
150. Antognini JF: Anaesthesia for Charcot-Marie-Tooth disease: a review of 86 cases. Can J Anaesth 39:398, 1992
151. Rosenbaum KJ, Neigh JL, Strobel GE: Sensitivity to nondepolarizing muscle relaxants in amyotrophic lateral sclerosis: report of two cases. Anesthesiology 35:638, 1971
152. Campbell AM, Finley GA: Anaesthesia for a patient with Friedreich's ataxia and cardiomyopathy. Can J Anaesth 36:89, 1989
153. Bell CF, Kelly JM, Jones RS: Anaesthesia for

Friedreich's ataxia. Case report and review of the literature. Anaesthesia 41:296, 1986
154. Kume M, Zin T, Oyama T: [Anesthetic experience with a patient with Friedreich's ataxia.] Masui 25:877, 1976
155. Drachman DB: Myasthenia gravis. N Engl J Med 330:1797, 1994
156. Hunter JM, Bell CF, Florence AM et al: Vecuronium in the myasthenic patient. Anaesthesia 40:848, 1985
157. Rolbin WH, Levinson G, Shnider SM, Wright RG: Anesthetic considerations for myasthenia gravis and pregnancy. Anesth Analg 57:441, 1978
158. Eisenkraft JB, Book WJ, Mann SM et al: Resistance to succinylcholine in myasthenia gravis: a dose-response study. Anesthesiology 69:760, 1988
159. Wainwright AP, Brodrick PM: Suxamethonium in myasthenia gravis. Anaesthesia 42:950, 1987
160. Baraka A: Suxamethonium block in the myasthenic patient. Correlation with plasma cholinesterase. Anaesthesia 47:217, 1992
161. Davies DW, Steward DJ: Myasthenia gravis in children and anaesthetic management for thymectomy. Can Anaesth Soc J 20:253, 1973
162. Eisenkraft JB, Sawhney RK, Papatestas AE: Vecuronium in the myasthenic patient, (letter). Anaesthesia 41:666, 1986
163. Ward S, Wright DJ: Neuromuscular blockade in myasthenia gravis with atracurium besylate. Anaesthesia 39:51, 1984
164. Blitt CD, Wright WA, Peat J: Pancuronium and the patient with myasthenia gravis. Anesthesiology 42:624, 1975
165. Macdonald AM, Keen RI, Pugh ND: Myasthenia gravis and atracurium. A case report. Br J Anaesth 56:651, 1984
166. Eisenkraft JB, Book WJ, Papatestas AE: Sensitivity to vecuronium in myasthenia gravis: a dose-response study. Can J Anaesth 37:301, 1990
167. Seigne RD, Scott RP: Mivacurium chloride and myasthenia gravis. Br J Anaesth 72:468, 1994
168. Baraka A, Dajani A: Atracurium in myasthenics undergoing thymectomy. Anesth Analg 63:1127, 1984
169. Engel AG: Myasthenic syndromes p. 1798. In Engel AG, Franzini-Armstrong C (eds): Myology: Basic and Clinical. 2nd Ed. McGraw-Hill, New York, 1994
170. Tsai SK, Huang SW, Lee TY: Neuromuscular interactions between suxamethonium and magnesium sulphate in the cat. Br J Anaesth 72:674, 1994
171. Dodson BA, Kelly BJ, Braswell LM, Cohen NH. Changes in acetylcholine receptor number in muscle from critically ill patients receiving muscle relaxants. Crit Care Med 23:815,1995
172. Giostra E, Magistris MR, Pizzolato G et al: Neuromuscular disorder in intensive care unit patients treated with pancuronium bromide. Occurrence in a cluster group of seven patients and two sporadic cases, with electrophysiologic and histologic examination. Chest 106:210, 1994
173. Fleming NW: Neuromuscular blocking drugs in the intensive care unit: indications, protocols, and complications. Semin Anesth 13:255, 1994
174. Danon MJ, Carpenter S. Myopathy with thick filament (myosin) loss following prolonged paralysis with vecuronium during steroid treatment. Muscle Nerve 14:1131, 1991
175. Rouleau G, Karpati G, Carpenter S et al: Glucocorticoid excess induces preferential depletion of myosin in denervated skeletal muscle fibers. Muscle Nerve 10:428, 1987
176. Genever EE: Suxamethonium-induced cardiac arrest in unsuspected pseudohypertrophic muscular dystrophy. Case report. Br J Anaesth 43:984, 1971
177. Linter SPK, Thomas PR, Withington PS, Hall MG: Suxamethonium associated hypertonicity and cardiac arrest in unsuspected pseudohypertrophic muscular dystrophy. Br J Anaesth 54:1331, 1982
178. Seay AR, Ziter FA, Thompson JA: Cardiac arrest during induction of anesthesia in Duchenne muscular dystrophy. J Pediatr 93:88, 1978
179. Rosenberg H, Gronert GA: Intractable cardiac arrest in children given succinylcholine, (letter). Anesthesiology 77:1054, 1992
180. Lee G, Antognini JF, Gronert GA: Complete recovery after prolonged resuscitation and cardiopulmonary bypass for hyperkalemic cardiac arrest. Anesth Analg 79:172, 1994
181. Hoffman EP, Fischbeck KH, Brown RH, et al: Characterization of dystrophin in muscle biopsy specimens from patients with Duchenne's or Becker's muscular dystrophy. N Engl J Med 318:1363, 1988
182. Richards WC: Anaesthesia and serum creatine phosphokinase levels in patients with Duchenne's pseudohypertrophic muscular dystrophy. Anaesth Intensive Care 1:150, 1972
183. Miller ED, Jr, Sanders DB, Rowlingson JC et al:

Anesthesia-induced rhabdomyolysis in a patient with Duchenne's muscular dystrophy. Anesthesiology 48:146, 1978
184. Solares G, Herranz JL, Sanz MD: Suxamethonium-induced cardiac arrest as an initial manifestation of Duchenne muscular dystrophy (letter). Br J Anaesth 58:576, 1986
185. Sethna NF, Rockoff MA, Worthen HM, Rosnow JM: Anesthesia-related complications in children with Duchenne muscular dystrophy. Anesthesiology 68:462, 1988
186. Kelly SS, Morgan GP, Smith JW: The origin of (+)-tubocurarine resistance in dystrophic mice. Br J Pharmacol 89:47, 1986
187. Munsat TL: Facioscapulohumeral disease and the scapuloperoneal syndrome. p. 1220. In Engel AG, Franzini-Armstrong C (eds): Myology: Basic and Clinical. 2nd Ed. McGraw-Hill, New York, 1994
188. Dresner DL, Ali HH: Anaesthetic management of a patient with facioscapulohumeral muscular dystrophy. Br J Anaesth 62:331, 1989
189. Harper PS, Rüdel R: Myotonic dystrophy. p. 1192. In Engel AG, Franzini-Armstrong C (eds): Myology: Basic and Clinical. 2nd Ed. McGraw-Hill, New York, 1994
190. Newberg LA, Lambert EH, Gronert GA: Failure to induce malignant hyperthermia in myotonic goats. Br J Anaesth 55:57, 1983
191. Heiman-Patterson T, Martino C, Rosenberg H et al: Malignant hyperthermia in myotonia congenita. Neurology 38:810, 1988
192. Heiman-Patterson TD, Rosenberg H, Fletcher JE, Tahmoush AJ: Halothane-caffeine contracture testing in neuromuscular diseases. Muscle Nerve 11:453, 1988
193. Phillips DC, Ellis FR, Exley KA, Ness MA: Dantrolene sodium and dystrophia myotonica. Anaesthesia 39:568, 1984
194. Boheimer N, Harris JW, Ward S: Neuromuscular blockade in dystrophia myotonica with atracurium besylate. Anaesthesia 40:872, 1985
195. Nightingale P, Healy TEJ: McGuinness K. Dystrophia myotonica and atracurium. A case report. Br J Anaesth 57:1131, 1985
196. Stirt JA, Stone DJ, Weinberg G et al: Atracurium in a child with myotonic dystrophy. Anesth Analg 64:369, 1985
197. Diefenbach C, Lynch J, Abel M, Buzello W: Vecuronium for muscle relaxation in patients with dystrophia myotonica. Anesth Analg 76:872, 1993
198. Buzello W, Krieg N, Schlickewei A: Hazards of neostigmine in patients with neuromuscular disorders. Report of two cases. Br J Anaesth 54:529, 1982
199. Castano J, Pares N: Anaesthesia for major abdominal surgery in a patient with myotonia dystrophica. Br J Anaesth 59:1629, 1987
200. Engel AG, Hohlfeld R, Banker BQ: The polymyositis and dermatomyositis syndromes. p. 1335. In Engel AG, Franzini-Armstrong C (eds): Myology: Basic and Clinical. 2nd Ed. McGraw-Hill, New York, 1994
201. Flusche G, Unger-Sargon J, Lambert DH: Prolonged neuromuscular paralysis with vecuronium in a patient with polymyositis. Anesth Analg 66:188, 1987
202. Saarnivaara LHM: Anesthesia for a patient with polymyositis undergoing myectomy of the cricopharyngeal muscle. Anesth Analg 67:701, 1988
203. Ganta R, Campbell IT, Mostafa SM: Anaesthesia and acute dermatomyositis/polymyositis. Br J Anaesth 60:854, 1988
204. Lehmann-Horn F, Engel AG, Ricker K, Rüdel R: The periodic paralyses and paramyotonia congenita. p. 1303. In Engel AG, Franzini-Armstrong C (eds): Myology: Basic and Clinical. 2nd Ed. McGraw-Hill, New York, 1994
205. Links TP, Zwarts MJ, Oosterhuis HJGH: Improvement of muscle strength in familial hypokalaemic periodic paralysis with acetazolamide. J Neurol Neurosurg Psychiatry 51:1142, 1988
206. Horton B: Anesthetic experiences in a family with hypokalemic familial periodic paralysis. Anesthesiology 47:308, 1977
207. Melnick B, Chang J-L, Larson CE, Bedger RC: Hypokalemic familial periodic paralysis. Anesthesiology 58:263, 1983
208. Rooney RT, Shanahan EC, Sun T, Nally B: Atracurium and hypokalemic familial periodic paralysis. Anesth Analg 67:782, 1988
209. Siler JN, Discavage WJ: Anesthetic management of hypokalemic periodic paralysis. Anesthesiology 43:489, 1975
210. Kim C, Fuke N, Martyn JAJ: Burn injury to rat increases nicotinic acetylcholine receptors in the diaphragm. Anesthesiology 68:401, 1988
211. Kim C, Martyn J, Fuke N: Burn injury to trunk of rat causes denervation-like responses in the gastrocnemius muscle. J Appl Physiol 65:1745, 1988
212. Mills AK, Martyn JAJ: Evaluation of atracurium

neuromuscular blockade in paediatric patients with burn injury. Br J Anaesth 60:450, 1988
213. Martyn JAJ, Matteo RS, Szyfelbein SK, Kaplan RF: Unprecedented resistance to neuromuscular blocking effects of metocurine with persistence after complete recovery in a burned patient. Anesth Analg 61:614, 1982
214. Laycock JR, Loughman E: Suxamethonium-induced hyperkalaemia following cold injury. Anaesthesia 41:739, 1986
215. Sarubin J, Gebert E: Serumkaliumanstieg nach depolarisierenden Muskelrelaxantien. I. Abhängigkeit von der Immobilisationsdauer. Anaesthesist 30:246, 1981
216. Cairoli VJ, Ivankovich AD, Vucicevic D, Patel K: Succinylcholine-induced hyperkalemia in the rat following radiation injury to muscle. Anesth Analg 61:83, 1982
217. Rao TLK, Shanmugam M: Succinylcholine administration—another contraindication? Anesth Analg 58:61, 1979
218. Sewall K, Flowerdew RMM, Bromberger P: Severe muscular rigidity at birth: malignant hyperthermia syndrome? Can Anaesth Soc J 27:279, 1980
219. Britt BA, Webb GE, LeDuc C: Malignant hyperthermia induced by curare. Can Anaesth Soc J 21:371, 1974
220. Waterman PM, Albin MS, Smith RB: Malignant hyperthermia: a case report. Anesth Analg 59:220, 1980
221. Harrison GG: Pancuronium and the triggering of malignant hyperthermia (letter). Anesth Analg 59:889, 1980
222. Bowman WC, Raper C: Spontaneous fibrillary activity of denervated muscle. Nature 201:160, 1964
223. McIntyre AR, King RE, Dunn AL: Electrical activity of denervated mammalian skeletal muscle as influenced by d-tubocurarine. J Neurophys 8:297, 1945
224. Chalstrey LJ, Edwards GB: Fatal hyperpyrexia following the use of pancuronium bromide in the pig. Br J Anaesth 44:91, 1972
225. Kaplan AM, Bergeson PS, Gregg SA, Curless RG: Malignant hyperthermia associated with myopathy and normal muscle enzymes. J Pediatr 91:431, 1977
226. King JO, Denborough MA: Anesthetic-induced malignant hyperpyrexia in children. J Pediatr 83:37, 1973
227. McPherson EW, Taylor CA, Jr: The King syndrome: malignant hyperthermia, myopathy, and multiple anomalies. Am J Med Genet 8:159, 1981
228. Eng GD, Epstein BS, Engel WK et al: Malignant hyperthermia and central core disease in a child with congenital dislocating hips. Arch Neurol 35:189, 1978
229. Frank JP, Harati Y, Butler IJ et al: Central core disease and malignant hyperthermia syndrome. Ann Neurol 7:11, 1980
230. Ginsburg R, Purcell-Jones G: Malignant hyperthermia in the Wolf-Hirschhorn syndrome. Anaesthesia 43:386, 1988
231. Gronert GA: Controversies in malignant hyperthermia (editorial). Anesthesiology 59:273, 1983
232. Caroff SN, Rosenberg H, Fletcher JE et al: Malignant hyperthermia susceptibility in neuroleptic malignant syndrome. Anesthesiology 67:20, 1987
233. Krivosic-Horber R, Adnet P, Guevart E et al: Neuroleptic malignant syndrome and malignant hyperthermia. *In vitro* comparison with halothane and caffeine contracture tests. Br J Anaesth 59:1554, 1987
234. Tollefson G: A case of neuroleptic malignant syndrome: *in vitro* muscle comparison with malignant hyperthermia. J Clin Psychopharmacol 2:266, 1982
235. Geiduschek J, Cohen SA, Khan A, Cullen BF: Repeated anesthesia for a patient with neuroleptic malignant syndrome. Anesthesiology 68:134, 1988
236. Shalev A, Munitz H: The neuroleptic malignant syndrome: agent and host interaction. Acta Psychiatr Scand 73:337, 1986
237. Patel P, Bristow G: Postoperative neuroleptic malignant syndrome. A case report. Can J Anaesth 34:515, 1987
238. Addonizio G, Susman VL: ECT as a treatment alternative for patients with symptoms of neuroleptic malignant syndrome. J Clin Psychiatry 48:102, 1987
239. George AL, Jr, Wood CA, Jr: Succinylcholine-induced hyperkalemia complicating the neuroleptic malignant syndrome (letter). Ann Intern Med 106:172, 1987
240. Sechi GP, Tanda F, Mutani R: Fatal hyperpyrexia after withdrawal of levodopa. Neurology 34:249, 1984
241. Edelstein G, Hirshman CA: Hyperthermia and ketoacidosis during anesthesia in a child with glycogen-storage disease. Anesthesiology 52:90, 1980

242. Katsuya H, Misumi M, Ohtani Y, Miike T: Postanesthetic acute renal failure due to carnitine palmityl transferase deficiency. Anesthesiology 68:945, 1988
243. Simmons PS, Smithson WA, Gronert GA, Haymond MW: Acute myelogenous leukemia and malignant hyperthermia in a patient with type 1b glycogen storage disease. J Pediatr 105:428, 1984
244. Morgan-Hughes JA: Mitochondrial diseases p. 1610. In Engel AG, Franzini-Armstrong C (eds). Myology: Basic and Clinical. 2nd Ed. McGraw-Hill, New York, 1994
245. Fishbein WN, Muldoon SM, Deuster PA, Armbrustmacher VW: Myoadenylate deaminase deficiency and malignant hyperthermia susceptibility: is there a relationship? Biochem Med 34:344, 1985

15 STEREOTACTIC SURGERY

WILLIAM J. PERKINS
PATRICK J. KELLY
RONALD J. FAUST
DUDLEY H. DAVIS

The term *stereotactic* is a composite of the Greek word *stereos*, which refers to the geometry of solid bodies, and the Latin word *tactus*, which signifies the sense of touch. Stereotactic neurosurgery makes detailed use of the relationship between the three-dimensional space occupied by intracranial structures or lesions and an extracranial reference system to guide instruments accurately and precisely to such targets.

Although the stereotactic methodology is not new, it experienced a renaissance due in large part to progress in noninvasive imaging technologies. Computed tomography (CT), magnetic resonance imaging (MRI), and digitally subtracted angiography (DSA) provide three-dimensional information about intracranial structures. Because of the increasing use of stereotactic neurosurgery and the need for anesthesia support this requires, both patient and surgical needs during such procedures should be understood.

CT AND STEREOTACTIC NEUROSURGERY

The introduction of CT and, in particular, its routine use in obtaining remarkably detailed images of the central nervous system (CNS) has made it possible for neurosurgeons to localize more precisely and treat surgically mass lesions. Although each CT slice is only two-dimensional, the series of slices that constitute the complete CT study taken together provide a three-dimensional image of the brain.[1] Shortly after the introduction of CT, stereotactic neurosurgeons made use of this imaging technology to guide the surgical approach to small, deep-seated lesions in the CNS. Stereotactic systems developed before this time (such as the Leksell, the Todd-Wells, the Riechert-Mundinger, and the Hitchcock systems) were adapted to make use of such CT data.[2] In addition, several new stereotactic systems were developed to make the fullest use of the three-dimensional database provided by CT.

Appreciation of the sequence of events beginning with the acquisition of raw CT data to the performance of the stereotactic procedures itself requires an understanding of some relatively basic principles and definitions. Each element in a CT image may be defined by a set of coordinates, X, Y, and Z, with respect to an orthogonal Cartesian three-axis system. In CT, these axes are conventionally defined as follows: the X axis signifies the left-right direction, the Y axis signifies the anterior-posterior (AP) direction, and the Z axis signifies the superior-inferior direction (Fig. 15.1). In some stereotactic literature, the orientations of the axes as defined before the advent of CT scanning are used. In this literature, the X, Y, and Z axes represent the AP, the superior-inferior, and the mediolateral directions,

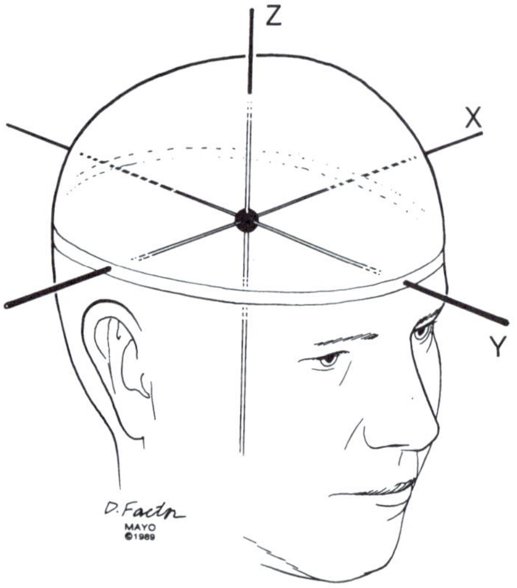

FIGURE 15.1 *Cartesian coordinate system as it applies to stereotactic neurosurgery. Note that the X, Y, and Z axes refer to the medial-lateral, anterior-posterior, and superior-inferior directions, respectively. (By permission of Mayo Clinic.)*

respectively. To avoid confusion, only the CT axis definitions will be followed throughout this chapter. Owing to the necessity of scanning in transverse planes, the individual CT slice provides information primarily in the X-Y plane. Each datum in this scan is referred to as a *pixel*. To obtain information along the Z axis, it is necessary to use a localizing system, that is, a system that measures the distance between the plane of the scan and a reference point or plane. In conventional CT, this information is obtained from a sagittal scout film, which shows the location of the slices with a series of transverse lines. The resulting three-dimensional information is composed of volume elements known as *voxels*, which have coordinates in three orthogonal planes and can be placed in a Cartesian coordinate system similar to that used for stereotactic coordinates. The resulting CT-derived intracranial images must then be transposed into stereotactic space (typically a polar-coordinate system that relates extracranial stereotactic elements, such as the stereotactic headframe and corresponding are quadrant frame, to an intracranial target). An intracranial target or targets must then be defined in the stereotactic coordinate system. Finally, a surgical trajectory is formulated that includes the point of entry and the depth at which the surgical target lies in relationship to the surgical instrument guide.

The major problem with calculating stereotactic coordinates from CT images is in the establishment of the vertical (Z) coordinate. Several different strategies have been adapted to establish the Z coordinate and have resulted in a variety of approaches to CT-guided stereotactic neurosurgery. Some cumbersome solutions to this problem even require performing the stereotactic surgical procedure in the CT scanner.

Perhaps the most flexible of the systems that transpose CT images into stereotactic space makes use of a relatively simple localizing device that can be attached to a stereotactic headframe, remains outside the image, and yet is included in the scan of each slice. A reference plane is fixed with two vertical rods connected by a diagonal rod (Fig. 15.2). The height above the reference plane of any point on the diagonal rod is a function of the ratio of the constant distance between the two vertical rods to the variable distance between one of the vertical rods and the diagonal rod. By combining three sets of these N-shaped localizing devices around or within a reference plane (often the base of the stereotactic headframe), three points in stereotactic space are demonstrated in the image plane. This fixes the position of the image with respect to the stereotactic headframe and allows the calculation of the AP, lateral, and vertical position of any other point in the image plane. Use of a reference ring that is fixed to the skull but positioned outside the scan image eliminates the need for a fixed relationship between the reference plane and the CT scanner gantry or table. A patient can thus move between scan slices without affecting the data acquisition. In addition, the CT scan image can be used to simply measure the AP and lateral coordinates of the image of the nine vertical and diagonal localizing rods and the target point. Computation of the coordinates of the target point can be accomplished independently of the data-processing capability of the scanner computer. Finally, because the localizing system

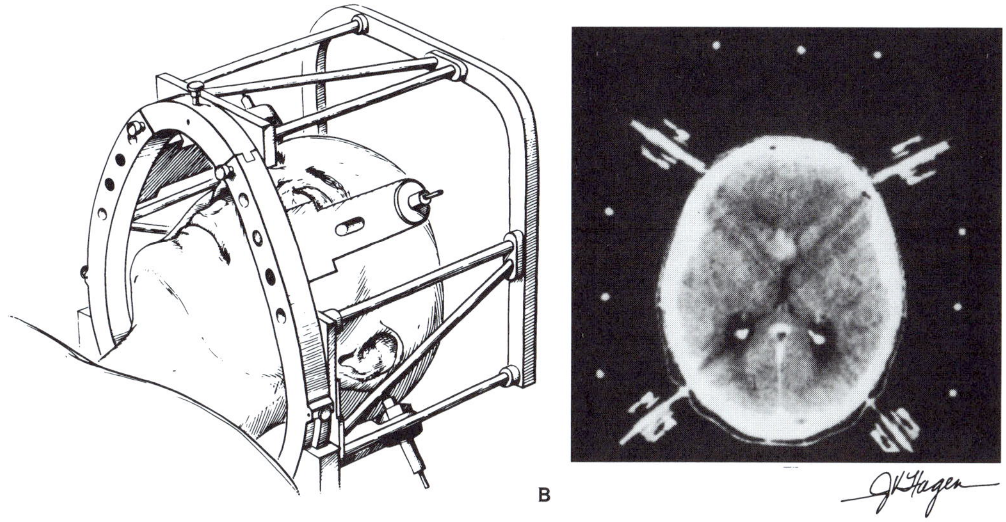

FIGURE 15.2 *(A) Localization system, consisting of three sets of three carbon-fiber rods arranged in an N-shaped configuration, attached to the modified Todd-Wells headframe. (B) The nine reference marks created by the system on a CT image may be used to calculate the position of an intracranial structure with respect to the headframe.*

fixes its reference plane to the skull alone via the stereotactic headframe, it may be used with any CT scanner. This localizing system also permits the neurosurgeon to perform data processing and surgery in either the operating room or the scanner facility. A similar localizing system may also be used to transpose both MRI- and DSA-acquired images into the stereotactic coordinate system.[3,4]

USE OF COMPUTERS IN STEREOTACTIC NEUROSURGERY

Bertrand and Olivier[5] were the first to make use of a computer as a stereotactic tool, performing the relatively simple task of simulating probe tracts on a stereotactic atlas. More recently, the computer has made possible the acquisition and storage of the vast quantities of data present in CT, MRI, and DSA images (for example, each CT image takes approximately 500,000 bytes of memory for storage). The CT image, often in conjunction with other imaging techniques, is an indispensable element of most contemporary stereotactic neurosurgery. Transformation of CT coordinates of a stereotactic system may be done either manually or with the use of a computer.[6–11] Computed transformation of CT coordinates typically makes use of either the CT scanner computer[12] or a computer system that is separate from the CT scanner.[11] The latter method permits integration of data from multiple imaging modalities into stereotactic space, intraoperative manipulation of data by the neurosurgeon at a site remote from the imaging location, high-resolution three-dimensional tumor volume reconstruction, and simulation of a variety of pertinent images in the operating room. In addition, a computer system can rapidly integrate intraoperative data collected from ultrasound, stereotactic radiographs, stereotactic ventriculograms, and neurophysiologic recordings into the stereotactic database. Furthermore, the computer can be used to solve for the target point, drive an automated positioning system to place the target point at the appropriate stereotactic location,[13] and monitor and control surgical instruments, such as a carbon dioxide laser,[3,4,14,15] in relationship to the stereotactic database.

The ability to integrate CT and/or MRI images with DSA images permits selection of trajectories to the target point that will avoid major cerebral vascular structures. Many of the abovementioned computer applications, however, are possibly of greater value for stereotactic resection of deep-seated brain tumors than for simpler intra-axial mass lesion biopsies. As computers continue to decrease in cost per megabyte and increase in speed and efficiency, it can be anticipated that their use in stereotactic neurosurgery will grow.

INDICATIONS FOR STEREOTACTIC NEUROSURGERY

Functional Procedures

Stereotactic techniques were initially developed to enable neurosurgeons to surgically approach intracranial structures deep to the cortical surface without damaging surrounding neurologic structures. These procedures are typically undertaken to alter the function of the nervous system and are thus termed *functional procedures*. Functional procedures frequently require interruption of a pathway by production of a lesion or pharmacologic manipulation and often make use of electrical recording techniques to identify the pathway of interest as well as surrounding structures.[16] The most common use of functional neurosurgery has been for the introduction of lesions in the basal ganglia, thalamus, or extrapyramidal pathways as a treatment for movement disorders. Other uses of functional neurosurgery include insertion of recording depth electrodes to evaluate patients being considered for surgical resection of seizure foci, treatment of pain by ablation of either lemniscal pathways in the midbrain or extralemniscal pathways within the thalamus, and treatment of intractable depression or obsessive-compulsive behavior by cingulotomy or dorsal median thalamotomy. Such procedures are not as amenable to conventional neurosurgical approaches owing to the risks of injury to adjacent or underlying structures.

Procedures Involving Mass Lesions

TUMOR RESECTION Although there are no widely accepted indications for stereotactic versus conventional neurosurgery, some guidelines have evolved in the neurosurgical literature. Conventional freehand resection of tumors deep in the brain relies on the surgeon's ability to ascertain the location and three-dimensional configuration of these lesions from several imaging modalities. This orientation becomes progressively more difficult as the procedure extends further below the cortical surface.[17,18] Such lesions are often irregularly shaped and necessitate some form of mechanical guidance to maintain an orientation adequate to locate and successfully resect the lesion. Hemispheric and deep-seated tumors are frequently located in functionally indispensable brain tissue. Surgeons may therefore be conservative in the management of intra-axial neoplasms and leave behind significant amounts of residual tumor.[19] Stereotactic methodology can provide the mechanical control that maintains surgical orientation during resection of tumors from neurologically important subcortical areas. Furthermore, deep intra-axial lesions can be treated by stereotactic interstitial brachytherapy or can be resected layer by layer using a computer-monitored, stereotactically directed carbon dioxide laser.[3,4,14,15,20] The presence of an intra-axial or deep midline tumor may therefore be considered a relative indication for a stereotactic neurosurgical procedure.

DIAGNOSTIC BIOPSY Though stereotactic techniques are used for the resection of neoplasms at some centers, they are most commonly used for obtaining diagnostic tissue samples from small (less than 1 cm in diameter) deep-seated mass lesions revealed by high-resolution imaging techniques. This is important because treatment, including chemotherapy and irradiation, is predicated on an accurate histologic diagnosis.[21] A diagnosis made on the basis of radiologic studies is not always reliable, particularly in distinguishing neoplastic from non-neoplastic disease. This is of particular relevance because as many as 18% of CT-demonstrated lesions have been histologically demonstrated to be non-neoplastic gliosis, infarct, radiation necrosis, infection, and arteriovenous malformation.[22] Clearly, patients with these lesions would not benefit from empiric radiation treatment or chemotherapy on the basis of a radiologic diagnosis. Bosch[23] has described several groups of patients who would benefit from stereotactic biopsy as opposed to open craniotomy. Resection of a tumor is central to the goal of reducing tumor burden and prolonging survival and should be done whenever possible on patients presenting with a new single intracerebral mass lesion and no previous history of tumor. When complete resection is impossible, as with certain midline tumors and in very large, diffusely growing hemispheric tumors, stereotactic biopsy is the procedure of choice. Patients without a previous history of tumor who present with multiple intracerebral lesions are commonly suspected of having a malignant tumor elsewhere in the body. When identification of the primary source of the tumor is not possible, stereotactic biopsy of one or more of the mass lesions is feasible when, because of the multiplicity of tumor locations, open craniotomy may not be ideal. Patients with a known primary tumor who present with an intra-axial mass lesion are also good candidates for stereotactic biopsy. Others have suggested that patients whose poor general medical condition makes a craniotomy a high-risk procedure should be candidates for stereotactic biopsy.

MORBIDITY AND MORTALITY OF STEREOTACTIC PROCEDURES

The morbidity and mortality associated with stereotactic neurosurgery are believed to be less than that associated with conventional or freehand neurosurgery.[17,22] In an excellent review, Ostertag[24] compiled the morbidity and mortality data for stereotactic biopsies from 15 major centers. With a total of 3,226 cases reported, the overall complication rate was 2.4%, ranging from 0 to 8%. The overall mortality in these series was only slightly greater than 1% with a range of 0 to 2.3%. Mundinger[25] has reported a 1% mortality rate in over 4,800 stereotactic procedures of various types. At the Mayo Clinic, the combined morbidity and mortality for 447 stereotactic biopsies was 1%.[22] The temptation to make a direct comparison between conventional and stereotactic procedures should be weighed against the fact that different brain areas are typically approached by the two methods.[23] A more appropriate comparison may be made between the freehand needle biopsy and stereotactic-directed biopsy, because both have been used to obtain tissue specimens from similar parts of the brain. Mortality rates as high as 13% have been reported for freehand biopsies in malignant gliomas,[26] results that may be attributable to an inability to select a trajectory to the lesion that avoids vascular structures. Hidden bleeding that cannot be easily stopped may then ensue.

When stereotactic angiographic studies are utilized before stereotactic biopsy, a trajectory can be chosen that will avoid any vessels between the brain surface and the lesion to be biopsied. Thus, the stereotactic method of biopsy that uses both angiographic and CT data to formulate a trajectory to a lesion has a lower associated morbidity and mortality than freehand needle biopsy. Stereotactic biopsies undertaken without the benefit of a cerebral angiogram or DSA study might be expected to carry a higher risk, although there are no data available in support of this. Stereotactic biopsies taken from such apparently high-risk areas as the brainstem and deep within the posterior fossa do not appear to have a higher morbidity and mortality[27,28] than those reported above. The morbidity (9.3%) but not the 30-day mortality (1%) may be higher for stereotactic volumetric tumor resection than for biopsy.[29]

Complications that have been reported after stereotactic biopsy include intracranial hematoma formation, neurologic deficit, infection, seizure, and infarction. Hemorrhage is the most frequent complication, accounting for more than one-half (55 to 73%) of the morbidity and mortality reported. Most hemorrhages were perilesional or intralesional and often were recognized on the immediate postoperative CT scan. Treatment was generally supportive, although at one center, as many as one-half of these patients were treated with an immediate craniotomy and evacuation of the hematoma.[30] Transient or permanent neurologic deficits ranging from mild hemiparesis to gait ataxia[17] are less common and may be the result of trauma or to edema formation in the functional tissue surrounding a biopsy site. Infection is an infrequent complication and occurs more often at the site of the burr hole than in the brain parenchyma.[30] Infarction of the posterior cerebral artery in association with perilesional edema has been reported in one case.[31]

Seizures are a very infrequent[22] but potentially devastating complication of stereotactic biopsy. This is particularly true of the awake patient undergoing stereotactic biopsy with local anesthetic infiltration of the scalp overlying the burr hole site. Access to the patient's airway can be extremely difficult owing to the presence of the headframe, and tracheal intubation may not be possible without the aid of a fiberoptic bronchoscope. Tonic-clonic seizure activity when the patient's head is in a stereotactic headframe affixed to a head holder could conceivably also result in cervical spine trauma. In addition, the pins that fix the position of the headframe with respect to the patient's skull may become displaced, lacerating the scalp or, less likely, penetrating the skull or eye. Finally, the acute changes in blood pressure that can occur during a seizure may increase the risk of intraparenchymal hemorrhage. Experience with two such cases of intraoperative seizures at the Mayo Clinic resulted in the use of general anesthesia for most stereotactic biopsies.

THE STEREOTACTIC HEADFRAME

The stereotactic headframe consists of a metal ring that serves as a base to which a localization system is attached during imaging studies (Fig. 15.3). Vertical supports fixed to the headframe are attached to the skull by either sharp metal or blunt carbon fiber pints. The headframe then serves as a reference point to which an arc quadrant system is attached, thus permitting surgical devices to be accurately directed to an intracranial target.

Application of the Headframe

The stereotactic headframe is applied just before imaging studies. Intravenous sedative and analgesic medications are administered to achieve moderate sedation yet maintain patient responsiveness. Combinations of fentanyl, midazolam, and/or propofol are used most often with local anesthesia. Patients that are unable to cooperate (i.e., patients less than 8 years of age or patients that are agitated or have a severe movement disorder) are given a general anesthetic for both the headframe application and the imaging studies. Oxygen saturation, blood pressure, electrocardiogram (ECG), and ventilation are monitored in all patients. Reapplication of the headframe just before the stereotactic procedure is usually performed with the patient under general anesthesia.

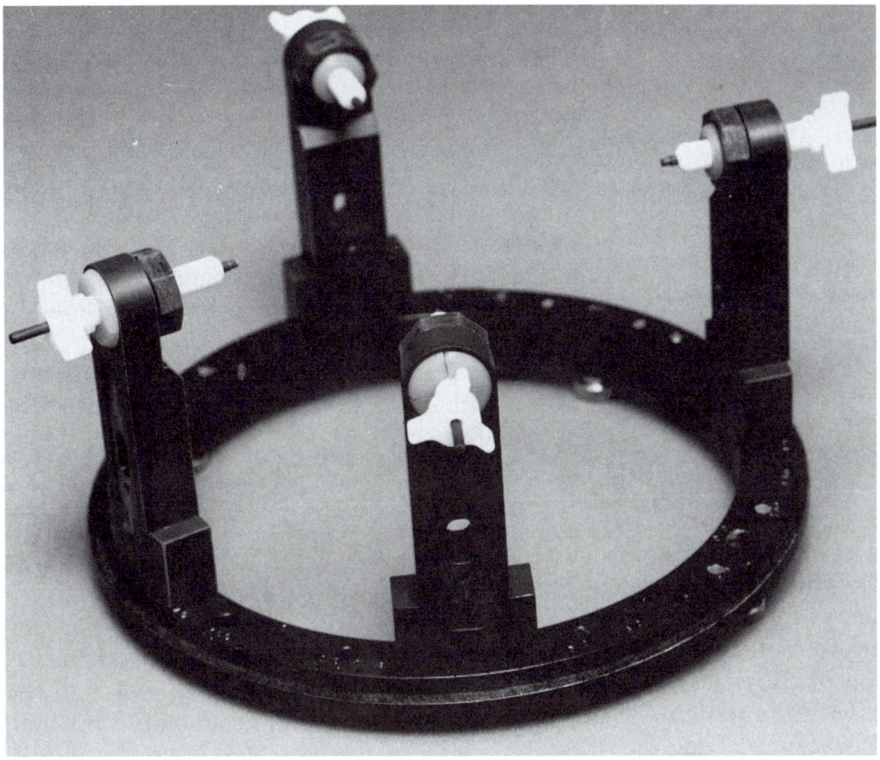

FIGURE 15.3 *Modified, CT-compatible Todd-Wells frame. The vertical supports are constructed of molybdenum disulfide and nylon, and the metal fixation screws have been replaced by carbon-fiber pins.*

Situations in Which Application of the Headframe Is Not Recommended

In stereotactic neurosurgery, the patient's skull must be firmly stationed and fixed in the frame throughout the procedure. Infants have relatively thin, compliant skulls with nonunited sutures and open fontanelles. Thus, tightening of fastening pins or rods with application of the headframe may result in intracranial hypertension,[32] skull fracture, or perforation of a fontanelle. Accordingly, patients under the age of 1 to 2 years only rarely undergo stereotactic neurosurgery. One group,[33] however, has developed a custom-fitted thermoplastic helmet that surrounds the infant's face and head and affords rigid protection of the skull. This device has been used successfully for a stereotactic biopsy in a 7-month-old boy, the youngest reported patient to undergo a stereotactic procedure.[33]

Other situations in which application of a stereotactic headframe would not be recommended are (1) a soft skull, as with tumor metastatic to the skull (e.g., multiple myeloma and breast carcinoma), Paget's disease, or severe osteoporosis; (2) a scalp infection in the area of an intended pin site; (3) a skull fracture near an intended pin site; and (4) a previous craniotomy or craniectomy near the pin site.[34] Careful attention to pin site selection will often permit headframe placement in spite of such abnormalities.

Potential Complications of Headframe Placement and Removal

Several complications are possible from placement and removal of a stereotactic headframe and have, in fact, been described in patients placed in a neurosurgical skull clamp. Because the pins used to fix the frame are embedded in the diploë, a potential communication between the diploic veins and the atmosphere is established. Venous air embolism is a well-recognized complication of the pin-type skull clamp,[35,36] and because the same type of venous-air communication is established with headframe application, the same risks or air embolism should be present. This complication is more likely to occur in patients in which the pins have been removed and reapplied. Patients at particular risk would be those undergoing stereotactic procedures in the sitting position or those in whom the headframe is removed with the patient sitting.[36] Whenever clinical evidence of air embolism appears in these patients (e.g., precordial Doppler evidence of air in the cardiac chambers, sudden decreased end-tidal carbon dioxide, the presence of end-tidal nitrogen, a sudden, otherwise inexplicable decrease in blood pressure, or the sudden appearance of a cardiac murmur and arrhythmias), the pin sites should be suspected. The possibility of this untoward event can be minimized by sealing the scalp around the pin sites with an antibacterial ointment. In addition, removal of the headframe with the patient in the supine position and immediate application of an antibacterial ointment-impregnated dressing to the pin sites should decrease the risk of air entrainment.

Perforation of the skull may also occur, particularly when drilling into the tabula externa or when hammering or tightening the pins to secure the headframe to the patient's skull. The complications of such a perforation may not become obvious until after removal of the headframe. For example, and epidural hematoma may develop if an underlying artery is perforated. If the dura is penetrated, a subdural hematoma, meningitis, or a cerebrospinal fluid fistula or leak may also occur. The latter complication can be treated without subsequent complications by simply oversewing the pin site at which the cerebrospinal fluid leak was observed. A traumatic middle meningeal arteriovenous fistula induced by a skull clamp pin has also been reported.[37] Rapid formation of a scalp hematoma or brisk hemorrhage from one or more pin sites occurs occasionally following headframe application and removal. Scalp bleeding occurs most frequently in the distribution of either the superficial temporal artery or occipital artery.

IMAGING STUDIES

A scanning table adaptation plate attaches to the gantry of the CT scanning unit. This device is similar in design to the receiving yoke on the Todd-Wells base unit and has a slot into which the base ring of the stereotactic headframe securely fits. The localization system described previously is attached to the headframe and creates nine reference points on each CT image (Fig. 15.2). The patient is then placed on the scanning table with the headframe secured on the adaptation plate. Stereotactic CT scanning is then performed using a 5-mm slice width and a 35-mm field of view format throughout the depth of the lesion.

Stereotactic digital angiography (DA) can enable the neurosurgeon to formulate a trajectory that avoids major vascular structures. DA is performed using a femoral catheterization technique. Four radiolucent plates, each containing an array of nine points, are attached to the stereotactic headframe bilaterally and together compose an angiographic reference system. The angiographic system creates 18 reference marks on each AP and lateral DA image. The mathematical relationships between the fiducial marks and their locations on the DA images are the basis from which stereotactic coordinates for intracranial vessels can be calculated. In addition, stereotactic target points derived from

CT and MRI studies can be displayed on the stereotactic DA images.[4,11]

The MRI-compatible stereotactic headframe is similar to that described for CT except that it is constructed entirely of carbon fiber and molybdenum disulfate and has no metal parts. The MRI localization system consists of nine capillary tubes containing copper sulfate solution arrayed in the same manner as in the CT localization system. These create nine reference marks on each MRI image. A multiplanar localization system may also be used that permits calculation of stereotactic coordinates from coronal, sagittal, and transverse images, thus making full use of the multiplanar imaging capabilities available using MRI. The patient is placed on the MRI scanning table with the stereotactic headframe and localization system in place. The patient is then advanced into the cavity of the magnet. Monitoring the patient in the MRI suite during scanning poses problems because ferrous material contained in most monitoring equipment can distort the magnetic field. In addition, ECG wires attached to the patient act as antennae for stray radiofrequency signals and may result in degradation of the MRI image or even skin burns under ECG pads. Use of ECG telemetry and a blood pressure cuff with plastic connectors and tubing has permitted monitoring of these critical vital signs.[38,39] Depending on the patient's condition, the anesthetist will observe the patient either in the MRI suite or just outside the scanning room, where the patient may be observed on a TV monitor and the patient's vital signs may be seen on a remote monitor screen. In the latter case, communication with the patient takes place through an intercom system.

Occasionally, a patient requiring an MRI study will be either unable to cooperate (e.g., the young patient, the patient with a severe movement disorder, or the agitated patient) or suffer from claustrophobia. When it is clear that the patient will be unable to undergo an MRI study while awake, the study can be performed with the patient either heavily sedated or under general anesthesia. A modified Bain circuit can be used for delivery of the volatile agent, nitrous oxide, and oxygen. After the patient has been positioned in the scanning apparatus, the anesthetist must remain as close to the patient as possible (during the actual MRI scan the anesthetist is at the patient's foot and observes the patient's face via a mirror placed inside the cavity of the magnet), controlling or assisting ventilation and monitoring the blood pressure and pulse oximetry. Although most pulse oximeters will function well in an MRI suite some may result in serious image degradation. The effect of a pulse oximeter on magnetic image quality must therefore be tested prior to routine use in an MRI suite.

The decision to administer a general anesthetic for headframe application and imaging studies is determined by the anesthesiologist. A general anesthetic is usually employed in the young patient. Although a child might be able to tolerate application of the headframe, the subsequent 1- to 2-hour period of immobility required for the imaging studies (if an MRI study is included) results in restlessness and anxiety. Other patients to whom we administer a general anesthetic are those whose mental status does not permit cooperation, those with a poorly controlled seizure disorder, those with a movement disorder that precludes laying still, and those with respiratory depression or failure. During transport to the imaging suites and for the duration of the imaging studies, anesthesia can be maintained with intravenous agents. If surgery is scheduled for the same day as the imaging studies, the patient is taken directly from the imaging suites to the operating room. If the patient is scheduled for surgery at a later date, the headframe is removed and the patient is observed while recovering from the general anesthetic. Reapplication of the headframe on the operative day is performed in the operating room after general anesthesia has been induced. Although the majority of headframe applications and imaging studies are performed with intravenous sedation at this institution, the ability to delivery a general anesthetic to some patient groups has been indispensable. Each imaging suite is fully equipped with appropriate monitoring equipment, an anesthesia machine, and the drugs and equipment necessary to induce general anesthesia should the need arise at any time during an imaging study.

Patients requiring only intravenous sedation for headframe application and imaging studies are taken to the recovery room. If surgery is scheduled for another day, the headframe is removed and the patient is discharged from the recovery room after an appropriate observation period. On the day of surgery, the headframe is reapplied after induction of general anesthesia. If surgery is scheduled for the same day, the headframe remains in place, and the patient awaits surgery in the recovery room, receiving further increments of intravenous sedation as required. These patients seem to tolerate the headframe well, requiring little or no additional sedative or narcotic for periods as long as several hours. Occasionally, the scalp around one or more pin sites is reinjected with local anesthetic for pain relief. Subsequent induction of general anesthesia in the awake patient with a headframe in place is described in a subsequent section.

THE STEREOTACTIC OPERATING ROOM

Two adjoining operating rooms (Fig. 15.4) are equipped for stereotactic surgery. A computer system (Data General MV 7800, SUN 3/260, and Vicom VME image processor) is located directly above the operating rooms. Display consoles are located in the treatment planning computer room and in an induction room between the operating rooms. Computer display monitors are suspended in both stereotactic operating rooms for display of stereotactic CT, MRI, and DA images. Displays of angiograms, scaled stereotactic atlas sections, tumor volumes, radionuclide-source isodose configurations, and reformatted target images may also be displayed. X-Ray tubes for 4-m teleradiography are suspended on a wormgear, servomotor-controlled slide system for collimation with the stereotactic headframe. A He-Ne laser beam coaxial with the central X-ray beam is used as a visual cue to facilitate collimation.

FIGURE 15.4 *Stereotactic operating suite. Note the presence of computer display monitors in each of the operating rooms.*

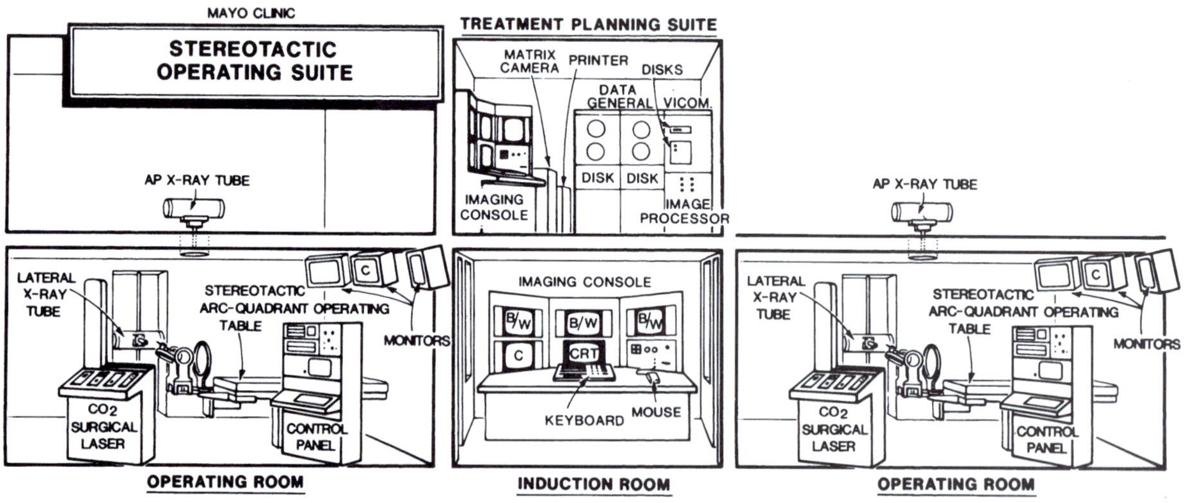

STEREOTACTIC DATA INPUT

After data acquisition, the archived data tapes from the CT, MRI, and DA examinations are read into the operating room computer system. The surgeon then views each of the CT and MRI images that encompass the lesion and digitizes the target.[8,11] The nine reference marks on each CT or MRI image are detected automatically by an intensity detection algorithm.[8] A complete series of images are thus used to create a three-dimensional stereotactic database, relating the location of intracranial structures to the stereotactic headframe and, ultimately, the stereotactic surgical apparatus. The outlines of the lesion defined by CT contrast enhancement or hypodensity and by the T_1- and T_2-weighted MRI images are then digitized by the surgeon with use of an interactive cursor system.[40] Each of these digitized contours is stored in a separate computer image matrix. A computer program interpolates intermediate contours at 1-mm intervals between each of the digitized contours.[40,41] The two-dimensional contour (Fig. 15.5A) or entire volume (Fig. 15.5B) of the lesion may thus be stored and displayed in the treatment planning room, the induction room, or on suspended computer display monitors in the stereotactic operating rooms. For stereotactic biopsy of a single lesion or multiple lesions, a single target point rather than the entire volume of the lesion is used. This point will then be placed at the center of the arc quadrant system and approached along a carefully selected trajectory. The mea-

FIGURE 15.5 *(A) Digitized contour of a mass lesion taken from a CT (white matter) and MRI (gray matter) image localized in stereotactic space. (B) By suspending CT and MRI data in a three-dimensional image matrix, the CT and MRI determined tumor volumes may be calculated and displayed. (By permission of Mayo Clinic.)*

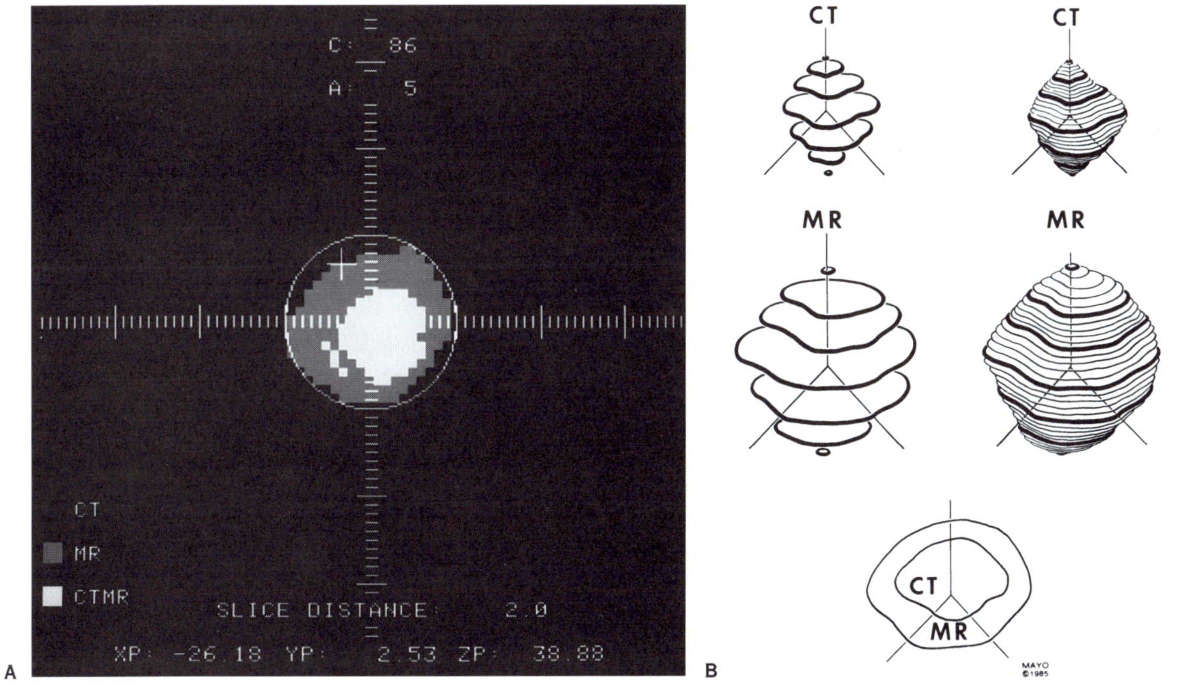

sured accuracy of this system for CT is ± 0.5 mm along the X (right-left) and Y (AP) axes and is within one-half the image thickness along the Z or vertical axis.[42] The tested accuracy of the MRI localization system is 1.1 mm in the X and Y axes and, again, one-half the image thickness along the Z axis.

The DA images may also be displayed on the viewing screen. After the surgeon digitizes all the 18 reference marks of the DA localization system, these images can be mathematically related to the coordinates established for CT and MRI.

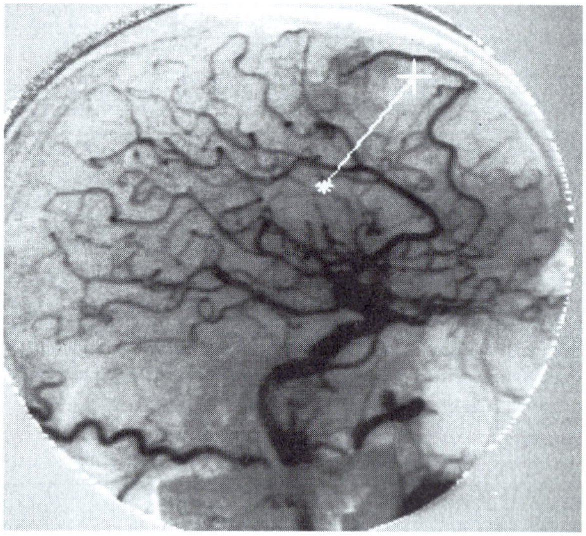

FIGURE 15.6 *Digital angiogram showing a simulated probe trajectory. This permits the surgeon to select a trajectory that avoids vascular structures.*

SELECTION OF THE SURGICAL APPROACH

After the stereotactic images have been transferred and transformed into stereotactic space, the trajectory (described in terms of arc and collar angles) or approach to the lesion is planned at the computer console. For a stereotactically guided tumor resection, the three-dimensional configuration of the tumor is analyzed and the approach is planned if possible along the long axis of the tumor volume. Whether a tumor resection or stereotactic biopsy is planned, the position of overlying cortical regions and critical surrounding subcortical structures and pathways are carefully noted. Using a mouse directed cursor and a simple-to-use computer program, the surgeon can simulate probe trajectories that are displayed as a line connecting the point of approach on the surface of the skull to the target point or tumor volume (Fig. 15.6). In addition, the surgeon can simulate the same trajectories on the arterial and venous phases of the DA.[4] Probe trajectories through contiguous CT and MRI images may also be displayed. After a trajectory has been selected that avoids critical neural tissue, bony structures, and blood vessels, the computer calculates the arc and collar settings that represent these approach angles on the stereotactic arc quadrant table. A phantom stereotactic headframe is then used to simulate the surgical approach to the target point. Any simple mechanical obstructions (i.e., a vertical support or carbon-fiber pin in the path of the trajectory) to the planned trajectory are thus observed before surgery and an alternative trajectory may be selected that avoids such pitfalls. Surgical instrumentation such as the circular trephine, the stereotactic cylindrical retractor,[43] side-biting biopsy forceps, the operating microscope, and the stereotactically directed carbon dioxide laser[8,9] are all directed to the surgical target along the line defined by the trajectory on the arc quadrant frame (Fig. 15.7).

PATIENT POSITIONING FOR STEREOTACTIC PROCEDURES

The position of the patient is determined by the trajectory the neurosurgeon has selected and may be at any headframe setting from 0° (supine) to 180° (prone) to 270° (left lateral decubitus). The high degree of variation in patient

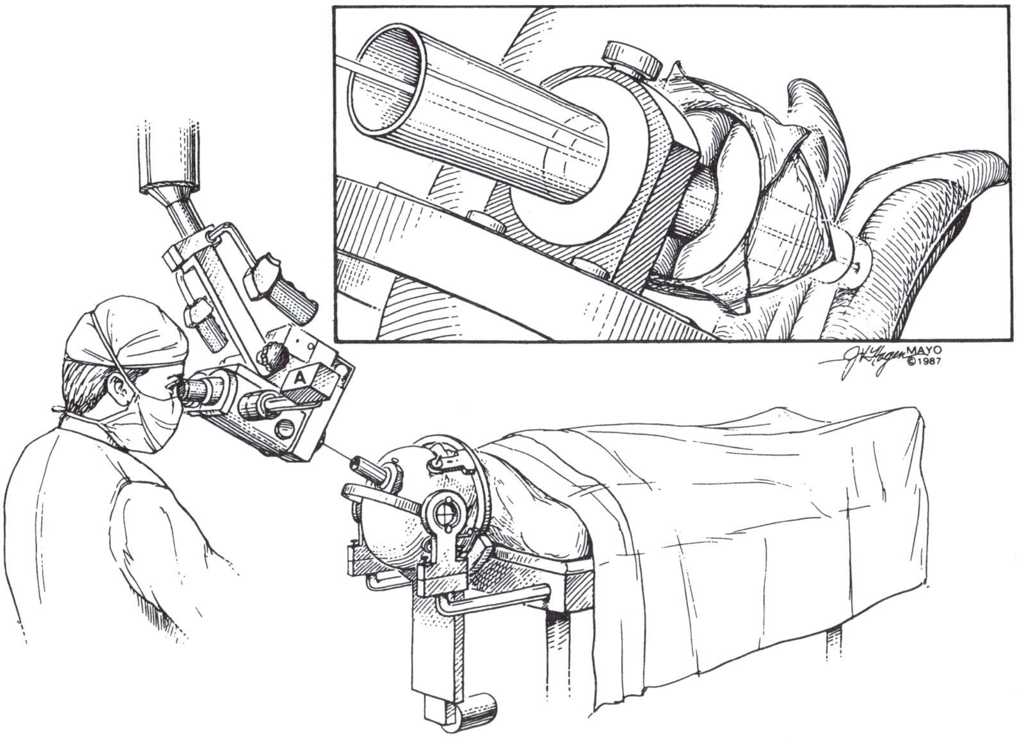

FIGURE 15.7 *Stereotactic cylindrical retractor mounted on the arc quadrant apparatus used to create a passage for the surgical laser. The surgeon views and directs the procedure through an operating microscope. (By permission of Mayo Clinic.)*

positioning for stereotactic procedures at this institution requires that the anesthesiologist be aware of the special requirements of several positions. The more common positions (other than supine) utilized are the prone, right and left lateral decubitus, and the semiprone positions, in which the patient's head, shoulders, and torso are no longer perpendicular to the operating table and the down arm rests behind rather than in front of the patient. Close attention to pressure points, excessive weight bearing on either the abdomen or portions of the chest wall, and traction along the neck, shoulders, hips, and upper and lower extremities has made anesthesia-related complications attributable to improper positioning extremely rare. Not uncommonly, the patient is positioned to face the side opposite that of the anesthesia machine and the anesthesiologist. Under such less than ideal circumstances, all connections in the anesthesia circuit are forcefully tightened and the endotracheal tube is carefully tested for stability after taping. Long anesthesia hoses are used and secured with tape to minimize traction on the endotracheal tube. Finally, after the patient has been draped, the anesthetist becomes familiar with an approach to the patient's airway such that a rapid response is possible in the event of an airway disconnection. The absence of breath sounds from the esophageal stethoscope and the airway circuit low-pressure alarm are the first indicators of a disconnection in the anesthesia circuit, which usually occurs at the connection between the endotracheal tube and the elbow connector. This is easily corrected by the anesthetist who is aware of a route of access to the airway beneath the drapes. Should the patient become extubated under such circumstances (an event that has not occurred at our institution), the surgical procedure would have to be stopped and the patient repositioned, ventilated via a mask, and reintubated.

Close attention must also be paid to the position of the stereotactic headframe base ring with respect to the patient's neck and shoulders. The edge of the base ring can forcefully encroach on the patient's neck and shoulder areas and could, conceivably, result in neuropraxia of the brachial plexus. This is particularly a problem in the stocky or obese patient with a relatively short neck and in the downward shoulder of patients placed in the lateral decubitus or semiprone position. Judicious placement of padding between the patient's neck and shoulders and the edge of the base ring is effective in preventing pressure sores. Care must also be taken when placing the base ring in the receiving yoke of the arc quadrant table. Folds of skin from the shoulder area may be entrapped and badly pinched between the yoke and the base ring. Careful examination of the yoke and base ring area during and just after securing the headframe will prevent this complication.

ANESTHETIC CONSIDERATIONS FOR STEREOTACTIC NEUROSURGICAL PROCEDURES

Local Anesthesia With Sedation Versus General Anesthesia

The majority of reported stereotactic neurosurgical procedures have been performed with infiltration of the scalp with local anesthetic and sedation obtained using neuroleptanalgesia, a benzodiazepine-narcotic combination, or narcotic alone. Exceptions to this have generally included children less than 6 years old, patients who are extremely restless and uncooperative, and patients requiring a transcerebellar stereotatic procedure (i.e., patients with lesions in the posterior cranial fossa).

Local anesthetic infiltration of the scalp has been used as the sole anesthetic for craniotomy in the awake patient.[44,45] In addition, infiltration of the scalp with either intermediate (lidocaine) or long-acting (bupivacaine) local anesthetic with and without epinephrine markedly attenuates or eliminates the arterial hypertension and tachycardia commonly observed following skull clamp placement, scalp incision, and craniotomy[46] in patients receiving general endotracheal anesthesia. Although it has not been systematically studied, at least 1 minute should elapse between the time of scalp infiltration with local anesthetic and placement of the stereotactic headframe. A mixture of 0.33% bupivacaine with epinephrine 1:200,000 reportedly provides adequate scalp anesthesia for 8 to 12 hours.[47] Plasma concentrations of the local anesthetics following infiltration of the scalp remain well below toxic levels.[48]

The success of local anesthetic infiltration in providing adequate anesthesia for placement of the stereotactic headframe and scalp incision is attributable to the mode of innervation of the scalp. The layers of the scalp, the skin, subcutaneous tissue, muscle, galea aponeurotica, and periosteum of the outer table of the skull are innervated by cutaneous nerves arising from the superficial ascending branches of the cervical plexus (the greater and lesser occipital nerves and the greater auricular nerve) and from branches of the three major divisions of the trigeminal nerve. Subcutaneous local anesthetic scalp infiltration either in the manner of a field block or over a specific sensory nerve branch thus blocks afferent sensory input from all the layers of the scalp.

The skull itself has no sensation and can be drilled, curetted, and sawed with little discomfort to the patient.[47,49] Unexpected pain may, however, occur when the bone is drilled, particularly as the tip of the drill bit or curette impinges on the dura. The intracranial dura mater is innervated by branches arising from all three divisions of the trigeminal nerve, a recurrent meningeal branch of the vagus nerve, and, possibly, branches from the upper two or three cervical roots. The sensitivity of the dura to painful stimuli is greatest in the distribution of the middle meningeal artery (i.e., in the middle or temporal fossa) but is also appreciable in proximity to the falx cerebri, particularly the posterior third, the tentorium, and the dural sinuses.[47,49–51] In the case of patients undergoing awake craniotomies, the dura has been successfully anesthetized by injection of local anesthetic between the dural leaflets before dural incision and reflection.[47] Although dural anesthesia for stereotactic procedures has not been reported or thought necessary, it would seem worth considering when a dural incision is necessary in proximity to a larger branch of the middle meningeal artery or in the posterior cranial fossa. The pia, the substance of the brain itself, and the cerebral vasculature are generally not sensitive to painful stimuli.[51]

The numbers and types of stereotactic procedures performed at our institution between July 1984 and July 1995 are shown in Table 15.1. Patients ranged from 3 months (with five patients less than 1 year old) to 84 years of age. Only ventral-lateral thalamotomies and some shunt placements are routinely performed using local anesthesia with sedation. All other procedures are performed using general endotracheal anesthesia. With the exception of very young patients, stereotactic biopsies were initially almost all performed using local anesthesia and intravenous sedation. Several patients, however, experienced prolonged seizures while undergoing stereotactic biopsy. Subsequent difficulties in management of the airway necessitated the rapid removal of the headframe. Stereotactic biopsies as well as most other stereotactic procedures have subsequently been performed using general anesthesia with endotracheal intubation.

Awake patients may arrive in the stereotactic operating room with or without the stereotactic headframe already in place. Those without the headframe in place are anesthetized before reapplication of the frame. The headframe is then reapplied and the patient is moved to the stereotactic operating table and positioned in such a way as to facilitate positioning of the target point in the center of the arc quadrant appara-

TABLE 15.1 *Stereotactic procedures and anesthetic used at the Mayo Clinic, July 1984 to July 1995*

PROCEDURE	NO. OF CASES	ANESTHESIA
Stereotactic biopsy	1,551	General/sedation
Third ventriculostomy	1,103	General
Thalamotomy	128	General/sedation
Cyst aspiration	108	Sedation
Amygdalohippocampectomy	114	General/sedation
Omaya reservoir placement	23	General
Interstitial radiation	29	General
^{32}P instillation	22	General
Shunt	21	Sedation
Adrenal medullary transplant	19	General
^{192}Ir instillation	8	General
Cingulotomy	6	General
Dentatotomy	4	General
Total	1	

tus. Patients that have been anesthetized for the imaging studies are often brought to the operating room while still anesthetized and with the headframe in place. These patients are simply transferred to the stereotactic operating table with continuation of general endotracheal anesthesia.

The awake surgical candidate with a headframe in place often has a decreased range of neck flexion and extension related to the position of the headframe with respect to the neck and shoulders. In addition, even when the anterior segment of the headframe is removable, access to the mouth is extremely limited. Accordingly, these patients are usually intubated with a small-diameter wire spiral endotracheal tube over a fiberoptic bronchoscope just before induction of general anesthesia. This is usually accomplished after topical application of 4% lidocaine spray to the larynx, possibly augmented by superior laryngeal nerve blocks or a transtracheal block. Patients are preoxygenated and monitored as described below before intubation and induction.

Monitoring

Routine monitoring for stereotactic procedures includes pulse oximetry, ECG, blood pressure cuff, precordial or esophageal stethoscope, and temperature probe. Respiratory gas monitoring is used to keep close control of patient's end-expired carbon dioxide level and the partial pressure of any volatile anesthetic being used. Even when a procedure is performed in an awake patient ventilation can be monitored by placing the tip of the mass spectrometer capillary gas sampling line in the patient's nostril. Direct arterial blood pressure monitoring is often used during stereotactic procedures performed under general endotracheal anesthesia to provide beat-to-beat blood pressure measurement and to facilitate arterial blood gas sampling. The latter are used to assess the patient's oxygenation and the gradient between the end-expired and arterial carbon dioxide.

Control of Blood Pressure

The incidence of postoperative intracranial hemorrhage is probably lower after stereotactic procedures than after open craniotomies because less brain tissue is incised. The risk of hemorrhage cannot be dismissed, however, as it is impossible for the neurosurgeons to see and cauterize all potential bleeding sites in the approach to and proximity of the surgical target. To decrease the risk of hemorrhage, it is crucial to prevent and aggressively treat marked elevations in the arterial blood pressure during and immediately after stereotactic procedures. α- and β-adrenergic receptor antagonists such as hydralazine, propranolol, esmolol, and labetalol, as well as direct arterial smooth muscle relaxants, such as sodium nitroprusside, can be used to treat and prevent hypertensive episodes.

Intracranial Hypertension

Increased intracranial pressure (ICP) can be more difficult to manage in a stereotactic procedure because the limited nature of the surgical exposure and resection often does little to relieve pressure caused by a mass lesion. Optimum elevation of the head to facilitate venous drainage may not be possible during a stereotactic procedure owing to restrictions placed on patient movement by stereotactic neurosurgical equipment. Steps that may be taken to lower ICP are described more fully in another chapter of this text (see Ch. 3). In the anesthetized patient, they include hyperventilation to a $PaCO_2$ of 25 mmHg, an immediate bolus of thiopental (1 to 3 mg/kg) or propofol (0.5 to 1 mg/kg)[52] to reduce the patient's cerebral blood volume quickly, and the administration of an osmotic diuretic (usually 0.25 to 1 g/kg mannitol)[53] with or without furosemide to decrease the brain water content. The effect of steroids is usually too slow in onset to be useful in treating intracranial hypertension intraoperatively.

SPECIFIC COMPUTER-ASSISTED STEREOTACTIC PROCEDURES

Stereotactic Thalamotomy

Parkinson's disease is a common condition, with a prevalence rate in Western societies as high as 180 per 100,000 population.[54] Before the introduction of levodopa in 1968 as a treatment, management of Parkinson's disease emphasized surgical treatment of tremor and rigidity. Despite the successes and advances in the pharmacologic treatment of Parkinson's disease, some patients with a severely disabling tremor fail to respond to medical management. An alternative treatment for disabling parkinsonian tremor is a thalamotomy, which, when performed in appropriately selected patients using stereotactic neurosurgical techniques, exposes the patient to no more morbidity and inconvenience than prolonged drug trials. The best surgical candidates are patients whose symptoms remain unilateral and who do not have speech and gait disturbances.[55] The improvement in tremor and rigidity following a stereotactic thalamotomy may be permanent on the side opposite the thalamotomy.[54,56]

For this procedure the stereotactic headframe is applied, and the patient undergoes stereotactic CT as described previously. In addition, a contrast ventriculogram is obtained by introduction of metrizamide into the lateral ventricle through a burr hole. Local anesthesia with very light sedation is utilized. It is important to make the patient as comfortable as possible to prevent disruption of the surgical field with tremor-related head movements and yet to keep the patient alert enough to answer questions and follow commands. Hypertension is treated aggressively. The coronal wound is reopened, and a bipolar concentric microelectrode[57] is introduced to permit somatotopic placement of a probe capable of introducing radiofrequency lesions. The microelectrode records electrical activity both aurally and visually. The background cellular activity increases as the electrode enters the nucleus ventralis posterior. When the procedure is being performed on the patient's dominant side, speech is tested intraoperatively after a test lesion is produced. If no adverse sequelae have resulted from the test lesion, the target lesion is produced by reheating the radiofrequency electrode tip. Excessive sedation at the time of or just following introduction of the test lesion would make it impossible to assess the effects of the test lesion on neurologic function.

Volumetric Stereotactic Surgical Resection of Intra-axial Brain Tumors

The methodology of computer-assisted stereotactic laser resection of intra-axial brain tumors was developed to facilitate an accurate and precise approach to brain tumors that lie below the cortical surface, often deep within the brain parenchyma. The precision afforded by stereotactic techniques offers more complete tumor removal with less destruction of surrounding brain tissue.

Anesthesia is induced with thiopental or propofol, and muscle relaxation is obtained with a nondepolarizing relaxant. Patients are hyperventilated before intubation and the introduction of volatile anesthetic agents. A second dose of intravenous anesthetic is often administered just before intubation, which is performed after loss of all four twitches following a train-of-four stimulus. Anesthesia is usually maintained with a mixture of isoflurane and nitrous oxide in oxygen and supplemented with intravenous fentanyl. After induction of anesthesia, the stereotactic headframe then is reapplied as described previously.

At the end of the surgical procedure, the stereotactic headframe is removed, and the patient is awakened and neurologically assessed in the operating room. If the patient's neurologic examination reveals no new or worsened deficits, the patient is transferred to the recovery room, where neurologic status is assessed frequently.

Gamma Knife Radiosurgery

Advancing technology has greatly improved the treatment options for patients with arteriovenous malformations (AVMs) of the brain. In addition to improved imaging techniques and new capabilities for staged endovascular embolizations, the introduction of the gamma knife (Electra Instruments, Atlanta, GA) has provided a significant therapeutic advance.[58] This instrument focuses radiation energy accurately from multiple directions onto a defined volumetric area to concentrate the highest doses possible on the AVM with minimal dose exposure to surrounding tissues. A number of other types of lesions also respond to radiosurgery. Radiosurgical therapy has led to the total obliteration of the AVM nidus in 72.1% of a series of 121 patients with lesions as large as 30 cm^3, including AVM considered surgically unresectable.[59] A stable or improved outcome was reported in 91.7% of patients in that series. Other series report angiographic complete obliteration rates ranging from 70 to 88%, although progressive AVM obliteration does not begin until 6 to 12 months after treatment.[59,60]

A stereotactic headframe is used to permit accurate AVM localization during angiography, MRI scanning, and the actual radiosurgical therapy in the gamma knife unit. For most adults, only mild sedation is needed for headframe placement, subsequent studies, and the actual period the patient is being irradiated, although the sequence of diagnostic and therapeutic steps necessitates the headframe to remain on the patient for 4 to 8 hours. General anesthesia would be indicated for children and for adults with motion disorders or severe claustrophobia.

Lesions Amenable to Radiosurgery

Most arteriovenous malformations
Skull-based meningioma
Metastatic neoplasms
Acoustic neuromas
Malignant skull-based tumors (i.e., glomus tumors)

THE FUTURE OF STEREOTACTIC NEUROSURGERY

The field of stereotactic neurosurgery is growing rapidly and will require the support of anesthesiologists familiar with its basic principles and instrumentation to better anticipate the needs of both the patient and the surgeon. Stereotactic-directed biopsies of brain lesions are becoming commonplace at some centers and will probably gain wider acceptance in the near future. The use of stereotactic techniques for the local introduction of irradiation,[61] chemotherapy, tumor-directed antibodies, and photo irradiation therapy to deep-seated brain tumors is another area of anticipated growth.[62]

The probable lower morbidity and mortality associated with the stereotactic approach to intra-axial brain structures compared with that of a conventional craniotomy makes the former the technique of choice for many types of neurosurgical procedures.

Frameless stereotactic surgery may become practical in the near future, which will obviate many of the headframe-related considerations described earlier.

References

1. Bergstrom M, Greitz T: Stereotaxic computed tomography. AJR 127:167, 1976
2. Kelly PJ: Introduction and historical aspects. p. 1.

In Tumor Stereotaxis. WB Saunders, Philadelphia, 1991
3. Kelly PJ: Computerized guidance for stereotactic treatment of brain tumors: From CT-guided biopsy to computerized resection. Neurosurg State Art Rev 2:165, 1987
4. Kelly PJ, Kall B, GoerssS, Alker GJ: A method of computed tomography-based stereotaxic biopsy with arteriographic control. Neurosurgery 14:172, 1984
5. Bertrand G, Olivier A: Computer display of stereotaxic brain maps and probe tracts. Acta Neurochir 21:235, 1974
6. Kall BA, Kelly PJ, Goerss SJ, Frieder G: Methodology and clinical experience with computed tomography and a computer-resident stereotactic atlas. Neurosurgery 17:400, 1985
7. Kall BA: The impact of computer and imaging technology on stereotactic surgery. Appl Neurophysiol 50:9, 1987
8. Kall BA, Kelly PJ, Goerss SJ: Interactive stereotactic surgical system for the removal of intracranial tumors utilizing the CO_2 laser and CT-derived database. IEEE Trans Biomed Eng 32:112, 1985
9. Kall BA, Kelly PJ, Goerss SJ: Stereotactic computer-aided neurosurgery. CO_2 laser resection of CNS tumors. IEEE Trans Biomed Eng 32:692, 1985
10. Kall BA, Kelly PJ, Goerss SJ: The computer as stereotactic surgical instrument. Neurosurg Res 8:201, 1986
11. Kall BA, Kelly PJ, Goerss SJ: Comprehensive computer-assisted data collection, treatment planning and interactive surgery. Soc Photo-Optical Instrument Eng 767:509, 1987
12. Gildenberg PL, Kaufman HH, Krishna Murthy KS: Calculation of stereotactic coordinates from the computed tomographic scan. Neurosurgery 10:580, 1982
13. Goerss SJ, Kelly PJ, Kall BA: Automated stereotactic positioning system. Appl Neurophysiol 50:100, 1987
14. Kelly PJ: The laser and stereotactic neurosurgery. Neurosurg State Art Rev 2:459, 1987
15. Kelly PJ, Kall BA, Goerss S, Alker GJ, Jr: Precision resection of intra-axial CNS lesions by CT-based stereotactic craniotomy and computer monitored CO_2 laser. Acta Neurochir 68:1, 1983
16. Feindel W: Wilder Penfield (1891–1976): A protagonist for functional neurosurgery. Appl Neurophysiol 50:347, 1987
17. Kelly PJ, Earnest F, Kall B et al: Surgical options for patients with deep-seated brain tumours. Mayo Clin Proc 60:223, 1985
18. Kelly PJ, Goerss S, Kall BA, Kispert DB: Computer tomography-based stereotactic third ventriculostomy: technical note. Neurosurgery 18:791, 1986
19. Kelly PJ, Kall BA, Goerss SJ, Cascino TL: Results of computer-assisted stereotactic laser resection of deep-seated intracranial lesions. Mayo Clin Proc 61:20, 1986
20. Kelly PJ: Volumetric stereotactic surgical resection of intra-axial brain mass lesions. Mayo Clin Proc 63:1186, 1988
21. Cascino TL: Treatment of patients with brain tumours. Mayo Clinic Proc 60:279, 1985
22. Davis DH, Kelly PJ, Marsh WR et al: Computer-assisted stereotactic biopsy of intracranial lesions. Appl Neurophysiol 50:172, 1987
23. Bosch DA: Indications for stereotactic biopsy in brain tumours. Acta Neurochir 54:167, 1980
24. Ostertag CB: Reliability of stereotactic brain tumor biopsy. p. 129. In Lunsford LD (ed): Modern Stereotactic Neurosurgery. Martinus Nijhoff Publishing, Boston, 1988
25. Mundinger F: Operable gehirnkrankheiten-stereotaktische Operationen. Z Allg Med 50:815, 1974
26. Marshall LF, Jennett B, Langfitt TW: Needle biopsy for the diagnosis of malignant glioma. JAMA 228:1417, 1974
27. Coffey RJ, Lunsford LD: Stereotactic surgery for mass lesions of the midbrain and pons. Neurosurgery 17:12, 1985
28. Kelly PJ, Kall BA, Goerss SJ: Computer-assisted stereotactic resection of posterior fossa lesions. Surg Neurol 25:530, 1986
29. Kelly PJ, Kall BA, Goerss SJ: Results of computed tomography-based computer-assisted stereotactic resection of metastatic intracranial tumors. Neurosurgery 22:7, 1988
30. Lunsford LD: Diagnosis and treatment of mass lesions using the Leksell stereotactic system. p. 145. In Lunsford LD (ed): Modern Stereotactic Neurosurgery. Martinus Nijhoff Publishing, Boston, 1988
31. Ostertag CB, Mennel HD, Kiessling M: Stereotactic biopsy of brain tumors. Surg Neurol 14:275, 1980
32. Nauta JH, Briner RP, Eisenberg HM: Computer tomogram-guided stereotactic brain biopsy in the pediatric patient. Pediatr Neurosci 12:63, 1986

33. Uematsu S, Rosenbaum AE, Abel DL et al: Helmet for infant skull fixation during stereotactic neurosurgery. Appl Neurophysiol 50:114, 1987
34. Reid SA, Grundy BL: The head-elevated positions. Surgical aspects: the neurosurgical skull clamp. p. 71. In Martin JT (ed): Positioning in Anesthesia and Surgery. WB Saunders, Philadelphia, 1987
35. Broere G: Complications of the Mayfield skull clamp. Anesthesiology 61:460, 1984
36. Wilkins RH, Albin MS: An unusual entrance site of venous air embolism during operations in the sitting position. Surg Neurol 7:71, 1977
37. Inagawa T, Takeda T, Taguchi H et al: Traumatic middle meningeal arteriovenous fistula caused by three-point skull fixation. J Neurosurg 60:853, 1984
38. Roth JL, Nugent M, Gray JE et al: Patient monitoring during magnetic resonance imaging. Anesthesiology 62:80, 1985
39. Jorgensen NH, Messick JM, Jr, Gray J et al: ASA monitoring standards and magnetic resonance imaging. Anesth Analg 79:1141, 1994
40. Kelly PJ, Kall BA, Goerss SJ: Transposition of volumetric information derived from computed tomography scanning into stereotactic space. Surg Neurol 21:465, 1985
41. Kelly PJ, Goerss SJ, Kall BA: Modification of Todd-Wells system for imaging data acquisition. p. 79. In Lunsford LD (ed): Modern Stereotactic Neurosurgery. Martinus Nijhoff Boston, 1988
42. Goerss SJ, Kelly PJ, Kall BA, Alker GJ: A computed tomographic stereotactic adaptation system. Neurosurgery 69:301, 1982
43. Kelly PJ, Goerss SJ, Kall BA: The stereotactic retractor in computer-assisted stereotaxic microsurgery. J Neurosurg 69:301, 1988
44. Varkey GP: Anesthetic Considerations for Craniotomy in Awake Patients. Little, Brown, Boston, 1986
45. Perkins WJ, Kelly PJ, Faust RJ: Stereotactic surgery. p. 379. In Cucchiara RF (ed): Clinical Neuroanesthesia. Churchill Livingstone, New York, 1990
46. Colley PS, Dunn R: Prevention of blood pressure response to skull-pin head holder by local anesthesia. Anesth Analg 58:241, 1979
47. Girvin JP: Neurosurgical considerations and general methods for craniotomy under local anesthesia. Int Anesthesiol Clin 24:89, 1986
48. Colley PS, Heavner JE: Blood levels of bupivacaine after injection into the scalp with and without epinephrine. Anesthesiology 54:81, 1981
49. Manninen P, Contreras J: Anesthetic considerations for craniotomy in awake patients. Int Anesthesiol Clin 24:157, 1986
50. Penfield W: Combined regional and general anesthesia for craniotomy and cortical exploration. Int Anesthesiol Clin 24:1, 1986
51. Penfield W, McNaughton F: Dural headache and innervation of the dura mater. Arch Neurol Psychol 44:43, 1940
52. Weglinski MR, Perkins WJ: Inhalational versus total intravenous anesthesia for neurosurgery: theory guides, outcome decides. J Neurosurg Anesth 6:290, 1994
53. Marshall LF, Smith RW, Rauscher LA, Shapiro HM: Mannitol dose requirements in brain-injured patients. J Neurosurg 48:169, 1978
54. Tasker RR: Tremor of parkinsonism and stereotactic thalamotomy. Mayo Clin Proc 62:736, 1987
55. Kelly PJ, Ahlskog JE, Goerss SJ et al: Computer-assisted stereotactic ventralis lateralis thalamotomy with microelectrode recording control in patients with Parkinson's disease. Mayo Clin Proc 62:655, 1987
56. Kelly PJ: Microelectrode recording for the somatotopic placement of stereotactic thalamic lesions in the treatment of parkinsonism and cerebellar intention tremor. Appl Neurophysiol 43:262, 1980
57. Kelly PJ, Derome PP, Guiot G: Thalamic spatial variability and the surgical results of lesions placed with neurophysiologic control. Surg Neurol 9:307, 1978
58. Leksell L: Stereotaxis and Radiosurgery. An Operative System. Charles C Thomas, Springfield, IL, 1971
59. Coffey RJ, Nichols DA, Shaw EG: Stereotactic radiosurgical treatment of cerebral arteriovenous malformations. Mayo Clin Proc 70:214, 1995
60. Lunsford LD: Stereotactic radiosurgical procedures for arteriovenous malformations of the brain (editorial). Mayo Clin Proc 70:305, 1995
61. Gutin PH, Edwards MSB, Wara WM et al: Preliminary experience with 125-I-brachytherapy of pediatric brain tumors. Concepts Pediatr Neurosurg 5:187, 1985
62. Kelly PJ: Presidential address: future possibilities in stereotactic surgery: where are we going? Appl Neurophysiol 50:1, 1987

Suggested Reading

Bosch DA: Stereotactic Techniques in Clinical Neurosurgery. Springer-Verlag, Wien, 1986

Lunsford LD (ed): Modern Stereotactic Neurosurgery. Martinus Nijhoff Publishing, Boston, 1988

Kelly PJ: Tumor Stereotaxis. WB Saunders, Philadelphia, 1991

Kelly PJ, Kall BA (eds): Contemporary Issues in Neurological Surgery: Computers in Stereotactic Neurosurgery. Blackwell Scientific Publications, Boston, 1992

16 PEDIATRIC NEUROANESTHESIA

RICHARD J. POLLARD

J. PARKER MICKLE

The goals of pediatric neuroanesthesia remain consistent and unchanged over time: to induce and maintain satisfactory anesthesia with amnesia, to reduce intracranial pressure (ICP), to optimize the surgical field, and to affect a quick postoperative recovery for early clinical evaluation. The subject matter contained in this chapter summarizes our experience and philosophy in attaining these goals.

The rapidity with which a child can deteriorate neurologically and systemically requires constant vigilance on the part of the attending physicians in the operating room, the pediatric intensive care unit, and on the standard pediatric floor. Nowhere in medicine is the team concept more appropriate and necessary than in retrieving a child from serious illness. An integral part of the health care team in these situations is often the family and its perception of the child's health and illness.

Some of the most serious illnesses affect the central nervous system (CNS), and three out of the four most serious threats to children (trauma, brain tumors, and congenital malformations) are cared for most directly by the pediatric neurosurgeon and pediatric neuroanesthesiologist. A working knowledge of the intricacies of the anatomy, physiology, and pathophysiology of the pediatric patient is essential for any anesthesiologist attending the pediatric neurosurgical patient. Just the mere size of these patients and the size of the equipment necessary to accomplish a successful anesthetic procedure are somewhat intimidating to most individuals inexperienced in this area. No major effort in pediatric neurosurgery can be considered without first-class pediatric neuroanesthesia and professional and experienced pediatric intensive care capability.

This chapter will attempt to define the most common entities encountered by the pediatric neurosurgeon and pediatric neuroanesthesiologist. Pediatric neuroanesthesia is changing rapidly because of new technical additions such as transcranial Doppler evaluation of cerebral blood flow (CBF) and electrophysiologic monitoring of various neurosystems during surgery. Controversies exist in virtually every area of clinical expertise summarized below. These controversies are simplified when approached from a base of strong and extensive clinical experience and supplemented with an investigative approach to problem solving. This technique of approaching each problem with a comprehensive differential diagnosis will often eliminate many of the problems associated with these patients.

PEDIATRIC ANATOMY AND PHYSIOLOGY

Neuroanatomy

The pediatric brain and CNS is the largest and fastest developing organ in the body. The neonatal brain at term weighs approximately 335 g and comprises 15 to 20% of total body weight. This more than doubles within the first year. By the age of 2 years, it has reached 80% of the adult weight. As the child ages, the rate of growth slows, and the disparity in size changes until the brain reaches approximately 1% of the body's weight by adulthood. The protection afforded the pediatric brain differs from the adult in that the bony skull is incomplete and the skull is pliable. Continued enlargement of the brain is allowed by growth of the nonfused cranial plates. These are easily identifiable in the neonate and infant population as are the anterior and posterior fontanelles. The posterior fontanelle closes by the second month, whereas the anterior fontanelle may remain open until the 19th month. These fontanelles allow for a mechanism of buffering of acute changes in intracranial volume and coincidentally provide easy sites for access to intracranial monitoring and rapid ultrasound imaging. This buffering mechanism along with the nonfused sutures allows for cranial expansion before ICP increases. These mechanisms, however, are not limitless as fibrous structures join the sutures and cover the fontanelles so limiting the potential for expansion.

In the embryo, the spinal cord extends the entire length of the vertebral canal. Because the vertebral column grows more rapidly than the spinal cord in the embryo and fetus, this relationship does not persist. In the newborn infant, the spinal cord terminates at L2 or L3, whereas in the adult, it usually ends at the inferior border of L1 vertebrae (Fig. 16.1). The meninges covering the spinal cord project to S3 or S4 in the infant, whereas in the adult, they extend only to S2.

FIGURE 16.1 *Development of the infant spinal cord showing relative locations at different stages of development. (A) 20 weeks gestation. (B) Birth, end of spinal cord at L3. (C) Adult location, spinal cord ends at L1. (Data from various sources.)*

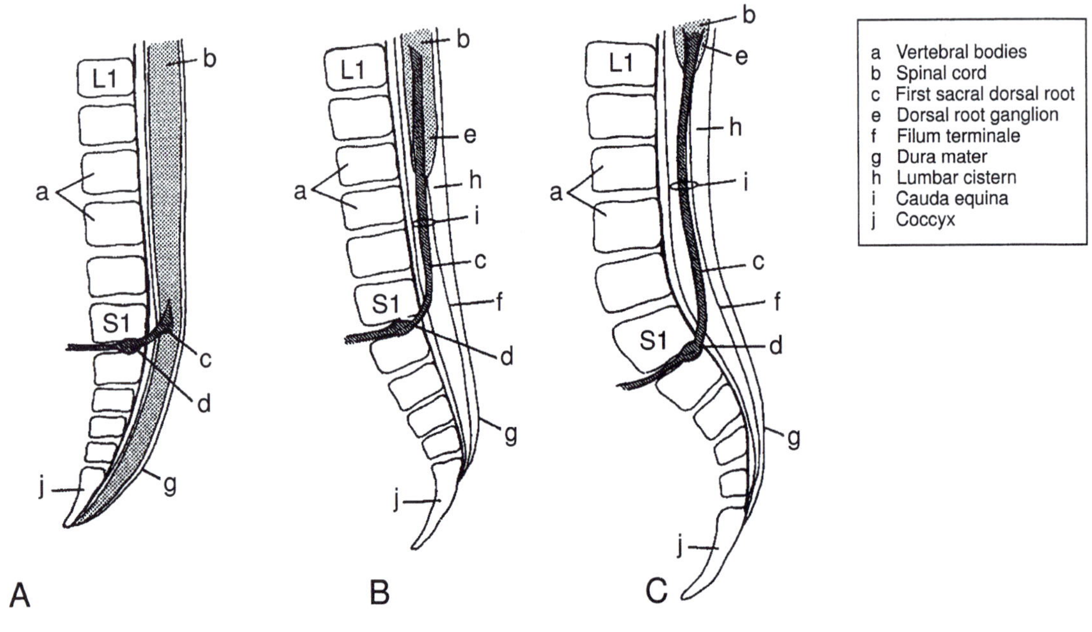

Neurophysiology

The intracranial contents of the normal pediatric patient are present in the same ratios as in the adult. The brain tissue and extracellular fluid occupy 80% of the volume with the cerebrospinal fluid (CSF) and the cerebral blood volume (CBV) comprising 10% each. CBF varies in the pediatric population. Blood flow is 50 ml/100 g/min in the adult, whereas in the premature infant, blood flow has been reported to be 12 ml/100 g/min and is 23 to 40 ml/100 g/min in the full-term neonate.[1–3] It has been noted that in the older pediatric population the CBF is greatly increased over that of adults. One study revealed a CBF of approximately 100 ml/100 g/min in the 3 to 11-year-old population.[4]

The cerebral metabolic rate for oxygen ($CMRO_2$) is also increased in the pediatric population. It has been shown that the $CMRO_2$ is 5.2 ml O_2/100 g/min in 3 to 11-year-old children versus adult values of 3.5 to 4.5 ml/100 g/min. The increased blood flow and oxygen consumption in children is not well understood, but the conclusion has been made that the pediatric brain is less tolerant to hypoxia than that of an adult. Cerebral autoregulation is normally intact in the pediatric patient, although the mean arterial blood pressure (MAPs) involved are lower (Fig. 16.2). Dog studies reveal that autoregulation occurs at 40 to 100 mmHg in puppies, whereas in adult dogs, it is shifted to 50 and 150 mmHg.[5] Cerebral perfusion pressure (CPP) is an indirect measurement of the perfusion pressure of the brain. It is derived from the MAP and ICP by the following equation: CPP = MAP − ICP. CPP increases with age, starting from 25 mmHg in neonates and increasing to 80 to 90 mmHg in adults.[6] The CBF, $CMRO_2$ and CBV are thought to be affected in the same manner as in the adult brain by physiologic and pharmacologic maneuvers. These elements are discussed in Chapter 1.

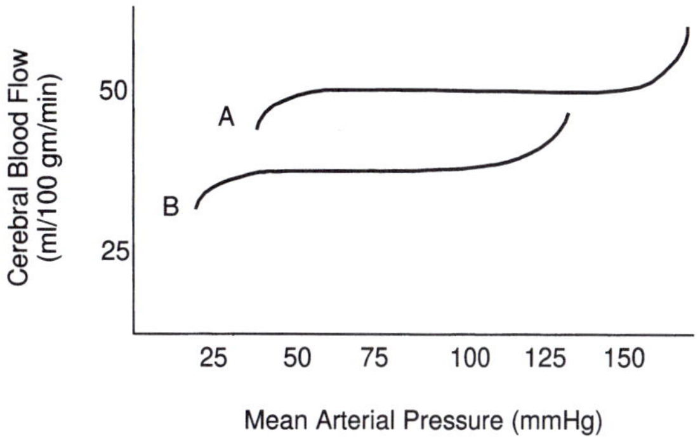

FIGURE 16.2 *Cerebral autoregulation in the adult (A) and the infant (B). The infant can maintain normal CBF at lower arterial pressures than the adult but may develop cerebral hyperemia from relatively modest increases in MAP. (From Harris,[119] with permission.)*

Neuropathophysiology

The mechanisms by which intracranial pathology occurs are numerous. However, they can be expressed in terms of primary and secondary injury. The primary injury involves the biomechanical effects of trauma to the brain tissue. This can occur due to a variety of insults, such as hemorrhage, impact, and mass effect. The secondary effects are those often preventable events that occur in response to the primary insult. For example, a primary insult may be the obstruction of the aqueduct of Sylvius by a tumor. The secondary result would be the ensuing increase in CSF volume with eventual intracranial hypertension (ICH).

The main concern for anesthesiologists is the consideration of ICH. The Monroe-Kellie hypothesis tells us that the sum of all the volume compartments must remain constant, except in instances where the cranium can expand to accommodate a larger volume. The pediatric population differs from that of an adult in that there is an additional compensatory mechanism via expansion of the cranium. A child with hydrocephalus may have a normal ICP, although the cranial circumference will be increased. If there is no obstruction of CSF circulation, non-CSF volume compartments mainly expand at the expense of the CSF volume. The pressure buffering capacity of the other compartments is minimal.

Measurement of ICP

The preoperative assessment is one of the best ways to find if the patient has ICH. Any gross alteration of behavior, sleeping or feeding problems, abnormal breathing patterns, nausea, and vomiting may be important in the history. Physical examination is inexact, as the classic signs of increased ICP such as papilledema and the Cushing's triad may be late findings. All techniques used to measure ICP in adults can, but are rarely, used in the pediatric population.[6] However, ventriculostomy is more difficult in the pediatric population due to the small size of the ventricles. Additionally a noninvasive transducer may also be applied to the open anterior fontanelle in infants, although the accuracy is somewhat in question.[7] Directly measured ICP is believed to be age related; the range is from 5.8 and 10.9 mmHg in toddlers and between 13 and 14.5 mmHg in older children and adolescents.

Treatment of ICH

The management of ICH is discussed elsewhere in this text. Similar techniques for the reduction of ICP in the adult population can be applied to the pediatric patient. Care should be exercised with mannitol as the infant has a limited cardiac reserve. This can be exceeded with osmotic diuretics and other fluid bolus techniques, leading to volume overload and pulmonary edema. Further discussion of this topic can be found in Chapter 3.

GENERAL ANESTHETIC CONSIDERATIONS

Preoperative Evaluation

The preoperative evaluation of the neurosurgical patient must include the usual history and physical examination seeking any conditions that require special concern with the anesthetic technique. Accurate assessment must be made of the patient's neurologic condition, including evidence of ICH, alteration in consciousness, and any local findings, particularly cranial nerve palsies. Bulbar palsies from brainstem pathology may be associated with reduced cough/gag reflex, leading to aspiration and its sequelae. Cranial nerve abnormalities, especially asymmetric abnormalities, indicate the probable presence of ICH. This may indicate the presence of intracranial pathology that may become exacerbated during the administration of anesthesia. The patient's level of consciousness should be evaluated using the Glasgow Coma Scale or the Children's Coma Scale (CCS) (Table 16.1). ICH can present as depressed consciousness, vomiting without nausea, lethargy, focal findings on

TABLE 16.1 *Children's coma scale (modified Glasgow Coma Scale)*

Eye Opening		
4	Spontaneous	
3	Reaction to speech	
2	Reaction to pain	
1	No response	
Best Motor Response		
6	Spontaneous	
5	Localizes pain	
4	Withdraws in response to pain	
3	Abnormal flexion in response to pain (Decorticate posture)	
2	Abnormal extension in response to pain (Decerebrate posture)	
1	No response	
Best Verbal Response		
5.	Smiles, oriented to sound, follows objects interacts	
	Crying	Interacts
4.	Consolable	Inappropriate
3.	Inconsistently consolable	Moaning
2.	Inconsolable	Irritable, restless
1.	No response	No response

(From Hahn et al.,[121] with permission.)

TABLE 16.2 *Pediatric vital signs (mean)*

AGE	WEIGHT (kg)	BLOOD PRESSURE (mmHg)	HEART RATE (bpm)	RESPIRATORY RATE (per min)
Premature	<2.5	50/30	140	35–80
Term neonate	>2.5	60/40	140	35–60
1 year	10	90/65	120	20–40
6 years	20	100/60	100	20–25
12 years	40	115/60	90	18–20

the neurologic exam, and any cranial nerve abnormalities. Some of these signs may not be evident to a physician seeing the patient for the first time, and so the family history in these areas will be invaluable.

ICH commonly presents in children as vomiting and may cause dehydration with hypovolemia, making the child liable to hypotension following induction. The fluid status of each patient should be assessed prior to induction and corrections made where appropriate. In children the mucus membranes, skin turgor, and capillary refill are a better indicator of fluid status than heart rate and blood pressure (Table 16.2). Cardiac and pulmonary auscultation will aid in identifying high-output congestive heart failure (CHF) due to a vein of Galen aneurysm. Electrolytes should be examined preoperatively and corrected as needed or indicated by the urgency of the condition. A hematocrit or hemoglobin level should be checked preoperatively and a type and screen or complete cross-match should be ordered if blood loss is expected to be great (Table 16.3). It is preferable that the computed tomographic (CT) or magnetic resonance image (MRI) scans be examined before induction and the operative technique and anticipated problems discussed with the neurosurgeon.

Unless the patient has been in a controlled environment, such as a hospital, there is a question as to whether the child has eaten. For patients undergoing emergent surgery for head trauma or acute intracranial bleeding a full stomach should be assumed. Those situations involving hydrocephalus due to blocked shunts or brain tumors can be associated with delayed gastric emptying, and so precautions should be taken.

One contraindication to elective neurosurgical procedures is the presence of fever. It is not worth the risk to the child of a major complication associated with a generalized infection or aberrant physiologic response to an anesthetic that can occur in the face of fever of unknown etiology. Even if the cause of the fever is identified, most often the procedure should be delayed.

Parents

The patient's parents are often the primary source of information on the course of the illness. It is important that the physician seek their

TABLE 16.3 *Normal and acceptable hematocrits in pediatric patients*

AGE	NORMAL HEMATOCRIT		ACCEPTABLE HEMATOCRIT
	MEAN	RANGE	
Premature	45	40–50	35–40
Newborn	54	45–65	35–40
3 months	36	30–42	25
1 year	38	34–42	20–25
6 years	38	35–43	20–25

(From Berry,[114] with permission.)

input when evaluating the child. This is especially important in the care of individuals who have hydrocephalus and an indwelling ventriculosystemic shunt. The parents understand the early significance of symptoms referable to shunt malfunction. They must be allowed access to understanding physicians equally sensitized to these symptom complexes and the potential clinical significance of early shunt malfunction.

The parents will also affect the disposition of their child when the time comes for an anesthetic. A parent who fully understands the planned procedure and is comfortable with the anesthesiologist will communicate this feeling to the patient. This in turn will often help comfort and relax the patient before induction.

Premedication

The use of premedication in the pediatric population must be considered carefully. Even though the use of premedication makes the experience of general anesthesia more pleasant, this must be balanced against the risk of exaggerated CNS response. There should be careful evaluation of the patient's mental status prior to commencement of anesthesia. Any evidence of impaired mental function or somnolence should be a contraindication for sedatives. Sedative medication should be used judiciously in those children undergoing intracranial surgery (Table 16.4). Children with ICH, especially those with blocked shunt systems, may appear well apart from complaining of headaches and vomiting. However, many of these children will have markedly raised ICP, and minor triggers such as sedation may cause difficulty. A decreased respiratory drive caused by most sedatives will increase the carbon dioxide tension and hence increase ICP. Children with intracranial pathology may also be more sensitive than usual to the usual doses of medications.

Narcotics are well known to cause respiratory depression in all age groups and hence should be avoided in all patients with known or suspected increased ICP. The use of barbiturates as a premedication is fraught with the same concerns as narcotics. Ketamine is notorious for increasing CBF and cerebral metabolic rate and as such has no place in the sedation of patients undergoing neurosurgical procedures. Although the combination of benzodiazepine and a narcotic can cause respiratory depression and even arrest in children,[8] benzodiazepines alone may be suitable for sedation of small children in that they induce sedation without respiratory depression.[9] However, benzodiazepines can have an effect on the monitoring of certain functions during the case (e.g., electromyographics [EMGs] in spinal surgery), and discussion with the neurosurgeon should be considered. For patients with ICH who remain inconsolable or in whom it is not possible to place an IV preoperatively, midazolam (0.3 to 0.5 mg/kg) may be given by mouth. This should be done in a location where careful monitoring of the patients' neurologic status may be carried out.

TABLE 16.4 *Pediatric premedication doses*

AGENT	DOSE (mg/kg)	ROUTE	ONSET (min)
Midazolam	0.3–0.5	PO	15–30
	0.02–0.1	IV	1–3
	0.2	IM	10
	0.3–1.0	PR	10–20
Methohexital	6–10	IV/IM	3–5
	20–35	PR	5–10
Thiopental	25–35	PR	5–10
Chloral hydrate	50–75	PO	30–60
Morphine	0.05–0.1	IV	3–10
	0.1–0.2	IM	30–45
Fentanyl	0.001–0.002	IV	1–3
Pentobarbital	2–3	IV	1–5

Abbreviations: PO, per oral; IV, intravenous; IM, intramuscular; PR, per rectum.
(Modified from Feychting,[115] with permission.)

Atropine (0.02 mg/kg; minimum dose, 0.2 mg) is often given to infants less than 6 months to aid with maintenance of heart rate. However, this agent can have CNS side effects as it crosses the blood-brain barrier, and caution should be exercised in its usage. A good alternative for this use as well as functioning as an antisialogogue is glycopyrrlate (0.005 to 0.01 mg/kg), which has no CNS effects. In cases of surgery on the brainstem, the changes of heart rate caused by encroachment can be a useful monitor of neural tissue damage. Hence the use of the above agents should be avoided as they may ablate this response intraoperatively.

The preoperative use of steroids or prophylactic seizure medications is often appropriate. Patients already on these medications should continue to receive their normal doses and may require a stress dose of steroids if therapy has been prolonged.

NPO Status

The perioperative fast is often an unpleasant experience for children. The purpose of an overnight fast is to reduce the risk of pulmonary aspiration of stomach contents by reducing the volume and content and increasing the pH of stomach fluids. Patients whose gastric contents are greater than 0.4 ml/kg or whose pH is less than 2.5 are believed to be at risk.[10] The necessary fast period in the pediatric population is controversial. It is commonly accepted that in the infant population a fast of 8 hours before an operation can cause severe dehydration and so complicate anesthetic management. Prolonged fasting does not decrease gastric volume.[11] A short fast after solid food increases gastric volume,[12] but a small drink of water 2 to 3 hours preoperatively decreases gastric volume.[13] It is customary to hold solid foods for at least 8 hours prior to the operation in all patients. Small children are permitted to drink clear liquids up to 3 hours prior to surgery, and some authors report that 2 hours is acceptable.[14]

Monitoring

Routine monitoring in all pediatric neurosurgery cases should include a precordial or esophageal stethoscope, electrocardiogram (ECG), pulse oximetry, noninvasive blood pressure, and end-tidal carbon dioxide or mass spectrometry monitoring. A case that will include a large amount of blood loss relative to blood volume or increased risk of venous air embolism (VAE) should require invasive monitoring. The intravascular volume of pediatric patients can be minuscule, demanding great expertise in gaining vascular access. In the premature and neonatal population, the umbilical circulation can be used as an excellent access route be physicians familiar with the procedure. Subclavian, external and internal jugular, and femoral lines can be placed but should not be used chronically for fear of infection and thrombosis. Care should be exercised with the neck lines for fear of compromising venous return from the brain. This complication can be minimized by neutral head positioning.

Esophageal or rectal temperature monitoring should be used in all cases. Urinary catheters or bags are required in long or complicated procedures or when large volumes of urine may cause fluid balance problems.

Evoked potential and electroencephalogram (EEG) monitoring can be utilized within the pediatric population if the situation warrants. Common procedures requiring monitoring are scoliosis correction, posterior fossa surgery, and dorsal rhizotomies. For a detailed description of these techniques, refer to Chapter 4.

Fluid Requirements

The mere size of the pediatric patient presents certain restrictions, and limitations are presented to the treating physician. Intravascular volume of these patients can be quite small, requiring great expertise in minimizing blood loss and maintaining adequate intravascular volume (Table 16.5). The cranium is very vascular and significant portions of the blood volume can be lost during exposure. Blood loss in neurosurgical cases is extremely difficult to measure in that a large amount of blood is on the floor and drapes instead of being located in readily measurable suction canisters and sponges. Maintenance fluids in children are commonly agreed to

TABLE 16.5 *Average pediatric blood volume*

AGE	BLOOD VOLUME (ml/kg)
Neonates	
Premature	95
Full term	85
Infants	80

Calculation of Allowable Blood Loss

1. Estimate the blood volume from table.
2. Estimate the red cell volume at the preoperative hematocrit ($RBCV_{preop}$).
3. Estimate the red cell volume at a hematocrit of 30% ($RBCV_{30\%}$), assuming a normal blood volume is maintained.
4. Calculate the red cell volume lost when the hematocrit is 30%; $RBCV_{lost} = RBCV_{preop} - RBCV_{30\%}$.
5. Allowable blood loss = $RBCV_{lost} \times 3$.

Example: A 10-kg patient has a preoperative hematocrit of 35%. How much blood loss will decrease the hematocrit to 30%?

Estimated blood volume = 85 ml/kg × 10 kg = 850 ml

$RBCV_{35\%}$ = 850 × 35% = 297.5 ml

$RBCV_{30\%}$ = 850 × 30% = 255 ml

Red cell loss at 30% = 297.5 − 255 = 42.5 ml

Allowable blood loss = 3 × 42.5 ml = 127.5 ml

(Adapted from Streitz,[116] with permission.)

be 4 ml/kg/h for the first 10 kg, 2 ml/kg/h for the next 11 to 20 kg, and then 1 ml/kg/h for each kilogram above 20 (Table 16.6). This means that for a 27-kg child the fluid requirement will be 67 ml/h. Surgery traumatizes tissue that in turn can sequester large amounts of fluid in the interstitial space. The degree of tissue trauma affects the increased amount of fluid required for maintenance. Minimal tissue trauma, such as occurs in craniotomies, can increase fluid requirements by perhaps 1 to 2 ml/kg/h. Moderate trauma (e.g., a tibial fracture) requires an additional 2 to 4 ml/kg/h. Severe trauma requires an additional 4 to 8 ml/kg/h. These requirements usually abate over hours.

Crystalloid solutions are primarily chosen for volume replacement and maintenance. Normal saline is the preferred crystalloid because the slightly hyperosomolar nature of this fluid (no free water) does not promote or aggravate cerebral edema. If the patient's sodium (Na) level is judged to be normal, then 3% saline may also be used judiciously to replete the intravascular space as needed. This hypertonic fluid will increase vascular volume and by creating an osmotic gradient between the normal brain and the intravascular space will help "shrink" the brain. Lactated Ringer's solution is somewhat hypoosmolar as it contains 100 mL free water/L. Further discussion of this topic can be found in Chapter 6.

There is a concern that children under 6 months or those with chronic debilitating conditions may require some form of glucose supplementation during the intraoperative period. Caution must be used in this replacement as hyperglycemia in the face of brain ischemia is known to be associated with an increase in neurologic injury.[14–17] Glucose supplementation should be used only where there is a concern for the child's metabolic stability.[18] Neonates or those children with inadequate metabolic reserves should receive supplemental glucose. Especially in such cases, care should be taken to measure the blood glucose levels to avoid hyper- or hypoglycemia.

TABLE 16.6 *Estimating pediatric maintenance fluid requirements*

WEIGHT	RATE (ml/kg/h)
For the first 10 kg	4
For the next 10–20 kg	Add 2
For each kg above 20 kg	Add 1

Example: What are the maintenance fluid requirements for a 25-kg child?

Answer: 40 + 20 + 5 = 65 ml/h

(Adapted from Gullen and Stoelting,[117] with permission.)

Intravascular expansion may be performed with hetastarch-containing fluids. This is especially useful in the case of emergent surgery in a hypovolemic patient. There has been evidence of clotting impairement with very large volumes of these compounds. Because intracranial hemorrhage has such a high morbidity, the clinician should carefully consider the utility of these agents in everyday practice.

The blood volume of infants and small children is such that the loss of a relatively small volume may cause hemodynamic instability. Pediatric patients do not usually show definite signs of hypovolemia until a critical state is reached, at which point profound hypotension will occur. It is vital to understand that rapid deterioration of physiologic parameters of the pediatric patient may occur with blood loss. It is therefore important to understand the usual formulas for replacement as well as having a rationale for such replacement. Knowledge of the blood volume can be used to estimate the acceptable blood loss before transfusion is needed (Table 16.4). Loss of less than the acceptable blood loss should be replaced with either a colloid or crystalloid solution as dictated by the hemodynamic parameters of the patient. Blood transfusion should be reserved for cases where the acceptable blood loss has been exceeded or rapid loss is likely to exceed such a value. The hematocrit of larger children can be allowed to fall lower than 30% if hemodynamics permit.

It should be noted that in the cases where large blood loss is expected, such as in craniofacial surgery, waiting for the hematocrit to fall will place the patient at risk. Hemorrhage in such a situation can be severe enough to cause vascular collapse in these patients. In this population it is wise to start volume replacement with blood products on incision. One clinical point of note is that it is wise to err on the side of overhydration early in case intravenous access is lost during the procedure. Some clinicians overhydrate such children by 20% of their blood volume and adjust fluids later in the case to compensate.

Induction

It is preferable that all patients with major medical problems, whether adults or children, should have an intravenous cannula before the induction of anesthesia. Because of the child's higher metabolic rate and lower functional residual capacity than adults, a critical situation can rapidly develop. In cases of ICH, the use of an inhalational technique can decrease the minute ventilation sufficiently to cause significant increases in ICP. Attempts to insert an intravenous catheter under emergency conditions during or after induction can be difficult. In cases of elective surgery, the use of Emla cream may facilitate intravenous access. If access looks tenuous then a 23- or 25-gauge butterfly can be placed intravenously and taped in place for induction. It should be mentioned that screaming and combativeness can elevate the ICP and so catheter placement should be avoided in this situation, and a secondary induction plan should be available. Those children with ICH are usually somnolent and lethargic and offer little resistance to placement of an intravenous catheter.

Inhalational induction can be used in children without intravenous access. The inhalational agents used can increase CBV and ICH and so must be used with caution. The usual pediatric practice of spontaneous ventilation until intravenous access is obtained is not always safe in the child with decreased intracranial compliance. Instead hyperventilation should be initiated in these cases as soon as the patient is unconscious.

If an intravenous catheter is in place, induction can proceed as with adults. In the case of increased ICP, voluntary hyperventilation with oxygen in the cooperative child as well as mannitol (0.5 to 1.0 mg/kg) can improve intracranial compliance.

Emergent intubation is sometimes performed in the neonatal population without anesthesia to ensure an adequate airway (Fig. 16.3). However, awake intubation in the neonate has been associated with significant increases in blood pres-

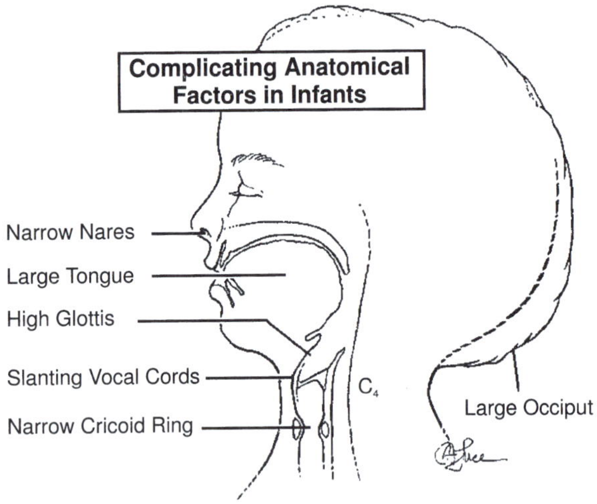

FIGURE 16.3 *Complicating anatomic factors in infants with regards to intubation. (From Berry,[120] with permission.)*

sure and ICP[14] and may be a contributing factor in the pathogenesis of intraventricular hemorrhage in premature babies.[20,21] By approximately 1 month of age, the infant is sufficiently vigorous to make awake intubation difficult unless the child is gravely ill. Older neonates and children must be assumed to have a full stomach in emergent situations and should receive a rapid sequence induction with a rapid-acting muscle relaxant, barbiturate, and cricoid pressure.

Maintenance

Ventilation is controlled in all infants. All halogenated inhalational anesthetics are cerebral vasodilators and should be used in low concentrations and coupled with hyperventilation when ICP is elevated until the dura is open. Isoflurane offers some theoretical advantages for neurosurgical cases in that it provides cardiovascular stability while provoking the smallest increase in CBF and the greatest decrease in $CMRO_2$. When used with hyperventilation, the effects on ICP are usually minimal. Enflurane should be avoided as it may be epileptogenic, especially when combined with hyperventilation. Additionally, enflurane may lead to an increase in CSF production, thereby increasing ICP in a manner unresponsive to hyperventilation.[22] A complete discussion of the effects of volatile agents on cerebral hemodyamics is found in Chapter 1.

TABLE 16.7 *Comparable safe doses of local anesthetics*

DRUGS	PLAIN (mg/kg)	WITH EPINEPHRINE (1 IN 200,000) (mg/kg)
2-Chlorprocaine	20	25
Procaine	14	18
Lidocaine	7	9
Etidocaine	4	4
Bupivicaine	2	2.5
Tetracaine	2	2

(Data from various sources.)

In our institution we favor a balanced anesthetic regimen using oxygen, air, low-dose inhalational agent, narcotics, and a muscle relaxant. The use of nitrous oxide is routinely avoided by preference. The narcotic is usually delivered in an infusion form, though for shorter cases a bolus on induction suffices.

The placement of the skull holder is stimulating and will require supplemental anesthesia with thiopental or fentanyl. Local anesthesia (0.25% bupivicaine) with epinephrine injected into the scalp and periosteum can minimize scalp blood loss and provide supplemental analgesia. The maximum bupivicaine dose is 3 mg/kg (Table 16.7).

Positioning

The pediatric patient must be positioned with the same care as the adult. There are still risks for nerve injury despite the small size and weight of the patient. Positioning should take into account three goals: comfort, safety, and exposure. Common to all operative positions is an elevated head position to minimize blood loss and promote drainage of CSF. Proper padding and positioning of all pressure points is crucial as is neutral head position. Positioning should be undertaken by the anesthesiologist and neurosurgeon. This part of the procedure carries with it the greatest risk of injury to the child as so many variables are involved. The head, inordinately heavy in a child, is perched on a flexible nonprotected spine. The eyes in a facedown position are at great risk unless skeletal fixation can be utilized. Small limbs distorted for intravenous access or hanging over the side of the table are at great risk for peripheral nerve injury (Fig. 16.4).

Macroglossia is one feared complication in the pediatric population that may result from either inadequate positioning of the head or excessive oral cavity manipulation.[23] It has been suggested that the oral airway not be left in place for extended periods; rather a soft bite block can be used. The head and neck must be checked for edema and ecchymoses as often as feasible, and the head must not be left in a position of extreme flexion.[24] In positioning of the head by the surgeons, the authors have found it useful to place two fingers between the jaw and chest to prevent extreme flexion. This motion is particularly important in smaller children whose airway is much more tenuous than adults[25] but is a useful guideline for all ages.

In our institution we rarely place patients in the sitting position for craniotomies. It is felt that the increased incidence of VAE, depression of cardiac output, hypotension, and cerebral ischemia secondary to a reduced CPP are sufficient to place patients in a more recumbent position. Instead, the supine, prone, and three-quarter lateral positions are used with the attention to positioning and pressure points that each entails.

Temperature Control

The surface area of the child's head represents 18% of the total body surface area, double that of an adult. In general children have a much larger surface-area-to-weight ratio than adults as well as less subcutaneous fat. Hence children are more at risk for dangerous drops in temperature than adults. Care must be taken to minimize losses of heat by conduction, convection,

FIGURE 16.4 *A patient with myelomeningocoele positioned for surgery. The abdomen is suspended free of the bed, and the extremities are padded and positioned.*

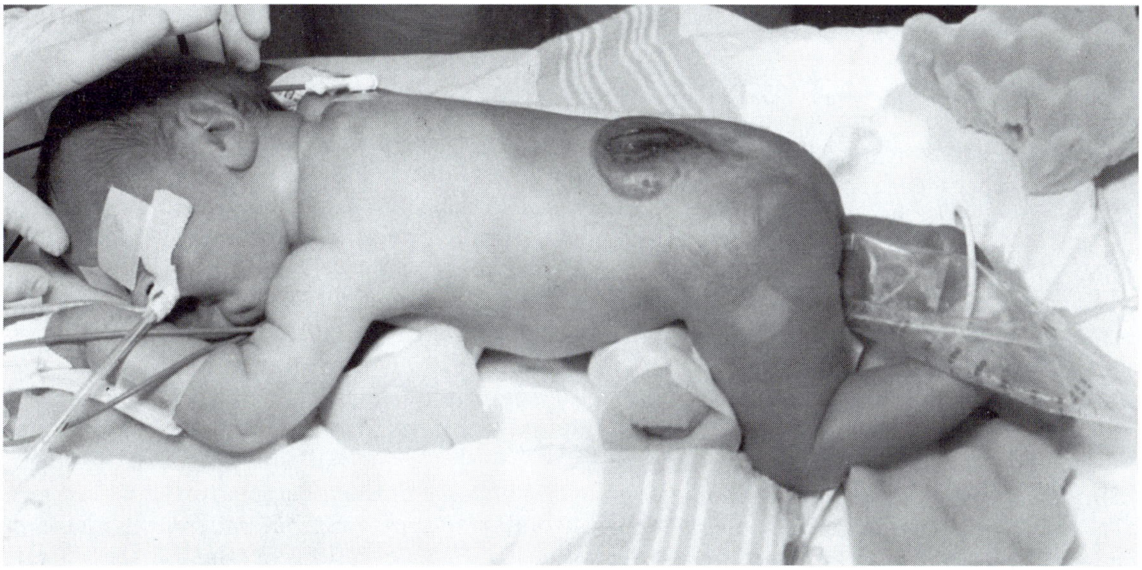

and radiation. It is suggested that the operating room be warmed to provide for the patient's comfort on induction and only be lowered as indicated by the patient's monitored temperature. Radiant heat should be carefully positioned to prevent thermal burns. These lamps should not be used to warm the patient once dura is exposed. Heated pediatric breathing circuits and intravenous fluids should be considered if the circumstances warrant.

Lowering patient temperature decreases the brain's metabolic demand for oxygen and is protective against ischemia. However, deleterious effects of shivering, metabolic acidosis, and dysrhythmias are well known. There are some surgical situations where a lower temperature may have a desirable protective effect. Temperatures about 34.5°C likely provide some cerebral protection without putting the child in jeopardy from cardiac arrhythmias and metabolic changes.[26] This can usually be accomplished by the removal of the heat-conserving measures and does not require active cooling.

Hyperthermia may also be counterproductive as increased body temperature increases cerebral metabolism. Postoperative hyperpyrexia is associated with surgery in craniopharyngioma resection, hypothalamic, pontine, and midbrain manipulations. The prognosis (if not treated) is uniformly poor especially if the temperature rises above 40.5°C. Active cooling methods include cooling blankets, increased use of cold intravenous fluids, and, if necessary, peripheral venodilation. If this is unsuccessful, then ice bags over the great vessels and liver as well a nasogastric lavage with cold fluid may be utilized. Pharmacologic treatment with acetaminophen (10 mg/kg per rectum) may also be used. This dose of medication does not have an adverse affect on platelet function.[27]

Emergence

The neurologic exam is the most useful means of assessing a neurosurgical patient in the postoperative period. An unexpected neurologic change can be successfully resolved if detected early. It is, therefore, desirable to have an awake and responsive patient at the completion of surgery. We have found that the use of a narcotic-based technique provides a smooth and rapid emergence.

Emergence is often associated with hypertension, coughing, gagging, and struggling. These factors can all cause a rise in ICP and encourage venous hemorrhage so great effort must be taken to avoid this in the patient with decreased intracranial compliance. These changes in blood pressure may be controlled with the use of short-acting antihypertensive such as esmolol and sodium nitroprusside. The continuation of muscle relaxation until the head clamp has been removed and bandaging commenced allows decrease of the level of anesthesia while still permitting control of patient movement. Coughing and gagging on the endotracheal tube may be controlled with the use of intravenous lidocaine (1 mg/kg), although it must be recognized that this can deepen the plane of anesthesia. The use of a narcotic-based anesthetic will often smooth the emergence so that excessive stimulation by the endotracheal tube will not be a factor.

Postoperative Care

All patients undergoing neurosurgical procedures should be monitored in an environment where health care professionals familiar with the care of these patients are readily available. The neurosurgical examination is the most important factor in assessing postoperative recovery. Deterioration in neurologic function is often a sign of intracranial bleeding. Therefore, it is usually desirable to have the child as fully alert as possible immediately following surgery. CT scans are extremely valuable in evaluating increasing ICP or deteriorating neurologic status to determine the presence of a surgically correctable cause. Cranial ultrasound techniques may also be useful in the case of open fontanelles. Routine postoperative ventilation is usually only used for those patients who have either had long operations or where there is a particular neurosurgical or airway indication such as brainstem glioma surgery. If prolonged ventilation is anticipated, then judicious sedation can be used so that neurologic examinations are not impeded.

Postoperative nausea may not be due to anesthesia and a search for possible increased ICP should be made. Antiemetic use should be limited to those agents with limited CNS side effects. The use of metoclopramide (0.15 mg/kg) or ondansetron (0.15 mg/kg) is indicated after initial evaluation.

Postoperative Pain

It is essential to control pain even in the smallest of individuals, and this should be done very aggressively. This is especially true after procedures that are notorious for causing significant pain and suffering, such as selective dorsal rhizotomy. Very specialized techniques can be used in this situation for early control of pain and spasms and facilitate early return to rehabilitation and physical therapy.

In the craniofacial area of pediatric neuroanesthesiology, we aggressively sedate the children postoperatively with phenobarbital and Tylenol/codeine for the first 3 days. Morphine (0.1 mg/kg) given intravenously is efficacious in the treatment of postoperative pain.

In the treatment of patients who have had a dorsal rhizotomy, we use an epidural catheter placed under direct vision in the operating room. This is then dosed with duramorph (30 to 40 μg/kg intraoperatively). Then an infusion of duramorph at a rate of 5 to 15 μg/kg/h is begun.

Venous Air Embolism

The concern of anesthesiologists for the occurrence of VAE is heightened in the pediatric population. VAE is caused by a Venturi effect of blood returning to the heart and drawing small air bubbles with it. Usually these small bubbles pass into the pulmonary circulation with no ill effects. Larger quantities can cause pulmonary vasoconstriction, increase pulmonary artery pressure, and can lead to right-sided heart failure or complete heart block.[28] The incidence of Doppler-detected VAE has been documented during 6 to 45% of sitting craniotomies.[29] The incidence of Doppler-detected VAE during seated pediatric cases is 33%.[30] Our institution has followed a national trend and use the sitting position for only specific infratentorial procedures. This, unfortunately, does not eliminate the risk of VAE as a 12% incidence of Doppler-detected air has been noted to occur in horizontal infratentorial cases.[31]

The pediatric population is often considered to be at increased risk from VAE. Because the neonatal population has a recently closed foramen ovale that, if the pressure in the right atrium exceeds that of the left atrium, predisposes to paradoxical air embolism. The risk of paradoxical air embolism is increased in the child with congenital heart defects. If preoperative echocardiography or intraoperative transesophageal echocardiography detects a patent foramen ovale, extra precautions should be taken to prevent a VAE. Unfortunately echocardiography detects a much lower incidence of patent foramen ovale than expected.[32,33] The child who presents with an undiagnosed murmur preoperatively should have some definitive evaluation to rule out possibility of intracardiac shunts.

Detection of VAE is best made by the use of precordial Doppler in the clinical setting. Other detection devices include transesophageal echocardiography, mass spectrometer detection of expired nitrogen, changes in end-tidal carbon dioxide tension, and the esophageal stethoscope. None of these monitors are completely reliable.

The treatment of VAE is a team approach and is discussed in detail in Chapter 10.

Latex Allergy

Unfortunately the population of pediatric neurosurgical patients contains one of the highest-risk groups for intraoperative reactions to latex products. The American College of Allergy and Immunology has identified patients with disorders such as spina bifida, myelomenigocoele, lipomyelomenigocoele, sacral/lumbar agenesis, and similar disorders as having an increased incidence of latex allergy.[34] Included in this group are orthopedic patients with spinal injury requiring multiple procedures and repetitive urinary instrumentation. The anesthesiologist becomes the physician responsible for the care of these children in the perioperative period and hence is responsible for the treatment of presumed or known latex allergy.

Latex or rubber products have been in use in the medical field since the late 1800s. Allergic reactions to these products were not reported until 1979.[35] Since that time, it has become well known that latex or rubber products can induce a type IV (delayed hypersensitivity) in the form of eczematous contact dermatitis. Over the past few years, there have been increasing numbers of reports in the literature of type I (anaphylactic) allergic reactions involving the use of latex-containing products.

The precise antigenic protein in latex has yet to be determined. Gonzalez[36] reported that there is a 30,000-molecular-weight protein within rubber that demonstrates a strong response to specific Immunoglobulen E (IgE) antibodies in a histamine release assay.

When an adaptive immune response occurs in an exaggerated or inappropriate form, causing tissue damage, the term *hypersensitivity* is applied.[37] Hypersensitivity is a characteristic of the individual and is manifested on second contact with a particular antigen. It has been classified into four types of reactions, type I and IV being the most common.

Type I hypersensitivity is characterized by allergic reactions that immediately follow contact with the antigen. The antigen stimulates the B cells, with T-cell help, to produce specific IgE. The antigen-specific IgE binds to mast cells via the Fc receptors thus sensitizing them. When the antigen subsequently reaches the sensitized mast cell, it cross-links surface-bound IgE and the cell degranulates, releasing mediators that cause the clinical symptoms. The level of symptoms depend upon the number of antibodies present, the affinity of the antigen for the antibody, and the number of mast cells affected. There are two main subtypes of mast cells; those found in the connective tissue, such as skin and peritoneum, and the mucosal mast cells found in high concentrations in the lung and the mucosa of the midgut.

The chemical mediators that cause the clinical manifestations include histamine, eosinophil chemotactic factor, and neutrophil-chemotactic factor of anaphylaxis. Also found are leukotrienes, prostaglandins, and kinins.

Anaphylaxis is a subtype of type I hypersensitivity.[38] This means that it is an exaggerated response to an antigen to which the host has been previously sensitized. The antigen enters the body (commonly through the skin, lungs, or gastrointestinal tract) and interacts with the IgE that is bound to mast cells, thereby causing a release of preformed mediators. These mediators consist of histamine, chemotactic factors of anaphylaxis, leukotrienes, prostaglandins, kinins, and platelet-activating factors.[39] As a group these mediators produce the increased capillary permeability, bronchoconstriction, smooth muscle constriction, vasodilation, coronary vasoconstriction, and myocardial depression seen in anaphylactic reactions (Table 16.8). The onset and severity of the reaction depends on the mediator's specific end organ effect. Antigenic

TABLE 16.8 *Signs of anaphylactic/anaphylactoid reaction*

SIGNS	PERCENTAGE OF PATIENTS INVOLVED
Tachycardia	94
Circulatory collapse	92
Widespread flushing, edema	79
Broncospasm	39
Cardiac arrest	14
Bradycardia	6
Dysrhythmias	4

(From Berry,[118] with permission.)

Preventing Anaphylaxis in Sensitive Individuals

PROTOCOL 1: TO BEGIN THE DAY BEFORE SURGERY

Prednisone 5–10 mg/kg q 6 hours for 24 h preoperatively

Diphenhydramine 0.5–1.0 mg/kg PO preop

Cimetidine 4–6 mg/kg PO preop

PROTOCOL 2: IF PATIENT HAS NOT BEEN PREPARED/EMERGENT SURGERY

Solucortef 25 mg/m^2 or 1 mg/kg IV preop, repeat 6 h postop

Diphenhydramine 1 mg/kg IV preop, then q 6 h for 4 doses

Ranitidine 0.5 mg/kg IV preop

challenge can result in immediate response in a sensitized individual, but the onset can be delayed for up to 30 minutes.

The diagnosis of latex allergy relies upon clinical history and/or a potentially hazardous skin test.[40] The evidence of an intraoperative allergic reaction in the past is definitive, but the physician should be suspicious of any child in the high-risk group. Specific questions should be asked about allergic reactions of any type. To date, no typical reactions that might indicate potential latex allergies in a sensitized group have been discovered. If the patient has known or suspected latex allergy, there are several treatment protocols that may be used. One study recommends a regimen consisting of diphenhydramine (mg/kg every 6 hours for four doses), ranitidine (2 mg/kg every 8 hours for three doses), and hydrocortisone (5 mg/kg every 6 hours for four doses) it is crucial to provide a latex-free environment for these children (Fig. 16.5). For the anesthesiologists the removal of all latex products can be problematic; however, the exposure can be minimized. The blood pressure cuff should not touch the skin directly. All latex products must be taped closed and only stopcocks used for injection. No cases of anaphylaxis have been shown to occur from syringes or medication vials.

FIGURE 16.5 *A flow chart for latex allergy treatment plan. (Courtesy of Dr. N. Setzer, Department of Anesthesiology, University of Florida.)*

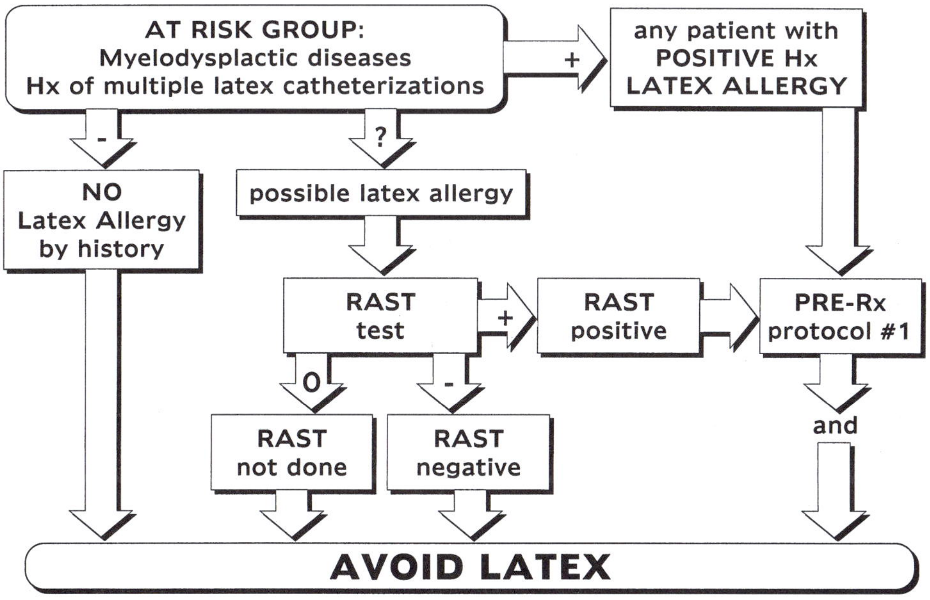

If, despite all precautions, an intraoperative anaphylactic reaction occurs, the following procedures should be followed. All latex products should be removed. The patient should be ventilated with 100% oxygen and all anesthetic agents should be discontinued. A bolus of fluid (10 to 20 ml/kg) should be administered along with an epinephrine bolus of 0.1 to 0.2 μg/kg for hypotension. Then the patient should be treated with diphenhydramine (0.5 to 1.0 mg/kg), hydrocortisone (4 to 8 mg/kg), and aminophylline (5 to 6 mg/kg) over 30 minutes as needed for continued bronchoconstriction. An epinephrine drip should be started and titrated to control blood pressure.

SPECIFIC CONDITIONS

Head Trauma

Unfortunately, head injury remains common in the pediatric patient. Head trauma in children remains one of the major causes of long-term disability in children, with about 95,000 children sustaining traumatic brain injuries each year.[41–43] Serious neurologic sequelae[44] and long-term neuropsychological deficits[45,46] have long been acknowledged consequences of even minor head trauma. The guidelines for treating children with head injuries remain unclear. Several authors have expressed dissatisfaction with the Glasgow Coma Scale and have proposed a modification to be used on children, especially those under 36 months.[47–49] This (CCS (Table 16.1) uses a modification of the best verbal response in order to more effectively categorize children. The scale utilizes the same 3 to 15 scale of adults, so that series from pediatric populations can be compared with an adult population. Studies seem to indicate that children with a CCS score of 8 or greater will have an excellent outcome.[50–51] This scale has provided clinicians with a greater ability to categorize the severity of children's head trauma as well as make improved estimates with regards to outcome.

The basic mechanism of injury in childhood is usually low-velocity deformational injuries in childhood (Table 16.9) Diffuse shearing and axonal injuries are the result of these forces in this age group, and significant intracranial hemorrhage is rare. Generally, for a given level of function at the time of presentation, the prognosis for pediatric head injury is better than for similar presentation in the adult population. Children, especially younger children, can present with unique symptoms following a head injury (Table 16.10). Often a presenting picture of labile mental status following a period of loss of consciousness can resolve within 24 hours without sequelae. Other children with a CCS score of less than 8 and fluctuating neurologic status and progressive decrease in consciousness require intubation and ventilation (Table 16.11). Head trauma can result in damage far beyond the initial insult. Secondary damage may result from cerebral edema, increased or decreased CBF, hypoxia, and general cerebral hyperemia.[52,53]

Infants have characteristic injury patterns. Children less than 6 months of age will suffer head injuries with more frequent tears in the subcortical white matter of the frontal and temporal lobes. Children with an open fontanelle can take the full force of impact on the brain tissue without some diminution of that force by the

TABLE 16.9 *Causes of pediatric head injury*

CAUSE	PATIENTS (n = 791)	
	NUMBER	%
Fall	513	65.0
Motor vehicle		
Pedestrian	123	15.5
Passenger	35	4.4
Bicycle	8	1.0
Assault	17	2.1
Abuse	17	2.1
Other	78	9.9
Total	791	100.0

(From Hahn and McLone,[49] with permission.)

TABLE 16.10 *Primary symptoms in pediatric minor head injury*

SYMPTOM	PATIENTS (n = 791) NUMBER	%
Loss of consciousness	338	42.7
Vomiting/nausea	122	15.4
Headache	121	15.3
Irritability	119	15.1
Seizure	47	5.9
Others	44	5.6
Total	791	100.0

(From Hahn and McLone,[49] with permission.)

cranial vault. These children are also unable to support their head, making them more susceptible to shearing forces. Therefore chronic subdural hematomas are more common in these young age groups.[54] In spite of the concern over the head trauma in the pediatric population, the overall outcome is better than for adults.[55]

Cervical injuries are common in children involved in motor vehicle accidents. The incidence has been reported to be as high as 17%.[56,57] In children sustaining severe head injury (Glasgow Coma Scale <7) following motor vehicle accidents, 16% had cervical spine injuries. Because of its unique mechanical and elastic properties, the immature cervical spine is especially susceptible to high cervical spine injuries such as fractures of the odontoid and subluxations at the atlanto-occipital, atlantoaxial, and C2-3 levels. In contrast, children over the age of 8 display an adult injury pattern characterized by fractures anywhere along the length of the cervical spine.[58] In suspected cases of spinal injury, high-dose methyl prednisolone should be instituted early, and careful sequential neurologic exams should be made.

TABLE 16.11 *Loss of consciousness and outcome in pediatric minor head trauma*

TIME PERIOD	OUTCOME GOOD (%)	POOR (%)	TOTAL (%)
0–15 min	780 (98.6)	—	780 (98.6)
> 15 min	9 (1.1)	2 (0.3)	11 (1.4)
Total	789 (99.7)	2 (0.3)	791 (100.0)

(From Hahn and McLone,[49] with permission.)

A special note should be made concerning the role of child abuse in head injury and spinal cord injury. This etiology is much more common than previously considered, and the diagnosis can be missed for an extended period of time, leaving the child at great risk. In every child with irritability and decreased level of consciousness, the etiology of significant head injury must be considered. Classically, in the case of child abuse, a CT scan demonstrates a swollen brain with evidence of subarachnoid hemorrhage, especially over the tentorium.

The treating physician needs to have an understanding of the mechanism of injury as well as the status of the cervical spine and volume status. The main concern for the anesthesiologist in cases of head trauma is to maintain adequate CPP while ensuring that an adequate airway is secured. There are many strategies to avoid cervical spinal injury during induction and positioning. The primary one is to ensure neutral positioning with neurosurgical assistance and proceed with oral intubation after oxygenation while providing cricoid pressure.[59,60] The decision of awake versus asleep intubation must be based on the patients physical and neurologic function as well as the emergent nature of such interventions.

Brain Tumors

Approximately 1,000 new pediatric brain tumors are diagnosed each year in the United States.[61] Although initially these tumors had a depressing outcome, over the past several decades the prognosis has begun to improve.[62] The most common brain tumors in childhood are located in the posterior fossa and present with progressive hydrocephalus, symptoms of ICH and lower brainstem dysfunction. These can present with nonspecific, nonlocalizing signs and can lead to a substantial delay in diagnosis with the child presenting as quite ill, dehydrated, and moribund. If diagnosed early, most of these tumors can be removed surgically, and only about 50% of these individuals require a shunt for the control of hydrocephalus following tumor removal. If the tumor is located within the brainstem, then total surgical excision is rarely possible but should be attempted in certain situations. Anesthetically, the physician should be prepared to monitor brainstem function, and in certain situations, cardiac pacing should be available.

CRANIOPHARYNGIOMAS Craniopharyngiomas are the most common suprasellar tumors in children. The origin of these tumors is thought to be from the vestige of Rathke's hypophyseal pharyngeal duct. They occur throughout childhood, but neonatal craniopharyngiomas are rare.[63] Typically this is a benign tumor composed of squamous epithelium and is often cystic and calcified. The location is invariably intrasellar or parasellar, although the cystic portion can extend into the basal cisterns, or can invaginate into the third ventricle or base of the brain, causing hydrocephalus.[64,65] The tumor may also impinge upon the hypophyseal-hypothalamic structures, the optic pathway, and/or the critical vasculature of the circle of Willis.[66]

The clinical picture at presentation is usually one of visual changes and headaches.[67,68] Advances in neuroimaging, including CT and MRI, have provided an accurate means of diagnosing craniopharyngiomas.[69,70] A combination of CT and MRI affords sufficient information as to the nature of the tumor to allow the surgeon to plan the eventual operation. These two modalities also answer questions the anesthesiologist will have with regards to involvement of hypophyseal-hypothalamic structures and the presence or absence of hydrocephalus.

During the preoperative assessment, the anesthesiologist should make every attempt to ensure there are no signs or symptoms of ICH or obstructive hydrocephalus. Examination of retinal fundi and a cautious questioning will be of assistance here. Diagnostic tests should include the CT and MRI scans as well as quantitative analysis of endocrine function. Growth hormone deficiency seems to be the most common endocrine abnormality. It has also been noted that 20% of patients will show evidence of diabetes insipidus (DI) preoperatively. The fluid and electrolyte status of a patient should be corrected prior to surgery. DI is generally well controlled with desmopressin acetate (DDAVP). The dose of DDAVP (1 to 4 μg per 12 hours) should have been carefully titrated preoperatively to correct electrolyte and fluid disturbances.

In craniotomy for recurrence, other endocrine abnormalities should be sought. DI is invariably present in patients in whom radical resection was attempted. As many as 80% may experience deficiencies of GH and thyroid-stimulating hormone. Seventy-five percent may show signs of adrenal insufficiency due to a lack of adrenocorticotropic or corticotrophin-releasing hormone. Clinical signs of inadequate cortisol replacement include fatigue, hypotension, diarrhea, vomiting, and dehydration. Stress dose steroids in addition to standard prednisone treatment (5 to 6 mg/m^2/day divided into two or three doses) should be considered. Cortisol replacement should be considered in those patients undergoing the stress of surgery. Thyroid deficiency is also a consideration in recurrent craniopharyngioma, and replacement therapy should be instituted.

Controversy exists as to the acceptable extent of surgical resection.[71] Some authors advocate complete radical resection[72,73] whereas others recommend limited surgical resections and radiotherapy (RT). In our institution we use the radical resection approach. The operative procedure is usually accomplished by frontal resection of the tumor. All patients receive a stress dose of cortisone acetate.[74] The intimate relationship of the craniopharyngioma to the optic nerve and chiasm, the hypothalmus, and the circle of Willis means that the utmost care and attention must be paid by the surgeon. The anesthesiologist can facilitate this by presenting the surgeon with a brain that is not tense. Some patients require initial shunts for hydrocephalus, but visual function may acutely deteriorate after bilateral shunt placement. This is thought to be due to acute decompression leading to upward herniation of the optic chiasm.

Induction is best accomplished via an intravenous technique. Most patients with this tumor should be treated as though they had decreased intracranial compliance. If nausea or vomiting was detected in the history, then a rapid sequence induction using cricoid pressure and rapid-acting muscle relaxants as indicated. An arterial catheter and central venous line should be placed after induction to facilitate fluid management. Mild hyperventilation should be used to produce an arterial partial pressure of carbondioxide ($PaCO_2$) between 25 and 30 mmHg. Arterial blood gas analysis should be used for examination of electrolyte and glucose status. In our institution anesthesia is maintained by a narcotic infusion. Amnesia is attained with the use of low end-tidal (0.5%) isoflurane and muscle relaxation is facilitated with pancuronium. Mannitol is not recommended due to difficulty in fluid management as well as difficulty in diagnosing DI during and after the surgery.[75] Intraoperative EEG monitoring may be useful in assessing adequate brain perfusion during manipulation of the vessels of the circle of Willis and cavernous sinus.

Intraoperative events of concern are DI, hemorrhage related to manipulation of large blood vessels of the anterior circle of Willis or the cavernous sinus, and hypothalamic dysfunction manifested primarily as poor temperature regulation. Occurrence of DI is evidenced by copious quantities of dilute urine of low specific gravity. Management is provided by injections of vasopressin (0.05 to 0.1 μg/kg) or DDAVP (1 to 4 μg per 12 hours). Hemorrhage may be treated by lowering of the MAP in order to facilitate surgical control of bleeding. This can be achieved via infusions of sodium nitroprusside or nitroglycerin to lower MAP.

Postoperative extubation of the child may proceed if the surgical course warrants. Evidence of cerebral edema or hemorrhage should be an indication for postoperative ventilation. The patient should be recovered in a pediatric intensive care unit or other facility where trained personnel can closely evaluate the patient. Postoperative visual disturbance is one of the most serious complications of radical tumor resection and can be noted in up to 40% of patients. Careful postoperative management should include vigilance for DI, endocrine abnormalities, hypothalamic disturbances, seizures, and possible subdural hematoma.

The recurrence of craniopharyngioma has been reported to be up to 17% after total resection.[76] Subtotal resection and RT has a recurrence rate of between 26 and 30% after 10 years.[77] These studies indicate that operative morbidity and mortality for recurrence, especially after RT, are significantly worse because of the difficulty of resection.

POSTERIOR FOSSA SURGERY Posterior fossa tumors are the most common solid tumor and the second most common malignancy of childhood.[78] Although most CNS tumors in adults are supratentorial, in children the majority are located in the posterior fossa. Brainstem tumors are a group that carry the worst prognosis for long-term survival. Until recently, the risk of significant morbidity and mortality has far outweighed the benefits of surgically debulking these tumors. RT was therefore the primary treatment. Unfortunately this only temporarily relieved the symptoms as 70% of children with these tumors died within 2 years of diagnosis.

The most common brain tumors in children are medulloblastomas, cerebellar astrocytomas, and brainstem gliomas. A large percentage of pediatric tumors arise in the posterior fossa near the fourth ventricle, the brainstem, and other midline structures, whereas 70% of adult tumors lie above the tentorium.[79] Posterior fossa masses can compress the brainstem or displace the tentorium upward into the cerebral hemispheres. In theory, transtentorial herniation can occur during hyperventilation if cerebral volume were reduced significantly,[80] but in practice this happens infrequently and requires drainage of large quantities of CSF. Brainstem structures vital to the control of respiration, heart rate, and blood pressure may be affected by surgical resection. Management of these physiologic variables during surgical resection can be challenging.

The initial symptoms of a CNS tumor can be subtle. Signs consistent with increased intracranial pressure may be the first to be noticed. Infants may present with an inappropriate increase in head circumference. Localizing signs of brainstem pathology may include cranial nerve palsies, ataxia, and nystagmus. The use of CT and MRI scans has greatly aided in the diagnosis and localization of these CNS tumors.

Perioperative assessment of patients for posterior fossa surgery should include a careful review of the medical history. These children frequently present with hydrocephalus. The baseline blood pressure, heart rate, respiratory rate, and temperature should be noted. The physical examination should include a thorough necrologic assessment. Focal signs such as motor weakness, gag reflex, and pupillary responsiveness and equality should be assessed. Symptoms of DI such as unexpected bed-wetting and nocturnal drinking should be noted. Preoperative laboratory studies should include a hematocrit, platelet count, and an examination of coagulation studies. Blood should be typed and crossed owing to the possibility of significant blood loss. In patients with tumors near the pituitary gland, it is important to have baseline values for serum electrolytes and osmolarity as well as urine osmolarity.

Children with intracranial tumors are often given steroids to reduce brain swelling. This is usually done with dexamethasone (1 mg/kg/day). This medication should be continued up to the day of surgery, although it only provides a short-term improvement.

The major anesthetic considerations in a patient with posterior fossa tumor are avoiding ICH, monitoring the competence of brainstem function as an indication of surgical transgression on vital structures, and preventing and, if necessary, treating a VAE. Premedication should be avoided in those patients with ICH. Those patients arriving for elective resection of posterior fossa tumors who do not have elevated ICP will benefit from preoperative midazolam (0.1 mg/kg IV, 0.3 mg/kg intranasal, 0.5 mg/kg PO). Precautions must be taken to avoid acute rises in ICP. This is best facilitated by intravenous induction, although mask induction with halothane until an intravenous line is obtained and pentothal is given is acceptable.

Standard monitoring for these cases should include a precordial and the esophageal stethoscope, ECG, temperature probe, noninvasive blood pressure monitor, pulse oximeter, and end-tidal capnograph. An arterial catheter should be inserted for continuous blood pressure monitoring and sampling of blood values. A 24 gauge catheter is appropriate for neonates and infants, whereas a 22-gauge catheter will be adequate for larger children. There is a risk of VAE in these patients, especially in the sitting position, and so the use of a central venous line should be considered along with the use of a precordial doppler.

Maintenance of the anesthetic may be performed with a standard narcotic technique utilizing low concentrations of inhalational agents. Muscle relaxation should be discussed with the neurosurgeon depending upon the location of the tumor. If cranial nerves V, VI, or XI are involved, the detection of muscle twitches by EMG may be a useful diagnostic modality. Most pediatric neurosurgeons position children prone for posterior fossa craniotomy. The sitting position is still occasionally utilized by some neurosurgeons, usually for small children older than 3 years of age with midline lesions. All pressure points must be padded, and the endotracheal tube must be secure and accessible.

Vital structures that can be injured or irritated during the procedure are located within the posterior fossa. Respiratory control centers can be damaged during surgical dissection.[81] Stimulation of the nucleus of cranial nerve V produces hypertension and tachycardia, whereas vagal nucleus stimulation induces bradycardia. Injury to the vagal nucleus can also result in postoperative vocal cord paralysis. Continuous blood pressure and ECG analysis are essential to detect irritation of these vital structures. The ready availability of a cardiac pacer should be checked for cases of severe bradycardia or cardiac arrest due to brainstem compression. Other cranial nerves that can be damaged include cranial nerves VII and XI as well as compression of the pons and medulla. Spontaneous respiration has been used as an indicator of the status of the brainstem, however, this means that the child will be expected to breathe against a large resistance imposed by the ventilatory apparatus. Such an imposed work of breathing could predispose the patient to respiratory fatigue and failure. Some authors also believe that this is not a sensitive indicator of brainstem well-being.[82]

Common postoperative problems include respiratory depression, fluid and electrolyte disorders, and arterial hypertension. Children with persistent vomiting should be evaluated for evidence of intracranial pathology. Pain is not usually a problem with this group of children, therefore potent narcotic analgesics are not usually required.

Intracranial Hypertension

HYDROCEPHALUS Hydrocephalus is one of the most frequent causes for pediatric neurosurgical intervention. Hydrocephalus is caused by a blockage of the CSF drainage and may be communicating or noncommunicating. The appearance of hydrocephalus is usually secondary to some initiating insult. Prenatal diagnosis is now common with ultrasound and antenatal surgery has been carried out in some centers. To reduce obstetric problems from the large head and to minimize permanent brain damage, many of these infants are electively delivered around 32 weeks when fetal lung maturity has been ensured. The advantages of this treatment modality must be weighed against the risk of prematurity in this population.

Although there has been a reduction in the number of infants with meningomyelocele being born, the numbers of very premature babies surviving neonatal intensive care and suffering from intraventricular hemorrhage have risen rapidly over the past two decades. The presenting feature of secondary hydrocephalus is increasing head circumference, crossing the standard growth chart lines. The clinical picture of a baby with a massively enlarged head, bulging fontanelles, engorged head veins, and sunsetting eyes is fortunately rarely seen.

Surgical treatment of hydrocephalus consists of some method of removal of the excess CSF from the ventricles. In the newborn the CSF has a high protein and cell count and after intraventricular hemorrhage remains viscous for some time. Until the protein and cell count return to normal, the patient is not suitable for shunt placement as the low flow rate and high viscosity will cause an unacceptably high valve blockage rate. Initial treatment in these cases is either by intermittent ventricular tapping via the anterior fontanelle or by insertion of a percutaneous drain.

When all other factors are considered suitable, a ventricular shunt is placed. The terminal end of this shunt can be placed in the atrium, the thorax, or more commonly the peritoneal cavity. The names of the various shunts denote their terminal portion. The shunt consists of a ventricular catheter, valve, and terminal catheter. Atrial shunts are rarely performed because of the rare but disastrous complications of infection, causing bacterial endocarditis and pulmonary emboli, leading to pulmonary hypertension. Ventriculoperitoneal shunting for hydrocephalus is the most commonly performed pediatric neurosurgical procedure.

Anesthetic considerations for this procedure should begin with a thorough assessment of the patient. Hydrocephalus is commonly associated with multisystem congenital defects, and those anomalies must be carefully sought. Many infants with hydrocephalus have associated meningomyelocele with partial or complete paraplegia. These infants are prone to urinary tract infections and impaired renal function.

Dehydration is common in these patients due to the depressed mental status leading to decreased oral intake. The degree of dehydration should be assessed by checking skin turgor, whether the eyes are sunken, urine output, and specific gravity. If severe dehydration is suspected then rehydration should be undertaken preoperatively if possible. Intravenous access must be obtained prior to induction. The preferred route is peripheral, but in cases of severe dehydration, this may be impossible and so central access must be obtained. First attempts should be made in the femoral vein since this is the site with the highest success rate. The jugular or subclavian route should only be attempted after ensuring which route the shunt will take. As a last resort, the intraosseous route may be chosen.[83] No sedative premedication should be ordered because it may cause further rise in ICP. These children may already be somnolent due to the intracranial pathology. This is most often seen in acute shunt malfunction.

In the critical situation of respiratory arrest due to raised ICP and tonsillar herniation, the trachea should be intubated immediately and the patient hyperventilated with 100% oxygen. A ventricular tap must be performed without delay.

The anesthetic requirements for shunt procedures are a rapid sequence induction to prevent aspiration, maintenance of anesthesia with stable cerebral and cardiovascular hemodynamics, and rapid emergence. After application of the standard monitors, the patient is preoxygenated. Muscle relaxation can be achieved with intravenous succinylcholine (2 mg/kg). Atropine may be administered prior to succinylcholine to prevent succinylcholine-induced bradycardia. In the presence of conditions where succinylcholine is contraindicated, the use of rocuronium (1.6 mg/kg) or vecuronium (0.4 mg/kg)[89] will achieve intubating conditions rapidly. Thiopental (4 to 5 mg/kg) decreases ICP and is the anesthetic agent of choice for induction.

Low concentrations of volatile anesthetics are convenient for maintenance because they are easily controllable, and recovery is usually rapid and predictable. All inhalational agents increase intracranial blood flow and ICP; however, the use of low concentrations together with mild hyperventilation minimizes the increase in ICP.[85] Supplementation with narcotics may also be used to lower the requirement of inhalational agents.

Intraoperative events of importance to the anesthesiologist include positioning and rapid decreases in ICP with placement of the ventriculostomy. This can cause systemic hypotension, and so care must be taken at this stage of the operation. The use of long-acting muscle relaxants is usually not needed for the case. At the end of the case, the patient should have anesthetic agents discontinued. Full reversal should be assured by the use of reversal with neostigmine (0.05 mg/kg) and glycopyrrlate (0.005 to 0.01 mg/kg).

SHUNT MALFUNCTION As has been mentioned above, the placement of a CSF shunt is the most commonly performed pediatric neurosurgical procedure. The revision rate for these shunts averages 2.6 operations per patient.[86] It has been reported that replacement of the entire shunt system, including the ventricular catheter, valve, and abdominal catheter, was required in 36% of ventriculoperitoneal shunt revisions.[87] The abdominal catheter alone was replaced in 24%, and the ventricular catheter alone was replaced in 20%.

The etiology of the hydrocephalus is related to the patency time of the shunt. Hydrocephalus caused by neoplasm has the shortest patency time and requires revision most frequently.

The patient presenting for shunt revision should not be treated in the same manner as a child arriving for treatment of hydrocephalus for the first time (Fig. 16.6). The child with a failed shunt will present with a much more acute onset of ICH symptoms than that of a child with hydrocephalus. Typically these patients are lethargic, and they frequently vomit during preoperative assessment. They can also have other signs of increased ICP. The elevated ICP of these patients is often associated with increased gastric acid secretion.[88] Once again a careful examination of the child and the history should be undertaken to rule out any complicating medical diagnoses. Anesthesia may be performed in the same manner as outlined above.

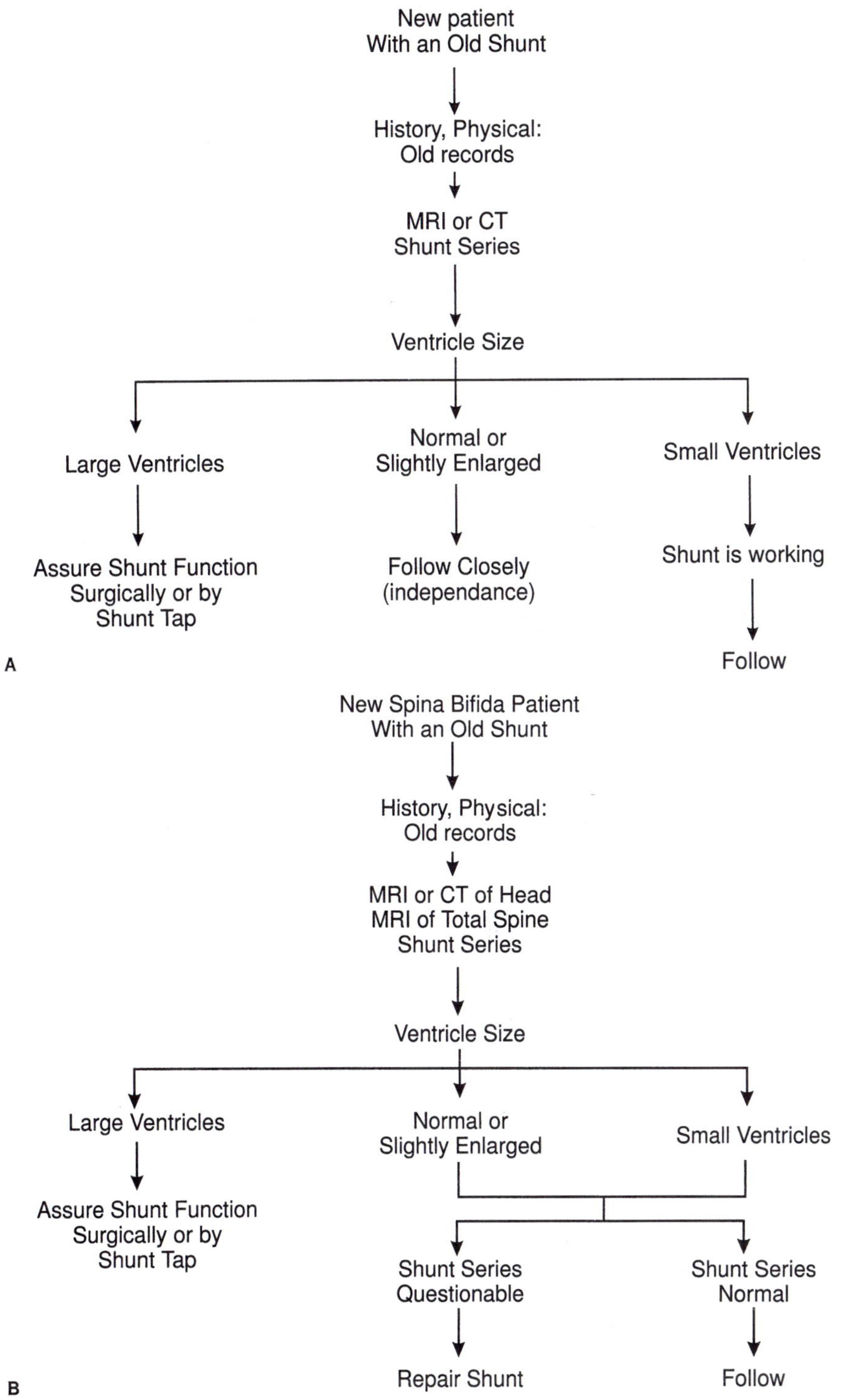

FIGURE 16.6 *An initial assessment of the shunted child without spina bifida by a new physician. (B) An initial assessment of the shunted child with spina bifida by a new physician. (Adapted from various texts.)*

Intracranial Vascular Malformations

Intracranial vascular malformations can include arteriovenous malformations (AVMs) and cavernous angiomas. These lesions can present in a variety of ways: acute or progressive neurologic deficits, seizures, irritability, or headaches. Frequently the AVMs can present as high-output CHF. Prior to any surgical resection, the size, location, arterial input, and venous drainage of these lesions must be delineated.

The most common cause of subarachnoid hemorrhage in the childhood population is AVMs. These lesions cause seizures and progressive neurologic deficits. The AVMs provide the anesthesiologist with a special challenge. Cerebral perfusion must be maintained, and at the same time, intravascular pressure must be maintained to minimize the chance of ICH. This may be best achieved with a narcotic anesthetic while maintaining the patient at normocapina. In the case of an intracranial aneurysm, the intracranial blood pressure may need to be controlled until the aneurysm is clipped and removed. Prevention of abrupt decreases in ICP will provide additional intracranial support of the vessels. The arterial and venous supplies of vascular malformations may be poorly defined. Consequently, unexpected bleeding is common, and the anesthesiologist may be asked to provide hypotension to decrease bleeding. Uncontrolled bleeding may require the patient to be placed in a pentobarbital coma to protect brain tissue. This can be achieved with an IV bolus of 10 mg/kg sodium thiopental then 10 mg/kg/h while monitoring of the EEG for burst suppression. Hypothermia is sometimes used to provide additional protection should the lesion be in a location where bleeding could be serious. Intravascular monitoring is essential in these cases.

The vein of Galen aneurysm is actually the result of increased flow usually due to a deeper AVM that drains into the vein of Galen or one of its tributaries.[89] This lesion, which represents about 1% of the AVMs in children, is almost uniformly fatal in the neonate whether medically or surgically managed. Recently developed techniques have permitted an improved survival in these infants by the use of embolization.[91] In this technique, the patient is placed under general anesthetic, and then embolic material is placed in to the aneurysmal dilatation of the vein of Galen to promote thrombosis of the vessel and reduction of the venous outflow (Fig. 16.7).

If presentation is later in life, surgical mortality drops significantly and is about 25% if surgical repair is undertaken after 1 year of age. This malformation can present as progressive heart failure, hydrocephalus, seizures, and subarachnoid hemorrhage. Cardiac death is the most frequent cause of morbidity. Aneurysmal dilatation of the vein of Galen provides a low-resistance pathway for blood within the brain (Figs 16.8 and 16.9). The torrential flow through these vessels often leads to high-output CHF.[91] CHF, usually present preoperatively, can also occur acutely during surgery as systemic vascular resistance abruptly increases with clipping of the aneurysm. Infarction may result from poor coronary perfusion. An arterial line and central line will facilitate the monitoring and control of blood pressure through the use of vasoactive medications. One means of assisting the neurosurgeon to determine if all the branches feeding the malformation have been isolated is to insert a catheter to monitor mixed venous oxygenation (SvO_2). As feeding vessels are clipped, cardiac output decreases, total systemic vascular resistance rises, and mixed venous oxygen saturation falls towards normal.

Cavernous angiomas are cavernous vessels with areas of marked proliferation of granulation tissue and partially re-endothelialized hemorrhage. Seemingly innocuous lesions (greater than 1 cm) should be excised because they can cause serious hemorrhage. Because lesions do bleed frequently and silently with hemorrhages of small volume and low pressure, surgical removal should be considered when the patient's clinical course is one of repetitive and progressive neurologic decline.

Progressive stroke in childhood can be caused by the syndrome Moya Moya disease, which has multiple etiologies. It results in progressive occlusion of the carotid arteries at the base of the

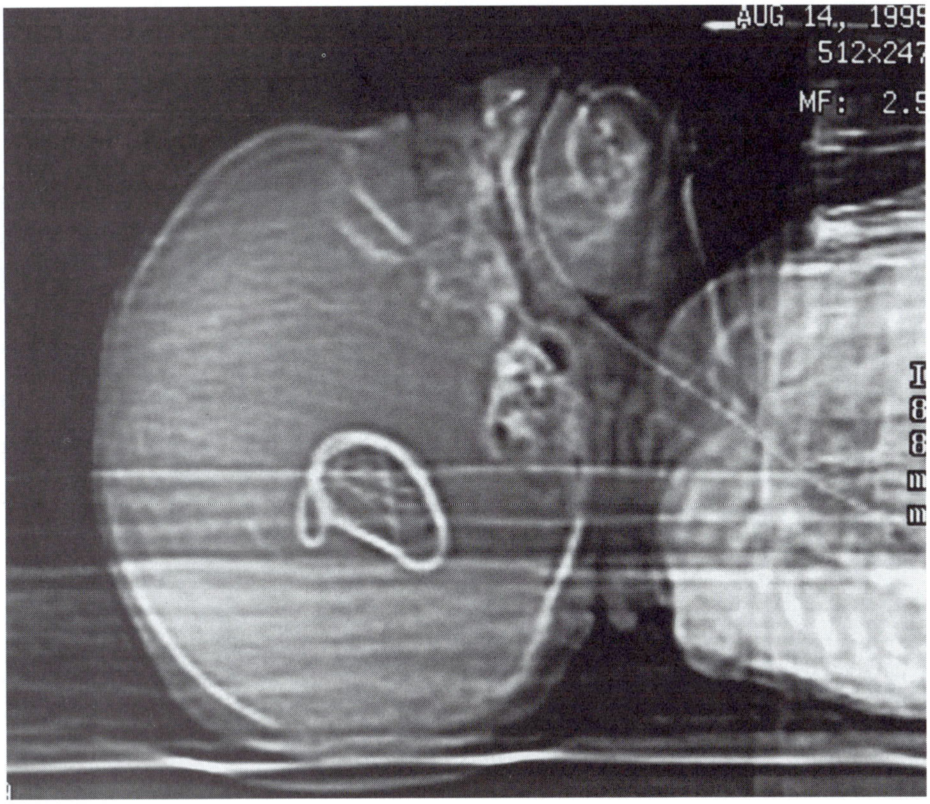

FIGURE 16.7 *A patient with a vein of Galen aneurysm after transtorcular occlusion with thrombogenic material.*

FIGURE 16.8 *An angiogram of vein of Galen aneurysm in a 4-day-old black male. Note widely dilated vein of Galen and straight sinus draining the aneurysm.*

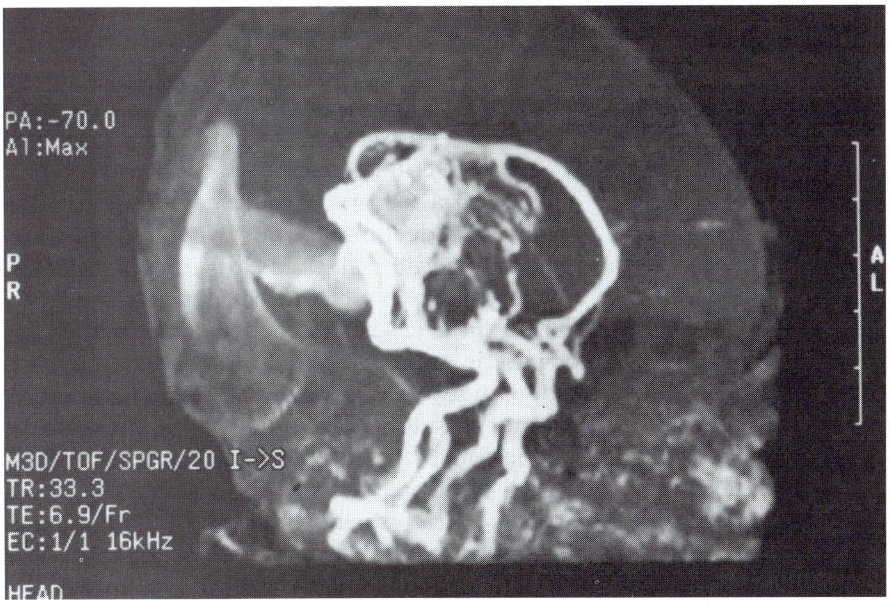

A B
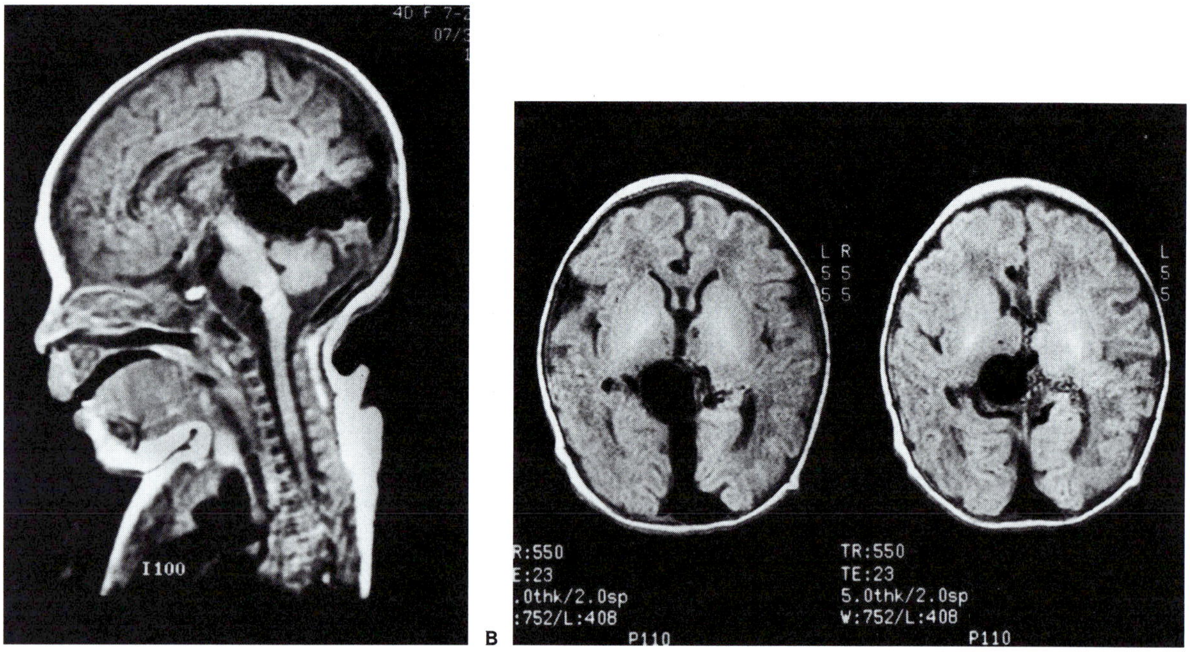

FIGURE 16.9 *A vein of Galen aneurysm; MRI studies. (A) The sagittal midline MRI view. Note the grossly dilated vein of Galen and straight sinus draining the aneurysm. (B) A transverse MRI examination of vein of Galen aneurysm.*

brain, with revascularization through collateral channels. These collaterals are insufficient to support the developing brain resulting in a progressive stroke syndrome. This can be extremely dangerous during surgery when cerebrovascular supply can be adversely affected during anesthesia, resulting in a neurologically compromised patient after emergence.

Congenital Malformations

ARNOLD-CHIARI MALFORMATION REPAIR The Arnold-Chiari malformation is a complex developmental abnormality frequently associated with meningomyelocele and other defects of the neural tube. Characteristics include the downward displacement of the inferior cerebellar vermis into the upper cervical spinal canal and elongation of the medulla oblongata and the fourth ventricle. This malformation may result in brainstem compression and lead to complete obstruction of the foramen of Luschka and Magendie with hydrocephalus and hydromyelia resulting. Brainstem compromise can produce apnea,[92] vocal cord paralysis, abnormal respiratory drive, autonomic instability, and spasticity.[93–95] The child presenting for repair often presents with a history of hydrocephalus that has required a decompressive ventriculostomy or ventriculoperitoneal shunt early in life. Occasionally, a child presents with stridor and bradycardia. In these cases, one or both vocal cords may be paretic or paralyzed, and the patient may present with severe upper airway obstruction and inspiratory stridor (occasionally with cyanosis). An evaluation by an otolaryngologist may be required in the preoperative period. Episodes of unexpected bradycardia unrelated to airway obstruction may occur in this syndrome. The hydromyelia may present in a variety of ways, depending on the location, extent, and frequent asymmetry of cord cavitation. The classic syndrome of brachial amyotrophy—beginning in the interossei and lumbricales muscles of the hand, the spreading proximally, with "capelike" suspended sensory loss—has been present in the majority of reported cases at the time of diagnosis.[96]

A history and physical examination will provide evidence for loss of airway reflexes or changes in phonation associated with vocal cord paralysis. Elective, awake tracheal intubation may be required to provide a safe airway during induction of anesthesia. These children have often had a decompressive procedure performed prior to their planned surgery, and in these cases shunt patency should be assessed before assuming the ICP is normal.

The treatment of the symptomatic Arnold-Chiari malformation requires a decompressive procedure. Posterior fossa craniotomy and upper cervical laminectomy for decompression of the hindbrain malformation is the most frequently performed surgical procedure for this repair. The goal of surgery is to restore to normal the circulation of CSF and remove further possibility of hindbrain compression. The child should be monitored as for the posterior fossa craniotomy mentioned above, and anesthesia induction and maintenance should proceed in the aforementioned fashion. Emphasis should be placed upon the changes in respiration and heart rate that surgical manipulation of the posterior fossa can evoke. Meticulous control of the airway is important in these patients if an artificial airway has not been established preoperatively. Failure of the decompressive procedure to ameliorate the vocal cord palsy may require elective tracheotomy to allow the child to grow and thrive.

Operative mortality after posterior fossa-hindbrain decompression ranges from 0 to 15% with recent series reporting less than 5%. The predominant cause of death was respiratory failure followed by postoperative hematoma, acute hydrocephalus, and medullary infarction from damage to the posterior inferior cerebellar artery. Morbidity includes aseptic meningitis, bradycardia, and respiratory dysfunction with apnea.[97]

Spasticity Procedures

Cerebral palsy is a common physical disability in childhood that results from a CNS injury during the perinatal period. Associated disorders such as hydrocephalus, seizures, and impairment of cognition, speech, vision, and hearing may occur in cerebral palsy; however, its primary manifestation is disturbance of motor function. The prevalence of cerebral palsy in industrialized nations has remained basically unchanged over the past 30 years at 2:1,000 live births.[98] The spastic type is common due to improved survival rates among low birth weight premature infants who are prone to develop spastic cerebral palsy. Clinically these patients develop contractures and bony deformities that are referred to the neurosurgeon and orthopedic surgeon for treatment. Techniques such as anterior rhizotomy, myelotomy, and implantation of cerebellar simulators have been used in an attempt to relieve spasticity with varying degrees of success. Posterior rhizotomy for reduction of spasticity began nearly 100 years ago and has been further developed over time to become a valuable tool for the management of selected patients with spastic cerebral palsy. In this procedure the excitatory input to lower extremities is decreased through division of posterior spinal nerve roots.

The surgical technique requires physiologic examination of the posterior or dorsal nerve roots of the spinal cord using EMG. In this technique the roots are divided into several fascicles. These fascicles are individually exposed to repetitive electrical stimulation and those showing inhibition of transmission are located. Stimulation of other fascicles may reveal either loss of inhibition or exaggeration of the motor responses (sustained responses or spread of responses to other muscle groups) (Figure 16.10). It is these fascicles of the dorsal roots that are believed to effect the spasticity noted in cerebral palsy. The normal response is characterized by single muscular contraction at 50 stimuli per second and no diffusion to other muscle groups, and abnormal response is defined as tetanic muscular contraction at 50 stimuli per second

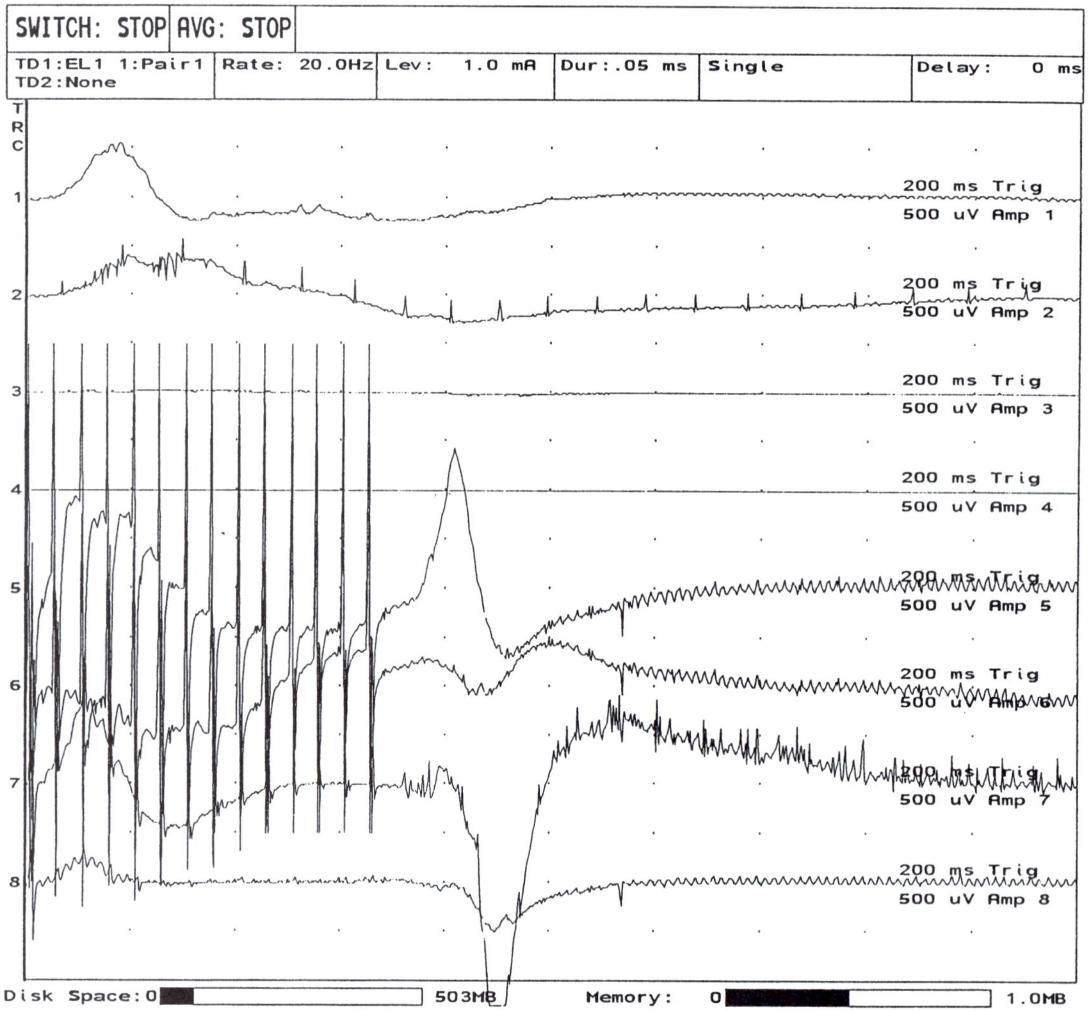

FIGURE 16.10 *Electromyography recording during selective dorsal rhizotomy. Surgical stimulation is occurring at a fascicle of the L3 nerve root on the right side. Recordings are made by needle electrodes placed in the muscle groups of the lower extremities. The waveforms shown represent EMG responses from; (1) left quadriceps, (2) left hamstrings, (3) left gastrocnemius, (4) left anterior tibialis, (5) right quadriceps, (6) right hamstrings, (7) right gastrocnemius, (8) right anterior tibialis. The figure shows an increased myographic response in leads 5, 6, 7, representing the right leg. There is also some spreading of response to the left side in lead 2. This response would be considered consistent with increased "abnormal" activity in response to stimulation, and this fascicle of the nerve root would be severed.*

with diffusion to other muscle groups.[100] The surgeon then divides the fascicles without inhibition and spares those with inhibition. In this way spasticity is reduced and sensation is maintained. Usually this means that 25 to 50% of the roots are divided.[101] For further discussion of this topic, refer to Chapter 4.

The anesthetic considerations include those of managing the induction and maintenance of anesthesia in a mentally retarded and possibly hypovolemic child as well as issues of volume replacement for laminectomy. The anesthetic chosen can alter the effectiveness of EMG recordings from the posterior roots. Muscle relaxants will prevent detection of muscle mass movement, and benzodiazepines can markedly decrease the sensitivity of EMG to detect excitatory and diffusion impulses in the roots.

Postoperatively, epidural narcotics and local anesthetics have been very important in controlling spasms and pain following this procedure. In older children, the patient-controlled analgesia pump, whether applied intravenously or epidurally, is an effective modality. Adequate control of pain and spasms following this procedure allows the child an early return to rehabilitation.

Epilepsy

The special pediatric neurosurgical requirements for epilepsy surgery entail the capability of performing awake surgery on a dominant temporal lobe patient, thereby minimizing the risk of significant injury to the speech apparatus during aggressive resections. Although this is rarely done in children, there are certain situations where it is indispensable for the control of the seizures, where the primary pathological process is a tumor. Again, the anesthetic has to be chosen to maximize the effectiveness of neurophysiologic monitoring needed for these resections. Many of these individuals can have seizures, either intraoperatively or immediately postoperatively, and this should be watched for very carefully by the anesthesiologist. Intraoperative seizures can be treated with the use of intravenous barbiturates and benzodiazepines as deemed fit, provided a patent airway is maintained (see Ch. 11).

SPINAL PROCEDURES

The major pathologic processes involving the spine include trauma, vascular malformations, tumors, and congenital malformations. It is important to realize that spinal trauma in childhood can result in major spinal cord injury, without bony injury. During the birthing process, the spinal cord is extremely vulnerable, especially at the craniocervical junction. Major spinal cord injury can be present and very difficult to diagnose, because the reflexive movements can mimic normal movements. If cervical injury is suspected, then early radiologic evaluation and immobilization is essential. Intubation in this situation can be very dangerous and requires special skills.

Tumors of the spinal cord can be intramedullary or extramedullary. The intramedullary tumors require extensive surgical exposure and prolonged anesthetics for total resection. Neurophysiologic monitoring is essential for safe removal of these tumors. The extrameduallry and epidural tumors can be malignant, and usually biopsy followed by radiation and chemotherapy is the treatment of choice. These tumors produce significant pain and require pharmacologic therapy for control.

Scoliosis

Scoliosis as a topic is covered elsewhere in the text and as such will receive only cursory mention in this chapter. The incidence of scoliosis is 1.8 per 1,000 with a heavy female preponderance. The sex difference is mainly due to the increased incidence of adolescent idiopathic curves in females, the commonest form of scoliosis.

Congenital scoliosis is frequently associated with other major abnormalities, especially cyanotic congenital heart disease or as a part of VATER syndrome with vertebral, anal, tracheoesophageal fistula, renal, radial, and cardiac abnormalities. Children with spina bifida who have severe scoliosis usually have major neurologic deficits.

Preoperative assessment includes detailed examination of the respiratory, cardiovascular, neuromuscular, and renal systems because of the high incidence of associated abnormalities. The two major factors that affect pulmonary function are the degree of curvature and neuromuscular dysfunction. Patients with idiopathic scoliosis rarely develop significant respiratory impairment unless the Cobb angle is greater than 65°. This gives a restrictive pattern with the greatest reduction occurring in vital capacity with smaller changes in total lung capacity and functional residual capacity. Ventilation-perfusion mismatch and alveolar hypoventilation result in early hypoxemia while carbon dioxide levels remain normal until late in the disease process. Those patients with a vital capacity of less than 30% of predicted values usually require postoperative ventilatory support.

The treatment of scoliosis is primarily a surgical one as plaster localizer casts and bracing are only used as a stop gap measure. There are two possible approaches to the spinal column. The anterior approach uses a thoracoabdominal incision in the lateral position. The procedure allows direct access to the vertebral bodies where removal of intervertebral discs results in a dramatic increase in spinal mobility. The complications of this approach result from the large thoracoabdominal wound and diaphragmatic disruption, causing severe postoperative pain and an increased incidence of postoperative ventilatory support. Posterior fusion is also an extensive procedure using a distraction rod applied to the concavity of the curve fixed at either end with hooks to the facet joints and usually stabilized with sublaminar wiring (Luque). There is extensive decortication of the vertebrae and application of bone graft from the iliac crest. These two operations are sometimes used in a two-stage procedure in cases where curvature is marked.

The main considerations for the anesthesiologist are respiratory status, blood loss, associated abnormalities, and intraoperative spinal cord monitoring. The respiratory status should be evaluated prior to induction and monitored prior to extubation. Because of the extensive nature of the surgery one of the major complications of spinal cord fusion is massive blood loss. Patients should be monitored with an arterial pressure and central venous catheters. Many factors affect blood loss, the first being the duration of surgery because of the large raw bony surface, and secondly, venous pressure in the vertebral veins. In those patients with fixed lordotic deformities, it may not be possible to place the patient in a position to facilitate venous drainage. The use of induced hypotension using a nitroprusside drip has the advantages of decreasing blood loss but can interfere with blood supply to the spinal cord in situations where circulation may be tenuous.

Spinal cord damage has been noted to occur in approximately 1% of patients undergoing scoliosis procedures.[101] Because of the potential risks of this type of surgery, intraoperative wake-up tests and electrophysiologic monitoring have become useful adjuncts to anesthetic techniques. The use of the wake-up test should be discussed with the patient in the preoperative period. This test is performed by "lightening" the depth of anesthesia sufficiently to allow the patient to follow commands. This is usually done as soon as all instrumentation is in place. The patient is first instructed to squeeze the hands, and then asked to move the feet and toes. If the patient is able to move the hands, but not the feet, the amount of spine distraction must be reduced until a safe degree of correction is achieved. As soon as the patient moves the feet, anesthesia is quickly deepened with small doses of benzodiazepine (e.g., midazolam, 0.2 to 0.2 mg/kg) or thiopental (1 to 1.5 mg/kg) and a muscle relaxant. Recall of intraoperative events is very unusual with this technique.

The use of intraoperative electrophysiologic monitoring (EP) means the anesthetic maintenance should be adjusted to allow for as little interference as possible. In our institution we use a narcotic-based technique without nitrous oxide and with the use of low levels of volatile inhalational agents. We use a 30 mg/kg IV bolus of methylprednisolone followed by a 5.5 mg/kg infusion for 24 hours for spinal cord protection. Other techniques for spinal cord protection are also used including CSF drainage, calcium channel blockers, and papaverine, but these modalities should only be used after discussion between the surgical and anesthesia teams.

Postoperative pain relief is very important after major surgery but will need to be administered cautiously in those patients with poor respiratory function. Patients with spasticity, especially those with cerebral palsy, experience extreme pain following all orthopedic procedures and have increased analgesic requirements.

Spinal Cord Tumors

Spinal cord tumors represent approximately 5 to 10% of CNS tumors within the pediatric group. Of these, approximately one-fourth are intramedullary tumors. Within the intramedullary group, the overwhelming majority of tumors belong to the glioma family. The usually benign nature of spinal cord tumors leads to an indolent history. The primary objective symptom is one of motor weakness in approximately 70% of patients. If present, then pain is initially localized to the epidural area. This is exacerbated by a recumbent position as a result of venous congestion.

In the past the anatomic complexity of the spinal cord along with the infiltrative nature of some tumors had led some authorities to advocate palliative treatment of spinal cord tumors. With the advancement of radiologic procedures as well as improvements in microsurgery, laser surgery and the use of a Cavitron have made the resection of tumors more successful. The use of somatosensory evoked potentials (SSEP's) has enabled the preservation of viable tissue during the resection. For further information on this topic, refer to Chapter 4.

The anesthetic considerations of spinal cord tumor surgery include psychological preparation of the family and patient. The induction and maintenance should be undertaken with a view to calm the fears of the child and provide a "pleasant" experience. The drugs used for maintenance should be tailored to minimize impact on the intraoperative monitoring of spinal cord function.

Congenital Deformities

SPINAL DYSRAPHISM Dysraphic lesions result from to failure of the neural tube to fully close during embryogenesis. This can lead to conditions incompatible with life, such as anencephaly. Meningomyelocele is a dysraphic condition of the spine. Meningomyelocele has a reported incidence of 20 per 100,000[102] and may be seen anywhere along the spinal cord, giving rise to a variety of neurologic deficits in the lower extremity, bowel, and bladder. This condition may have the Arnold-Chiari malformation associated with it.

A child born with a significant myelomeningocele does not require emergency surgery, and delays up to a week while the family is learning to deal with the situation is acceptable. However, early closure of these defects is recommended to minimize the risks of infection and other potential complications. Positioning of the child may be difficult due to the presence of exposed meninges; a donut may be formed to cushion the defect (Fig 16.11). Anesthesia may be induced with volatile anesthetics once the presence of intracranial hypertension has been ruled out. Facilitation of intubation may be provided with succinylcholine because it does not cause an increase in potassium release in these patients.[103]

Closure of the defect requires attention during the anesthetic period to blood and evapora-

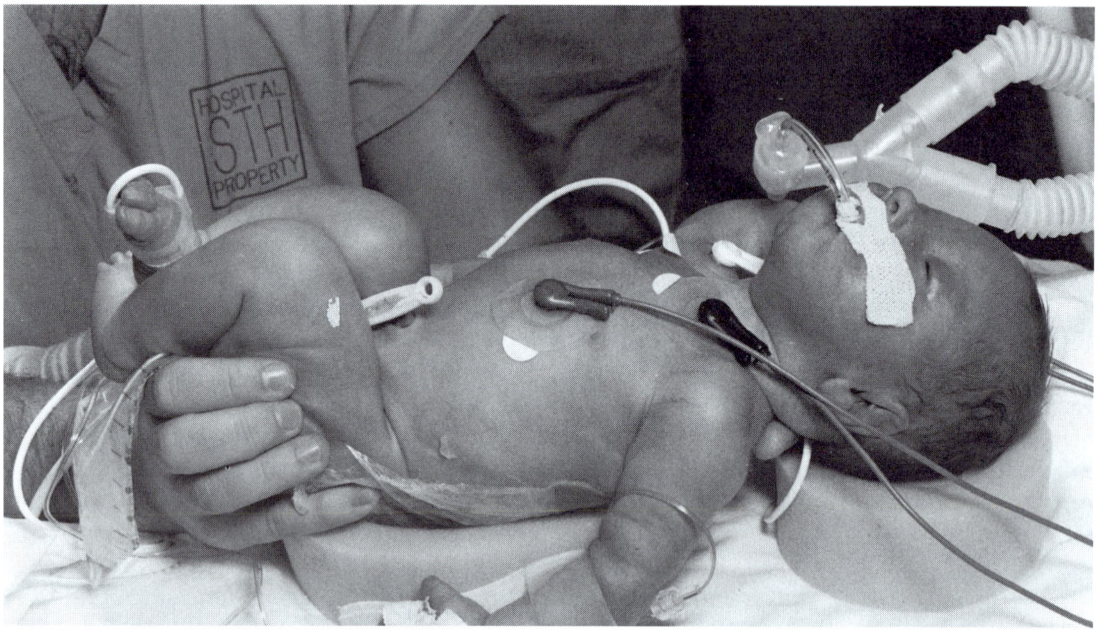

FIGURE 16.11 *The position for intubation of a patient with a meningomyelocoele. The patient is positioned with the spinal defect kept clear of the bed with a donut and hands. Other options for intubation include lateral intubation.*

tive fluid loss, neonatal fluid requirements, temperature maintenance, prone positioning, and securing of the endotracheal tube. If the surgeon plans to use a nerve stimulator, neuromuscular blockade should be carefully monitored or avoided altogether.

TETHERED CORD Until the third month of fetal life, the spinal cord and the spinal canal are of equal length. Thereafter the more rapid longitudinal growth of the vertebral column is such that the tip of the conus usually lies opposite L3 at birth. Abnormal fixation of the conus either directly or via the cauda equina may result in tethering of the cord such that its "ascent" is impeded and so remains at a lower vertebral level and may be under tension. The majority of these patients also have abnormalities of the lumbar spine, ranging from a single-level spina bifida occulta to the much more widespread neural arch abnormalities. Cutaneous stigmata over the back such as hairy patches are common, and an associated progressive kyphoscoliosis or scoliosis is common in the growing child. Pain is a frequent presenting symptom. Neurologic deterioration can occur if the defect is not treated.[104]

LIPOMYELOMENINGOCELE Lipomyelomeningocele presents a complex problem associated with the dysraphic process, producing not only the bony canal deformities of spina bifida, but also a subcutaneous lumbosacral lipoma, which communicates through a dural defect with an abnormal and tethered spinal cord. The lipoma is often intimately related to the abnormally low conus. Surgical repair is usually attempted at less than 6 months of age, as this is before the presentation of neurologic deficits.[105] Anesthesia for this procedure should be similar to other spinal surgery cases in which there is the possibility of intraoperative monitoring of EMGs.[106]

SYRINGOMYELIA Syringomyelia and hydromyelia are not synonymous. Hydromyelia is dilation of the central canal of the cord. Syringomyelia constitutes the formation of cavities within the actual parenchyma of the spinal cord. The consequent destruction of neural elements and their replacement by gliosis and cavitation leads to the associated neurologic disturbance. The walls of a syringomyelic cavity, or syrinx, include degenerate and edematous tissue with overgrowth of glia and obliteration of some blood vessels. The disease primarily affects the cervical cord but can extend to the thoracic spine.[107] The cavity lies mainly in the gray matter to the central canal, extending posteriorly to the dorsal columns. There are several theories of production of these cavities, but most seem to include the abnormal passage of CSF from the fourth ventricle to the central canal. However, a spinal cord tumor must be ruled out.

The classic picture of syringomyelia is that of a stepwise though persistent deterioration culminating in a picture of dissociated sensory loss, lower motor neuron damage in the upper limbs, upper motor neuron changes affecting the lower limbs, and trophic skin changes.

The ideal treatment of this disorder is not yet known. Surgical treatment includes posterior fossa decompression combined with an upper cervical laminectomy and cyst drainage. Anesthetic considerations should be the same as those in posterior fossa decompressions but with SSEP monitoring.

Traumatic Spinal Cord Injury

One of the chief anesthetic concerns when managing a patient with an acute spinal injury is preventing progression of the neurologic injury. Securing an airway in the patient with a cervical spine injury must be accomplished with minimal neck movement. A team approach is particularly helpful, with the anesthesiologist attending to the airway and the surgeon maintaining head and neck position with axial traction throughout airway management, tracheal intubation, and patient positioning.

Awake fiberoptic tracheal intubation techniques are frequently the best method of securing an airway, but topical anesthesia in a well-sedated patient is imperative to prevent excessive coughing and movement when the tracheal tube is placed in the sensitive glottis and trachea. In pediatric patients this technique may be impossible due lack of patient cooperation. An alternative solution is fiberoptic intubation through a laryngeal mask airway. This technique will provide a secure airway in a manner that may prevent spinal movement.

In acute spinal cord injury above T6, the abrupt disruption of sympathetic innervation to the vasculature produces venodilatation and hypotension. When cord dysfunction extends higher than T1, sympathetic control of heart rate is also interrupted, leading to bradycardia. Venous capacitance vessels dilate, and compensatory baroreceptor responses to decreased vascular volume are lost. Position changes, such as moving from supine to prone for surgery and positive pressure ventilation, frequently aggravate hypotension in patients with "spinal shock." Cardiac responses to increased ventricular volume are also altered in spinal-cord-injured patients, and small changes in intravascular volume can lead to pulmonary edema. As spinal shock resolves 24 to 72 hours postinjury, a return of sympathetic tone may result in a shift in blood volume from the dilated venous capacitance vessels to the central circulation.

In patients with chronic high spinal cord injury, severe hypertension and bradycardia due to hyperreflexia may occur. This is usually initiated by visceral or somatic stimulation from below the level of the lesion. General or regional anesthesia is often required to control this autonomic response in susceptible patients who require surgery. The incidence of this syndrome has been reported at 66% to 85% in the spinal cord injury population.[108] An additional concern in paraplegia is the hyperkalemic response to succinylcholine. This can occur 24 hours after the lesion, and remain for greater than 6 months. Avoidance of this potassium release can be attained by using short-onset muscle relaxants, such as rocuronium and mivacurium on intubation.

As mentioned elsewhere SSEPs can be used to identify and monitor potentially reversible neurologic lesions during operations on the spinal cord.

Vascular Disorders of the Spine

The major vascular disorders of the spine include AVMs, vertebral angioma, and extradural hematoma. Although AVM may occur anywhere throughout the length of the spinal cord, it occurs more frequently in the caudal area. The majority of AVMs arise form the posterior circulation, and in many cases the site of the true fistula may not be intradural with fistulous communication in the extradural space and the cord vessels merely being the draining vessels. Even true posteriorly situated AVMs do not necessarily penetrate the cord or implicate its blood supply but rather seem to invaginate it.

Clinically, AVMs may present at any age. Intramedullary varieties tend to present early and have a higher incidence of subarachnoid hemorrhage, whereas the other types tend to present later in life with a progressive neurologic deficit. The commonest clinical presentation of a spinal AVM is with a progressive, usually episodic, spastic paraparesis and hemorrhage.

Localization of the AVM with the use of CT, MRI, and spinal angiography enables the surgical team to localize the main branches of the AVM and plan a complete resection. The anesthetic considerations should be to maintain a stable blood pressure to prevent the premature rupture or hemorrhage of the malformation prior to resection.

SPECIAL REQUIREMENTS

Those procedures involving the cranium and face are becoming more common and are being performed earlier for optimum results. The special neuroanesthetic requirements for these procedures are the establishment and maintenance of a safe airway and the careful monitoring of blood loss. VAE is a risk to the child undergoing these procedures, because major dural sinuses and the capacious diploe of the skull are at risk for pulling air into the vascular space. The biggest risk, however, is blood loss and postoperative infection. Total vascular collapse from inadequate blood replacement can occur precipitously. Even in the simplest situations in craniofacial surgeries, such as single-suture resection and cranial shaping, blood loss can be significant. The average blood loss over a 24-hour period in a child with single-suture resection is 80 to 100 ml of blood.

Craniosynostosis

Craniosynostosis results from the premature fusion, usually in utero, of the cranial sutures. One or more of the sutures may be involved, and the end result is a malformed skull and face, which can impede normal brain growth. Most commonly only one of the sutures is involved, and the problem is essentially cosmetic. Elevated ICP is prevented by expansion of the skull at the unfused suture sites. The incidence of this condition is approximately 12,000 patients.[109] Craniosynostosis covers a wide range of deformities ranging from single-suture fusion to multiple-suture fusion with associated craniofacial abnormalities. Multiple synostoses are associated with increased ICP and, if not treated, can lead to retardation and optic atrophy. The primary site of involvement is the sagittal suture.

Brain growth, which is the normal stimulus for expansion and shaping of the head, occurs very rapidly in infancy. Brain size doubles in the first 6 months of life and reaches 80% of the adult weight by 2 years of age. Surgical intervention is usually recommended at 4 to 6 weeks of age to achieve the greatest cosmetic benefit in single-suture fusion and cases of ICH.[110]

Surgery for this disorder is usually carried out in infancy. Because the fusion can occur in utero and may involve multiple sutures, it may be an emergent procedure in the immediate postpartum period due to brain constriction. Up to 20% of these patients will have associated hydrocephalus, although this is usually in those with associated craniofacial abnormalities. Thorough understanding of the lesion involved must be obtained prior to induction. If craniofacial abnormalities exist, the intubation may be difficult and the patient may benefit from remaining ventilated at the conclusion of the procedure.

Anesthetic considerations during this procedure concern mainly the volume status of the child. The scalp is a very vascular structure, and significant blood loss can be expected during these procedures. Occasionally blood loss can be massive if a sinus is accidentally opened. The physician should ensure that a complete type and cross-match has been performed and that the blood is in the room prior to induction. Vascular access should be a primary consideration for this case. Not only should an arterial line be placed, but a central venous line may be utilized for following volume status and fluid replenishment. Intubation should be performed using an armored or oral RAE tube as the airway will be very close to the surgical field. The tube should be secured firmly in place as there will be extensive manipulation of the head and tube during the operation. For operations in the prone position, the head rest should be adequately padded to prevent necrosis of pressure points, and the head should be lifted periodically during the surgery to relieve pressure.

Monitoring should include the items as mentioned above as well as a urinary catheter for assessment of adequate output. Regular blood samples should be sent for hemoglobin and electrolyte levels. This operation is usually performed in the supine, head-elevated position, and there is a risk of VAE.[111] A precordial Doppler has been shown to be effective in detecting air embolism in children[31] and should be utilized in this case. The likelihood of VAE is increased if fluid replacement lags behind blood loss. Treatment for VAE should be as mentioned earlier.

The vault of the skull is removed during surgery and so some manipulation of the brain is unavoidable. The use of dexamethasone (0.2 mg/kg) should be considered for the minimizing of cerebral edema. Standard procedures should be used to improve the surgical field. Hyperventilation and mannitol are frequently used to reduce brain bulk. Due to the application of brain retractors, it is inadvisable to utilize controlled hypotension for blood loss control to reduce the risk of tissue ischemia.

Craniofacial Deformities

Craniofacial repair involves the cosmetic restoration of congenital or acquired bony abnormalities of the skull and face. Craniosynostosis has been mentioned above, and this section will focus on the concerns of facial reconstruction. Anesthetic considerations for craniofacial surgery (i.e., hypertelorism, craniodacialdysotoses, and facial clefts or asymmetries) include hemorrhage, elevated ICP, airway difficulties, VAE, hypothermia, and coagulopathies. Airway complications are common because of abnormal anatomy such as mandibular hypoplasia as well as scar tissue after repeat surgeries. The anesthesiologist should have a fiberoptic bronchoscope available on induction as well as a surgeon standing by to perform a tracheotomy if endotracheal intubation is impossible. Once intubation is achieved, accidental extubation is common due to close proximity of the surgical field. Nasal intubation and securing the endotracheal tube to the teeth has minimized the risk of extubation but does not completely remove it. Constant monitoring of breath sounds via an esophageal stethoscope is the recommended way of ensuring airway patency.

Massive hemorrhage in the face of extensive surgery is possibly the greatest single risk to the patient. Blood loss is continuous during the procedure but is especially high during any cranial osteotomy. The use of an arterial line, frequent hematocrit determinations, central venous pressure, and urine output as a gauge of adequate intravascular volume is suggested. In general, massive blood replacement is complicated by dilutional thrombocytopenia, coagulopathy,[112] and calcium-mediated hypotension.[113] An adequate volume of blood and blood products should be cross-matched preoperatively, although controlled hypotension, autologous blood transfusion, hemodilution, and red cell saving devices may be used to reduce blood loss and limit reliance on the blood bank.

Neuroradiologic Procedures

Often the pediatric neuroanesthesiologist is asked to participate in off-site anesthetic procedures, especially in neuroradiology. The anesthesiologist is called in as the patient is unable to tolerate the procedure under "light" sedation. (Fig. 16.12). These procedures are usually delayed until the afternoon because of primary commitments to the operating theater. This results in children who are frightened and dehydrated.

Managing children for neurodiagnostic imaging demands special vigilance and attention because unexpected neurologic deterioration, oversedation, airway obstruction, drug reactions, and respiratory arrest are common in this setting. Equipment should be available in all locations where the anesthesiologist is present to provide for a safe general anesthetic should the need arise.

The older healthy child may require little more than simple assurance from the physician or nearby parent. Other children, especially those involved in protracted or uncomfortable procedures, will require sedation or more likely general anesthesia. Infants, toddlers, uncooperative, or retarded children may require general anesthesia. The use of sedation should be carefully weighed against the possibility of losing the patient's airway in a situation where intubation is difficult.

FIGURE 16.12 *A patient intubated for radiosurgery on a nonoperable brain tumor. (Courtesy of Dr. Mendenhall, Department of Radiation Therapy, University of Florida.)*

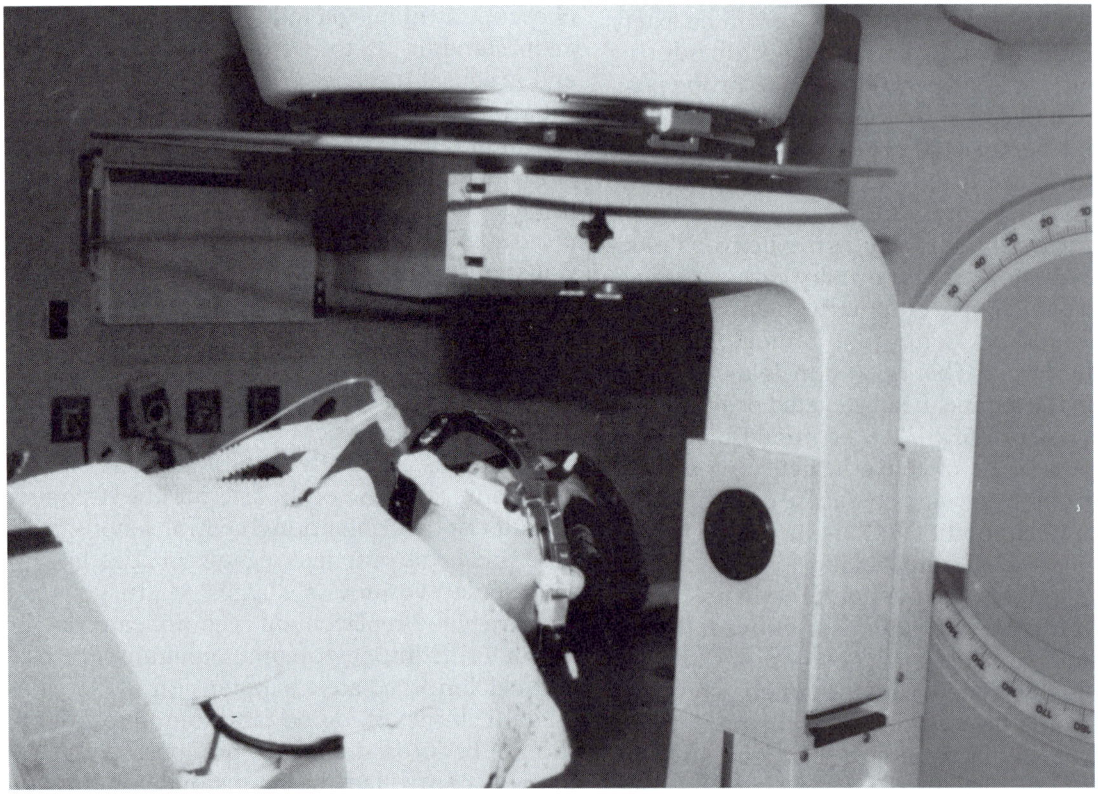

The issue of general anesthesia in the magnetic resonance imager (MRI) should be addressed. The magnetic filed generated by the machine will render most of the anesthesia equipment routinely used useless or, in worst cases, lethal. The use of ferromagnetic material in the vicinity of the coil is impossible as they degrade and distort the magnetic filed and also may be turned into projectiles by the magnetic field. Consequently, manufactures have developed nonferromagnetic anesthesia equipment for use in this theater. Prior to attempting anesthesia coverage in the MRI unit, all equipment should be checked to make sure it is MRI compatible. Further discussion of this topic occurs in Chapter 17.

SUMMARY

This chapter contains our own philosophy for the treatment of pediatric neurosurgical patients. Certainly the management of these patients requires extraordinary cooperation between the neurosurgeon and anesthesiologist. A frank and open discussion of the expectations of both will provide the best care for the child. The patient population has unique attributes that require specialized training from the anesthesiologist in order to prevent disastrous consequences.

References

1. Griesen G: Cerebral blood flow in preterm infants during the first week of life. Acta Paediatr Scand 75:43, 1986
2. Fetis-Hansen B: Perinatal brain injury and cerebral blood flow in newborn infants. Acta Paediatr Scand 74:323, 1985
3. Younkin DP, Levich M, Jaggi J et al: Noninvasive mechanism of estimating human newborn regional blood flow. J Cereb Blood Flow Metab 2:415, 1982
4. Kennedy C, Sokoloff L: An adaptation of the nitrous oxide method to the study of the cerebral circulation in children: normal values for cerebral blood flow and cerebral metabolic rate in childhood. J Clin Invest 36:1130, 1937
5. Hernandez MJ, Brennan RW, Bowman GS: Autoregulation of cerebral blood flow in the newborn dog. Brain Res 184:199, 1980
6. Newton RW: Intracranial pressure and its monitoring in childhood: a review. J R Soc Med 80:566, 1987
7. Bunegin L, Albin MS: Pitfalls encountered in relating anterior fontanelle pressure to intracranial pressure. Anesth Analg 66:1196, 1987
8. Bailey P, Pace N, Ashburn M et al: Frequent hypoxia and apnea after sedation with midazolam and fentanyl. Anesthesiology 73:826, 1990
9. Feld L, Negus J, White P: Oral midazolam preanesthetic medication in pediatric outpatients. Anesthesiology 73:831, 1990
10. Roberts RB, Shirley MA: Reducing the risk of acid aspiration during cesarean section. Anesth Analg 53:859, 1974
11. Sutherland AD, Stock JG, Davies JM: Effects of preoperative fasting on morbidity and mortality and gastric contents in patients undergoing day-stay surgery. Br J Anaesth 58:876, 1986
12. Meakin G, Dingwall AE, Addison M: Effect of fasting and oral premedication on the pH and volume of gastric aspirates in children. Br J Anaesth 59:678, 1987
13. Sutherland AD, Maltby JR, Sale JP, Reid CRG: The effect of perioperative oral fluid and ranitidine on gastric fluid volume and pH. Can J Anaesth 34:117, 1987
14. Schreiner MS, Triebwasser A, Keon TP: Ingestion of liquids compared with preoperative fasting in pediatric outpatients. Anesthesiology 72:593, 1990
15. Seiber FE, Smith DS, Traystman RJ, Wollman H: Glucose: a reevaluation of its intraoperative use. Anesthesiology 67:72, 1987
16. Drummond JC, Moore SS: The influence of dextrose administration in the rabbit. Anesthesiology 70:64, 1989.
17. Pulsinelli WA, Levy DE, Singsbee B et al: Increased damage after ischemic stroke in patients with hyperglycemia with or without established diabetes mellitus. Am J Med 74:540, 1983
18. Mikawa K, Mackawa N, Goto R et al: Effects of exogenous intravenous glucose on plasma glucose and lipid homeostasis in anesthetized children.
19. Marshall TA Oecder R, Pai S et al: Physiologic changes associated with endotracheal intubation in preterm infants. Crit Care Med 12:501, 1984

20. Pasternak JF, Grouthuis DR, Fisher JM, Fisher DP: Regional cerebral blood flow in the beagle puppy model of neonatal intraventricular hemorrhage: studies during systemic hypertension. Neurology 33:559, 1983
21. Wimberly PD, Low HC, Pedersen H et al: Hypertensive peaks in the pathogenesis of intraventricular hemorrhage in the newborn: abolition by phenobarbitone sedation. Acta paediatr Scand 71:537, 1982
22. Jones RM: Clinical comparison of inhalational anesthetic agents. Br J Anaesth 56:57S, 1984
23. McAllister RG: Macroglossia: a positional complication. Anesthesia 40:199, 1974
24. Haynes RH, Gramling-Babb P, Baker DJ: Fatal outcome of postoperative macroglossia as a complication of a craniotomy. Am J Anesthesiol 22:41, 1995
25. Mayhew JF, Milner M, Katz J: Macroglossia in a 16-month-old child after a craniotomy. Anesthesiology 64:845, 1986
26. Brentman L, Welsh FA, Harp JR: Cerebral protective effect of low-grade hypothermia. Anesthesiology 55:495, 1981
27. Miller LG, Prichard JG: Current issues in NSAID therapy. Primary Care 17:589, 1990
28. English JB, Westernskow D, Hodges MR et al: Comparison of venous air embolism monitoring methods in supine dogs. Anesthesiology 48:425, 1978
29. Albin MS, Caroll RG, Maroon JC: Clinical considerations concerning detection of venous air embolism. Neurosurgery 3:380, 1978
30. Cucchiara RF, Bowers B: Air embolism in children undergoing suboccipital craniotomy. Anesthesiology 57:338, 1982
31. Black S, Ockert DB, Oliver WC, Cucchiara RF: Comparison of outcome following posterior fossa craniectomy done in either a sitting or horizontal position. Anesthesiology 69:49, 1988
32. Lechat PH, Mas JL, Lascault G et al: Prevelance of patent foramen ovale in patients with stroke. N Engl J Med 318:1148, 1988
33. Kronik G, Mosslacher H: Positive contrast echocardiography in patients with patent foramen ovale and normal right heart hemodynamics. Am J Cardiol 49:1806, 1982
34. American College of Allergy and Immunology Task Force on Latex Hypersensitivity: Interim recommendations to health professionals and organizations regarding latex allergy precautions. American College of Allergy and Immunology, 1992
35. Nutter AF: Contact uticaria to rubber. Br J Dermatol 101:597, 1979
36. Gonzalez E: Latex hypersensitivity: a new and unexpected problem. Hosp Pract Off 27:32, 1992
37. Riott IM: Hypersensitivity – Type I. p. 19.1 In: Immunology. CV Mosby, St Louis, C 1985
38. Levine SJ, Shelhamer JH: Anaphylaxis. p. 1477. In Civetta JM, Taylor RW, Kirby RR (eds): Critical Care. 2nd Ed. JB Lippincott, Philadelphia, 1992
39. Levy JH: The allergic response. p. 1379. In Barash PG (ed): Clinical Anesthesia. JB Lippincott, Philadelphia, 1989
40. Kerner MM: Diagnosis and management of latex allergy in surgical patients. Am J Otolaryngol 14:440, 1993
41. Klonoff H, Low MD, Clark C: Head injuries in children: a prospective five year follow-up. J Neurol Neurosurg Psychiatry 40:1211, 1977
42. Haller JA: Pediatric trauma: the no. 1 killer of children. JAMA 249:47, 1983
43. Mayer T, Walker ML, Johnson DG et al: Causes of morbidity and mortality in severe pediatric trauma. JAMA 245:719, 1981
44. Singer HS, Freeman JM: Head trauma for the pediatrician. Pediatrics 62:819, 1978
45. Klauber MR, Marshall LF, Luersen TG et al: Determinants of head injury mortality: importance of the low risk patient. Neurosurgery 24:31, 1989
46. Langfitt TW, Bruce DA: Microcirculation and brain edema in head injury, p. 133. In Viken PJ, Bruyn GW (eds): Handbook of Clinical Neurology. Vol. 23. North-Holland, Amsterdam, 1978
47. Hahn YS, Chyung C, Barthel MJ et al: Head injuries in children under 36 months of age. Childs Nerv Syst 4:34, 1988
48. Leih-lai MW, Theodorou AA, Sarnaik AP et al: Limitations of the Glasgow Coma Scale in predicting outcome in children with traumatic brain injury. J Pediatr 120: 195, 1992
49. Hahn YS, McLone DG: Risk factors in the outcome of children with minor head injury. Pediatr Neurosurg 19:135, 1993
50. Bruce DA, Raphaely RC, Goldbert AI et al: Pathophysiology, treatment and outcome following severe head injury in children. Childs Brain 5:174, 1979
51. Humphreys RP, Jaimovich R, Hendrick EB, Hoffman H: Severe head injury in children. P

1910. In Raimondi AJ (ed): In Concepts in Pediatric Neurosurgery. Vol 3. Karager, Basel, 1983
52. Bruce DA, Alavi A, Bilaniuk L et al: Diffuse cerebral swelling following head injuries in children: the syndrome of "malignant brain edema." J Neurosurg 54:170, 1981
53. Ishige N, Pitts LH, Berry I: The effects of hypovolemic hypotension on high-energy phosphate metabolism of traumatized brain in rats. J Neurosurg 68:129, 1988
54. Langfitt TW: Measuring the outcome from head injuries. J Neurosurg 48:673, 1978
55. Luerssen TG, Klauber MR, Marshall LF: Outcome from head injury related to patient's age. J Neurosurg 68:409, 1988
56. Bayless P, Ray VG: Incidence of cervical spine injuries in association with blunt head trauma. Am J Emerg Med 7:139, 1989
57. Mackenzie CF, Shin B, Fisher R et al: Four year mortality of trauma victims admitted directly from the accident by helicopter. Anesthesiology 57:A96, 1982
58. Hill SA, Miller CA, Kosnik EJ et al: Pediatric neck injuries. J Neurosurg 60:700, 1984
59. Yearly DM, Cantees KK, Verdile VP et al: Emergency airway management in trauma patients with suspected spinal cord injuries. Anesth Analg 68:415, 1989
60. Grande CM, Barton CR, Stene JK: Appropriate techniques for airway management of emergency patients with suspected spinal cord injury. Anesth Analg 67:714, 1988
61. Hoffman HJ, Becker L, Craven MA: A clinically and pathologically distinct group of benign brainstem gliomas. Neurosurgery 7:243, 1980
62. Epstein F, Wisoff J: Surgical management of brainstem tumors of childhood and adolescence. Neurosurg Clin North Am 1:111, 1990
63. Azar-Kia B, Krishman UB, Schecter MM: Neonatal craniopharyngioma. A case report. J Neurosurg, 42:91, 1975
64. Shillito J: Treatment of craniopharyngioma. Clin Neurosurg 33:533, 1986
65. Yasargil MG, Curcic M et al: Total removal of craniopharyngiomas: approaches and long-term results in 144 patients. J Neurosurg 73:3, 1990
66. McLone DG, Raimondi AJ, Naidich TP: Craniopharyngiomas. Childs Brain 9:188, 1982
67. Tomitta T, McLone D: Radical resections of childhood craniopharyngiomas. Pediatr Neurosurg 19:6, 1993
68. Baskin DS, Wilson CB: Surgical management of craniopharyngiomas: a review of 74 cases. J Neurosur 66:22, 1986
69. Pusey E, Kortman KE, Flannigan BD et al: MR of craniopharyngiomas: tumor deliniation and characterization. AJR 149:383, 1987.
70. Pigeau I, Sigal R, Halmi P et al: MRI features of craniopharyngiomas at 1.5 tesla: a series of 13 cases. J Neuroradiol 15:276, 1988
71. Tomitta T: Management of craniopharyngiomas in children. Pediatr Neurosci 14:204, 1988
72. Hoffman HJ, De Silva M, Humphreys RP et al: Aggresive surgical management of craniopharyngiomas in children. J Neurosurg 76:47, 1992
73. Yasargil MG, Curcic M, Kis S et al: Total removal of craniopharyngiomas: approaches and long-term results in 144 patients. J Neurosurg 73:3, 1990
74. Green OC: Endocrinology: hormonal involvement in children p. 785. In Amador LV (ed): Brain Tumors in the Young. Charles C Thomas, Springfield, 12, 1983
75. Tomitta T, McLone DG: Radical resections of childhood craniopharyngiomas. Pediatr Neurosurg 19:6, 1993
76. Amacher L: Craniopharyngioma; the controversy regarding radiotherapy. Childs Brain 6:57, 1980
77. Sung DI, Chang CH, Harisiadis L, Carmel PW: Treatment results of craniopharyngiomas. Cancer 47:847, 1981
78. Epstein F, Wisoff J: Brainstem tumors in childhood: surgical indications. p. 357. In: Pediatric Neurosurgery: Surgery of the Developing Nervous System. WB Saunders, Philadelphia, 1989
79. Milhort TA: Pediatric Neurosurgery. FA Davis, Philadelphia, 1978
80. Swedlow DB: Anesthesia for neurosurgical procedures. p. 961. In Gregory GA (ed): Pediatric Anesthesia. 2nd Ed. Churchill Livingstone, New York, 1989
81. Artru AA, Cucchiara RF, Messick JM: Cardiorespiratory and cranial-nerve sequelae of surgical procedures involving the posterior fossa. Anesthesiology. 52:83, 1980
82. Mahla ME: Spontaneous ventilation is not a sensitive indicator of brainstem well-being. J Neurosurg Anesthesiol 7:58, 1995
83. Fiser DH: Intraosseous infusion. N Engl J Med 322:1579, 1990
84. Sloan MH, Lerman J, Bissonette B: Pharmacodynamics of high-dose vecuronium in children

during balanced anesthesia. Anesthesiology 74:656, 1991
85. Gordon E, Lagerkranser M, Rudehill A et al: The effect of isoflurane on cerebrospinal fluid pressure in patients undergoing neurosurgery. Acta Anaesthesiol Scand 32:108, 1988
86. Serlo W, Fernell E, Heikkinen E et al: Functions and complications of shunts in different etiologies of childhood hydrocephalus. Chil Nerv Syst 6:92, 1990
87. Liptak GS, McDonald JV: Ventriculoperitoneal shunts in children: factors affecting shunt survival. Pediatr Neurosci 12:289, 1985
88. Mulvihill SJ, Pappas TN, Debas HT: Effect of increased intracranial pressure on gastric acid secretion. Am J Surg 151:110, 1986
89. Lasjaunias P, Tcr Brugge K, Lopez Ibor L et al: The role of dural anomalies in vein of Galen aneurysms: report of six cases and review of the literature. AJNR 8:185, 1987
90. Mickle JP, Quisling RG: Vein of Galen fistulas. Neurosurg Clin north 5:529, 1994
91. Long DM, Seljeskog EL, Chou SN et al: Giant arteriovenous malformations of infancy and childhood. J Neurosurg 40:304, 1974
92. Cochrane DD, Adderley R, White CP et al: Apnea in patients with myelomeningocele. Pediatr Neurosurg 16:232, 1990–1991
93. Ishak BA, McClone D, Seleny FL: Intraoperative autonomic dysfunction associated with Arnold-Chiari malformation. Am J Dis Child 140:221, 1986
94. Oren J, Kelly DH, Todres ID et al: Respiratory complications in patients with myelodisplasia and Arnold-Chiari malformation. Childs Brain 7:146, 1980
95. Park TS, Cail WS, Maggio WM et al: Progressive spasticity and scoliosis in children with myelomeningocoele. J Neurosurg 62:367, 1985
96. Cahan LD, Bentson JR: Consideration in the diagnosis and treatment of syringomyelia and the Chiari malformation. J Neurosurg 57:24, 1982
97. Wisoff JH, Epstein F: Management of hydromyelia. Neurosurgery 25:562, 1989
98. Paneth N, Kiely J: The frequency of cerebral palsy: a review of population studies in industrialized nations since 1950, p. 35. In Stanely F, Alderman E (eds): The Epidemiology of the Cerebral Palsies. Clinics in Developmental Medicine. JB Lippincott, Philadelphia, 1984
99. Peacock WJ, Staudt LA: Selective psoterior rhizotomy: evolution of theory and practice. Pediatr Neurosurg 17:128, 1991–1992
100. Fasano VA, Barolat-Romana G, Zeme S, Sguazzi A: Electrophysiologic assesment of spinal circuits in spasticity by direct dorsal root stimulation. Neurosurgery 4:146, 1979
101. MacEwan GD, Bunnell WP, Sriram K: Acute neurological complications in the treatment of scoliosis. A report of the Scoliosis Research Society. J Bone Joint Surg [Am] 57:404, 1975
102. Stein SC, Feldman JG, Friedlander M: Is myelomeningocoele a disappearing disease? Pediatrics 69:511, 1982
103. Dierdorf SF, McNiece WL, Chalapathi CR et al: Failure of succinylcholine to alter plasma potassium in children with myelomeningocele. Anesthesiology 64:272, 1986
104. Becker K, Enck P, Wilhelm K et al: Colonic and anorectal dysfunction in a patient with the tethered cord syndrome. Am J Gastroenterol 89:1564, 1994
105. Kaneu PM, Lemire RJ, Loser JD, Berge F MS: Management and long-term follow up of children with lipomyelomeningocele, 1852–1987. J Neurosurg 73:48, 1990
106. Kothbauer K, Schmid UD et al: Intraoperative monitoring of the cauda equina. Neurosurgery 34:702, 1994
107. Charry O, Koops S, Winter R et al: Syringomyelia and scoliosis: a review of twenty-five pediatric patients. J Pediatr Orthop 14:309, 1994
108. Lambert DH, Deane RS, Mazuzan JE: Anesthesia and the control of blood pressure in patients with spinal cord injury. Anesth Analg 61:344, 1982
109. Hockley AD, Wake MJ, Goldin H: Surgical management of craniosynostosis. Br J Neurosurg 2:307, 1988
110. DiRocco C, Iannelli A, Verladi F: Early diagnosis and surgical indication in craniosynostosis. Childs Brain 6:175, 1980
111. Harris MM, Strafford MA, Rowe RW et al: Venous air embolism and cardiac arrest during craniectomy in a supine infant. Anesthesiology 65:547, 1986
112. Hewson JR, Neame PB, Kumar N et al: Coagulopathy related to dilution and hypotension during massive transfusion. Crit Care Med 13:387, 1985
113. Cote CJ, Drop LJ, Hoaglin DC et al: Ionized

hypocalcemia after fresh frozen plasma administration to thermally injured children. Anesth Analg 67:152, 1988
114. Berry FA: Practical aspects of fluid and electrolyte therapy. p. 106. In: anesthetic management of the difficult and Routine Pediatric Patients. 2nd Ed. Churchill Livingstone, New York, 1990
115. Feychting H: Psychological preparation for surgery and promedecation. p. 19. In Summer E, Hatch DJ (eds): Textbook of Paediatric Anaesthetic. Balliere Tindall, Philadelphia, 1989
116. Streitz SL: Anesthesia for pediatric surgery. p. 398. In Firestone LL (ed): Clinical Anesthesia: Procedures of the Massachusetts General Hospital. Little, Brown, Boston, 1988
117. Gullen BF, Stoelting RK: Pediatric anesthesia. p. 405. In Barash PG, (eds): Handbook of Clinical Anesthesia. 2nd Ed. JB Lippincott, Philadelphia, 1984
118. Berry FA: p. 75. In: Anesthetic Management of the Difficult and Routine Patients. 2nd Ed. Churchill Livingstone, New York,1990
119. Harris MM: Pediatric neuroanesthesia. p. 345. In Berry FA (ed): Anesthetic Management of the Difficult and Routine Patients. Churchill Livingstone, New York, 1990
120. Berry FA: Physiology and surgery of the infants. p. 127. In: Anesthetic Management of the Difficult and Routine Patients. Churchill Livingstone, New York, 1990
121. Hahn YS, Chyung C et al: Head injuries in children under 36 months of age. Child's Nerv Syst 4:34, 1988

17 CENTRAL NERVOUS SYSTEM TRAUMA

JOHN L.D. ATKINSON

RONALD J. FAUST

The symbiosis between the anesthesiologist and the neurosurgeon must interact to the fullest during emergent or urgent surgery for central nervous system trauma. This requires the anesthesiologist to be familiar with the objectives and therapeutic aims of the neurosurgeon but also requires the neurosurgeon to understand neuroanesthetic principles and techniques. Optimal interaction for patient care requires clear communication during the preoperative, intraoperative, and postoperative phases. Because the management of central nervous system trauma is on the verge of an explosive accumulation of pharmacologic and physiologic information, continual reassessment and interactive communication between the two specialities should take place on a regular basis. This chapter summarizes some fundamental concepts with respect to central nervous system trauma and the neurosurgical treatment objectives. Hopefully, this will enable the reader to better understand neurosurgical goals in the urgent or emergent trauma setting.

HISTORY

The most significant gains in the treatment of central nervous system trauma have occurred primarily from the development of the emergency medical system and its continued improvement and the identification and removal of space-occupying lesions affecting the central nervous system. The emergency medical system has evolved over the past several decades and has dramatically affected not only neurosurgical intervention, but intervention for the multiple trauma patient in general.[1] Fifty percent of multiple-trauma patients will die of their head injury, and therefore, any discussion involving the treatment of central nervous system injury requires a philosophic understanding of the general treatment of the whole trauma patient.[2] Rapid resuscitation of the patient at the scene and expedient transfer of the patient to a facility equipped to manage such patients has made a marked improvement not only in survival, but in diminished morbidity as well. With the evolution of computed tomography (CT) in the mid-1970s, the rapid identification of space-occupying lesions and their expedient evacuation and reversal of herniation and compressive syndromes, have markedly improved the outlook for central nervous system trauma patients.[3] The evolution of both the emergency medical system and expedient detection of space-occupying lesions continue today with faster generation imaging techniques and better management and treatment of patients at the scene of injury and on route to treatment centers.

It could be stated that the modern era of physiologic understanding with respect to head injury began with the continuous intracranial monitoring by Lunderberg.[4] It had been known for decades that herniation syndromes were ultimately fatal and that uncontrollable intracranial pressure (ICP) frequently led to herniation.[5] The Monro-Kellie doctrine has been known conceptually since its first written description by Alexander Monro in 1783.[6] Subsequently, George Kellie further substantiated Monro's theory, and though neither factored in cerebrospinal fluid as part of the enclosed intracranial space, the premise was founded and remains the fundamental concept for treatment to this date.[7] This concept espouses that brain, blood, and spinal fluid are composed primarily of water and being relatively incompressible sustain a constant intracranial volume. The addition of any further volume to the intracranial contents requires buffering or pressure will increase within the closed cranial vault. Normal physiologic buffers are already in place. Fluid-filled cavities, such as the ventricles or various cisterns at the base of the brain, allow cerebrospinal fluid to be displaced into the spinal canal and the venous system of the brain will buffer mass effect by shifting parenchymal and large-channel venous blood supply elsewhere. However, these physiologic buffers at some point reach their limit, and further addition of volume to the closed intracranial vault will result in diminished brain perfusion locally, regionally, or globally, depending on the mechanisms of elevated ICP.[8] The fundamental target therapy of all acute central nervous system injury is prevention of postinjury ischemia by maintaining cerebral and spinal cord blood flow. This central tenant is critical to understanding and treating central nervous system injury. Ischemia in the acute setting involves either diminished blood flow, diminished oxygen, or both and can be focal, regional, or global in distribution.[9]

The current rationale of treatment for severe head injury requires knowledge of the ICP. Any management of central nervous system trauma and elevated ICP is based on removal of space occupying lesions, and knowledge of the patient's ICP affects all current therapeutic aims.

PATHOPHYSIOLOGY OF CENTRAL NERVOUS SYSTEM INJURY

Blood flow regulation to the central nervous system is extremely complex but perhaps best generalized as three types of control: pressure autoregulation, metabolic vasoreactivity, and carbon dioxide vasoreactivity (see also Chapter 1, "Cerebral Blood Flow and Metabolism").

Pressure autoregulation, or the Bayliss effect, has been known for over 100 years.[10] Every organ system in the body autoregulates blood supply to blood pressure. Some organs autoregulate better than others, and the brain is exceptional in this respect. Pressure autoregulation depicts that blood flow to an organ remains relatively constant regardless of blood pressure changes within certain parameters. For the central nervous system, normal flow is maintained by vessel constriction or relaxation to keep cerebral blood flow constant at mean arterial pressures of 50 to 150 mmHg. Under normal circumstances, if mean arterial blood pressure falls below 50 mmHg, then central nervous system blood flow becomes passively dependent on pressure as maximal vasodilatation has occurred within the arterial system.[11] At mean arterial pressures above 150 mmHg, blood flow will increase as intraluminal pressures fatigue larger vessel walls and then subsequently medium-sized and smaller vessel walls, which drives the increased arterial pressure into the small metarterioles and capillaries. These structures are ill equipped to handle these significantly increased pressures, and as a result, the cerebrovascular volume is markedly increased and the blood-brain barrier becomes disrupted. If the pressure remains markedly elevated above mean arterial systolic pressure of 150 Torr, then cerebral swelling and/or hemorrhages occur.

This is clinically described as *malignant hypertension syndrome*.[12] It is of note that pressure autoregulation of the central nervous system blood flow can become markedly abnormal or even abolished experimentally with trauma, ischemic injury, hypercarbia, seizures, or pharmacologic manipulation. Pressure autoregulation after severe head injury may be abnormal in a significant number of severely head-injured patients.[13] This point becomes important when considering etiologic factors evoking intracranial hypertension following severe head injury and directing therapeutic options.

Metabolic vasoreactivity is a focal and a global phenomenon within the central nervous system. The brain and the heart at rest consume large quantities of total body energy substrate for their well-being.[14] All organ systems increase their blood flow by an increase in metabolic demand, but in the brain, this process is tightly coupled. In fact, an increase in central nervous system blood flow occurs almost instantaneously with an increase in metabolism. Current theories have evoked metabolic end products such as adenosine, but in fact the increase in blood flow may occur so rapidly that there is a strong suggestion central nervous system tissue by its very nature may innervate and regulate its own blood supply. This theory purports that as groups of neurons increase function their electrical conductivity is channeled to blood vessels by innervation and synaptic transmission with resultant vasodilatation and increased blood flow. Whatever the mechanism, the coupling of central nervous system blood flow and metabolism is well described. By the same logic, when metabolism is markedly impaired, as in severe head or spinal cord injury or coma from any cause, blood flow may remain coupled to metabolism and diminish accordingly. This is compatible with the diminished synaptic activities of neurons. For unknown reasons, blood flow may also become uncoupled from metabolism and increase over and above the depressed metabolic demands. This is called *hyperemia*, which results from an increase in blood flow above metabolic requirements, and may add to cerebral vascular volume. This may become important as an etiology of elevated ICP. Uncoupling of blood flow from metabolism in the central nervous system is poorly understood but can be simply considered a dysregulation phenomenon as a result of neuronal depression from injury.[15–17]

Carbon dioxide vasoreactivity is a physiologic process separate from metabolic vasoreactivity or pressure autoregulation. Carbon dioxide is perhaps the most potent vasodilator of the central nervous system circulation known. Elevated arterial carbon dioxide tension will dilate vasculature and will override pressure autoregulation and metabolic vasoreactivity. There is evidence that carbon dioxide has an intrinsic effect on arteries themselves but probably plays its major dilatory role by its free diffusion across vessels and conversion by carbonic anhydrase to hydrogen ion and bicarbonate. Hydrogen ion concentration $[H^+]$ is an extremely potent vasodilator to any arterial bed.[18] There is some evidence that elevated levels of carbon dioxide will dilate capillaries as well and considering the surface area of capillaries within the brain; small incremental dilations at the capillary level would add significantly to the cerebrovascular volume of the brain.[19] Control of cerebral vascular volume is an important concept in the management of elevated ICP.

All of the aforementioned mechanisms of vasoreactivity in the brain are important to understanding the treatment of elevated ICP. Elevated ICP may be elevated due to an increase in cerebrospinal fluid, such as in hydrocephalus; an increase in cerebrovascular volume, such as malignant hypertension or hypercarbic syndromes; an increase in cerebral interstitial edema, as in breakdown of the blood-brain barrier; and an increase in cellular or cytotoxic edema, resulting from the inability of cells to maintain ionic integrity due to loss of metabolic substrate and ischemic injury. These concepts formulate the basis in medical management of elevated ICP. Therapy is based on preventing or improving ischemia by improving blood flow, and an important component of this is to diminish elevated

ICP by targeting therapy to the mechanism or mechanisms involved.[20] Isolated spinal cord injury therapy is based on maintaining spinal cord blood flow, prevention of ischemic complications, and decompression of spinal cord impingement in surgically appropriate patients.[21,22]

HEAD INJURY

The Biomechanics of Head Injury

There are three distinct varieties of head injury, and components of each may be present in any single head injury. They include skull fractures, focal central nervous system injury, and diffuse central nervous system injuries. These mechanisms occur with the ictus of the head injury, but associated pathophysiology may evolve or accelerate for an extended period of time after injury.

Two basic mechanisms of injury occur with trauma. *Contact injuries* are physical forces delivered at focal regions. Examples would be projectiles or other penetrating types of injuries and blows or forces delivered to points of the skull or spine evoking injury to the underlying central nervous system. *Acceleration and deceleration injuries* are evoked when the brain rapidly changes its momentum. Because of the different mass densities that make up the constituents of the brain, these different components accelerate or decelerate at different rates for the same forces applied. Injury may be evoked at stress points within the brain or at points of contact between the brain and the anatomy of the skull or its dural divisions.[23] High stress points within the brain are primarily precipitated as axons traverse acute angles around nuclear or other structures, and it is these areas that are most involved in the pathologic process called *diffuse axonal injury*. Povlishock has found that visual identification of these lesions may take hours after injury and suggests there may be a therapeutic window at prevention or halting progression. However, this remains speculative and may in fact be pathology destined to occur regardless of treatment.[24,25] Areas of the brain accelerated or decelerated into components of the skull or dural separation are also prone to injury, particularly the roughened surface of the skull base. These injuries can produce massive contusions of the surface and deeper structures of the brain depending on the forces involved.

Skull fractures may be classified as linear fractures, depressed fractures, or basilar skull fractures. In and of themselves, they may or may not produce neurologic injury. Emergency surgery is almost always necessary in the setting of a concomitant hematoma or significant mass effect from a contused brain beneath or associated with the fracture.

Focal brain injuries are associated with four major categories—epidural, subdural, parenchymal, and subarachnoid hemorrhages—that may be found individually or collectively in head-injured patients (Figs. 17.1 to 17.4). As you may surmise, isolated epidural hematomas have a better prognosis than acute parenchymal and subdural hematomas in any clinical setting. The decision to operate on any of these lesions is based on neurosurgical principles.[26] Treatment until surgical evacuation of space-occupying lesions can be achieved focuses on maintaining cerebral perfusion to compressed or herniating brain tissue and decreasing intracranial hypertension. Generally, after evacuation of hematomas, the initially compressed brain becomes hyperemic and focal or regional swelling may become a problem in the postoperative period.[27] Head injury is the most common presentation of subarachnoid hemorrhage and is of concern because it connotes the severity of injury and also, as with aneurysmal subarachnoid hemorrhage, is associated with cerebral vasospasm. Posttraumatic vasospasm may occur in as many as 40% of severe head-injured patients, although the spasm may not acquire the intensity associated with aneurysmal subarachnoid hemorrhage. A transcranial Doppler in the Intensive Care Unit setting may suggest the presence of vasospasm on serial studies. The time course associated with this vasospasm appears to be shorter than that of aneurysmal subarachnoid hemor-

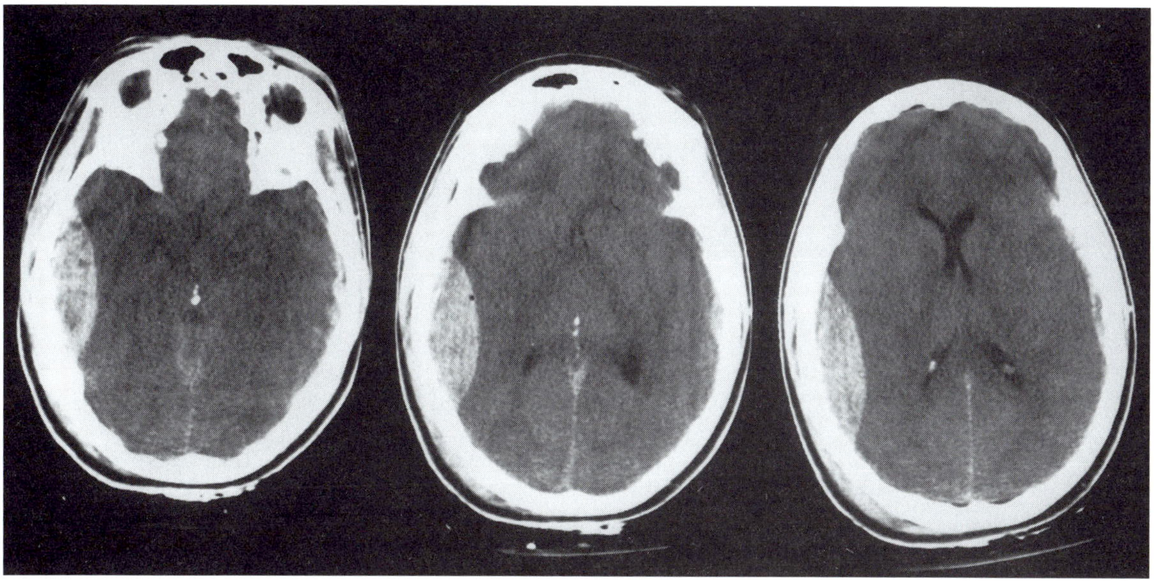

FIGURE 17.1 *Right temporal epidural hematoma with mild hemisphere shift in a confused patient. Rapid deterioration during examination necessitated emergent evacuation with excellent results.*

rhage. Its contribution to morbidity and mortality from head injury is currently unknown.[28]

Diffuse brain injuries are acceleration or deceleration injuries and are termed *diffuse axonal injury* as discussed above. These injuries are major contributors to elevated ICP and the significant morbidity and mortality associated with head injury.

Ischemic regions in the brain associated with severe head injury have been identified for

FIGURE 17.2 *Large right subfrontal epidural hematoma in a comatose patient. Emergent evacuation produced good outcome after rehabilitation.*

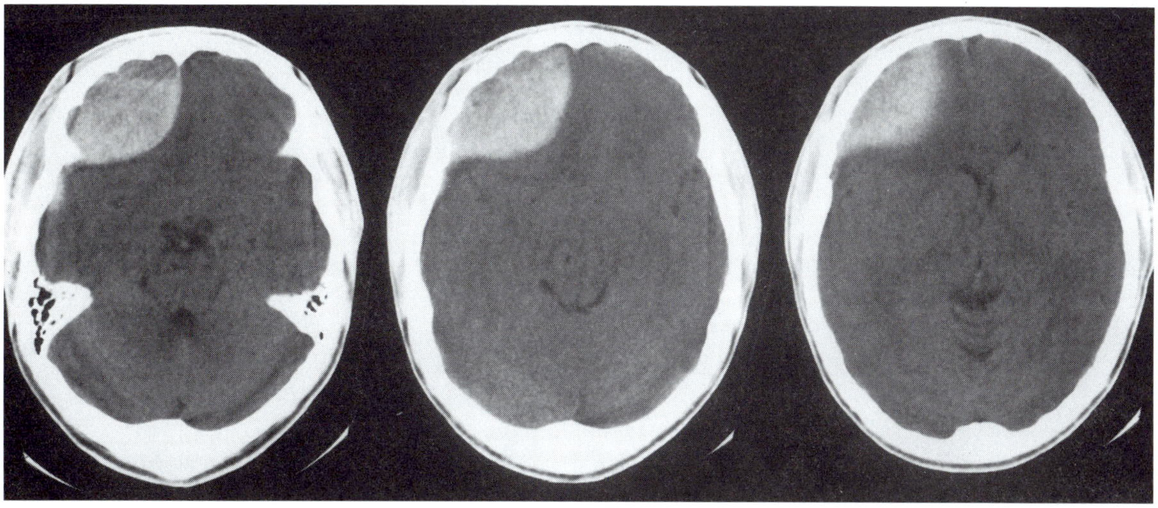

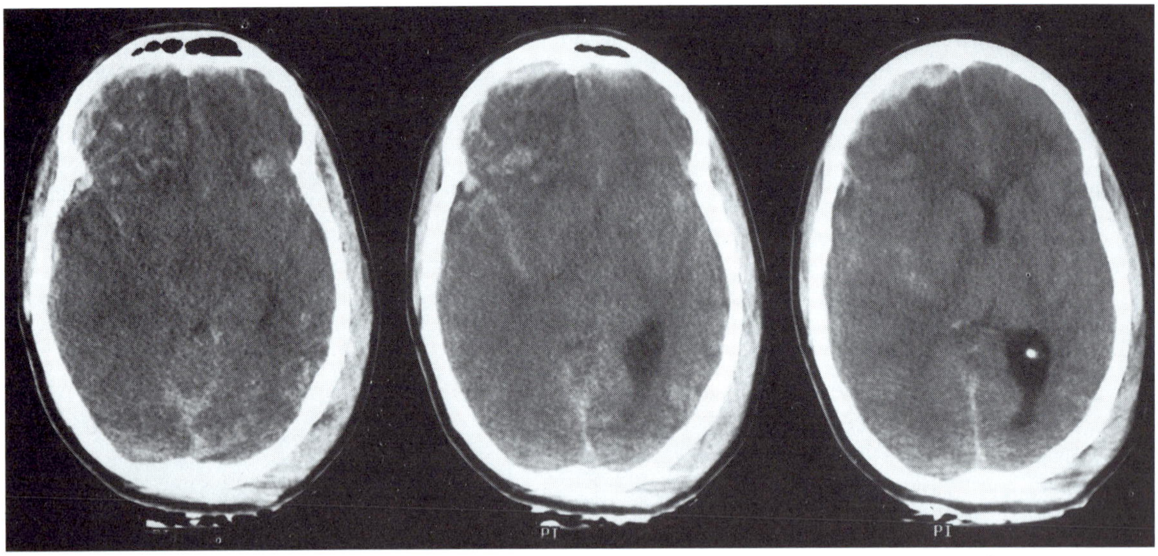

FIGURE 17.3 *Extensive hemispheric swelling associated with thin-rim subdural hematoma. The loss of basal cisterns and brain shift predicts elevated ICP. Despite aggressive management, the patient subsequently died.*

FIGURE 17.4 *Extensive diffuse basal brain contusions with subarachnoid hemorrhage. The loss of basal cisterns suggest an elevated ICP, and diffuse subarachnoid hemorrhage may predispose to subsequent post-traumatic vasospasm.*

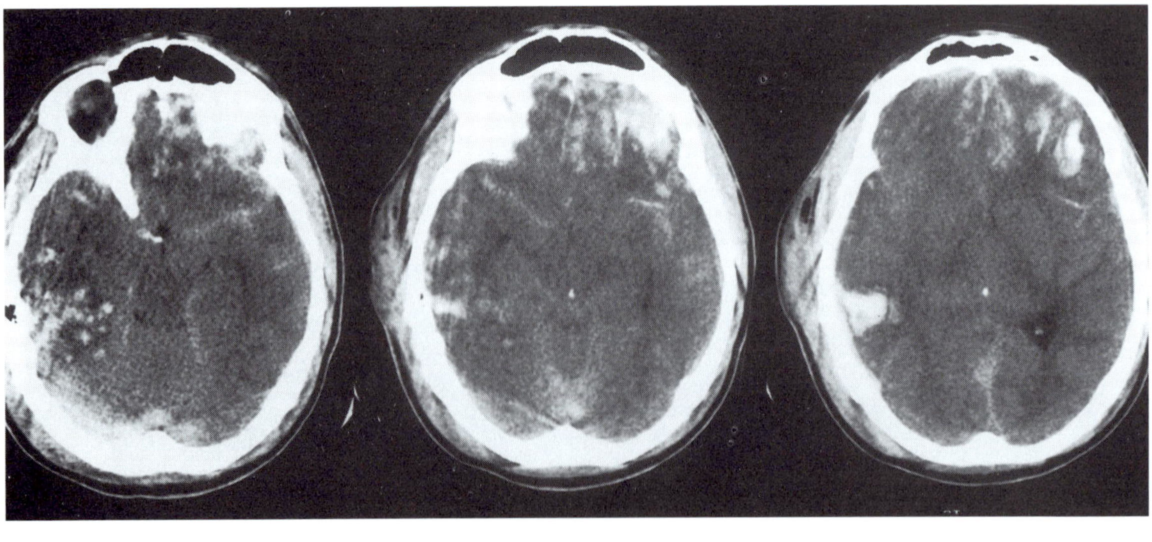

decades.[29,30] The exact mechanisms of this ischemia remain unclear, although it is felt that the majority of this pathophysiology occurs within the first several hours of head injury.[31] It is of note that apnea is associated with every concussive head injury. This apnea and subsequent respiratory dysfunction are dependent upon the magnitude of head injury and the forces transmitted to brainstem regions.[32,33] Recent work in our laboratory (unpublished) has revealed a linear correlation with post–head-injury apneic respiratory dysfunction and the severity of head injury in animals. Head injury in the laboratory setting is associated with the rapid onset of hypertension due to systemic epinephrine surge. In the setting of the injured brain, there is apnea and subsequent inadequate ventilation with resultant hypoxia and, more importantly, hypercarbia. Severe head injury often impairs pressure autoregulation, resulting in vessels passively dilated by any blood pressure surge. Hypertension then occurs seconds after head injury in a paralyzed dilated cerebrovascular bed and the result is increased cerebrovascular volume and increased edema formation translated as diffuse brain swelling. Theoretically, therefore, the sequence of events after severe head injury are apnea and hypertension followed by inadequate ventilation for possibly minutes with resultant hypoxia and hypercarbia. Vasodilatation from hypercarbia and impaired autoregulation allows transmission of the hypertensive blood pressure surge to cerebral small arteries and capillaries that are overwhelmed. The result is hypoxic induced ischemic brain injury and a generalized increase in cerebral vascular volume and edema formation (Fig. 17.5). Patients with severe head injury who present soon after injury with massively swollen brains and elevated ICP remain the most difficult to treat. In the Traumatic Coma Data Bank series of patients, hypoxia was strongly associated with diffuse brain swelling on patient admission to the emergency room. CT scans associated with diffuse brain swelling are high prognostic indicators for elevated ICP, as are focal brain shifts due to space-occupying lesions and loss of basal cisterns from swollen or shifted

FIGURE 17.5 *A graph depicting rat blood pressure tracing (superior) and respirometer tracing (inferior) followed by fluid percussion injury of three atmospheres. Note hypertensive surge and apnea with ictus followed by spontaneous dysrhythmic and inadequate respirations. If the animal is not rescued with mechanical ventilation, respirations remain inadequate to sustain life 15 minutes later.*

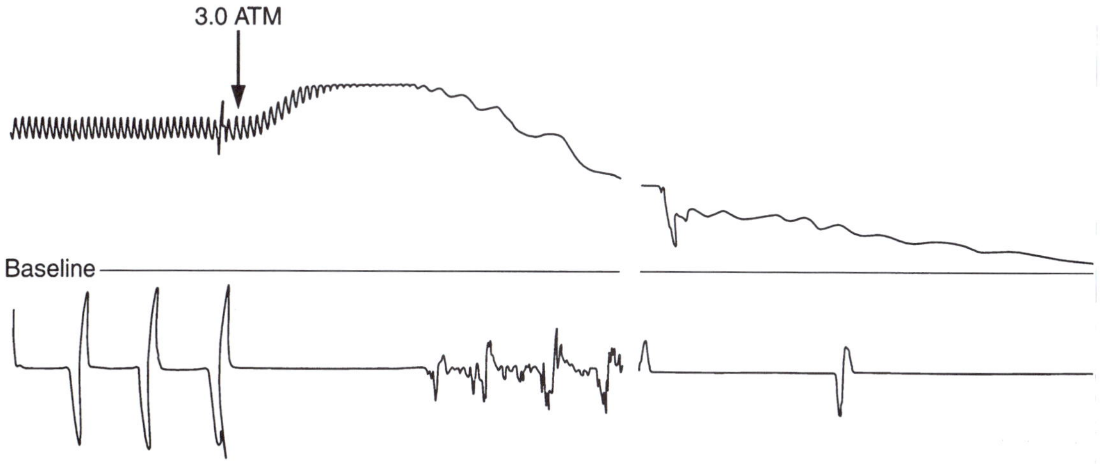

brain tissue.[34,35] Swollen or shifted brain compromises vascular perfusion of the brain, and treatment is aimed at maintaining this perfusion status by lowering elevated ICP medically and/or surgically and maximizing perfusion without contributing further to an increase in cerebrovascular volume or edema formation.

Therapeutic Principles of Head Injury

Anesthetic techniques are based on the fundamentals applied to the setting of central nervous system mass lesions and elevated ICP, the primary reasons for neurosurgical intervention. All emergent treatment is based on principles of advanced trauma life support resuscitation. This involves ensuring an airway, ventilation, and circulation support if necessary. As many as 50% of multiple systemic trauma deaths have associated severe head injury and neurosurgical principles are based on euvolemic patients and normalization of blood pressure.[2,36] This cannot be overstated, and the old days of "drying a patient out" have fallen into disfavor. Current traumatic management of the central nervous system is the same resuscitation given other organ systems, that is, restoration of normal blood flow and metabolic parameters. However, within this setting, special techniques are also utilized because, unlike other organs, the brain is encased within an enclosed cranial vault and methods to improve or maintain perfusion are parallel with methods to diminish or protect against intracranial hypertension.

There are many techniques to measure cerebral blood flow directly and indirectly, which is the target manipulation of all directed therapy. In the acute setting, many of these studies are impractical, and because they lack real time information, the ability to guide therapy acutely is impaired. Therefore, in the patient whose management may be changing minute by minute, certain guidelines must be applied. Cerebral perfusion pressure management is one such guideline.[1] Most head-injured patients are hypertensive or at least normotensive on arrival to the emergency room. If hypotension is seen in a head-injured patient, it strongly suggests either end-stage cerebral failure or secondary to other injuries. Cerebral perfusion pressure has in principle been utilized in the management of head-injured patients for decades. However, emphasis in past years has been placed on diminishing ICP perhaps at the expense of circulating volume as the primary mode of treatment to improve cerebral perfusion.

Current management principles are based on both diminishing ICP and improving cerebral perfusion by maintaining adequate blood pressure. Previous clinical and laboratory studies suggesting blood pressure elevations escalated elevated ICP and associated herniation syndromes were based on relatively high blood pressure levels. Therefore, conclusions were reached that blood pressure should be lowered to protect against cerebral swelling. However, there is now good evidence that blood pressure maintained in normal to mildly high ranges enhances cerebral perfusion and may even lower elevated ICP if pressure autoregulation is still present by causing a reflex vasoconstriction and decreasing cerebral vascular volume.[37] Caution must be utilized, however, as severe hypertension in a dysautoregulatory brain may precipitate brain swelling from increased cerebral vascular volume and edema formation.[38]

Blood pressure therapy in brain injury attempts to maintain a cerebral perfusion pressure at least 70 mmHg, although this must be individualized for each patient. It must be kept in mind that cerebral perfusion pressure (CPP) roughly equals mean arterial pressure (MAP) minus ICP ($CPP = MAP - ICP$) and does not equate with cerebral blood flow. The cerebrovascular resistance is unknown, and cerebral perfusion pressure is simply an indirect method of indicating to some degree that blood pressure is adequate for brain perfusion but does not assure perfusion is actually taking place focally, regionally, or globally within the central nervous system. Therefore, maintaining adequate cerebral perfusion pressure is an indirect target therapy in the acute head injury setting, and knowledge of ICP is essential in this management.[1]

As stated above, most head-injured patients have normal or elevated blood pressure on arrival to emergency rooms and use of pharmacologic agents to elevate blood pressure should be individualized in the volume resuscitated euvolemic hypotensive patient. After the patient has been stabilized, neurologic evaluation dictates whether the patient will undergo any efforts to decrease presumed elevated ICP. The neurologic evaluation is essential on arrival to the emergency room and after resuscitation as well. Patients with evidence of elevated ICP, such as a deteriorating neurologic examination or lateralized findings during a pupillary or motor examination, move directly to CT head scanning at the earliest possible time. After the neurological examination and CT head findings, the patient either moves directly to surgery for evacuation of intracranial space-occupying lesions or will not require immediate neurosurgical intervention but may require further systemic or spinal assessment or surgery for other systemic injuries or will be transported to the intensive care unit. The timing of neurosurgical intervention concomitant with other surgical injuries is based on coordinated efforts between other trauma surgeons and neurosurgeons present in the emergency room.[36]

The following principles apply to the management of elevated ICP due to head injury with or without mass lesion before, during, or after any surgical intervention systemically or intracranially. Again, the basis of treatment is prevention of cerebral ischemia, a secondary manifestation of head injury, by improving arterial input and diminishing ICP. In the emergency room setting, the emphasis is on resuscitation, detection of intracranial mass effect, and elevated ICP. A general algorithm is depicted in Figure 17.6.

Head elevation is relatively simple and ensures adequate venous egress from the cranial vault. Arguments have been made recently that head elevation diminishes cerebral perfusion, and perhaps maintaining the patient at 0° elevation, or even in some cases Trendelenburg, would aid cerebral perfusion. Head elevation will lower cerebral perfusion to some degree, but most studies suggest that elevation of the head of the bed up to 30° significantly improves venous outflow and diminishes ICP as well. Most head injury centers continue to maintain some elevation of the head of the bed with 0° rotation to avoid angulation of the jugular veins for optimal venous outflow.[39]

An agitated patient with expanding mass lesion and/or significant intracranial hypertension will often require sedation for optimal capture and treatment of ICP. Short-acting benzodiazopines, such as midazolam or other short-acting agents, are usually titrated to effect. This is also necessary in the setting of agitated head trauma in the emergency room and the requisite need to obtain adequate radiologic evaluation.[40] Muscular paralysis can also be utilized but should not be generally given until a neurologic examination has been performed. In the Traumatic Coma Data Bank series, long-term patients managed in the intensive care unit with paralysis had increased risks of complications and no significant improvement in outcome. Therefore, sedation should be used for agitation as needed, and paralysis should only be used as necessary to optimize radiographic studies or for surgical management.[41]

Mean arterial blood pressure should be kept at greater than or equal to 90 mmHg in accordance with advanced trauma life support measures.[36] In the acute setting of head injury alone, this is rarely a problem. However, concomitant systemic injury may predispose to hypotension, and rapid restoration of blood pressure and hypovolemia should be undertaken. Fluids normally utilized are isosmotic, but there is some evidence that hypertonic fluids may improve outcome in the laboratory setting, although this remains to be proven clinically.[42] Once the ICP is known, then efforts to maintain a cerebral perfusion pressure of approximately 70 mmHg or greater has some clinical efficacy, although the effect of this treatment on long-term outcome remains unproven.[1] However, current evidence

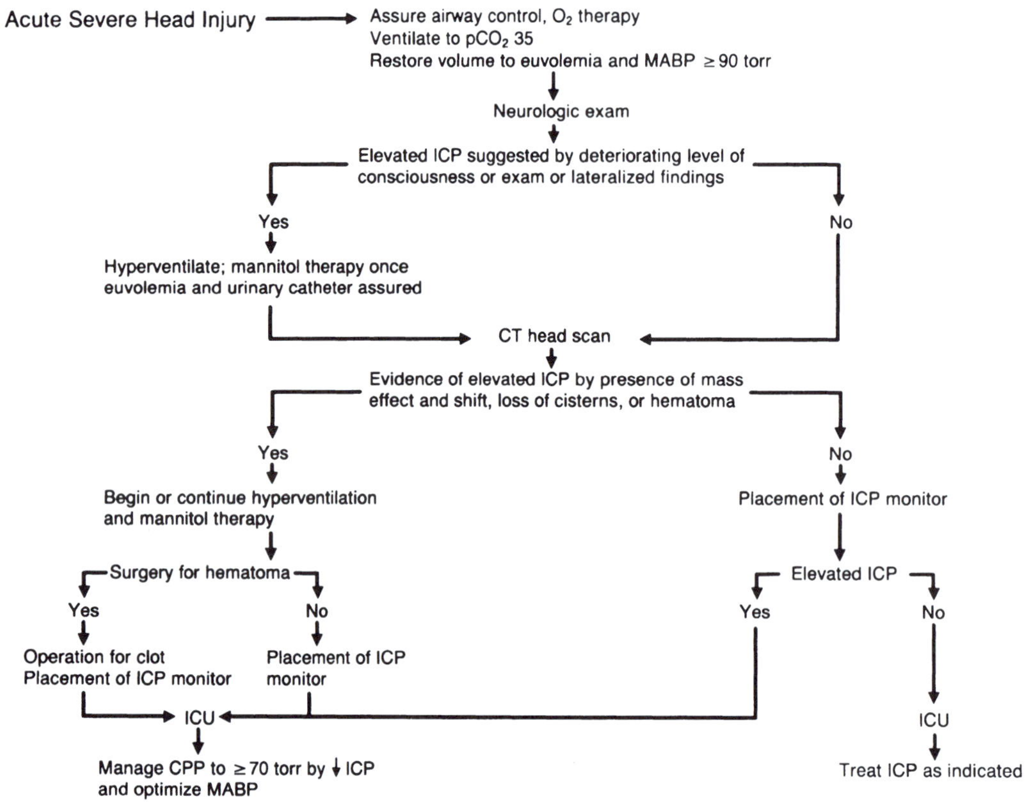

FIGURE 17.6 *A general algorithm for emergency management of severe head injury.*

supports cerebral perfusion pressure therapy as long as blood pressures are not significantly elevated in a dysautoregulatory injured brain.[38]

Mannitol is the most commonly used diuretic for elevated ICP. Its mechanisms of action are probably two: (1) an immediate effect at lowering ICP, probably by improving blood rheology by lowering blood viscosity and possibly a reflex vasoconstriction by the same mechanism,[43] and (2) a later effect by osmotically drawing any interstitial fluid accumulation within the brain back into the vasculature and reducing cerebral edema.[44] There is some evidence that multiple doses of mannitol may predispose to rebound elevation of ICP by spillage of mannitol across a dysfunctional blood-brain barrier and thereby acting as an osmotic gradient within a previously injured brain.[45] Thus, mannitol should be used sparingly and in boluses as low as possible to produce the desired effect. Evidence suggests that a 0.25 g/kg dose may be as effective as a 1 g/kg dose.[46] Its maximal effect requires that the patient remain euvolemic, and therefore, mannitol should always be used with a urinary catheter for obvious reasons but also replacement of diuresed urinary output with intravenous fluids should follow to maintain euvolemia. Mannitol will have little effect intracranially in hypovolemic patients, and as the serum osmolality increases to more than 320 mosm/dl, mannitol should be withheld or risk precipitating renal injury.[47]

Hyperventilation is described as therapy for elevated ICP when in fact it is the pharmacologic manipulation of arterial carbon dioxide, one of the most potent cerebrovasodilators known. In the treatment of elevated ICP, ventilation parameters should be utilized only in reference to the level of carbon dioxide desired. There is substantial evidence over the last several decades that hyperventilation induced effects of vasoconstriction due to hypocarbia fatigues over 12 to 48 hours.[48] This means that vasoconstriction and decreased cerebrovascular volume occur initially by lowering the carbon dioxide tension in the arterial system; however, the vasculature slowly dilates over hours to a day or two to allow levels of previously normal cerebral blood flow.[49] This is important for several reasons:

1. The effects of lowering ICP by lowering carbon dioxide tension are transient and, therefore, should only be considered as a transient therapy.
2. If vasoconstrictive therapy is necessary for treatment of refractory ICP, then serially lowering carbon dioxide tension in a sequence of small steps will produce a desired result over a longer period of time even though fatigue and increased blood flow will follow several hours after each step.

When weaning a patient from hypocarbia to normocarbia, it must be considered that the longer the patient has remained in the hypocarbic state, the more likely cerebral blood flow has normalized and raising carbon dioxide tension will cause blood flow to markedly overshoot normal parameters. This is of concern as cerebral vascular volume will increase with vasodilation and could exacerbate and elevate ICP. The vasoconstriction fatigue is primarily chemically mediated due to cerebrospinal fluid accumulation of bicarbonate buffer, which interacts with the hydrogen ion produced from carbon dioxide interaction with carbonic anhydrase.[18,49]

There is some concern in the literature that profound hyperventilation and hypocarbia may exacerbate any ischemia in head injury by further causing vasoconstriction in ischemic areas and exacerbating low-flow phenomena. However, hypocarbia remains a powerful tool against elevated ICP, and, if used appropriately for its transient effects, can markedly help control refractory intracranial hypertension sequelae. There is no significant evidence in the laboratory or clinical setting that moderate hypocarbia (i.e., 28 to 32 mmHg), will exacerbate ischemia. In fact, areas of brain ischemia usually override the effect of hypocarbia, and vessels supplying regions of ischemic brain will remain dilated despite hypocarbia. This has been shown to be present in profound hypocarbia as well, provided that anemia is not coexistent. Reverse steal may be of concern because normal brain will vasoconstrict and ischemic brain will vasodilate, resulting in shunting of blood to ischemic regions. This could be utilized as a mechanism for improving blood flow to ischemic regions. However, if blood flow is markedly increased through these areas of vasoparalysis with dysfunctional blood-brain barrier, then cerebrovascular volume and edema formation may be increased as well.[50] A prospective randomized trial has suggested that patients randomly assigned to 5 days of profound hyperventilation do worse than patients mildly hyperventilated over a period of 5 days.[51] This has been used for evidence that ischemia may be produced or exacerbated by the hyperventilation, which worsened outcome in the profound hypocarbia group. However, not addressed was hypocarbic vasoconstriction fatigue and possible resultant increased cerebral blood flow that may also have played a role in a worse outcome in this group by subacutely increasing cerebral vascular volume. We currently use moderate hyperventilation specifically to control elevated ICP in the emergency and acute care setting and in the post-traumatic or postoperative period for refractory elevations of ICP. We do not use hyperventilation on a routine basis, and we never use it prophylactically in severe head injury. However, it remains a valuable method of treatment and recent evidence suggests that it may improve brain metabolism if used selectively.[52]

Barbiturates are used as a last medical resort to capture refractory ICP and are not used on a routine basis. Barbiturates will lower ICP by lowering cerebral blood flow, and this is brought about by lowering the cerebral metabolic rate of the brain and also to some degree by inducing hypotension, which at times may be very difficult to treat.[53] Because of this, they are almost always used in conjunction with intravenous pressor agents in the intensive care setting and can be titrated to ICP effect or to electroencephalographic depiction of burst suppression. The cerebral metabolic rate cannot be lowered further after burst suppression is achieved by barbiturates, and theoretically, ICP will be at its lowest barbiturate-induced level when burst suppression is achieved. Barbiturates in the head-injured adult population are rarely used. Pediatric patients with refractory elevation of ICP have been treated.[54,55]

Seizure prophylaxis for severe head injury will not prevent the incidence of late seizure disorder. However, seizures in the acute phase of head injury may be diminished in frequency with antiepileptic medication. Seizures by their very metabolic nature significantly elevate cerebral blood flow and in a patient whose ICP is marginally controlled may increase cerebral blood volume and worsen management. Those brain injuries with the highest frequency of seizure, such as subdural hematomas or parenchymal hematomas in regions of epileptogenic brain, are often prophylactically treated. Therefore, the mechanism of injury would suggest use of antiepileptic medication, although improvement in clinical outcome has yet to be determined.[56,57]

Steroids have not proven efficacious in the treatment of head injury and are not currently recommended unless there is concomitant hypothalamic or pituitary injury and dysfunction.[58]

Surgical therapy for elevated ICP centers primarily on removing space-occupying lesions, such as frank hematomas or contused swollen brain; it is a neurosurgical decision alone. Other surgical measures that can be utilized to diminish elevated ICP involve drainage of cerebrospinal fluid primarily through exteriorized ventricular drains. There are a multitude of different ICP-measuring modalities on the market. However, the exteriorized ventricular drain remains the most commonly utilized and yields the singular advantage of ability to measure as well as treat elevated ICP by removal of cerebrospinal fluid. Massively swollen cerebral lobes or hemispheres with herniation syndromes may be subjected to subtemporal decompressions or frank lobectomies in hopes of salvaging select patients. These latter are usually last resort measures, although good results have been reported in select patients.[59]

Anesthetic Management of Head Injury

The anesthetic management of central nervous system trauma can be divided into preoperative, intraoperative, and postoperative phases.

Preoperative evaluation is concerned with the injury status of the patient with respect to systemic and/or central nervous system injury. Pulmonary, cardiovascular, and renal function along with metabolic laboratory parameters are essential and require rapid assessment in the emergency setting. A decision to move the patient to surgery may be for systemic injury, central nervous system injury, or any combination. All therapy is initiated within the guidelines of advanced trauma life support measures, including assurance of adequate airway and intravascular volume repletion for cardiovascular status.[36]

If ventilation is compromised by partial airway obstruction or central nervous system depression due to the trauma, early intubation is critical; hypercarbia must be prevented to avoid its deleterious effects on ICP. Because cervical trauma is frequently associated with head trauma, the method of intubation is critical. If time permits, cervical fractures and instability should be first ruled out with radiographs of the cervical spine. When airway compromise necessitates intubation before the cervical spine is "cleared," the airway must be secured while avoiding excessive cervical manipulation. Awake fiberoptic intubation is the theoretical ideal method, but this technique may be impossible due to upper airway bleeding, an uncooperative patient, or a lack of equipment. Direct laryngoscopy after rapid sequence induction can be more expedient and can be performed safely if the head and neck are stabilized by traction or an assistant. Although nasal intubation can be advantageous for long-term management of a comatose patient, airway control should not be delayed if there is any difficulty with a nasal intubation. It is possible to introduce an endotracheal or nasogastric tube through a basilar skull fracture into the brain; hence, attempted nasal intubation and nasogastric tube placement are contraindicated when there is the possibility of a basilar skull fracture.

If the neurologic evaluation suggests elevated ICP either by examination, such as unilateral findings on motor or pupillary examination or deterioration in the level of consciousness, emergent medical treatment such as elevation of the head of the bed, ensuring adequate arterial blood pressure and hyperventilation, are initiated as soon as possible. Mannitol is given as soon as the patient is volume resuscitated. Subsequent studies are obtained rapidly and in rare cases may be simply postponed in order to expedite surgical intervention. Patients who do not exhibit evidence of herniation syndromes or CT evidence of elevated ICP are managed by general resuscitation measures with target carbon dioxide levels of 35 mmHg and a mean arterial blood pressure more than 90. Mannitol and hyperventilation are no longer routinely administered in severe head injury but only initiated with an examination or CT scan suggesting elevated ICP or an ICP monitor measuring elevated ICP.

Intraoperative management is based on these same principles. Premedication can add to the risk of hypoventilation and impair neurologic evaluation in a patient with elevated ICP any small increase in cerebral blood volume may markedly affect an elevated ICP. If a patient meets criteria for ICP monitoring and is taken to the operating room for other systemic surgery, then an intracranial monitor should be placed prior to or during the surgical procedure for rational treatment by cerebral perfusion pressure management. This would also be true in emergency surgery for non-neurosurgical injuries in any patient with a decreased level of consciousness and no time for CT head scan. ICP monitoring can be helpful in this setting as well for anesthesia management during other types of surgery.

The patient with closed head trauma who is undergoing an emergency non-neurosurgical procedure should be hyperventilated intraoperatively to decrease ICP. Anesthetic techniques employing barbiturates, propofol, narcotics, and isoflurane are referable to those employing halothane because it is more difficult to control anesthetic effects on cerebral blood flow if halothane is employed. Ketamine would be contraindicated due to its ability to increase cerebral blood flow and ICP.

When access to the face is possible, the pupils can be monitored intraoperatively; development of anisocoria could signal the intraoperative development of a lateralizing intracranial space-occupying lesion. Although control of hemorrhage and repair of intra-abdominal injuries would still have to be completed first, neurosurgical evaluation and intervention would take precedence over continuation of a prolonged procedure for distal orthopedic injuries. The anesthesiologist and neurosurgeon must set priorities in the care of the patient with closed head trauma and multiple injuries. If elevated ICP is suggested preoperatively by neurologic examination or CT scan, then an ICP monitor should be placed concominantly during other emergent surgery to optimize intraoperative management. In the setting of significant closed head injury without preoperative evidence of an elevated ICP, an ICP monitor should be considered in cases expected to last for hours and/or expectations of significant fluid shifts during any surgical procedure. If there is doubt as to the ICP status with closed head injury during any surgery, ICP monitoring should be considered.

An early wakeup should also be a goal when any patient with closed head injury is anesthetized so that complete neurologic evaluation can be performed in the early postoperative period. When there is any chance of hypoventilation or partial airway obstruction, endotracheal intubation must be continued.

The anesthetic techniques discussed above apply as well to patients undergoing neurosurgical procedures for central nervous system trauma. Control of ventilation is critical. Hyperventilation down to an arterial $PaCO_2$ of 25 mmHg will decrease ICP and might prevent herniation of brain tissue intraoperatively. Neuromuscular blockers are important to prevent coughing, as increases in venous pressure transmitted from the chest to the head can lead to acute, severe increases in ICP. Direct arterial monitoring is used to achieve beat-to-beat control of the blood pressure so that extreme hypo- and hypertension can be treated quickly and aggressively.

Postoperatively, attempts to maintain ICP at controlled levels are undertaken as the patient emerges from anesthesia. Again, emphasis is placed on maintaining adequate cerebral perfusion and minimizing the effects of elevated ICP. Currently, the state of ICP can only be determined by monitoring, and rational treatment of elevated ICP requires its use.

SPINAL CORD INJURY

Acute spinal cord injury remains a difficult therapeutic arena to date. Primary injury transmitted to the spinal cord from compressive forces is as yet treated best through prevention. However, there may be resultant secondary injury mechanisms occurring over hours after ictus that may allow timely therapeutic intervention. One such window of opportunity was defined in the laboratory and subsequently found in the second National Acute Spinal Cord Injury Study that outcome in spinal cord injury was improved by using specific methylprednisolone dosing within 8 hours of injury.[60] Although the qualitative improvement in outcome may be debated, a 30 mg/kg intravenous loading dose followed by 5.4 mg/kg/h intravenously for 23 hours was found to significantly improve outcome in all follow-up studies to date.[61] Therefore, with any acute spinal cord injury, methylprednisolone dosing is now a standard of care.

Therapeutic goals of spinal cord injury are the same as for any other organ system in that assuring perfusion of tissue is critically important. This is best accomplished through volume resuscitation and maintaining adequate blood pressure. Aggressive hemodynamic therapy utilizing pulmonary artery catheter monitoring is used at some centers but has not yet been shown to improve outcome.[22] Prevention of further spinal cord injury by spinal immobilization remains a cornerstone of treatment.[21]

Surgical intervention may vary between medical centers; however, the only clear indication for emergent surgery is a deteriorating neurologic examination despite otherwise adequate intervention. The timing of surgery for any other reason, such as stabilization, is surgeon dictated, but the general trend in uncomplicated patients without significant systemic injury is for early surgery in hopes of allaying the complications of prolonged recumbency. Anesthetic goals during surgery are prevention of further spinal cord injury by optimizing physiologic parameters of spinal cord perfusion and maintaining spine immobilization during surgery. Assuring that the spinal cord has not been further injured by positioning or by surgical instrumentation may necessitate awake fiberoptic intubation and neurologic examination after positioning or 'wake-up tests' in which the patient is awakened during surgery for retesting the neurologic examination. Physiologic monitoring such as sensory evoked potentials may also be utilized.[62]

THE FUTURE

The target of directed therapy for head injury is optimizing cerebral blood flow to the injured brain. Many head injury centers routinely measure cerebral blood flow on severely head-injured patients, but these techniques may be inaccurate, time-consuming, and intermittently applied so that guiding acute therapy may be difficult. Methods of real time global cerebral blood flow measurement are currently being developed that can also visualize the intracranial contents at the bedside for developing mass lesions, brain swelling, or ventricular dilatation. It is hoped this will better define acute surgical and medical management and also diminish the necessity of serial CT head scanning. If cerebral blood flow can be determined accurately on a real time basis, then it may obviate the necessity of ICP monitoring.

Pharmacologic treatment of spinal cord injury to prevent secondary ischemic injury will continue. Future controlled studies will clarify the optimal timing of surgery with respect to outcome. Techniques for injured spinal cord healing may be developed over time.

Evolution in the treatment of central nervous system injury develops management principles that are applied to a multitude of central nervous system pathologies. Over time we can and will improve on the current abysmal severe head and spinal cord injury statistics and apply these evolving therapeutic methods to other disease processes of the central nervous system.

References

1. Rosner MJ, Daughton S: Cerebral perfusion management in head injury. J Trauma 30:933, 1990
2. Anderson DW, McLaurin RL: The national head and spinal cord injury survey. J Neurosurg 53:S1, 1980
3. Becker DP, Miller JD, Ward JD et al: The outcome from severe head injury with early diagnosis and intensive management. J Neurosurg 47:491, 1977
4. Lundberg N: Continuous recording and control of ventricular fluid pressure in neurosurgical practice. Acta Psychiat Kbh, supple. 149:1, 1960
5. Miller JD, Becker DP, Ward JD et al: Significance of intracranial hypertension in severe head injury. J Neurosurg 47:503, 1977
6. Monro A: In Observations on the Structure and Functions of the Nervous System. Creech, Johnson (eds): Edinburgh, 1783
7. Kellie G: Appearances observed in the dissection of two individuals; death from cold and congestion of the brain. Trans Med Chir Soc Edinburgh 1:84, 1824
8. Weed LH: Some limitations of the Monro-Kellie hypothesis. Arch Surg 18:1049, 1929
9. Chan K-H, Dearden WM, Miller JD et al: Multimodality monitoring as a guide to treatment of intracranial hypertension after severe brain injury. Neurosurgery 32:547, 1993
10. Bayliss WM: On the local reaction of the arterial wall to changes of internal pressure. J Physiol (Lond) 28:220, 1902
11. Paulson DB, Strandgaard S, Edvinsson L: Cerebral autoregulation. Cerebrovasc Brain Metab Rev 2:161, 1990
12. Kontos HA, Wei EP, Navari RM et al: Responses of cerebral arteries and arterioles to acute hypotension and hypertension. Am J Physiol 234:H371, 1978
13. Bouma GJ, Muizelaar JP: Relationship between cardiac output and cerebral blood flow in patients with intact and with impaired autoregulation. J Neurosurg 73:368, 1990
14. Green HD, Rapela CE: Blood flow in passive vascular beds. Circ Res, suppl. 1 (14/15):I11, 1964
15. Kuschinsky W, Wahl M: Local chemical and neurogenic regulation of cerebrovascular resistance. Physiol Rev 58:656, 1978
16. Reis DJ, Iadecola C: Regulation by the brain of its blood flow and metabolism: role of intrinsic neuronal networks and circulating catecholamines. p. 129. In: Owman C, Harbedo JE (eds): Neuronal Regulation of the Brain Circulation. Elsevier, Amsterdam, 1986,
17. Uddman R, Edvinsson L: Neuropeptides in the cerebral circulation. Cerebrovasc Brain Metab Rev 1:230, 1989
18. Edvinsson L, MacKenzie ET, McCulloch J: Changes in arterial gas tensions. p. 524. In: Cerebral Blood Flow and Metabolism. Cippincott-Raven, Philadolphia, 1993
19. Atkinson JLD, Anderson RE, Sundt TM, Jr: The effect of carbon dioxide on the diameter of brain capillaries. Brain Res 517:333, 1990
20. Marmarou A, Maset AL, Ward JD et al: Contribution of CSF and vascular factors to elevation of ICP in severely head injured patients. J Neurosurg 66:883, 1987
21. Ducker TB, Salcman M, Daniel HB: Experimental spinal cord trauma. III. Therapeutic effect of immobilization and pharmacologic agents. Surg Neurol 10:71, 1978
22. Levi L, Wolf A, Belzberg H: Hemodynamic parameters in patients with acute cervical cord trauma: description, intervention, and prediction of outcome. Neurosurgery 33:1007, 1993
23. Gennarelli TA, Thibault LE: Biomechanics of head injury. p. 1531. In Wilkins RH, Rengachary

SS (eds): Neurosurgery. McGraw-Hill: New York, 1985
24. Povlishock JT, Becker DP: Fate of reactive axonal swellings induced by head injury. Lab Invest 52:540, 1985
25. Povlishock JT: Traumatically induced axonal injury: pathogenesis and pathobiological implications. Brain Pathol 2:1, 1992
26. Sakas DE, Bullock MR, Teasdale GM: One-year outcome following craniotomy for traumatic hematoma in patients with fixed dilated pupils. J Neurosurg 82:961, 1995
27. Langfitt TW, Obrist WD: Cerebral blood flow and metabolism after intracranial trauma. Prog Neurol Surg 10:14, 1981
28. Martin NA, Doberstein C, Zane C et al: Posttraumatic cerebral arterial spasm: transcranial doppler ultrasound, cerebral blood flow, and angiographic findings. J Neurosurg 77:575, 1992
29. Graham DI, Adams JH, Doyle D: Ischemic brain damage in fatal non-missile head injuries. J Neurol Sci 39:213, 1978
30. Graham Di, Ford I, Adams JH et al: Ischemic brain damage is still common in fatal non-missile head injury. J Neurol Neurosurg Psychiat 52:346, 1989
31. Bouma GJ, Muizelaar JP, Stringer WA et al: Ultra-early evaluation of regional cerebral blood flow in severely head-injured patients using xenon-enhanced computerized tomography. J Neurosurg 77:360, 1992
32. Miller JD: Head injury and brain ischemia — implications for therapy. Br J Anaesth 57:120, 1985
33. Price JE, Murray A: The influence of hypoxia and hypotension on recovery from head injury. Br J Accid Surg 3:218, 1972
34. Marmarou A, Anderson RL, Ward JD et al: The Traumatic Coma Data Bank: impact of ICP instability and hypotension on outcome in patients with severe head trauma. J Neurosurg 75:S59, 1991
35. Marshall LF, Gautille T, Klauber MR et al: The Traumatic Coma Data Bank: the outcome of severe closed head injury. J Neurosurg 75:S28, 1991
36. Alexander RH, Proctor HJ: Head Trauma. p. 159. In Alexander RH, Proctor HJ (eds): Advanced Trauma Life Support Program for Physicians. 5th Ed. American College of Surgeons, Chicago, 1993
37. Rosner MJ, Becker DP: Origin and evolution of plateau waves. Experimental observations and a theoretical model. J Neurosurg 60:312, 1984
38. Bouma GJ, Muizelaar JP: Cerebral blood flow, cerebral blood volume, and cerebrovascular reactivity after severe head injury. J Neurotrauma, suppl. 9:S333, 1992
39. Feldman Z, Kanter MJ, Robertson CS et al: Effect of head elevation on intracranial pressure, cerebral perfusion pressure, and cerebral blood flow in head injured patients. J Neurosurg 76:207, 1992
40. Chiolero RL: Sedatives and antagonists in the management of severely head injured patients. Acta Neurochir (Wien), suppl. 55:43, 1992
41. Hsiang JK, Chesnut RM, Crisp CB et al: Early, routine paralysis for intracranial pressure control in severe head injury: is it necessary? Crit Care Med 22:1471, 1994
42. Shackford SR, Zhuang J, Schmoker J: Intravenous fluid toxicity: effect on intracranial pressure, cerebral blood flow, and cerebral oxygen delivery in focal brain injury. J Neurosurg 76:91, 1992
43. Muizelaar JP, Lutz HA, Becker DP: Effect of mannitol on ICP and CBF and correlation with pressure autoregulation in severely head injured patients. J Neurosurg 61:700, 1984
44. Bell BA, Smith MA, Kean DM et al: Brain water measured by magnetic resonance imaging: correlation with direct estimation and change after mannitol and dexamethasone. Lancet 1:66, 1987
45. Kaufmann AM, Cardoso ER: Aggravation of vasogenic cerebral edema by multiple dose mannitol. J Neurosurg 77:584, 1992
46. Marshall LF, Smith RW, Rauscher LA: Mannitol dose requirements in brain injured patients. J Neurosurg 48:169, 1978
47. Feig PU, McCurdy DK: The hypertonic state. N Engl J Med 297:1449, 1977
48. Christensen MS: Prolonged artificial hyperventilation in cerebral apoplexy. Acta Anaesthesiol Scand, suppl. 62:6, 1976
49. Muizelaar JP, Van Der Poel HG, Li Z et al: Pial arteriolar vessel diameter and CO_2 reactivity during prolonged hyperventilation in the rabbit. J Neurosurg 69:923, 1988
50. Darby JM, Yonas H, Marion DW, Latchaw RE: Local "inverse steal" induced by hyperventilation in head injury. Neurosurgery 23:84, 1988
51. Muizelaar JP, Marmarou A, Ward JD et al: Adverse effects of prolonged hyperventilation in patients with severe head injury: a randomized clinical trial. J Neurosurg 75:731, 1991

52. Cruz J: An additional therapeutic effect of adequate hyperventilation in severe acute brain trauma: normalization of cerebral glucose uptake. J Neurosurg 82:379, 1995
53. Kassell NF, Hitchon PW, Gerk MK et al: Alterations in cerebral blood flow, oxygen metabolism, and electrical activity produced by high-dose thiopental. Neurosurgery 7:598, 1980
54. Nordstrom CH, Messeter K, Sundbarg G et al: Cerebral blood flow, vasoreactivity and oxygen consumption during barbiturate therapy in severe traumatic brain lesions. J Neurosurg 68:424, 1988
55. Ward JD, Becker DP, Miller JD et al: Failure of prophylactic barbiturate coma in the treatment of severe head injury. J Neurosurg 62:383, 1985
56. Dikmen SS, Temkin NR, Miller B et al: Neurobehavioral effects of phenytoin prophylaxis of posttraumatic seizures. JAMA 265:1271, 1991
57. Young B, Rapp RP, Norton JA et al: Failure of prophylactically administered phenytoin to prevent late posttraumatic seizures. J Neurosurg 58:231, 1983
58. Giannotta SL, Weiss MH, Apuzzo MLJ, Martin E: High dose glucocorticoids in the management of severe head injury. Neurosurgery 15:497, 1984
59. Litofsky NS, Chin LS, Tang G et al: The use of lobectomy in the management of severe closed-head trauma. Neurosurgery 34:628, 1994
60. Bracken MB, Shepard MJ, Collins WF et al: A randomized, controlled trial of methylprednisolone or naloxone in the treatment of acute spinal cord injury. N Engl J Med 322:1405, 1990
61. Bracken MB, Shepard MJ, Collins WF et al: Methylprednisolone or naloxone treatment after acute spinal cord injury: one year follow-up data. J Neurosurg 76:23, 1992
62. Levi L, Wolf A, Rigamonte D et al: Anterior decompression in cervical spine trauma: does the timing of surgery affect outcome? Neurosurgery 29:216, 1991

18 NEUROINTENSIVE CARE

A. JOSEPH LAYON

JOSEPH B. STACHNIAK

ARTHUR L. DAY

The field of intensive care medicine has undergone tremendous change and growth over the past 30 years. Groups such as the Society for Critical Care Medicine have taken an active role in education, clinical practice, and research. Tertiary care centers, in particular, have seen increases in intensive care unit (ICU) beds; this has created a requirement for intensivists and nurses trained in critical care medicine. Unfortunately, this need has often surpassed the resources of adequately trained personnel. In the area of neurointensive care, with its many unique problems, this issue seems to us of signal importance.

Although traditionally organized under the administrative umbrella of neurologists and neurosurgeons, the advent of increasingly complex technology, both in the operating room (OR) and in the ICU, and improved initial survival of neurologically injured patients requires the neuro-ICU medical staff to have formal training and/or extensive experience in both neurophysiology/pathophysiology and critical care medicine. Thus, in the modern neurointensive care unit, a collaborating team of multidisciplinary physicians and specially trained nurses care for complex, critically ill patients.

To the resident beginning a neurointensive care unit rotation or to the anesthesiologist long out of critical care practice, we offer this chapter. We only briefly discuss basic physiologic principles, as they are covered elsewhere in this text; the remainder of the chapter deals with problems seen in critically ill, neurologically impaired patients.

GENERAL CONCEPTS

Cerebral Blood Flow

Maintenance of constant cerebral blood flow (CBF) is a critical aspect of the brain's homeostasis (see also ch 00). Normal CBF ranges between 45 and 67 ml/100 g/min,[1–5] and in a normocarbic state, CBF in gray matter (cortical flow) is slightly increased compared with that of white matter. In pathologic states, reduction of CBF to levels between 15 and 18 ml/100 g/min results in a loss of electroencephalographic (EEG) activity.[6,7] At this level, cellular viability is maintained, but no synaptic transmission occurs, and there appears to be no differential of the ischemic threshold between gray and white matter.[6] CBF decreased to levels at or below 10 ml/100 g/min results in ionic pump failure and cell death.[8]

CBF is normally tightly maintained by the process of autoregulation, primarily through changes in arteriolar smooth muscle tone. Autoregulation maintains normal CBF between 60 and 150 mmHg mean arterial pressure (MAP) and drops off or increases linearly in direct proportion to blood pressure outside this range (Fig. 18.1). Mechanisms controlling autoregulation are not instantaneous, usually requiring

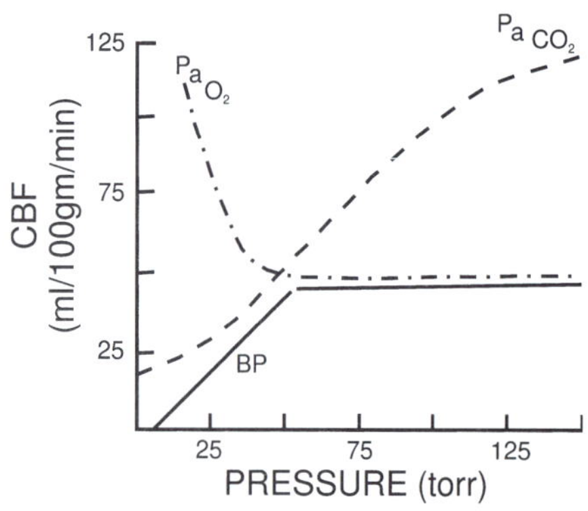

FIGURE 18.1 *Autoregulation maintains normal cerebral blood flow (CBF) between 60 and 150 mmHg MAP. Note the effects of $PaCO_2$ on CBF. (From Shapiro,[28] with permission.)*

several minutes to alter the cerebrovascular resistance. These vasoactive responses are extremely sensitive to changes in the arterial partial pressure of carbon dioxide ($PaCo_2$), primarily mediated through changes in the cerebrospinal fluid (CSF) hydrogen ion concentration. In the range between 20 and 80 mmHg (the physiologic range), each 1 mmHg change in $PaCO_2$ results in an approximate 2% linear change in CBF. The arterial partial pressure of oxygen (PaO_2) has little effect on CBF in the physiologic range. Below 50 mmHg, however, the PaO_2 increases CBF, and in hyperbaric ranges, it decreases CBF.

Cerebral perfusion pressure (CPP) is strongly correlated to CBF and is a more accessible and easily measurable indicator of cerebral perfusion, particularly in the head-injured patient. CPP is normally equal to MAP except under conditions of increased intracranial pressure (ICP) when CPP = MAP – ICP.

Cerebral Metabolism

Cerebral oxygen consumption and metabolism ($CMRO_2$) is tightly coupled to CBF, and the brain regulates utilization (focally or globally) based on demand (see Ch. 1). The normal $CMRO_2$ is 3.8 ± 0.55 ml/100 g/min,[2,3] accounting for about 20% of total body oxygen consumption. Under normal circumstances, the brain is exclusively dependent on the aerobic metabolism of glucose to provide its energy requirements. During starvation, ketone bodies can provide an alternative energy source.

Under aerobic conditions, the brain extracts up to 38 moles of adenosine triphosphate (ATP) per mole of glucose to sustain its activities. In the anaerobic state, however, the efficiency of glucose metabolism is greatly reduced, and the brain is only able to extract about 2 moles of ATP per mole of glucose. In anaerobic conditions, glucose resources are rapidly consumed within 4 to 5 minutes, leading to irreversible neuronal damage and death.

Intracranial Pressure

The normal adult human brain weighs about 1,400 g, and its parenchymal bulk occupies the great majority of the intracranial space (see ch 00). Blood (primarily within the venous system) and CSF each occupy an additional 75 ml of space. Because the skull is a closed, inelastic space, expanding the volume of brain, CSF, or blood will initially be followed by reciprocal decreases in one of the other constituents (the Monro-Kelly doctrine).[9,10] Thus, small additions of volume (i.e., from cerebral edema, expanding hematoma, hydrocephalus, or neoplasm) are initially well tolerated. Once spatial compensation is exceeded, however, further small increases in intracranial volume result in rapid and significant increases in ICP (see pressure-volume curve, Fig. 18.2). Normal ICP is low, ranging between 2 and 10 mmHg. As the ICP increases, CPP becomes adversely affected (CPP = MAP – ICP), and therapy aimed at reducing total intracranial volume must be considered; selecting an appropriate method (i.e., hyperventilation, osmotic diuresis, CSF drainage, and evacuation of mass) depends on the underlying pathophysiology.

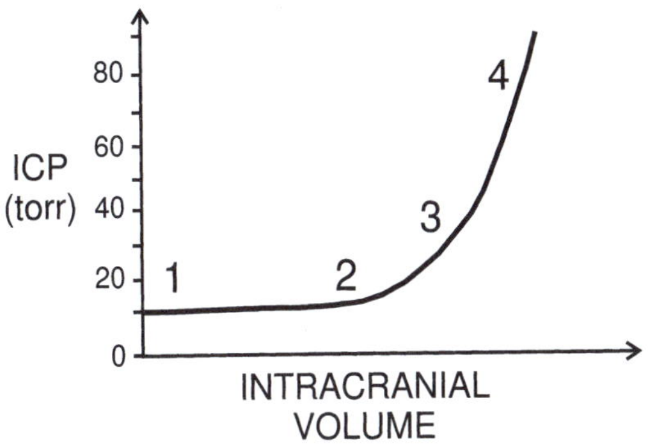

FIGURE 18.2 *Idealized relationship of intracranial volume and ICP. (From Burchiel et al.,[23] with permission.)*

Neuroimaging

Advances in neuroimaging have greatly improved neurologic diagnostic capabilities, particularly in acutely critically injured patients (Table 18.1) (see Ch. 4). Noncontrast computed tomography (CT) provides a rapid, accessible, and relatively inexpensive method of diagnosing life-threatening injuries. Bone window images usually show fractures of the skull or spine, and three-dimensional formatting provides details of complex fractures useful in surgical planning. Soft tissue windows provide accurate images of parenchymal damage or acute hemorrhage. Debris or metal fragments, problematic in magnetic resonance imaging (MRI), are inconsequential obstacles to this modality. Contrast utilization improves the characterization of tumors, infectious processes, and stroke in evolution. Combined with myelography, CT is very useful in clarifying spinal cord compression for surgical decompression.

MRI is particularly useful in diagnosing soft tissue injuries to the brain, spinal cord, or peripheral nerves. Tumors, congenital defects, certain vascular lesions (especially cavernous malformations), traumatic lesions to the brachial or lumbar plexus, and demyelinating diseases are particularly well visualized with this modality. Gadolinium enhancement can provide further details about stroke, infectious processes, and tumors. MRI angiography provides rapid information about vascular lesions such as arteriovenous malformations (AVMs), arterial dissections, aneurysms, or major trunk stenosis or thrombosis (arterial or venous). Although not as detailed as traditional arteriography, MRI angiography is quicker, less invasive, and less expensive and can serve as a good screening tool, especially in certain critically ill patients.

Arteriography continues to be the gold standard for the detailed imaging of most vascular lesions, especially aneurysms and AVMs. Digital

TABLE 18.1 *MRI compared with CT: advantages and disadvantages*

	ADVANTAGES	DISADVANTAGES
MRI	Enhanced soft tissue resolution MR-angiography capability for evaluation of vascular lesions Ability to image in different planes (e.g., sagittal, coronal, axial) Good screening tool for spinal axis	Expensive Poor for trauma evaluation Ferromagnetic implants or devices prevent usage Poor evaluation of bony changes or acute hemorrhage
CT	Fast and relatively inexpensive Excellent for evaluation of trauma and bony lesions	Relatively poor soft tissue resolution

Abbreviations: MRI, magnetic resonance imaging; CT, computed tomography.

subtraction techniques can further improve visualization in areas obscured by artifact or bone. Arteriography is particularly useful in evaluating the ICU patient declining from vasospasm following an aneurysmal subarachnoid hemorrhage (SAH).

Multiple imaging modalities have been developed to measure CBF, including Technetium-99 (^{99}Tc), single-photon emission computed tomography (SPECT), xenon CT, and positron-emission tomography (PET). Each has its own particular advantages and limitations. ^{99}Tc scans are useful for brain death determinations and are discussed in a later section. SPECT can provide imaging of hypoperfused areas, but it is costly and provides poor spatial resolution. Xenon CT has similar problems with spatial resolution and accuracy, and its use in severely head-injured and hyperventilated patients can cause a transient but clinically significant increase in ICP (6.9 ± 7.7 mmHg).[11] PET provides useful information about CBF, $CMRO_2$, and regional glucose utilization, but its cost limits its availability to only a few centers.

Neuromonitoring

Neuromonitoring in the ICU and OR has become important to the care of neurologically impaired patients. Devices commonly used include ICP monitors, EEG, evoked potentials, transcranial Doppler (TCD), and jugular venous oxygen saturation monitoring.

Multiple ICP monitoring devices exist, including ventriculostomies, subarachnoid catheters, subdural bolts, and fiberoptic cables. Although usually used supratentorially, it was recently shown that infratentorial monitoring can also be safely accomplished after tumor resections by appropriate placement of a subdural catheter.[10] Although initially at variance with one another by as much as 50%, after 48 hours, supratentorial and infratentorial pressures had equilibrated.

Ventriculostomy catheters are historically the gold standard for ICP monitoring, as they are accurate, easily rezeroed, and allow the removal of CSF. Disadvantages include the risk of hemorrhage or parenchymal injury with passage of the catheter, infection,[12,13] the need to keep the head at a constant level relative to the transducer, and placement difficulty in patients with small ventricles. A subarachnoid catheter is placed after creating a small hole in the skull. The dura and arachnoid membranes are opened so the device is coupled to the CSF. This provides a safe, reliable, and minimally invasive method for monitoring ICP. The subdural (Richmond) bolt is placed after making a 1/4-in. hole in the skull and opening the dura. This technique provides an easy method to measure ICP and does not require invasive passage through the brain. It can, however, become clogged and dysfunctional and also requires frequent rezeroing with change in head position. A recent comparison study with ventriculostomy and subarachnoid catheters suggest that the subdural bolt is significantly less reliable than the other two modes.[14]

Fiberoptic ICP monitoring is versatile in that it can be placed in the ventricle is subdural space or into parenchyma. Although drift (± 2.1 mmHg) tends to develop after 5 days,[9] the fiberoptic device is reliable and provides relatively rapid access to ICP monitoring. Codman, Incorporated recently developed a new system that utilizes dual microprocessors at the end of a thin cable. This system is more versatile and durable than the fiberoptic system. As the cable is not fiberoptic, it can be bent or kinked without resultant system damage. There is also less drift, the portable monitor is half the size of the fiberoptic system, and the system may be coupled with bedside ICU monitors. The Codman device may be placed in the subdural or subarachnoid spaces or inserted through a ventriculostomy catheter.

An important initial issue relative to ICP monitoring is determining which patients require monitoring. Although use criteria continue to evolve, we generally monitor patients with a Glasgow Coma Scale (GCS) of less than 8, patients with a severe injury as shown by CT scan (i.e., epidural hematoma, subdural hematoma, or evidence of extensive cerebral edema), patients who have received neuromuscular or sedating agents that compromise the examination, and patients with mild to moderate injuries who will have general anesthesia for treatment of other traumatic, non-neurologic injuries.

TCD measures blood flow velocity in large vessels and thus provides indirect information about CBF. Ultrasound penetrates the skull and comes in contact with moving red blood cells. This movement causes a Doppler shift, which is detected by the probe, and velocity is calculated based upon this shift. Because worsening of cerebral vasospasm causes a higher mean velocity that, at least in the middle cerebral artery territory, correlates well with regional CBF,[15] TCD can be used to follow patients with this ischemic pathology. TCD can also be used for evaluation of head injury, as a progressive increase in the TCD pulsatility index occurs as CPP decreases below 70 mmHg[16] (pulsatility index = peak systolic TCD velocity – end-diastolic velocity ÷ timed mean velocity). Interestingly, when increases in ICP were not associated with CPP decrement, no changes in TCD velocity or pulsatility index were noted.

Somatosensory and brainstem auditory evoked responses are the most commonly used evoked potentials in the ICU. These may be particularly helpful in patients with depressed levels of consciousness, those who are deeply sedated or paralyzed, or those in a barbiturate coma. In such individuals, the neurologic examination is lost, and evoked potentials can provide important information. For example, grossly abnormal or absent evoked potentials can be a reliable predictor of poor outcome (false pessimism in 5 of 1,023 cases). Normal evoked potentials are less predictive of a good final outcome.[17,18]

Pulmonary Care

Neurologically impaired patients may suffer from a variety of airway or pulmonary parenchymal problems. Head-injured patients may suffer airway obstruction in the field, with resultant hypoxia and worsening of the initial injury. These patients may also suffer midfacial trauma, making bag-valve-mask ventilation difficult and thus necessitating tracheostomy or cricothyrotomy. Pulmonary aspiration of gastric contents, rib fractures, pulmonary contusion, hemothorax, pneumothorax, or flail chest may be present and should be evaluated with physical examination and chest radiography. The respiratory synchrony, rate, and paradoxical motion of spontaneously breathing patients should be noted, because endotracheal intubation may be required for primary pulmonary problems and/or to treat elevated ICP. Initial analysis of arterial blood to assess adequacy of ventilation and oxygenation should be performed.

Following skull base or posterior fossa surgery, patients may have cranial nerve deficits that compromise the gag reflex and airway. Lengthy spinal procedures or other procedures that require a prolonged period in the prone position and significant fluids may cause extensive facial swelling. These patients should be left with a protected airway overnight or until the swelling begins to abate and a leak is auscultatable around the endotracheal tube when the cuff is deflated. Patients who have undergone extensive anterior neck dissection may also require 12 to 96 hours of endotracheal intubation, as swelling can lead to acute loss of the airway with early extubation.

Controversy has existed for years over whether positive end-expiratory pressure (PEEP) or continuous positive airway pressure (CPAP) used with mechanical ventilation is safe in patients with elevated ICP. There is concern that intrathoracic pressure, which is elevated with PEEP/CPAP, could be transmitted to the draining veins, causing venous engorgement and a resultant further increase in ICP. Actually, the physiology is a bit more complicated, as venous valves, particularly at the thoracic inlet, prevent retrograde flow and impede pressure transmission. Additionally, cerebral veins act as resistors, partially collapsing as a patient's head is elevated.[19,20] The same resistor effect limits augmentation of already elevated ICP when PEEP/CPAP is applied to the lungs.[19] Early studies by Apuzzo et al.[21] and Frost[22] exemplify this controversy as the former showed that PEEP/CPAP elevated ICP, whereas the latter suggested that it had no effect at various levels. Part of the controversy was resolved with the understanding that extensive lung injury decreases pulmonary compliance, causing less intrathoracic pressure to be transmitted to the head. It is impossible to determine the degree of lung injury in the patients of Apuzzo's et al., whereas 5 of 7 of Frost's patients had severe lung injury (PaO_2:FIO_2 = 175; FIO_2, fraction of inspired oxygen); PEEP/CPAP was being used therapeutically in the latter group. Burchiel et al. noted that the degree of intracranial injury, as documented by an abnormal volume-pressure response (VPR), and the degree of pulmonary injury as documented by pulmonary compliance are useful in determining the risk for elevation of the ICP with PEEP/CPAP.[23] Patients with normal VPR and either normal or decreased compliance or abnormal VPR and decreased compliance will show no elevation in ICP with the addition of expiratory pressure. Cooper et al. suggest that increases in ICP with PEEP/CPAP are based on hemodynamic and respiratory factors such as cardiac output, shunt, peak inspiratory pressure (PIP), and changes in $PaCO_2$, but his data are incomplete and thus difficult to interpret.[24] We use the lowest PEEP/CPAP possible that allows a nontoxic FIO_2 of less than 0.5 to achieve an arterial saturation of greater than or equal to 93 to 95%; head elevation is kept at 30°. Neuromuscular blocking agents, sedatives, and pressure preset ventilation with prolonged inspiratory time are used as needed.[25] Careful attention is paid to ICP and CPP.

Abnormal Breathing Patterns

One of several abnormal breathing patterns may, if present, provide information on the severity and/or level of an injury. Cheyne-Stokes breathing, alternating hyperpnea with decremental hypoventilation ending in a respiratory pause, usually occurs with subcortical or midbrain level injury.[26] This pattern is thought to occur secondary to altered responsivity to CO_2 and medullary output.[27] *Central hyperventilation* is associated with a midbrain lesion resulting in decreased hemispheric inhibition. *Apneustic* breathing is associated with prolonged end-inspiratory pauses[26] and occurs with a middle or caudal pontine lesion, presumably with loss of input from the parabrachial and Kölliker-Fuse nuclei.[28] Ataxic breathing is a shallow, irregular pattern associated with a medullary injury.

Central neurogenic hyperventilation (CNH) is a rare disorder[26] most often associated with brainstem tumors, the most common of which are lymphomas and astrocytomas, although CNH has occurred with lymphoid granulomatosis, medulloblastoma, and metastatic disease. The exact etiology of the disorder is unknown but is likely due to loss of cortical inhibitory respiratory control from a mesencephalic lesion.[28] The diagnosis should be one of exclusion, for it is relatively common for neurologically injured patients to hyperventilate from pulmonary problems such as pneumonia. In CNH, the tachypnea is sustained even at night, and the patient has no volitional control over the pattern. $PaCO_2$ is markedly depressed, even to single digits, with a corresponding alkalosis. There may or may not be any presenting neurologic deficits. The differential diagnosis includes a variety of different pathologies including drug intoxication (salicylates, cyanide), metabolic disorders (hepatic encephalopathy), anxiety, and sepsis, all which may result in prolonged hyperventilation. There are no definitive therapies available, but narcotics have been used to depress respiratory drive with some success.[29]

Neurogenic Pulmonary Edema

Neurogenic pulmonary edema is primarily associated with a large catecholamine surge associated with SAH.[30] Therapy for this disorder is as for noncardiogenic pulmonary edema of any etiology. A complete discussion is found in Chapter 8.

Gastrointestinal Care

Healthy patients who are immediately postoperative seem to do well without food for 3 or 4 days. However, those with postsurgical complications and/or prolonged hospital stays may be nutritionally depleted as the primary caregivers concentrate on the neurologic injury; these individuals should be fed as soon as possible. Endotracheally intubated patients or those unable to take nutrition by mouth should have a small-bore feeding tube placed distal to the pylorus. They should also have a nasogastric tube so that residual/regurgitated feeding volumes can be checked to minimize the incidence of pulmonary aspiration of gastric (especially refluxed from the feeding tube) contents. When enteral or parenteral feeding is needed, we first estimate the caloric needs of a patient. This may be done using the Harris-Benedict equation to calculate the resting metabolic expenditure (RME) derived from, respectively, 136 and 103 normal adult men and women. This is done as follows:

RME (kcal/day) =
Men: 66.473 + 13.7516(weight) + 5.0033 (height) − 6.755 (age)
Women: 65.595 + 9.563(weight) + 1.8496 (height) − 4.6756(age)

Weight is in kilograms, height is in centimeters, and age is in years. From this calculation, you obtain the RME, which must be multiplied by a factor to account for the metabolic stress of illness/injury, for example: 1.4 to 2 for a major head injury in which steroids are used as part of the treatment regimen, 1.4 for a major head injury in which steroids are not used, 1.4 to 1.8 for sepsis, 1.2 to 1.5 for peritonitis, 1.0 to 1.3 in the normal state, and so forth. Indirect calorimetry, in which the O_2 consumption and CO_2 production are measured, may also be used. A microcomputer in the metabolic cart uses the Weir calculation to obtain kilocalories per minute from these values and then multiplies this number by 1,440 min/day. The modified Weir calculation is as follows:

$$\text{kcal/min} = 3.9(O_2 \text{ consumption}) + 1.1(CO_2 \text{ production})$$

Both O_2 consumption and CO_2 production are in liters per minute. A total requirement of 1.3 to 1.5 times that calculated via the modified Weir equation may be necessary to account for nutritional repletion and metabolic stress. Finally, you may simply approximate the caloric needs as shown in Table 18.2. After the initial estimate, follow-up nitrogen balance calculation or, preferably, measurement of a rapidly turned over visceral protein should be measured once or twice weekly (Table 18.3). When parenteral hyperalimentation is utilized, calories and protein are provided in a ratio such that amino acids are not consumed for fuel. This is done by ensuring a calorie:nitrogen ratio of from 115:1 to 300:1. Calories are calculated from the glucose, (4 kcal/g,) and fat, (9 kcal/g,) one is planning to administer. The nitrogen is calculated by dividing the amino acid to be administered in a day (in grams) by 6.25. You thus have the total number of carbohydrate and fat calories as well as the amount of nitrogen to be administered. The calorie:nitrogen ratio is then calculated by dividing the nitrogen into the total calories. Whenever possible, it is our preference to administer enteral feeding as, in addition to providing the calories necessary for healing and recovery, enteral nutrition may help prevent sepsis by eliminating or decreasing translocation of bacteria across the gut wall. Some controversy exists regarding translocation in humans.[31] In a prospective, randomized study of patients having suffered severe head injury (GCS 5 to 7 on admission), Grahan found that the group enter-

TABLE 18.2 *Caloric intake that will satisfy the needs of most patients*

CLINICAL STATUS	KILO CALORIES PER KILOGRAM IDEAL BODY WEIGHT
Basal state	25–30
Maintenance (ambulatory)	30–35
Mild stress and malnutrition	40
Severe injuries and sepsis	50 to 60
Extensive burns	80

(From Silberman,[283] with permission.)

TABLE 18.3 *Visceral proteins useful in nutritional assessment*

	HALF-LIFE	NORMAL LEVELS
Albumin	18 days	3.5 to 5.5 g/dl
Transferrin	8 days	200 to 400 mg/dl
Thyroxine-binding prealbumin	2 days	15.7 to 29.6 mg/dl
Retinol-binding protein	12 h	2.6 to 7.6 mg/dl

1. Nitrogen intake (g) = protein intake (g) ÷ 6.25
2. Nitrogen balance (g) = 24-h nitrogen intake − (24-h urinary nitrogen + 1.5)

OR: Nitrogen balance (g) = 24-h nitrogen intake − (1.2 × 24-h urinary urea nitrogen + 1.5)

(From Silberman,[284] with permission.)

ally fed early (less than or equal to 36 hours after admission) had a shorter length of ICU stay and fewer infectious complications than did the group enterally fed later (greater than or equal to 72 hours).[32]

The severely neurologically injured patient, like any critically ill individual, is at risk for stress ulceration; additionally, these patients are often on intravenous steroids to treat intracranial swelling. Thus, stress ulcer prophylaxis is required. Currently, we use H_2-antagonists either orally or intravenously until patients are off steroids and out of the ICU. Work done some years ago suggests that duodenojejunal enteral feeding helps in the prophylaxis of stress ulceration, likely by increasing gastric inhibitory polypeptide levels.[33] In that study, patients receiving enteral feeding as opposed to duodenojejunal saline required fewer aliquots of antacid to keep gastric pH above 4; further, serum gastric inhibitory polypeptide levels were increased in the patients given nutrition.

Glucose control is significant in light of recent studies suggesting that supranormal glucose may worsen ischemia and stroke. Lam et al. retrospectively studied patients with severe head trauma (29 of 32 males; closed head injury in 31 of 32 patients) and found this to be true if serum glucose was greater than 150 mg/dl[34]. Especially in the setting of transient focal ischemia, glucose is converted to lactate in the brain; this is believed to be involved in secondary neuronal injury. It may be, however, that benefits of tight glucose control occur secondary to insulin, as it shares significant homology with nerve growth factor and may aid in the repair of neuronal membranes.[35] Two animal studies evaluating outcome in complete[36] or incomplete[37] cerebral ischemia suggest that fluid replacement with solutions containing glucose results in significantly worse neurologic outcome than does replacement with a crystalloid without glucose. Finally, Ashwal and colleagues suggest that elevated blood glucose levels as well as reduced CBF measured by the stable xenon technique correlate with poor outcome.[38] Thus, our initial solution for emergency resuscitation is 0.9% saline. Glucose is not utilized unless the measured blood glucose is subnormal.

Cardiac Care

As with any preoperative patient, those undergoing neurosurgical interventions require a thorough cardiac history and review of symptomatology as well as a complete general examination before surgery. Cardiac events should be documented and records obtained. Exercise tolerance should be assessed, and any history of angina pectoris (including its duration and location and whether it occurs at rest or with exertion) should be noted. A chest radiograph and electrocardiogram (ECG) may be obtained if clinically indicated.

ECG abnormalities may occur in patients with SAH, stroke, head injury, tumors, or meningitis. Thirty-five to 95 percent of patients who suffer a SAH have ECG abnormalities,[39,40] which can include inverted T- waves, ST-T segment abnormalities, shortened PR intervals, QT_c prolongation, and peaked P, U, and Q waves. Multiple dysrhythmias may occur, including premature atrial contractions, premature ventricular contractions, supraventricular and ventricular tachycardia, atrial fibrillation, Torsade de Pointes, and heart block. ECG changes tend to occur in the first 48 hours but can occur after this time. Although elevation of cardiac enzymes and abnormal ECGs may all be seen in the initial 48 hours,[39–41] enzyme elevation is not usually as high as that seen with transmural myocardial infarction. The cardiac alterations are likely secondary to the large catecholamine output (primarily from the hypothalamus), which results in myocardial stunning. Currently, limited information exists on the precise risk of surgery; however, it appears that patients with SAH are at relatively low risk (see Chs. 3 and 8).

In general, patients are at increased cardiac risk if there is evidence of unstable angina, poorly controlled hypertension, congestive heart failure, an ejection fraction less than 40%, left ventricular end-diastolic pressure greater than 18 mmHg, cardiac index less than 2 L/min/m^2, or multiple areas of ventricular dyskinesia.[42] Current estimates on relative risk for reinfarction are variable, depending upon how long after myocardial infarction the surgery occurs. Estimates for risk up to 3 months range from 4 to 37%; 4 to 6 months, 0 to 16%; and after 6 months, all studies suggest a 1 to 6% reinfarction rate.[43–46]

Fluid and Electrolyte Imbalance

Neurologically injured patients are at risk for alterations of fluids and electrolytes. Further, after multiple trauma, patients may have extensive muscle injury and develop myoglobinuria, which can lead to acute renal failure. Patients with increased ICP may require dehydrating agents (e.g., mannitol), which can predispose to renal failure. This section will focus primarily on the three relatively common electrolyte disorders seen in neurologically injured patients: the syndrome of inappropriate secretion of antidiuretic hormone (SIADH), cerebral salt wasting (CS), and diabetes insipidus (DI).

PHYSIOLOGY The body attempts to maintain normal serum sodium at 135 to 145 mEq/L and osmolarity at 275 to 295 mOsm/kg H_2O[47] through a variety of mechanisms, including the secretion of antidiuretic hormone (ADH), aldosterone, and angiotensin. Prohormone is produced in two hypothalamic neuron clusters, the supraoptic and paraventricular nuclei. It is then transported down the long axons to the posterior pituitary and after glycosylation, modified to yield three molecules: ADH, neurophysin, and vasopressin glycopeptide.[48] Hypothalamic baroreceptors are sensitive to as little as a 1% increase in serum osmolarity with a resultant increase in ADH release.[49] When the serum osmolarity is less than 280, ADH release is normally inhibited; above this level, ADH secretion increases at a rate linear with osmolarity.[48,50] As osmolarity increases above 280 mOsm/kg H_2O, ADH release is incrementally stimulated; however, the thirst mechanisms are not activated until 290 to 295 mOsm/kg H_2O. Thirst is also an important, but insensitive mechanism for responding to osmolar change. Volume receptors (high-pressure baroreceptors in the carotid sinus and aortic arch; low-pressure volume receptors in the left atrium and lung) are less sensitive than osmoreceptors in altering ADH release, as a 10 to 15% volume change must occur prior to increased ADH release.[48,51] Once stimulated, though, ADH release is brisk. ADH released by these mechanisms binds to receptors on renal collecting tubules and increases free water absorption; a pressor response to ADH is not commonly seen.[50]

Because water freely moves across the blood-brain barrier along osmotic gradients,[52] the brain is particularly sensitive to changes in serum sodium (actually body water concentration) and osmolarity. Normally, the intracranial contents can increase by only about 10% prior to life-threatening increases in ICP. When serum sodium is decreased, the relative increase in free water causes the brain to swell. Although a 10% decrease in serum sodium corresponds roughly to 127 mEq/L, patients frequently have serum sodium levels below this value without life-threatening sequelae.[52] The basis for this tolerance relates to the brain's ability to adapt to sodium and osmolar changes at both a macro and cellular level. At a macrolevel, acute cerebral edema results in displacement of CSF out of the intracranial space within minutes; this excess CSF then enters the systemic circulation. Cellular adaptation is slower, requiring 3 to 4 hours to begin, with maximal effect at 24 hours.[53–56] Initially, outward potassium flux increases; later, neurons extrude organic solutes such as phosphocreatine myoinositol, glutamate, taurine, and glutamine. The intracellular concentrations of these osmotically active molecules, once termed *idiogenic osmoles*, vary during the adaptation process to either hypo- or hypernatremia.[53,57,58]

Some Causes of Hyponatremia

NONHYPOTONIC

- Hyperglycemia
- Hypertonic mannitol infusion
- Postprostatectomy
- Pseudohyponatremia
  - Hypertriglyceridemia
  - Multiple myeloma
  - Macroglobulinemia

HYPOTONIC

- Intact diluting function
  - Psychogenic polydipsia
  - Beer potomania
- Impaired diluting function
  - Normal ADH secretion
    - Oliguric renal failure
    - Thiazide diuretics (some cases)
  - Abnormal ADH secretion
    - Abnormal hemodynamic parameters
      - Volume depletion
      - Edematous conditions
        - Congestive heart failure
        - Cirrhosis
        - Nephrotic syndrome
      - Thiazide diuretics (some cases)
      - Adrenal insufficiency
      - Cerebral salt wasting
    - Normal hemodynamic parameters
      - SIADH
        - Ectopic (tumor) ADH production
        - CNS disorders
        - Pulmonary disease
        - Postsurgical
        - Nausea
        - Drug induced
      - Hypothyroidism

Abbreviations: ADH, antidiuretic hormone; SIADH, syndrome of inappropriate ADH secretion; CNS, central nervous system.
(From Sterns,[52] with permission.)

SIADH AND ACUTE WATER INTOXICATION SYNDROME Postoperative patients may exhibit decreased urine output shortly after their return to the ICU. If bedside clinical assessment is not helpful in sorting out the cause of this, an assessment of serum and urine osmolarity and the fractional excretion of sodium may be helpful. A normal serum and elevated urine osmolarity, together with a fractional excretion of sodium less than or equal to 1%, suggest hypoperfusion of the kidney. In this situation, fluid replacement may be indicated. If hypovolemia/hypoperfusion is not the cause of the decreased urine output, other etiologies must be investigated. For example, in the patient who has undergone multiple surgical procedures or one who is suffering from recent head or multiple traumas, urine must be assessed for myoglobin. If positive, the patient is at risk of developing acute renal failure. Treatment entails alkalinized intravenous fluids, a urine output of 1.5 to 2 ml/kg ideal body weight/h, and a urine pH of greater than or equal to 6. This is continued until myoglobin is no longer present in the urine. If there is evidence of hyponatremia, a history must be obtained to determine its chronicity. Acute hyponatremia, developing at a rate of greater than 0.5 mEq/L/h, must be differentiated from chronic hyponatremia.[52,54] Acute hyponatremia tends to become symptomatic if the serum sodium decreases to less than or equal to 120 to 125 mEq/L.[52,53] Chronic hyponatremia develops over greater than or equal to 48 hours and is usually asymptomatic until the serum sodium decreases to less than or equal to 115 mEq/L.[52]

Causes of hyponatremia are many; some important ones are listed in the accompanying box. Postpituitary resection, patients are often encouraged to drink copious clear liquids to regulate fluid balance. However, if intake of free water becomes excessive, acute water intoxication may develop. Minor symptoms include headache, nervousness, nausea, emesis, disorientation, and stupor. Serious sequelae include seizures, coma, or death. These more serious signs are usually associated with an acute drop in serum sodium to less than 120 to 125 mEq/L.[52,53] If secondary to excessive free water intake, restricting fluids and determining serial serum sodium levels may be all that is necessary.

Decreased urine output in conjunction with decreased serum sodium may be secondary to SIADH. Potential causes of SIADH include brain tumors, the postsurgical state, and drugs such as vincristine, carbamazepine, clofibrate, chlorpropamide, nonsteroidal anti-inflammatory agents, and morphine. In SIADH, free water continues to be reabsorbed even though serum osmolarity has dropped below its narrow window of normality of 282 to 292 mOsm/kg. Additionally, urine osmolarity will be normal or elevated instead of dilute as would be expected by way of compensation.

Correction of chronic hyponatremia must be slow or the patient may be left with serious neurologic deficits. The need for slow correction is related to the brain's compensatory mechanisms for edema and hyponatremia. Organic solutes, extruded during the development of the hyponatremia syndrome as a means to prevent cerebral edema, are slow to reaccumulate as the serum sodium normalizes.[56,57] Intracellular osmolar normalization must be allowed to occur or the cell will become dehydrated.[54]

TREATMENT OF HYPONATREMIA

Treatment of hyponatremia begins with volume restriction, usually to between 1,000 to 1,500 ml/day. Fluid restriction decreases intravascular volume, which decreases renal blood flow and glomerular filtration rate, and increases sodium resorption in the proximal tubule. Further, increased aldosterone secretion enhances distal tubular sodium resorption. Furosemide is an excellent first-line treatment for SIADH, as it impairs the ability of the kidney to concentrate urine and thus increases free water loss. Three percent NaCl solution may be used to initiate correction of critically low serum sodium levels in those patients refractory to first-line treatment or in symptomatically hyponatremic patients. Although there is some controversy (see below) we generally begin 3% NaCl if the serum sodium has acutely dropped to less than or equal to 120 to 125 mEq/L. Conversely, we worry much less about the complications of hyponatremia once the serum sodium is greater than or equal to 125 mEq/L. If the patient is having a seizure or is comatose, 3% NaCl can be infused at 1 to 2 ml/kg/h for 2 to 3 hours. Although this is not likely to correct the serum sodium to normal, it should take the patient to a value of approximately 125 mEq/L, out of the range of acute danger. In all events, we try to avoid an increase in serum sodium of greater than 0.5 mEq/L/h if possible. In chronic refractory hyponatremia, 3% NaCl solution infused initially at a rate of 15 to 25 ml/h is helpful. We follow serum sodium levels every 1 to 2 hours until the serum sodium is out of the danger range, then every 4 hours; Hourly urine output, specific gravity, and serum osmolarity should be closely followed every 6 to 8 hours, particularly over the first 24 hours. We emphasize that it is never necessary to raise the sodium level to normal in a rapid manner. Even our preferred "safe" value of 125 mEq/L should not be attempted if this requires a correction of greater than 10 to 12 mEq/L/day. Sterns points out that an increase in serum sodium of only 6 to 12 mEq/L can be expected to virtually eliminate cerebral edema due to hyponatremia.[52]

Although quite rare, osmotic demyelination syndrome may occur one to several days after the serum sodium has normalized. Initially, patients begin to exhibit behavioral changes, movement disorders, or seizures.[52,54] Thereafter, pseudobulbar palsy, quadriparesis, and coma may develop, and pontine demyelination may be seen on autopsy or MRI.[53,60,61] This is thought to be due to rapid correction of hyponatremia. Thus, although there is controversy,[42] we believe that the serum sodium should be aggressively corrected to 125 mEq/L no faster than 12 mEq/L/day (0.5 to 1 mEq/L/h), particularly if the patient is an alcoholic or has other debilitating diseases. Thereafter, normalization can safely be allowed to occur over several days.

An intriguing disorder termed the cerebral salt wasting (CSW) syndrome has been described in patients who have suffered SAH.[63] This syndrome has some characteristics similar to those of SIADH; specifically, serum sodium is low and urine sodium is high, although in SIADH, urine sodium is usually in the 20 to 30 mEq/L range, whereas in CSW it may be as high as 150 to 200 mEq/L. The main difference between these syndromes is that in CSW, the patient is hypovolemic and the plasma atrial natriuretic factor is elevated, whereas in SIADH, the patient's volume status is normal to increased and vasopressin levels are increased. This difference is critical because if hypovolemic SAH patients are not provided with adequate volume replacement, pre-existing vasospasm could worsen, resulting in a stroke.

Some Causes of Hypernatremia

HYPOVOLEMIC/EUVOLEMIC HYPERNATREMIA

- Impaired thirst
  - Coma
- Nonrenal water loss
  - Skin (thermal injury, sweating)
  - Gastrointestinal tract (diarrhea)
  - Respiratory (febrile state)
- Renal water loss
  - Diabetes insipidus
  - Diuretics
  - Osmotic diuresis (glucose, mannitol)
  - Renal disease (diuretic phase of acute renal failure)
  - Postobstructive diuresis
  - Adrenal failure
  - Osmoreceptor failure
  - Reset osmostat

HYPERVOLEMIC HYPERNATREMIA

- Iatrogenic
  - Hypertonic sodium solution
- Mineralocorticoid excess
  - Hyperaldosteronism
  - Cushing disease
  - Congenital adrenal hyperplasia
  - Exogenous

(From Civetta et al.,[282] with permission.)

DIABETES INSIPIDUS DI involves an excessive loss of free water as a result of inadequate secretion or action of ADH, with resultant high urine output that can lead to hyperosmolarity and elevated serum sodium. The symptoms usually associated with DI are polydipsia in the awake individual and production of copious, dilute urine (polyuria). Other general symptoms may include impaired mentation, obtundation, weakness, lethargy, coma, seizures, and intracranial bleeding secondary to excessive dehydration. Twenty-five percent of adult DI cases are idiopathic, 13% are associated with intracranial malignancies,[64] and only 15% are associated with hypophysectomy.[65] Central nervous system (CNS) tumors that may result in DI include craniopharyngioma, pinealomas, meningiomas, dysgerminomas, and pituitary tumors.[66] Metastatic lesions can also cause DI; in one series these were reported to be the cause of 14% of the total cases.[64] Tumor types causing DI are small-cell lung cancer, leukemia, lymphoma, breast cancer, adenocarcinoma, and leiomyosarcoma.[64] Patients who have undergone craniotomy for tumor must be watched carefully, as they frequently have depressed mental status and may be unable to regulate their volume status with oral fluid intake. Other causes of hypernatremia are to be found in the accompanying box.

There are three distinct patterns of DI following surgery.[67] The most common, occurring in 50 to 60% of patients who develop DI, consists of acute onset polyuria within 24 hours of surgery, with resolution in 3 to 5 days. This is the usual pattern associated with posthypophysectomy patients, occurring in 10 to 20% of patients whose pituitary adenoma is confined to the sella.[67] The second most common pattern is permanent DI associated with 30 to 40% of trauma and neurosurgical cases in which proximal injury to the pituitary stalk, median eminence, or hypothalamus occurs. The third pattern, occurring in no more than 5 to 10% of all cases of DI, involves a triphasic response. The initial phase is evidenced by abrupt onset of polyuria. This is followed by cessation of diuresis after several days that lasts up to 2 weeks. The second stage is believed secondary to inappropriate release of ADH from injured neurohypophyseal tissue.[68] During the second stage, the patient is at risk for development of hyponatremia and water intoxication. After this, the standard picture of DI returns, reflecting the death of magnocellular neurons by retrograde degeneration.[50]

Prior to the initiation of therapy for DI, assessment of the free water deficit should be made as follows:

$$\textit{free } H_2O \textit{ deficit} = \frac{\textit{actual Na} - 140}{140 \times 0.6 \textit{ body weight (kg)}}$$

Treatment begins with isotonic fluid to reverse any hypovolemia that may be present. If elevated urine output persists, and the urine has a specific gravity of 1.000 to 1.005, then hypotonic intravenous fluids (0.45% saline solution, lactated Ringer's solution) should be initiated after a baseline serum sodium and osmolarity have been obtained. In a patient not yet hypovolemic, our practice is to replace urine output greater than 1.5 to 2 ml/kg ideal body weight via intravenous fluids. If the patient has a free water deficit requiring correction, replacement of urine output is begun. We avoid the use of free water (5% dextrose in H_2O = D5W) if at all pos-

TABLE 18.4 *Drugs used to treat diabetes insipidus*

DRUG	DOSE	ROUTE	ONSET (h)	DURATION (h)
Central Diabetes Insipidus				
Aqueous vasopressin	5–10 U	SC,IM	0.5–1.0	4–6
Vasopressin tannante	2–5 U	SC,IM	2–4	24–72
8-Lysine vasopressin	5–10 U[a]	Nasal	0.5–1.0	4–6
DDAVP (desmopressin)	5–20 μg[a]	Nasal	0.5–1.0	12–24
	2–4 μg	IV,SC	0.05–0.1	12–24
Partial and Nephrogenic Diabetes Insipidus				
Hydrochlorothiazide	50–100 mg daily	Oral		12–24
Chlorpropamide	250–750 mg daily	Oral		24–36
Clofibrate	250–500 mg every 6 to 8 h	Oral		6–8
Carbamazepine	100–400 mg daily	Oral		12–24

Abbreviations: SC, subcutaneously; IM, intramuscularly; IV, intravenously; DDAVP, deamino-8-D-arginine vasopressin.

[a] One or two sprays each nostril.

(From Civelto et al.,[285] with permission.)

sible. Frequently, DI is diagnosed very rapidly after onset, so drastic measures such as the utilization of D5W are only rarely necessary. Only with a serum sodium greater than or equal to 160 mEq/L or osmolarity greater than or equal to 320 mOsm/kg would we consider rapid correction of the free water deficit. About 25% of the calculated free water deficit is rapidly replaced; once the serum sodium is approximately 155 mEq/L, we correct more gradually.

When possible, patients should be allowed to control fluid intake themselves with hypotonic oral fluids; this may not be immediately possible in the postoperative period due to altered mental status, such as in the postcraniotomy patient. If drug therapy is required, multiple options exist (Table 18.4). We most frequently use the deamino-8-D-arginine vasopressin (DDAVP) subcutaneously or intravenously and obtain serial serum sodium values to follow progress. This is well tolerated and very effective in treating DI, as onset is within about 1 hour and duration may be as long as 24 hours.

CARE OF SPECIFIC TYPES OF DISORDERS

Particular Problems in the Early Postoperative Period

AIRWAY PROBLEMS We usually attempt to decannulate the airway of our neurosurgical patients at the end of the surgery while the patient is still in the OR. Early extubation allows the neurosurgeons an opportunity to examine the patient for neurologic deficits as well as allowing for more extensive serial examinations in the ICU, so that neurologic changes are noted immediately. If gas exchange is acceptable while the patient is spontaneously breathing, SpO_2 should be greater than or equal to 93%; FIO_2 less than or equal to 0.5; and pH greater than or equal to 7.2 but less than or equal to 7.45. Criteria for airway decannulation include a 10-second head lift, a negative inspiratory force of less than –20 cm H_2O, a full train-of-four without fade on tetanic stimulation, and the ability to follow commands. At times, we extubate as the patient is emerging from anesthesia so there is no bucking against the endotracheal tube, which results in elevated blood pressure and ICP. There are patients who should be kept intubated longer, including those who have undergone extensive skull base procedures or posterior fossa resections in which either the tumor was intimately involved with the brainstem or with the lower cranial nerves, which could compromise their respiratory drive or ability to protect the airway. Other patients who should be kept intubated longer are those given large amounts of sedating drugs or those in whom facial swelling makes extubation a high-risk procedure. In the subgroup of patients requiring more prolonged endotracheal intubation and mechanical ventilation, it has become our practice not just to evaluate for adequate strength and acceptable gas exchange (see above), but to ensure that there is minimal glottic edema (a leak around the endotracheal tube when positive pressure is administered after the cuff has been deflated), adequate respiratory muscle endurance (the ability to double, on command, the spontaneous minute volume without pressure support ventilation assistance, even for overcoming imposed work of breathing), that there is a gag reflex present, and that suctioning of the airway is required no more frequently than every 2 hours.

SLOW EMERGENCE FROM ANESTHESIA Patients may arrive in the ICU sedated secondary to medications such as droperidol, barbiturates, or anticonvulsants, which are given near the end of the case, or from the residual effects of high-dose narcotics used intraoperatively. Unless the patient is unresponsive, postoperative sedation should not precipitate immediate administration of narcotic or benzodiazepine antagonists, as they may create an unpleasant wakeup with dangerous increases in blood pressure. Naloxone, if used, is administered in small intravenous doses of 20 to 40 μg every 3 to 5 minutes. Fully reversed neuromuscular blockade is easily confirmed by a full train-of-four and a 100-Hz tetanic stimulus without fade. Slow emergence should prompt discussion between the neurosurgeon, anesthesiologist, and intensivist as to pertinent patient history or intraoperative difficulties that may explain the phenomenon. For example, patients who have recently suffered a cerebrovascular accident may have recrudescence of stroke residua temporarily after anesthesia; hypothermia between 30 and 35°C may be an alternative explanation. Serum electrolytes, glucose, anticonvulsant levels, and arterial blood gas analysis must be evaluated for abnormalities. If, after evaluation, the etiology of the slow emergence is still unclear, the patient will require a CT scan of the head to rule out postoperative hemorrhage or pneumocephalus; additionally, an EEG may be needed to rule out subclinical status epilepticus.

BLOOD PRESSURE CONTROL We must first point out that our recommendations for levels of blood pressure control are just that, recommendations based upon an extensive clinical experience. There are no studies providing unambiguous data on where and for how long blood pressure should be controlled. Patients with no history of hypertension should maintain a systolic blood pressure in the "normal range" of 110 to 140 mmHg. Control is more tightly maintained in the 110 to 120 mmHg range after, for example, posterior fossa tumor resection, as a bleed there may be catastrophic. Supratentorial resection allows for slightly more lenient systolic blood pressure parameters of from 140 to 160 mmHg. Nausea and pain after craniotomy can be potent stimuli for elevation of blood pressure and should be treated accordingly (see below). If the patient is comfortable, but blood pressure remains elevated, it should be treated initially with intravenous continuous sodium nitroprusside and then intermittently with the intravenous α- and β-blocker labetalol. This drug has an intermediate half-life, does not cross the blood-brain barrier, and has minimal effect on CPP.[69] Doses are given intravenously starting at the lowest dose every 5 to 10 minutes until the desired blood pressure is achieved. After this point, when redosing is required, the first redose given is the labetalol dose just below the one at which blood pressure control was achieved. Thus, in a patient in whom 0.8 mg/kg ideal body weight labetalol was required, redosing will begin at 0.4 mg/kg. Our dosing protocol is shown in Table 18.5. Because sodium nitroprusside may augment ICP in a low intracranial compliance state,[70] we switch to labetalol as rapidly as possible after arrival in the ICU.

Although labetalol usually provides adequate control, if the blood pressure remains high, sodium nitroprusside infusion may need to be reinstituted for a short time. When used at high doses (greater than or equal to 10 μg/kg/min) or for prolonged periods (usually days), the administration of sodium nitroprusside may result in lactic acidosis or renal failure, weakness, and mental status changes due to accumulation of thiocyanate, a metabolic intermediate. If nitroprusside is required for more than 24 hours, we add another agent such as intravenous enalapril to allow elimination of the nitroprusside. Enalapril is begun at a dose of 0.625 mg intravenously every 6 hours and titrated up to a maximum of 5 mg every 6 hours.

Patients with chronic arterial hypertension shift the cerebral autoregulation curve to the right; their brains require a significantly higher CPP to maintain normal function. We therefore keep the systolic blood pressure of these patients in the range of 140 to 160 mmHg range with agents as described above. We prefer to place the patient back on original medications as soon as

TABLE 18.5 *Labetalol dosing protocol*

	DOSE (mg/kg ideal body weight)
1.	0.1
2.	0.2
3.	0.4
4.	0.8
5.	1.6[a]

[a] The 1.6 mg/kg dose may be administered a total of three times, 5 to 10 min apart, in an attempt to achieve blood pressure control. If, after the third dose of 1.6 mg/kg, control is not obtained, another agent will be required.

possible, especially if they are agents associated with rebound hypertension after withdrawal.

SEDATION AND PAIN CONTROL Prior to the advent of the CT scanner, neurosurgeons had to rely exclusively on the neurologic examination for evaluation of impending problems. Therefore, postoperative craniotomy patients were forced to endure pain without adequate analgesia. Pain associated with a craniotomy is primarily derived from trauma to the scalp and muscle. Traditionally, our patients are treated with codeine (15 to 30 mg intramuscularly) in the initial postoperative period since this agent causes minimal sedation. Unfortunately, it is also a poor analgesic. After uneventful craniotomies in which the patient's respiratory drive is uncompromised, low-dose morphine (0.05 mg/kg ideal body weight intravenously every 2 to 4 hours) may be used effectively. Generally, we prefer not to sedate our patients; however, if intracranial and other pathologies have been ruled out and analgesic control is not in question, then propofol is an excellent choice because of its pharmacokinetic properties. The rapidity of offset is due to the drug's rapid redistribution when discontinued, so careful attention must be paid to level of consciousness when administration is continuous.

ANTIEMETIC THERAPY Even though postoperative nausea is a common problem, particularly after posterior fossa surgery, little data exist comparing the various antiemetic agents. The desirable agent should be effective, provide minimal sedation, and not affect the seizure threshold. We do not use promethazine (Phenergan) because of its sedative and seizure threshold lowering effects. Instead, benztropine (Emeticon), 25 to 50 mg intramuscularly every 4 to 6 hours, has been the agent of choice. Unfortunately, it is not very effective in controlling postoperative nausea and, additionally, is administered as a painful intramuscular injection. The recent availability of the 5-hydroxytryptamine antagonist ondansetron provides a powerful agent for postoperative use. This drug does not lower the seizure threshold and is not very sedating; its primary drawback is high cost. Ondansetron has been used successfully in patients receiving chemotherapy. A recent double-blinded study comparing ondansetron to droperidol and metoclopropamide suggested that the former was more effective in treating postanesthetic nausea after dilation and curettage to terminate pregnancy.[71] Although it has not been studied extensively in neurosurgical patients, we have recently begun using it for all of our posterior fossa cases. In these patients, it has been more effective in controlling nausea than benztropine. Dosage of ondansetron is 4 to 8 mg (about 50 μg/kg[72]) intravenously[73] after induction of anesthesia.

Strokes

Cerebrovascular accidents (strokes) follow ischemic heart disease and cancer as the third leading cause of death in the United States, with 500,000 new cases reported annually.[74,75] Most strokes arise from disease of the arterial system and can be broadly divided into two types. In ischemic stroke (85% of total), a vessel is obstructed, usually by arteriosclerosis or an embolus, and the brain becomes damaged due to loss of blood supply. In hemorrhagic stroke (15% of total), loss of arterial wall integrity results in "leaks," allowing blood to extravasate into surrounding structures (the subarachnoid space or brain parenchyma). The 1 month mortality rate has been reported to be between 15 and 33% for ischemic stroke and between 31 and 84% for hemorrhagic stroke.[76–79] Since 1972, particularly due to improvements in treating hypertension and in general medical care, the age-adjusted mortality rate for stroke has decreased by 53%.[75] Despite this reduction in mortality, little progress has been made for the 2.9 million people who survive stroke but who are left with major residual neurologic disabilities.[74] Attempts are now being made to educate the public towards considering stroke with the same urgency that they react to chest pain and heart attack. Adoption of this concept of "brain attack" will hopefully allow early intervention within a therapeutic window during which permanent damage can be reduced or avoided.

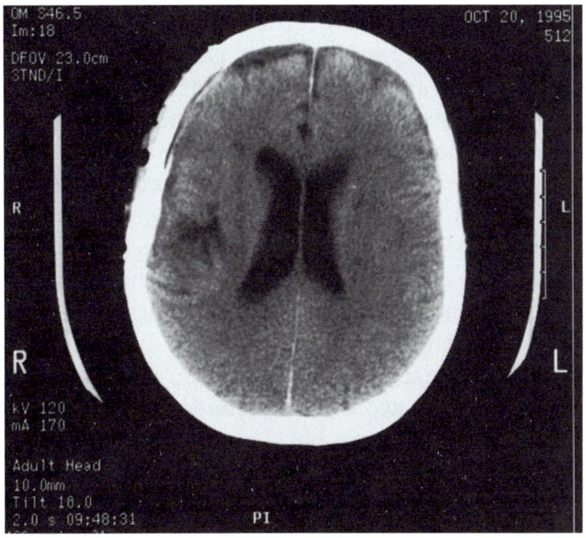

FIGURE 18.3 *A CT scan of a right temporoparietal ischemic stroke. No mass effect is present. The distribution suggests an embolic source.*

ISCHEMIC STROKES Patients at risk of developing ischemic strokes (Fig. 18.3) invariably have many associated and identifiable risk factors that promote arterial disease, including strong genetic tendencies toward arteriosclerosis, diabetes mellitus, cardiac disorders, peripheral vascular disease, hypertension, and smoking history. Up to 85% of all strokes are ischemic, and most arise in association with obstructive cervical carotid artery disease or from embolic sources originating from the heart.[80–82] Signs and symptoms of ischemic cerebrovascular disease include (1) asymptomatic bruits from the turbulence created within the artery by arteriosclerosis (usually within the internal carotid artery just above the cervical carotid bifurcation) (2) transient ischemic attacks (TIAs) that typically last only a few seconds, minutes, or hours; (3) reversible ischemic neurologic deficits that last longer than 24 hours; and (4) completed strokes, which are accompanied by permanent neurologic deficits.

The reduced CBF associated with ischemic strokes may be focal or global, depending on the site and cause of the circulatory abnormality. If they are caused by a small embolus that lodges distally in the cerebral circulation, focal strokes may be small and limited to a peripheral end-artery infarction. Conversely, if a major trunk (i.e., internal carotid or middle cerebral artery) is obstructed, focal strokes may be large and involve most of a cerebral hemisphere. Global ischemia is caused by low systemic blood flow (hypotension or anoxia following cardiac arrest) or hypoxic insults (near drowning or carbon monoxide intoxication). The damaged area includes a region of central infarction and necrosis surrounded by an ischemic penumbra in which the injury may be reversible. As the duration of symptoms before treatment increases, the likelihood of permanent infarction-related deficits increases greatly, and the ability to "retrieve" the penumbra is correspondingly reduced.

Initial care is supportive, with protection of the airway, ventilation (if required), and careful monitoring of vital signs. The maintenance of euvolemia and adequate renal function, vigilance for infection, deep-vein thrombosis prophylaxis, adequate nutrition, and good skin care are also obvious requirements of good medical care. Many of these patients have concurrent heart disease, and any ECG changes, cardiac laboratory abnormalities, or suspicious symptoms should receive a thorough work-up. New onset cardiac arrhythmias are identified in approximately 77% of hemorrhagic stroke patients and in 22% of ischemic stroke patients.[83] Some patients, particularly those with intracranial hemorrhage, will exhibit a "stunned" myocardium, presumably from a hyperadrenergic state associated with hypothalamic injury.

Many strokes occur at night, presumably when the resting blood pressure decreases below the level necessary to maintain perfusion. Broderick and colleagues found spontaneous systolic blood pressure reductions of 29 ± 22 mmHg in approximately one-third of stroke patients examined early after the onset of symptoms.[84] Because patients with long-standing hypertension may have right-shifted autoregulatory curves and require higher pressures to maintain normal cerebral perfusion, abnormalities should be judiciously corrected. Depending on the severity of the hypertension, we prefer to maintain systolic blood pressures in the range of 140 to 160 mmHg.

Medical Management. Anticoagulation would appear to be an obvious mainstay for the acute treatment of thromboembolic disease. However, several large studies failed to demonstrate a significant benefit to heparin use in acute ischemic stroke patients.[85,86] Duke and colleagues[85] found that 17% of patients given heparin within 48 hours of symptom onset exhibited neurologic deficit progression after treatment compared with 19.5% in the control group. One-year mortality was higher in the treatment group (17 vs. 8 deaths) but appeared to be unrelated to the anticoagulation. A recent study, however, demonstrated clear effectiveness of acute anticoagulation using low-molecular-weight heparin for specific patients with ischemic stroke symptoms.[87] On the recommendations of the cerebral embolism study group, full heparinization should be considered for nonhemorrhagic stroke, particularly for patients with stroke in evolution or those seen within 6 hours of symptom onset. Heparin should also be considered in patients with TIAs from a cardiac source or those with high-grade carotid stenosis whose symptoms continue despite antiplatelet therapy.[80] Long-term anticoagulation with coumadin has clearly been effective in reducing the ischemic stroke rate in patients with atrial fibrillation or valvular disease. A short course (3 to 12 months) may be similarly effective in recently postmyocardial infarction patients.

Intravenous thrombolytic therapy using urokinase, streptokinase, or tissue plasminogen activator theoretically provides a direct method for recanalization of an affected vessel. Initial studies with these agents demonstrated a high rate of intracranial hemorrhage.[88,89] More recent studies, however, have shown significant beneficial effects, particularly when the agents are delivered soon after symptom onset. Pilot data suggest that infusion of tissue plasma activator within 90 minutes of symptoms led to rapid improvement in 30% of patients,[90] whereas therapy begun between 91 and 180 minutes after the ischemic episode was less effective.[91] If initiated within 8 hours of the ischemia, thrombolytic treatment can lead to angiographic recanalization of 26% of obstructed proximal vessels and 38% of middle cerebral artery occlusions.[92] Hemorrhage was reported in 31% of study subjects and was more frequent if the drug was delivered later after symptom onset. Drug dosage appeared unrelated to the incidence of hemorrhagic transformations. Recent long-term studies have demonstrated a 30% improvement in the number of high-quality functional survivors among patients who receive intravenous thrombolytic therapy within 3 hours of symptom onset compared with those receiving best medical care only.[93]

Other therapeutic interventions that have been tried or are under consideration include hemodilution, hypothermia, and specific drug therapies. Hemodilution theoretically and experimentally improves the rheologic aspects of blood flow. However, even though initial reports were favorable,[94] this methodology did not significantly improve outcome in a large follow-up study of 1,254 patients.[95] Hypothermia can improve ischemic tolerance by decreasing the cerebral metabolic rate and inhibiting the release of excitatory amino acids. Significant hypothermia can cause cardiac arrhythmias, however, and is difficult to maintain without cardiac bypass.

Calcium channel blockers are believed to limit the secondary neuronal injury that accompanies ischemia. Some data suggest that male patients with moderate deficits treated with nimodipine within 24 hours of ischemic stroke have decreased mortality and improved overall quality outcomes at 6 months.[96] However, the American Nimodipine Study Group series,[97] which enrolled 1,064 patients in a double-blinded study, failed to show any differences between nimodipine and placebo groups. Thus, the role of calcium channel blockers for acute ischemia remains unclear.

Excitatory amino acids such as glutamate appear to be major contributors to secondary neuronal injury through the process known as excitotoxicity. Extensive animal research suggests that glutamate receptor blockade (using *N*-methyl-D-aspartate [NMDA] and amino-3-hydroxy-5-methyl-isoazole antagonists) or free radical scavengers (superoxide dismutase and 21-aminosteroids) may reduce stroke volumes by maintaining viability within the ischemic penumbra.[98] In the future, these agents or their relatives may demonstrate significant clinical benefits.

Surgical Management. Surgical intervention for ischemic stroke has been controversial for many years. Recent prospective, double-blinded, randomized studies, however, have clarified the merits of carotid endarterectomy as an effective stroke preventative treatment. The North American Symptomatic Carotid Endarterectomy Trial (NASCET)[99] demonstrated that carotid endarterectomy reduces the incidence of all ipsilateral strokes by nearly three-fourths (17% actual risk reduction over 18 months) in patients with symptomatic, high-grade (70% or greater) cervical carotid arteriosclerotic obstruction. The risks of all ipsilateral major or fatal strokes are similarly reduced (11% actual reduction). Both the NASCET and the European Carotid Surgery Trialists' Collaborative Group investigators continue to evaluate the appropriateness of symptomatic moderate stenosis (30 to 69%) for carotid endarterectomy.

Urgent or emergent carotid endarterectomy is indicated for patients with crescendo TIAs or persistent symptoms on full heparin therapy. The value of emergent endarterectomy for any other reason, however, is not as clear, as surgery for patients with moderate or severe acute deficits carries much higher risks.[80] Carotid arteries recently occluded (within 48 hours) can usually be reopened safely. Longer-standing obstructions may occasionally be reopened days to weeks later, especially if the patient has been treated with anticoagulation during the interval.[100–104]

Some patients with very high-grade stenosis will have lost autoregulation of the affected hemisphere, and the rapid restoration of blood flow to chronically dilated (and transiently unreactive) cerebral vessels may promote intracerebral hemorrhage through a phenomena called *normal perfusion pressure breakthrough*. The postoperative blood pressure in individuals at risk must be carefully controlled at the lower end of the normal range for several days after surgery until the arterioles regain their capacity to vasoconstrict.

Arterial embolectomy for acutely occluded intracranial vessels has been largely replaced by the use of thrombolytic agents but may still be indicated in certain instances, most commonly to retrieve errant balloons or other devices deployed during interventional radiological procedures. Patients with the best outcome are those with good collateral circulation who were reopened within a few hours after onset of the neurologic deficit.[80]

HEMORRHAGIC STROKES Depending on the source and site of the bleeding, intracranial hemorrhage can be divided into several broad categories, including (1) intraparenchymal, (2) subarachnoid, (3) subdural, and (4) epidural varieties. Combinations of clot locations within several intracranial spaces are not infrequent. Subdural and epidural bleeding are most commonly caused by head trauma and will be discussed more fully in the section on Traumatic Brain Injury (see below). The term *hemorrhagic stroke* is herein confined to include only nontraumatic intraparenchymal or subarachnoid bleeding.

Intraparenchymal Hemorrhage. Most hemorrhagic strokes have been classically attributed to the effects of hypertension on small, deep-penetrating vessels (Fig. 18.4). Long-standing exposure of these arteries to increased blood pressure promotes the formation of microscopic degenerative aneurysms (Charcot-Bouchard) that rupture into the intracranial parenchyma to produce deep and often quite large hematomas. Areas commonly affected include the putamen, globus pallidus, and thalamus (65%), the subcortical white matter (15%), the cerebellum (10%), and the brainstem (10%).[80,105]

Surgical management of deep basal ganglia or thalamic hemorrhages is controversial and has generally been discouraged since McKissock's studies demonstrated no improvement in either morbidity or mortality.[106] The volume of the hematoma has a direct influence on outcome, with mortality rates ranging from 5% for clots less than 30 ml in volume to 85% for clots greater than 50 ml.[107] Several recent Japanese studies have indicated that microsurgical clot evacuation undertaken within 6 hours

A

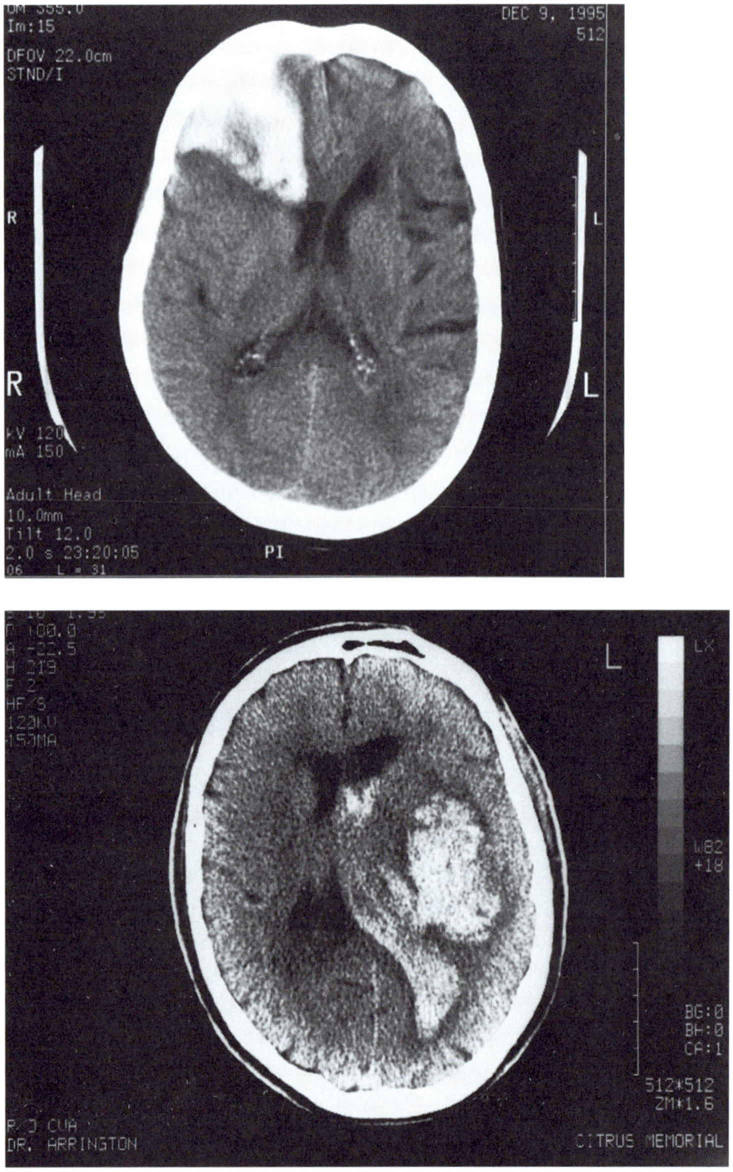

B

FIGURE 18.4 *(A) A CT scan of a spontaneous right frontal hemorrhagic stroke. Note the mass effect exhibited by midline shift. Distribution and lack of subarachnoid blood make aneurysm unlikely. (B) A CT scan of a large, left-sided, deep basal ganglion intracerebral hemorrhage with extension into the ventricular system. Mass effect present is causing transfalcine herniation. This is characteristic of a hypertensive bleed.*

of the hemorrhage can allow 50% of patients to return to independent life and 15% to have a complete recovery.[108] However, several other randomized, prospective studies have not corroborated such favorable results.[109–112] Stereotactic clot aspiration combined with urokinase instillation has been attempted, but the effectiveness of such intervention currently remains unproven.[113]

Cerebellar hemorrhages, on the other hand, are often very effectively treated with surgical clot evacuation as long as the intervention is undertaken before the patient becomes comatose from brainstem compression. Alert patients with hematomas less than 3 cm and no brainstem compressive signs can be treated conservatively while being carefully observed in the ICU. Hematomas larger than 3 cm, however, should always be treated with emergent craniotomy and evacuation regardless of the patient's neurologic status.[80] Many such patients also require a ventriculostomy to prevent obstructive hydrocephalus from causing further increases in ICP.

Intraparenchymal bleeding may also develop in patients on chronic anticoagulation therapy or in those with other bleeding disorders. Obviously, normal clotting must be re-established before any surgical therapy can be considered, so such patients are managed medically until that time. Amyloid angiopathy associated with aging and Alzheimer's disease may also predispose to intraparenchymal bleeding, particularly in the subcortical regions of the frontal, parietal, and occipital lobes of the cerebrum.[107] Primary tumors (gliomas, meningiomas, and pituitary adenomas) and metastasis (most commonly, melanoma, renal cell carcinoma, lung cancer, and choriocarcinoma) may also spontaneously bleed into the head. Indications for surgery are individually determined based on the size and site of the clot, the neurologic status of the patient, and the future expectations of the underlying disease.

Subarachnoid Hemorrhage. Spontaneous isolated bleeding into the subarachnoid space or ventricular system is typically caused by structural abnormalities of the intracranial arteries, such as aneurysms (Fig. 18.5) or AVMs, until proven otherwise by high-quality cerebral arteriography. The resultant blood deposited in the CSF may lead to acute hydrocephalus or may cause delayed ischemia secondary to cerebral vasospasm. Parenchymal blood may destroy critical brain areas and/or may raise ICP to life-threatening levels. Therapy in the ICU is aimed at the control of these conditions while avoiding rebleeding until the structural abnormality and any associated mass effect can be controlled with surgery or interventional radiologic techniques. An algorithm for the management of patients with acute subarachnoid bleeding is shown in Figure 18.6. The critical care management of aneurysms and AVMs can be quite different and challenging, and the problems associated with each entity are discussed independently below.

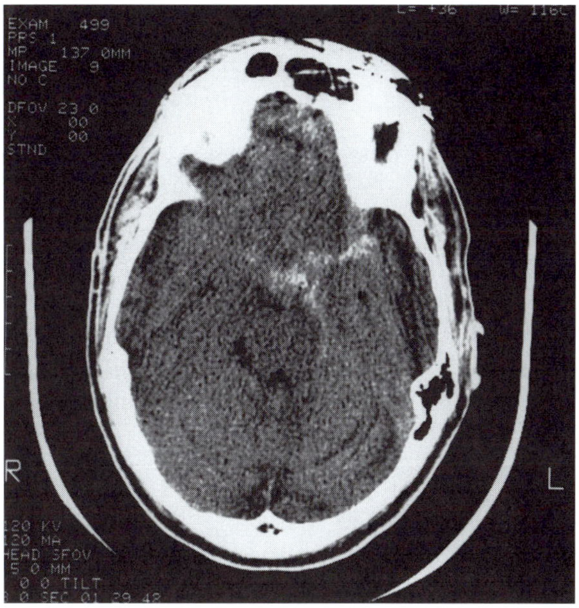

FIGURE 18.5 *A CT scan of a left-sided SAH involving the basilar and sylvian fissure cisterns. This is due to a basilar apex aneurysm.*

Aneurysms. See Chapter 8.

Arteriovenous Malformations and Fistulae. AVMs are congenital lesions in which there is an

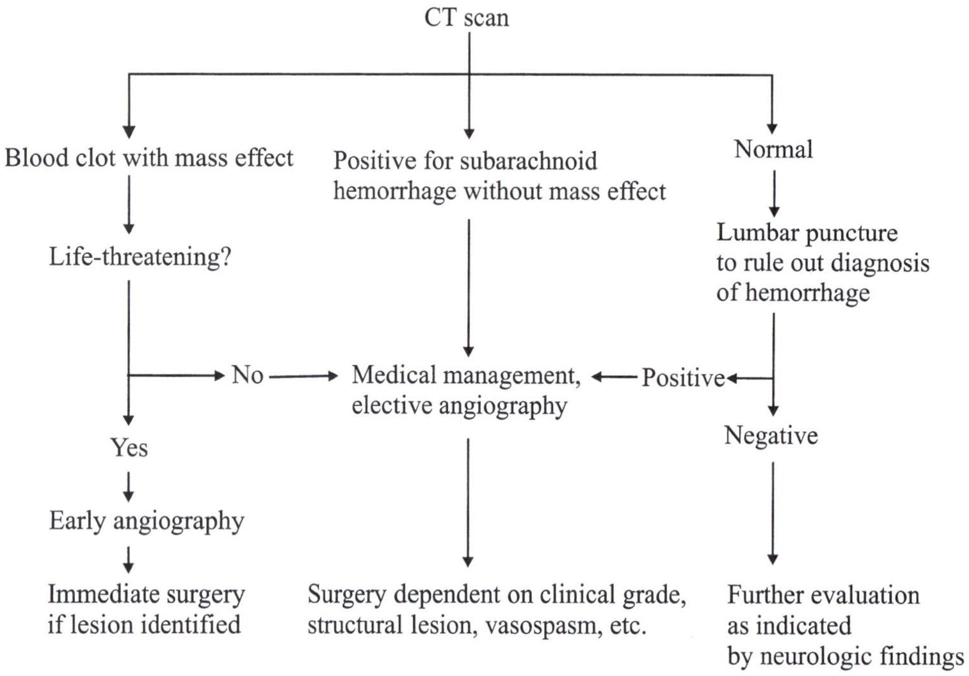

FIGURE 18.6 *An algorithm for decision making and treatment of patients with SAH and cerebral vasospasm.*

abnormal connection between the arterial and venous system without an intervening capillary bed (Fig. 18.7) (see also Ch. 8). This direct communication leads to a transfer of arterial blood into adjacent veins, which are not normally constructed to withstand such pressures. The net result is an engorgement of the local or distant venous system, which may then promote headaches, seizures, or hemorrhage (subarachnoid, intraventricular, or intraparenchymal). Most AVMs are located superficially in the cerebral cortex, although some are positioned in the brainstem, cerebellum, or ventricular system.

Arteriovenous fistulae (AVFs) may also be congenital, but most are acquired lesions that develop following spontaneous thrombosis of a major dural venous sinus. The body's attempts at recanalization or rerouting of sinus flow can result in a fistula being established between small dural arteries and the dural sinus adjacent to the site of thrombosis. In most instances, the arterialized blood is diverted into large venous dural sinuses that can withstand the pressures without significant bleeding risks. If the arterialized flow is shunted into parenchymal vessels, however, these lesions carry the same or higher hemorrhagic and surgical risks as AVMs.

In the past, many AVMs and AVFs were considered inoperable and untreatable. Improved understanding of anatomy and physiology, combined with new surgical, radiosurgical, and interventional neuroradiologic techniques, now allows most of these lesions to be treated safely. The primary ICU responsibility for these lesions involves the tight control of systemic blood pressure during the immediate postoperative or postembolization period aimed at the prevention of destructive edema and hemorrhage.

Spetzler and Martin have developed a grading system to evaluate AVMs for associated surgical risks and outcome by assigning risk points based on size, location, and venous drainage patterns (Table 18.6).[114] These points are then added to create a score for a particular lesions: grade I, 1 point; grade II, 2 points; grade III, 3 points, grade IV, 4 points; and grade V, 5 points. Retro-

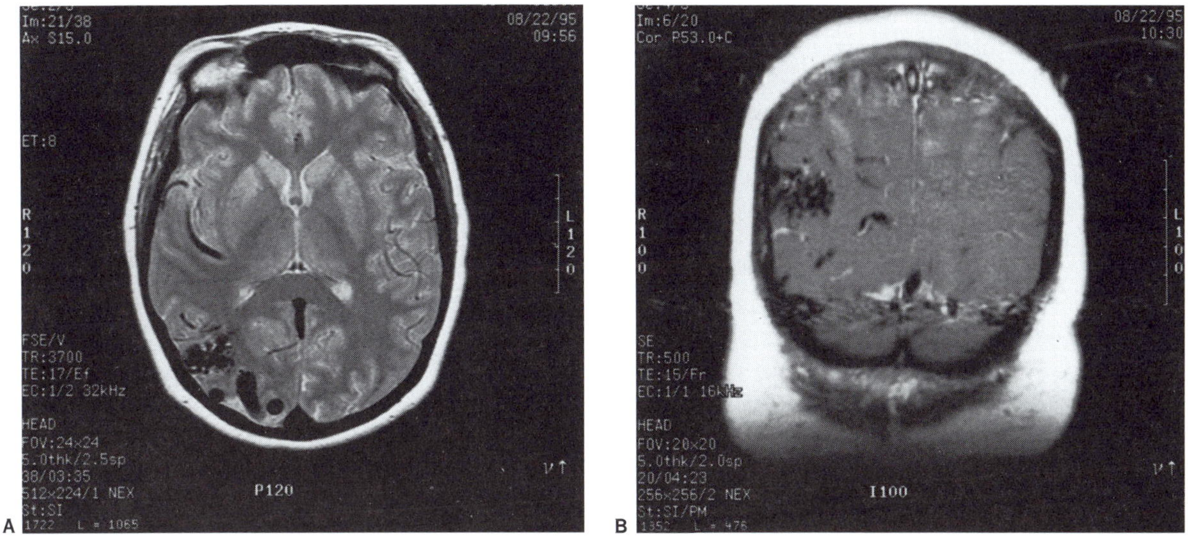

FIGURE 18.7 *(A) An MRI of right-sided parietotemporo-occipital AVM showing a large posterior draining vein (B) An MRI showing coronal section of a right-sided parietotemporo-occipital AVM. Note nidus of malformation and dilated venous drainage.*

spective analysis of resected AVMs using this grading system shows good correlation between higher grades and increased perioperative complications.[115,116]

The cause of these complications is often related to perilesional cerebral edema and hemorrhage from the bed of the resected malformation. The shunting of arterialized blood away from parenchyma adjacent to the malformation creates an abnormal state of autoregulation, during which the vessels become chronically dilated in an attempt to overcome a relatively ischemic state.[117] After AVM resection, restoration of normal perfusion to these areas can produce further congestion of these dilated vessels, leading to increased parenchymal edema or hemorrhage in up to 6% of patients.[117–119] Stagnant flow in the coagulated arterial feeders, venous outflow obstruction, and engorgement of the drained tissue can further amplify these risks. This phenomenon can reach critically significant proportions in up to 10% of patients and is much more common in high flow or larger lesions.[119,120]

At our institution, patients at high risk of these problems (high flow or large AVMs) have their systemic blood pressure decreased by 20 to 30% from baseline, usually via sodium nitroprusside or labetalol, for the first several days af-

TABLE 18.6 *Arteriovenous malformation grading chart*

FEATURE	POINTS
Size (cm)	
<3	1
3–6	2
>6	3
Eloquence of adjacent brain	
Noneloquent	0
Eloquent	1
Venous drainage pattern	
Superficial	0
Deep	1

(From Spetzler and Martin,[114] with permission.)

ter surgical treatment. During this period, patients are watched for neurologic changes and are maintained in a euvolemic state to reduce the risk of thrombosis of critical draining veins. After 48 hours, the blood pressure is slowly allowed to return toward normal. Despite these measures, some cases of delayed hemorrhage still occur and may be catastrophic, so patients are kept in the ICU for several days for continued close monitoring and observation. If serial or continuous CBF data were available, it might be possible to assess exactly when normal autoregulation and flow has been restored. Systemic blood pressure control could then be relaxed without increased edema or hemorrhage risks. Xenon CT,[121] TCD,[122–124] SPECT, or laser flow Doppler[125] have been investigated, but unfortunately, there is presently no specific monitoring system that is ideal for this task.

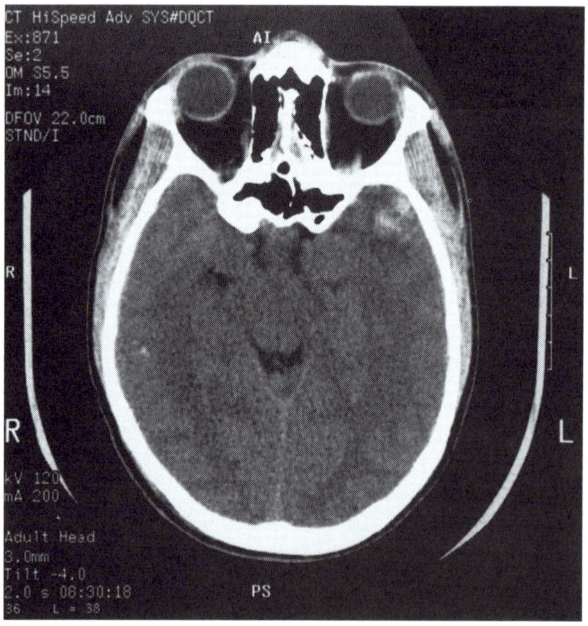

FIGURE 18.8 *A CT scan of a post-traumatic left-sided temporal polar contusion.*

Traumatic Brain Injury

Traumatic brain injury (Fig. 18.8) represents a significant problem in the United States, with an estimated 2 million people affected annually. Of these, 500,000 require hospitalization, 70,000 to 90,000 experience long-term disability, and 2,000 live in a persistent vegetative state.[126]

The initial evaluation involves a prioritization of all injuries to decide if a surgically treatable intracranial lesion exists. The patient is usually seen by multiple specialists, with general surgeons and neurosurgeons providing management direction. If the patient has a life-threatening abdominal or thoracic problem, neurologic management must obviously be secondary. If there are no life-threatening general surgical problems, but physical findings suggest a surgically correctable neurologic injury, an emergent CT scan of the head should be obtained. The patient without a surgically treatable injury is stabilized and transported to the ICU.

A thorough evaluation must be performed by the neurointensivist, as significant injuries may be missed in the flurry of emergency department activity. The airway should be reassessed to determine stability; endotracheal tubes may hang precariously on arrival at the ICU. If the patient has an adequate airway, spontaneous ventilatory status should be assessed with a visual observation for rate, synchrony, and evidence of flail chest. Arterial blood should be sent for gas analysis. The cardiac rhythm, rate, and evidence for hemodynamic instability should be re-evaluated and treated if appropriate. Intravenous fluids may have been running at high rates, and the intensivist must be mindful of iatrogenically worsened cerebral edema after traumatic brain injury. A thorough neurologic examination should be performed to determine if the patient's neurologic status has changed. A detailed general physical examination should be performed to elucidate any injuries missed in the emergency department. If the patient is determined to be at risk for elevated ICP, management should commence immediately to prevent further injury and possible herniation (Fig. 18.9).

Treatment of elevated ICP begins with simple modes of intervention. For many years, it was uncontested dogma that elevation of the head

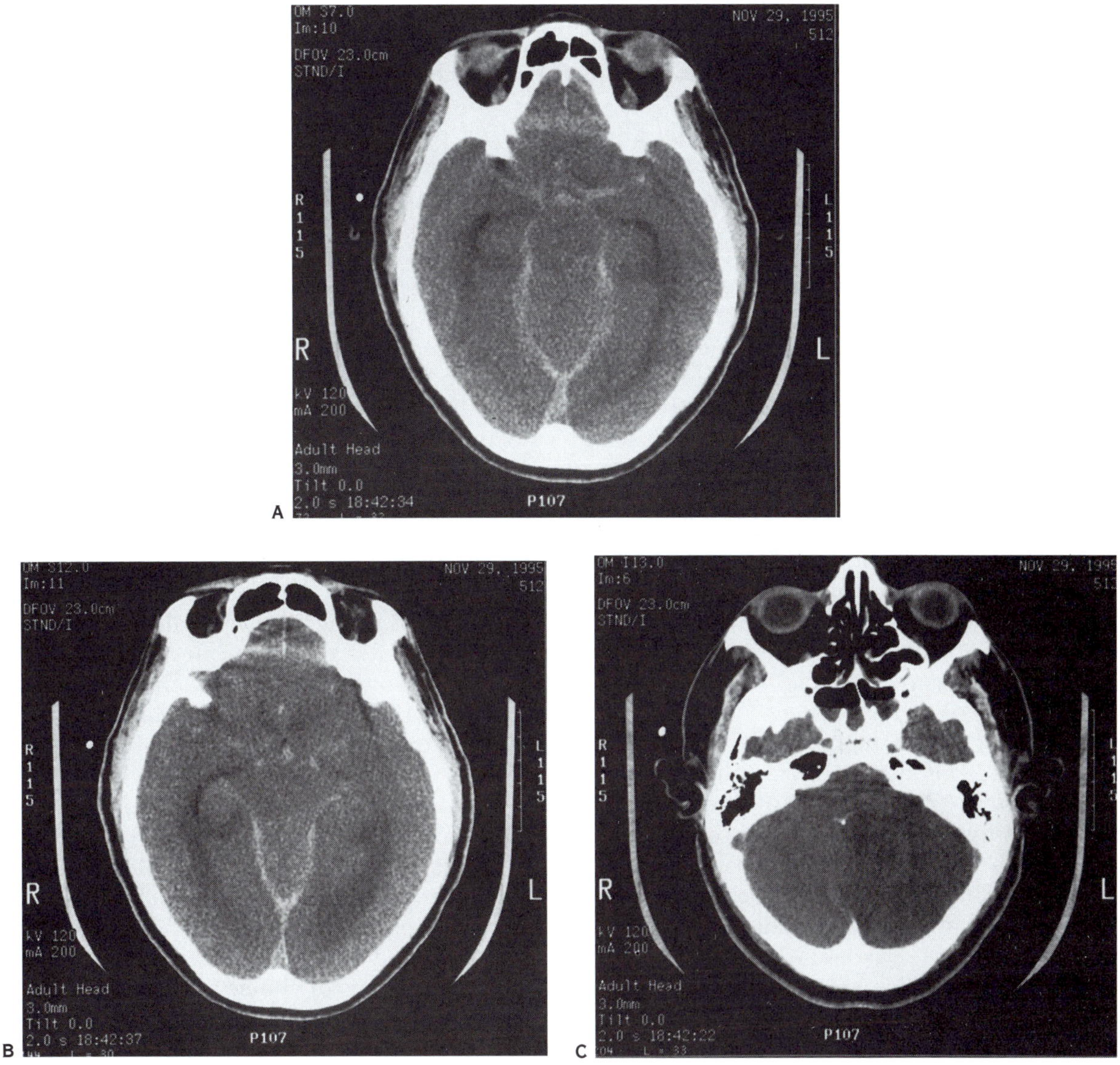

FIGURE 18.9 *(A & B) CT scans showing transtentorial herniation. Note the complete obliteration of the perimesencephalic cisterns secondary to bilateral cerebral swelling and incisural compromise, (C) The same case as Figs. A and B, showing medullary herniation with obliteration of the fourth ventricle and posterior fossa compression, implying tonsillar herniation. Note the glassy appearance of the posterior fossa contents, implying diffuse swelling.*

was the best initial treatment for elevated ICP. Although head elevation clearly decreases ICP, not until recently did researchers consider the negative impact on CPP. Rosner's studies found that the best treatment for ICP was to keep the head flat; this was refuted subsequently in a series of studies examining the effect of head position on CPP and ICP.[127–129] The best data suggest that mild head elevation to 15° to 30° has beneficial effects on ICP with no significant detrimental effects on CPP. The head should also be kept neutral (i.e., not turned to the left or right) to minimize decreases in jugular venous outflow, which could further elevate ICP.

Fluid management may dramatically affect ICP. Careful records of hourly intake and output should be kept to maintain the patient's euvolemic status. Animal studies have suggested that hypertonic fluids are superior to isotonic or hypotonic mixtures for preventing or treating elevated ICP.[130–133] Hypertonic (7.5% NaCl) saline has even been shown to be as effective as mannitol in treating increased ICP.[134] Hypertonic fluids may also simultaneously improve any prerenal failure caused by dehydrating agents such as furosemide and mannitol.[135] Recent studies suggest that there are no benefits to using colloid solutions.[136] Few organized studies have examined the effects of hypertonic fluids on cerebral water content in humans. A multicenter group (the Consortium for Brain Injury) is currently prospectively examining whether hypertonic fluids are beneficial for treating head injury.

Hypothermia may provide a noninvasive method for cerebral protection in head trauma patients, as every 1°C decrease in core body temperature is associated with an approximate 7% decrease in cerebral oxygen consumption.[137] The outpouring of catecholamines that occurs with the stress of trauma can cause elevations in core temperature, particularly if there is hypothalamic injury. Recent studies suggest that moderate hypothermia (32 to 33°C[138] or 34°C[139] core temperature) induced with cooling blankets and iced gastric lavage can decrease ICP and CBF (40% and 26 to 45%, respectively) and ultimately improve outcome. Karibe et al. showed that hypothermia experimentally decreased postischemic hyperperfusion and delayed hypoperfusion, the extent of blood-brain barrier disruption, the volume of brain edema, and neuronal damage.[140] The mechanism may be prevention of glutamate and aspartate buildup, the absence of which prevents NMDA channel-mediated calcium influx.[138,141] The lack of calcium entry through the NMDA channel may then inhibit the marked augmentation in nitric oxide synthase activity usually seen with ischemia.[142]

Patients with traumatic brain injury may have infections from a variety of sources, including pulmonary aspiration of gastric contents and intra-abdominal or extremity wounds. Although appropriate workup of infection must be instituted, the patient should be treated to prevent prolonged periods of temperature elevation. Although acetaminophen or ibuprofen may suffice, our experience suggests that a fan blowing air over alcohol–tepid water-soaked towels placed on the patient will cause the temperature to rapidly revert toward normal.

Sedation and analgesia are important cornerstones of elevated ICP control. Traumatic brain injury patients often have multiple additional painful injuries that, left untreated, can elevate ICP. The endotracheal tube and mechanical ventilation may also be uncomfortable, resulting in the patient "fighting" the ventilator and elevating ICP. Sedation may be accomplished by titrating short-acting agents such as propofol, (starting at 10 $\mu g \cdot kg^{-1} min^{-1}$) or midazolam, (1 to 2-mg intravenous bolus doses with initial infusion of 0.5 to 2 mg/h). Neuromuscular blockade, although occasionally needed in patients who are difficult to ventilate and oxygenate, is seldom used in our unit in neurologically injured patients. These agents should be used only in conjunction with appropriate neuromuscular monitoring and in the presence of adequate sedation. Our agents of choice are mivacurium or atracurium. We titrate the neuromuscular blocking agent infusion so that 1 of 4 twitches of a train-of-four is always present. The key concept with sedation in the patient with traumatic brain injury is to be able to lighten sedation rapidly so that hourly neurologic examinations may be performed. The number of elective interventions such as turning or suctioning should be minimized. Lidocaine can be placed in the endotracheal tube, but our experience suggests that this stimulates coughing. Intravenous administration 90 seconds prior to suctioning can be more effective.

Hyperventilation has been the traditional treatment for increased ICP but has recently become controversial because of suggestions that it causes deleterious ischemia. Hyperventilation causes a decrease in the $PaCO_2$, which subsequently causes cerebral vasoconstriction. Because the CBF varies to the fourth power with diameter, a 20% change in vessel size can lead to a 60% decrease in CBF.[143] Patients are at greatest risk for problems with ischemia in the first 24 hours after the injury. Severely head-injured patients initially may have depressed CBF with a low arteriovenous oxygen difference ([a-v]DO_2). With hyperventilation, CBF decreases further, but [a-v]DO_2 increases, suggesting worsening ischemia. Xenon CBF studies have also shown that an "inverse steal" may occur with hyperventilation. Normal brain areas with intact autoregulation shunt blood to injured areas that have less CO_2 reactivity, thereby worsening edema.[144] Muizelaar and colleagues have performed several studies examining the beneficial effects of trishydroxyaminomethane (THAM) on patients being hyperventilated after head injury.[145] Although the initial study suggested improved outcome, this was not found in a follow-up study, which showed improved control of the ICP and less requirement for barbiturates but no effect on ultimate outcome.[146] In an animal study, THAM compromised MAP and CPP when compared with bicarbonate.[147] Thus, the overall benefits of THAM remain questionable. It appears, in general, that hyperventilation, although effective at lowering ICP, may cause serious ischemic problems and should therefore be limited to a $PaCO_2$ of between 25 and 30 mmHg.

Mannitol or other dehydrating agents represent another treatment option for elevated ICP. In brains with an intact blood-brain barrier, mannitol acts via its hyperosmolarity, by moving water from the intracellular space into the vascular space The subsequent decrease in ICP results in improved CPP. Mannitol is also a oxygen free-radical scavenger and may therefore prevent secondary neuronal injury.[143] The usual starting dose is 0.25 to 0.5 g/kg followed by an infusion of 20% solution at 0.06 to 0.12 g/kg/hr. Disadvantages of mannitol use include rebound edema with discontinuation and hyperosmolar-induced renal failure if the serum osmolarity surpasses 320 mOsm/kg H_2O; these are minor in comparison to its benefits. Mannitol may also be used in conjunction with furosemide, resulting in a synergistic diuresis with prolongation of the reversal of the blood-brain osmotic gradient.[148] The dose of furosemide used (0.7 mg/kg) is too small to impair CSF formation.

Barbiturates have traditionally been used as a last-ditch effort to treat uncontrolled ICP. In 1979, Marshall et al. reported one of the first trials showing barbiturates could control ICP. Several other small and/or retrospective studies and only three controlled randomized ones have looked at this issue.[149] Eisenberg and colleagues evaluated barbiturate use in patients with severe head injury (69 of 73 with closed head injury), comparing it with equally aggressive (except for barbiturates) therapy.[150] Although ICP was more effectively treated with barbiturates, it did not appear to improve outcome or mortality. Ward and co-workers examined the effectiveness of prophylactic barbiturates in patients with severe head injury and failed to show an improvement in either outcome or mortality, although some of their patients may not have actually required barbiturate therapy and a treatment response may have been diluted.[151] Schwartz and the Toronto Head Injury Group compared mannitol and barbiturates in patients with severe closed head injury and elevated ICP.[152] No improvement in ICP control was noted with barbiturates as compared to mannitol; mortality was higher in the barbiturate group. Most recently, barbiturates were given in conjunction with hyperventilation to assess whether there was a synergistic improvement in ICP relative to hyperventilation alone. In this animal study, barbiturate administration was no more effective in controlling ICP than was hyperventilation alone.[153]

Because the brain has essentially no oxygen reserve, adequate oxygen delivery is critical for brain function. When delivery is inadequate, anaerobic metabolism begins, resulting in the accumulation of lactic acid. Hyperbaric oxygen therapy provides a means of supplying supranormal amounts of oxygen and, because of the vasoconstrictive effects of hyperoxia, helps treat elevated ICP. The vasoconstricting effect is seen at a depth of 1.5 atms. A recent randomized and controlled study of traumatic brain injury patients treated hyperburic oxygen (1.5 atm) showed that mortality but not outcome quality were improved with this therapy.[154] Several randomized and/or prospective trials strongly suggest that steroids (high or low dose) have no benefit in the treatment of traumatic brain injury.[155–157]

Spinal Cord Injury

Despite years of research, spinal cord injuries continue to be a devastating problem. The complexity of these injuries mandate that critical care begin in the field, with referral to a tertiary care center for acute care and finally to a spinal cord rehabilitation center for subacute/chronic therapy.

PREHOSPITAL CARE Patients with spinal cord injury, particularly those with a high cervical injury, frequently have airway compromise, difficulty breathing spontaneously, and hemodynamic instability. Initial assessment of the airway, breathing rate and pattern, and hemodynamic stability should be followed by a brief neurologic examination to detect obvious neurologic deficits. The neck and spine should be securely immobilized with a hard collar and tape, the patient secured to a backboard, and, as soon as vital signs are stable, transported emergently to the hospital. Airway compromise may be in evidence due to facial trauma, putting the patient at risk of obstruction and/or aspiration. If there is any question about airway security or patency or respiratory distress supervenes, the patient should have an endotracheal tube placed. Orotracheal insertion is preferable, using a jaw thrust to minimize the cervical spine hyperextension. Tracheostomy or cricothyrotomy may be necessary but are not preferred as they may complicate future anterior stabilization procedures. Patients displaying neurogenic shock may be supported with combinations of fluids (0.9 or 3% saline) and/or pressors (phenylephrine or epinephrine); significant bradycardia may be treated with intravenous bolus doses of atropine (0.5 to 2 mg). Glucose-containing solutions are not used unless hypoglycemia is present. We aggressively control serum glucose, beginning on arrival to the emergency department, to between 80 and 150 mg/dl, based upon data suggesting a correlation between hyperglycemia and neurologic injury in head-injured patients.[34]

EMERGENCY DEPARTMENT AND ICU CARE Once in the emergency department, the patient requires a thorough general and neurologic examination as well as radiographic studies (including a lateral cervical spine, Fig. 18.10); other studies are dependent upon the mechanism of injury and associated injuries. Ultimately, the patient will need a full cervical spine series and, particularly if the mechanism of injury was motor vehicular with ejection, a full spine and long bone series. If a cervical fracture is present, traction will be required for reduction using Gardner-Wells tongs or a halo applied to the skull just above the pinna. Traction is applied with the addition of 2.5-lb to 5-lb weights, with the general rule of 5-lb per cervical spine level. If traction is required, it is critical to perform serial neurologic examinations and serial cervical spine films to assess the alignment and amount of distraction. The presence of a neurologic deficit requires, in addition to bony stabilization, the immediate administration of methylprednisolone bolus followed by infusion (see below).

In the emergency department, after other injuries have been assessed, their priority may be determined. If the patient has no other significant injuries, he/she can be transported to the ICU. Hourly, serial neurologic examinations are critical to evaluate for development of any neurologic deficit progression.

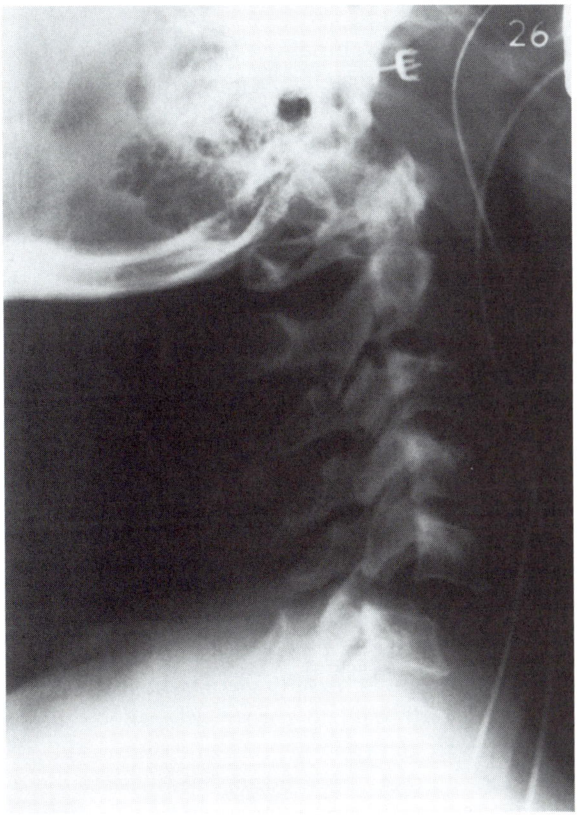

FIGURE 18.10 *A lateral radiograph of a post-traumatic C5-6 bilateral facet fracture dislocation producing quadriplegia.*

PULMONARY CARE The injured but stable, intubated cervical-spine–injured patient must be closely observed for the slow development of respiratory failure secondary to fatigue of the diaphragm and/or secretion aspiration. Many patients require endotracheal intubation after several days of stability, ultimately requiring lengthy periods of ventilatory support. The mechanism for this delayed deterioration may involve edema of the spinal cord in the area around the initial injury.

Pulmonary function is evaluated and followed by continuous pulse oximetry, intermittent arterial blood gas analysis, negative inspiratory force, respiratory rate, forced vital capacity, and maximal voluntary ventilation. Patients should also have a suction device available to them; a handheld device is acceptable for a paraplegic patient. A mounted device accessible by head movement is required for the quadriplegic. Periodic (every 2 to 4 days if the patient is stable) chest radiograms is helpful to follow development of atelectasis or aspiration. Pulmonary toilet is critical, as these patients may develop micro- or macroatelectasis. If aggressive pulmonary toilet does not result in re-expansion, the patient may benefit from lavage and suction via bronchoscopy.

Normal respiratory function is accomplished primarily with the diaphragm. Extradiaphragmatic muscles (intercostal, abdominal, and accessory muscles [sternocleidomastoid, trapezius, and scalenes]) contribute about 12% toward resting ventilation and 25% at maximal levels of tidal ventilation.[158] The diaphragm, innervated via C-3, C-4, and C-5 level input, is composed of three fiber types: high-oxidative slow twitch (type I fiber, 55% of total), high-oxidative fast twitch (type IIa, 21%), and low-oxidative fast twitch (type IIb, 24%).[158] A cervical cord lesion may compromise some of these and increase the importance of the accessory musculature. In vitro studies show that after 10 minutes of stimulation, the tension generated by a diaphragmatic muscle strip is primarily due to high-oxidative slow-twitch fibers.[158] Although parameters such as respiratory rate, negative inspiratory force, and forced vital capacity have been used to determine the readiness of a patient for endotracheal decannulation, these measurements are primarily measures of strength and utilize mostly low-oxidative, fast-twitch fibers.[159] However, spinal cord injury patients may have difficulties with endurance as well as strength. This is evaluated using maximal voluntary ventilation, which appears to evaluate primarily high-oxidative, slow-twitch fibers. Recently, the ability to measure clinically the work of breathing has become available. Work performed by the patient and by the ventilator are measurable; such measurements may allow more rapid ventilator weaning in some patients. A recent study evaluating the ability to rapidly wean by clinical versus work of breathing crite-

TABLE 18.7 *Major morbidity associated with unfractionated heparin*

	% CASES SEEN
Hemorrhage	
Major	1–33%
Fatal	0.5%
Thrombocytopenia	
Mild[a]	2–5%
Severe	Rare
Other	
Osteoporosis	Rare
Spontaneous vertebral fractures	Rare
Hyperkalemia[b]	Rare

[a] Two to fifteen days after drug initiation.

[b] Secondary to aldosterone synthesis inhibition.

ria showed that in a medical ICU population, clinical criteria led to more prolonged weaning than did work of breathing criteria.[160] Further study is needed in this area.

The risk of deep venous thrombosis and pulmonary embolus in this subset of neurosurgical patients not receiving prophylaxis is of concern, with a recorded clinical incidence from 13 to 84% (untreated) and 4 to 15%[161–163] in the prophylactically treated groups. As the diagnosis of deep venous thrombosis and pulmonary embolus can be quite difficult and therapy with full-dose heparin carries significant morbidity and mortality (Table 18.7), emphasis should be placed on prevention. Thus, patients should be prophylactically treated with pneumatic compression stockings and subcutaneous heparin; the latter is dosed at 5,000 units every 8 to 12 hours. Recent data suggest that low-molecular-weight heparin may be more effective than traditional unfractionated forms[164,165]; the dose for this agent is 50 to 70 units/kg administered subcutaneously every day.[165]

CARDIOVASCULAR PROBLEMS Patients with acute spinal cord injury generally require continuous cardiac monitoring. Neurogenic shock occurs secondary to loss of descending sympathetic innervation, resulting in decreased vascular tone and vagal input to the heart, causing decreased cardiac output and bradycardia. These negative responses may initially be treated with fluids or relatively low-dose β-agonists, such as dopamine, 3 to 5 μg/kg/min. Significant bradycardia can be treated with intravenous glycopyrrolate or atropine, 0.2 to 0.4 mg. Alternatively, an external pacemaker may be used in urgent situations. If large amounts of intravenous fluids are required for blood pressure maintenance, invasive monitoring with a balloon flotation pulmonary artery catheter should be considered. Cardiac instability may last for several weeks, necessitating ICU care during this period.

GASTROINTESTINAL PROBLEMS Patients with spinal cord injury may have profound problems with the ileus shortly after the accident, resulting in delayed gastric emptying and increasing the risk of pulmonary aspiration of gastric contents. Initially, a nasogastric tube that can be removed after 2 to 5 days should be placed. Serial abdominal examinations should be performed to determine whether the patient is becoming more distended; abdominal radiography may help determine the etiology. A bowel regimen, utilizing daily stool softeners and, when needed, enemas, should be started early and can prevent the unpleasant problem of impaction. These patients are also at risk for pancreatitis, cholestasis, and gastrointestinal bleeding. Unfortunately, their ability to sense abdominal pain is compromised and the problem may not be obvious until quite advanced. Serial hematocrits and intermittent stool guaiac studies will help identify occult blood loss; intermittent serum liver function studies and amylase and lipase determination may assist in the diagnosis of pancreatitis.

Early feeding, preferably utilizing the gut, is important due to the large caloric demands imposed by severe injury. These demands may reach 30 to 40 kcal/kg ideal body weight. We initiate feeding by assuming a requirement of about 30 kcal/kg and an approximate 1 g/kg amino acid need. If possible, all feedings are enteral, using a small bowel feeding tube. As feeding is begun, a metabolic cart for caloric expenditure is obtained, as is serum prealbumin ($T_{1/2}$ 2 days); the latter is followed twice weekly to ensure progressive anabolism. If the serum prealbumin decreases or does not increase to the normal range, calorie/protein requirements are re-evaluated.

GENITOURINARY COMPLICATIONS Urosepsis is one of the leading causes of death in patients with severe cervical spine injuries. The injury results in bladder atony with incomplete emptying and may require either chronic indwelling or intermittent catheterization. If the residual urine volume following reflex emptying is greater than or equal to 100 ml, catheterization will likely be necessary. High-pressure reflex voiding may sometimes be improved using α-adrenergic blocking and antispasticity agents.[166] Bacterial colonization of urine is quite common, but antibiotic therapy is withheld unless patients become symptomatic with fever, pyuria, leukocyte casts, or more than 10^5 bacteria/ml in the urine. The use of prophylactic antibiotics selects for resistant microorganisms and is therefore infrequently recommended.

SKIN CARE Pressure sores are one of the most common causes of morbidity in spinal-cord–injured patients.[166] Proper skin care, involving padding of contact points with the bed, traction apparatus, and halo vest, and changing the patient's body position every 15 minutes to 2 hours are of great significance in the critically ill, neurologically injured patient. The sores begin as areas of erythema in the location of pressure points and progress to deep ulcers if not rapidly treated. Superficial damage can be protected with an occlusive barrier; a deeper wound may require wet to dry gauze dressings several times daily. If not controlled, skin breakdown may ultimately require debridement and skin grafting or tissue flaps. The cost of surgical treatment of a pressure sore is reported to be in excess of $50,000.[166]

CONSERVATIVE VERSUS OPERATIVE CARE Some patients with spine fractures and spinal cord injury should be treated conservatively with a halo or other external orthosis, whereas others require surgical decompression and stabilization. Prior to current technology, investigators showed that conservative therapy could improve the patient's clinical status.[167–170] Others have felt that surgical decompression and more accurate anatomical correction should naturally provide the best outcome. Some studies have suggested that early surgical stabilization has a beneficial effect on hospital cost, length of stay, and residual spinal deformity.[171,172] Marshall et al.[173] and Heidan et al.,[174] treating all levels of spinal trauma, respectively found an approximate 3% increase in neurologic deterioration when surgery was performed within 5 days of cervical spine fracture, with a significantly increased risk of pulmonary complications.[173,174] Similar rates of deterioration were not noted when surgery was performed after the fifth postinjury day. Other series have also noted the potential for deterioration after surgical correction of spinal trauma.[175,176]

In another study of 14 patients with thoracic spine fracture and spinal cord injury, however, surgical decompression and stabilization improved final outcome by 2.2 Frankel grades.[177] Donovan reviewed the literature and found that considerations of the patient's general medical condition, coexisting trauma, degree of instability, and the degree of incompleteness of the neurologic injury all impacted on surgical decision making.[178] He felt that surgery was indicated in patients who deteriorated neurologically or who had incomplete neurologic injuries. Surgical intervention also allowed these patients access to earlier and more aggressive rehabilitation.

PREVENTION OF SECONDARY SPINAL INJURY Several different compounds have been examined and others are currently being investigated in clinical trials for secondary protection after spinal cord injury. The most successful agent is methylprednisolone, used extensively in animal and human trials. The NASCIS

II trial examined methylprednisolone and naloxone after spinal cord injury, finding that the former agent, given as a bolus dose of 30 mg/kg within 8 hours of the injury and followed by a 5.4 mg/kg/h infusion for the following 23 hours, significantly improved motor outcomes at 6 weeks, 6 months, and 1 year[179]; naloxone therapy showed no benefit. A phase III study is now underway examining the effect of the current methylprednisolone-dosing regimen against methylprednisolone therapy extended for 48 hours and methylprednisolone bolus, 30 mg/kg, followed by tirilazad, a 21-aminosteroid, 2.5 mg/kg, for 48 hours. The outcome of the phase III studies are critical, because even though methylprednisolone treatment is the standard of care for spinal cord injury patients, many investigators remain skeptical about its effectiveness.

Tirilazad is a 21-aminosteroid that functions through inhibition of iron-mediated lipid peroxidation, which may protect neuronal membranes from oxygen free-radical–induced secondary injury.[180,181] The protective effects of tirilazad have been suggested in a large ongoing study of SAH patients. An advantage of the 21-aminosteroid is its lack of adverse glucocorticoid effects, including glucose intolerance, immune suppression, and aseptic bone necrosis.

Polyethylene glycol conjugated superoxide dismutase, a free-radical scavenger, displays an extended half-life and has been used in animal studies of aortic occlusion with some initial positive effects.[182] Another agent, GM1 ganglioside, appears to function through augmentation of neurite outgrowth and restoration of neuronal function. In a phase I trial, 34 spinal cord injury patients began therapy within 48 hours of injury and continued for 26 days. The data suggest significant improvement in the treatment group compared with the control patients.[183] This work requires further elaboration.

Many of the theories of secondary injury include increased calcium influx as a mechanism for neuronal death. Although the calcium channel blocker nimodipine has been used in animal studies of thoracic aorta cross-clamping with some positive effects,[184] other work using flunarizine was equivocal.[185] An alternative mode of therapy involves intrathecal infusion of substances such as papaverine to dilate the longitudinal spinal arteries. This agent is thought to work via blockade of calcium channels and impairment of free-radical formation. Initial studies in patients undergoing aortic operations suggest that papaverine may protect the spinal cord.[184]

Seizures

Seizures are a serious problem, particularly in the ICU. For example, recognition of seizures or new neurologic deficits in the immediate postoperative period may be delayed due to residual anesthetic agent. The seizure may affect the airway or cause the patient to suffer injuries to the extremities resulting from uncontrolled movements during the ictal episode. Seizures may also cause structural brain injury, predisposing the patient to further seizures.[186] Status epilepticus carries a serious risk of death ranging as high as 20%. Seizures may put the postoperative patient at increased risk of cerebral acidosis, cerebral edema, and increased ICP.[187]

Patients with a preoperative history of seizure are at greatest risk for early postoperative (within 48 hours) ictal activity (27.7% vs. 10.6% without previous history of seizures).[188] The extent of cortical injury and postoperative metabolic derangements—primarily hypoxia, hypernatremia, hyponatremia, hyperglycemia, and acidosis—also increase seizure risk. Surgical retraction can also be associated with risk for postoperative seizures. Extra-axial lesions, such as aneurysms, have a postoperative risk of seizure activity from 3 to 4%.[188,189] Anticonvulsant levels are also of critical importance. North and colleage found that inadequate phenytoin levels were seen in 89% of seizures occurring in patients treated with the anticonvulsive agent postoperatively.[90]

Certain tumor types have an increased risk of associated postoperative seizures. Benign lesions are associated with a higher relative incidence of seizures: oligodendroglioma, 50 to 81%; astrocytoma, 40 to 66%; ependymoma, 33 to 50%; glioblastoma, 30 to 42%; meningioma, 30 to 40%; and metastatic lesions, 19 to 26%.[186] The increased frequency of seizures seen with benign tumors may be related to the longer life span of those with nonmalignant lesions. The series of Fukamachi et al. showed the incidence of immediate postoperative seizures to be highly associated with meningiomas followed by glioblastomas and benign astrocytomas.[188]

As expected, supratentorial tumors are associated with higher risks of seizure activity, with an incidence between 35 and 80%.[186,191] The specific location of the tumor is also a critical factor.[186] Tumors in close proximity to the motor strip appear to be highly susceptible to epileptic activity.[186] Correcting for orientation to the motor strip results in a particularly high seizure incidence: ictal activity is seen in 83% of oligodendroglioma/astrocytomas, 71% of meningiomas, and 53% of glioblastomas. In a study of tumor patients with preoperative seizures, Mahaley and Dudka showed that frontal, temporal, and parietal lesions all had a seizure incidence of 41 to 45%, whereas that for occipital lesions was 14%.[192] Ramamurthi et al. examined 127 patients with meningioma and found that, of the 37 (29%) patients with preoperative seizures, 27 (73%) had frontal or parietal lesions, whereas only 10 (27%) patients with temporal, occipital, posterior fossa, and miscellaneous locations had seizures.[193] Although posterior fossa tumors are associated with a decreased incidence of early seizure activity (1.8%), an increased incidence (7%) has been noted with medulloblastoma.[194]

Although seizure type may vary by tumor location, the preponderance of data suggests that seizure qualities are the same pre- and postoperatively.[188,193] Time to onset of seizure is brief, usually occurring in the immediate postoperative period. Two series suggest that 25 to 38% of all seizures will occur in the first 24 to 72 hours,[190,194] 45% within the first week, and 64% within the first month.[190]

Deutschman and Haines reviewed several series that strongly point to the benefits of preoperative initiation of prophylactic anticonvulsives, usually phenytoin.[186] Their review of both efficacy and complications (10 to 15% were serious enough to change therapy) suggests that prophylactic therapy of up to 16 weeks of, initiated preoperatively and in which therapeutic anticonvulsant levels are maintained, is likely to lower risks. Phenytoin dosing schedules have been suggested: 15 mg/kg (about 1 g) over the 20 minutes prior to wound closure followed by 5 to 6 mg/kg/day (in three divided doses) postoperatively.[187] Our policy is similar; however, we give phenytoin at the beginning of the case, as late administration of anticonvulsants may delay emergence from anesthesia. Therapeutic levels of 10 to 20 μg/ml are achieved.

Approximately 5,000 new cases of post-traumatic epilepsy occur annually and can be divided into three categories: early onset (within 24 hours of the traumatic event), delayed onset (within 1 to 7 days), and late onset (more than 7 days).[126] Early or delayed seizures occur in 3.6 to 14% and late seizures occur in 10 to 27% of head-injured patients.[195–197] The major predisposing factors responsible for development are penetrating head trauma, focal neurologic deficits, hematoma formation, depressed skull fracture, post-traumatic amnesia, CNS infection, and loss of consciousness for greater than 1 hour.[198]

Results of double-blinded studies evaluating the prophylactic use of antiseizure medication post-trauma are somewhat equivocal. Tempkin et al. suggest that phenytoin is an effective prophylactic treatment for seizures in the first week postinjury, but other studies have failed to find any benefit.[195–197] Even in controlled trials, it may be difficult to obtain compliance in this population, so assessment of the true benefit of these medications is difficult. Generally, we suggest that phenytoin, 10 mg/kg load followed by 5 to 7 mg/kg/day in three divided doses and aiming for a level of between 10 and 20 μg/ml, or some other anticonvulsant be continued at least 2 weeks after the injury if there has been no seizure activity. If a seizure occurs, drug therapy should be continued for a year postevent, and an EEG should be obtained prior to slow taper of the medication. A retrospective study carried out for the years 1984 to 1988 showed that patients undergoing supratentorial procedures who were treated intraoperatively with penicillin had almost twice the incidence of early postoperative seizures as those not given this class of antibiotics.[199]

Infections of the CNS

The neurointensivist may be faced with a wide variety of primary CNS infections, including meningitis, encephalitis, postoperative neurosurgical infections, and traumatic CNS infections. Human immunodeficiency disease (HIVD), in particular, has resulted in the emergence or re-emergence of previously rare infectious entities. The unifying theme in dealing with all these problems is thorough evaluation and rapid treatment.

Meningitis

Bacterial meningitis represents a deadly problem. Mortality can range from 6 to 34%, depending on the availability of medical care and antibiotics.[200,201] Morbidity, which is related to bacterial cell wall components stimulating the production of tumor necrosis factor, IL-1, and IL-6, in addition to platelet-activating factor, prostaglandins, and other eicosanoids, can be significant and, ironically, worsened by antimicrobial therapy.[202] The most common neonatal pathogens are group B streptococci, *Escherichia coli*, and *Listeria monocytogenes*. *Hemophilus influenzae* and *Neisseria meningitides* in childhood and *Streptococcus pneumoniae* and *N. meningitides* in adulthood are the predominant organisms. The source of infection may be from bacteremia, endocarditis, pulmonary infection, or local extension from sinusitis, otitis media, mastoiditis, or osteomyelitis. Classically, patients present with high fever, meningismus, and, later, altered mental status. Patients with *N. meningitides* infection may also have a petechial rash. In clinical practice, however, signs and symptoms may vary, especially if the patient is elderly or immunosuppressed. Findings in the CSF may include opening pressure greater than or equal to 400 mm H_2O in 20% of patients, a white blood cell count of greater than or equal to 100 cells/ml in 80 to 90%, protein greater than 45 mg/dl in 96%, and glucose less than 20 mg/dl in 45 to 50%.[201] Latex agglutination and counterimmunoelectrophoresis tests for *H. influenzae*, *N. meningitides*, and *S. pneumoniae* may also be helpful. The latter study has an accuracy of about 80%.[203] Neonatal meningitis is usually treated with ampicillin and gentamicin or a combination of these with a third-generation cephalosporin. Childhood meningitis may be treated with ceftriaxone, as it sterilizes the CSF faster than cefuroxime.[204] Meningitis in adults may also be treated with ceftriaxone or, if the pathogen is *S. pneumoniae*, with penicillin. Close attention must be paid to culture and antimicrobial sensitivity results and therapy altered accordingly. The use of steroids to decrease morbidity remains controversial.[202]

Fungal meningitis is rare except in immunosuppressed individuals such as those with HIVD and in transplant patients. *Cryptococcus neoformans* and *Coccidioides immitis* are the most common fungal agents causing meningitis. *C. neoformans* has four capsular antigen types, of which serotype A is most common in the United States. This agent is usually associated with pigeon droppings but can also be found in fruit, vegetables, milk, and soil.[205,206] The organism is usually inhaled and initially causes a pulmonary infection that is asymptomatic or self-limited. Days to weeks later, patients begin to complain of mild headache and show signs of minimal fever and personality changes. The meninges and brain, primarily perivascular cortical gray matter and basal ganglia, become inflamed and edematous. CSF shows normal to slightly elevated opening pressure, elevated protein, depressed glucose, and a predominantly lymphocytic pleocytosis.[206] India ink stain will be positive in 50% of non-HIVD and 75% of HIVD patients.[207,208] Culture is positive in 95% of cases[206]; latex agglutination detection of capsular antigen is highly sensitive and specific. A 6-week course of intravenous amphotericin B is standard therapy.

Patients with HIVD may benefit from flucytosine plus amphotericin B,[205] and will need chronic suppressive therapy with daily fluconazole or weekly amphotericin B.[206]

Coccidioides immitis is most common in the arid climate of the southwestern United States. As with *C. neoformans*, *C. immitis* begins as a mild pulmonary infection that disseminates to the CNS; only about 1% with primary disease will develop disseminated coccidioidomycosis.[204] The infection is usually subacute with the development of low-grade fever, headache, and mental status changes. Nausea, vomiting, focal neurologic deficits, and seizures may develop, but signs of meningeal irritation are uncommon. *C. immitis* tends to affect the basal meninges with granulomatous changes and therefore mimics tuberculous meningitis. CSF studies are similar to those seen in cryptococcal disease, but the organism is cultured from CSF in only about 50% of patients. Amphotericin B is the drug of choice, although intrathecal therapy is required for meningeal involvement. Therapy may be required for years.

Candida albicans is the most commonly isolated fungus in humans because it is a commensal organism. However, even with disseminated candidiasis, meningitis is uncommonly diagnosed in the antemortem state. In an autopsy series, *Candida* was the most common fungal agent infecting the CNS.[204] *Candida* meningitis tends to occur in immunosuppressed patients and causes multiple parenchymal microabscesses. Histoplasmosis, blastomycosis, and mucormycosis can all cause infections in the CNS but are relatively uncommon. Amphotericin B is currently the drug of choice for all of these organisms.

Aseptic meningitis is often associated with viral meningitis and can have a variety of etiologies, including nonpolio enterovirus (42%), polio virus (12%), mumps (22%), lymphocytic choriomeningitis virus (12%), leptospirosis (5%), herpes simplex (2%), arbovirus (1%), and others (2%).[209] Other agents, such as HIV and the Lyme agent, can also cause aseptic meningitis. As many as 8,300 to 12, 700 cases of aseptic meningitis are reported annually, but many cases are thought to go unreported.[210–216]

Enterovirus infection is the most common cause of aseptic meningitis, occurring most often in the warmer months of the year. Infants and young children are frequently affected with this self-limited disease. Presenting signs include headache, pharyngitis, low-grade fever, malaise, and nausea and vomiting. The CSF usually shows mild lymphocyte pleocytosis, but in the acute phase, polymorphonuclear cells may predominate. Protein levels are normal or slightly elevated. Glucose is usually normal but in about 20% of patients will be decreased. Other than supportive care, there is no specific treatment. Except for infants who may have ataxia, weakness, paralysis, or perceptive language deficits,[209] most individuals are ultimately left without residual.

Poliovirus, a member of the enterovirus family, is rarely symptomatic, with only 4 to 8% of the patients developing aseptic meningitis, and no more than 1 to 2% developing paralytic polio.[217] Mumps (paramyxovirus) may also cause aseptic meningitis, which, although usually benign and self-limited, can sometimes be associated with encephalitis, seizures, polyradiculitis, polyneuritis, cranial nerve palsies, myelitis, Guillain-Barré syndrome, and death. Transient bilateral deafness is seen in 1 to 5% of patients, with residual unilateral deafness occurring in less than 1 in 30,000 cases.[209] CSF findings are similar to those in enterovirus infection.

Lymphocytic choriomeningitis, an arenavirus transmitted to humans by contact with rodents or their excreta,[209] is a another benign form of aseptic meningitis that develops subacutely and has symptoms reflecting meningeal irritation. It is most often self-limited, lasts 1 to 4 weeks, and requires only supportive care.

Mycobacteria may cause aseptic meningitis-like symptoms. Primarily affecting the basal meninges, it may present with cranial nerve deficits, altered mental status, or SIADH. Chlamydia, *Mycoplasma pneumoniae*, and spirochetal infection may also resemble aseptic meningitis.

Differential Diagnosis of the Acute Aseptic Meningitis Syndrome: Noninfectious Diseases or Diseases of Unknown Etiology

- Lymphomatous meningitis
- Carcinomatous meningitis
- Leukemia
- Intracranial tumors/cysts
  - Craniopharyngioma
  - Dermoid/epidermoid cyst
  - Pituitary adenoma
  - Astrocytoma
  - Glioblastoma multiforme
  - Medulloblastoma
  - Pinealoma
  - Ependymoma
  - Teratoma
- Medications
  - Trimethoprim
  - Sulfamethoxazole
  - Trimethoprim-sulfamethoxazole
  - Ibuprofen
  - Sulindac
  - Naproxen
  - Tolmetin
  - OKT3
  - Azathioprine[a]
  - Isoniazid
  - Cytosine arabinoside (high dose)
  - Carbamazepine[a]
  - Immune gobulin
  - Phenazopyridine
  - Penicillin
- Serum sickness
- Heavy metal poisoning: lead, arsenic
- Systemic illnesses
  - Systemic lupus erythematosus
  - Sarcoidosis
  - Behçet's disease
  - Sjogren's syndrome
  - Mixed connective tissue disease
  - Rheumatoid arthritis
  - Polymyositis
  - Wegener's granulomatosis
  - Polyarteritis nodosa
  - Granulomatous angiitis
  - Other cerebral vasculitides
  - Familial Mediterranean fever
  - Kawasaki's syndrome
  - Vogt-Koyanagi-Harada syndromes
- Procedure related
  - Postneurosurgery
  - Spinal anesthesia
  - Intrathecal injection of air, dyes, isotopes, antibiotics, antineoplastics, steroids, serum
  - Chymopapain injection
  - Pleocytosis postseizure
  - First presentation of recurrent benign meningitis (Mollaret's meningitis)

[a] In patients with connective tissue disorders.
(From Connolly and Hammer,[209] with permission.)

Noninfectious causes of aseptic meningitis include medications such as ibuprofen, naproxen, tolmetin, sulindac, and trimethoprim-sulfamethoxazole.[209] Tumors may cause aseptic meningitis either through direct infiltration of leukemia, lymphoma, or metastatic disease or via release of irritating substances from dermoid/epidermoid tumors, craniopharyngiomas, or infarcted pituitary tumors. Vasculitic or connective tissue diseases such as sarcoidosis, systemic lupus erythematosus, or Behçet's disease may all cause a form of aseptic meningitis. These patients often respond favorably to treatment with steroids. Postoperative neurosurgical patients, particularly those who have undergone posterior fossa procedures, are at risk for aseptic meningitis secondary to irritation from blood.[203]

Aseptic meningitis may mimic bacterial meningitis, creating a dilemma for the physician. Although some advocate close observation and repeat lumbar puncture in patients with recent exposure to community viral outbreaks who appear well, the risk associated with missing a bacterial infection is so great that most physicians, ourselves included, start antibiotics and await culture results. Serial cultures that return consistently negative then lead to consideration of discontinuing the antibiotic regimen.

HIVD-Related Infections

HIVD/acquired immunodeficiency syndrome (AIDS) is a problem of epidemic proportions, with many related infectious complications affecting the CNS. AIDS dementia complex (ADC) caused by HIV infection of the CNS encompasses cognitive motor and behavioral changes. Patients become forgetful and have slowed mentation. Other signs, which may be progressive, include difficulty with balance and lower extremity weakness. These individuals may appear depressed, are socially withdrawn and apathetic, or, conversely, may appear manic or psychotic.[218] Although possibly an underestimate of the true incidence, as this diagnosis is not usually seen until late in the disease and CDC data are based upon presenting problems,[219] 1992 statistics suggest that 7.3% of AIDS patients have ADC. There are no good studies available to make the diagnosis of ADC, although there are attempts to correlate the amount of atrophy relative to the severity of the clinical condition.

HIV likely reaches the CNS via infected macrophages or T cells.[218,220] There is no evidence of neuronal infection, but nonproductive infection occurs in astrocytes.[221] HIV infection appears to occur primarily in the subcortical white and deep gray nuclei. Neuronal death, presumably the cause of the dementia, is likely secondary to indirect mechanisms. Studies have suggested that secondary injury to neuronal elements may occur through changes in calcium flux[222] or cytokines,[223,224] or through activation of NMDA receptors.[225] Treatment with the antiretroviral agent zidovudine has been controversial and may only be effective at higher doses of 1,000 mg/day.[218,226]

Cerebral toxoplasmosis is the most common cerebral mass lesion, occurring in 3 to 40% of patients with HIVD/AIDS.[218] Cerebral toxoplasmosis tends to be multifocal and has a predisposition for the choroid plexus, suggesting hematogenous spread.[227,228] The disorder tends to be seen late in the course of HIVD/AIDS when $CD4^+$ counts are less than 200 cells/μl.[229] Although common symptoms are headache, confusion, and fever, patients may also have lethargy, seizures, or focal neurologic deficits. CT or MRI scans of the head may identify the lesions of cerebral toxoplasmosis; addition of contrast may improve detection. Although absence does not rule out the disease, immunoglobulin G (IgG) antibody to *Toxoplasma* is present in about 80% of patients.[229] Therapy is classically composed of oral pyrimethamine, 200 mg as a load followed by 50 to 75 mg/day, and sulfadiazine, 4 to 6 g/day in four divided doses. Folinic acid is given to prevent the hematologic toxic effects of pyrimethamine.[227] Alternatively, pyrimethamine and clindamycin have also been shown to be an effective treatment.[227] Stereotactic biopsy may be required if the patient fails to improve within 1 to 2 weeks.[230]

Although prior to the HIVD/AIDS epidemic, primary CNS lymphoma was relatively rare, the incidence of this malignancy in non-HIVD patients has significantly increased over the past 20 years for reasons that are unknown.[231] In the HIVD population, it generally occurs late in the disease when the $CD4^+$ count is less than 100 cells/μl.[218] Epstein-Barr virus appears to be highly associated with these tumors.[218,232] Patients may present with signs and symptoms similar to toxoplasmosis, and imaging studies may be similar, resulting in a diagnostic dilemma. A single lesion on a CT or MRI scan and negative *Toxoplasma* titers suggests consideration of CNS lymphoma; stereotactic biopsy may be required and will result in a definitive diagnosis in 85 to 90% of cases. The prognosis of CNS lymphoma has generally been poor, with an untreated survival time of less than 1 month, and 4 to 6 months with radiation.[231] However, the quality of life is improved in over 75% of patients so treated.

Progressive multifocal leukoencephalopathy

occurs from an infection with the human papillomavirus. One study reported the incidence of this disease in AIDS patients at 4%, with 29% having this disorder as the AIDS indicator disease.[233] Patients present with weakness, visual loss, cognitive dysfunction, limb incoordination, dysarthria, and other focal neurologic deficits.[233] Neuropathologically, the infection causes a pronounced white matter demyelinating process, especially at the gray-white matter junction and in the cortical gray matter. The lesions appear as multiple white matter plaques usually in the parieto-occipital area on T2-weighted MRI scans. $CD4^+$ counts will be less than 100 cells/μl on presentation.[233,234] Median survival is usually 2 to 4 months, but approximately 10% of patients will survive longer. Although some groups have attempted high-dose zidovudine and cytarabine therapy, this has not been particularly successful.[234,235]

Infections Related to Neurosurgical Intervention

Postcraniotomy infections are uncommon because of the extreme care taken by neurosurgeons in preincision skin preparation and the use of sterile technique. The overall infection rate for clean cases, shown in several studies, is between 2 (with perioperative antibiotics) and 6% (without antibiotics).[203] Factors that may increase infection risk are length of the procedure, reoperations, increased patient age, and postoperative CSF leak. Although gram-positive or negative organisms may be involved, *Staphylococcus* species are commonly isolated. Wound examination often is the only diagnostic study required, but neuroimaging and/or measurements of an elevated erythrocyte sedimentation rate or C-reactive protein may occasionally be helpful. Treatment involves wound drainage, culture and Gram's stain of drained material, and broad-spectrum antibiotics. At our institution, vancomycin and ceftazidime are the antibiotics most commonly used initially. When culture and sensitivity results become available, the antibiotic regimen is tailored accordingly.

Ventriculostomy infections may be life threatening in patients otherwise recovering uneventfully from surgery. In a series of 256 patients, Ohrstrom et al. reported an 11% infection rate, although they comment that rates as high as 27% have been noted.[236] The traditional dogma that ventriculostomies need weekly changing stems from the study of Mayhall et al. suggesting a significant increase in the infection rate after 5 days.[13] However, other work gave a more evenly distributed infection rate and suggested that increasing the frequency of change might increase the rate of infection.[236] Our procedure is to change ventriculostomies weekly. Ventriculitis, once initiated, becomes a difficult infection to eradicate. *Staphylococcus epidermidis* and *Staphylococcus aureus* are the most common agents noted, but other gram-positive or -negative organisms are seen.[234] Ventricular infection causes changes in the choroid plexus that results in decreased (by 50 to 67%) CSF production.[237] The most important associated factor for infection was the presence or absence of a CSF leak around the ventricular catheter; incidence of infection was 2% without a leak and 13% with a CSF leak.[238]

Therapy for shunt-associated ventriculitis involves removal of the infected catheter and treatment for 2 weeks with intravenous and intrathecal[239] antibiotics. As CSF vancomycin levels may not be adequate despite meningeal inflammation,[240] intraventricular vancomycin and/or gentamicin may provide important adjunctive therapy, particularly in serious infections. In one study of ventriculitis associated with shunts or external drains, 22 of 24 cases were cured (two were lost to follow-up) when systemic and ventricular antibiotics and shunt removal were used as therapy.[241] Although the standard dose of intraventricular vancomycin is 20 mg daily, this may need adjusting for ventricular size. Nonetheless, despite high doses, there were no problems noted with intraventricular administration of vancomycin.

Guillain-Barré Syndrome

Guillain-Barré syndrome, an immune-mediated subacute demyelinating polyneuropathy, causes peripheral nerve damage that can lead to cranial neuropathies, quadriparesis, and respiratory failure. It is the most common cause of acute flaccid paralysis in previously healthy people, occurring at a rate of 0.6 to 1.9 cases per 100,000 people per year.[242] There is usually a history of recent viral respiratory or gastrointestinal infection, cytomegalovirus infection, or immunization prior to the onset of symptoms. The disease progresses over several days to 3 weeks and then slowly improves. Patients usually notice lower extremity paresthesias followed by weakness. Sensory deficits are variable. Cranial neuropathies may occur first or may follow the lower extremity changes. Although most patients have a functional recovery, approximately 15% have residual deficits and about 5% remain disabled.

Electromyographic and nerve conduction velocity studies typically show a pattern of multifocal demyelination with Guillain-Barré syndrome, including reduced conduction velocity, partial motor conduction block, prolongation of distal sensory and motor latencies, and delayed or absent F or H responses.[242] Analysis of the CSF usually shows a paucity of cells, although a mild mononuclear pleocytosis may be seen; the protein content is frequently elevated. Thorough medical evaluation accompanies the standard neurologic examination as approximately 65% of patients have some autonomic dysfunction.[243] These may include blood pressure, lability, arrhythmias (especially bradycardia and heart block), urinary retention, sweating abnormalities, and gastrointestinal dysfunction. Patients are at risk for respiratory failure and should be followed every 4 to 6 hours with a bedside assessment of pulmonary function. Patients who generate a negative inspiratory force of greater than –20 cm H_2O and a forced vital capacity of less than 12 ml/kg, who also have hypoxia and difficulty clearing secretions should be prophylactically intubated prior to clinical respiratory failure.[244,245] These parameters may be assessed at regular intervals to evaluate for return of function. Intubation for several weeks without ability to wean may require a tracheostomy. Approximately 60% of patients may temporarily need a tracheostomy.[244,245]

Cardiovascular lability usually warrants continuous blood pressure and ECG monitoring; bradycardia or heart block may benefit from glycopyrrolate or atropine.[243] Nutritional needs are often considerable and are handled as described above. It is our preference to provide enteral feeds so as to maintain a functional and trophic small bowel and, thus, possibly help to prevent bacterial translocation. Gastric emptying is often delayed, so continuous feeding distal to the pylorus is preferable. Metoclopropamide should not be used as it may cause a dystonic reaction.[242] General care for mobility of joints and prevention of skin breakdown is crucial, as is psychosocial support. This disease can be devastating for both the patient and family, so good communication, counseling, and, occasionally, the addition of antidepressants are of significant help.

Definitive treatment for Guillain-Barré syndrome is still debatable. Attempts to use methylprednisolone 500 mg daily for 5 days, exclusively, failed to show superiority over a placebo.[244] A large multicenter study compared what had been the traditional treatment, plasma exchange, with intravenous human IgG, 0.4 g/kg/day, and found that the latter was at least as good and perhaps superior.[247] This was confirmed by a recent retrospective pediatric study showing shorter duration to improvement and fewer days of mechanical ventilation in the intravenous IgG group.[248] Plasma exchange is believed to work by removing pathogenic antibodies. The mechanism of action for intravenous IgG is less clear and may work by anti-idiotypic Ab effect, complement absorption, downregulation of immunoglobulin production, receptor blockade, virus neutralization, enhancement of suppressor cells, and/or inhibition of lymphocyte proliferation.[249] These results, however, are tempered by the fact that there is tremendous variability in presenting symptoms and severity of Guillain-Barré syndrome in different patients. There also have been several reports of patients relapsing after intravenous IgG and subsequently improving with plasma exchange.[250–252] The Dutch Guillain-Barré study group is now studying the effect of combined methylprednisolone and intravenous IgG with initial favorable results.[253]

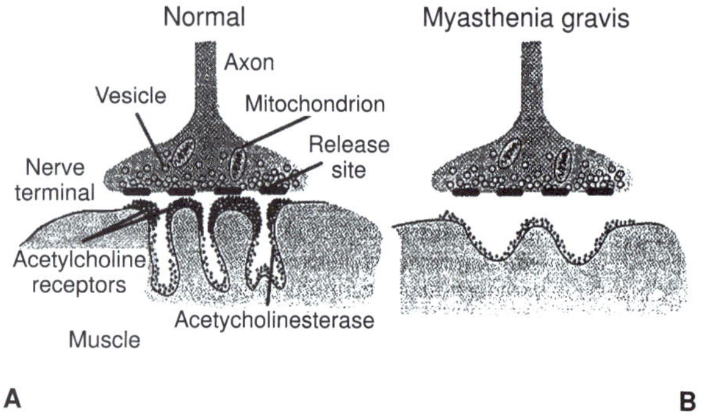

FIGURE 18.11 *Normal (A) and myasthenic (B) neuromuscular junctions. (From Drachman,[254] with permission.)*

Myasthenia Gravis

Myasthenia gravis, a disease resulting from antibody-mediated autoimmune attack against the acetylcholine receptors at neuromuscular junctions, has a prevalence of 5 to 12.5 cases per 100,000 people.[254] The disease is age and gender related, with one peak between the second and third decades affecting mostly females and a second peak between the sixth and seventh decades involving primarily men. Fluctuating muscle weakness, occurring in the eye, face, oropharynx, neck, or limbs, is common on presentation. Crisis occurs when oropharyngeal and respiratory muscle weakness leads to respiratory failure and the need for mechanical ventilation. Diagnosis is based on the tetrad of history, electrophysiologic abnormality at the neuromuscular junction (i.e., decremental response with repetitive stimulation), presence of antinicotinic acetylcholine receptors (AChRs), antibodies, and response to cholinergic drugs (i.e., clinical improvement with a test dose of 10 mg of edrophonium). Changes seen at the neuromuscular junction—fewer AChRs, simplification of the pattern of postsynaptic folding, and the increased gap between nerve terminal and postsynaptic membrane (Fig. 18.11)—fully account for the clinical and electrophysiologic findings of myasthenia gravis.[254]

A classification system has been developed for myasthenia gravis: grade I, ocular signs and symptoms only; grade IIA, generalized mild muscle weakness; grade IIB, generalized moderate weakness and/or bulbar dysfunction; grade III, severe generalized disease; grade IV, a crisis with life-threatening respiratory impairment. Several subtypes of the disease also exist.[255] A *neonatal* form occurs in 15 to 20% of babies born to myasthenic mothers. Antibody is passed to the newborn infant. This form is short term and resolves spontaneously within 2 to 4 weeks. A *congenital* form has onset between birth and 2 years, no history in the mother, and may occur in siblings; this nonfluctuating variant is compatible with long-term survival. The *juvenile* form occurs between the ages of 2 and 20 years and has a high association with anti-AChR antibody. Although there is slower progression and more frequent remissions, it is much like the adult form. There is a 4:1 female:male predominance.

Additional subtypes include drug-induced myasthenia gravis, primarily associated with D-penicillamine therapy, and a related disorder, Eaton-Lambert syndrome, a paraneoplastic syndrome associated primarily with small-cell carcinoma of the lung and having manifestations similar to myasthenia gravis. Eaton-Lambert syndrome patients tend to be 50 to 70 years of age and may complain of limb girdle muscle weakness. It is suggested that an IgG cross-reacts with presynaptic calcium channels, resulting in decremental and quantal release of acetylcholine.[255] Electromyographic findings show incremental improvement with repetitive stimulation, unlike myasthenia gravis. Electromyographic findings fail to improve with anticholinesterase agents.

Medical therapy for myasthenia gravis usually begins with acetylcholinesterase inhibitors such as pyridostigmine. The usual starting dose of this agent is 60 mg four times a day; the maximal useful dose rarely exceeds 120 mg every 3 hours.[254] Tremendous variation exists in the severity of symptomatology in myasthenia gravis patients, possibly necessitating a slow-release version of pyridostigmine for evening doses. Because of this variation, patients must be warned about the signs of cholinergic (overdosing) or myasthenic (insufficient dosing) crisis. If crisis does occur, acetylcholinesterase drugs should be withheld until the definitive cause can be determined.

Thymectomy has proven to be very effective in improving the condition of patients with myasthenia gravis.[256] Related factors that improve the effectiveness of thymectomy include the presence of thymoma rather than hyperplasia, female gender, age less than 45 years, and a higher grade of myasthenia gravis.[256] Ocular and juvenile myasthenia gravis represent mild versions of the disease for which surgery is still controversial.[254]

Plasmapheresis provides an excellent mode of therapy for acute exacerbations or crisis. It effectively lowers antibody levels and improves clinical status for 4 to 6 weeks.[257] Unfortunately, plasmapheresis may cause a rebound antibody synthesis and, thus, is more effective if used in conjunction with steroids. Plasmapheresis is particularly effective in treating ill patients prior to thymectomy as it helps decrease the incidence of postoperative pulmonary problems.

Second-line therapy involves the use of immunosuppressive drugs, steroids, azathioprine, cyclophosphamide, cyclosporin, and intravenous IgG. Steroids have traditionally been used first with considerable success. Several studies investigating the effectiveness of steroids have shown improvement in 63 to 82% of patients.[258,259] Unfortunately, these were not blinded and randomized studies; this is significant given the fluctuating nature of the disease. The decision to begin steroids is a serious one as it often means committing patients to long-term drug therapy. The starting dose of prednisone is between 15 and 100 mg/day titrated to effect[257]; titration down must be performed over weeks. Patients beginning steroid therapy should be hospitalized as increased weakness including respiratory failure may occur 48 hours after initiation of therapy. Multiple side effects have been associated with steroid therapy and include problems related to bacterial infection and cushingoid features.[260]

Azathioprine, metabolized to 6-mercaptopurine and acting primarily on T cells, can be used alone or in conjunction with steroids with effective results.[260,261] Beneficial results have a latency of 3 to 12 months with a peak at 1 to 6 years.[261] The usual starting dose is 100 mg/day (1.5 to 3 mg/kg total [not lean] body weight). In one study, therapy had a mean duration of 7 years.[262] Important side effects include pancytopenia, hepatic dysfunction, and opportunistic infections.

Intravenous IgG is an effective therapeutic agent for helping patients through periods of increased myasthenic weakness. Two to five courses are given at the onset of an exacerbation.[254,257] This drug causes no significant drop in anti-AChR antibody and does not lose efficacy with repeated use.[263] Although expensive, it is popular and effective as a treatment for acute decline.

Cyclosporin provides an additional treatment option for immunosuppression via inhibition of cytokine expression, primarily IL-2. Initially used in elderly, nonthymectomized patients who had not previously received immune suppressive therapy, it resulted in clinical improvement in many of the patients; there was, however, substantial nephrotoxicity. In a follow-up study, severely ill myasthenia gravis patients who failed treatment with thymectomy, previous long-term (more than 3 years) steroids, and azathioprine therapy benefited from treatment with cyclosporin and steroids for up to 2 years.[264] At 6 months, there was a 15% decrease in antibody titers, a 40% decrease in steroid dosage, and improvement in the quantified myasthenia gravis score.[264] Although 10% of patients suffered nephrotoxicity, an additional 45% had protocol violations or other side effects that caused them to leave the study. Currently, cyclosporin is considered effective for refractory myasthenia gravis patients; unfortunately, its price limits availability.

An alternative form of treatment for severely ill myasthenia gravis patients refractory to immunosuppression and thymectomy is total body irradiation. A recent study with a 4-year follow-up examined 12 patients with severe myasthenia gravis and exposed them to low-dose (1 to 2 Grays) total body irradiation in single 0.1-Gray doses 2 or 3 times per week during the study. Six of the 12 patients had objective clinical improvement, with a long-lasting decrease in $CD4^+$ cells, stable $CD8^+$ cells, and a decrease followed by an increase in $CD16^+$ (natural killer) and $CD20^+$ cells. Antibody titers against AChR were also decreased.[265]

Respiratory failure represents a serious complication of myasthenia gravis. In particular, patients have problems with sleep apnea and hypoventilation primarily during rapid eye movement sleep.[266] Patients at greatest risk include older patients and those with increased body mass, abnormal lung volumes, and abnormal daytime arterial blood gas values.[266] Patients with myasthenia gravis often have facial weakness and, thus, may not show the usual signs of respiratory distress.[257] Arterial blood gas analysis must be carefully watched as changes in $PaCO_2$ may occur late, and patients should have intervention at an early stage. The best noninvasive studies are forced vital capacity, negative inspiratory pressure, and maximal expiratory pressure.[267] The forced vital capacity decreases 50% when the patient has 30% of normal muscle strength. Residual volume is increased secondary to inability to exhale. Maximum voluntary ventilation is decreased by 50% in patients with respiratory failure.[257] Patients suffering from myasthenia gravis usually require only short-term ventilation, so tracheostomy is rarely required.

Patients with myasthenia gravis who do require surgery, however, have special anesthetic considerations. They have variable response to succinylcholine and often require larger doses for depolarization of the end plate. On the other hand, nondepolarizing agents have increased effect and patients often need only one-tenth the normal dose. Because these patients are so sensitive to neuromuscular blocking agents, anesthesiologists frequently prefer to use deep inhalational anesthesia with halothane.[254] Also, because these patients frequently have limited respiratory reserves, preoperative anxiolytics should be kept to low doses or withheld completely. Preoperative placement of an epidural lumbar catheter for postoperative narcotic administration has been shown to improve immediate postoperative pain control and maximize initial recovery of forced vital capacity after thymectomy via median sternotomy.[268]

Brain Death and Withdrawal of Care

The diagnosis of brain death and the ultimate withdrawal of care represent difficult emotional and ethical decisions for the intensivist (see Ch. 21). However, organ transplantation requires rapid diagnosis and appropriate care after diagnosis of brain death so that useful organs can be removed in a timely fashion. Prior to the advent of sophisticated ICU technology, pronouncement of death simply meant documenting the absence of cardiac and respiratory function. Now intensivists are faced with the requirement of determining brain death in patients who are mechanically ventilated with stable cardiac function. This problem was simplified by the President's Commission for the study of Ethical Problems in Medicine. The commission's definition of death is (1) irreversible cessation of circulatory and respiratory function, or (2) irreversible cessation of all functions of the entire brain including the brainstem.[269] The determination requires a recent history of a devastating brain injury; with sophisticated neuroimaging such as CT and MRI, this is usually well documented. There should be no recent history of drug intake (e.g., narcotics or barbiturates), which might affect the physical examination or monitoring findings. If such medications have been used, subtherapeutic drug levels or a sufficient waiting period must intervene to eliminate the confounding factors. Patients should be normothermic and have normal laboratory studies prior to determination of death.

A thorough neurologic examination must then document the absence of brain function. There should be no evidence of spontaneous respirations, and the patient should not react in any way to noxious stimulation. Brainstem examination must show fixed and dilated pupils, with no evidence of reaction to light, no corneal reflex, no gag, and no evidence of an intact oculocephalic reflex. The oculovestibular reflex should be tested with the patient's head elevated 30°. Ice water is then instilled with the use of a syringe and flexible catheter tip. This should be performed carefully so the tympanic membrane is not perforated; the brain dead patient will show no evidence of tonic deviation or nystagmus. Once these tests have verified no evidence of brain function, an apnea test can be performed.

The apnea test is performed once the patient is normothermic and has no significant metabolic derangement. First, the patient is placed on 100% oxygen and the ventilator rate is adjusted so the patient becomes normocarbic. During apnea, the $PaCO_2$ usually increases 4 mmHg in the first minute and 3 mmHg every minute afterward, so it is easy to calculate the amount of time required to reach a $PaCO_2$ of 60 mmHg. This level of CO_2 will maximally stimulate the medullary brainstem to incite breathing. The test is performed with the patient on 100% oxygen without ventilation. Apneic oxygenation, except in the presence of significant pulmonary dysfunction, prevents desaturation. After the $PaCO_2$ reaches greater than or equal to 60 mmHg without any attempt at spontaneous respiration, and in the presence of the above neurologic examination, the patient has a positive apnea test.[270] It is important that the decision to perform the apnea test be discussed with the family so that all parties are in agreement. The family should not be present at the final physical examination or during the apnea test, because Lazarus signs have been recorded, with the patient demonstrating flexion or extension reflexive movements with noxious stimuli. These findings are hypothesized to be due to remaining viable cervical neurons.[271]

Many facilities, ours included, will consider a positive apnea test in conjunction with a compatible physical examination sufficient to proclaim brain death. However, in infants, patients who have suffered extensive facial trauma, or patients who have been in barbiturate coma, ancillary studies may be necessary. The "gold standard" has traditionally been cerebral angiography,[272] but critics suggest that it is invasive, logistically difficult—requiring transport to radiology—and expensive. Alternative options, used in conjunction with clinical findings, include TCD,[273–275] evoked potential monitoring,[276,277] EEG, ^{99}Tc blood flow scans[278,279] (Fig. 18.12), and possibly[31] magnetic resonance spectroscopy.[280]

Withdrawal of care represents a difficult decision for both the family and physicians. Often, physicians feel they have failed when a patient is declared brain dead or that they will be open to medicolegal sanction if care is withdrawn when the patient is declared dead. The family may

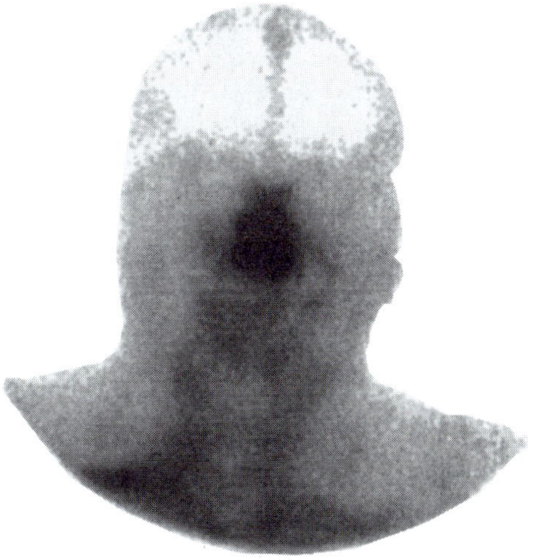

FIGURE 18.12 *HMPAO-^{99}Tc scan showing no blood flow to the brain diagnostic of brain death.*

have difficulty with this decision as they may feel responsible for the death. Thus, the declaration of brain death is a decision made with the input of all parties involved. We find it particularly helpful to have our social worker involved early with the family of the severely neurologically injured, possibly dying patient. Nonetheless, although we prefer to have family involvement and agreement, brain death is not a state that requires democratic input to be diagnosed. Education regarding advanced directives has helped both physicians and family members to understand the desires of the patient. This can also be an important legal aid as the courts usually desire to act in favor of the patient's desires or presumed desires relative to death.

References

1. Cohen PJ, Alexander SC, Smith TC et al: Effects of hypoxia and normocarbia on cerebral blood flow and metabolism in conscious man. J Appl Physiol 23:183, 1967
2. Lassen NA, Feinberg I, Lane MH: Bilateral studies of cerebral oxygen uptake in young and aged normal subjects and in patients with organic dementia. J Clin Invest 39:491, 1960
3. Schienberg P, Stead EA, Jr: The cerebral blood flow in male subjects as measured by the nitrous oxide technique: normal values for blood flow, oxygen utilization, glucose utilization, and peripheral resistance, with observations on the effect of tilting and anxiety. J Clin Invest 28:1163, 1949
4. Sokoloff L, Perlin S, Kornetsky C, Kety SS: The effects of D-lysergic acid diethylamide on cerebral circulation and overall metabolism. Ann N Y Acad Sci 66:468, 1957
5. Kety SS, Schmidt CF: The determination of cerebral blood flow in man by the use of nitrous oxide in low concentrations. Am J Physiol 143:53, 1945
6. Morawetz RB, Crowell RH, DeGirolami U et al: Regional cerebral blood flow thresholds during cerebral ischemia. Fed Proc 38:2493, 1979
7. Sharbrough FW, Messick JM, Sundt TM, Jr: Correlation of continuous electroencephalograms with cerebral blood flow measurements during carotid endarterectomy. Stroke 4:674, 1973
8. Astrup J, Siesjo BK, Symon L: Thresholds in cerebral ischemia—the ischemic penumbra. Stroke 12:723, 1981
9. Takizawa H, Gabra-Sanders T, Miller JD: Analysis of changes in intracranial pressure and pressure-volume index at different locations in the craniospinal axis during supratentorial epidural balloon inflation. Neurosurgeryery 19:1, 1986
10. Rosenwasser RH, Kleiner LI, Krzeminski JP, Buchheit WA: Intracranial pressure monitoring in the posterior fossa: a preliminary report. J Neurosurg 71:503, 1989
11. Plougmann J, Astrup J, Pedersen J, Gyldensted C: Effect of stable xenon inhalation on intracranial pressure during measurement of cerebral blood flow in head injury. J Neurosurg 81:822, 1994
12. Kanter RK, Weiner LB: Ventriculostomy-related infections (letter). N Engl J Med 311:987, 1984
13. Mayhall CG, Archer NH, Lamb VA et al: Ventriculostomy-related infections: a prospective epidemiologic study. N Engl J Med 310:553, 1984
14. Mollman HD, Rockswold GL, Ford SE: A clinical comparison of subarachnoid catheters to ventriculostomy and subarachnoid bolts: a prospective study. J Neurosurg 68:737, 1988
15. Grosset DG, Straiton J, du Trevou M, Bullock R: Prediction of symptomatic vasospasm after subarachnoid hemorrhage by rapidly increasing transcranial Doppler velocity and cerebral blood flow changes. Stroke 23:674, 1992
16. Chan KH, Miller JD, Dearden NM et al: The effect of changes in cerebral perfusion pressure upon middle cerebral artery blood flow velocity and jugular bulb venous oxygen saturation after severe brain injury. J Neurosurg 77:55, 1992
17. Goodwin SR, Friedman WA, Bellefleur M: Is it time to use evoked potentials to predict outcome in comatose children and adults? Crit Care Med 19:518, 1991
18. Barelli A, Valente MR, Clemente A et al: Serial multimodality-evoked potentials in severely head-injured patients: diagnostic and prognostic implications. Crit Care Med 19:1374, 1991
19. Luce JM, Huseby JS, Kirk W, Butler J: A Starling resistor regulates cerebral venous outflow in dogs. J Appl Physiol 53:1496, 1982
20. Toung T, Ngeow YK, Long DL et al: Comparison of the effects of positive end-expiratory pressure and jugular venous compression on canine cerebral venous pressure. Anesthesiology 61:169, 1984

21. Apuzzo JL, Weiss MH, Petersons V et al: Effect of positive end-expiratory pressure ventilation on intracranial pressure in man. J Neurosurg 46:227, 1977
22. Frost EA: Effects of positive end-expiratory pressure on intracranial pressure and compliance in brain-injured patients. J Neurosurg 47:195, 1977
23. Burchiel KJ, Steege TD, Wyler AR: Intracranial pressure changes in brain-injured patients requiring positive end-expiratory pressure ventilation. Neurosurgery 8:443, 1981
24. Cooper KR, Boswell PA, Choi SC: Safe use of PEEP in patients with severe head injury. J Neurosurg 63:552, 1985
25. Blanch PB, Jones M, Layon AJ, Camner N: Pressure-preset ventilation, 1. Physiologic and mechanical considerations. Chest 104:590, 1993. 2: Mechanics and safety. Chest 104:904, 1993
26. Plum F, Posner JB: The diagnosis of stupor and coma. Contemp Neurol Ser 10:1, 1972
27. Cherniack NS, von Euler C, Homma I, Kao FF: Experimentally induced Cheyne-Stokes breathing. Respir Physiol 37:185, 1979
28. Hodge CJ, Primrose D: Physiological considerations. p. 1572. In Apuzzo MLJ (ed): Brain Surgery: Complication Avoidance and Management. Churchill Livingstone, New York, 1993
29. Jaeckle KA, Digre KB, Jones CR et al: Central neurogenic hyperventilation: pharmacologic intervention with morphine sulfate and correlative analysis of respiratory, sleep, and ocular motor dysfunction. Neurology 40:1715, 1990
30. Mackersie RC, Christensen JM, Pitts LH, Lewis FR: Pulmonary extravascular fluid accumulation following intracranial injury. J Trauma 23:968, 1983
31. Lipman TO: Bacterial translocation and enteral nutrition in humans: an outsider looks in. J Parenter Enteral Nutr 19:156, 1995
32. Grahm TW, Zadrozny DB, Harrington T: The benefits of early jejunal hyperalimentation in the head-injured patient. Neurosurgeryery 25:729, 1989
33. Layon AJ, Florete OG, Jr, Day AL et al: The effect of duodenojejunal alimentation on gastric pH and hormones in intensive care unit patients. Chest 99:695, 1991
34. Lam AM, Winn HR, Cullen BF, Sundling N: Hyperglycemia and neurological outcome in patients with head injury. J Neurosurg 75:545, 1991
35. White BC: Free radical mediated brain injury. Presented at the Neurotrauma Conference: Current Practice and Emerging Therapies, Detroit, MIC, June 11, 1992
36. Lanier WL, Stangland KJ, Scheithauer BW et al: The effects of dextrose infusion and head position on neurologic outcome after complete cerebral ischemia in primates: examination of a model. Anesthesiology 66:39, 1987
37. Hoffman WE, Braucher E, Pelligrino DA et al: Brain lactate and neurologic outcome following incomplete ischemia in fasted, nonfasted, and glucose-loaded rats. Anesthesiology 72:1045, 1990
38. Ashwal S, Schneider S, Tomasi L, Thompson J: Prognostic implications of hyperglycemia and reduced cerebral blood flow in childhood near-drowning. Neurology 40:820, 1990
39. Pollick C, Cujec B, Parker S, Tator C: Left ventricular wall motion abnormalities in subarachnoid hemorrhage: an echocardiographic study. J Am Coll Cardiol 12:600, 1988
40. Szabo MD, Crosby G, Hurford WE, Strauss HW: Myocardial perfusion following acute subarachnoid hemorrhage in patients with an abnormal electrocardiogram. Anesth Analg 76:253, 1993
41. Kono T, Morita H, Kuroiwa T et al: Left ventricular wall motion abnormalities in patients with subarachnoid hemorrhage: neurogenic stunned myocardium. J Am Coll Cardiol 24:636, 1994
42. Stoelting RK, Dierdorf SF: Anesthesia and Co-Existing Disease. 3rd Ed. Churchill Livingstone, New York, p. 3
43. Tarhan S, Moffit EA, Taylor WF, Giuliani ER: Myocardial infarction after general anesthesia. JAMA 220:1451, 1972
44. Steen PA, Tinker JH, Tarhan S: Myocardial reinfarction after anesthesia and surgery. JAMA 239:2566, 1978
45. Shah KB, Kleinman BS, Sami H et al: Reinfarction following anesthesia in patients with myocardial infarction. Anesth Analg 71:231, 1991
46. Rao TLK, Jacobs EH, El-Etr AA: Reevaluation of perioperative myocardial infarction. Anesthesiology 59:499, 1983
47. Robertson GL: Abnormalities of thirst regulation. Kidney Int 25:460, 1984
48. Robinson AG: Regulation and pathophysiology of posterior pituitary function. p. 65. In Collu R, Brown GM, Van Loon GR (eds): Clinical Neuroendocrinology. Blackwell Scientific, Boston, 1988
49. Baylis PH, Robertson GL: Plasma vasopressin response to hypertonic saline infusion to assess

posterior pituitary function. J R Soc Med 73:255, 1980
50. Ober KP: Endocrine crises: diabetes insipidus. Crit Care Clin 7:109, 1991
51. Robinson AG: Disorders of antidiuretic hormone secretion. Clin Endocrinol Metab 14:55, 1985
52. Sterns RH: The management of hyponatremic emergencies. Crit Care Clin 7:127, 1991
53. Berl T: Treating hyponatremia: damned if we do and damned if we don't (clinical conference). Kidney Int 37:1006, 1990
54. Sterns RH: Neurological deterioration following treatment for hyponatremia. Am J Kidney Dis 13:434, 1989
55. Sterns RH, Spital A: Disorders of water balance. p. 139. In Kokko JP, Tannen RL (eds): Fluids and Electrolytes. 2nd Ed. WB Saunders, Philadelphia, 1990
56. Sterns RH, Thomas DJ, Herndon RM: Brain dehydration and neurologic deterioration after rapid correction of hyponatremia. Kidney Int 35:69, 1989
57. Thurston JH, Hauhart RE, Nelson JS: Adaptive decreases in amino acids (taurine in particular), creatine, and electrolytes prevent cerebral edema in chronically hyponatremic mice: rapid correction (experimental model of central pontine myelinolysis) causes dehydration and shrinkage of brain. Metab Brain Dis 2:223, 1987
58. Lien YH, Shapiro JI, Chan L: Effects of hypernatremia on organic brain osmoles. J Clin Invest 85:1427, 1990
59. Cluitmans FH, Meinders AE: Management of severe hyponatremia: rapid or slow correction? Am J Med 88:161, 1990
60. Sterns RH, Riggs JE, Schochet SS, Jr: Osmotic demyelination syndrome following correction of hyponatremia. N Engl J Med 314:1535, 1986
61. Brunner JE, Redmond JM, Haggar AM et al: Central pontine myelinolysis and pontine lesions after rapid correction of hyponatremia: a prospective magnetic resonance imaging study. Ann Neurol 27:61, 1990
62. Layon AJ, Bernards WC, Kirby RR: Fluids and electrolytes in the critically ill. p. 457. In Civetta JM, Taylor RW, Kirby RR (eds): Critical Care. 2nd Ed. JB Lippincott, Philadelphia, 1992
63. Wijdicks EF, Ropper AH, Hunnicutt EJ et al: Atrial natriuretic factor and salt wasting after aneurysmal subarachnoid hemorrhage. Stroke 22:1519, 1991
64. Kimmel DW, Oneil BP: Systemic cancer presenting as diabetes insipidus: clinical and radiologic features of 11 patients with a review of metastatic-induced diabetes insipidus. Cancer 52:2355, 1993
65. Moses AM, Miller M, Streeten DH: Pathophysiologic and pharmacologic alterations in the release and action of ADH. Metabolism 25:697, 1976
66. Vokes TJ, Robertson GL: Disorders of antidiuretic hormone. Endocrinol Metab Clin North Am 17:281, 1988
67. Verbalis JG, Robinson AG, Moses AM: Postoperative and post-traumatic diabetes insipidus. Front Horm Res 10:163, 1982
68. O'Connor WJ: The normal interphase in the polyuria which follows section of the supraoptic-hypophyseal tracts in the dog. Q J Exp Physiol 37:1, 1952
69. Gandhi P, Cottrell JE, Scialabba FP, Shwiry B: Deliberate hypotension with labetalol in neurological patients, abstracted. Anesthesiology 59:A360, 1983
70. Davis RF, Douglas ME, Heenan TJ, Downs JB: Brain tissue pressure measurement during sodium nitroprusside infusion. Crit Care Med 9:17, 1981
71. Alon E, Himmelseher S: Ondansetron in the treatment of postoperative vomiting: a randomized, double-blind comparison with droperidol and metaclopropamide. Anesth Analg 75:561, 1992
72. Watcha MF, Bras PJ, Cieslak GD, Pennant JH: The dose-response relationship of ondansetron in preventing postoperative emesis in pediatric patients undergoing ambulatory surgery. Anesthesiology 82:47, 1995
73. Khalil SN, Kataria B, Perason K et al: Ondansetron prevents postoperative nausea and vomiting in women outpatients. Anesth Analg 79:845, 1994
74. American Heart Association: Heart and Stroke Facts. p. 7. The American Heart Association, Bethesda, MD, 1992
75. White MF: Reducing cardiovascular risk factors in the United States: an overview of the national educational programs. Cardiovasc Risk Factors 1:277, 1991
76. Silver FL, Norris JW, Lewis AJ, Hachinski VC: Early mortality following stroke: a prospective review. Stroke 15:492, 1984
77. Matsumoto N, Whisnant JP, Kurland LT,

Okazaki H: Natural history of stroke in Rochester, Minnesota, 1955 through 1969: an extension of a previous study, 1945 through 1954. Stroke 4:20, 1973
78. Sacco RL, Wolf PA, Kannel WB, NcNamara PM: Survival and recurrence following stroke: the Framingham study. Stroke 13:290, 1982
79. Douglas MA, Haerer AF: Long-term prognosis of hypertensive intracerebral hemorrhage. Stroke 13:488, 1982
80. Camarata PJ, Heros RC, Latchaw RE: "Brain attack": the rationale for treating stroke as a medical emergency. Neurosurgery 34:144, 1994
81. Mohr JP, Caplan LR, Melski JW et al: The Harvard Cooperative Stroke Registry: a prospective registry. Neurology 28:754, 1978
82. Cerebral Embolism Task Force: Cardiogenic brain embolism. Arch Neurol 46:727, 1989
83. Hachinski VC: The clinical problem of brain and heart. Stroke 24(suppl. I):I1–2, 1993
84. Broderick J, Brott T, Barsan W et al: Blood pressure during the first minutes of focal cerebral ischemia. Ann Emerg Med 22:1438, 1993
85. Duke RJ, Bloch RF, Turpie AG et al: Intravenous heparin for the prevention of stroke progression in acute partial stable stroke. Ann Intern Med 105:825, 1986
86. Cerebral Embolism Study Group: Immediate anticoagulation of embolic stroke: a randomized trial. Stroke 14:668, 1983
87. Kay R, Wong KS, Yu YL et al: Low-molecular-weight heparin for the treatment of acute ischemic stroke. N Engl J Med 333:1588, 1995
88. Hass WK, Clauss RH, Goldberg AF et al: Special problems associated with surgical and thrombolytic treatment of strokes. Arch Surg 92:27, 1966
89. Meyer JS, Gilroy J, Barnhart MI, Johnson JF: Anticoagulants plus streptokinase therapy in progressive stroke. JAMA 189:373, 1964
90. Brott TG, Haley EC, Jr, Levy DE et al: Urgent therapy for stroke. I. Pilot study of tissue plasminogen activator administered within 90 minutes. Stroke 23:632, 1992
91. Haley EC, Jr, Levy DE, Brott TG et al: Urgent therapy for stroke. II. Pilot study of tissue plasminogen activator administered 180 minutes from onset. Stroke 23:641, 1992
92. del Zoppo GJ, Poeck K, Pessin MS et al: Recombinant tissue plasminogen activator in acute thrombotic and embolic stroke. Ann Neurol 32:78, 1992
93. The National Institute of Neurologic Disorders and Stroke Study Group: Tissue plasminogen activator for acute ischemic stroke. N Engl J Med 333:1581, 1995
94. Strand T, Asplund K, Eriksson S et al: A randomized controlled trial of hemodilution therapy in acute ischemic stroke. Stroke 15:980, 1984
95. Italian Acute Stroke Study Group: The Italian hemodilution trial in acute stroke. Stroke 18:670, 1987
96. Gelmers HJ, Gorter K, DeWeerdt CJ, Wiezer HJ: A controlled trial of nimodipine in acute ischemic stroke. N Engl J Med 318:203, 1988
97. The American Nimodipine Study Group: Clinical trial of nimodipine in acute ischemic stroke. Stroke 23:3, 1992
98. Clark WM, Hotan T, Lauten JD, Coull BM: Therapeutic efficacy of tirilazad in experimental multiple cerebral emboli: a randomized, controlled trial. Crit Care Med 22:1161, 1994
99. North American Symptomatic Carotid Endarterectomy Trial Collaborators: Beneficial effect of carotid endarterectomy in symptomatic patients with high-grade carotid stenosis. N Engl J Med 325:445, 1991
100. Mentzer RM, Jr, Finkelmeier BA, Crosby IK, Wellons HA, Jr: Emergency carotid endarterectomy for fluctuating neurologic deficits. Surgery 89:60, 1981
101. McCormick PW, Spetzler RF, Bailes JE et al: Thromboendarterectomy of the symptomatic occluded internal carotid artery. J Neurosurg 76:752, 1992
102. Meyer FB, Sundt TM, Jr, Piepgras DG et al: Emergency carotid endarterectomy for patients with acute carotid occlusion and profound neurologic deficits. Ann Surg 203:82, 1986
103. Goldstone J, Effeney DJ: The role of carotid endarterectomy in the treatment of acute neurologic deficits. Prog Cardiovasc Dis 22:415, 1980
104. Walters BB, Ojemann RG, Heros RC: Emergency carotid endarterectomy. J Neurosurg 66:817, 1987
105. Heiskanen O: Treatment of spontaneous intracerebral and intracerebellar hemorrhages. Stroke 24(suppl. I):I94, 1993
106. McKissock W, Richardson A, Taylor J: Primary intracerebral hemorrhage: a controlled trial of surgical and conservative treatment in 180 unselected cases. Lancet 2:221, 1961

107. Weir B: The clinical problem of intracerebral hematoma. Stroke 24(suppl. I):193, 1993 1993
108. Kaneko M, Tanaka K, Shimada T et al: Long-term evaluation of ultraearly operation for hypertensive intracerebral hemorrhage in 100 cases. J Neurosurg 58:838, 1983
109. Kanno T, Sano H, Shinomiya Y et al: Role of surgery in hypertensive intracerebral hematoma: a comparative study of 305 nonsurgical and 154 surgical cases. J Neurosurg 61:1091, 1984
110. Kanno T, Nagata J, Nonomura K et al: New approaches in the treatment of hypertensive intracerebral hemorrhage. Stroke 24(suppl. I):196, 1993
111. Batjer HH, Reisch JS, Allen BC et al: Failure of surgery to improve outcome in hypertensive putaminal hemorrhage: a prospective randomized trial. Arch Neurol 47:1103, 1990
112. Auer LM, Deinsberger W, Niederkorn K et al: Endoscopic surgery versus medical treatment for spontaneous intracerebral hematoma: a randomized study. J Neurosurg 70:530, 1989
113. Kaufman HH: Treatment of deep spontaneous intracerebral hematomas. Stroke 24(suppl. I):1101, 1993
114. Spetzler RF, Martin NA: A proposed grading system for arteriovenous malformations. J Neurosurg 65:476, 1986
115. Heros RC, Korosue K, Diebold PM: Surgical excision of cerebral arteriovenous malformations: late results. Neurosurgery 26:577, 1990
116. Sundt TM, Piepgras DG, Stevens LN: Surgery for supratentorial arteriovenous malformations. Clin Neurosurg 37:49, 1990
117. Spetzler RF, Wilson CB, Weinstein P et al: Normal perfusion pressure breakthrough theory. Clin Neurosurg 25:651, 1978
118. Parkinson D, Bachers G: Arteriovenous malformations. Summary of 100 consecutive supratentorial cases. J Neurosurg 53:285, 1980
119. Al-Rodhan NR, Sundt TM, Jr, Piepgras DG et al: Occlusive hyperemia: a theory for the hemodynamic complications following resection of intracerebral arteriovenous malformations. J Neurosurg 78:167, 1993
120. Miyasaka Y, Yada K, Ohwada T et al: An analysis of the venous drainage system as a factor in hemorrhage from arteriovenous malformations. J Neurosurg 76:239, 1992
121. Batjer HH, Purdy PD, Giller CA, Samson DS: Evidence of redistribution of cerebral blood flow during treatment for an intracranial arteriovenous malformation. Neurosurgery 25:599, 1989
122. Chioffi F, Pasqualin A, Beltramello A, DaPian R: Hemodynamic effects of preoperative embolization in cerebral arteriovenous malformations: evaluation with transcranial Doppler sonography. Neurosurgery 31:877, 1992
123. Petty GW, Massaro AR, Tatemichi TK et al: Transcranial Doppler ultrasonographic changes after treatment for arteriovenous malformations. Stroke 21:260, 1990
124. Kader A, Young WL, Pile-Spellman J et al: The influence of hemodynamic and anatomic factors on hemorrhage from cerebral arteriovenous malformations. Neurosurgery 34:801, 1994
125. Rosenblum BR, Bonner RF, Oldfield EH: Intraoperative measurement of cortical blood flow adjacent to cerebral AVM using laser Doppler velocimetry. J Neurosurg 66:396, 1987
126. Goldstein M: Traumatic brain injury: a silent epidemic (editorial). Ann Neurol 27:327, 1990
127. Rosner MJ, Coley IB: Cerebral perfusion pressure, intracranial pressure, and head elevation. J Neurosurg 65:636, 1986
128. Durward QJ, Amacher AL, Del Maestro RF, Sibbald WJ: Cerebral and cardiovascular responses to changes in head elevation in patients with intracranial hypertension. J Neurosurg 59:938, 1983
129. Feldman Z, Kanter MJ, Robertson CS et al: Effect of head elevation on intracranial pressure, cerebral perfusion pressure, and cerebral blood flow in head-injured patients. J Neurosurg 76:207, 1992
130. Prough DS, Johnson JC, Poole GV, Jr et al: Effects on intracranial pressure of resuscitation from hemorrhagic shock with hypertonic saline versus lactated Ringer's solution. Crit Care Med 13:407, 1985
131. Prough DS, Johnson JC, Stump DA et al: Effects of hypertonic saline versus lactated Ringer's solution on cerebral oxygen transport during resuscitation from hemorrhagic shock. J Neurosurg 64:627, 1986
132. Prough DS, Whitley JM, Taylor CL et al: Regional cerebral blood flow following resuscitation from hemorrhagic shock with hypertonic saline. Anesthesiology 75:319, 1991
133. Todd MM, Tommasino C, Moore S: Cerebral effects of isovolemic hemodilution with a hypertonic saline solution. J Neurosurg 63:944, 1985
134. Freshman SP, Battistella FD, Matteucci M Wis-

ner DH: Hypertonic saline (7.5%) versus mannitol: a comparison for treatment of acute head injuries. J Trauma 35:344, 1993
135. Worthley LI, Cooper DJ, Jones N: Treatment of resistant intracranial hypertension with hypertonic saline. Report of two cases. J Neurosurg 68:478, 1988
136. Zhuang J, Shackford SR, Schmoker JD, Pietropaoli JA, Jr: Colloid infusion after brain injury: effect on intracranial pressure, cerebral blood flow, and oxygen delivery. Crit Care Med 23:140, 1995
137. Rosomoff HL, Holaday DA: Cerebral blood flow and cerebral oxygen consumption during hypothermia. Am J Physiol 179:85, 1954
138. Marion DW, Obrist WD, Carlier PM et al: The use of moderate therapeutic hypothermia for patients with severe head injuries: a preliminary report. J Neurosurg 79:354, 1993
139. Shiozaki T, Sugimoto H, Taneda M et al: Effect of mild hypothermia on uncontrollable intracranial hypertension after severe head injury. J Neurosurg 79:363, 1993
140. Karibe H, Zarow GJ, Graham SH, Weinstein PR: Mild intraischemic hypothermia reduces postischemic hyperperfusion, delayed postischemic hypoperfusion, blood-brain barrier disruption, brain edema, and neuronal damage volume after temporary focal cerebral ischemia in rats. J Cereb Blood Flow Metab 14:620, 1994
141. Illievich UM, Zornow MH, Choi KT et al: Effects of hypothermia or anesthetics on hippocampal glutamate and glycine concentrations after repeated transient global cerebral ischemia. Anesthesiology 80:177, 1994
142. Kader A, Frazzini VI, Baker CJ et al: Effect of mild hypothermia on nitric oxide synthesis during focal cerebral ischemia. Neurosurgery 35:272, 1994
143. Muizelaar JP, Schröder ML: Overview of monitoring of cerebral blood flow and metabolism after severe head injury. Can J Neurol Sci 21:S6, 1994
144. Darby JM, Yonas H, Marion DW, Latchaw RE: Local "inverse steal" induced by hyperventilation in head injury. Neurosurgery 23:84, 1988
145. Muizelaar JP, Marmarou A, Ward JD et al: Adverse effects of prolonged hyperventilation in patients with severe head injury: a randomized clinical trial. J Neurosurg 75:731, 1991
146. Wolf AL, Levi L, Marmarou A et al: Effect of THAM upon outcome in severe head injury: a randomized prospective clinical trial. J Neurosurg 78:54, 1993
147. Duthie SE, Goulin GD, Zornow MH et al: Effects of THAM and sodium bicarbonate on intracranial pressure and mean arterial pressure in an animal model of focal cerebral injury. J Neurosurg Anesthesiol 6:201, 1994
148. Pollay M, Fullenwider C, Roberts PA, Stevens FA: Effect of mannitol and furosemide on blood-brain osmotic gradient and intracranial pressure. J Neurosurg 59:945, 1993
149. Marshall LF, Smith RW, Shapiro HM: The outcome with aggressive treatment in severe head injuries. J Neurosurg 50:20, 1979
150. Eisenberg HM, Frankowski RF, Contant CF et al: High-dose barbiturate control of elevated intracranial pressure in patients with severe head injury. J Neurosurg 69:15, 1988
151. Ward JD, Becker DP, Miller JD et al: Failure of prophylactic barbiturate coma in the treatment of severe head injury. J Neurosurg 62:383, 1985
152. Schwartz ML, Tator CH, Rowed DW et al: The University of Toronto head injury treatment study: a prospective, randomized comparison of pentobarbital and mannitol. Can J Neurol Sci 11:434, 1984
153. Louis PT, Goddard-Finegold J, Fishman MA et al: Barbiturates and hyperventilation during intracranial hypertension. Crit Care Med 21:1200, 1993
154. Rockswold GL, Ford SE, Anderson DC et al: Results of a prospective randomized trial for treatment of severely brain-injured patients with hyperbaric oxygen. J Neurosurg 76:929, 1992
155. Dearden NM, Gibson JS, McDowall DG et al: Effect of high-dose dexamethasone on outcome from severe head injury. J Neurosurg 64:81, 1986
156. Cooper PR, Moody S, Clark WK et al: Dexamethasone and severe head injury: a prospective double-blind study. J Neurosurg 51:307, 1979
157. Gudeman SK, Miller JD, Becker DP: Failure of high-dose steroid therapy to influence intracranial pressure in patients with severe head injury. J Neurosurg 51:301, 1979
158. Lieberman DA, Faulkner JA, Craig AB, Jr, Maxwell LC: Performance and histochemical composition of guinea pig and human diaphragm. J Appl Physiol 34:233, 1973
159. Banner MJ, Kirby RR, Kirton OC et al: Breathing frequency and pattern are poor predictors of

work of breathing in patients receiving pressure support ventilation. Chest 108:1338, 1995
160. Gluck EH, Barkoviak MJ, Balk RA et al: Medical effectiveness of esophageal balloon pressure manometry in weaning patients from mechanical ventilation. Crit Care Med 23:504, 1995
161. DeVivo MJ, Kartus PL, Stover SL et al: Cause of death for patients with spinal cord injuries. Arch Intern Med 149:1761, 1989
162. Gruber UF, Thoni F: Prevention of thrombo-embolic complications in paraplegics, abstracted. Paraplegia 23:124, 1985
163. Myllynen P, Kammonen M, Rokkanen P et al: Deep venous thrombosis and pulmonary embolism in patients with acute spinal cord injury: a comparison with non-paralyzed patients immobilized due to spinal fractures. J Trauma 25:541, 1985
164. Turpie AG, Levine MN, Hirsh J et al: A randomized controlled trial of a low-molecular weight heparin (enoxaparin) to prevent deep-vein thrombosis in patients undergoing elective hip surgery. N Engl J Med 315:925, 1986
165. Green D, Twardowski P, Wei R, Rademaker AW: Fatal pulmonary embolism in spinal cord injury. Chest 105:853, 1994
166. Ditunno JF, Jr, Formal CS: Chronic spinal cord injury. N Engl J Med 330:550, 1994
167. Morgan TH, Wharton GW, Austin GN: The results of laminectomy in patients with incomplete spinal cord injuries. Paraplegia 9:14, 1971
168. Bedbrook GM: Use and disuse of surgery in lumbo-dorsal fractures. J West Pac Orthopaed Assoc 3:5, 1969
169. Frankel HL, Hancock DO, Hyslop G et al: The value of postural reduction in the initial management of closed injuries of the spine with paraplegia and tetraplegia. I. Paraplegia 7:179, 1969
170. Burke DC, Murray DD: The management of thoracic and thoraco-lumbar injuries of the spine with neurologic involvement. J Bone Joint Surg Br 58:72, 1976
171. Jacobs RR, Asher MA, Snider RK: Thoracolumbar spinal injuries: a comparative study of recumbent and operative treatment in 100 patients. Spine 5:463, 1980
172. Hardy AG: The treatment of paraplegia due to fracture-dislocation of the dorsolumbar spine. Paraplegia 3:112, 1965
173. Marshall LF, Knowlton S, Garfin SR et al: Deterioration following spinal cord injury: a multicenter study. J Neurosurg 66:400, 1987
174. Heiden JS, Weiss MH, Rosenberg AW et al: Management of cervical spinal cord trauma in southern California. J Neurosurg 43:732, 1975
175. Roberts JB, Curtiss PH, Jr. Stability of the thoracic and lumbar spine in traumatic paraplegia following fracture or fracture-dislocation. J Bone Joint Surg Am 52:1115, 1970
176. Bohlman HH, Freehafer A, Dejak J: The results of treatment of acute injuries of the upper thoracic spine with paralysis. J Bone Joint Surg Am 67:360, 1985
177. Krengel WF III, Anderson PA, Henley MB: Early stabilization and decompression for incomplete paraplegia due to a thoracic-level spinal cord injury. Spine 18:2080, 1993
178. Donovan WH: Operative and nonoperative management of spinal cord injury: a review. Paraplegia 32:375, 1994
179. Bracken MB, Shepard MJ, Collins WF, Jr et al: Methylprednisolone or naloxone treatment after acute spinal cord injury: 1-year follow-up data. Results of the second National Acute Spinal Cord Injury Study. J Neurosurg 76:23, 1992
180. Fowl RJ, Patterson RB, Gewirtz RJ, Anderson DK: Protection against postischemic spinal cord injury using a new 21-aminosteroid. J Surg Res 48:597, 1990
181. Francel PC, Long BA, Malik JM et al: Limiting ischemic spinal cord injury using a free radical scavenger 21-aminosteroid and/or cerebrospinal fluid drainage. J Neurosurg 79:742, 1993
182. Agee JM, Flanagan T, Blackbourne LH et al: Reducing postischemic paraplegia using conjugated superoxide dismutase. Ann Thorac Surg 51:911, 1991
183. Geisler FH, Dorsey FC, Coleman WP: Recovery of motor function after spinal-cord injury: a randomized, placebo-controlled trial with GM-1 ganglioside. N Engl J Med 324:1829, 1991
184. Schittek A, Bennink GB, Cooley DA, Langford LA: Spinal cord protection with intravenous nimodipine: a functional and morphologic evaluation. J Thorac Cardiovasc Surg 104:1100, 1992
185. de Mol B, Hamerlijnck R, Janssen T, Jagenau A: Infrarenal aortic occlusion in the rabbit to assess the effect of flunarizine in the prevention of ischemic spinal cord injury. Thorac Cardiovasc Surg 39:36, 1991
186. Deutschman CS, Haines SJ: Anticonvulsant pro-

phylaxis in neurological surgery. Neurosurgery 17:510, 1985
187. Lee ST, Lui TN, Chang CN et al: Prophylactic anticonvulsants for prevention of immediate and early postcraniotomy seizures. Surg Neurol 31:361, 1989
188. Fukamachi A, Koizumi H, Nukui H: Immediate postoperative seizures: incidence and computed tomographic findings. Surg Neurol 24:671, 1985
189. Kvam DA, Loftus CM, Copeland B, Quest DO: Seizures during the immediate postoperative period. Neurosurgery 12:14, 1983
190. North JB, Penhall RK, Hanieh A et al: Phenytoin and postoperative epilepsy: a double blind study. J Neurosurg 58:672, 1983
191. Sachs E, Furlow LT: The significance of convulsion in the diagnosis of brain tumors. J Mo State Med Assoc 33:121, 1936
192. Mahaley MS, Jr, Dudka L: The role of anticonvulsant medications in the management of patients with anaplastic gliomas. Surg Neurol 16:399, 1981
193. Ramamamurthi B, Ravi B, Ramachandran V: Convulsions with meningiomas: incidence and significance. Surg Neurol 14:415, 1980
194. Lee ST, Lui TN, Chang CN, Cheng WC: Early postoperative seizures after posterior fossa surgery. J Neurosurg 73:541, 1990
195. Temkin NR, Dikmen SS, Wilensky AJ et al: A randomized, double-blind study of phenytoin for the prevention of post-traumatic seizures. N Engl J Med 323:497, 1990
196. Young B, Rapp RP, Norton JA et al: Failure of prophylactically administered phenytoin to prevent early posttraumatic seizures. J Neurosurg 58:231, 1983
197. Young B, Rapp RP, Norton JA et al: Failure of prophylactically administered phenytoin to prevent late posttraumatic seizures. J Neurosurg 58:236, 1983
198. Feeney DM, Walker AE: The prediction of posttraumatic epilepsy: a mathematical approach. Arch Neurol 36:8, 1979
199. Michenfelder JD, Cucchiara RF, Sundt TM, Jr: Influence of intraoperative antibiotic choice on the incidence of early postcraniotomy seizures. J Neurosurg 74:311, 1991
200. Schlech WF III, Ward JI, Band JD et al: Bacterial meningitis in the United States, 1978 through 1981: the National Bacterial Meningitis Surveillance Study. JAMA 253:1749, 1985
201. Durand ML, Calderwood SB, Weber DJ et al: Acute bacterial meningitis in adults: a review of 493 episodes. N Engl J Med 328:21, 1993
202. Hart CA, Cuevas LE, Marzouk O et al: Management of bacterial meningitis. J Antimicrob Chemother 32(suppl. A):49, 1993
203. Kaufman BA, Tunkel AR, Pryor JC, Dacey RG, Jr: Meningitis in the neurosurgical patient. Infect Dis Clin North Am 4:677, 1990
204. Schaad UB, Suter S, Gianella-Borradori A et al: A comparison of ceftriaxone and cefuroxime for the treatment of bacterial meningitis in children. N Engl J Med 322:141, 1990
205. Armstrong D. Problems in management of opportunistic fungal diseases. Rev Infect Dis 11 (suppl. 7):S1591, 1989
206. Treseler CB, Sugar AM: Fungal meningitis. Infect Dis Clin North Am 4:789, 1990
207. Chuck SL, Sande MA: Infections with Cryptococcus neoformans in the acquired immunodeficiency syndrome. N Engl J Med 321:794, 1989
208. Dismukes WE, Cloud G, Gallis HA et al: Treatment of cryptococcal meningitis with combination amphotericin B and flucytosine for four as compared with six weeks. N Engl J Med 317:334, 1987
209. Connolly KJ, Hammer SM: The acute aseptic meningitis syndrome. Infect Dis Clin North Am 4:599, 1990
210. Centers for Disease Control: Annual summary 1982: reported morbidity and mortality in the United States. MMWR 31(54):1, 1983
211. Centers for Disease Control: Annual summary 1983: reported morbidity and mortality in the United States. MMWR 32:3, 1984
212. Centers for Disease Control: Annual summary 1984: reported morbidity and mortality in the United States. MMWR 33(54):1, 1986
213. Centers for Disease Control: Summary of notifiable diseases in the United States, 1985. MMWR 34(54):1, 1985
214. Centers for Disease Control: Summary of notifiable diseases in the United States, 1986. MMWR 35(55):1, 1986
215. Centers for Disease Control: Summary of notifiable diseases in the United States, 1987. MMWR 36(54):1, 1987
216. Centers for Disease Control: Summary of notifiable diseases in the United States, 1988. MMWR 37(54):1, 1988
217. Cherry JD: Enteroviruses: polioviruses (poliomyelitis), coxsackieviruses, echoviruses, and enteroviruses p. 1729. In Feigin RD, Cherry JD

(eds): Textbook of Pediatric Infectious Diseases. 2nd Ed. WB Saunders, Philadelphia, 1987

218. Simpson DM, Tagliati M: Neurologic manifestations of HIV infection. Ann Intern Med 121:769, 1994
219. Janssen RS, Nwanyanwu OC, Selik RM, Stehr-Green JK: Epidemiology of human immunodeficiency virus encephalopathy in the United States. Neurology 42:1472, 1992
220. Peluso R, Haase A, Stowring L et al: A Trojan Horse mechanism for the spread of visna virus in monocytes. Virology 147:231, 1985
221. Tornatore C, Chandra R, Berger JR, Major EO: HIV-1 infection of subcortical astrocytes in the pediatric central nervous system. Neurology 44:481, 1994
222. Dreyer EB, Kaiser PK, Offermann JT, Lipton SA: HIV-1 coat protein neurotoxicity prevented by calcium channel antagonists. Science 248 (4953):364, 1990
223. Grimaldi LM, Martino GV, Franciotta DM et al: Elevated alpha-tumor necrosis factor levels in spinal fluid from HIV-1-infected patients with central nervous system involvement. Ann Neurol 29:21, 1991
224. Griffin DE, McArthur JC, Cornblath DR: Neopterin and interferon-gamma in serum and cerebrospinal fluid of patients with HIV-associated neurologic disease. Neurology 41:69, 1991
225. Lipton SA: Models of neuronal injury in AIDS: another role for the NMDA receptor? Trends Neurosci 15:75, 1992
226. Schmitt FA, Bigley JW, McKinnis R et al: Neuropsychological outcome of zidovudine (AZT) treatment of patients with AIDS and AIDS-related complex. N Engl J Med 319:1573, 1988
227. Luft BJ, Remington JS: Toxoplasmic encephalitis in AIDS. Clin Infect Dis 15:211, 1992
228. Falangola MF, Petito CK: Choroid plexus infection in cerebral toxoplasmosis in AIDS patients. Neurology 43:2035, 1993
229. Porter SB, Sande MA: Toxoplasmosis of the central nervous system in the acquired immunodeficiency syndrome. N Engl J Med 327:1643, 1992
230. Luft BJ, Hafner R, Korzun AH et al: Toxoplasmic encephalitis in patients with acquired immunodeficiency syndrome. N Engl J Med 329:995, 1993
231. Galetto G, Levine A: AIDS-associated primary central nervous system lymphoma. JAMA 269:92, 1993
232. Rosenberg NL, Hochberg FH, Miller G, Kleinschmidt-DeMasters BK: Primary central nervous system lymphoma related to Epstein-Barr virus in a patient with acquired immune deficiency syndrome. Ann Neurol 20:98, 1986
233. Berger JR, Kaszovitz B, Post MJ, Dickinson G: Progressive multifocal leukoencephalopathy associated with human immunodeficiency virus infection: a review of the literature with a report of sixteen cases. Ann Intern Med 107:78, 1987
234. von Einsiedel RW, Fife TD, Aksamit AJ et al: Progressive multifocal leukoencephalopathy in AIDS: a clinicopathologic study and review of the literature. J Neurol 240:391, 1993
235. Portegies P, Algra PR, Hollak CEM et al: Response to cytarabine in progressive multifocal leukoencephalopathy in AIDS (letter). Lancet 337:680, 1991
236. Ohrstrom JK, Skou JK, Ejlertsen T, Kosteljanetz M: Infected ventriculostomy: bacteriology and treatment. Acta Neurochir (Wien) 100:67, 1989
237. Breeze RE, McComb JG, Hyman S, Gilles FH: CSF production in acute ventriculitis. J Neurosurg 70:619, 1989
238. Bogdahn U, Lau W, Hassel W et al: Continuous-pressure controlled, external ventricular drainage for treatment of acute hydrocephalus: evaluation of risk factors. Neurosurgery 31:898, 1992
239. Gerner-Smidt P, Stenager E, Kock-Jensen C: Treatment of ventriculostomy-related infections. Acta Neurochir (Wien) 91:47, 1988
240. Young EJ, Ratner RE, Clarridge JE: Staphylococcal ventriculitis treated with vancomycin. South Med J 74:1014, 1981
241. Bayston R, Hart CA, Barnicoat M: Intraventricular vancomycin in the treatment of ventriculitis associated with cerebrospinal fluid shunting and drainage. J Neurol Neurosurg Psychiatry 50:1419, 1987
242. Hund EF, Borel CO, Cornblath DR et al: Intensive management and treatment of severe Guillain-Barré syndrome. Crit Care Med 21:433, 1993
243. Zochodne DW: Autonomic involvement in Guillain-Barré syndrome: a review. Muscle Nerve 17:1145, 1994
244. Ropper AH, Kehne SM: Guillain-Barré syndrome: management of respiratory failure. Neurology 35:1662, 1995
245. Sunderrajan EV, Davenport J: The Guillain-Barré Syndrome: pulmonary-neurologic correlations. Medicine 64:333, 1995

246. Guillain-Barré Syndrome Steroid Trial Group: Double-blind trial of intravenous methylprednisolone in Guillain-Barré syndrome. Lancet 341:586, 1993
247. van der Meche FG, Schmitz PI, the Dutch Guillain-Barré Study Group: A randomized trial comparing intravenous immune globulin and plasma exchange in Guillain-Barré syndrome. N Engl J Med 326:1123, 1992
248. Vajsar J, Sloane A, Wood E, Murphy EG: Plasmapheresis vs intravenous immunoglobulin treatment in childhood Guillain-Barré syndrome. Arch Pediatr Adolesc Med 148:1210, 1994
249. Thornton CA, Griggs RC: Plasma exchange and intravenous immunoglobulin treatment of neuromuscular disease. Ann Neurol 35:260, 1994
250. Castro LH, Ropper AH: Human immune globulin infusion in Guillain-Barré syndrome: worsening during and after treatment. Neurology 43:1034, 1993
251. Irani DN, Cornblath DR, Chaudhry V et al: Relapse in Guillain-Barré syndrome after treatment with human immune globulin. Neurology 43:872, 1993
252. Kleyweg RP, van der Meche FG: Treatment related fluctuations in Guillain-Barré syndrome after high-dose immunoglobulins or plasma-exchange. J Neurol Neurosurg Psychiatry 54:957, 1991
253. The Dutch Guillain-Barré Study Group: Treatment of Guillain-Barré syndrome with high-dose immune globulins combined with methylprednisolone: a pilot study. Ann Neurol 35:749, 1994
254. Drachman DB: Myasthenia gravis. N Engl J Med 330:1797, 1994
255. Baraka A: Anaesthesia and myasthenia gravis. Can J Anaesth 39:476, 1992
256. Frist WH, Thirumalai S, Doehring CB et al: Thymectomy for the myasthenia gravis patient: factors influencing outcome. Ann Thorac Surg 57:334, 1994
257. Verma P, Oger J: Treatment of acquired autoimmune myasthenia gravis: a topic review. Can J Neurol Sci 19:360, 1992
258. Evoli A, Batocchi AP, Palmisani MT et al: Long-term results of corticosteroid therapy in patients with myasthenia gravis. Eur Neurol 32:37, 1992
259. Cosi V, Citterio A, Lombardi M et al: Effectiveness of steroid treatment in myasthenia gravis: a retrospective study. Acta Neurol Scand 84:33, 1991
260. Gajdos P, Elkharrat D, Chevret S et al: A randomized clinical trial comparing prednisone and azathioprine in myasthenia gravis: results of the second interim study. J Neurol Neurosurg Psychiatry 56:1157, 1993
261. Mertens HG, Hertel G, Reuther P, Ricker K: Effect of immunosuppressive drugs (azathioprine). Ann N Y Acad Sci 377:691, 1981
262. Fonseca V, Havard CW: Long term treatment of myasthenia gravis with azathioprine. Postgrad Med J 66:102, 1990
263. Arsura EL, Bick A, Brunner NG et al: High-dose intravenous immunoglobulin in the management of myasthenia gravis. Arch Intern Med 146:1365, 1986
264. Tindall RS, Phillips JT, Rollins JA et al: A clinical therapeutic trial of cyclosporine in myasthenia gravis. Ann N Y Acad Sci 681:539, 1993
265. Durelli L, Ferrio MF, Urgesi A et al: Total body irradiation for myasthenia gravis: a long-term follow-up. Neurology 43:2215, 1993
266. Quera-Salva MA, Guilleminault C, Chevret S et al: Breathing disorders during sleep in myasthenia gravis. Ann Neurol 31:86, 1992
267. Gracey DR, Divertie MB, Howard FM, Jr: Mechanical ventilation for respiratory failure in myasthenia gravis: two year experience with 22 patients. Mayo Clin Proc 58:597, 1993
268. Kirsch JR, Diringer MN, Borel CO et al: Preoperative lumbar epidural morphine improves postoperative analgesia and ventilatory function after transsternal thymectomy in patients with myasthenia gravis. Crit Care Med 19:1474, 1991
269. President's Commission for the Study of Ethical Problems in Medicine and Biomedical and Behavioral Research: Guidelines for the determination of death. JAMA 246:2184, 1981
270. Earnest MP, Beresford HR, McIntyre HB: Testing for apnea in suspected brain death: methods used by 129 clinicians. Neurology 36:542, 1986
271. Ropper AH: Unusual spontaneous movements in brain-dead patients. Neurology 34:1089, 1984
272. Greitz T, Gordon E, Kolmodin G, Widen L: Aortocranial and carotid angiography in determination of brain death. Neuroradiology 5:13, 1973
273. Petty GW, Mohr JP, Pedley TA et al: The role of transcranial Doppler in confirming brain death: sensitivity, specificity, and suggestions for performance and interpretation. Neurology 40:300, 1990

274. Payen DM, Lamer C, Pilorget A et al: Evaluation of pulsed Doppler common carotid blood flow as a noninvasive method for brain death diagnosis: a prospective study. Anesthesiology 72:222, 1990
275. Feri M, Ralli L, Felici M et al: Transcranial Doppler and brain death diagnosis. Crit Care Med 22:1120, 1994
276. Machado C, Valdes P, Garcia-Tigera J et al: Brainstem auditory evoked potentials and brain death. Electroencephogr Clin Neurophysiol 80:392, 1991
277. Besser R, Dillmann U, Henn M: Somatosensory evoked potentials aiding the diagnosis of brain death. Neurosurg Rev 11:171, 1988
278. de la Riva A, Gonzalez FM, Llamas-Elvira JM et al: Diagnosis of brain death: superiority of perfusion studies with^{99m}Tc-HMPAO over conventional radionuclide cerebral angiography. Br J Radiol 65:289, 1992
279. Reid RH, Gulenchyn KY, Ballinger JR: Clinical use of technetium-99m HM-PAO for determination of brain death. J Nucl Med 30:1621, 1989
280. Kato T, Tokumaru A, O'uchi T et al: Assessment of brain death in children by means of P-31 MR spectroscopy: preliminary note. Radiology 179:95, 1991
281. Shapiro HM: Intracranial hypertension: therapeutic and anesthetic consideration. Anesthesiology 43:445, 1975
282. Civetta J, Taylor R, Kirby R: p. 449. In: Critical Care. 2nd Ed. JB Lippincott, Philadelphia, 1992
283. Silberman H: p. 95. In: Parenteral and Enteral Nutrition. 2nd Ed. Appleton & Large, Stamford, CT 1989
284. Silberman H: p. 36. In: Parenteral and Enteral Nutrition. 2nd Ed. Appleton & Large, Stamford, CT, 1989
285. Civetta J, Taylor R, Kirby R: p. 455. In: Critical Care. 2nd Ed. JB Lippincott, Philadelpia, 1992

19 TRANSESOPHAGEAL ECHOCARDIOGRAPHY

THOMAS J. LOSASSO

Transesophageal echocardiography (TEE) has found application in the anesthetic and surgical management of neurosurgical patients. Specifically, TEE has clinical application in the following intraoperative settings:

1. Detection of venous air embolism (VAE).
2. Identification of patients with a patent foramen ovale (PFO) who are at significant risk for VAE.
3. Detection of paradoxical (or arterial) air embolism during episodes of VAE.
4. Localization of the distal end of a right atrial (RA) catheter at the junction of the superior vena cava and right atrium.
5. Localization of the distal end of a ventriculoatrial (VA) shunt at the cavoatrial junction of the heart during surgical placement.

PRINCIPLES OF TEE

Echocardiography probes transmit sound waves with a frequency in excess of 1 MHz. An ultrasound transducer emits the sound waves in a narrow beam during an active transmission mode and then "listens" for the ultrasound wave that is reflected from cardiac tissues or other echogenic surfaces while in a detection mode. Each cycle of transmission/detection is approximately 250 microseconds in duration, with transmission time taking less than 1 microsecond.[1] The time delay between the emitted sound and the received echo indicates the *distance* between the echocardiography probe and the cardiac structure. The intensity of the reflected echo indicates the *density* of the cardiac structure. Using Doppler principles, the frequency shift between the emitted and reflected wave determines the *velocity* of the cardiac structure or other echogenic surface. Using these principles, the technology of echocardiography reproduces a real time image of the heart and its contents.

INTRAOPERATIVE DETECTION OF VAE

VAE is a well-recognized complication of neurosurgical procedures performed upon patients while in the sitting position. Previous studies indicate that the incidence of Doppler-detected VAE is approximately 10% during cervical laminectomy and approximately 45% during posterior fossa surgery that is performed with patients in the sitting position.[2,3] In addition, in patients undergoing posterior fossa surgery in nonsitting positions (i.e., supine, prone, park bench, and lateral), the incidence of VAE is approximately 12%.[3] The most important factors that limit morbidity and mortality secondary to

VAE are early diagnosis and prompt treatment. At the present time, the most sensitive monitors for intraoperative detection of VAE are the precordial Doppler and TEE. In a dog model of VAE, audible changes in the Doppler and the appearance of echogenic densities in the right atrium on the TEE are found to occur almost simultaneously during episodes of VAE.[4,5] Interestingly, although nitrous oxide can increase the volume of compliant air-containing cavities in the body such as intravascular air bubbles, the sensitivity of the TEE and Doppler were found to be unaffected by the presence of nitrous oxide.[5] Some TEE probes, such as the Aloka SSD-870, are equipped with a Doppler sensor at the distal end of the probe. This allows for Doppler ultrasound monitoring for VAE in addition to visual monitoring for VAE with the same piece of equipment. Potential advantages in the use of the transesophageal (TE) sensor as opposed to a precordial Doppler sensor are the following: (1) one is able to confirm the area within the heart that is being monitored by Doppler ultrasound and (2) the quality of the Doppler signal is independent of external body habitus with the TE Doppler sensor in contrast to the precordial Doppler with which signal quality is very dependent upon external body habitus. In a human study comparing the sensitivity of the precordial Doppler, TEE, and TE Doppler to detect microair bubbles injected through a RA catheter, both the TEE and TE Doppler were found to be more sensitive than the precordial Doppler in detecting VAE.[6] The authors suggested that the increased sensitivity of the TE Doppler compared to the precordial Doppler may be related to its ability to remove chest wall configuration and lung volumes as confounding factors in the transmission of an ultrasonic signal.

Based upon the animal and human data cited above, TE Doppler is of greater sensitivity and TEE is of equal or slightly greater sensitivity than precordial Doppler in detecting VAE. Although there is a statistically significant difference in the sensitivity of these monitors to detect VAE, this difference is small and is likely to be clinically insignificant. Therefore, in neurosurgical patients at risk for VAE, it is unlikely that use of TEE or TE Doppler instead of a properly placed precordial Doppler will reduce the already extremely low morbidity and mortality due to VAE.

PATIENTS WITH A PFO

Preoperative Identification of PFO

Paradoxical (or arterial) air embolism is a rare complication in patients undergoing neurosurgi-

TABLE 19.1 *Detection of PFO using two-dimensional contrast echocardiography and provocative maneuvers*

REFERENCE	PATIENTS (N)	INCIDENCE (DETECTION RATE) OF PFO (%)	ECHOCARDIOGRAPHY TECHNIQUE
Lynch et al.[11]	96	18	Precordial
Guggiari et al.[12]	211	10	Precordial
Black et al.[13]	101	6	Precordial
	51	8	Transesophageal
Konstadt et al.[16]	50	22	Transesophageal
Jaffe et al.[21]	33	10	Transesophageal
Losasso et al.[15]	280	17	Transesophageal
Schwartz et al.[14]	285	25	Precordial

Abbreviation: PFO, patent foramen ovale.

cal procedures in the sitting position. However, when paradoxical air embolism occurs, the results can be devastating.[7] It has been postulated that the presence of a PFO predisposes patients to development of paradoxical air embolism during episodes of VAE. Venous air entering the pulmonary circulation results in an increase in pulmonary artery pressure secondary to obstruction to pulmonary arterial blood flow and reflex pulmonary vasoconstriction. The resultant pulmonary hypertension may yield increases in RA and right ventricular pressures relative to left-sided pressures. Consequently, a right-to-left atrial pressure gradient can occur that would predispose a patient to development of paradoxical air embolism if a PFO exists.

Autopsy studies indicate that a probe PFO is present in approximately 25 to 35% of patients with no history of cardiac disease.[8,9] TEE may be used preoperatively to identify patients with a PFO, thus alerting the clinician to the potential increased risk of paradoxical air embolism. However, the limitations of this diagnostic tool in detecting a PFO must be understood in order to best apply information gained to the clinical setting. Several studies have reported varying success rates when utilizing two-dimensional contrast echocardiography to detect a PFO in the presurgical period (Table 19.1). Detection rates vary between 6 and 25% for precordial echocardiography and between 8 and 22% for TEE. It appears as though detection rates for PFO are comparable with precordial and TEE, although TEE may provide a better "window" to view the relevant cardiac chambers in a patient with unusual body habitus. Studies using two-dimensional contrast precordial echocardiography in otherwise healthy patients have identified a PFO in 10 to 18% of subjects.[10,11] Preoperatively, two-dimensional contrast precordial echocardiography in the evaluation of patients scheduled to undergo neurosurgical procedures in the sitting position identified a PFO in 6 to 25% of subjects.[12–14] Similarly, in anesthetized patients scheduled to undergo neurosurgical procedures in the sitting position, two-dimensional contrast TEE detected a PFO in 8 to 17% of subjects.[13,15] In anesthetized patients scheduled to undergo cardiac surgery, 2-D contrast precordial echocardiography was able to detect a PFO in 22% of subjects (26% of subjects with the addition of color flow Doppler techniques).[16] Interestingly, in a study of patients with an angiographically identified PFO, 2-D contrast precordial echocardiography successfully identified a PFO in only 64% of the patients using both a Valsalva maneuver and cough to facilitate right-to-left shunting.[17]

In summary, these results suggest that even in the hands of cardiologists experienced in echocardiography, preoperative echocardiography will reliably detect only a portion of patients with a PFO. Preoperative detection of a PFO suggests that the patient is at increased risk for paradoxical air embolism during surgical procedures associated with a significant risk of VAE. However, failure to detect a PFO does not eliminate the possibility that the patient will develop paradoxical air embolism should VAE occur.[13,18,19]

The Methodology Identifying a PFO

Agitated saline contains microbubbles that show up as small echogenic densities on the TEE when injected into the right atrium. In patients with a PFO, these echogenic densities should be observed to cross from the RA to left atrial chambers if the RA pressure exceeds the left atrial pressure during the injection of agitated saline. Optimizing the chances of detecting a PFO requires the use of some type of provocative maneuver that will transiently increase RA pressure relative to left atrial pressure during the examination. Provocative maneuvers include a Valsalva maneuver in an awake patient or the transient application and sudden release of positive end-expiratory pressure (PEEP) in an anesthetized patient. It is well documented that these provocative maneuvers will dramatically and significantly increase the detection rate for PFO.[11,12,13,16]

TEE can be used after induction of anesthesia but prior to beginning the surgical procedure to identify patients with a PFO. In anesthetized patients, PEEP release is the provocative maneuver. Our current practice is to induce anesthesia and subsequently place a multiorificed RA catheter at the superior aspect of the right atrium with electrocardiographic guidance. The TEE probe is positioned so as to obtain a biatrial or four-chamber view of the heart with special attention paid to the interatrial septum. Twenty to thirty centimeter of H_2O PEEP is applied for 10 to 15 seconds. Immediately after the PEEP is removed, RA pressure transiently exceeds left atrial pressure (Fig. 19.1).[20] Simultaneous with the release of PEEP, 10 ml of agitated saline (with microbubbles) is injected into the right atrium via the RA catheter. The microbubbles appear on the TEE as echogenic densities in the right atrium. Under optimal test conditions, enough microbubbles are injected so as to opacify the right atrium transiently but completely. The left atrium is examined for the presence of microbubbles. If the microbubbles are observed to pass from the right-to-left atrium, a PFO is presumed to be present. In patients with an intact interatrial septum, the most likely etiology of a right-to-left shunt at the atrial level is a PFO. Figure 19.2 shows sequential echocardiograms obtained during performance of a PEEP test in a patient with a PFO. Microbubbles are best generated using a two-syringe technique as shown in Figure 19.3.

Patients With a PFO: Now What Do We Do?

In patients scheduled to undergo neurosurgery in the sitting position, we now have the ability to identify most patients with a PFO prior to beginning the operative procedure. This raises new questions concerning choice of position and intraoperative monitoring for paradoxical air embolism. In order to arrive at meaningful recommendations, you need to determine the risk of paradoxical air embolism during episodes of VAE in patients with a PFO.

We can calculate the maximum theoretical risk of paradoxical air embolism during sitting neurosurgical procedures simply by multiplying the incidence of Doppler-detected VAE (10% during cervical laminectomy, 45% during craniotomy) by the incidence of PFO in the general population (25%). This calculation suggests a theoretical risk of paradoxical air embolism in up to 2.5% of cervical laminectomies and 11% of craniotomies performed in the sitting position. These numbers are inconsistent with the reported clinical experience in which clinically symptomatic paradoxical air embolism is an extremely rare event.

We have experience with TEE monitoring to identify patients with a PFO and to monitor for intraoperative paradoxical air embolism during episodes of VAE in 280 patients scheduled for neurosurgery in the sitting position at the Mayo Clinic (Table 19.2). Consistent with the litera-

Positioning of Patients With a PFO: Recommendations

1. The decision concerning positioning should be made jointly between the anesthesiologist and neurosurgeon.
2. Consider performing the procedure in an alternative horizontal position with a lower risk of VAE and, therefore, a theoretically lower risk of paradoxical air embolism.
3. If there is a justifiable reason to perform the procedure in the sitting position (such as improved surgical exposure and/or operating conditions), this can be done with what appears to be a low risk of TEE-detected paradoxical air embolism.
4. Regardless of the position selected, the patient may benefit from intraoperative TEE monitoring for paradoxical air embolism.
5. In the event that TEE-detected paradoxical air embolism occurs intraoperatively and the source of air entrainment cannot be identified, be prepared to alter the surgical position and/or prematurely terminate the surgical procedure and close the surgical site in order to prevent further air entrainment.

Abbreviations: PFO, patent foramen ovale; VAE, venous air embolism; TEE, transesophageal echocardiography.

TABLE 19.2 *TEE monitoring for PFO and intraoperative paradoxical air embolism in 280 patients scheduled for neurosurgery in the sitting position at the Mayo Clinic*

	SITTING PATIENTS WITH PFO	SITTING PATIENTS WITHOUT PFO	HORIZONTAL PATIENTS WITH PFO
Patients[a] (n)	42	230	8
Surgical procedure			
CRAN (n)	24	130	6
CSS (n)	18	100	2
Patients with VAE	13	73	0
Episodes of VAE	31	167	0
Episodes of paradoxical air embolism	2[b]	1[c]	0
Paradoxical air embolism during VAE (% of episodes of VAE)	6.5%	0.6%	—

Abbreviations: TEE, transesophageal echocardiography; PFO patent foramen ovale; CRAN, craniotomy; CSS, cervical spine surgery; VAE, venous air embolism.

[a] Includes one patient with PFO in whom surgery was canceled.

[b] One episode in each of two patients. The source of VAE was identified promptly, and surgery was completed without difficulty. No morbidity or mortality from paradoxical air embolism.

[c] Transpulmonary passage of air. Source of air entrainment not identifiable. The surgical procedure was terminated prematurely and the surgical site was closed in expeditious fashion. No morbidity or mortality from paradoxical air embolism.

(From Losasso et al.,[15] with permission.)

FIGURE 19.1 *The relationship between right atrial (RA) and left atrial (LA) pressure following the release of PEEP. Immediately following the release of PEEP, RA pressure transiently exceeds LA pressure. Injection of agitated saline into the right atrium simultaneous with PEEP release should allow TEE detection of microbubbles in the left atrium in patients with a PFO. (From Black et al.,[20] with permission.)*

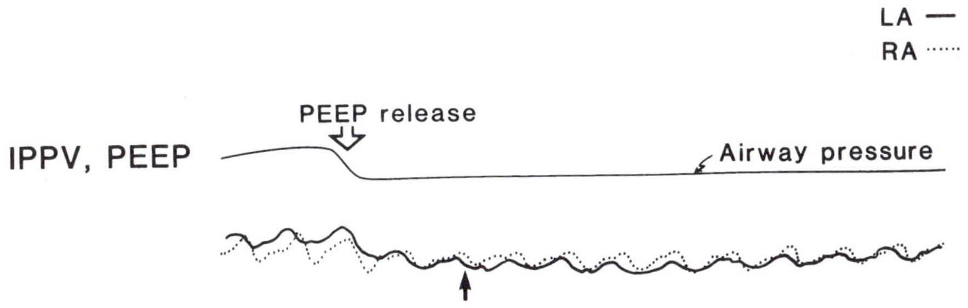

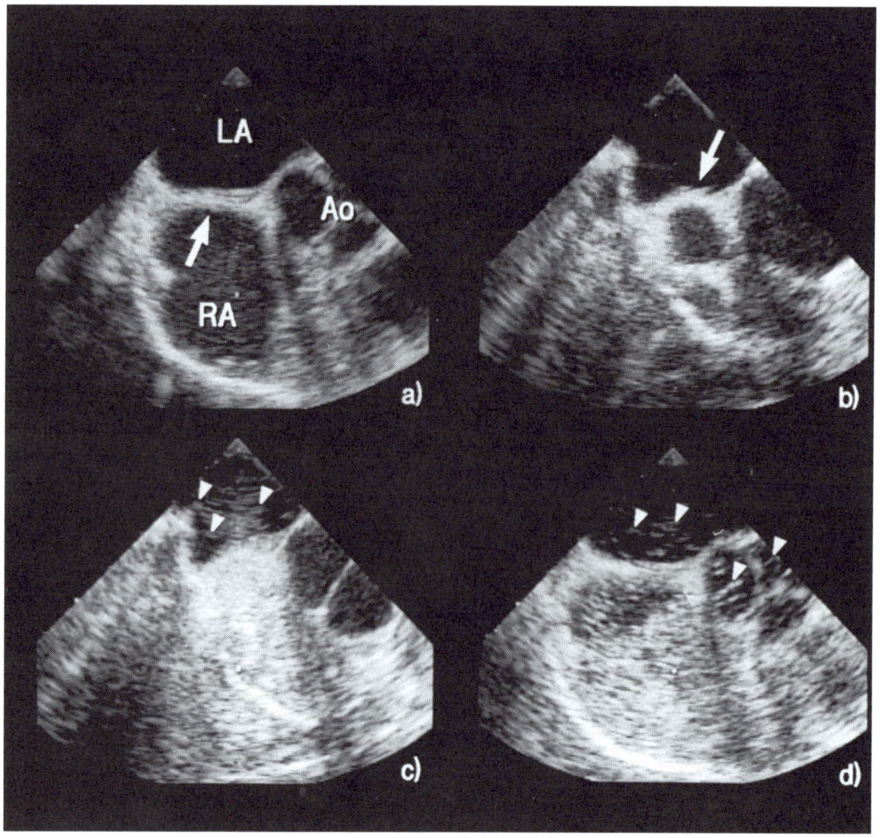

FIGURE 19.2 *Sequential echocardiograms obtained during performance of a PEEP test in a patient with a PFO. The left atrium (LA), right atrium (RA), and aortic valve (Ao) are shown. The interatrial septum is identified by the large arrow, whereas the small arrows indicate microbubbles. (A) A baseline echocardiogram. (B) Conditions following 15 to 20 seconds of PEEP with RA pressure presumably exceeding LA pressure as indicated by the interatrial septum bulging from right to left. With PEEP release and injection of agitated saline (C), microbubbles are noted to opacify the RA. Additionally, some microbubbles are seen to have crossed into the LA through a PFO (C) and slightly later are seen passing into the aorta at the level of the aortic valve (D).*

ture, we identified a PFO prior to beginning the operative procedure in 50 of 280 patients (17%). In seven cases, surgical positioning was changed to an alternative horizontal position, and in one case, the procedure was canceled. In these horizontal patients, there were no episodes of VAE and consequently no episodes of paradoxical air embolism. In 42 patients with a PFO, surgery was performed as originally planned in the sitting position. There was a total of 31 episodes of VAE in these 42 patients. Paradoxical air embolism occurred during only 2 (or 6.5%) of these 31 episodes of VAE. One episode of TEE-detected paradoxical air embolism occurred in each of two patients with a PFO. In each case, the source of VAE was identified promptly, surgery was completed without difficulty, and no morbidity or mortality occurred from paradoxical air embolism. In 230 sitting patients without a PFO, there was a total of 167 episodes of VAE and only one episode of TEE-detected paradoxical air embolism. In this one instance, paradoxical air embolism resulted from transpulmonary passage of air.[18] The source of air entrainment could not be identified, the surgical procedure was prematurely terminated, and the surgical site was closed in an expeditious fashion. Again, no morbidity or mortality occurred from paradoxical air embolism.

Consistent with expectations, these data suggest that the incidence of TEE-detected detected paradoxical air embolism during VAE is greater in patients with a PFO compared to patients without a PFO (6.5% vs. 0.6% of episodes of VAE, respectively). Additionally, and again as would be expected, operating upon patients with a PFO in a horizontal position compared to the sitting position reduces the risk of VAE and consequently the risk of paradoxical air embolism. More importantly, however, these data suggest that in sitting neurosurgical patients with a PFO, paradoxical air embolism during VAE is an infrequent occurrence (6.5% of episodes of VAE). This finding may be explained, at least in part, by the fact that (1) most episodes of Doppler-detected VAE are associated

FIGURE 19.3 *The two-syringe technique to create microbubbles. Agitated saline is created by vigorously exchaning saline between syringes interconnected with a three-way stopcock. This is a superior technique to produce a solution with a high concentration of microbubbles for injection.*

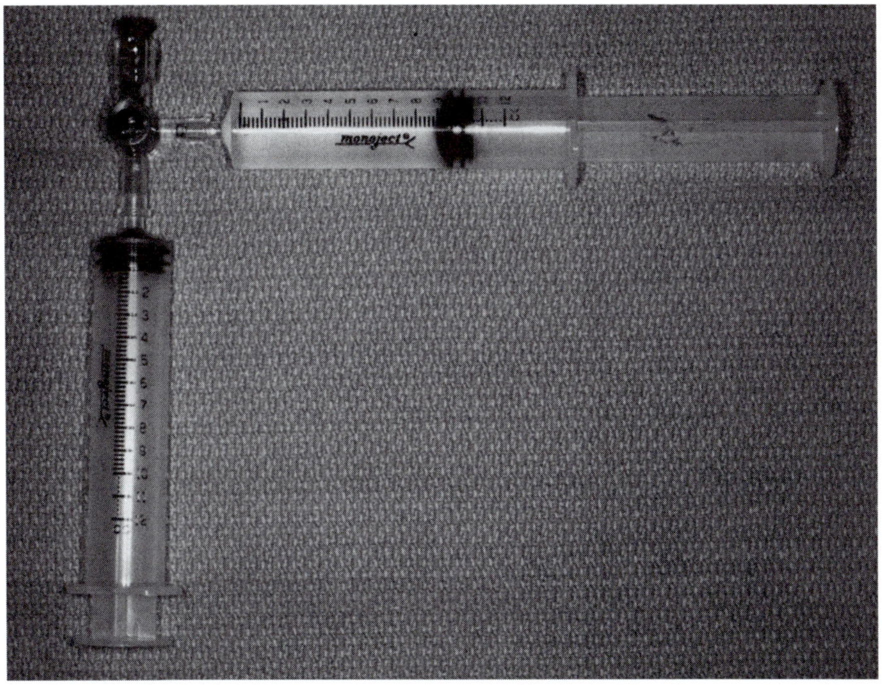

with small amounts of entrained air and (2) due to the complaint nature of the right atrium and the presence of competent tricuspid and pulmonary valves in most patients, RA pressure does not increase appreciably during most clinical episodes of VAE. It is likely that there is a critical "opening pressure" (i.e., right-to-left interatrial pressure gradient) that is necessary to open a PFO and that this opening pressure is not exceeded during most clinical episodes of VAE.[21]

Based upon these data, the accompanying box lists some recommendations for positioning of patients in whom a PFO is identified prior to beginning the surgical procedure. It should be noted that these recommendations apply specifically to patients with a PFO and not to patients with an atrial septal defect (ASD). We must be careful to differentiate between patients with a PFO (which in most cases is only a *potential* right-to-left shunt) and patients with an ASD (which are associated with *actual* bidirectional shunts). Undoubtedly, the risk of paradoxical air embolism during VAE is greater in patients with an ASD compared to patients with a PFO.

INTRAOPERATIVE MONITORING FOR PARADOXICAL AIR EMBOLISM

At the present time, TEE is the most sensitive and reliable monitor available for intraoperative detection of paradoxical air embolism. Failure to detect a PFO prior to surgery does not eliminate the risk of paradoxical air embolism. During an episode of VAE, a paradoxical air embolism can occur through a previously unidentified PFO (i.e., a patient with a false-negative PEEP test) or via transpulmonary passage of air emboli.[13,15,18,19] However, the sensitivity of the TEE to detect paradoxical air embolism during episodes of VAE is high so that it is extremely unlikely that clinically significant paradoxical air embolism can occur without appearing on the TEE.

Although it is unproven at this time, it is logical to assume that the TEE can do for the problem of paradoxical air embolism what the precor-

TABLE 19.3 *The Mayo Clinic experience of sitting neurosurgical patients with intraoperative TEE-detected paradoxical air embolism*[a]

REFERENCE	PATIENTS WITH INTRAOPERATIVE TEE-DETECTED PARADOXICAL AIR EMBOLISM (n)	NO. OF PATIENTS CLINICALLY SYMPTOMATIC
Cucchiara et al.[23]	1	0
Cucchiara et al.[24]	1	0
Cucchiara et al.[19]	2	0
Black et al.[13]	1	0
Losasso et al.[15]	2	0
Bedell et al.[18]	1	0
Total	8	0

Abbreviation: TEE, transesophageal echocardiography.

[a] In all cases, either the source of air entrainment was promptly identified and surgery completed as planned or the source of air entrainment could not be identified, surgery was prematurely terminated, the surgical site was closed, and the patient was allowed to emerge from anesthesia. No morbidity or mortality occurred secondary to paradoxical air embolism.

dial Doppler has done for the problem of VAE. By allowing for early detection and prompt treatment, intraoperative monitoring with TEE may minimize if not eliminate significant morbidity and mortality resulting from paradoxical air embolism. The threshold for "safe" volumes of paradoxical air in humans is unknown and is likely to never be known. Any amount of paradoxical air should be considered as potentially dangerous because it is not only the volume, but also the ultimate destination that contribute to organ dysfunction and serious morbidity and mortality.

It is important to distinguish between clinically significant paradoxical air embolism and TEE-detected paradoxical air embolism. The goal of TEE monitoring is to detect paradoxical air embolism early so as to allow the clinician to intervene and to make appropriate decisions intraoperatively. When paradoxical air embolism is detected, identification of the source of air entrainment must be aggressively pursued. Experience shows that if the source is promptly identified and the episode is brief, TEE-detected paradoxical air embolism is likely to be limited to a subclinical event with the patient sustaining no injury.[13,15,18,19,22–24] Table 19.3 reviews the Mayo Clinic experience of sitting neurosurgical patients with TEE-detected paradoxical air embolism. In all cases (N = 8), either the source of air entrainment was immediately identified and

FIGURE 19.4 *An intraoperative TEE image obtained in a patient undergoing VA shunt insertion. The distal end of the catheter (indicated by the small arrow) is localized to the junction of the superior vena cava (SVC) and right atrium (RA). The right pulmonary artery (RPA) is labeled.*

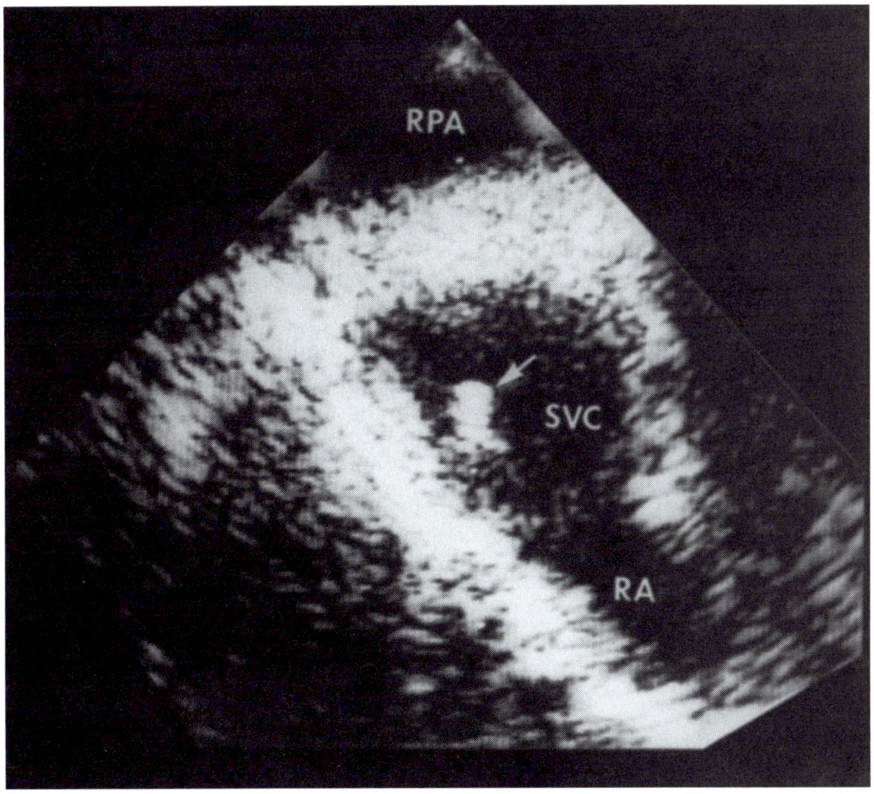

the surgery completed as planned or the source of air entrainment could not be identified, surgery was prematurely terminated, the surgical site was closed in an expeditious fashion, and the patient was allowed to emerge from general anesthesia. No paradoxical air embolism-related morbidity or mortality occurred in any of the eight patients.

The goal of TEE monitoring is to prevent a subclinical event (i.e., TEE-detected paradoxical air embolism) from becoming clinically significant. It is difficult to prove that TEE monitoring reduces morbidity and mortality from paradoxical air embolism in sitting neurosurgical patients. However, it is logical that a monitor that provides for early detection of paradoxical air embolism and permits prompt intervention may limit morbidity and mortality. The data presented in Table 19.3 are consistent with this theory.

INTRAOPERATIVE PLACEMENT OF RA CATHETERS

In a canine model of VAE, Artru demonstrated improved survival in animals with an RA catheter in place from which air could be aspirated from the central circulation compared to animals in which air was not removed from the central circulation.[25] Laboratory data and clinical experience suggest that the proximal port of a multiorificed RA catheter (or tip of a single-lumen catheter) should be localized to the superior vena cava-right atrial (SVC-RA) junction in order to optimize aspiration of air from the central circulation during episodes of VAE.[26,27]

TEE can be used intraoperatively to guide and confirm proper placement of the RA catheter at the SVC-RA junction. RA catheters are frequently positioned using electrocardiographic guidance. However, it has been demonstrated that intravenous electrocardiography may not accurately localize the proximal port of multiorificed RA catheters.[28] Additionally, RA catheters can migrate during patient positioning or during the operative procedure.[29] Catheter migration can compromise efforts to aspirate air during clinical episodes of VAE due to suboptimal or incorrect catheter tip location.

We have found the TEE useful in the following circumstances: (1) to localize the RA catheter tip in patients in whom intravenous electrocardiography is technically difficult, (2) to monitor for catheter tip migration associated with patient positioning, and (3) to monitor periodically for catheter tip migration throughout the operative procedure. Prospective studies are necessary to determine if air retrieval during episodes of VAE is improved with RA catheters that are positioned with TEE versus electrocardiographic guidance.

INTRAOPERATIVE PLACEMENT OF VA SHUNTS

Ventriculoperitoneal (VP) shunts have become the mainstay of hydrocephalus treatment in children and adults because of their ease of insertion and long-term function.[30] A commonly used alternative to the VP shunt is the VA shunt. Accurate placement of the distal end of a VA shunt near the SVC-RA junction is important for long-term shunt function as well as for avoiding cardiac arrhythmias, thrombus formation, and damage to myocardial tissue.[31] Standard methods of intraoperative localization of distal catheter placement include electrocardiographic guidance, chest x-ray, and/or pressure measurement. However, these techniques can result in inaccurate and unreliable catheter localization.

Intraoperatively, TEE can be used to localize the distal end of the VA shunt catheter near the SVC-RA junction.[32] Figure 19.4 shows the TEE image obtained in a patient undergoing VA shunt placement. During the past several years we have used this technique to place more than 10 VA shunts at the Mayo Clinic. A chest x-ray obtained perioperatively confirmed proper positioning in all patients. Prospective studies are necessary to determine whether intraoperative

TEE localization is superior to previously employed methods.

References

1. Thys DM, Konstadt S, Hillel Z: Perioperative echocardiography. In: Clinical Monitoring. WB Saunders, Philadelphia, Chap 9, p 149–171, 1994
2. Losasso TJ, Muzzi DA, Dietz NM, Cucchiara RF: Fifty percent N_2O does not increase the risk of venous air embolism in neurosurgical patients operated upon in the sitting position. Anesthesiology 77:21, 1992
3. Black S, Ockert DB, Oliver WC, Cucchiara RF: Outcome following posterior fossa craniectomy in patients in the sitting or horizontal positions. Anesthesiology 69:49, 1988
4. Glenski JA, Cucchiara RF, Michenfelder JD: Transesophageal echocardiography and transcutaneous O_2 and CO_2 monitoring for detection of venous air embolism. Anesthesiology 64:541, 1986
5. Losasso TJ, Black S, Muzzi DA et al: Detection and hemodynamic consequences of venous air embolism: does N_2O make a difference? Anesthesiology 77:148, 1992
6. Muzzi DA, Losasso TJ, Black S, Nishimura R: Comparison of a transesophageal and precordial ultrasonic doppler sensor in the detection of venous air embolism. Anesth Analg 70:103, 1990
7. Gronert GA, Messick JM, Michenfelder JD: Paradoxical air embolism from a patent foramen ovale. Anesthesiology 50:548, 1979
8. Thompson T, Evans W: Paradoxical embolism. Q J Med 23:135, 1930
9. Hagen PT, Scholz DG, Edwards WD: Incidence and size of patent foramen ovale during the first 10 decades of life: an autopsy study of 965 normal hearts. Mayo Clin Proc 59:17, 1984
10. Lechat PH, Mas JL, Lascault G et al: Prevalence of patent foramen ovale in patients with stroke. N Engl J Med 318:1148, 1988
11. Lynch JJ, Schuchard GH, Gross CM, Wann LS: Prevalence of right to left atrial shunting in the healthy population. Am J Cardiol 52:1478, 1984
12. Guggiari M, Lechat PH, Garen-Colonnec C et al: Early detection of patent foramen ovale by two-dimensional contrast echocardiography for prevention of paradoxical air embolism during the sitting position. Anesth Analg 67:192, 1988
13. Black S, Muzzi DA, Nishimura RA, Cucchiara RF: Preoperative and intraoperative echocardiography to detect right to left shunt in patients undergoing neurosurgical procedures in the sitting position. Anesthesiology 72:436, 1990
14. Schwarz G, Fuchs G, Weihs W et al: Sitting position for neurosurgery: experience with preoperative contrast echocardiography in 301 patients. J Neurosurg Anesth 6:83, 1994
15. Losasso TJ, Muzzi DA, Weglinski MR: The risk of paradoxical air embolism in sitting neurosurgical patients with and without a demonstrable right-to-left shunt. Anesthesiology 77:A198, 1992
16. Konstadt SN, Louie EK, Black S et al: Intraoperative detection of patent foramen ovale by transesophageal echocardiography. Anesthesiology 74:212, 1991
17. Kronik G, Mosslacher H: Positive contrast echocardiography in patients with patent foramen ovale and normal right heart hemodynamics. Am J Cardiol 49:1806, 1982
18. Bedell EA, Berge KH, Losasso TJ: Paradoxic air embolism during venous air embolism: transesophageal echocardiographic evidence of transpulmonary air passage. Anesthesiology 80:947, 1994
19. Cucchiara RF, Nishimura RA, Black S: Failure of preoperative echo testing to prevent paradoxical air embolism. Anesthesiology 71:604, 1989
20. Black S, Cucchiara RF, Nishimura RA, Michenfelder JD: Parameters affecting occurrence of paradoxical air embolism. Anesthesiology 71:235, 1989
21. Jaffe RA, Pinto FJ, Schnittger I et al: Aspects of mechanical ventilation affecting interatrial shunt flow during general anesthesia. Anesth Analg 75:484, 1992
22. Furuya H, Okumura F: Detection of paradoxical air embolism by transesophageal echocardiography. Anesthesiology 60:374, 1984
23. Cucchiara RF, Nugent M, Seward JB, Messick JM: Air embolism in upright neurosurgical patients: detection and localization by two-dimensional transesophageal echocardiography. Anesthesiology 60:353, 1984
24. Cucchiara RF, Seward JM, Nishimura RA et al: Identification of patent foramen ovale during sitting position craniotomy by transesophageal echocardiography with positive airway pressure. Anesthesiology 63:107, 1985
25. Artru AA: Modification of a new catheter for air retrieval and resuscitation from lethal venous air embolism: effect of N_2O on air retrieval. Anesth Analg 75:226, 1992

26. Bunegin L, Albin MS, Helsel PE et al: Positioning the right atrial catheter: A model for reappraisal. Anesthesiology 55:343, 1981
27. Michenfelder JD: Central venous catheters in the management of air embolism: whether as well as where. Anesthesiology 55:339, 1981
28. Artru AA, Colley PS: The site of origin of the intravascular electrocardiogram recorded from multiorificed intravascular catheters. Anesthesiology 69:44, 1988
29. Lee DS, Kuhn J, Shaffer MJ, Weintraub HD: Migration of tips of central venous catheters in seated patients. Anesth Analg 63:649,1984
30. Chapman PH: Hydrocephalus in childhood. p. 1236. In Youmans JR (ed): Neurological Surgery. 3rd Ed. Vol. 2. WB Saunders, Philadelphia, 1990
31. Illingsworth RD, Logue V, Symon L et al: The ventriculo-caval shunt in the treatment of adult hydrocephalus. Results and complications in 101 patients. J Neurosurg 35:681, 1977
32. McGrail K, Muzzi DA, Losasso TJ, Meyer FB: Ventriculo-atrial shunt distal catheter placement using transesophageal echocardiography. J Neurosurg 30:747, 1992

20 CHRONIC AND INTERVENTIONAL PAIN MANAGEMENT

PETER R. WILSON

ORLANDO G. FLORETE, JR.

DANIEL S. ROWE, JR.

Chronic pain is a significant cause of cost and impairment in the community, as affected patients suffer reduction in quality of life and decreased productivity while and requiring use of medical services and thus facing increased expense—a "silent epidemic."[1] The patient's family, significant others, employer, and society are all adversely affected in addition to the patient. This chapter cannot be a definitive review of all chronic pain syndromes but serves as a guide to resources and certain management principles. The problems of acute and cancer-related pain management have been adequately addressed by practice guidelines promulgated by the Agency for Health Care Policy and Research (AHCPR).[2]

There are significant difficulties in deriving scientific bases for any discussion about acute, chronic, and terminal pain. The epidemiologic studies are sparse and suspect, and there are few therapeutic trials that satisfy the usual requirements for scientific rigor; for example, there are more than 60 different published treatments for reflex sympathetic dystrophy (RSD), all of which claim 60 to 100 percent success. Not one of these is a controlled, blinded, objective long-term study. It is clearly necessary to base treatment recommendations on valid studies and to use an evidence-based model. When this approach is used, the result is dismal, as most of the literature comprises case reports and uncontrolled, open-label trials. The pain syndromes themselves are usually poorly defined, and outcome measures are rarely objective. For example, many studies use "50 percent reduction in pain" as the criterion of success. If a 10-cm visual analog scale is used, for example, a reduction from 10 cm to 5 cm is regarded as equivalent to a reduction from 2 cm to 1 cm. There are very few studies that use objective criteria, such as return to work, medication use, or cost of medical care, as outcome measures. In addition, good long-term studies (greater than 3 months) are also rare. There are difficulties in follow-up and an assumed tendency of the chronic pain to return to baseline over time, whatever the intervention.

This chapter therefore attempts to present evidence-based recommendations for the diagnosis and treatment of nociceptive and neuropathic pain syndromes and gives examples of each. It also reviews the therapeutic modalities likely to be used by the readers and indicates the validity of each. It draws on the literature review performed for the American Society of Anesthesiologists by Dr. Richard Connis,[3] in which only 376 papers were used from an original database of more than 3,000 reviewed.

DEFINITION

Chronic pain is often defined as pain that has lasted for more than an arbitrary time (e.g., 3 months).[4] However, it might also be defined in terms of a duration longer than the expected healing time, with no apparent biologic warning function and with significant adverse biopsychosocial consequences. It may occur as the continuation of acute pain of nociceptive origin or as the result of damage or malfunction of peripheral nerves or their central connections (neuropathic pain). There may be components of both types of pain in the same syndrome. It is important both from a diagnostic and therapeutic point of view to distinguish these components, as the prognosis and therapy may be quite different. There are also psychogenic pain syndromes, with no evidence of nociceptive or neuropathic mechanisms, but with evidence of psychologic or psychiatric pathology. This is also beyond the scope of this chapter.

NOCICEPTIVE PAIN

Nociception is the sum of the neurophysiologic processes that are involved in the detection of potentially tissue-damaging stimuli. However, nociception is not pain until it reaches consciousness and evokes the unpleasant sensory and emotional experiences that define pain.

Nociceptors supply all structures of the body (except the brain itself) with A δ and C fibers, which may have specific or nonspecific peripheral terminals (although named receptors, to be distinguished from neurochemical receptors). Nociceptive endings respond variably to mechanical, thermal, and chemical stimulation. They exhibit sensitization (i.e., an increase in response with repeated applications of a particular stimulus). This sensitization is composed both of peripheral and central mechanisms, mediated by different neurochemicals. The rate and extent of sensitization may be altered by manipulation of these chemicals (with anti-inflammatory agents), and the resulting pain may be reduced. Similarly, it is theoretically possible to modify the gain of the transmission system (with opioids, serotonin, or norepinephrine reuptake inhibitors), reduce "wind-up" in the spinal cord (with *N*-methyl-D-aspartate [NMDA] antagonists), and block neural transmission in the periphery or centrally with local anesthetics.

It can be seen that the nociceptive component of an acute or chronic or terminal pain syndrome is amenable to treatment with presently available pharmacologic agents. However, it is imperative that the contribution of this mechanism be appropriately determined in each case. Therapeutic trials of pharmacologic agents may be necessary, at all times being aware of the placebo effect of any treatment.

There is considerable controversy surrounding the relationship between depression and pain, particularly chronic pain. It is apparent that there is an association between the two, but it is not yet clear from the literature whether there is a cause-effect relationship. The picture is further confounded because pharmacologic treatments for depression (with agents having a serotonin and norepinephrine reuptake inhibition) have an independent effect on nociception at the spinal cord level.

There are other alterations in sensory perception, often related to tissue damage, of peripheral and/or central processing of the stimuli. These terms have been defined by the International Association for the Study of Pain (IASP).[2] They are not regarded as pain but may have important implications in the diagnostic process. For example, the presence of allodynia is suggestive of a neuropathic component, with peripheral or central amplification of the signal.

Suffering is an experience that does not necessarily require nociceptive pain for initiation or maintenance. Loss of bodily or mental function, social support or status, personal identity, or psychological health may all produce suffering. The simple relief of physical pain might achieve

Definitions of Pain and Pain-Related Sensory Perception

Pain: an unpleasant sensory and emotional experience, usually associated with tissue damage or described in terms of such damage

Dysesthesia: unpleasant sensation, often with "electric" characteristics

Paresthesia: unpleasant electrical sensation in the distribution of a peripheral nerve

Hyperpathia: unpleasant dysesthesia with an exaggerated pain perception after noxious or non-noxious stimuli

Hyperalgesia: increased pain response to a noxious stimulus

Hyperesthesia: increased sensitivity to non-noxious stimulation

Allodynia: perception of pain evoked by a normally non-noxious stimulus

(The terms *hypalgesia* and *hypesthesia* have not been endorsed by the IASP Committee on Taxonomy.)

little in the overall relief of such suffering. The careful evaluation of all nonphysiologic responses is an essential component of comprehensive and humane pain management.

The accompanying box indicates some of the neurochemicals implicated in dorsal horn nociceptive function (for a more complete list, see ref. 5). Some of these chemical activities can be altered by systemic or spinal administration of the appropriate agonists or antagonists. Unfortunately, the roles of these chemicals in the transduction and transmission processes and in defining the characteristics and intensity of the nociception are still unclear. It is also not clear whether these are the only chemicals involved in nociception. There is still much to be learned about the relationships between nociception and the experience of pain. There are many pain syndromes with little evidence of nociception and without experimental models (e.g., most of the neuropathic pain syndromes).

Treatment of nociceptive pain therefore depends on accurate diagnosis of the mechanisms and reducing neurologic activity at the peripheral detectors, peripheral fibers, and central relays.

Partial Listing of Neurochemicals Implicated in Dorsal Horn Nociceptive Function

PEPTIDES

Atrial natriuretic factor
Angiotensin II
Bombesin
Cholecystokinin
Calcitonin gene-related peptide
Neuropeptide Y
Neurotensin
Oxytocin
Prodynorphins
Proenkephalins
Somatostatin
Tachykinins (including substance P)
Vasoactive intestinal peptide

EXCITATORY AMINO ACIDS

Aspartate
Glutamate

INHIBITORY AMINO ACIDS

GABA
Glycine

MONOAMINES

Dopamine
Epinephrine
Histamine
Norepinephrine
Serotonin

MISCELLANEOUS

Acetylcholine
ATP

NEUROPATHIC PAIN

Neuropathic pain refers to pain that is apparently generated within the nervous system, in the absence of other tissue damage. The abnormal generator(s) of the neuropathic pain can be structural damage to neural tissue or chemical malfunction within the nervous system. The damage/malfunction can be within the central nervous system (CNS), the peripheral nervous system, or in both, with or without involvement of the sympathetic nervous system. The mechanisms have been summarized by Casey[6] and Portenoy[7] and in the accompanying box.

It may be assumed that neuropathic pain results from activation of abnormal generators, abnormal "amplification" of normal signals, or abnormal reduction or absence of normal inhibitory mechanisms. Therapy of neuropathic pain states has therefore been directed toward these putative mechanisms and neurochemicals. Categories of therapeutic agents include (singly and in combination): opioids, antidepressants, NMDA antagonists, membrane stabilizers, benzodiazepines, and substance P depleters. Unfortunately, there are few neuropathic states that respond reliably to pharmacotherapy.

Sympathetically maintained pain (SMP) is an operational definition of pain that is accompanied by signs of sympathetic dysregulation in the area of the pain and that responds favorably to sympathetic blockade. Although animal models of nerve damage mimic some of the characteristics of SMP, there are no convincing models of this clinical condition.

Neuropathic Pain

CENTRAL PAIN GENERATOR

Hypersensitivity to nociceptive and non-nociceptive inputs

Ectopic impulse generation

Changes in receptive fields

Loss of central inhibitory processes

e.g., Deafferentation pain

  Sympathetically maintained pain

PERIPHERAL PAIN GENERATOR

Sensitization of primary afferents

Neuroma formation

Ephapses

Other sources of ectopic impulses

e.g., Painful polyneuropathies

  Painful mononeuropathies

    "Lancinating neuralgias"

    Nerve compression or inflammation

    Nerve transection

  Sympathetically maintained pain

COMBINED GENERATORS

e.g., Sympathetically maintained pain

COMPLEX REGIONAL PAIN SYNDROME—REFLEX SYMPATHETIC DYSTROPHY

RSD is a clinical diagnosis of great antiquity, but one that has even yet not been defined adequately. Attempts have been made to clarify the clinical criteria and understand the pathophysiologic mechanisms. The whole subject has been recently revisited by an international committee, whose report is now available.[8] The committee recommended that a clinical condition "complex regional pain syndrome (CRPS) type I" be used to describe variants of the condition formerly known as RSD and type II be used to describe "causalgia." The accompanying boxes indicate the characteristics of CRPS(I) and criteria for the diagnosis of SMP. It is important to recognize that SMP and sympathetically independent pain can occur separately or together. It must also be recognized that some therapeutic interventions will be more effective in one case or the other.

Treatment of RSD, as reported in the literature, has successfully used at least 60 modalities, ranging from acupuncture to Zen. Unfortunately, in the absence of consensus regarding di-

Complex Regional Pain Syndrome (I) (RSD)

PAIN

CRPS is a pain syndrome

The characteristics of the pain vary with the initiating event, extent of neuropathic involvement

Extent of sympathetic involvement varies from 0 to 100 percent

The pain is often described as burning, spontaneous, or evoked, often related to hyperalgesia or allodynia

HISTORY

Often develops after a noxious event or immobilization

Usually unilateral extremity onset (often spreads)

Usually develops within 1 month after injury

EXCLUSIONS

Major nerve injury—CRPS (II)—causalgia

No other demonstrable pathology to account for the symptoms

SYMPTOMS

Pain, spontaneous or evoked, burning, aching or throbbing

Hyperalgesia or allodynia (mechanical or thermal, superficial or deep)

Associated (minor) symptoms:

- Swelling/edema
- Temperature/color asymmetry and instability
- Sweating asymmetry and instability
- Trophic changes of skin, hair, nails

SIGNS

Hyperalgesia and/or allodynia

Edema (unilateral—no other causes)

Vasomotor changes

Sudomotor changes

Trophic changes (hair, skin, nails, joints)

CRITERIA

Sympathetically Maintained Pain

1. Peripheral skin temperature asymmetry and difference >1°C
2. Resting or evoked sweat asymmetry
3. Appropriate response to technically adequate local anesthetic sympathetic blockade
4. Appropriate response to adequate alpha receptor blockade (placebo-controlled)

TESTS OF UNKNOWN SENSITIVITY AND SPECIFICITY

Three-phase bone scan

Patchy demineralization

Tourniquet ischemia test

Cutaneous blood flow (laser Doppler)

Somatosensory evoked potential/electromyography

Intravenous regional sympathetic blockade

Pain that remains after adequate sympathetic blockade must be sympathetically independent pain.

agnostic criteria and objective outcome measures, there are no robust studies to direct either the workup or therapy. It would be reasonable to assume that general principles of pain management apply and that a multidisciplinary approach with emphasis on rehabilitation would be the most effective. However, the anesthesiologist is uniquely equipped to facilitate physical therapy with the judicious application of appropriate neural blockade. Unfortunately (again), there are no valid studies to indicate the type of block, agent, frequency, or adjuvant pharmacologic therapy.

MANAGEMENT STRATAGEMS

All pain syndromes comprise elements of nociceptive pain, neuropathic pain, and psychosocial factors that contribute to the total experience. It is therefore necessary to define, as accurately as possible, the relative contributions of these factors.

History and Examination

The comprehensive evaluation of a patient with pain necessarily includes the following elements:

1. A complete general medical history; history of the present and previous pain complaints; information about previous tests and therapies; the quality, intensity, distribution, duration, affective components, and exacerbating and relieving factors. Documentation of this baseline information is essential to follow the results of therapy and measure outcome.
2. Psychosocial information must include the presence of psychological symptoms (e.g., anxiety, depression, anger), coping mechanisms, and the meaning of the pain. Social effects of the pain (withdrawal, loss of employment) and direct and indirect costs are important in defining the impact of the pain. These measures may also be used as outcome measures.
3. Physical examination usually involves a directed neurologic and orthopaedic evaluation, with assessment of disability and impairment, if appropriate.
4. Differential diagnosis of the pain syndrome, including underlying pathologies and consequences of the pain, is necessary to define potential therapies.
5. Treatment options must be developed with input from the patient, other involved professionals, and other involved individuals (e.g., significant other, rehabilitation and vocational counselors).

Diagnostic Evaluation

There is widespread acceptance for the use of diagnostic imaging (computed tomography, magnetic resonance imaging, myelography, facet arthrography, discography) for defining anatomic abnormalities. However, the relationship between structural abnormalities and clinical status is not well defined in many cases.[9] However, there may be a relationship between "functional" diagnostic blocks and the pain syndrome[10] in some specific cases. However, the "differential block"[11] has never been validated. Sympathetic blockade is used to define SMP. Local anesthetic somatic blockade may be useful in the definition of the anatomic component of the nociceptive pain. Autonomic blocks may be useful in other pain syndromes and may predict the response to chemical or surgical sympathectomy. Unfortunately, the scientific bases for these practices is not robust.

Multidisciplinary Pain Management

The scientific evidence relating to chronic pain management is strongest in the field of multidisciplinary management. There is no standard definition of multidisciplinary care, although the Commission on Accreditation of Rehabilitation Facilities (which accredits pain programs) indicates that a "core team" comprises the patient, pain physician, and members from three other disciplines including psychology. The composition of the team is dictated by the needs of the patient ("person served"). Successful programs emphasize improvement of functional status, quality of life, return to work, reduction in medication intake, and reduction in pain behaviors.[12,13]

Opioid Therapy

The use of opioids for the management of acute and cancer/terminal pain is well established and well understood. However, opioid use in long-term pain in controversial, both medically and legally. Portenoy[14] reviewed the pharmacology of opioids, indicating the efficacy and potency of the different compounds. He defined the correct and appropriate use of the terms *tolerance*, *dependence*, and *addiction*. Tolerance is the biochemical phenomenon of decreasing effect of constant doses or the requirement for increasing doses to obtain a constant effect. Associative tolerance refers to a change in effect due to operant conditioning. Pharmacologic tolerance may be dispositional (pharmacokinetic) or pharmacodynamic (presumably at the receptor level). Addiction usually refers to a behavioral state of compulsive use resulting in physical, psychologic, or social harm, continuing despite that harm.[15] There is concern that the use of opioids in non-nociceptive pain will lead to the development of tolerance, dependence, and addiction.

Considerations in the Management of Chronic Pain with Opioids

1. Only after failure of all other reasonable therapies
2. Single physician/prescriber, in consultation with pain consultant
3. Written, informed consent, including

Agreement on responsible, compliant behavior

Recognition of potential adverse cognitive, pharmacologic, and behavioral effects

Likelihood of physical dependence and withdrawal potential

4. Written contract defining patient's responsibilities regarding the treatment program
5. Long-acting oral opioid on a fixed schedule
6. "Rescue" doses only as agreed in advance
7. Regular (at least monthly) review
8. Written monitoring of efficacy criteria:

Analgesia

Side effects

Functional status

Aberrant behaviors

Portenoy lists aberrant behaviors that raise concerns about the development of addiction, including selling, stealing, or borrowing drugs, forging or losing prescriptions, multiple sources of prescriptions, multiple emergency department attendances, and evidence of social and psychological deterioration.

There are controversies surrounding the efficacy of opioids in chronic (nonmalignant) pain[16] and concerns by licensing bodies of malfeasance among prescribers (including diversion). Consequently, "contracts" have been developed for the protection of both the patient and prescriber, elucidated by Portenoy and summarized in the accompanying box, which was adapted from his Table 11-9.

Spinal Pain

Back and neck pain constitute an incalculable cost to society in terms of individual suffering, direct medical costs, and indirect costs related to decreased productivity. However, in most cases, no structural abnormality can be found. The problem is of such magnitude that the AHCPR developed guidelines for the management of acute low back problems in adults.[17] The subject was deliberately restricted to the first 12 weeks of symptoms. In all, more than 10,000 abstracts were reviewed, 3,918 papers evaluated, and 360 papers finally used to draft the guidelines. The final guidelines reflect the paucity of scientifically valid data available.

In the patient guide, published as an educational tool for patients, "proven treatments" are listed as medicine (over-the-counter or prescription), heat or cold, and spinal manipulation. The following treatments "may give relief for a short time, none have been found to speed recovery or keep acute back problem from returning. They may also be expensive: traction, TENS, massage, biofeedback, acupuncture, injections into the back, back corsets, ultrasound." The use of epidural corticosteroids was not found to have sufficient published evidence to be recommended. There was similar lack of support for other commonly used interventions such as

AHCPR Acute Low Back Guidelines

1. Initial assessment focuses on the detection of "red flags" (indicators of potentially serious spinal pathology or other nonspinal pathology)
2. In the absence of red flags, imaging studies and specific testing are not helpful during the first 4 weeks
3. Relief of discomfort can be accomplished most safely with nonprescription medication and/or spinal manipulation
4. Some limitation of activity may be necessary, but bedrest of >4 days is not helpful and may further debilitate the patient
5. Low-stress aerobic activities can be safely started in the first 2 weeks, but trunk conditioning exercises may be delayed at least 2 weeks
6. Early return to work or normal daily activity should be encouraged
7. Further investigation may be necessary if symptoms persist
8. Patients with sciatica recover more slowly, but further evaluation can be safely delayed
9. Within the first 3 months of low back symptoms, only patients with evidence of serious spinal pathology or severe debilitating sciatica or physiologic evidence of specific nerve root compromise corroborated on imaging studies can be expected to benefit from surgery
10. With or without surgery, 80 percent of patients with sciatica recover eventually
11. Nonphysical factors (e.g., psychological or socioeconomic problems) may be addressed in the context of discussing reasonable expectations for recovery

facet injections and trigger-point injections. Patients should probably be informed of the guideline and given the option to defer such treatment (as the guideline did not examine treatment beyond 12 weeks).

Cervical facet pain, however, has been subjected to much more rigorous scrutiny, particularly by Lord and colleagues.[18] The anatomy, symptomatology, diagnosis, and therapy of pain arising from these joints have been clearly and methodically documented.[18,19] Unfortunately, this has not been done for the lumbar or thoracic facets.

INTERVENTIONAL PAIN MANAGEMENT

One of the more recent advances in the management of chronic pain syndromes is the application of implantation technology for totally implantable drug administration systems as well as spinal cord stimulator implantation. The use of implantable infusion devices provide the clinician with an accurate and safe means of delivering long-term infusion of intraspinally administered drugs. Like the implantable drug infusion pump, the use of a spinal cord stimulator is reserved for those patients who are nonresponsive to standard therapy.

Intraspinal Drug Delivery Systems

Intraspinal administration of drugs such as narcotics or an intrathecal muscle relaxant such as baclofen has been effectively used in the management of pain or muscle spasticity, respectively, that is not amenable to more conservative therapies. Opiate receptors have been found to be highly concentrated in the cerebral cortex, midbrain, and spinal cord. The opiate receptor system in the spinal cord is located in the dorsal areas of the gray matter, close to the surface, and in the region where sensory impulses feed into the complex spinal circuitry that is responsible for pain transmission and modulation.[21] Blockade of these receptors results in significant analgesia.[22]

INDICATIONS Specific indications for the insertion of an implantable pump (Figs. 20.1 and 20.2) include

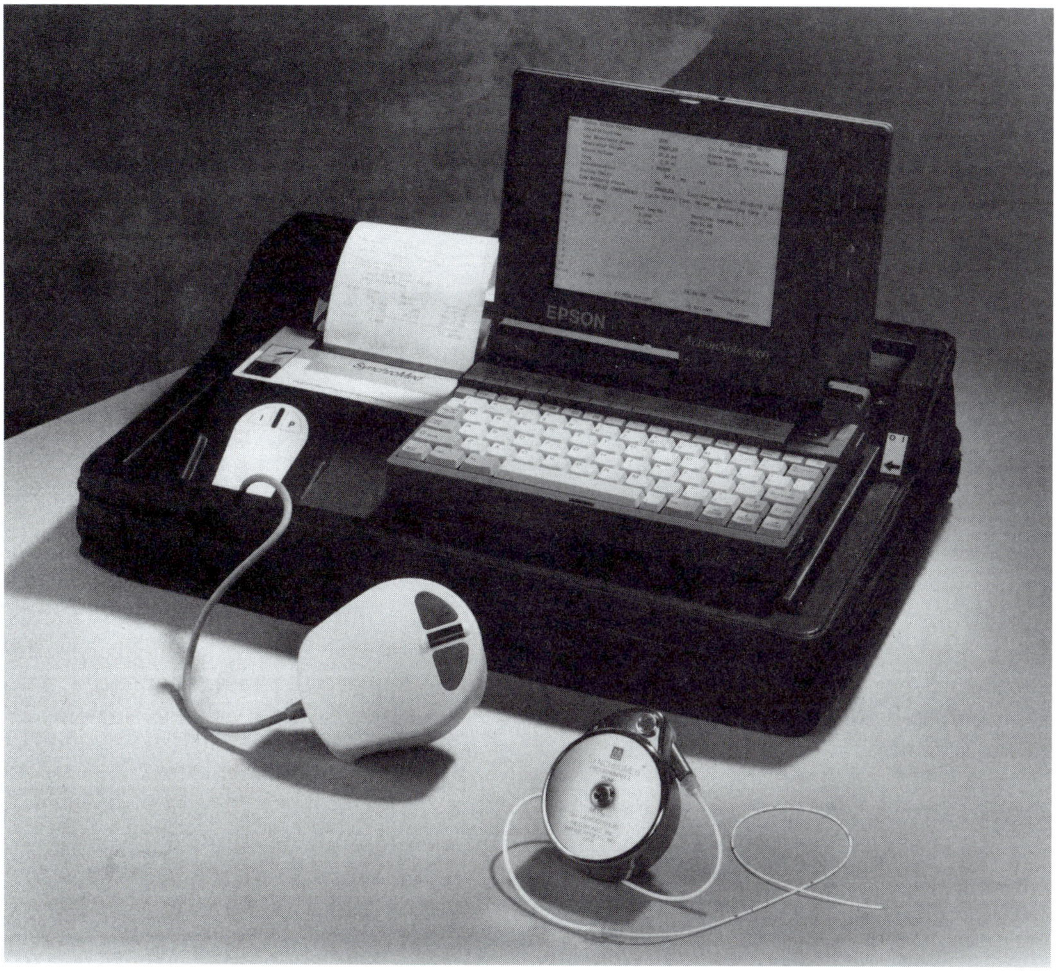

FIGURE 20.1 *The Synchromed infusion system, consisting of an implantable drug pump and a desktop programmer. Once implanted, the pump is externally programmed via radio signals to dispense a drug through a catheter to a specific site in the body with precise timing and accuracy. (Courtesy of Medtronic, Inc.)*

1. Intrathecal opioid is indicated in incomplete pain relief from aggressive oral or transcutaneous opioid analgesia or relief that is accompanied by opioid side effects that limit the patient's desired activity level. Intrathecal baclofen is indicated in the management of spasticity of spinal cord origin in patients who are unresponsive to oral baclofen or experience intolerable CNS side effects at effective doses.
2. In both pain and spasticity, implantable pumps may be indicated when neurodestructive and neurosurgical procedures are not deemed to be clinically indicated.

Additional criteria for patient selection include the absence of any serious untreated drug habituation. Appropriate psychologic evaluation and "clearance" and no medical contraindications to implantation, such as sepsis, coagulopathy, or localized infection, are present. The patient must also undergo a successful trial of

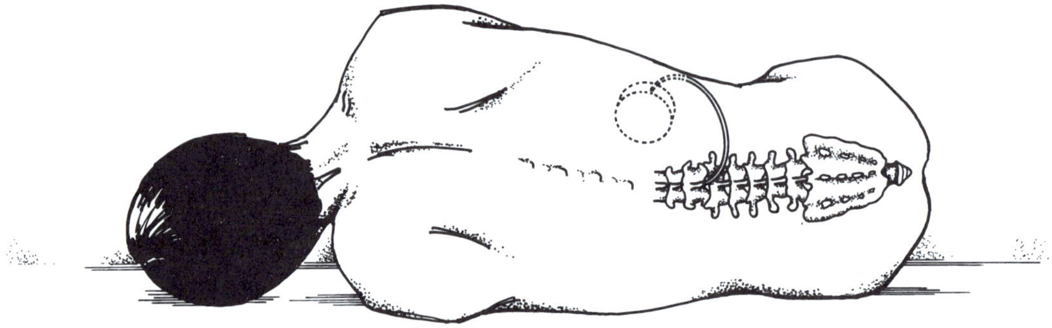

FIGURE 20.2 *In the treatment of chronic pain or severe spaccity of spinal cord origin, the round pump of the Medtronic Synchromed infusion system is implanted surgically, usually in the abdominal region as shown here. A catheter is tunneled under the skin from the pump to the spinal cord. Tiny, precisely controlled doses of medication are delivered from the pump to the area surrounding the spinal cord.*

intrathecal drug administration. The facilities, equipment, and professional support personnel required for the proper diagnosis, treatment training, and follow-up of the patient must be available in the institution where implantation is to be performed.

The final decision to insert the drug infusion pump is made within the context of a treatment pyramid, using first the most noninvasive conservative therapy before proceeding to the more invasive, costly procedures as shown in the accompanying box.

Pyramid Scheme of Pain Management

* Nonprescription medications
* Nonsteroidal anti-inflammatory drugs
* Muscle relaxants
* Coanalgesic adjuvants
* Physical/occupational therapies, manipulation
* Psychologic management
* Diagnostic and therapeutic nerve blocks
* Surgery
* Opioids of increasing potency
* Spinal cord stimulation
* Intraspinal drug administration
* Destructive neuroablative technique

(Modified from Krames,[42] with permission.)

DELIVERY SYSTEMS The intraspinal drug administration as a method of pain or spasticity relief uses the concept of "focused drug delivery," defining a goal of limiting drug action to specific receptor sites within certain organs or specific tissues to cause a discrete physiologic action. By binding to opioid and GABA receptors in the spinal cord at the level of injection, neuraxial opioid or baclofen administration can produce analgesia or muscle relaxation at doses that, if applied systematically, would have a small and transient effect.

DELIVERY SYSTEMS There are several approaches to intraspinal drug delivery systems available including the following:

Temporary Epidural Catheter System. This is used most commonly for control of acute pain. It is easy to place, economical, reliable and cheap and has a low infection risk. However, it can be easily displaced, and its use is limited to days (5 to 10 days). It makes showering or bathing difficult, and the tape can be uncomfortable and irritating.

Tunneled Percutaneous. "Semipermanent" Epidural/Intrathecal System (DuPen catheter). This is most commonly used in cancer pain that is not responsive to a standard analgesic regimen and in which life expectancy is limited. It requires minimal surgical intervention and relatively low cost in comparison with programmable implantable pumps and is usually reliable for weeks to months. Unfortunately, it can be readily displaced or disconnected. Skin infection can develop through skin tracts, so the care of the catheter requires intensive nursing care and may be physically/psychologically burdensome for some patients. It also requires frequent injection or attachment to an external pump.

Fully Implanted Epidural/Intrathecal Port Systems These can be used in patients who have cancer pains and are expected to have a longer life expectancy. It requires minimal surgical intervention, is less expensive than programmable implantable pumps, and is reliable for months. It is easier to maintain compared with the percutaneous system, but it also requires frequent percutaneous injection or external pump attachment. Problems include the possibility of catheter occlusion or leaks.

Fully Implanted Intrathecal Continuous Infusion Pumps. These are indicated in chronic pain that is nonresponsive to conventional therapy. The pump can either be gas-powered, fixed-flow intrathecal pump (Shiley-Infusaid), or an electronic programmable infusion rate intrathecal delivery pump (Medtronic SynchroMed infusion system). The pump requires minimal maintenance, has a low infection risk, is reliable and easy to use, and has programming flexibility. The pump itself is expensive, requires more extensive surgery, has a limited volume capacity if tolerance develops, and if programmable, requires an expert to change the dosage.

The Shiley-Infusaid system is a similar pump used for chemotherapy in other clinical settings. It uses freon gas to compress the fluid in the reservoir to 1.4 atmosphere of pressure. The fluid flows through a metal tube with high resistance delivering a volume of approximately 1 to 3 ml per 24 hours. A fixed volume is delivered, and by changing drug concentration, the dose can be altered depending on the patient's need. This pump is simple, highly reliable, but more bulky.

The Synchromed MedTronic infusion system is more complicated and uses a battery-operated rotary pump that is computer-driven. The computer, in turn, receives instruction from a radiofrequency link outside the patient. This allows regulation of flow and doses without invasively accessing the system nor altering drug concentration. We prefer to use this system because of ease of usage and because it allows a much longer period of time between refills of the reservoir than with the Infusaid device.

IMPLANTATION TECHNIQUE COMPONENTS. The Medtronic system consists of an implantable programmable pump, an intrathecal catheter, and an external programmer with a printer and a programming head. The pump is small (approximately 3 in. in diameter) and contains a miniature battery-powered peristaltic roller pump. The drug reservoir is self-contained within the pump. It is refilled by inserting a Huber needle through the drug reservoir port. The pump also contains a bacterial filter and audible alarm system. An electronic module controls the pump, and an antenna allows telemetry to the electronic module. Newer models have a catheter access port that allows injection or removal of fluid directly from the intrathecal space. Caution should be observed when this port is accessed because direct injection into the catheter through this port may cause a life-threatening overdose.

PROGRAMMING AND PREPARATION. To analyze and program the pump, communication is established by radio-telemetry link between an external programmer and the pump. The rate, mode, and pattern of infusion over time can be selected and altered according to patient's need. Dosage titration and schedule revision can be done by noninvasively reprogramming the pump.

The pump is usually refilled percutaneously every 4 to 12 weeks, depending on the drug and the dose that is necessary for a particular patient. The residual drug is removed by using a sterile refill kit and pressure monitor. The new drug solution is then injected into the reservoir.

Depending on the drug and its concentration, programming allows usage of the solution without any further dilution and minimizes the potential for contamination. The dosage pattern is entered into the programmer and communicated to the pump using telemetry.

Before implanting the pump, we require the patient to undergo psychological testing to be sure that the patient is in the proper frame of mind to handle an implantable system that may stay in place throughout his or her entire lifespan. The presence of any underlying major psychologic problem is a contraindication for pump implantation. Also, the patient is required to see a neurosurgeon to rule out any correctable neurosurgical problems and to allow the patient to be familiarized with the surgeon who will be working in conjunction with the algologist during pump insertion.

PROCEDURE. Once psychologic and neurosurgical consultation are obtained, the patient is admitted to the hospital for screening by administration of single-dose intrathecal morphine or baclofen. For chronic pain, 0.75 to 1.0 mg of preservative-free morphine is injected intrathecally, and the patient is observed for the next 23 hours for effectiveness of the drug and monitoring of adverse side effects. Patients with spasticity are also admitted, intrathecal baclofen at a single dose of 50 to 100 μg is administered, effectiveness of therapy is observed, and side effects are observed for the next 23 hours. If the patient has a positive response (i.e., significant analgesia or relief or spasticity with minimal or no side effects), the patient is then considered for a permanent pump implantation. A second intrathecal injection containing saline is generally carried out in the trial period to rule out placebo effect. In the future, we may be able to avoid a second intrathecal puncture by inserting a continuous intrathecal catheter and administering the active drug and placebo at timed intervals.

The pump is implanted using general anesthesia. The distal catheter is placed into the intrathecal space through a 16-gauge Touhy needle. Proper placement is confirmed using fluoroscopy. The subcutaneous pump pocket is created in one side of the abdomen, usually the lower outer quadrant. The proximal catheter is then tunneled from the pump pocket site to the back and connected to the distal catheter. The pump is primed for implantation, connected to the catheter, and inserted into the pump pocket. Both incisions are then closed. Generally, it takes 2 to 4 hours to perform the procedure. The patient is maintained on bedrest in the hospital for 3 to 4 days to decrease the incidence of cerebrospinal fluid (CSF) leakage.

Once the pump is in place, it is our aim to discontinue or significantly reduce concomitant oral pain medications or muscle relaxants to avoid possible overdose or adverse side effects. Gradual reduction in dosage is done to prevent symptoms of withdrawal.

The patient is followed up 1 week later to determine effectiveness of treatment and check for complications. Subsequent dosage adjustment is based on the degree of pain relief for intrathecal opioid or muscle relaxation for intrathecal baclofen, the presence of adverse drug effects, and the presence of disease progression or patient-related condition such as an infection. If the patient experience loss of effect, the pump is checked for patency or failure.

The pump can be set in different types of modes. Initially, a simple continuous infusion mode can be used. Depending on the patient needs, the pump can be reprogrammed to a complex continuous infusion mode to allow drug delivery to meet the patient's demand.

In addition to relief of symptoms, the effective use of intrathecal pump delivery system results in secondary benefits to the patient. The patient becomes more independent, the quality of life improves, and the accompanying depression is generally alleviated. Approximately two-thirds or more of the patients get adequate pain relief.[22]

Fully Implanted Intrathecal Patient-Controlled Pumps. These have the same indication as the fully implanted intrathecal continuous infusion pumps. They are currently considered investigational devices within the United States but are available in Canada and Europe. The pump may have a fixed infusion volume, variable concentration, and no lock-out periods (Cordis pumps), or it may have a 1-hour lock-out period (patient-activated reservoir). The pump requires minimal maintenance and is more economical compared with electronic or other mechanical devices. It is reliable for long-term use and has a low infection risk, and some models have a large volume reservoir needing infrequent refills. Implantation of the pump requires more extensive surgery and has a higher risk of occlusion or leak due to fibrosis around the catheter, and refill requires expert assistance.

Long-term use of neuraxial opioid has been advocated for chronic patients with regionalized pain below T-1 who have failed adequate trials of several different treatment modalities including conservative pharmacotherapy that includes systemic narcotics, surgery, physical therapy, and psychotherapy.

MECHANISM OF PAIN RELIEF The discovery of opioid receptors and endogenous opioid compounds in the spinal cord provides a rationale for attempts to deliver intrathecal opioids. Radiolabeled opiate ligands localize almost exclusively in the substantia gelatinosa of the spinal cord. Opioids preferentially depress C and A-δ fiber-evoked activation of wide dynamic range interneurons. The effect is dose-dependent and is naloxone-reversible. Spinal opiate receptor subtypes include kappa receptors, which may directly inhibit presynaptic release of substance P by blocking calcium influx required for neurotransmitter release. Another opiate receptor, the mu, facilitates the postsynapting coupling of mu receptor and G-effector proteins. This leads to inhibition of cyclic AMP with increased potassium conductance and postsynaptic neuronal hyperpolarization. Pain relief is therefore due to selective spinal analgesia with maintenance of an ample analgesic reservoir in the CSF at both the spinal cord and brainstem level.

COMPLICATIONS Complications can be divided into either system, drug-, or patient-related problems. The most common system complications are catheter kinks and dislodgments. Surgical intervention is required to correct these problems. The most common drug-related problems for opioid use include sedation, pruritus, constipation, urinary retention, nausea, and vomiting. For baclofen, the most commonly associated adverse drug effects include drowsiness, weakness, and dizziness. The most common patient-related complication for chronic intraspinal drug therapy is skin and subcutaneous tissue infection around the catheter exit site. Epidural hematoma, abscess, and meningitis are less common complications. Overdose of either drug may result in loss of consciousness and requires intubation, mechanical ventilation, and supportive care, usually for a period of 24 to 36 hours until recovery. The pump is turned off, and antidotes are administered. To reverse the effects of the narcotic, either naloxone or nalmefene is used as direct antidotes. For baclofen, physostigmine is used.

Tolerance does not seem to develop any more rapidly than with systemic opioid. Slow tolerance usually develops over weeks to months.[24] Failure of intraspinal opioid analgesia may be due the presence of neuropathic or incident pain, failure of the delivery system, inadequate dose, incorrect prescription. Obstructed CSF mechanics, psychoemotional decompensation, and development of drug tolerance.

Stimulation-Produced Analgesia

Spinal cord stimulation has been used as one of the novel modalities in treatment of chronic pain. It was first introduced in 1967 by Dr. Norman Shealy and colleagues for the clinical control of pain and provided the first clinical evidence of electrical stimulation–produced analgesia.[25] The authors believed that electrical stimulation worked only at the dorsal horn of the spinal cord; the treatment modality was called *dorsal column stimulator*. It is now known that analgesia can be achieved by electrical stimulation anywhere in the spinal cord; hence the more accurate term *spinal cord stimulation* is generally used.

INDICATIONS Spinal cord stimulation is indicated when more conservative therapies have failed, further surgical intervention is not indicated, no serious drug habituation exists untreated, psychologic evaluation for implantation has been obtained, trial has been successful, and no medical contraindication to implantation exists (e.g., sepsis, coagulopathy, infection at the insertion site). It is most appropriately used in patients with a single unilateral pain focus. Similar to the implantation of a drug infusion device, the treatment protocol is within the context of the pyramid scheme in the management of pain. This method of analgesia is an implantable technology that requires the insertion of epidural electrodes over the spinal cord area needed to be stimulated. If pain relief is achieved during a trial of cord stimulation, implantation of a permanent neuropulse generator is conducted.

This method of pain relief is effective in the management of persistent back pain/arachnoiditis (74 percent success rate),[25–27] ischemic pain secondary to peripheral vascular disease of vasospastic or microvascular origin (83 to 87 percent),[25,28,29] amputation pain, either phantom limb or stump pain (68 to 85 percent), neuropathic pain syndrome such as diabetic neuropathies, sympathetically mediated pain, postherpetic neuralgia, and other deafferentation pain, as well as painful spasms from torticollis, cerebral palsy, multiple sclerosis, and dystonia.[25,30–32]

MECHANISMS OF ACTION Its mechanisms of action include the following:

1. *Blockade of impulse transmission in the spinothalamic tract*: spinal cord stimulation blocks actual transmission of electrical impulses anywhere in the spinothalamic tract. Larson et al. [33] showed a reduction in pain, joint rotation, and touch sensation on application of electrical current on the dorsal column of 11 of 18 patients with cancer and intractable pain. Neurologic status returned to baseline 1 hour after cessation of stimulation. Dorsal column stimulation was also applied to 15 monkeys over the lower, middle, and upper thoracic spinal cord, the ventral posterior lateral nucleus, and the sensory motor cortex. Application of current resulted in blockage of neuronal transmission by producing local changes in the spinal cord.

2. *Supraspinal pain inhibition*: Larson et al.[33] also suggested that stimulation of the dorsal column produce changes in the supraspinal neurons effecting pain. Others believe that pain relief is due to activation of supraspinal pain modulating centers after showing that antidromic activation of dorsal column stimulation was prevented by dorsal column cuts caudal to the stimulating electrodes in rats.[34]

3. *Activation of central inhibitory mechanisms influencing sympathetic efferent neurons*: during spinal cord stimulation, vasodilation is also observed in addition to analgesia. Spinal cord stimulation may directly modify central sympathetic efferent outflow from the spinal cord or inhibits B and C afferent nerve fibers by antidromic conduction to produce this vasodilatory effect. Linderoth et al.[35] observed this change after dorsal column stimulation of the proximal ends of the cut dorsal root innervating the hind limb of rat models. No change was observed after stimulation of the distal end of the same cut nerve roots. They concluded that spinal cord stimulation antidromically activates a central loop and not small afferent fibers for poststimulation vasodilation to occur.[35] Another possible cause for vasodilation during spinal cord stimulation is the release of vasoactive substances such as va-

soactive peptide, substance P, or calcitonin gene-related peptide, although the data are still inconclusive.[36]

4. *Also cause segmental antidromic activation of large nerve fibers (type A-δ afferent neurons), which closes the gate to reception of small unmyelinated C-fiber (pain) information:* Foreman et al.[37] found that dorsal column stimulation in anesthetized monkeys suppressed the activity of the spinothalamic tract cells on the ipsilateral dorsal column as well as depression of response to electrical stimulation of peripheral nerves and mechanical stimulation of cutaneous nociceptors. Lesioning the dorsal columns eliminated this depression by dorsal column stimulation below the lesion, but lesioning of the lateral columns had no effect.

5. *Activation of putative neurotransmitters or neuromodulators, which can modify pain transmission*: the theory is based on the clinical observation in patients that pain relief often outlasts actual electrical stimulation of the spinal cord by minutes, hours, or even days. An increase in various neurotransmitters in the CSF had been reported after spinal cord stimulation including epinephrine,[38] substance P,[39] endorphins,[40] and serotonin and its metabolite, 5-hydroxy indole acetic acid.[41]

IMPLANTATION TECHNIQUE For a spinal cord stimulator to work (Figs. 20.3 and 20.4), concordant stimulation paresthesia must be present in the area of pain. Either quadripolar or octipolar epidural electrodes are placed either directly under minilaminotomy or percutaneously into the epidural space over the spinal cord area to be stimulated. The successful placement of this implantable device is ensured by initially doing a trial of spinal cord stimulation before actual implantation of a permanent neuropulse generator.

As with implantation of drug infusion pump, the patient undergoes psychologic assessment and neurosurgical consultation before being considered a candidate for this procedure. Once the patient is deemed suitable for implantation, we perform stage 1 of the procedure: the placement of the epidural electrode, connecting it to an external neuropulse generator. The patient is usually admitted for a 23-hour stay in the hospital, and the stimulator is programmed to cover the area of pain. If the patient achieves adequate pain coverage, he or she returns within 1 week for the permanent placement of a neuropulse generator (stage II).

The stage I procedure is performed in the operating room under monitored anesthesia care. Sterile technique is observed, and fluoroscopy is mandatory. Before implantation, the patient receives a prophylactic parenteral antibiotic. The patient is placed in the prone position, and the epidural space into which the epidural electrode will be inserted is identified under fluoroscopic guidance. The skin and underlying soft tissue are infiltrated with generous amounts of local anesthetic, and the epidural space is entered with a 16-gauge Touhy needle by using the loss of resistance technique. Proper placement is confirmed by injecting 2 to 3 ml of Omnipaque radioactive contrast. Preservative-free saline 3 to 5 ml is then injected through the needle to flush the dye and observe its characteristic distribution ("railroad tracking or butterfly pattern") into the epidural space. A guide wire is then inserted into the needle, and a tract is created in the epidural space up to the highest point of the desired area of the spinal cord to be stimulated. The guide wire is removed, and the epidural electrode is inserted into the desired area to be stimulated. It is then connected to a temporary extender cable that is attached to an external pulse generator. The spinal cord is stimulated, and once the desired concomitant paresthesia is deemed adequate to cover the area of pain, a 3-cm incision below and 2 cm above the Touhy needle is made after adequate local anesthesia is administered. Dissection is made until a pocket is created just above the supraspinous ligament. An extender cable is tunneled subcutaneously, exiting out of a mid-flank puncture wound. The cable is again connected to the external pulse generator, and stimulation is again repeated to ensure that the electrode is still in place. Fluo-

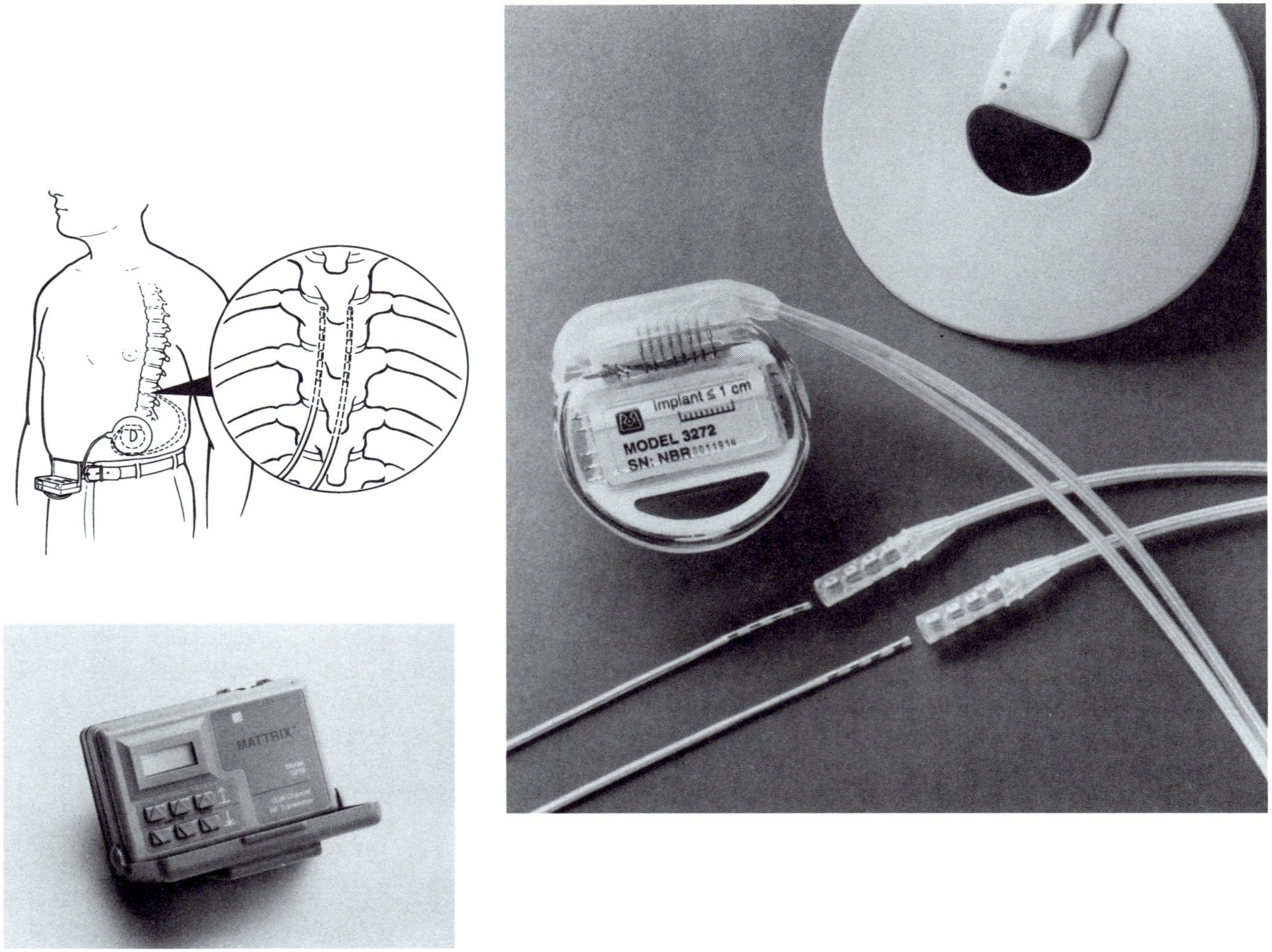

FIGURE 20.3 *The Medtronic Mattrix neurostimulation system used during stage 1 implantation. (Right) The two stimulation leads of the Mattrix system are shown with the receiver (left center), which is implanted under the skin. The external antenna (upper right) is affixed to the skin over the receiver. The belt-mounted transmitter (lower left) is easily adjusted by the patient with parameters set by the clinician to deliver stimulation impulses via the antenna to the receiver (upper left) and then through the leads to the spinal column (inset). Dashed lines indicate implanted receiver and leads.*

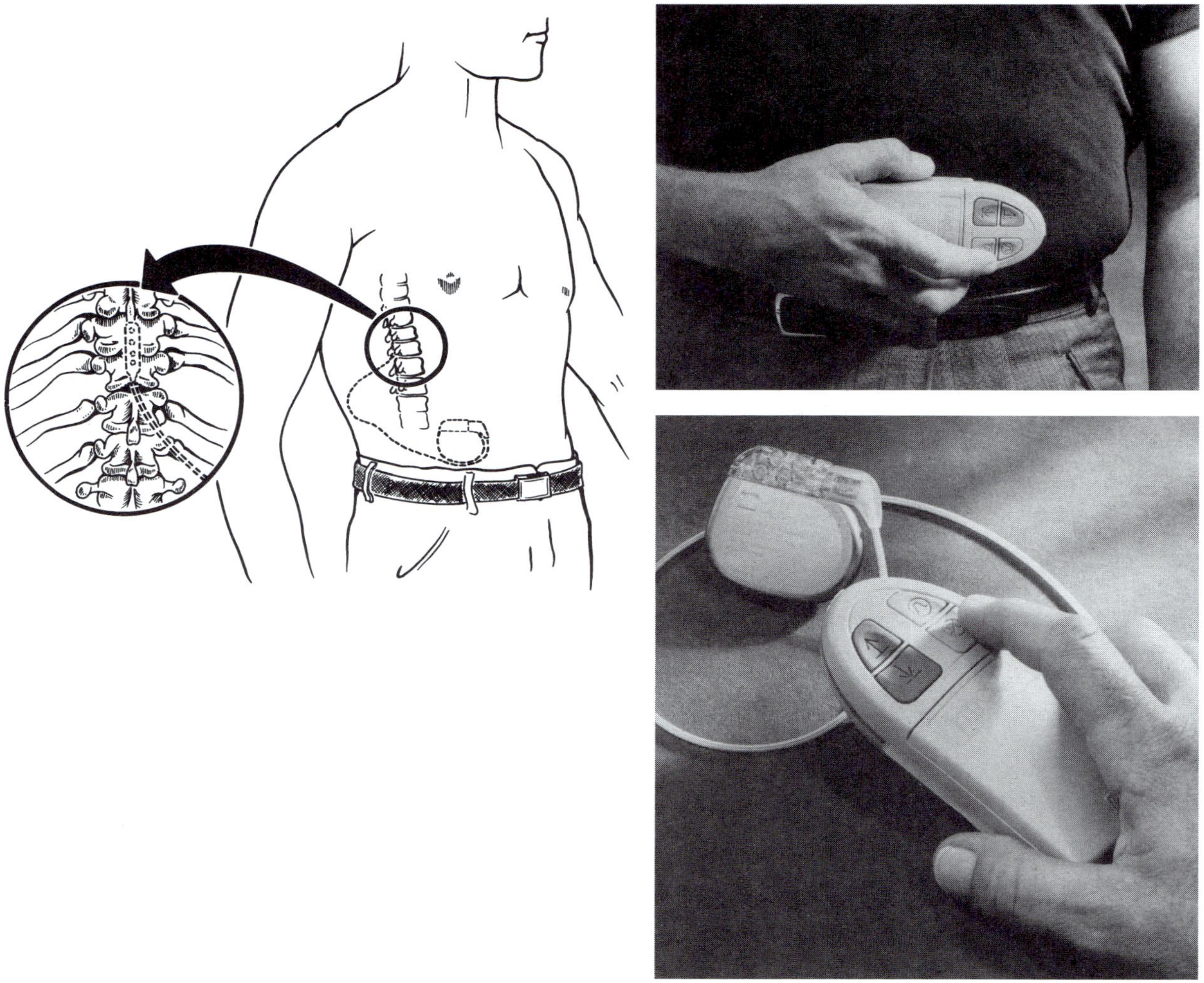

FIGURE 20.4 *Typical implanted permanent spinal cord stimulator and hand-held programmer (Medtronic Intrel 3 neurostimulation system). (Left, inset) Posterior view of the spine indicating lead placement. (Top right) The EZ patient programmer used by the patient to adjust therapy between parameters set by the clinician. (Lower right) The EZ programmer with the implantable Intrel 3 neurostimulation device.*

roscopy is used to guide and confirm electrode placement. The electrode is secured to the extender cable by a plastic connector and is sutured to the underlying tissue with a winged plastic stabilizer or anchor. The anchor is usually sutured to the supraspinous ligament to ensure that the electrode does not move. The wound is then closed and covered aseptically. The patient is transferred to the PACU for observation and thoracolumber radiographs (anterior-posterior and lateral views) are taken for confirmation of electrode placement. Subsequently, the patient is discharged the next day. The trial with the external pulse generator usually lasts for 3 to 5 days before a decision is made to proceed to stage II.

The criteria for a successful stage I trial is a reduction in pain greater than 60 percent during spinal cord stimulation. The patient is instructed to physically challenge the pain during the trial period to ensure coverage even during activity. If the patient receives greater than 60 percent pain relief, we proceed to stage II implantation.

Stage II involves placement of the permanent neuropulse generator in a subcutaneous pocket in either side of the abdomen. We prefer inserting a permanently placed electrode during stage I so that a new electrode need not be replaced during stage II. Some algologists prefer using a temporary quadripolar electrode called "Pisces" during stage I, remove it after successful trial, and place a permanent quadripolar disk-like epidural cord stimulating electrode called "Resume" through a minilaminotomy incision.

The second stage procedure is usually performed under general anesthesia. The back wound is reopened, and the temporary extender cable is disconnected from the electrode and removed through the flank wound. A subcutaneous pocket is made at a site according to patient's preference, either at the lower quadrant of the abdomen, directly over the rib cage, the mid-flank region, or buttocks. A permanent cable is tunneled through the pocket and connected to the epidural electrode.

The cable is connected to the neuropulse generator, which is then implanted in the subcutaneous pocket. After the permanent electrodes are anchored in place, the wounds are closed creating a completely implanted spinal cord stimulating system.

COMPLICATIONS Problems associated with the implantation procedure include wound infection, subcutaneous infections, epidural abscess, meningitis, surgical bleeding, and inadvertent dural puncture with postpuncture spinal headache.

References

1. Wall PD, Jones M: Defeating Pain. The War against a Silent Epidemic. Plenum Press, New York, 1991
2. Acute Pain Management Guideline Panel: Acute Pain Management: Operative or Medical Procedures and Trauma. Clinical Practice Guideline Agency for Health Care Policy and Research, Rockville, MD, 1992
3. Connis R: Report of a Task Force on Chronic Pain Management of the American Society of Anesthesiologists. House of Delegates Report. 1996
4. Merskey H, Bogduk N (eds): Classification of Chronic Pain. 2 Ed. IASP Press, Seattle, WA, 1994
5. Portenoy RK: Basic mechanisms. P. 19. In Portenoy RK, Kanner RM (eds): Pain Management: Theory and Practice. Contemporary Neurology Series 48, 1995
6. Casey KL: Pain and central nervous system disease: a summary and overview. In Casey KL (ed): Pain and Central Nervous System Disease: The Central Pain Syndromes. Raven Press, New York, 1991
7. Portenoy RK: Neuropathic pain. p. 83. In: Pain Management: Theory and Practice. Contemporary Neurology Series 48, 1996
8. Janig W, Stanton-Hicks M (eds): Reflex Sympathetic Dystrophy: A Reappraisal. Progress and Management. Vol. 6. IASP Press, Seattle, WA, 1996
9. Jackson RP, Jacobs RR, Montesana PX: Facet Joint injection in low back pain: a prospective statistical study. Spine 13:966, 1988
10. Barnsley L, Bogduk N: Medial branch blocks are specific for the diagnosis of cervical zygapophyseal joint pain. Reg Analesth 18:343, 19xx
11. Winnie AP, Collins VJ: The pain clinic. 1. Differential neural blockade in pain syndromes of questionable etiology. Med Clin North Am 52:123, 1968

12. Maruta T, Swanson DW, McHardy MJ: Three year follow-up of patients with chronic pain who were treated in a multidisciplinary pain management center. Pain 41:47, 1990
13. Ralphs JA, Wiliams AC, Richardson PH et al: Opiate reduction in chronic pain patients: a comparison of patient-controlled reduction and staff-controlled cocktail methods. Pain 56:279, 1994
14. Portenoy RK: Opioid analgesics. P. 248. In Portenoy RK, Kanner RM, (eds): Pain Management: Theory and Practice. Contemporary Neurology Series 48, 1996
15. Rinaldi RC, Steindler EM, Wilford BB et al: Clarification and standardization of substance abuse terminology. JAMA 259:555, 1988
16. Schofferman J: Long-term use of opioid analgesics for the treatment of chronic pain of non-malignant origin. J Pain Symptom Manage 8:279, 1993
17. Bigos, Brower O, Braen G et al: Acute low back problems in adults: clinical practice guideline 14. AHCPR Publication 95-0642, Rockville, MD, 1994
18. Lord SM, Barnsley L, Wallis BJ, Bogduk N: Percutaneous radiofrequency neurotomy for the treatment of cervical zygapophyseal joint pain—a caution. Neurosurgery 36:732, 1995
19. Barnsley L, Lord SM, Bogduk N: Clinical review: whiplash injury. Pain 58:283, 1994
20. Yaksh TL: Opioid receptor systems and the endorphins: a review of their spinal organization. J Neurosurg 67:157, 1987
21. Onofrio BM, Yaksh TL, Arnold PG: Continuous low dose intrathecal morphine administration in the treatment of chronic pain of malignant origin. Mayo Clin Proe 55:469, 1981
22. Coombs DW et al: Relief of continuous chronic pain by intraspinal narcotic infusions via an implanted reservoir. JAMA 250:2336, 1983
23. Shetter AG, Handley MN, Wilkinson E: Administration of intraspinal morphine sulfate for treatment of intractable cancer pain. Neurosurgery 18:740, 1986
24. Shealy CN, Mortimer, JT, Reswick J: Electrical inhibition of pain by stimulation of the dorsal column, preliminary clinical reports. Anesth Analg 46:489, 1967
25. Barolat G: Current status of epidural spinal cord stimulation. Neurosurg Q 5:98, 1995
26. North RB, Kidd DH, James C, Long DM: Spinal cord stimulation for chronic intractable pain: experience over two decades. Neurosurgery 2:384, 1993
27. Blume H, Richardson R, Rojas C: Epidural nerve stimulation of the lower spinal cord and cauda equina for the relief of intractable pain in failed back surgery. Appl Neurophysiol 5:456, 1982
28. Broseta J, Barbara J, de Vera et al: Spinal cord stimulation in peripheral arterial disease. A cooperative study. J Neurosurg 64:71, 1986
29. Broggi G, Servello D, Franzini A et al: Spinal cord stimulation for treatment of peripheral vascular disease. Appl Neurophysiol 50:431, 1987
30. Spiegelmann R, Friedman WA: Spinal cord stimulation: a contemporary series. Neurosurgery 8:65, 1991
31. Koeze TH, Williams AC, Reiman S: Spinal cord stimulation and the relief of chronic pain. J Neurol Neurosurg Psychiatry 50:1424, 1987
32. Robaina F, Dominguez M, Diaz M et al: Spinal cord stimulation for relief of chronic pain in vasospastic disorders of the upper limbs. Neurosurgery 24:63, 1989
33. Larson SJ et al: Neurophysiological effects of dorsal column stimulation in man and monkey. J Neurosurg 41:217, 1975
34. Saade E et al: Supraspinal modulation of nociception in awake rats by stimulation of the dorsal column nuclei. Brain Res 369:307, 1986
35. Linderoth B, Fedorcsak I, Meyerson BA: Is vasodilatation following dorsal column stimulation mediated by antidromic activation of small diameter fibers? Acta Neurochir Suppl 46:99, 1989
36. Broseta J, Barbera J, de Vera JA et al: Spinal cord stimulation in peripheral arterial disease. J Neurosurg 64:71, 1986
37. Foreman RD et al: Effects of dorsal column stimulation on primate spinothalamic tract neurons. J Neurophysiol 39:534, 1976
38. Levin BE, Hubschmann OR: Dorsal column stimulation: effect on human cerebrospinal fluid and plasma catecholamines. Neurology 30:65, 1980
39. Meyerson BA, Brodin E, Linderoth B: Possible neurohumoral mechanisms in CNS stimulation for pain suppression. Appl Neurophysiol 48:175, 1985
40. Tonelli L, Setti T, Falasca A et al: Investigation on cerebrospinal fluid opioids and neurotransmitters related to spinal cord stimulation. Appl Neurophysiol 51:324, 1988
41. Richardson DE, Dempsey CW: Monoamine turnover in CSF of patients during spinal cord stimulation for pain control. Pain, suppl. 2:223, 1984
42. Krames ES: When to Pump, when to Stimulate. Osler Institute Pain Review Course Manual. 1994

21 COMA AND BRAIN DEATH

HIROSHI TAKESHITA

Clinical interest lies not in the state of preservation of isolated cells but in the fate of a person.

Declaration of Sydney, 1968

COMA

Altered Consciousness

Altered consciousness is a feature of many neurologic and neurosurgical patients and is one of the most important neurologic symptoms. One of the grades of altered consciousness, *coma* means advanced brain failure. It is well recognized that the longer such brain failure lasts, the narrower the margin becomes between recovery and the development of permanent neurologic sequelae. At best, comatose patients recover without any appreciable mental and neurologic dysfunction. At worst, they irreversibly lose all brain function, that is, brain death. Coma from any cause necessitates admission to an intensive care unit (ICU), where monitoring and possibly respiratory and circulatory support become mandatory. The diagnosis and treatment of comatose patients in the ICU requires an understanding of coma as an extreme of altered consciousness. A detailed discussion of the diagnosis and treatment of coma caused by a variety of diseases, however, is not the purpose of this chapter; rather it addresses the general concept of coma and a practical approach to evaluating and managing comatose patients.

Definition of Coma

According to Plum and Posner[1] consciousness is the state of awareness of the self and the environment, and coma is its opposite. In other words coma is a state of the total absence of awareness of self and environment, even when the subject is externally stimulated. There are a wide variety of acutely and chronically altered states of consciousness between the state of full consciousness and coma.

States of altered consciousness, particularly those caused by an acute process, can be categorized into several stages: clouded consciousness, confusional state, delirium, stupor, and coma. Conscious behaviour necessitates the presence of both functioning cerebral cortex and the activating system of the upper brainstem, hypothalamus, and thalamus with their relatively intact functional areas that interact extensively with each other. It has been generally accepted that the state of consciousness has two components, arousal and content (cognitive and affective mental function), and that brain diseases affect each component differently.

Arousal depends on the functional integrity of the reticular formation and other structures that lie in the upper brainstem and arise from the middle of the pons to the hypothalmus. Decreased arousal states include drowsiness and stupor, from which patients can be briefly aroused, but these may develop into coma and brain death. In contrast, the cognitive *content* of consciousness disappears if the cerebral cortex is totally or nearly totally obliterated, even in the absence of brainstem lesions. An altered content of consciousness is often found as a confusional state in patients with focal cortical lesions. However, a confusional state and delirium usually combine with an alteration in the content of consciousness, with at least some reduction in total arousal. Thus it is difficult to set the different stages of altered consciousness on a single, straight continuum. Chronically altered states of consciousness may be described as dementia, hypersomia, vegetative state, akinetic mutism, apallic syndrome, and locked-in syndrome. These states are comparatively described in Plum and Posner's well-known text.[1]

Cause of Coma

Coma results from either bilateral cerebral disturbances or involvement of the brainstem reticular activating system by a pathologic process. There are many causes of unconsciousness. These can be divided into primary and secondary types or into structural and metabolic types. In the former, brain damage is caused from an intracranial process, whereas the latter is caused secondarily from respiratory and circulatory failure and systemic diseases including hepatic coma, uremia, and diabetic coma. Causes of coma are also divided into four major categories: structural (traumatic, vascular, infective), metabolic (renal, hepatic, endocrine, hypothermia), epilepsy, and drug intoxication.[2] However, it must be kept in mind that more than one cause may contribute to coma.

Neurologic Examination

The neurologic examination provides information important for localizing the process within the nervous system and often contributes valuable information regarding the etiology of coma. Coma of unknown cause in a previously healthy patient, especially with sudden onset, may be due to drug poisoning, subarachnoid hemorrhage, or head trauma. In elderly patients, acute coma may be due to brainstem hemorrhage or infarction. Patients with supratentorial mass lesions or metabolic encephalopathy develop symptoms more gradually. Drugs may be the primary cause of coma or only an aggravating factor. Toxicologic tests may confirm a suspicion of metabolic or drug factors as a cause of coma. Focal neurologic signs will indicate structural brain damage, which can be best determined by computed tomography (CT).

Examination begins with assessment of the patients' spontaneous activity, if any, and their response to environmental stimuli. Neuro-ophthalmologic examination constitutes a major part of the clinical examination. Pupil size, equality, and reaction should be tested with a bright light. Eye opening indicates activity of the reticular activating system. Differentiation of coma from other unresponsive states depends essentially on eye opening. Deeply comatose patients may have no spontaneous eye movements. In postcardiac arrest coma, ocular bobbing of the eyes has been described that is characterized by spontaneous downward deviation, which is more rapid than the upward component. Another variant is ocular dipping, which consists of slow downward deviation followed by rapid upward movement.[3] Eye movements are tested either with a doll's head maneuver or ice water calories. When brainstem gaze mechanisms are intact but the cortical influences are depressed, the head can be rotated horizontally to one side, causing the eyes to deviate conjugately to the opposite side. Brisk back-and-forth eye movements are characteristic of metabolic coma. When the doll's eyes are absent, it becomes necessary to apply the ice water caloric test. When cortical influences on the oculovestibular pathways are absent but the brainstem pathway is intact, ice water produces tonic deviation of the eyes toward the irrigated ear. The caloric response can be obtained in comatose patients by irrigating the tympanum with about 50 ml of ice water. The patient must be placed in a supine position with head elevation of 30°. It must be remembered that labyrinthine disease, drug-induced coma (e.g., phenytoin overdosage), and brainstem lesions eliminate the caloric response.

Body movement should be described as purposeful or reflex. Because observers may differ in interpretation of such movements, the nature and location of the noxious stimulus as well as the response should be noted. Reflex asymmetries and Babinski reflexes may indicate focal central nervous system (CNS) pathology.

Respiratory patterns contribute important diagnostic information. Cheyne-Strokes respiration may be caused by either toxic-metabolic or structural pathology. Hyperventilation occurs in the early phase of hepatic coma and occasionally with brainstem lesions. Disordered respiratory patterns may also be seen with brainstem lesions.

Grading of Coma

After the initial examination and treatment has begun, it is essential to monitor the changes in the state of consciousness since these are the most important and sensitive clinical signs in evaluating response to treatment, progression of brain pathology, development of new complications, and prediction of outcome. Laboratory tests, which include routine EEG, evoked responses, and CT, cannot substitute for clinical observation of the level of consciousness.

Simple methods of monitoring changes in the level of consciousness that can be easily and frequently performed by junior staff and nurses are desirable. The Glasgow group has developed a practical scale that provides both a useful bedside monitor and a means of categorizing the degree of coma in numerical terms (Table 21.1).[4] The numerical system facilitates identification of changes in the level of consciousness and permits comparison between groups of patients. Using this scale the Glasgow group defined coma as the inability to obey commands, utter recognizable words, or open the eyes. If any of these could be appropriately achieved, the patient was regarded as not in coma. All patients with a coma score of less than 7 should be regarded as comatose. The reliability of this coma scale has been proved by multi-institutional studies and it has been strongly recommended for worldwide use. Even with the recent introduction of a new hierarchical scale called the reaction level scale, the Glasgow Coma Scale seems to remain as the most widely used numerical system for the grading of level of consciousness.[5]

Eye opening may occur spontaneously: only when the patient is spoken to, when a painful stimuli is applied, or not at all.

Motor response can be assessed by applying a painful stimulus (e.g., nailbed pressure or supraorbital pressure). The response is recorded as localizing if the hands move above the chin toward the stimulus; less directed flexion than that is recorded as flexor withdrawal. Experienced observers may readily distinguish between normal and abnormal flexion. Different responses may be obtained from each of the limbs. In this case it is recommended to take the best response during the examination of the best limb.

Verbal response indicates hemispheric func-

TABLE 21.1 *Glasgow coma scale*

FINDING	RATE
Eye opening	
Spontaneous	4
To speech	3
To pain	2
Nil	1
Motor response	
Obeys	6
Localizes	5
Withdraws (flexion)	4
Abnormal flexion	3
Extensor response	2
Nil	1
Verbal response	
Oriented	5
Confused conversation	4
Inappropriate words	3
Incomprehensible sounds	2
Nil	1

(From Jennett and Teasdale,[4] with permission.)

tion. If the patient can conduct a conversation but is disoriented, the response is called *confused*. If the patient utters only occasional expletives but does not carry on a conversation, the response is called *inappropriate words*. *Incomprehensible sounds* refers to wordless grunts and groans.

In addition, it is useful to record pupil size and reaction, eye movement, any abnormal pattern of motor responses in all four limbs, cardiopulmonary features, and other organ functions that may be affected in comatose patients.

Anoxic Coma

The term *anoxic coma* as used clinically indicates the state of coma due to any form of inadequate oxygen delivery to the brain, including both hypoxemia and ischemia. Coma after cardiac arrest deserves specific comment because anesthesiologists play an important role in resuscitation of cardiac victims in emergency rooms and ICUs. Brain anoxia of brief duration can be well tolerated, and the patient may awaken promptly. In the patient with a slightly longer duration of anoxia, coma, if present, lasts usually less than 12 hours. In these patients, transient confusion and/or amnesia may continue for days, but the outcome is essentially good. Damage to highly vulnerable areas, including the hippocampus, may be responsible for the development of amnesia.[6] Clinically available neurologic and neuroradiologic examinations, however, usually cannot detect lesions in these areas. Patients in whom coma lasts longer than 12 hours may present a variety of symptoms including amnesia, dementia, focal signs, seizures, myoclonus, and ataxia. Ataxia may also be caused by lesions in another vulnerable area, the cerebellum.

An ischemic infarct concentrated in the boundary zones of the territories of the major arteries is another pathologic process that appears following cardiac arrest or profound hypotension of longer duration. In the cerebral cortex such boundary zone infarcts are often hemorrhagic and most severely affect the parieto-occipital regions. Selective distribution of infarcts provokes the speculation that the deleterious effects of reduced oxygen and glucose supply are maximal in boundary zones most distant from the origin of major arteries, although experimental studies have not consistently shown focal infarcts in those areas.[7] Rarely, patients exhibit a progressive neurologic deterioration after they recover from the immediate effects of anoxic brain insults.[8] Histopathologic examination in this event has revealed lesions primarily restricted to the deep white matter of the parietal and occipital lobes. It is perhaps surprising that this delayed anoxic leukoencephalopathy in cardiac arrest victims was first reported in the 1960s. Recent investigations also revealed that delayed neuronal death occurs 2 days to 1 week after cerebral ischemia in experimental animals, although the site of pathology is not primarily in the white matter. It is uncertain whether the delayed derangement observed in the clinical setting is equivalent to the delayed neuronal death observed in animals.

Management of patients in coma after cardiopulmonary resuscitation consists of maintenance of cardiopulmonary function and neurologic intensive care. The latter includes repeat neurologic examinations and, if indicated, monitoring with electroencephalogram (EEG), evoked potentials, and CT. Therapeutic measures are directed at reduction of intracranial pressure (ICP) if intracranial hypertension is present, control of seizures, and avoidance of hyperthermia. Unfortunately, no effective delayed therapy has yet been established, although animal studies have revealed several pathophysiologic processes that contribute to the development of neuronal death and may be amenable to therapy. Disturbance of calcium homeostasis, an excessive release of excitatory neurotransmitters, cerebral acidosis, and a profuse production of free radicals have all been implicated.[9]

Outcome Assessment

There are increasing concerns about the assessment and prediction of outcome in comatose patients. When intensive care medicine was introduced it was expected that this discipline would greatly reduce mortality and morbidity. However, there is no well-controlled study proving the effectiveness of intensive care for comatose patients. Jennett[2] has estimated, extrapolating from previous reports, an incidence of 14,000 new patients in the United States each year with permanent brain damage after acute insults leading to coma. Nearly one-half of these patients will live for many years, and this population of brain-damaged patients is the price paid for the patients who make a good recovery. A Japanese survey has revealed that two-thirds of a series of more than 100 vegetative patients were still alive after more than 3 years.[10] However, the duration of survival depends on whether a decision has been made to withdraw some of the therapeutic interventions.

It is essential to clarify the terms that describe the state of patients; otherwise it is difficult to compare reports from different institutions or to evaluate the effectiveness of management. For this reason the Glasgow outcome scale has been proposed.[11] The *severely disabled* are those who are conscious but dependent; the latter is defined as needing the attention of another person for some part of every 24 hours. *The moderately disabled* are independent but disabled; they can live on their own, can organize their lives, and are capable of work, although not necessarily the work they previously did. *Good recovery* describes those who have minor residual sequelae but are able to participate in all previous occupational and social activities.

One problem encountered when assessing the patient is the timing of the evaluation. Early assessment—for example, at the time of discharge from ICU or from the hospital—is not meaningful. Outcome assessment at 6 months has been considered useful timing in assessing head-injured patients.

Predictability of outcome in comatose patients depends on the individual disease processes, and it is not possible to cover all of these processes in this chapter. As far as anoxic coma is concerned, Levy et al.[12] have reported that early clinical signs were useful in predicting outcome. Briefly, patients with evidence of brainstem dysfunction and/or neurologic signs of multifocal patterns have poor prognosis. Intact brainstem functions at the time of initial examination and some evidence of cortical function at 1 day or later indicates good recovery. In addition to neurologic findings, somatosensory and auditory evoked responses also offer a relatively accurate prognosis.

BRAIN DEATH

Recent advances in resuscitative and life support technology have stimulated a refinement of the traditional concepts that are used to determine death of the individual. Even when all brain function has completely ceased, cardiovascular, pulmonary, and other functional systems may be maintained by artificial means or may still be viable. Irreversible loss of all brain function is called *brain death*. It is an increasingly important clinical diagnosis in the ICU because patients with brain death are often considered as donor candidates for organ transplantation. Clinically, the most relevant definition of brain death is the irreversible loss of all integrated neuronal functions.[13] In this situation there is widespread devastating brain damage. The term *integrated* is essential because recovery of some metabolic and electric activity occurring in certain brain regions after prolonged total ischemia has been reported, even with irreversible loss of the functional integrity of the brain.

Philosophically, to view brain death as the death of the individual is appropriate because (1) the brain is the essential site where human personality exists as well as the origin of integrated function of the organism as a whole; (2) brain death inevitably leads to cessation of vital functions, usually within 2 weeks of the cardiac arrest, unless extraordinary means have been taken[14,15], and (3) virtually all vital organs can be artificially maintained and/or replaced in humans except for the brain. These considerations have led to the belief that death of the brain is equivalent to death of the individual.

When brain death is discussed, it is apparent

that the terminology is vague and confusing. The term *brain death* has been used as synonymous with irreversible coma, cerebral death, and cortical death. This has led to enormous confusion not only in the medical community, but also in the legal community and for the lay public.[16] This situation was further complicated when the concept of brainstem death was introduced by British neurologists.[17,18]

The remainder of this chapter deals with definitions of brain death terminology, the historic development of brain death criteria, ancillary tests, and basic principles of brain death criteria. Legal aspects are beyond the scope of this chapter.

Definition of Brain Death

Brain death is defined as irreversible loss of all brain function, which includes brainstem function; spinal cord function may be present. Using this definition, the term *brain* obviously includes both the cerebral hemispheres (cortex and deep structure) as well as the cerebellum and brainstem. It seems generally accepted that brain function represents the presence of life, whereas persistent cardiopulmonary function with no brain function does not. The traditional definition of death also implies brain death, because the cessation of cardiopulmonary function inevitably leads to brain death within minutes. Thus there are not two different concepts of death; death and brain death are equivalent. Rather, there are two different sets of criteria that may be used to diagnose death.

Terminologic Problems

IRREVERSIBLE COMA Perhaps the Harvard criteria[19] for the determination of irreversible coma (Ad Hoc Committee) are the first that used the term *irreversible coma* as equivalent to brain death. Their concept is exactly the same as the present definition of brain death. However, the use of the term *irreversible coma* created confusion in terminology after it had been published. Irreversible coma may include not only brain death, but a wide variety of unconscious states such as persistent vegetative state or irreversible noncognitive state. As will be discussed later, the Harvard criteria for irreversible coma are an historical milestone that first proposed new criteria for defining death. However, the 1968 proposal avoided the term *brain death* because their concept did not conflict with the traditional concept of death (cardiac arrest) if the heartbeat is considered to be artificially maintained by means of artificial ventilation.

BRAINSTEM DEATH These criteria for brain death were proposed by Mohandas and Chou[20] in 1971. They thought that irreversible damage of the brainstem was the point of no return in patients with known but irreparable intracranial lesions. The concept was further elaborated by Pallis,[17] who conceived of human death as a state in which there is irreversible loss of consciousness combined with irreversible loss of respiration. Both capacities essentially represent brainstem function at different ends of the brainstem. In such patients irreversible loss of brainstem function inevitably leads to cessation of cardiac rhythm.

CEREBRAL DEATH Unfortunately, the term *cerebral death* has been used synonymously with *brain death*. Anatomically, however, it does not indicate irreversible loss of function of the structures in the posterior fossa. This is a grammatical problem. In order to use more precise terminology, cerebral death should not be used as equivalent to brain death. In cerebral death, the brainstem, pons, midbrain, and cerebellum may still function at least in part. This condition may be called *apallic syndrome*, *persistent vegetative state*, or *neocortical death*. At present, there are very few who accept the belief that irreversible loss of function of the cerebrum is equivalent to death of the individual.

PERSISTENT VEGETATIVE STATE Patients in a persistent vegetative state have diverse and irreversible pathologic features, survive from months to many years, and show some form of cephalic reflexes, spontaneous respirations, and EEG activity. Their anatomic substrates of damage include bilateral destruction of the cortex, basal ganglia, thalamus, and reticular formation and their combinations. This state must be clearly differentiated from brain death. In these patients, the personality of the individual may or may not be destroyed. Irreversibility of the loss of neuronal function in these patients is still difficult to demonstrate with currently available techniques, and there is difficulty in predicting the prognosis. Patients in a persistent vegetative state have never been considered brain dead.

Historic and Representative Brain Death Criteria

For practical purposes, this section reviews historic and representative brain death criteria developed in various countries that have had a strong impact on the diagnosis of brain death and/or are being widely used. The essences of these criteria are described, but you should refer to the original article when establishing criteria for testing for and declaring brain death. Because brain death is a clinical diagnosis, no guidelines can replace the physician's judgement in individual cases. They are neither intended to encourage the use of resources in establishing the diagnosis of brain death nor to indicate the physician's role once the diagnosis has been made.

HARVARD CRITERIA (1968) The Harvard criteria[19] were the first and therefore remain the most important published criteria for brain death, although they caused some confusion in terminology by defining brain death as irreversible coma. However, their statement was the first to indicate that brain death means the death of the individual. The Harvard criteria defined irreversible coma as follows:

1. *Unreceptivity and unresponsivity*. A total unawareness to even the most intensely painful stimuli.
2. *No movements or breathing*. Observation covering a period of at least 1 hour by physicians is adequate to satisfy the criteria of no spontaneous muscular movements or spontaneous respiration or response to stimuli. The total absence of spontaneous breathing may be established by turning off the respirator for 3 minutes.
3. *No reflexes*. The pupils will be fixed and dilated and will not respond to a direct source of bright light. Ocular movement (doll's eye maneuver and ice water caloric test) and blinking are absent. There is no evidence of postural activity (decerebrate or decorticate). Swallowing, yawning, and vocalizing are in abeyance. Corneal and pharyngeal reflexes are absent. As a rule the stretch or tendon reflexes cannot be elicited.
4. *Isoelectric EEG*. The flat or isoelectric EEG is of great confirmatory value.

All of the above tests shall be repeated at least 24 hours later with no change. The validity of such data depends on the exclusion of two factors: hypothermia (temperature below 32.2°C [90°F]) or CNS depressants such as barbiturates. In situations in which EEG monitoring is not available, the absence of cerebral function has to be determined by purely clinical signs. However, subsequent reports communicated criteria that were less rigid; using them, the EEG was not considered essential for the diagnosis of brain death.[21] Spinal reflexes are known to be irrelevant to the diagnosis.

MINNESOTA CRITERIA (1971) The Minnesota criteria are unique in that the emphasis is more upon clinical judgement. Mohandas and Chou[20] who formulated the criteria, stated that in patients with known but irreversible intracranial lesions determination of brain death can be based solely on clinical grounds.

Minnesota criteria are as follows:

1. No spontaneous movement.
2. No spontaneous respiration when tested for a period of 4 minutes at a time.
3. Absence of brainstem reflexes.
   a. Dilated and fixed pupils.
   b. Absent corneal reflexes.
   c. Absent ciliospinal reflexes.
   d. Absent doll's eye phenomenon.
   e. Absent gag reflex.
   f. Absent vestibular response to caloric stimulation.
   g. Absent tonic neck reflex.
4. A status in which all of the findings above remain unchanged for at least 12 hours.
5. Brain death can be pronounced only if the pathologic processes responsible for status 1 to 4 above are deemed irreparable with presently available means.

The authors believed that the EEG was unnecessary and the presence of spinal reflexes had no bearing on the question of brain death. However, they cautiously emphasized that their criteria could be applied only to patients in whom the definitive etiology and the degree of damage to vital centers of the CNS could be established beyond reasonable doubt.

UNITED KINGDOM CRITERIA (1976)

The United Kingdom brain death criteria[22] are based on the concept of brainstem death as judged by clinical examination, with emphasis on the prerequisites, that is, absence of brainstem reflexes and apnea, not requiring the EEG. Although this concept of brain death is different in detail from the criteria currently accepted in the United States, they both yield the same diagnosis.

According to the United Kingdom criteria, brain death should be considered under the following conditions:

1. The patient is deeply comatose.
   a. There should be no suspicion that this state is due to depressant drugs.
   b. Primary hypothermia as a cause of coma should be excluded.
   c. Metabolic and endocrine disturbances that can be responsible for or contribute to coma should be excluded.
2. The patient is being maintained on a ventilator because spontaneous respiration is inadequate or has ceased altogether.
   a. Relaxants—and other drugs—are excluded as a cause of respiratory inadequacy or failure.
3. There should be no doubt that the patient's condition is due to irreversible structural brain damage. The diagnosis of a disorder that can lead to brain death is fully established.

Their diagnostic tests for the confirmation of brain death include the following indications that all brainstem reflexes are absent:

1. The pupils are fixed in diameter and do not respond to abrupt changes in the intensity of incident light.
2. There is no corneal reflex.
3. The vestibulo-ocular reflexes are absent.
4. No motor responses within the cranial nerve distribution can be elicited by adequate stimulation of any somatic area.
5. There is no gag reflex or reflex response to bronchial stimulation by a suction catheter passed down the trachea.
6. No respiratory movements occur when the patient is disconnected from the mechanical ventilator for long enough to ensure that the arterial carbon dioxide tension rises above the threshold for stimulation of respiration.

Other considerations in the diagnosis of brain death under these criteria include:

1. *Repetition of testing*. The interval between tests must depend upon the primary pathology and the clinical course of the disease. In some conditions the outcome is not so clear, and in these it is recommended that the tests should be repeated. The interval between tests depends on the progress of the patient and might be as long as 24 hours. This is a matter of medical judgment.
2. *Integrity of spinal reflexes*. It is well established that spinal cord function can persist after insults that irreversibly destroy brainstem function.
3. *Confirmatory investigations*. The EEG is not necessary for the diagnosis of brain death. Other investigations such as cerebral angiography or cerebral blood flow (CBF) measurements are not required for the diagnosis of brain death.
4. *Body temperature*. The body temperature in these patients may be low because of depression of central temperature regulation by drugs or by brainstem damage; it should be more than 35°C before the diagnosis of brain death is made.

A decision to withdraw artificial support should be made after all the criteria presented above have been fulfilled and can be made by any of the following combination of doctors:

1. A consultant who is in charge of the case and one other doctor.
2. In the absence of a consultant, his deputy, who should have been registered for five years or more and who should have had adequate previous experience in the care of such cases, and one other doctor.

THE COLLABORATIVE STUDY (NATIONAL INSTITUTES OF HEALTH, 1977) Based on the findings in a National Institutes of Health (NIH)[23] collaborative study of 503 comatose and apneic patients, the below criteria were developed for the determination of brain death. At least 6 hours must be allowed for therapeutic measures to be completed, remediable causes to be eliminated, and the cardiovascular system to be stabilized. The following criteria were adopted:

Prerequisite. All appropriate diagnostic and therapeutic procedures have been performed.

Criteria (to be present for 30 minutes at least 6 hours after the onset of coma and apnea) are as follows:

1. Coma with cerebral unresponsiveness.
2. Apnea.
3. Absent cephalic reflexes and dilated pupils.
4. Electrocerebral silence.

The report indicated that four-vessel angiography, commonly used to demonstrate CBF, is invasive and requires complicated radiologic techniques, which are impractical for routine use in critically ill patients. Walker[24] suggested that if any of these criteria were equivocally met, the diagnosis should be validated by the demonstration of absence of CBF; and that should be accomplished using a simple, minimally traumatic, and reliable technique that includes isotope angiography together with the gamma camera, cerebral isotope bolus, and enhanced CT.

THE PRESIDENT'S COMMISSION FOR THE STUDY OF ETHICAL PROBLEMS IN MEDICINE AND BIOMEDICAL AND BEHAVIORAL RESEARCH (1981) The criteria enumerated by the President's Commission for the Study of Ethical Problems in Medicine and Biomedical and Behavioral Research[25] should be considered definitive today for the diagnosis of brain death. The guidelines begin by stating that an individual who has sustained either (1) irreversible cessation of circulatory and respiratory functions or (2) irreversible cessation of all functions of the entire brain, including the brainstem, is dead.

The full criteria are listed below.

A. An individual with irreversible cessation of circulatory and respiratory functions is dead.

1. Cessation is recognized by appropriate clinical examination.
2. Irreversibility is recognized by persistent cessation of functions during an appropriate period of observation or trial of therapy.

B. An individual with irreversible cessation of all functions of the entire brain including the brainstem is dead. It is important to note that the functions of the entire brain that are relevant to the diagnosis are those that are clinically ascertainable.

1. Cessation is recognized when evaluation discloses findings of items a and b.
   a. Cerebral functions are absent, and there must be deep coma, cerebral unreceptivity, and unresponsivity.
   b. Brainstem functions are absent.

      Pupillary light, corneal, oculocephalic, oculovestibular, oropharyngeal, and respiratory reflexes are absent. Adequate testing for apnea is very important and should be done by ventilating the patient with pure oxygen or an oxygen and carbon dioxide mixture for 10 minutes. The ventilator should then be withdrawn, followed by passive flow of oxygen. Hypercarbia adequately stimulates respiratory effort within 30 seconds when arterial partial pressure of carbon dioxide ($PaCO_2$) is greater than 60 mmHg.

2. Irreversibility is recognized when evaluation discloses findings of items a, b, and c as follows:
   a. The cause of coma is established and is sufficient to account for the loss of brain functions.
   b. The possibility for recovery of any brain function is excluded.
   c. The cessation of all brain functions persists for an appropriate period of observation of trial of therapy.

The duration of the observation period is a matter of clinical judgment, and some physicians recommend shorter or longer periods than those given here. Except for patients with drug intoxication, hypothermia, or shock or patients of young age, no cases of brain function returning following a 6-hour cessation, documented by clinical examination and confirmatory EEG, have been reported. In the absence of confirmatory tests, a period of observation of at least 12 hours is recommended. For anoxic brain damage, in which the extent of damage is more difficult to ascertain, observation for 24 hours is generally desirable. The observation period may be reduced if a test shows cessation of CBF or if an EEG shows electric silence in an adult patient without drug intoxication, hypothermia, or shock.

Complicating conditions that may invalidate the usual criteria and require special examinations to establish brain death are (1) drug and metabolic intoxication, (2) hypothermia, (3) age under 1 year, and (4) shock.

The dual definition of death seems particularly acceptable to the general public. EEG and blood flow studies may also be required, depending on the circumstances. The minimum time required for declaration is 6 hours, which is the time generally required for initial resuscitation and evaluation. In a normothermic adult with a known cause of coma, no drug intoxication or shock, and one isoelectric EEG, brain death can be declared at this time. If cerebral angiography or radioisotope techniques show circulatory cessation to the brain for 10 minutes, brain death can be declared without a 6-hour waiting time.

If neither EEG nor angiography is used, an observation period of 12 hours is suggested.

SWEDISH CRITERIA (THE SWEDISH MINISTRY OF HEALTH AND SOCIAL AFFAIRS, 1984) These Swedish criteria[26] are influenced by the implication of cerebral death as total cerebral infarction as described by Ingvar and Widen,[27] and hence emphasize cerebral angiography.

A. The cause of the condition is known. Intoxication and hypothermia are excluded.

1. A clinical neurologic examination, carried out on at least two occasions with an interval of 2 hours shows
   a. Unconsciousness without reaction to spoken command, touch, or pain (spinal reflexes can exist).
   b. Pupils unreactive to light and in most cases dilated.
   c. Loss of corneal reflexes, blink reflexes (e.g., response to light), pharyngeal reflexes, and vestibulo-ocular reflexes.
   d. Absence of spontaneous movement of muscles innervated by the cranial nerves (no ocular movements or movements of the jaw, face, tongue, or pharynx).
   e. Absent cardiac cerebral reflexes (the cardiac rhythm cannot be influenced by pressure on the eyeballs or massage of the carotid sinus)
   f. Complete cessation of spontaneous respiration, established by disconnecting the respirator for 10 minutes.
2. Supplementary EEG. The EEG can be used to supplement the clinical examination. The EEG must show a complete cessation of electrical activity in the cerebral cortex.

B. Other cases. Cerebral (aortocranial) angiography performed on two occasions with an interval of about 30 minutes. Radiographic observation of the intracranial vessels, showing that the brain lacks circulation during the specified period, and the existence of sufficient grounds for diagnosis, regardless of any suspicion of intoxication or hypothermia.

In Scandinavia, patients with known primary or secondary brain lesions who are in unresponsive coma with apnea, absence of all cerebral functions including brainstem reflexes, and a single isoelectric EEG are diagnosed as brain dead. It must be stressed that these criteria use cerebral angiography when the cause of the condition is unknown.

JAPANESE CRITERIA (BRAIN DEATH STUDY GROUP, MINISTRY OF HEALTH AND WELFARE, 1987) In 1983, a new brain death study group was organized in Japan under the sponsorship of the Ministry of Health and Welfare[28] to re-evaluate previously adopted criteria. Previous criteria were applied only to cases of acute primary brain lesions and consisted of deep coma, apnea, bilateral dilated pupils, absent pupillary and corneal reflexes, persistent hypotension, isoelectric EEG, and the presence of all the preceding for at least 6 hours.

Re-evaluation of these criteria by a new brain death study group led to the introduction of revised criteria for the determination of brain death as outlined below.

Prerequisite. A known irreparable organic brain lesion detected by CT.

Exclusion. Children under 6 years, hypothermia, drug intoxication, or endocrine and metabolic disorders.

The new Japanese criteria are as follows:

1. *Deep coma*. Three hundred Japan Coma Scale (patient does not arouse to stimulation, does not respond to pain) and 3 Glasgow Coma Scale (patient does not open eyes, vocalize, or have motor function).
2. *Apnea confirmed by apnea test*. The inspired oxygen concentration should be 100% for 10 minutes before the test. The $PaCO_2$ should be more than 40 mmHg. To increase $PaCO_2$, ventilatory volume should be decreased or 5% carbon dioxide should be added to the inspiratory gases for 5 minutes before the ventilation is stopped. The ventilator is stopped for 10 minutes with 6 L/min of 100% oxygen insufflation through the endotracheal tube.
3. *Absence of brainstem reflexes*. Bilaterally fixed pupils larger than 4 mm in diameter. Absent corneal, ciliospinal, oculo-

cephalic, vestibular, pharyngeal, and cough reflexes.

4. *Isoelectric EEG*. An accurate recording of the EEG is essential, using 4 leads at least for over 30 minutes.

The preceding criteria must be present for a 6-hour period or longer if necessary and must include a second EEG. With secondary brain lesions or in children over 6 years old, a longer observation period is necessary.

These criteria emphasize the use of CT for confirming organic lesions in the brain regardless of brain pathology and strongly recommend blood gas analysis during the apnea test.

Determination of Brain Death in Children

The diagnosis of brain death in young children is difficult compared with adults.[29] It is generally believed that the child's brain is more resistant to insults that lead to death, although this belief lacks convincing clinical documentation.[30,31]

A task force for the determination of brain death in children proposed the following criteria[29]:

1. Coma and apnea must coexist. The patient must exhibit complete loss of consciousness, vocalization, and volitional activity.
2. Absence of brainstem function is established as defined by
   (a). Midposition or fully dilated pupils that do not respond to light.
   (b). Absence of spontaneous eye movements, including those induced by oculocephalic and oculovestibular testing.
   (c). Absence of movement of bulbar musculature, including facial and oropharyngeal muscles. The corneal, gag, cough, sucking, and rooting reflexes are absent.
   (d). Respiratory movements are absent with the patient off the ventilator. Apnea testing using standardized methods can be performed but is done only after the other criteria are met.[32,33]
3. The patient must not be significantly hypothermic or hypotensive.
4. Flaccid tone and absence of spontaneous or induced movements, excluding spinal cord events such as reflex withdrawal or spinal myoclonus, should exist.
5. The examination should remain consistent with brain death throughout the observation and testing period.

The recommended observation period depends on the age of the patient and the available laboratory tests.

Age 7 days to 2 months. Two examinations including the EEG separated by at least 48 hours.

Age 2 months to 1 year. Two examinations including the EEG separated by at least 24 hours. A repeat examination and EEG are not necessary if a concomitant radionuclide angiographic study demonstrates no visualization of cerebral arteries.

Over 1 year of age. When an irreversible cause exists, laboratory testing is not required, and the observation period is at least 12 hours.

The extent and reversibility of brain damage caused by hypoxia/ischemia is difficult to assess, particularly in young children. Thus a more prolonged period of at least 24 hours of observation has been highly recommended in this situation. The observation period, however, may be shortened if the EEG shows electrosilence or angiography does not visualize cerebral arteries.

LABORATORY TESTING

EEG. In small children it may be impossible to meet the standard requirement for 10-cm electrode separation. The interelectrode distance should be decreased proportional to the child's head size. The value of angiography in infants under 2 months is under investigation.

Angiography. Demonstration of arrested carotid circulation at the base of the skull and absence of intracranial arterial circulation with a cerebral radio-nuclide angiogram can be considered confirmatory of brain death, even though there may be some visualization of the intracranial venous sinuses.[34-36] Other ancillary tests similar to those used in adults are still investigational.

Basic Principles of Brain Death Criteria

PREREQUISITES Before the declaration of brain death is considered, there are essential prerequisites. First, the cause of coma should be clarified. Without knowing the cause, the diagnosis of brain death should never be made. There should be no doubt that the patient's condition is due to irremediable structural brain damage. In this regard, conditions under which the diagnosis of brain death should be considered are well described in the report by the Conference of Royal Colleges and Faculties of the United Kingdom.[22] All the other published criteria stress prerequisites similar to those of the British criteria. In essence, the patient must be in an unresponsive coma and dependent on a ventilator because spontaneous respiration is inadequate or absent. All criteria require normothermia and the absence of both sedative drug intoxication and cardiovascular shock. When the brainstem and hypothalamic centers are damaged, thermal regulation and vasomotor control may be impaired.

After reviewing these criteria, it is clear that brain death is a clinical concept that can be diagnosed with clinical findings and appropriate ancillary tests if necessary.

In many of these criteria, *coma* refers to a state of total unreceptivity and un-responsivity in which the patient is totally unaware of externally applied stimuli. However, it remains difficult to define the term *coma* precisely. If you include in the term the absence of spontaneous movement, fixed dilated pupils, and the absence of all reflexes, it soon becomes apparent that the clinical approach has several limitations in that it cannot distinguish cerebral, cerebellar, brainstem, or spinal cord functions. Thus most brain death criteria depend on ancillary tests such as EEG and CBF examination to confirm the absence of cerebral function.

ABSENCE OF BRAINSTEM REFLEX

Brainstem reflexes reflect brainstem function, involving pathways from the midbrain to the lower medulla.[1] Total absence of brainstem reflexes indicates marked dysfunction of the cranial CNS. Although respiration is one of the most important brainstem reflexes, determination of irreversible loss of spontaneous respiration deserves separate discussion. Brain death is clearly different from the vegetative state, because the former requires the absence of all brainstem reflex. In the vegetative state and the apallic syndrome, brainstem reflexes are often present and their presence excludes the diagnosis of brain death.

Brainstem reflexes have varying significance in diagnosis. Therefore in diagnosing brain death, the individual brainstem reflexes differ in their importance as indicators of the brainstem functions as suggested by Walker.[24] The single most important brainstem reflex is pupillary. Other reflexes of importance include the oculocephalic, oculovestibular, and cough reflexes. As previously mentioned, the concept of brainstem death emphasizes the absence of brainstem reflexes. Although the tests for brainstem reflexes enable the functional integrity of the brainstem to be determined, there are several conditions under which brainstem reflexes have to be carefully evaluated. Anticholinergic drugs and ganglion blocking agents may dilate and fix the pupils. Oculovestibular reflexes can be modified by the presence of ototoxic agents such as antibiotics, antidepressants, and anticonvulsants.

ABSENCE OF SPONTANEOUS RESPIRATION Confirmation of apnea is the most essential test in diagnosing brain death, and anesthesiologists must fully understand the ap-

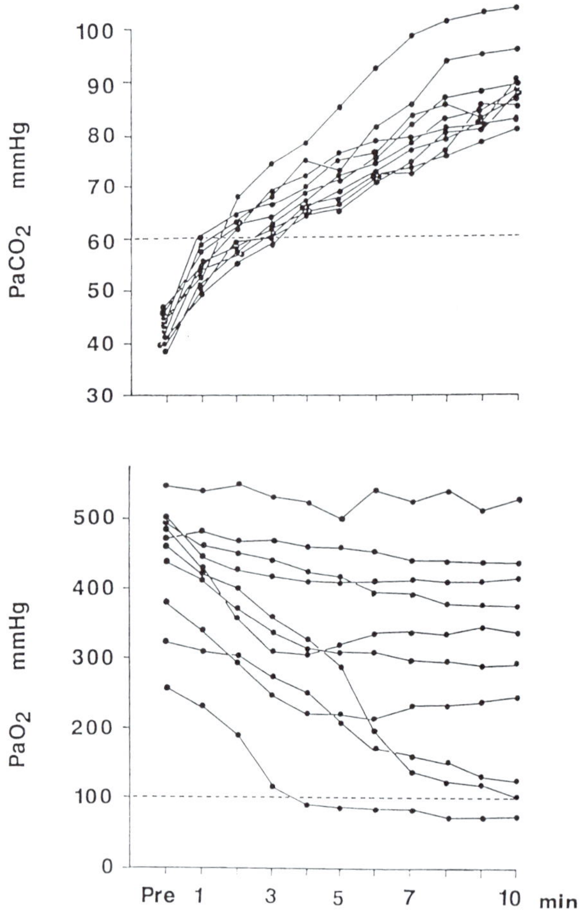

FIGURE 21.1 *Changes in $PaCO_2$ (A) and (B) PaO_2 during apnea test in 10 brain-dead patients. Before disconnection from the ventilator, 100% oxygen was given at a rate of 6 L/min insufflated through a catheter. In one case, PaO_2 decreased to 80 mmHg at the end of the test at 10 minutes. In most of the patients, body temperature was within normal range, but in the case with the highest $PaCO_2$, the body temperature was 39°C.*

nea test. Apnea is an early indication of impending brain death, usually being present before signs of circulatory impairment appear. In this situation respiration becomes entirely dependent on mechanical ventilation. The apnea test should be performed without subjecting the patient to an anoxic risk after all other criteria have been met. The principles of apneic oxygenation have been known in anesthetic practice since the 1950s. However, this technique has become popular only recently in the apnea test. The goal of the apnea test is to increase the $PaCO_2$ sufficiently to stimulate the medullary respiratory centers while maintaining arterial pressure of oxygen (PaO_2) at a safe level.[37] The level of $PaCO_2$ sufficient for inducing respiratory effort is at 55 to 60 mmHg.[38,39] During the apnea test, repeated blood gas analysis is strongly recommended; usually the $PaCO_2$ increases approximately 2.5 to 4.3 mmHg/min.[40] The examiners must be aware that the increase in $PaCO_2$ depends in part on the body temperature. Figure 21.1 shows PaO_2 and $PaCO_2$ changes after disconnecting the ventilator from brain-dead patients. Ten minutes is more than sufficient to raise the $PaCO_2$ above 55 mmHg. For the maintenance of oxygenation, it is recommended that 100 % oxygen be insufflated with a flow rate of more than 6 L/min via a catheter, the tip of which is placed 2 cm above the carina. If maintenance of PaO_2 above 100 mmHg during the apnea test is difficult, positive and expiratory pressure of about 10 cm water and monitoring arterial saturation with pulse oximetry are highly recommended.

Table 21.2 summarizes the published recommended apnea tests. In reviewing these criteria, it should be noted that the Harvard criteria were the first to describe the apnea test, and they required that the ventilator be disconnected for 3 minutes after the patient has been breathing room air for 10 minutes with a normal $PaCO_2$. Today the apnea test must be rigorous because of its importance in meeting the brain death criteria.[46] It should as a general rule include preoxygenation with 100% oxygen and a normal level of $PaCO_2$ before disconnection followed by oxygen insufflation during a 10-minute period with blood gas analysis before and during the apnea test. The time necessary for the apnea test depends in part on the previous state of oxygenation and the body temperature.

Ropper reported movements of the arm, shoulder, and thorax, during apneic testing, that resembled respiratory movements in five brain dead patients (Lazarus's sign).[47] These move-

TABLE 21.2 *Methods of apnea testing*

REFERENCE	PREOXYGENATION	APNEIC OXYGENATION	DURATION OF APNEA (min)
Royal Colleges and Faculties of the U.K.[22]	100% O_2 for 10 min (preoxygenation), then with 5% CO_2 in O_2 for 5 min	Delivering O_2 at 6 L/min through a catheter into the trachea	10
Schafer and Coronna[39]	100% O_2 for 10 min (control $PaCO_2$ to normal range)	100% O_2 at a rate of 6 L/min through an endotracheal tube	10
Pitts et al.[41]	100% O_2 for 5 min ($PaCO_2$ 30 ~ 35 mmHg)	100% O_2 at a rate of 4 L/min through a catheter down the endotracheal tube, approximately to the carina	>15
Milhaud et al.[42]	100% O_2 for more than 1 h (denitrogenation)	100% O_2 at a rate of 4 or 5 L/min through a catheter introduced into the tracheal tube	>15
President's Commission[25]	100% O_2 or O_2 and CO_2 mixture for 10 min	Passive flow of O_2	10
Ropper et al.[38]	100% O_2 for 5 min	Tracheal catheterization with 10–12 L/min	10
Pallis[17]	100% O_2 for 10 min	Delivering O_2 at 6 L/min by a catheter down the trachea	10
Perel et al.[43]	100% O_2 for 15 min	High fresh gas flow of 100% O_2 with PEEP of 4–8 cm water	3
Rowland et al.[32]	100% O_2 for 10 min	100% O_2 at 6 L/min through a catheter into the length of endotracheal tube	15
Outwater and Rockoff[33]	100% O_2 for 5 min	A continuous flow of O_2 via the endotracheal tube	5
Belsh et al.[44]	100% O_2 for at least 30 min ($PaCO_2$: greater than or equal to 36 mmHg)	Delivering O_2 (6 L/min) into the endotracheal tube via a T piece	10
van Donselaar et al.[45]	100% O_2 for 10 min	100% O_2 at a rate of 6 L/min through an endotracheal tube	14

Abbreviation: PEEP, positive end-expiratory pressure.

ments were believed to be elicited at the level of the spinal cord and may still be consistent with the diagnosis of brain death.

ANCILLARY TESTS FOR BRAIN DEATH

Among the many ancillary tests, the EEG and cerebral angiography are the most commonly used. Nonfilling angiography was stressed by European investigators. It must be noted that any ancillary tests should be used in conjunction with appropriate clinical criteria and should be based on clinical judgment. No single test for the diagnosis of brain death is available at present or will likely ever emerge.

Electroencephalogram. As mentioned before, some of the published criteria clearly indicated that the EEG is unnecessary for the diagnosis of brain death. However, the EEG is perhaps the most commonly used ancillary procedure in the diagnosis of brain death. It has been reported that 17% of brain-dead patients will have activity on their EEGs if the Minnesota criteria are followed.[48] Isoelectric or electric silence can be defined when the EEG shows the following condition: there is no evidence of electric activity over 2 μV when it is recorded from scalp electrode pairs 10 or more cm apart, with interelectrode impedance between 100 and 10,000 ohms. In addition, for the diagnosis of brain death, it may be necessary to sustain this for a period of 30 minutes. Electrocerebral silence may indicate irreversible dysfunction of the cerebrum if the cause of coma is not intoxication or metabolic disturbances that may be reversible. The American EEG Society[49] has proposed the following guidelines for EEG recording.

1. A minimum of eight scalp electrodes should be used.
2. Interelectrode impedance should be under 10,000 ohms but over 100 ohms.
3. The integrity of the entire recording system should be tested.
4. Interelectrode distances should be at least 10 cm.
5. Sensitivity must be increased from 7.0 μV/mm to at least 2 μV/mm for at least 30 minutes of the recording.
6. Filter setting should be appropriate for the assessment of electrocerebral silence.
7. Additional monitoring techniques should be employed when necessary (e.g., electrocardiograph.).

FIGURE 21.2 *Somatosensory evoked response in a normal adult (28-year-old man). The left median nerve was stimulated at the wrist. The arrow indicates stimulation. N9, Erb's potential (brachial plexus); N13, potentials arise from cervical spinal cord and dorsal column nuclei; N19(20), potentials arise from thalamocortical projections or the sensory cortex. In brain death, N19(20) is abolished.*

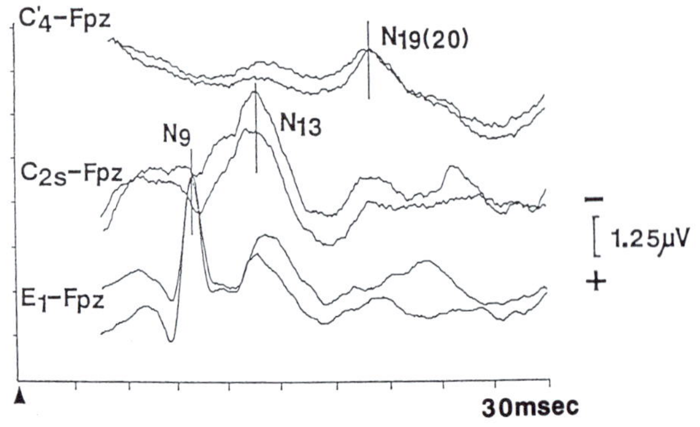

If the absence of both cortical and brainstem function is required for the diagnosis of brain death an isoelectric EEG is an important adjunct. However, whether or not the EEG is necessary remains controversial. I believe that a well-executed and reliably read EEG is a useful adjunct in the diagnosis of brain death, if loss of both cortical and brainstem function are required in the diagnosis of brain death.

Evoked Responses. There are a variety of tests that are designed to stimulate afferent pathways entering the brainstem and subcortical structures. Evoked neuronal responses are recorded by a computer-averaged technique.[50–52] This electrophysiologic technique can be used as an appropriate ancillary test for the diagnosis of brain death.

Somatosensory Response. The somatosensory response to median nerve stimulation in normal subject elicits Erb's potential (N9), N13, and N20 (Fig. 21.2). In brain death, N20 is abolished, whereas N13 is frequently present. Erb's potential (N9) is usually seen and the presence of this potential serves to confirm an intact peripheral pathway. Preservation of N13 suggests that the function of the upper cervical spinal cord and the dorsal column nuclei are preserved. Loss of somatosensory responses usually precedes establishing the clinical criteria for brain death.[53]

Auditory Brainstem Response. Although somatosensory stimuli are usually recorded as in-

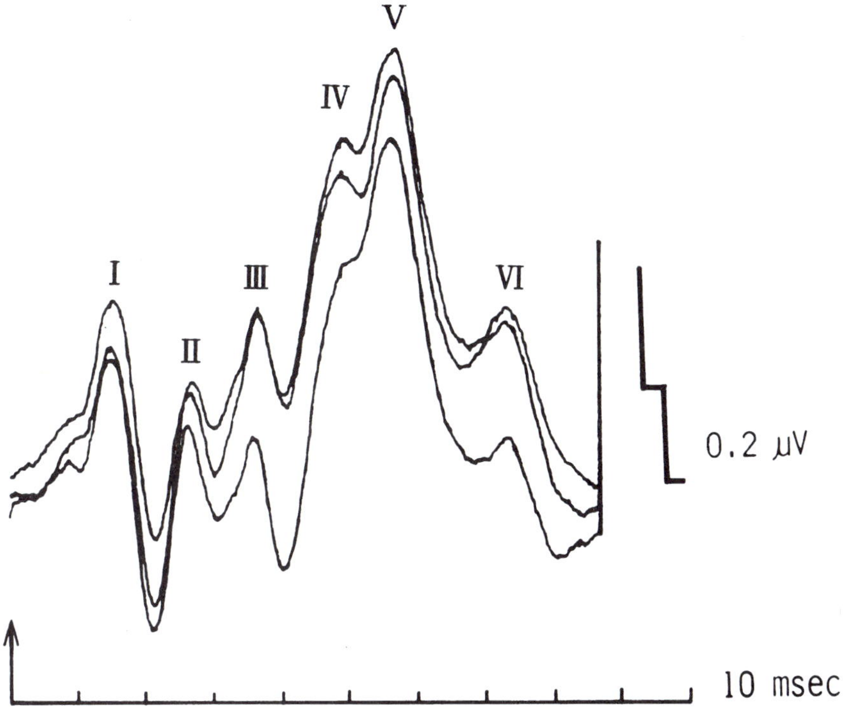

FIGURE 21.3 *An ABR in a normal adult (25-year-old man). Possible generators of the waves are I, acoustic nerve; II, cochlear nucleus; III, superior olivary complex and trapezoid body; IV, lateral lemniscus at the pontine level; V, inferior colliculus; VI, not well defined. The arrow indicates stimulation.*

dicators of cerebral activity, auditory brainstem response (ABR) is considered an indicator of the functional integrity of the brainstem. ABR has been found to be of considerable value in differentiating metabolic or toxic comas from organic brainstem lesions. Waveforms in a normal subject and a brain dead patient who fulfilled the Japanese criteria are shown in Figures 21.3 and 21.4, respectively. Waves I and II may remain in a patient who has been diagnosed clinically as brain dead. However, absence of wave I may not be an indication of brain death, because wave I is derived from the acoustic nerve and may not be elicitable due to pre-existing traumatic damage to the peripheral auditory structures. Wave II may arise from the proximal portion of the acoustic nerve[54] It can be seen that the ABR was present upon initial examination of the patient but subsequentially was abolished as the pathophysiology progressed rostrocaudally[55] A similar progression is seen in Figure 21.5. The ABR may be present in brainstem lesions that do not involve the auditory tract. The value of this electrophysiologic measure of brainstem function is apparent. However, the limitations include the requirement of specific equipment and experience.

Tests of CBF in Diagnosing Brain Death

ANGIOGRAPHY Some believe that serial cerebral angiography is the definitive method for diagnosing brain death. Particularly in Scandinavia, confirmation of arrested circulation in cerebrum, brainstem, and posterior fossa was considered to be essential for the diagnosis of brain death, based on the concept of total brain

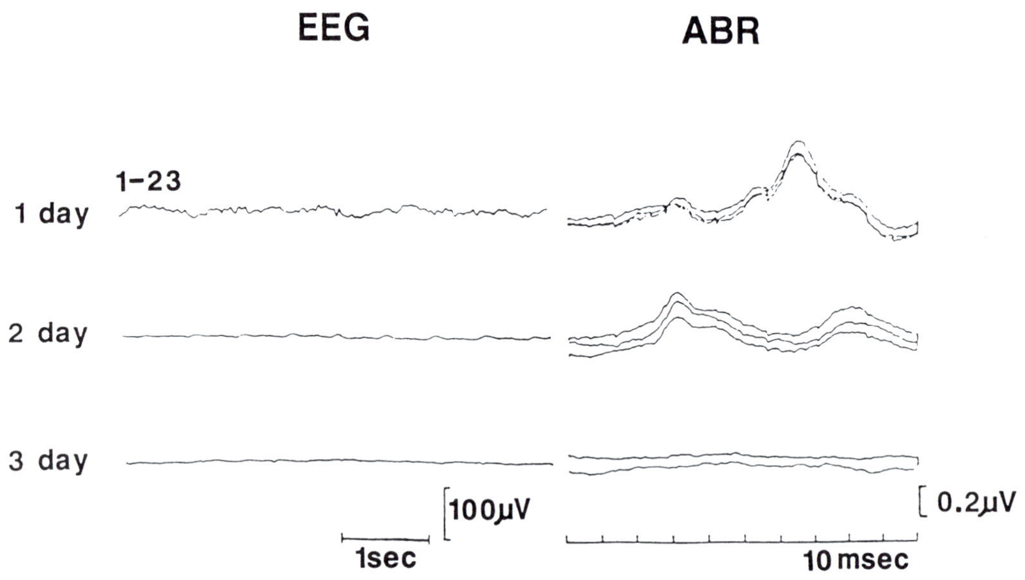

FIGURE 21.4 *Conventional EEG and ABR in a head-injured patient (19-year-old man). On the first day after the insult, the EEG showed predominant slow wave activity and the ABR was deteriorated. On the third day, the patient was in coma and all brainstem reflexes were abolished. The apnea test revealed no respiratory movement. Both the EEG and the ABR became isoelectric.*

infarction.[27] There is little doubt that the complete cessation of brain blood flow over 20 minutes inevitably leads to neuronal death in the adult human at normothermia. Carotid angiography alone does not visualize the circulation of the brainstem and posterior fossa structures and hence is inappropriate for testing for the cessation of blood flow to the whole brain. However, we frequently use carotid angiography at the bedside in the ICU as an ancillary test because of its simplicity (Fig. 21.6). Demonstration of both the carotid and vertebrobasilar systems requires four-vessel angiography. Commonly, selective catheterization of the neck vessels is performed via the femoral arteries with radiographic control. The dye is usually injected under maximal pressure, and serial films must be taken over a longer period of time than usually required for cerebral angiography under normal conditions. Absent cerebral circulation is defined as absence of filling of the venous system. Some believe that this technique has limited diagnostic capabilities and is undesirable because it is invasive and introduces the difficulties of transporting a comatose and artificially ventilated patient to the radiographic suites. In addition, the need for expert interpretation and the possibility of hypotension or arrhythmia induced by the procedure must be considered as limitations as well.[56]

As the pathologic processes associated with brain death progress and ICP increases, visualization of the intracranial vascular system progressively diminishes until an arrested dye column at the skull base eventually occurs. Angiographic findings of brain death are commonly characterized by fairly abrupt block of the dye column at the skull base or in the carotid siphon. Rarely, there may be a tapering of the dye column and nonfilling "pseudo-occlusion" in the cervical portion of the internal carotid artery.[57] In all cases, there may be excellent visualization of the external carotid vessels, but the intracranial venous phase is never observed. The dye column in the vertebral artery is usually

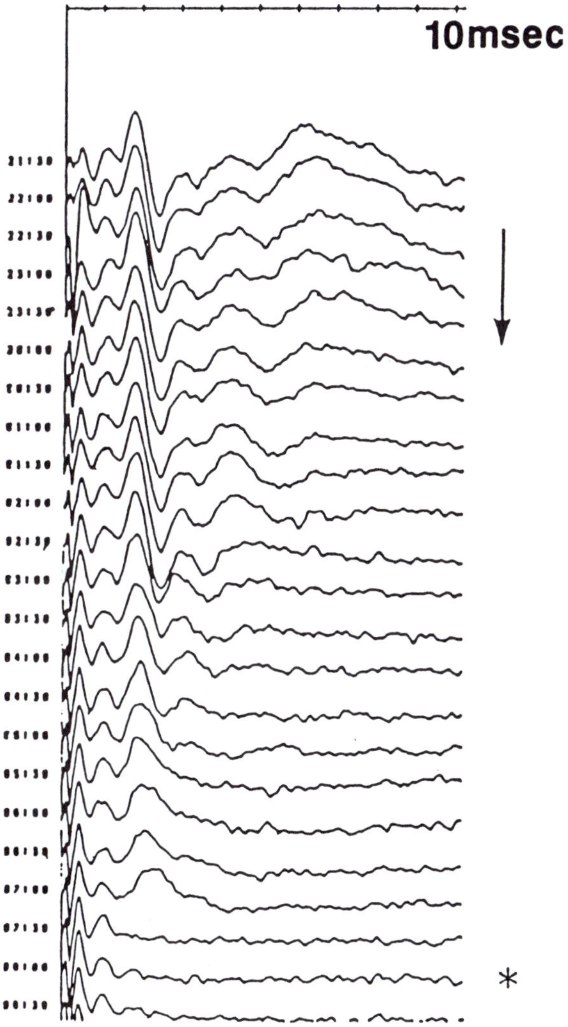

FIGURE 21.5 *ABR taken every 30 minutes in a 68-year-old woman after a subarachnoid hemorrhage. The first deflections are stimulus artifact. With time, wave V was abolished. Wave I remained in the last recording. The asterisk shows the time clinical brain death was confirmed using Japanese criteria. Four hours after the last recording, four-vessel angiography revealed nonfilling.*

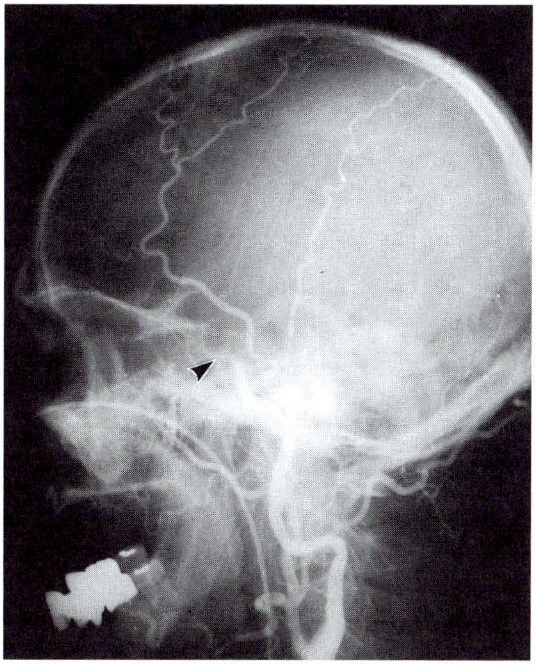

FIGURE 21.6 *Carotid angiogram using direct puncture method in a patient with clinical brain death (55-year-old man, head injury). There is no visualization of the intracranial vessels. Extracranial vessels are clearly seen. The dye column was arrested at the skull base (arrowhead).*

arrested at the atlanto-occipital junction, less often, intracranially. Variations in filling patterns of the anterior and posterior circulation during angiography have been reported.[58] The blood flow in the carotid and basilar systems may cease concurrently, but usually the vertebrobasilar circulation is seen for several hours after the cessation of carotid flow. Four-vessel angiography seems to have special value in cases of suspected drug intoxication and hypothermia. In these patients clinical findings and the EEG may be misleading.

Digital subtraction angiography has also been recommended as a method that can directly assess intracranial circulation with fewer cardiopulmonary side effects than conventional contrast angiography[59,60] (Fig. 21.7).

Radioisotope angiography with intravenous injection of technetium-labeled albumin and subsequent cranial scanning has also been used to demonstrate absent CBF. This procedure can be done at the bedside if portable imaging equipment is available[61] A limitation of this technique

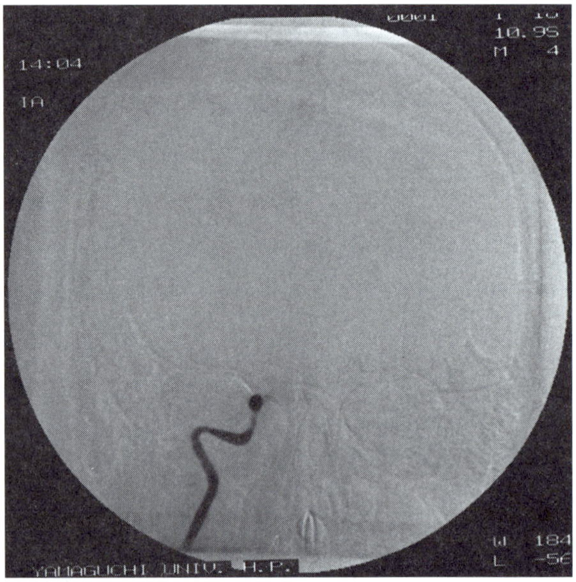

FIGURE 21.7 *Digital subtraction angiogram in a patient with clinical brain death (56-year-old man, cardiac arrest due to traumatic asphyxia). The arrested dye column at the level of skull base is clearly seen.*

FIGURE 21.8 *Transcranial Doppler ultrasonogram of the middle cerebral artery with time in a 46-year-old man after cardiac arrest due to subarachnoid hemorrhage. (A) Two hours after cardipulmonary resuscitation, normal pattern. (B) Five hours after, diastolic flow velocity was decreased and all brainstem reflexes were absent, but pupillary size was 1.5 mm in diameter. No spontaneous respiration. (C) Eight hours after, diastolic flow velocity was nearly zero. (D) Sixteen hours after clinical brain death, biphasic patterns were observed. The EEG and ABR were isoelectric.*

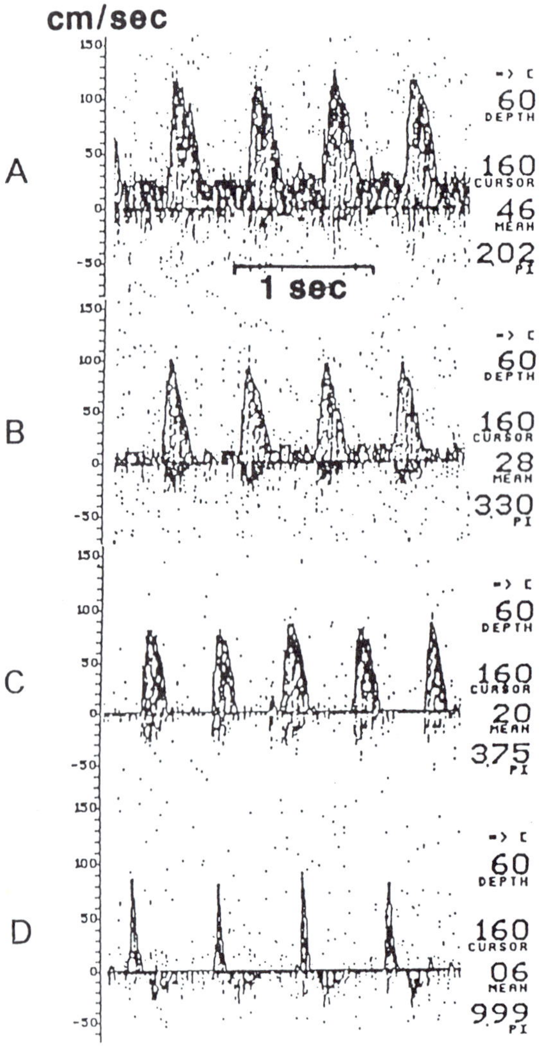

is that the vertebral system is not visualized. Variations in isotope flow patterns have also been reported.[62]

TRANSCRANIAL DOPPLER Transcranial Doppler ultrasound may also be used as an ancillary test. With this technique, Hassler et al.[63] examined patients suffering from intracranial hypertension with subsequent brain death and found that with increasing ICP, the waveform exhibited different characteristic high-resistance profiles, with first low, then zero, then reversed diastolic flow velocities, depending on the relationship between ICP and blood pressure. Figure 21.8 illustrates wave patterns observed in clinical brain death. This technique is readily available at the bedside and makes it possible to assess the intracranial circulation in patients who met clinical criteria. Disadvantages of this method are the requirement of technical expertise and occasional false-positive or false-negative results.[64]

COMPUTED TOMOGRAPHY CT may visualize indirectly the presence of intracranial blood flow, allowing evaluation of the appearance of intravenous contrast material on rapidly sequenced scans.[65,66] This method appears to be increasingly more available and hence may become useful in diagnosing brain death.

SUMMARY

The various brain death criteria established by authorized organizations do not offer important divergent differences in fundamentals. They have three major components: coma, absence of brainstem reflexes, and absence of spontaneous respiration. These components can be evaluated chiefly with clinical examination at the bedside and do not necessitate sophisticated equipment. However, if there is any doubt based on clinical examination, ancillary tests such as the EEG and blood flow studies must be added for confirmation. Among these ancillary tests, the EEG is the most widely used in the world.

References

1. Plum F, Posner JB: The diagnosis of stupor and coma. 3rd Ed. FA Davis, Philadelphia, 1980
2. Jennett B: Altered consciousness and coma. p. 267. In Cottrell JE, Turndorf H (eds): Anesthesia and Neurosurgery. CV Mosby, St. Louis, 1980
3. Ropper AH: Ocular dipping in anoxic coma. Arch Neurol 38:297, 1981
4. Jennett B, Teasdale G: Aspect of coma after severe head injury. Lancet 1:878, 1977
5. Starmark J-E, Stalhammar D, Holmgren E: A comparison of the Glasgow coma scale and the reaction level scale (RLS85). J Neurosurg 69:699, 1988
6. Petito CK, Feldmann E, Pulsinelli WA et al: Delayed hippocampal damage in humans following cardiorespiratory arrest. Neurology 37:1281, 1987
7. Miller JR, Myeres RE: Neuropathology of systemic circulatory arrest in adult monkeys. Neurology 22:888, 1972
8. Ginsberg MD: Delayed neurological deterioration following hypoxia. p. 21. In Fahn S, Davis JN, Rowland LP (eds): Advances in Neurology. Vol. 26. Raven Press, New York, 1979
9. Siesjö BK, Katsura K, Kristián T: The biochemical basis of cerebral ischemic damage. J Neurosurg Anesthesiol 7:47, 1995
10. Higashi K, Sakata Y, Hatano M: Epidemiological studies on patients with a persistent vegetative state. J Neurol Neurosurg Psychiatry 40:876, 1977
11. Jennett B, Bond MR: Assessment of outcome after severe brain damage. Lancet 1:480, 1975
12. Levy DE, Caronna JJ, Singer BH et al: Predicting outcome from hypoxic-ischemic coma. JAMA 253:1420, 1985
13. Polacek DJ, Grenvik A: Medical aspects of brain death. p. 1390. In Shoemaker WC, Ayres S, Grenvik A et al (eds): Textbook of Critical Care. 2nd Ed. WB Saunders, Philadelphia, 1989
14. Jennett B, Gleave J, Wilson P: Brain death in three neurosurgical units. Br Med J 282:533, 1981
15. Pallis C: Prognostic significance of a dead brain stem. Br Med J 286:123, 1983
16. Korein J: The problem of brain death: Development and history. NY Acad Sci 215:19, 1978
17. Pallis C: ABC of brain stem death, diagnosis of brain stem death. II. Br Med J 285:1641, 1982
18. Korein J: Brain death: interrelated medical and social issues. Ann NY Acad Sci 315:62, 1978
19. Definition of irreversible coma: report of ad hoc committee of Harvard Medical School to examine definition of brain death. JAMA 205:85, 1968
20. Mohandas A, Chou SN: Brain death: a clinical and pathological study. J Neurosurg 35:211, 1971
21. A report by the task force on death and dying of the institute of society, ethics, and the life sciences: refinements in criteria for the determination of death: an appraisal. JAMA 221:48, 1972
22. Royal Colleges and Faculties of the United Kingdom: Diagnosis of brain death. Br Med J 2:1187, 1976
23. Collaborative Study: An appraisal of the criteria of cerebral death—a summary statement. JAMA 273:982, 1977
24. Walker AE: Cerebral Death. 3rd Ed. Urban & Schwarzenberg, Baltimore, 1985
25. President's Commission for the Study of Ethical Problems in Medicine and Biomedical and Behavioral Research: Defining Death: Medical, Legal, and Ethical Issues in the Determination of Death. U.S. Government Printing Office, Washington, 1981
26. Report of the Swedish Committee on Defining Death: The Concept of Death Summary. The Swedish Ministry of Health and Social Affairs, Stockholm, 1984

27. Ingvar DH, Widen L: Brain death: summary of a symposium. Lakartidningen 34:3804, 1972
28. Takeuchi K, Takeshita H, Takakura K et al: Evolution of criteria for determination of brain death in Japan. Acta Neurochir (Wien) 87:93, 1987
29. Task force for the Determination of Brain Death in Children: Guidelines for the determination of brain death in children. Neurology 37:1077, 1987
30. Schwartz JA, Baxter J, Brill DR: Diagnosis of brain death in children by radionuclide cerebral imaging. Pediatrics 73:14, 1984
31. Moshe SL, Alvarez LA: Diagnosis of brain death in children. J Clin Neurophysiol 3:239, 1986
32. Rowland TW, Donnelly JH, Jackson AH: Apnea documentation for determination of brain death in children. Pediatrics 74: 505, 1984
33. Outwater KM, Rockoff MA: Apnea testing to confirm brain death in children. Crit Care Med 12:357, 1984
34. Goodman JM, Heck LL, Moore BD: Confirmation of brain death with portable isotope angiography: a review of 204 consecutive cases. Neurosurgery 16:492, 1985
35. Drake B, Ashwal S, Schneider S: Determination of cerebral death in the pediatric intensive care unit. Pediatrics 78:107, 1986
36. Holzman BH, Curless RG, Sfakianakis GN et al: Radionuclide cerebral perfusion scintography in determination of brain death in children. Neurology 33: 1027, 1983
37. Marks SJ, Zisfein J: Apneic oxygenation in apnea tests for brain death. Arch Neurol 47:1066, 1990
38. Ropper AH, Kennedy SK, Russell L: Apnea testing in the diagnosis of brain death: clinical and physiological observations. J Neurosurg 55:942, 1981
39. Schafer JA, Caronna JJ: Duration of apnea needed to confirm death. Neurology 28: 661, 1978
40. Fujii Y, Takeshita H, Yokota K et al: Relationship between body temperature and arterial carbon dioxide tension during apnea test in brain death. J Int Care Med 12:1011, 1988
41. Pitts LH, Kaktis J, Caronna J et al: Brain death, apneic diffusion oxygenation, and organ transplantation. J Trauma 18:180, 1978
42. Milhaud A, Riboulot M, Gayet H: Disconnecting tests and oxygen uptake in the diagnosis of total brain death. p. 241. In Korein J (ed): Braindeath: Interrelated Medical and Social Issues. Ann NY Acad Sci Vol. 315, 1978
43. Perel A, Berger M, Cotev S: The use of continuous flow of oxygen and PEEP during apnea in the diagnosis of brain death. Int Care Med 9:25, 1983
44. Belsh JM, Blatt R, Schiffman PL: Apnea testing in brain death. Arch Intern Med 146:2385, 1986
45. van Donselaar C, Meerwaldt J, Gijn JV: Apnea testing to confirm brain death in clinical practice. J Neurol Neurosurg Psychiatry 49:1071, 1986
46. Earnest MP, Beresford HR, McIntyre HB: Testing for apnea in suspected brain death: methods used by 129 clinicians. Neurology 36:542, 1986
47. Ropper AH: Unusual spontaneous movement in brain-dead patients. Neurology 34:1089, 1984
48. Grigg MM, Kelly MA, Celesia GC et al: Electroencephalographic activity after brain death. Arch Neurol 44:948, 1987
49. American EEG Society: Guideline three: minimum technical standards for EEG recording in suspected cerebral death. J Clin Neurophysiol 3:144, 1986
50. Hall JW, Machey-Hargadine JR, Kini E: Auditory brainstem response in determination of brain death. Arch Otolaryngol 111:613, 1985
51. Goldie WD, Chiappa KH, Young RR et al: Brainstem auditory and short-latency somatosensory evoked responses in brain death. Neurology 31:248, 1981
52. Pfurtscheller G, Schwartz G, List W: Brain death and bioelectrical brain activity. Int Care Med 11:149, 1985
53. de la Torre JC: Evaluation of brain death using somatosensory evoked potentials. Biol Psychiatry 16:931, 1981
54. Garg DP, Markland ON, Bustion TF: Brainstem auditory evoked responses in hereditary motor-sensory neuropathy: site of origin of wave II. Neurology 32: 1017, 1982
55. Stockard JE, Stockard JJ, Kleinberg F et al: Prognostic value of brainstem auditory evoked potentials in neonates. Arch Neurol 40:360, 1983
56. Powner DJ: The diagnosis of brain death in adult patient. J Intensive Care Med 2:181, 1987
57. Hazratji SM, Singh BM, Strobos RJ: Angiography in brain death. NY State J Med 1:82, 1981
58. Kricheff II, Pinto RS, George AE et al: Angiographic findings in brain death. Ann NY Acad Sci 315:168, 1978
59. Vatne K, Nakstad P, Lundar T: Digital subtraction angiography in the evaluation of brain death. Neuroradiology 27:155, 1985
60. Gomes AS, Hallinan JM: Intravenous digital subtraction angiography in the diagnosis of brain death. AJNR 4:21, 1983
61. Schwartz JA, Baxter J, Brill D et al: Radio nuclide cerebral imaging confirming brain death. JAMA 249:246, 1983

62. Brill DR, Schwartz JA, Baxter JA: Variant flow patterns in radionuclide cerebral imaging performed for brain death. Clin Nucl Med 10:346, 1985
63. Hassler W, Steinmetz H, Gawlowski J et al: Doppler ultrasonography in raised intracranial pressure and in intracranial circulatory arrest. J Neurosurg 68:745, 1988
64. Petty GW, Mohr JP, Pedley TA et al: The role of transcranial Doppler in confirming brain death: sensitivity, specificity, and suggestions for performance and interpretation. Neurology 40:300, 1990
65. Handa J, Matsuda M, Matsuda I, et al: Dynamic computed tomography in brain death. Surg Neurol 17:417, 1982
66. Arnold H, Kuhne D, Rohr W et al: Contrast bolus technique with rapid CT scanning—a reliable diagnostic tool for determination of brain death. Neuroradiology 22:129, 1981

INDEX

Page numbers followed by f indicate figures; those followed by t indicate tables.

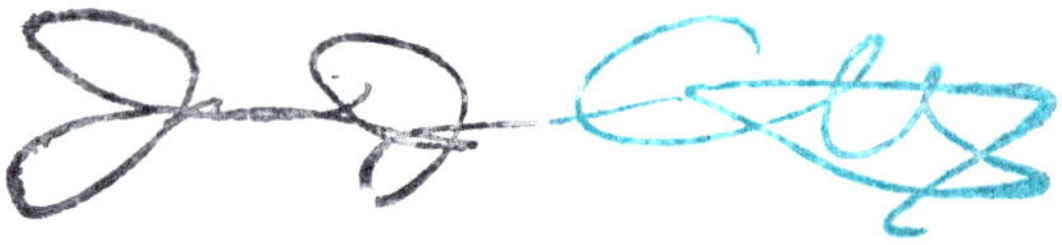